D

New Therapeutic Agents in Thrombosis and Thrombolysis

FUNDAMENTAL AND CLINICAL CARDIOLOGY

Editor-in-Chief

Samuel Z. Goldhaber, M.D.
*Harvard Medical School and Brigham
and Women's Hospital, Boston,
Massachusetts, U.S.A.*

New Therapeutic Agents in Thrombosis and Thrombolysis

Third Edition

Edited By

Jane E. Freedman
Boston University School of Medicine
Boston, Massachusetts, USA

Joseph Loscalzo
Brigham and Women's Hospital
Harvard Medical School
Boston, Massachusetts, USA

informa
healthcare

New York   London

Informa Healthcare USA, Inc.
52 Vanderbilt Avenue
New York, NY 10017

International Standard Book Number-10: 1-4200-6923-3 (Hardcover)
International Standard Book Number-13: 978-1-4200-6923-5 (Hardcover)

Library of Congress Cataloging-in-Publication Data

New therapeutic agents in thrombosis and thrombolysis / edited by Jane E.
Freedman, Joseph Loscalzo. – 3rd ed.
    p. ; cm. – (Fundamental and clinical cardiology ; 65)
  Includes bibliographical references and index.
  ISBN-13: 978-1-4200-6923-5 (hardcover : alk. paper)
  ISBN-10: 1-4200-6923-3 (hardcover : alk. paper) 1. Thrombolytic therapy.
2. Fibrinolytic agents. 3. Thrombosis. I. Freedman, Jane E. II. Loscalzo, Joseph.
III. Series: Fundamental and clinical cardiology ; v. 65
  [DNLM: 1. Thrombolytic Therapy. 2. Fibrinolytic Agents–therapeutic use.
3. Hemostasis–drug effects. 4. Platelet Aggregation Inhibitors–therapeutic use.
5. Thrombosis–drug therapy. W1 FU538TD v.65 2009 /
QZ 170 N532 2009]
  RC694.3.N49 2009
  616.1'3506–dc22

                                         2008042440

For Corporate Sales and Reprint Permissions call 212-520-2700 or write to: Sales Department, 52 Vanderbilt Avenue, 16th floor, New York, NY 10017.

Visit the Informa Web site at
www.informa.com

and the Informa Healthcare Web site at
www.informahealthcare.com

Series Introduction

Informa Healthcare has developed various series of beautifully produced books in different branches of medicine. These series have facilitated the integration of rapidly advancing information for both the clinical specialist and the researcher, especially in the area of cardiovascular medicine.

Jane E. Freedman, MD, and Joseph Loscalzo, MD, PhD, serve as editors of the third edition of the masterpiece, *New Therapeutic Agents in Thrombosis and Thrombolysis, Third Edition*. As editor-in-chief of the Fundamental and Clinical Cardiology Series, I am proud to tell you that this book has been one of our most successful. And because knowledge in the field of new antithrombotic agents and thrombolytics has escalated almost exponentially, the demand for a contemporary, totally rewritten and updated book has emerged. Together, Freedman and Loscalzo have crafted a timely textbook, with the latest information to evaluate hot topics such as novel anticoagulants, targets for antiplatelet drugs, and the evolution of thrombolytic agents as their use matures.

The third edition emphasizes topics such as pharmacogenomics, biomarkers, proteomics, as well as new anticoagulants such as oral direct factor Xa inhibitors, direct thrombin inhibition, and factor IX inhibitors. The rest of the text is devoted to new antiplatelet agents and thrombolytics.

My goal as editor-in-chief of the Fundamental and Clinical Cardiology Series is to assemble the talents of world-renowned authorities to discuss virtually every area of cardiovascular medicine. We have achieved this objective with *New Therapeutic Agents in Thrombosis and Thrombolysis, Third Edition*. Future contributions to this series will include books on molecular biology, interventional cardiology, and clinical management of such problems as chronic coronary artery disease, venous thromboembolism, peripheral vascular disease, and cardiac arrhythmias.

Samuel Z. Goldhaber, MD
Professor of Medicine
Harvard Medical School
Senior Staff Cardiologist
Brigham and Women's Hospital
Boston, Massachusetts, U.S.A.

Editor-in-Chief
Fundamental and Clinical Cardiology Series

Preface

As our understanding of hemostasis and thrombosis continues to evolve, so does the development of agents directed toward treating relevant cardiovascular and thromboembolic diseases. This development continues to be fueled by scientific discovery, the growing number of patients and indications for antithrombotics, as well as unmet medical needs with currently available therapies. This evolution is particularly notable since the publication of the second edition of *New Therapeutic Agents in Thrombosis and Thrombolysis* six years ago. In that span of time, we have continued to define the molecular details of the hemostatic and thrombotic pathways and uncover their therapeutic relevance. There has been ongoing progress in the area of coagulation inhibitors with new intravenous formulations being developed. Oral thrombin inhibitors have progressed with both successes and failures. Targets for antiplatelet drugs continue to be defined, leading to novel therapies as well as the development of additional agents in existing successful classes. While there has been less growth in the area of thrombolytic agents, their use continues to evolve with additional clinical functions described.

As with the previous editions, this book is divided into four parts. Because of the continuing evolution in the development of therapeutic agents aimed at treating thrombosis, we have reorganized and redistributed the specific sections. The first section has been expanded to include the background on biomarkers, testing, and pharmacogenomics. The second section continues to examine the specific areas of development for heparins and thrombin inhibitors, with the addition of new targets for antithrombotics, including aptamers and other inhibitors. The third section, on antiplatelet therapies, reflects the decreasing use of GPIIb/IIIa as a specific target and the development of novel classes of platelet inhibitors. The final section, on thrombolytic agents, updates the therapies in development and adds sections on evolving clinical uses, including ischemic stroke and venous thrombosis.

We are indebted to our distinguished section editors: we would like to thank our new section editor Roger Lijnen; Robert Giugliano, who assisted in the second edition; and Jeffrey Weitz, who has assisted in all three editions. We also thank Stephanie Tribuna, our editorial assistant, for her tireless efforts. Lastly, we are grateful to Sandra Beberman, vice president and publishing director, Informa Healthcare, for her assistance with this third edition.

Jane E. Freedman
Joseph Loscalzo

Contents

**PART I. OVERVIEW OF THE INVESTIGATION
AND REGULATION AND THROMBOSIS**
Jane E. Freedman

Contributors

Sonia S. Anand   CIHR and Department of Medicine, McMaster University, Hamilton, Ontario, Canada

Elliott M. Antman   Cardiovascular Division, Department of Medicine, Brigham and Women's Hospital, Harvard Medical School, Boston, Massachusetts, U.S.A.

Lina Badimon   Cardiovascular Research Center of Barcelona, CSIC-ICCC, Hospital de la Santa Creu i Sant Pau (UAB) and CIBEROBN (06/03), Instituto Salud Carlos III, Barcelona, Spain

Wadie F. Bahou   Department of Medicine, State University of New York, Stony Brook, New York, U.S.A.

Shannon M. Bates   Department of Medicine, McMaster University and Henderson Research Centre, Hamilton, Ontario, Canada

Kristian C. D. Becker   Department of Molecular Biology, Cell Biology and Biochemistry, Boston University, Boston, Massachusetts, U.S.A.

Richard C. Becker   Department of Medicine, Divisions of Cardiology and Hematology, Duke University Medical Center, Duke University School of Medicine, and Duke Clinical Research Institute, Durham, North Carolina, U.S.A.

Rohit Bhatheja   Gill Heart Institute and Division of Cardiovascular Medicine, University of Kentucky, Lexington, Kentucky, U.S.A.

Price Blair   Department of Medicine and Pharmacology, Boston University School of Medicine, Boston, Massachusetts, U.S.A.

Paul F. Bray   The Cardeza Foundation for Hematologic Research and the Department of Medicine, Jefferson Medical College, Philadelphia, Pennsylvania, U.S.A.

Harry R. Büller   Department of Vascular Medicine, Academic Medical Center, Amsterdam, The Netherlands

Marco Cattaneo Unità di Ematologia e Trombosi, Ospedale San Paolo, Dipartimento di Medicina, Chirurgia e Odontoiatria, Università degli Studi di Milano, Milan, Italy

Erdal Cavusoglu Division of Cardiology, Department of Medicine, SUNY Downstate Medical Center, Brooklyn, New York, U.S.A.

Anthony K.C. Chan Department of Pediatrics, McMaster University, Hamilton; Career Investigator Heart and Stroke Foundation of Canada, Coagulation Laboratory, The Hospital for Sick Children, Toronto, Ontario, Canada

Mark Chan Department of Medicine, Divisions of Cardiology and Hematology, Duke University Medical Center, Duke University School of Medicine, and Duke Clinical Research Institute, Durham, North Carolina, U.S.A.

Mark A. Crowther Department of Medicine, St. Joseph's Hospital, McMaster University, Hamilton, Ontario, Canada

Gregory J. del Zoppo Department of Medicine (in Hematology), Department of Neurology, University of Washington, Seattle, Washington, U.S.A.

John W. Eikelboom Department of Medicine, McMaster University, Thrombosis Service, Hamilton General Hospital, Hamilton, Ontario, Canada

Charles T. Esmon Howard Hughes Medical Institute, Oklahoma Medical Research Foundation, Oklahoma City, Oklahoma, U.S.A.

Jane E. Freedman Department of Medicine and Pharmacology, Boston University School of Medicine, Boston, Massachusetts, U.S.A.

David Gailani Departments of Pathology and Medicine, Vanderbilt University, Nashville, Tennessee, U.S.A.

Robert P. Giugliano Cardiovascular Division, Brigham and Women's Hospital, Harvard Medical School, Boston, Massachusetts, U.S.A.

Dmitri V. Gnatenko Department of Medicine, State University of New York, Stony Brook, New York, U.S.A.

Samuel Z. Goldhaber Cardiovascular Division, Department of Medicine, Brigham and Women's Hospital, Harvard Medical School, Boston, Massachusetts, U.S.A.

Andras Gruber Departments of Biomedical Engineering and Medicine, Oregon Health and Science University, Portland, Oregon, U.S.A.

Paul A. Gurbel Sinai Center for Thrombosis Research, Sinai Hospital of Baltimore and Johns Hopkins University School of Medicine, Baltimore, Maryland, U.S.A.

Melkon Hacobian Venous Thromboembolism Research Group, Cardiovascular Division, Brigham and Women's Hospital, Harvard Medical School, Boston, Massachusetts, U.S.A.

Hussam Hamdalla Gill Heart Institute and Division of Cardiovascular Medicine, University of Kentucky, Lexington, Kentucky, U.S.A.

Robert A. Harrington Division of Cardiovascular Medicine, Duke University Medical Center and Duke Clinical Research Institute, Durham, North Carolina, U.S.A.

Emily L. Howard Department of Pathology, College of Medicine, University of Arkansas for Medical Sciences, Little Rock, Arkansas, U.S.A.

Pieter W. Kamphuisen Department of Vascular Medicine, Academic Medical Center, Amsterdam, The Netherlands

Jason N. Katz Division of Cardiovascular Medicine, Duke University Medical Center and Duke Clinical Research Institute, Durham, North Carolina, U.S.A.

Suzanne M. Leal Department of Human and Molecular Genetics, Baylor College of Medicine, Houston, Texas, U.S.A.

Agnes Y. Lee Department of Medicine, McMaster University and Hamilton Health Sciences, Henderson Hospital, Hamilton, Ontario; and Department of Medicine, University of British Columbia and Vancouver Coastal Health, Vancouver, British Columbia, Canada

Edward N. Libby Division of Hematology/Oncology, University of New Mexico Cancer Center, Albuquerque, New Mexico, U.S.A.

H. Roger Lijnen Center for Molecular and Vascular Biology, Katholieke Universiteit Leuven, Leuven, Belgium

Joseph Loscalzo Department of Medicine, Brigham and Women's Hospital, Harvard Medical School, Boston, Massachusetts, U.S.A.

Geert Maleux Department of Interventional Radiology, University Hospitals of Leuven, Leuven, Belgium

Catherine McGorrian Department of Medicine, McMaster University, Hamilton, Ontario, Canada

Simon J. McRae Institute of Medical and Veterinary Science, The Queen Elizabeth Hospital, South Australia, Australia

Alan D. Michelson Center for Platelet Function Studies, Departments of Pediatrics, Medicine, and Pathology, University of Massachusetts Medical School, Worcester, Massachusetts, U.S.A.

David J. Moliterno   Gill Heart Institute and Division of Cardiovascular Medicine, University of Kentucky, Lexington, Kentucky, U.S.A.

Paul T. Monagle   Department of Pediatrics, University of Melbourne, and Department of Hematology, Royal Children's Hospital, Melbourne, Victoria, Australia

Shaker A. Mousa   The Pharmaceutical Research Institute, Albany College of Pharmacy/Medicine, Albany, New York, U.S.A.

Srikanth Nagalla   The Cardeza Foundation for Hematologic Research and the Department of Medicine, Jefferson Medical College, Philadelphia, Pennsylvania, U.S.A.

Menaka Pai   Department of Adult Hematology, Princess Margaret Hospital, University of Toronto, Toronto, Ontario, Canada

Gregory Piazza   Cardiovascular Division, Department of Medicine, Beth Israel Deaconess Medical Center, Harvard Medical School, Boston, Massachusetts, U.S.A.

Nahid Qushmaq   Department of Medicine, Henderson Research Centre and McMaster University, Hamilton, Ontario, Canada

Thomas Renné   Institute of Clinical Biochemistry and Pathobiochemistry, Julius-Maximilians-University of Würzburg, Würzburg, Germany

Christopher P. Rusconi   Regado Biosciences, Inc., Durham, North Carolina, U.S.A.

Andrew I. Schafer   Department of Medicine, Weill Cornell Medical College, New York-Presbyterian Hospital Weill Cornell, New York, New York, U.S.A.

Robert G. Schaub   Preclinical Research and Development, Archemix Corporation, Cambridge, Massachusetts, U.S.A.

Sam Schulman   Department of Medicine, McMaster University, Hamilton, Ontario, Canada

Lisa Senzel   Department of Pathology, State University of New York, Stony Brook, New York, U.S.A.

Steven R. Steinhubl   Gill Heart Institute and Division of Cardiovascular Medicine, University of Kentucky, Lexington, Kentucky, U.S.A.

Udaya S. Tantry   Sinai Center for Thrombosis Research, Sinai Hospital of Baltimore, Baltimore, Maryland, U.S.A.

Alexander G. G. Turpie   Department of Medicine, Hamilton Health Sciences, Ontario, Canada

Raymond Verhaeghe   Department of Vascular Medicine and Haemostasis, University Hospitals of Leuven, Leuven, Belgium

Peter Verhamme   Department of Vascular Medicine and Haemostasis, University Hospitals of Leuven, Leuven, Belgium

Gemma Vilahur   Cardiovascular Research Center of Barcelona, CSIC-ICCC, Hospital de la Santa Creu i Sant Pau (UAB) and CIBEROBN (06/03), Instituto Salud Carlos III, Barcelona, Spain

Theodore E. Warkentin   Department of Pathology and Molecular Medicine, and Department of Medicine, Michael G. DeGroote School of Medicine, McMaster University, Transfusion Medicine, Hamilton Regional Laboratory Medicine Program, Hamilton Health Sciences, Hamilton General Site, Hamilton, Ontario, Canada

Jeffrey I. Weitz   Department of Medicine, Henderson Research Centre and McMaster University, Hamilton, Ontario, Canada

Harvey D. White   Green Lane Cardiovascular Service, Cardiology Department, Auckland City Hospital, Auckland, New Zealand

James T. Willerson   Health Science Center at Houston, The University at Texas, Cullen Cardiovascular Research Laboratories at Texas Heart Institute, Baylor College of Medicine, and The University of Texas M.D. Anderson Cancer Center, Houston, Texas, U.S.A.

Stephen D. Wiviott   Cardiovascular Division, Department of Medicine, Brigham and Women's Hospital, Harvard Medical School, Boston, Massachusetts, U.S.A.

Cheuk-Kit Wong   Department of Medical and Surgical Sciences, Dunedin School of Medicine, University of Otago, Dunedin, New Zealand

1

Overview of Hemostasis and Fibrinolysis

Andrew I. Schafer

Department of Medicine, Weill Cornell Medical College, New York-Presbyterian Hospital Weill Cornell, New York, New York, U.S.A.

INTRODUCTION

The human hemostatic system has evolved as an exquisitely orchestrated mechanism to preserve blood fluidity throughout the circulation under normal circumstances. At the same time, it is capable of responding instantaneously to injury to form a protective hemostatic plug that is precisely localized and limited to the site of vascular damage. Hemostasis involves the balance and dynamic interplay between three major components: (*i*) the vessel wall, (*ii*) blood platelets, and (*iii*) the coagulation proteins (i.e., clotting and fibrinolytic factors).

The intimal surface of the entire circulatory tree is carpeted by a monolayer of endothelial cells. Endothelial cells are therefore the only stationary, anchored cells that components of flowing blood ever normally encounter. As such, we now understand that endothelial cells serve much more than a simple barrier function to separate blood from the rest of the vessel wall. They continuously elaborate substances that maintain blood fluidity, keeping circulating platelets inactive and minimizing the formation of thrombin and deposition of fibrin in the microvasculature. There is endothelial cell heterogeneity in different regions of the circulatory tree, and hemostasis is differentially regulated between blood vessel types and organs (1).

At a site of vessel wall injury, the thromboresistant (antithrombotic) properties of endothelium are locally lost and prothrombotic substances in the vessel wall beneath the endothelial monolayer become exposed to blood. This leads to the rapid, focal activation of platelets and the coagulation system and the formation of a hemostatic plug, which is composed of platelets anchored by a fibrin mesh. This is the *physiological* process of "hemostasis," a desirable, protective response that is designed to prevent exsanguination. The hemostatic plug is localized in this case because the normal endothelial lining immediately adjacent to the site of damage prevents propagation of the clot. Following stabilization of the hemostatic plug, local reparative processes restore normal vascular architecture and the fibrinolytic system reestablishes patency of the vascular lumen.

In contrast, intrinsic abnormalities of the vessel wall (e.g., atherosclerosis) can cause arterial thrombosis, while abnormalities in blood flow (e.g., stasis) or blood composition (e.g., hypercoagulability) can cause venous thrombosis. Thus, while "hemostasis" is a protective, physiological response, "thrombosis" is a deleterious, *pathological* process of clot formation.

The mechanisms of platelet activation, coagulation, and fibrinolysis are summarized separately below, but it should be kept in mind that these are not independent, sequential events. They are completely interdependent processes that are modulated by the balance of activities of thrombin, the pivotal enzyme of the coagulation system, and the antithrombotic properties of endothelium. In this overview, the normal mechanisms of hemostasis will be discussed as a background for the chapters on antithrombotic and fibrinolytic pharmacotherapies for thrombotic disorders.

PLATELET ACTIVATION

Several platelet-inhibitory activities of endothelium act in concert constitutively to maintain circulating platelets in their inactive form under normal conditions (2). They contribute to the thromboresistant properties of the normal vascular intimal surface. Prostacyclin (prostaglandin I_2, PGI_2) is the major oxygenation product of arachidonic acid in endothelial cells, synthesized via the sequential actions of aspirin-inhibitable cyclooxygenase (which in endothelial cells is predominantly the inducible form of the enzyme, COX-2) and prostacyclin synthase. Prostacyclin inhibits platelet activation by platelet receptor–coupled activation of adenylyl cyclase, thereby raising intra-platelet levels of cyclic adenosine monophosphate (cAMP). Nitric oxide (NO) is a product of NO synthase–mediated metabolism of L-arginine in endothelial cells. It inhibits platelet activation by diffusing into the platelet cytosol, where it binds to the heme activator site of soluble guanylyl cyclase, thereby raising intra-platelet levels of cyclic guanosine monophosphate (cGMP). Prostacyclin and NO are also released by intact endothelium abluminally, raising cAMP and cGMP levels, respectively, in vascular smooth muscle cells. Both cAMP and cGMP induce smooth muscle cell relaxation. Thus, the net effects of endothelium-derived prostacyclin and NO are to maintain blood fluidity through their combined platelet-inhibitory and vasodilatory actions. Other platelet-inhibitory and vasodilatory properties of endothelial cells are (*i*) carbon monoxide (CO), a product of heme oxygenase–mediated heme catabolism, which, like NO, acts via a cGMP-mediated mechanism, and (*ii*) ADPase (CD39), an ectonucleotidase that hydrolyzes and inactivates platelet-stimulatory ADP on the endothelial surface.

At a site of loss of thromboresistant endothelium, platelets adhere to the injured intimal surface primarily by the binding of von Willebrand factor (vWf), a large, multimeric protein, to its receptors on platelet-surface glycoprotein (GP) Ib, part of the platelet-membrane GP Ib/V/IX complex. vWf is synthesized by endothelial cells (as well as megakaryocytes) and secreted into both plasma and the extracellular matrix of the subendothelial vessel wall. Large vWf multimers serve as the major molecular "glue" (ligand) for the attachment of platelets to the damaged vessel wall, with sufficient strength to withstand the varying levels of shear stress in the circulation that would tend to detach them and sweep them back into flowing blood. In fact, the higher shear stresses in the arterial side of the circulation actually promote the interaction between vWf and platelet-membrane GP Ib. This is the process of "platelet adhesion," which is further reinforced by collagen binding to several platelet-membrane collagen receptors, including GP Ia and GP VI.

Following adhesion of a monolyarer of platelets to the extracellular matrix of the damaged vascular intimal surface, the adherent platelets are activated by a combination of platelet-derived stimuli such as ADP, serotonin, and thromboxane A_2 and extraplatelet activators such as epinephrine, thrombin, and collagen (also see ch. 2). These autocrine and paracrine mediators generally activate platelets through G-protein-coupled receptors and recruit additional platelets from the circulation into a growing hemostatic plug (3,4). Several of these mediators can activate platelets synergistically and may also act in concert with the shear forces they simultaneously encounter.

The interaction of platelets with other platelets within the developing hemostatic plug ("platelet aggregation") is mediated by the binding of bivalent fibrinogen to the heterodimeric platelet-surface integrin, GP IIb/IIIa (αIIbβ3). The GP IIb/IIIa complex as a functional fibrinogen receptor is expressed only on the surfaces of activated platelets. Under conditions of high shear stress (e.g., in diseased coronary arteries), multivalent vWf replaces fibrinogen as the major GP IIb/IIIa-binding ligand. The occlusive platelet plug thus created at the site of vascular injury becomes anchored by a mesh of fibrin, which is simultaneously formed as the final product of the coagulation system described below.

COAGULATION

Coagulation refers to the conversion of soluble plasma fibrinogen into insoluble fibrin (5). This process occurs by way of a series of linked reactions in which the enzymatically active product of each reaction converts the next downstream inactive plasma protein precursor (zymogen) into another active serine protease. Each of the zymogen-protease transitions occurs by the hydrolysis of peptide bonds. This sequence (or "cascade") of coagulation reactions is a powerful biochemical amplifier in which a small initiating stimulus can explosively generate relatively large amounts of the end product, fibrin. Fibrin is then deposited precisely at the site of vascular injury (Fig. 1).

The transmembrane receptor tissue factor (TF) is constitutively expressed by certain cells in the vessel wall beneath endothelium, such as vascular smooth muscle cells and

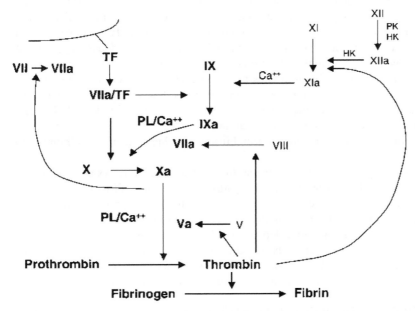

Figure 1 Coagulation pathways. Roman numerals denote specific coagulation factors which, when followed by an "a," indicate their active forms. The dominant pathways of coagulation activation are depicted in larger, bolder type; the other reactions are considered to serve more of an amplification role. *Abbreviations*: TF, tissue factor; PK, prekallikrein; HK, high-molecular-weight kininogen; PL, membrane (acidic) phospholipids; Ca^{++}, free ionized calcium.

fibroblasts, but it is not normally expressed by intact endothelial cells (6). The coagulation cascade is initiated primarily by vascular injury that exposes TF to flowing blood. Plasma factor VII, presumably associated with trace amounts of activated Factor VII (FVII/VIIa) is the ligand for TF. The binding of FVII/VIIa to newly exposed TF at the site of damage leads to rapid, autocatalytic conversion of FVII to FVIIa, amplifying this coagulation-initiating reaction. The TF-FVIIa complex then activates downstream FX to FXa. Alternatively, and possibly preferentially, the complex can indirectly activate FX by initially converting FIX to FIXa, which then activates FX in conjunction with its cofactor, FVIIIa. (Blood-borne TF in the form of cell-derived microparticles may play a role in the amplification of the coagulation cascade. Furthermore, under *pathological* conditions, TF is also expressed by leukocytes, platelets, and endothelial cells.)

FXa, in conjunction with its cofactor, FVa, converts the inactive plasma zymogen prothrombin to thrombin. Thrombin, the pivotal protease of the coagulation system (see below), converts soluble plasma fibrinogen to insoluble fibrin, which then polymerizes through an orderly process of intermolecular associations. Thrombin also activates FXIII (fibrin-stabilizing factor) to FXIIIa, a transglutaminase that covalently cross-links and thereby stabilizes the fibrin clot.

The so-called intrinsic or contact activation pathway of coagulation, involving prekallikrein, high-molecular-weight kininogen, FXII and FXI (Fig. 1), which was formerly considered to be an alternative pathway for activation of FX, is now viewed as only a possibly ancillary and amplifying system for the TF-FVIIa-initiated coagulation cascade.

Physiological hemostasis requires fibrin to be formed rapidly and to be precisely localized to the site of vascular injury along with the platelet plug it anchors. Therefore, the sequential activation of coagulation proteins requires their coordinated spatial and temporal assembly, which occurs most efficiently on cell membrane surfaces rather than in fluid-phase plasma. Membrane phospholipids, especially acidic phospholipids, link coagulation proteins through their calcium-binding sites (vitamin K-dependent γ-carboxyglutamic acid residues) to the membrane. Importantly, quiescent cell membranes expose insufficient acidic phospholipids on their surfaces to promote coagulation. Following endothelial cell or platelet activation, however, critical surface concentrations of these surface-binding sites are exposed to blood, and assembly of the so-called tenase (Xase) and prothrombinase complexes is facilitated. Factor Xa, generated by the activated membrane–associated tenase complex (consisting of FIXa, FVIIIa, and FX), diffuses from the complex along the membrane surface to form the prothrombinase complex (consisting of FXa, FVa, and prothrombin), which then converts prothrombin to thrombin.

Coagulation is regulated by several physiological antithrombotic systems, including antithrombin (AT; also known as ATIII), TF pathway inhibitor (TFPI), the protein C/protein S pathway, and, to a lesser extent, heparin cofactor II and protein Z–dependent protease inhibitor (7). These factors normally act in concert to limit thrombin generation. In addition, as with the endothelium-dependent platelet inhibitors (see above), these anticoagulant systems depend generally on the presence of intact endothelial cells. Normal endothelium thus provides a thromboresistant surface to prevent the activation of both platelets and the coagulation system where hemostasis is not required.

CENTRAL ROLE OF THROMBIN IN HEMOSTASIS

Thrombin serves as the central serine protease of the coagulation cascade (8). Diffusion of thrombin from the membrane site of its generation into blood both converts fibrinogen into fibrin monomers and activates platelets. The activated platelet then provides a

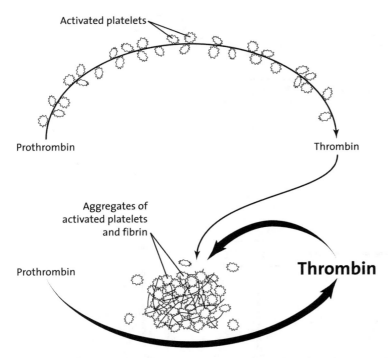

Figure 2 Platelet activation and thrombin generation are reciprocally amplified in the localized formation of a hemostatic plug. Conversion of prothrombin to thrombin is accelerated on activated platelet surfaces (*top*). Thrombin thus generated further activates platelets and induces their aggregation, providing increased and localized platelet surface for further thrombin generation (*bottom*).

membrane surface to further activate the coagulation cascade, generate more thrombin, and thereby amplify and localize the formation of the hemostatic plug (Fig. 2). In addition, thrombin sustains the coagulation cascade by feedback activation of other coagulation factors (Fig. 1).

Thrombin is unique amongst the activated coagulation proteinases in that, once formed, it loses those of its domains that are required for initial recognition and activation reactions, allowing thrombin to diffuse freely to interact with its numerous substrates (9). At sites where normal endothelium is lost, free thrombin acts primarily on substrates that function in concert to rapidly promote the formation of a stable hemostatic clot. These include (*i*) protease activated receptors and GP V on the platelet surface (to activate platelets), (*ii*) fibrinogen (to catalyze its conversion to fibrin), (*iii*) FVIII and FV (to activate these cofactors to FVIIIa and FVa, and thereby accelerate the generation of FXa and thrombin, respectively), (*iv*) FXIII (to catalyze FXIIIa-mediated fibrin cross-linking), (*v*) FXI (to amplify the coagulation cascade via the intrinsic pathway), and (*vi*) thrombin-activatable fibrinolysis inhibitor, TAFI (to stabilize the fibrin clot).

Once the hemostatic clot has occluded the damaged site, it begins to encroach upon the adjacent endothelium (9). Here, the procoagulant actions of thrombin must be shut down to prevent propagation of the clot beyond the site of injury. Therefore, in the presence of normal endothelial cells, the substrate specificity of thrombin is redirected from procoagulant to anticoagulant reactions (Fig. 3). First, free thrombin generated adjacent to intact endothelium is removed from the circulation by binding in a high-affinity complex to the glycoprotein thrombomodulin (TM) on the endothelial surface (10).

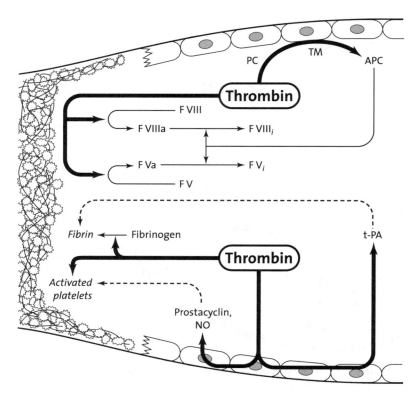

Figure 3 Central role of thrombin in hemostasis. Intact endothelium (contiguous to an area of vascular injury, vasoconstriction and clot formation) converts the prothrombotic actions of thrombin (fibrin formation and platelet activation) to antithrombotic actions, including generation of APC from PC on endothelial surface TM, and stimulation of prostacyclin, NO and t-PA production. Dashed lines represent inhibitory effects. *Abbreviations*: APC, activated protein C; PC, protein C; TM, thrombomodulin; NO, nitric oxide; t-PA, tissue-type plasminogen activator.

Second, thrombin bound to TM activates protein C (APC). APC is an anticoagulant protease that, with its cofactor protein S, proteolytically inactivates FVIIIa and FVa. Thus, APC downregulates further thrombin generation in the presence of intact endothelium. Finally, as shown in Figure 3, free thrombin stimulates endothelial cells to release anti-platelet prostacyclin and NO, as well as the plasminogen activators that are discussed below.

FIBRINOLYSIS

The fibrinolytic system (Fig. 4) represents another important endothelium-dependent mechanism for limiting fibrin accumulation (11). The central molecule of fibrinolysis is the serine protease plasmin, which is formed from the plasma zymogen plasminogen by the action of endothelial cell–derived plasminogen activators (12). Two naturally occurring plasminogen activators exist: tissue-type plasminogen activator (t-PA) and urokinase-type plasminogen activator (u-PA). These enzymes themselves exist in relatively inactive zymogen precursor forms: t-PA as a single-chain species and u-PA as prourokinase. Following the conversion of single-chain t-PA to a two-chain form or of urokinase to a high-molecular-weight or low-molecular-weight two-chain form, these

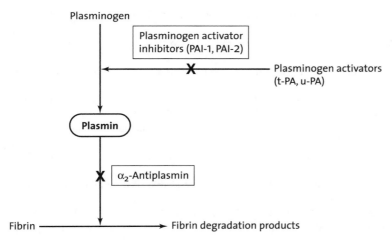

Figure 4 Fibrinolysis. *Abbreviations*: t-PA, tissue-type plasminogen activator; u-PA, urokinase-type plasminogen activator; PAI-1, plasminogen activator inhibitor-1; PAI-2, plasminogen activator inhibitor-2.

enzymes convert plasminogen to plasmin, likewise a two-chain molecule, by a single peptide bond cleavage. Whereas the enzyme-active site of plasmin resides in its light (or B) chain, its heavy (or A) chain contains lysine-binding sites that permit it to bind to fibrin. The fibrin specificity of physiological fibrinolysis is further enhanced by the several hundredfold catalytic efficiency of t-PA after binding to fibrin. Specific cell-surface membrane receptors also facilitate plasminogen activation by t-PA and u-PA and, in this way, promote degradation of the fibrin clot from the microenvironment of the endothelial cell, macrophage, or platelet surface.

Plasmin, once formed, degrades fibrin (and fibrinogen) into smaller-sized soluble fibrin(ogen) degradation fragments (FDPs). FDPs themselves have antithrombotic activity owing to their ability to compete with fibrin monomer for fibrin polymer–binding sites and with fibrinogen for platelet-surface GP IIb/IIIa-binding sites. When plasmin acts on covalently cross-linked fibrin, the FDPs released are D-dimers, which can be measured in plasma as a relatively specific test of fibrin (rather than fibrinogen) degradation.

Plasminogen activation and plasmin activity are regulated by other serine protease inhibitors (serpins). α_2-Antiplasmin and plasminogen activator inhibitors (PAI-1 and PAI-2) inhibit plasmin and plasminogen activators, respectively, by forming one-to-one stoichiometric complexes with the active enzymes. Further control of fibrinolysis occurs via TAFI, which provides a direct molecular link between the coagulation and fibrinolytic systems (13).

In summary, the delicate balance that maintains the human hemostatic system preserves blood fluidity throughout the circulation under normal circumstances. Although it is capable of responding instantaneously to injury to form a protective hemostatic plug, deregulation of this system may result in thrombotic occlusion. Specifically targeting the pathways discussed in this chapter has led to evolving development of antithrombotics (part 2) and fibrinolytics (part 4).

REFERENCES

1. Aird WC. Vascular bed-specific thrombosis. J Thromb Haemost 2007; 5(suppl 1):283–291.
2. Jin RC, Voetsch B, Loscalzo J. Endogenous mechanisms of inhibition of platelet function. Microcirculation 2005; 12:247–258.

3. Davi G, Patrono C. Platelet activation and atherothrombosis. N Engl J Med 2007; 357:2482–2494.

4. Offermanns S. Activation of platelet function through G protein-coupled receptors. Circ Res 2006; 99:1293–1304.

5. Mosesson MW. Fibrinogen and fibrin structure and functions. J Thromb Haemost 2005; 3:1894–1904.

6. Mackman N, Tilley RE, Key NS. Role of extrinsic pathway of blood coagulation in hemostasis and thrombosis. Arterioscler Thromb Vasc Biol 2007; 27:1687–1693.

7. Rau JC, Beaulieu LM, Huntington JA, et al. Serpins in thrombosis, hemostasis and fibrinolysis. J Thromb Haemost 2007; 5(Suppl 1):102–115.

8. Bode W. The structure of thrombin: a janus-headed proteinase. Semin Thromb Hemost 2006; 32(suppl. 1):16–31.

9. Crawley JTB, Zanardelli S, Chion CKNK, et al. The central role of thrombin in hemostasis. J Thromb Haemost 2007; 5(suppl 1):95–101.

10. Van de Wouwer M, Collen D, Conway EM. Thrombomodulin-protein C-EPCR system: integrated to regulate coagulation and inflammation. Arterioscler Thromb Vasc Biol 2004; 24:1374–1383.

11. Cesarman-Maus G, Hajjar KA. Molecular mechanisms of fibrinolysis. Br J Haematol 2005; 129:307–321.

12. Longstaff C, Thelwell C. Understanding the enzymology of fibrinolysis and improving thrombolytic therapy. FEBS Lett 2005; 579:3303–3309.

13. Willemse JL, Hendriks DF. A role for procarboxypeptidase U (TAFI) in thrombosis. Front Bioscie 2007; 12:1973–1987.

2

Overview of Platelet-Dependent Thrombosis

Jane E. Freedman and Price Blair
Department of Medicine and Pharmacology, Boston University School of Medicine, Boston, Massachusetts, U.S.A.

Joseph Loscalzo
Department of Medicine, Brigham and Women's Hospital, Harvard Medical School, Boston, Massachusetts, U.S.A.

INTRODUCTION

Thrombosis can cause occlusion of either the venous or arterial circulation and is a major cause of morbidity and mortality in various diseases. Typically, hemostasis carefully balances pro- and antithrombotic factors in the vasculature, while thrombosis reflects a pathological imbalance that favors prothrombotic factors. Advances in understanding the mechanisms of platelet-dependent thrombosis, as well as discovery of new targets, have led to the development of novel classes of antithrombotic drugs.

Thrombus formation within a vessel is the precipitating event in many common distinct vascular diseases, including thrombotic cerebrovascular events, myocardial infarction, and venous thrombosis; however, the pathophysiological processes regulating these diseases are not the same. In venous thrombosis, primary hypercoagulable states reflecting defects of the proteins of coagulation and fibrinolysis or secondary hypercoagulable states involving abnormalities of blood vessels and blood flow lead to thrombosis. By contrast, the vessel wall and platelet typically play a greater role in arterial thrombosis. After platelet adherence to the vessel wall, a thrombus forms as platelets aggregate via the binding of fibrinogen to the glycoprotein (GP) IIb-IIIa complex. The regulation of platelet adhesion, activation, aggregation, and recruitment will be described in further detail below. Many processes in platelets are similar to common pathways other cell types such as housekeeping enzymes and signal transduction components; however, unlike most cells, platelets lack a nucleus and are unable to adapt to changing biological settings by altered transcription. Platelets sustain limited protein synthetic capacity from megakaryocte-derived mRNA, but most of the molecules needed to respond to various stimuli are maintained in storage granules and membrane compartments. While the primary function of platelets is regulation of hemostasis, our understanding of their role in other processes, such as immunity and inflammation, continues to expand.

Initially, characterization of arachidonic acid metabolism in platelets furthered an understanding of the therapeutic utility of cyclooxygenase inhibitors (such as aspirin) in cardiovascular disease. The study of platelet receptors, including adenosine diphosphate (ADP) receptors and GPIIb/IIIa (see chaps. 25, 27, and 28), has been associated with the development of additional classes of antiplatelet drugs, such as thienopyridine derivatives and GPIIb/IIIa receptor antagonists, respectively. As receptor pathways continue to be defined, additional inhibitors are being developed, including inhibitors of platelet adhesion (chap. 26), and protease activation receptor-1 (PAR1) inhibitors (chap. 30). Equally important, as platelet function testing is refined (chap. 7), the relative role of many of these therapies in the clinical setting will be delineated. Lastly, additional understanding of platelet pharmacogenomics (chap. 5) and platelet proteomics/transcriptomics (chap. 8) will yield novel antithrombotic targets and greatly assist with individualized therapy and dosing.

OVERVIEW OF THE PLATELET

Platelets are disk-shaped and very small anucleate cells (1–5 μm in diameter; Fig. 1). In humans, platelets circulate in the bloodstream at concentrations of 200 to 400,000/μL, with an average life span of 7 to 10 days. Owing to their size compared with that of erythrocytes, platelets in whole blood are displaced toward the vessel wall under laminar flow conditions. In this location, they are optimally positioned to detect changes in and respond to the endothelium, the contiguous layer of cells that line the lumen of the blood vessel.

Platelet Granules

Platelet granules are synthesized in megakaryocytes prior to thrombopoiesis and contain an array of pro-thrombotic, pro-inflammatory, and antimicrobial mediators. The two major types of platelet granules, α and dense, are distinguished by their size, abundance,

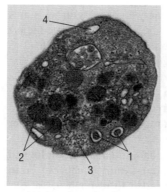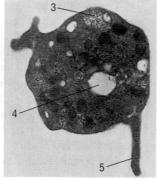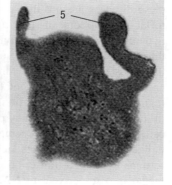

(A) Resting platelet   (B) Activated platelet (3 min)   (C) Activated platelet (20 min)

Figure 1   Changes in platelet structure and granule content in (**A**) a resting platelet, (**B**) 3 minutes after thrombin (0.1 U/mL) stimulation, and (**C**) 20 minutes after thrombin (0.1 U/mL) stimulation by transmission electron microscopy (1. Dense granules; 2. α-Granules; 3. Glycogen; 4. Canalicular system; 5. Pseudopodia. Pictures courtesy of O. Vitseva).

and granular content (Fig. 1). α-Granules are the larger and more abundant granules ($\sim$80/platelet), and they contain soluble coagulation proteins, adhesion molecules, growth factors, integrins, cytokines, and inflammatory modulators. Prototypical α-granule proteins include P-selectin (CD62P), platelet factor-4 (PF-4), von Willebrand factor (vWF), platelet-endothelial cell adhesion molecule (PECAM), GPIb, integrin $\alpha_{IIb}\beta_3$, and fibrinogen. While the majority of these proteins are synthesized in megakaryocytes, some proteins, such as fibrinogen, are incorporated from the plasma by receptor-mediated endocytosis (1). α-Granule proteins are either secreted into the local environment, or, as with P-selectin and integrin $\alpha_{IIb}\beta_3$, redistributed to the platelet plasma membrane. Platelet-dense granules are smaller than α-granules and one-tenth as abundant ($\sim$7–8/ platelet) (2). While α-granules contain proteins that may be more important in the inflammatory response, dense granules are packed with high concentrations of small molecules influencing platelet aggregation. These small molecules include nucleotides such as ADP, ions such as calcium and magnesium, and platelet ligands such as serotonin. Dense granules are secreted within two to five seconds after stimulation, and their contents, especially ADP, act locally to stimulate other platelets.

Platelets are derived from megakaryocytes. Found primarily in the bone marrow, megakaryocytes are polyploidal hematopoietic cells whose sole function is to produce platelets (3). Upon stimulation with thrombopoietin (TPO), the primary regulator of platelet biogenesis, megakaryocytes transcribe RNA, synthesize platelet-specific proteins, assemble organelles, and package these elements for incorporation into platelets. The mechanism by which megakaryocytes produce and release fully formed platelets is unclear, but the process likely involves formation of proplatelets, pseudopod-like structures generated by the evagination of the cytoplasm (4,5). In culture, TPO-stimulated megakaryocytes form one to many of these microtubule-rich extensions, the surface of which is covered by platelet-sized extrusions. In vivo, it is believed that proplatelets extend into the vascular sinusoids of the bone marrow, where they branch and bifurcate until individual platelets fragment from the ends (5), Nitric oxide may also play a role in thrombopoiesis (6).

PLATELET ADHESION AND THE INITIATION OF THROMBUS FORMATION

The formation of a thrombus and the process of hemostasis are initiated by the adherence of platelets to the damaged vessel wall. This damage exposes subendothelial components responsible for triggering platelet reactivity, and includes different types of collagen, vWF, fibronectin, and other adhesive proteins, such as vitronectin and thrombospondin. The specific hemostatic response may vary depending on the extent of damage, the specific proteins exposed, as well as flow conditions. There are specific collagen-binding proteins expressed on the platelet surface that subsequently regulate collagen-induced platelet adhesion, particularly under flow conditions and include GPIV, GPVI, and integrin $\alpha_2\beta_1$. These receptors are thought to interact in a synergistic way, depending on the flow conditions and relative exposure of specific types of collagen or extracellular matrix proteins (7).

Glycoprotein Ib-IX-V (GPIb-IX-V) complex adhesive receptor is central to both platelet adhesion and initiation of platelet activation. Damage to the blood vessel wall exposes subendothelial vWF and collagen to the circulating blood. The GPIb-IX-V complex found on the platelet surface binds to the exposed vWF, causing platelets to adhere to the injured subendothelium (Fig. 2). In addition, the engagement of the

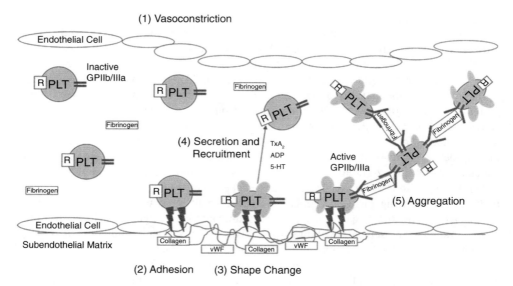

Figure 2 Platelet function in hemostasis and thrombosis. Disk-shaped platelets circulate in an inactive state in the bloodstream. Upon damage to the endothelium, the vessel wall constricts and platelets adhere to exposed subendothelial collagen and vWF via specific surface receptors. This event triggers platelet shape change, in addition to synthesis and secretion of TXA_2, ADP, and serotonin (5-HT). Release of these prothrombotic mediators causes activation of various platelet receptors (R). These events lead to a conformational change in integrin $\alpha_{IIb}\beta_3$ (Glycoprotein IIb/IIIa), enabling the high-affinity binding of fibrinogen. A stable platelet thrombus forms as recruited platelets adhere to one another via fibrinogen bridges. *Abbreviations*: vWF, von Willebrand factor; TXA_2, thromboxane.

GPIb-IX-V complex causes a transduction of signals, which leads to platelet activation. von Willebrand factor–bound GPIb-IX-V induces a conformational change in the GPIIb/IIIa receptor, transforming it from an inactive low-affinity state to an active receptor. This active receptor binds additional vWF or fibrinogen with high affinity. Given the central role of the GPIb-IX-V complex in platelet adhesion and aggregation, it has become an attractive target for the development of antiplatelet drugs (chap. 27).

Signaling Mechanisms Regulating Platelet Adhesion and Shape Change

Platelet shape change is largely regulated by receptor-mediated changes in intracellular calcium concentration. Collagen ligation of GPVI results in Src-kinase-dependent activation of phospholipase C (PLC), an enzyme that hydrolyzes polyphosphoinositide $PI_{4,5}P_2$ to 1,4,5-IP_3 and diacylglycerol (DAG) (8,9). DAG acts as a second messenger to activate the serine/threonine kinase, protein kinase C (PKC), while IP_3 stimulates calcium release from intracellular stores and triggers calcium influx across the platelet plasma membrane (10). During this process, cytosolic calcium concentration increases from 100 nM to over 1 μM—a 10-fold change (10). This rapid increase activates calcium-sensitive gelsolin, a regulatory protein that cleaves actin filaments and thus allows for rearrangement of the platelet cytoskeleton (11,12).

Ligation of platelet adhesion receptors also activates other signaling molecules, including phosphoinositide 3-kinase (PI3-K) (12). PI3-K is a lipid kinase, abundantly expressed in platelets and known to regulate a variety of functional responses in hematopoietic cells (13). The major class of PI3-Ks, class IA, are heterodimers consisting of a regulatory (p85) and a catalytic subunit (p110). PI3-K catalyzes the phosphorylation of phosphoinositides, and its main product, PtdIns (3–5)P3—commonly known as PIP3—activates protein kinase B/Akt, PLC, some isoforms of PKC, and a host of other targets. PI3K is known to bind, via its p85 subunit, to the cytoplasmic tail of receptors possessing either tyrosine kinase activity or receptors coupled to Src-type protein tyrosine kinases. Although the platelet GPIb-IX-V receptor has no known tyrosine kinase activity, vWF ligation of this receptor has been shown to activate PI3-K (14). Animal studies have demonstrated that platelet adhesion responses are impaired in p85-deficient mice (12), but the downstream targets of PI3-K signaling that promote platelet adhesion have yet to be established.

PLATELET RECEPTORS AND ACTIVATION

The activation of platelets is regulated by distinct surface receptors that subsequently regulate various functions. These receptors are engaged by a wide variety of agonists (stimulants) and adhesive proteins. In summary, the stimulation or engagement of platelet receptors triggers two distinct processes: (*i*) activation of specific and numerous internal signaling pathways that lead to further platelet activation, often associated with granule release; and (*ii*) the capacity of the platelet to bind to other platelets or adhesive proteins, which causes hemostasis or thrombus formation. As both of these processes may lead to vessel occlusion, many of these receptors have been and are being examined as targets for preventing and treating thrombus formation and are discussed in other chapters. While there are many families and subfamilies of receptors found on platelets known to regulate platelet functions, only those of major therapeutic relevance will be considered below.

Transmembrane Receptors

The seven transmembrane receptor family is the primary agonist-stimulated receptor family. There are several seven transmembrane receptors found on platelets, including ADP receptors, the thrombin receptor, lipid receptors, prostaglandin receptors, and chemokine receptors.

Thrombin Receptors

Thrombin receptors comprise the major seven transmembrane receptor class found on platelets. The first identified was the PAR1 (15,16). This group of receptors (the PAR class) have a distinct mechanism of activation that involves specific cleavage of the N-terminus, which acts as a ligand to the receptor. Other PAR receptors are present on platelets, including PAR2 (not activated by thrombin) and PAR4.

ADP Receptors

Adenosine receptor inhibitors have been successfully used in the treatment of stroke and prevention of thrombosis after cardiac intervention, and there continues to be great interest in these receptor pathways. Erythrocytes and endothelial cells secrete ADP that contributes to hemostasis, thrombus formation, and vascular occlusion by stimulating platelet aggregation. In addition, ADP secreted from the dense granules of stimulated platelets acts to potentiate platelet aggregation (17–19). In the platelet, ADP induces an influx of calcium, mobilizes calcium from intracellular stores, and attenuates the inhibition of adenylyl cyclase. These signals involve the binding of ADP to puringeric receptors on the platelet surface. There are several distinct ADP receptors, classified as $P2X_1$, $P2Y_1$, and $P2Y_{12}$ (Fig. 2) (18–22). ADP stimulation of the $P2Y_1$ G_q-coupled receptor activates PLC, leading to internal calcium mobilization (22,23). Activation of the $P2Y_1$ receptor is thought to be responsible for mediating ADP-induced platelet shape change (23) in addition to ADP-induced platelet aggregation.

Activation of both the $P2Y_{12}$ and $P2Y_1$ receptors is needed for ADP-induced platelet aggregation (23,24). The activation of the platelet $P2Y_1$ receptor mediates the initial rapid response to ADP, defining the maximal rate of ADP-induced platelet aggregation (24). The degree of sustained platelet aggregation, however, is primarily due to ADP activation of the $P2Y_{12}$ receptor (24). Selective antagonism of the $P2Y_{12}$ receptor demonstrates that it plays a role in sustaining and amplifying ADP-induced aggregation (25). The antiplatelet effect of thienopyridine derivatives is due to irreversible inhibition of ADP binding to platelet purinergic receptors (26,27).

Integrins

Integrin receptors are adhesive and signaling molecules that consist of noncovalently associated heterodimers of α and β subunits, and typically exist in either a low- or high-affinity state. In unstimulated platelets, the major platelet integrin GPIIb/IIIa ($\alpha_{IIb}\beta_3$) is maintained in an inactive conformation and functions as a low-affinity adhesion receptor for fibrinogen (28). This integrin is only expressed on platelets. After activation, the interaction between fibrinogen and GPIIb/IIIa forms intracellular bridges between platelets, leading to platelet aggregation (Fig. 2).

After engagement, the GPIIb/IIIa receptor serves as a bidirectional conduit with GPIIb/IIIa-mediated signaling (outside-in signaling) occurring immediately after the binding of fibrinogen and initiating intracellular signaling that further stabilizes the platelet aggregate. The initial phase of outside-in signaling contributes to further activate the integrin GPIIb/IIIa because of the formation of a complex network of signaling proteins and alterations in structural cytoskeletal proteins. Subsequently, calcium mobilization, tyrosine phosphorylation, and activation of phosphoinositide metabolism result from the activation of the GPIIb/IIIa complex. These complex series of events transform platelet aggregation from a reversible to an irreversible process.

PLATELETS AND INFLAMMATION

Inflammation plays an important role during the acute thrombotic phase of unstable coronary syndromes. Patients with acute coronary syndromes have not only increased interactions between platelets (homotypic aggregates), but also increased interactions between platelets and leukocytes (heterotypic aggregates). These heterotypic aggregates form when platelets are activated and undergo degranulation, after which they adhere to circulating leukocytes and potentially contribute to the atherothrombotic process. Platelets bind via P-selectin (CD62P) expressed on the surface of activated platelets to the leukocyte receptor P-selectin glycoprotein ligand-1 (PSGL-1) (29). This interaction leads to increased expression of CD11b/CD18 (Mac-1) on leukocytes (30), which itself supports interactions with platelets. Platelet leukocyte binding in unstable coronary syndromes highlights the interaction between inflammation and thrombosis in atherothrombotic disease. Plaque rupture promotes activation of inflammatory responses, and increased expression of tissue factor (TF) initiates the coagulation cascade. In addition, the expression of TF on both endothelial cells and monocytes is partially regulated by proinflammatory cytokines, including tumor necrosis factor-α and IL-1 (31).

Given that platelets are the first blood cells to accumulate at sites of vascular damage, their involvement in the inflammatory process is entirely logical. From an evolutionary standpoint, hemostasis and inflammation have always been coupled. In many lower organisms (i.e., invertebrates and lower), the cells involved in hemostasis also fulfill roles in host defense and wound repair. Although mammalian platelets have evolved as specialized hemostatic cells, they retain many features of inflammatory cells and contribute to inflammation in two fundamental ways: (*i*) by secreting pro-inflammatory mediators; and (*ii*) by interacting synergistically with other vascular cells, such as leukocytes and endothelial cells (32–34).

Platelet Secretion of Pro-inflammatory Mediators

A recent study suggests that activated platelets secrete over 300 different types of proteins (35). While many of these peptides are prothrombotic mediators, much of the platelet secretome comprise adhesion proteins, growth factors, chemokines, and cytokines. These proteins, in collaboration with platelet-derived small molecules, influence inflammation by concertedly regulating cell recruitment, cell adhesion and aggregation, cell survival and proliferation, and proteolysis. Platelet-α granules store and release the majority of platelet-derived inflammatory peptides. Platelet-derived growth factor (PDGF) stimulates smooth muscle cell proliferation and is chemoattractant to leukocytes. RANTES (regulated upon activation, normal T cell expressed and secreted) is involved in chemotaxis and activation of numerous leukocytic cell types, including basophils, eosinophils, and monocytes (36). Neutrophils, in particular, are the cellular target of many platelet-derived inflammatory mediators. PF-4 and β-thromboglobulin (β-TG), both protypical α-granule peptides, are chemoattractant to neutrophils (37). PF-4, which is the most abundant protein secreted from activated platelets, also directly stimulates neutrophils, inducing both degranulation and adhesion to endothelial cells (37). Platelet-derived transforming growth factor-β (TGF-β), neutrophil-activating peptide 2 (NAP-2), and even ADP also stimulate neutrophil chemotaxis, degranulation, and oxidative burst. Additionally, activated platelets release soluble CD40 ligand (sCD40L), which generates an inflammatory response in endothelial cells through its interaction with the CD40 receptor. CD40L-stimulated endothelial cells upregulate production of chemotactic proteins [monocyte chemoattractant protein-1 (MCP-1)], adhesive proteins [intercellular adhesion molecule-1 (ICAM-1), $\alpha_v\beta_3$], proteolytic compounds [matrix metalloproteinases (MMPs)], and prothrombotic mediators TF (38). Platelet-derived CD40L also plays a role in lymphocyte stimulation and downstream activation of the adaptive immune system (39).

Pro-inflammatory Interactions with Leukocytes and Endothelial Cells

As discussed, platelet-derived peptides and small molecules stimulate leukocytes, lymphocytes, and endothelial cells, inducing a pro-inflammatory response in these cells. In addition, activated platelets influence inflammation by directly interacting with blood cells. This interaction results in the mutual activation of each cell, thereby amplifying the inflammatory response. Leukocyte-activated platelets secrete prothrombotic and pro-inflammatory mediators, while platelet-activated leukocytes secrete or expose various chemokines, cytokines, coagulation factors, adhesive proteins, and proteolytic compounds.

As an example, formation of platelet-neutrophil heterotypic aggregates has been shown to increase platelet release of sCD40L and neutrophil production of superoxide (40).

In addition to forming co-aggregates with circulating leukocytes, activated platelets directly interact with endothelial cells. As discussed, under normal settings, endothelial secretion of NO and prostacyclin (PGI_2) inhibits platelet adhesion to the vessel wall. Moreover, endothelial cells express surface enzymes with ecto-ADPase (CD39) activity, which prevents platelet activation by free ADP. Inflamed endothelial cells upregulate a number of receptors that actively promote platelet adhesion. P-selectin, which is stored in endothelial Weibel-Palade bodies, rapidly translocates to the endothelial surface in response to inflammatory stimuli. Platelets also express PSGL-1, and interactions between endothelial P-selectin and platelet PSGL-1 are sufficient to induce platelet rolling on the endothelial monolayer. Similar to platelet-leukocyte aggregates, platelets and endothelial cells become mutually activated by their interactions. Platelet-endothelial interactions are particularly important for the recruitment of leukocytes to sites of vascular inflammation. Although activated leukocytes are able to bind to inflamed endothelial cells through receptor-ligand interactions, adherent platelets provide a sticky surface to recruit leukocytes and facilitate their transmigration across the vessel wall. Thus, through their secretion of inflammatory mediators and their synergistic interactions with vascular cells, platelets play a central role in the initiation and propagation of the inflammatory process.

CONCLUSION

Advances in the understanding of the mechanisms of platelet activation, as well as the development of new techniques for studying platelet function, have led to greater insight into the formation of a thrombus and have supported the development of new classes of platelet-inhibiting drugs. Initially, characterizing arachidonic acid metabolism in platelets furthered an understanding of the utility of cyclooxygenase inhibitors, most notably aspirin. The discovery and characterization of the panoply of platelet receptors, such as ADP receptors and GPIIb/IIIa, have been associated with the development of novel classes of antiplatelet drugs such as thienopyridine derivatives and GPIIb/IIIa receptor antagonists, respectively. Future examination of receptor pathway inhibitors, including GPIb-IX and collagen-GPVI (41), as well as further understanding of P2Y12 inhibitors (42) and other antiplatelet agents will lead to additional pharmacological development in the field of antithrombotics. As the coagulation and platelet-dependent pathways are also intimately tied to the atherosclerotic process, future knowledge may also affect our view of the normal, global, and diseased states of the vasculature as well as lead to the development of therapeutic approaches that protect vessel patency and limit vascular disease.

REFERENCES

1. Harrison P, Wilbourn B, Debili N, et al. Uptake of plasma fibrinogen into the alpha granules of human megakaryocytes and platelets. J Clin Invest 1989; 84:1320–1324.
2. Baumgartner HR, Born GV. Effects of 5-hydroxytryptamine on platelet aggregation. Nature 1968; 218:137–141.
3. Ogawa M. Differentiation and proliferation of hematopoietic stem cells. Blood 1993; 81:2844–2853.
4. Italiano JE Jr., Lecine P, Shivdasani RA, et al. Blood platelets are assembled principally at the ends of proplatelet processes produced by differentiated megakaryocytes. J Cell Biol 1999; 147:1299–1312.

5. Patel SR, Hartwig JH, Italiano JE Jr. The biogenesis of platelets from megakaryocyte proplatelets. J Clin Invest 2005; 115:3348–3354.
6. Battinelli E, Willoughby SR, Foxall T, et al. Induction of platelet formation from megakaryocytoid cells by nitric oxide. Proc Natl Acad Sci U S A 2001; 98:14458–14463.
7. Hugel B, Socie G, Vu T, et al. Elevated levels of circulating procoagulant microparticles in patients with paroxysmal nocturnal hemoglobinuria and aplastic anemia. Blood 1999; 93:3451–3456.
8. Jones ML, Craik JD, Gibbins JM, et al. Regulation of SHP-1 tyrosine phosphatase in human platelets by serine phosphorylation at its C terminus. J Biol Chem 2004; 279:40475–40483.
9. Poole A, Gibbins JM, Turner M, et al. The Fc receptor gamma-chain and the tyrosine kinase Syk are essential for activation of mouse platelets by collagen. EMBO J 1997; 16:2333–2341.
10. Sage SO, Rink TJ. The kinetics of changes in intracellular calcium concentration in fura-2-loaded human platelets. J Biol Chem 1987; 262:16364–16369.
11. Hartwig JH, Kung S, Kovacsovics T, et al. D3 phosphoinositides and outside-in integrin signaling by glycoprotein IIb-IIIa mediate platelet actin assembly and filopodial extension induced by phorbol 12-myristate 13-acetate. J Biol Chem 1996; 271:32986–32993.
12. Watanabe N, Nakajima H, Suzuki H, et al. Functional phenotype of phosphoinositide 3-kinase p85alpha-null platelets characterized by an impaired response to GP VI stimulation. Blood 2003; 102:541–548.
13. Hirsch E, Katanaev VL, Garlanda C, et al. Central role for G protein-coupled phosphoinositide 3-kinase gamma in inflammation. Science 2000; 287:1049–1053.
14. Yin H, Stojanovic A, Hay N, et al. The role of Akt in the signaling pathway of the glycoprotein Ib-IX induced platelet activation. Blood 2008; 111:658–665.
15. Hung DT, Vu TK, Wheaton VI, et al. Cloned platelet thrombin receptor is necessary for thrombin-induced platelet activation. J Clin Invest 1992; 89:350–1353.
16. Vu TK, Hung DT, Wheaton VI, et al. Molecular cloning of a functional thrombin receptor reveals a novel proteolytic mechanism of receptor activation. Cell 1991; 64:1057–1068.
17. Clutton P, Folts JD, Freedman JE. Pharmacological control of platelet function. Pharmacol Res 2001; 44:255–264.
18. Cattaneo M, Lombardi R, Zighetti ML, et al. Deficiency of (33P)2MeS-ADP binding sites on platelets with secretion defect, normal granule stores and normal thromboxane A2 production. Evidence that ADP potentiates platelet secretion independently of the formation of large platelet aggregates and thromboxane A2 production. Thromb Haemost 1997; 77:986–990.
19. Gachet C, Cattaneo M, Ohlmann P, et al. Purinoceptors on blood platelets: further pharmacological and clinical evidence to suggest the presence of two ADP receptors. Br J Haematol 1995; 91:434–444.
20. Daniel JL, Dangelmaier C, Jin J, et al. Role of intracellular signaling events in ADP-induced platelet aggregation. Thromb Haemost 1999; 82:1322–1326.
21. Daniel JL, Dangelmaier C, Jin J, et al. Molecular basis for ADP-induced platelet activation. I. Evidence for three distinct ADP receptors on human platelets. J Biol Chem 1998; 273:2024–2029.
22. Fagura MS, Dainty IA, McKay GD, et al. P2Y1-receptors in human platelets which are pharmacologically distinct from P2Y(ADP)-receptors. Br J Pharmacol 1998; 124:157–164.
23. Jin J, Kunapuli SP. Coactivation of two different G protein-coupled receptors is essential for ADP-induced platelet aggregation. Proc Natl Acad Sci U S A 1998; 95:8070–8074.
24. Jarvis GE, Humphries RG, Robertson MJ, et al. ADP can induce aggregation of human platelets via both P2Y(1) and P(2T) receptors. Br J Pharmacol 2000; 129:275–282.
25. Storey RF, Sanderson HM, White AE, et al. The central role of the P(2T) receptor in amplification of human platelet activation, aggregation, secretion and procoagulant activity. Br J Haematol 2000; 110:925–934.
26. Savi P, Pereillo JM, Uzabiaga MF, et al. Identification and biological activity of the active metabolite of clopidogrel. Thromb Haemost 2000; 84:891–896.
27. Savi P, Combalbert J, Gaich C, et al. The antiaggregating activity of clopidogrel is due to a metabolic activation by the hepatic cytochrome P450-1A. Thromb Haemost 1994; 72:313–317.
28. Savage B, Ruggeri ZM. Selective recognition of adhesive sites in surface-bound fibrinogen by glycoprotein IIb-IIIa on nonactivated platelets. J Biol Chem 1991; 266:11227–11233.

29. Rinder HM, Bonan JL, Rinder CS, et al. Dynamics of leukocyte-platelet adhesion in whole blood. Blood 1991; 78:1730–1737.
30. Neumann FJ, Zohlnhofer D, Fakhoury L, et al. Effect of glycoprotein IIb/IIIa receptor blockade on platelet-leukocyte interaction and surface expression of the leukocyte integrin Mac-1 in acute myocardial infarction. J Am Coll Cardiol 1999; 34:1420–1426.
31. Shebuski RJ, Kilgore KS. Role of inflammatory mediators in thrombogenesis. J Pharmacol Exp Ther 2002; 300:729–735.
32. Lindemann SW, Yost CC, Denis MM, et al. Neutrophils alter the inflammatory milieu by signal-dependent translation of constitutive messenger RNAs. Proc Natl Acad Sci U S A 2004; 101:7076–7081.
33. Weyrich AS, Lindemann S, Zimmerman GA. The evolving role of platelets in inflammation. J Thromb Haemost 2003; 1:1897–1905.
34. Weyrich AS, Zimmerman GA. Platelets: signaling cells in the immune continuum. Trends Immunol 2004; 25:489–495.
35. Coppinger JA, Cagney G, Toomey S, et al. Characterization of the proteins released from activated platelets leads to localization of novel platelet proteins in human atherosclerotic lesions. Blood 2004; 103:2096–2104.
36. von Hundelshausen P, Weber KS, Huo Y, et al. RANTES deposition by platelets triggers monocyte arrest on inflamed and atherosclerotic endothelium. Circulation 2001; 103:1772–1777.
37. Petersen F, Bock L, Flad HD, et al. Platelet factor 4-induced neutrophil-endothelial cell interaction: involvement of mechanisms and functional consequences different from those elicited by interleukin-8. Blood 1999; 94:4020–4028.
38. May AE, Langer H, Seizer P, et al. Platelet-leukocyte interactions in inflammation and atherothrombosis. Semin Thromb Hemost 2007; 33:123–127.
39. Sprague DL, Sowa JM, Elzey BD, et al. The role of platelet CD154 in the modulation in adaptive immunity. Immunol Res 2007; 39:185–193.
40. Vanichakarn P, Blair P, Wu C, et al. Neutrophil CD40 enhances platelet-mediated inflammation. *Thrombosis Research* 2008; 122(3):346–358.
41. Gruner S, Prostredna M, Aktas B, et al. Anti-glycoprotein VI treatment severely compromises hemostasis in mice with reduced alpha2beta1 levels or concomitant aspirin therapy. Circulation 2004; 110:2946–2951.
42. Gachet C. ADP receptors of platelets and their inhibition. Thromb Haemost 2001; 86:222–232.

3

Design Issues in Clinical Trials of Thrombolytic and Antithrombotic Agents

Robert P. Giugliano
Cardiovascular Division, Brigham and Women's Hospital, Harvard Medical School, Boston, Massachusetts, U.S.A.

INTRODUCTION

Prior to the 1990s, there were only a limited number of choices of antithrombotic agents available to the clinician. However, rapid advances in the next two decades resulted in the introduction of a plethora of agents into clinical practice, including a variety of antiplatelet, anticoagulant, and fibrinolytic agents with differing targets, modes of administration, and pharmacokinetic properties. In parallel, a number of challenges have arisen in the clinical development of such novel agents. In this chapter, I discuss the three broad themes of complexity (involving human biology, therapies, and patients), the high bar that exists for new agents owing to the prior successes, and practical drug development issues that must be addressed in the designs of modern clinical trials of novel thrombolytic and antithrombotic agents. The final section of this chapter explores some potential solutions to these challenges.

According to the Old Testament (1), King Nebuchadnezzar II inadvertently initiated what was arguably the first clinical trial in recorded history in the 6th century B.C. when he ordered that a strict diet of meat and wine be followed for three years by his servants-in-training. Daniel and three other children convinced their guard that they should test vegetables and water instead, and then compare their results with those of the other children. After only 10 days, Daniel and his friends appeared healthier and better nourished, and Nebuchadnezzar's guard was so convinced of the difference that he took away the meat and wine diet from the others.

This "trial" shares some of the features with observational studies that were common in earlier medical eras and textbooks. Indeed, another careful observation in the late 1940s by Dr. Lawrence Craven (2) led to the use of aspirin, a drug that had been available for nearly a half century already, to prevent myocardial infarction (MI). He noticed that 400 men prescribed aspirin for rheumatologic conditions rarely suffered heart attacks, thus he began recommending aspirin to prevent MI. However, it took another 26 years before the first clinical trials of aspirin to prevent MI were published (3).

Case studies and observational reports have now been supplanted by the randomized controlled trial (RCT)—the current gold standard for assessment of new medical therapies. RCTs of thrombolytic and antithrombotic therapies began in the mid-1980s. The GISSI-1 study (Table 1) (4) was the first large randomized trial that definitively showed that intravenous thrombolytic therapy with streptokinase improved survival. This trial ushered in an era of large-scale multicenter RCTs in acute MI (AMI) that initially focused on thrombolytic therapy, but also soon spread to antiplatelet and anticoagulant agents. In fact, the ISIS-2 trial (5) published just two years after GISSI-1 was a landmark 2 × 2 factorial study that established the independent and additive

Table 1 Trial Acronyms

ADVANCE MI	Addressing the value of facilitated angioplasty after combination therapy or eptifibatide monotherapy in acute myocardial infarction
BRAVO	Blockade of the glycoprotein IIb/IIIa receptor to avoid vascular occlusion
CHARISMA	Clopidogrel for high atherothrombotic risk and ischemic stabilization management and avoidance
COMMIT/CCS-2	Clopidogrel and metoprolol in myocardial infarction trial/Chinese cooperative study-2
CONSORT	Consolidated standards of reporting trials
CRUSADE	Can rapid risk stratification of unstable angina patients suppress adverse outcomes with early implementation of the ACC/AHA guidelines
EPIC	Evaluation of 7E3 for the prevention of ischemic complications
ESTEEM	Efficacy and safety of the oral direct thrombin inhibitor ximelagatran in patients with recent myocardial damage
EXCITE	The evaluation of xemilofiban in controlling thrombotic events
GISSI-1	Gruppo Italiano per lo studio della strepochinasi nell' infarto Miocardio-1
GRACE	Global registry of acute coronary events
GUSTO	Global use of strategies to improve outcomes
IMPACT-II	Integrilin to minimize platelet aggregation and coronary thrombosis
INTEGRITI	Integrilin and tenecteplase in acute myocardial infarction
ISAR-REACT 2	Intracoronary stenting and antithrombotic regimen: rapid early action for coronary treatment 2
ISIS-2	International study of infarct survival-2
PROTECT	Randomized trial to evaluate the relative protection against post-PCI microvascular dysfunction and post-PCI ischemia among anti-platelet and anti-thrombotic agents
PURSUIT	Platelet glycoprotein IIb/IIIa in unstable angina: receptor suppression using integrilin therapy
OPUS	Oral glycoprotein IIb/IIIa inhibition with orbofiban in patients with unstable coronary syndromes
REPLACE-2	Randomized evaluation in PCI linking angiomax to reduced clinical events-2
SYMPHONY	Sibrafiban vs. aspirin to yield maximum protection from ischemic heart events post-acute coronary syndromes
SYNERGY	Superior yield of the new strategy of enoxaparin, revascularization and glycoprotein IIb/IIIa inhibitors
TARGET	Do Tirofiban and ReoPro give similar efficacy trial
TIMI	Thrombolysis in myocardial infarction

benefits of streptokinase and aspirin by randomizing 17,187 patients with AMI to either aspirin, streptokinase, both, or neither.

However, the rapid introduction of a number of new fibrinolytic, antiplatelet, and anticoagulant agents for the treatment of AMI and other atherosclerotic conditions soon led to several major challenges that continue even today. These challenges to new drug development can be grouped under the broad thematic issues of complexity, prior success, and practicality.

Complexity

Clinical trials of antithrombotic agents face complexity at a number of levels, including the complexity of human biology, the growing number of concomitant therapies and their combinations that are used in clinical practice, and the diversity of the large number of patients that must be enrolled in current clinical trials to adequately evaluate safety and efficacy.

Complexity of Human Biology

Unlike a highly controlled physics experiment performed in a vacuum, studies comprising human biology involve a magnitude of variables that interact in many ways that are often unpredictable. While highly schematic views of biologic systems, such as the role of platelets in the coagulation system are easy to remember and explain, these are highly simplified representations. The redundancy of human biology is far richer than can be represented by a simple figure. Indeed, even the notion that platelets and clotting factors operate independently is an oversimplification, as more modern schemas incorporate both into a cell-based model of coagulation (Fig. 1) (6).

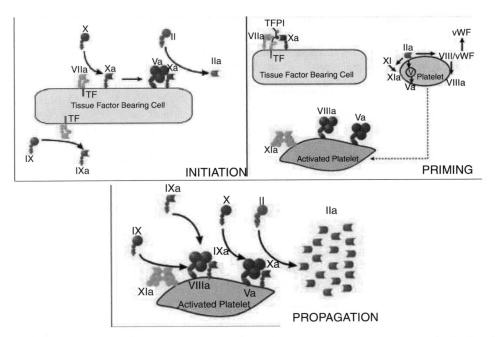

Figure 1 Cell-based model of coagulation. Since neither the coagulation factors nor platelet-based clotting systems act independently, more recent models of coagulation incorporate both systems in a cell-based model that more accurately depicts their interaction (6).

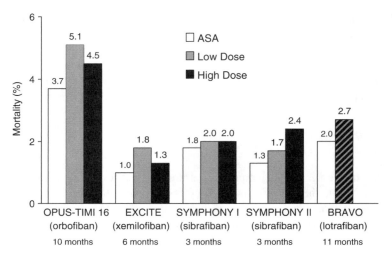

Figure 2 First generation oral GP IIb/IIIa inhibitor phase III trials. Each of these five large studies demonstrated a higher rate of mortality with an oral GP IIb/IIIa inhibitor compared with aspirin monotherapy (8) *Abbreviation*: GP, glycoprotein. The hatched bar at the far right represents the one dose of lotrafiban studied in BRAVO.

This rich complexity of human biologic systems should not be underestimated. Our simplified notions of how therapies work can lead us astray or sometimes to an unexpected serendipitous discovery. For example, intravenous glycoprotein (GP) IIb/IIIa antagonists have been demonstrated to reduce death and ischemic complications following percutaneous coronary interventions (PCI) (7). Clearly then, should not oral forms of these drugs be similarly safe and effective? Yet, the five large randomized clinical trials of oral GP IIb/IIIa antagonists surprisingly showed higher mortality with these agents compared with placebo (Fig. 2) (8). In an example of unforeseen interactions between complex systems, a recent study of proximal inhibitors of the coagulation cascade (monoclonal antibody to tissue factor) was associated with "platelet-type" mucosal hemorrhage most typically observed with antiplatelet drugs (9). A second proximal anticoagulant targeting the tissue factor/factor VIIa complex was very effective in preventing de novo thrombus formation as demonstrated by dose-dependent reduction in F1.2, but was associated with thrombotic complications in 5 of 26 patients undergoing interventional procedures (10). Lastly, while "on-target" effects of novel therapies are often the focus of interest, there may be "off-target" effects that are of equal or greater clinical importance. For example, the oral direct thrombin inhibitor ximelagatran reduced death or recurrent ischemic complications by 24% (95% CI 2–41%) following MI in the ESTEEM trial (11), however, there was a 6.2-fold (95% CI 3.8–10.0) excess in the odds of elevated liver function tests and rare, but sometimes fatal hepatic failure, that ultimately led to the termination of this drug's development program. These observations serve to underscore the importance of formal, rigorous evaluation of new therapies in large-scale RCTs since our simplified conceptions and intuitions may be misleading or incomplete.

Complexity of Therapies

Prior to 1990, there were two each of thrombolytic (streptokinase, urokinase), antiplatelet (aspirin, dipyridamole), and anticoagulant (heparin, warfarin) agents commonly used in clinical practice. Assuming that a clinician may want to use neither, either one, or both of

The Professor's Cube
282,870,942,277,741,856,536,180,333,107,150,328,293,127,731,985,
672,134,721,536,000,000,000,000,000,000 different combinations

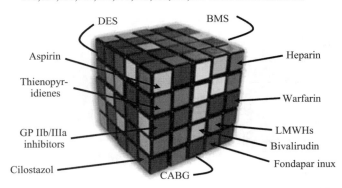

Figure 3 Cardiology's Rubik cube. There are a vast number of possible combinations of antiplatelet, anticoagulant, and revascularization strategies that could be used in clinical practice. As the number of potential choices increase, the complexity of finding the ideal solution increases, similar to that of a multicolored Rubik's cube.

each of these three classes of drugs yields a total of 64 different combinations. Yet, the rapid introduction of new thrombolytics (tPA then followed by 2 bolus fibrin-specific agents), antiplatelets (thienopyridines, GP IIb/IIIa antagonists, newer COX and phosphodiesterase inhibitors), and anticoagulants (low-molecular-weight heparins, direct thrombin inhibitors, factor Xa inhibitors) over the next two decades led to many more combinations than could ever be tested (Fig. 3). While not all combinations may be rationale and/or deserve evaluation, newer agents do need to be studied in a greater number of larger studies to establish their optimal role in current practice. Even well-established therapies can become quickly outdated if they are not continually reevaluated in contemporary studies as newer agents are introduced.

Complexity of Patients

While a good clinical trial evaluates a therapy in a well-defined cohort, the effect of the intervention may not be uniform across the population tested, and the risks or benefits cannot be easily generalized to other patients who differ from the population studied. Yet there is often considerable variability among patients with respect to clinical diagnosis, level of risk, and individual response to therapy, which makes sweeping generalizations treacherous.

Large studies increase the chances of a definitive conclusion and provide a better estimate of adverse effects. However, larger trials are less likely to enroll a homogeneous patient population, and these heterogeneities in clinical presentation can result in important differences in the response to therapies. In the CHARISMA trial (12) that evaluated long-term clopidogrel versus placebo in addition to aspirin, patients with a qualifying diagnosis of atherosclerosis (involving either the coronary, cerebrovascular, or peripheral vascular arterial bed) demonstrated a 12% risk reduction ($p = 0.046$) in the primary composite endpoint, but all other patients in the trial (who were eligible on the basis of the presence of multiple risk factors for atherosclerosis) showed no benefit (20% relative increase, $p = 0.20$) with a significant interaction ($p = 0.045$) between these two prespecified subgroups (Fig. 4).

Primary Efficacy Results (MI/Stroke/CV Death) by Pre-Specified Entry Category in the CHARISMA Trial

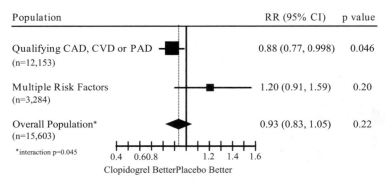

Population	RR (95% CI)	p value
Qualifying CAD, CVD or PAD (n=12,153)	0.88 (0.77, 0.998)	0.046
Multiple Risk Factors (n=3,284)	1.20 (0.91, 1.59)	0.20
Overall Population* (n=15,603)	0.93 (0.83, 1.05)	0.22

*interaction p=0.045

0.4 0.60.8   1.2 1.4 1.6

Clopidogrel BetterPlacebo Better

Figure 4 Primary endpoint results of the CHARISMA trial (12). Patients who had CAD, CVD, or peripheral vascular disease diagnoses prior to randomization had a 12% relative risk reduction ($p = 0.046$) in the primary efficacy composite of cardiovascular death, myocardial infarction or stroke with aspirin + clopidogrel compared with aspirin + placebo. There was no benefit (with a weak trend toward harm) for 20% of patients without established atherosclerosis (multiple risk factor subgroup). In the overall population, there was no statistical benefit of dual antiplatelet therapy (RR 0.93, $p = 0.22$). *Abbreviations*: CAD, coronary artery disease; CVD, cerebrovascular disease

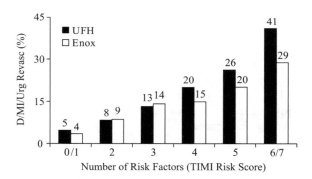

Figure 5 Enoxaparin is more efficacious in higher risk patients. In the TIMI 11b trial (13), patients with unstable angina/non-ST-elevation MI with a TIMI risk score ≥ 4 demonstrated increasing benefit with enox compared with UFH. There was no apparent benefit of enox over UFH at lower TIMI risk scores. *Abbreviations*: UFH, unfractionated heparin; D, death; MI, myocardial infarction; Urg Revasc, urgent revascularization; enox, enoxaparin.

Even within the same clinical diagnosis, a spectrum of risks exists (13). More importantly, careful assessment of the risks of the patients can identify those patients more likely to benefit from aggressive therapies. For example, patients in the TIMI 11b trial (14) randomized to enoxaparin overall experienced a reduction in death or major ischemic complications (RRR 0.84, $p = 0.048$), however, the benefit was most apparent in those of moderate to high risk (13) (Fig 5). As a single risk feature in patients with non-STE-ACS, an elevated troponin level is among the most important as it both identifies a high-risk patient and is also useful in identifying patients who benefit from more intensive therapy. In the ISAR-REACT 2 trial, patients with a positive baseline troponin experienced a 28% relative reduction ($p = 0.02$) in death or in MI when abciximab was added to aspirin + 600 mg clopidogrel, while there was no benefit (0% RR, $p = 0.98$) of abciximab in the troponin-negative cohort (15).

Lastly, individual patients exhibit important differences in drug absorption, distribution, metabolism, and excretion that can result in unpredictable clinical effects. One of the most widely studied recent examples is the variable response to the standard clopidogrel regimen of a 300-mg loading dose followed by 75 mg daily. Several studies demonstrated a variable response in the degree of platelet inhibition, but more importantly, recent data (16–18) have linked less effective inhibition of the platelet with an increase in adverse thrombotic complications. As further research identifies important pharmacogenetic differences between patients [such as differences in warfarin metabolism that have been associated with increased bleeding risk (19)], increased individualization of therapies will surely follow.

Prior Success

Prior to the 1960s, the rate of early mortality following acute MI was approximately 30%. With the advent of cardiopulmonary resuscitation, defibrillation, and introduction of the coronary care unit, 30-day mortality was halved over the next decade. During the subsequent 40 years, we have witnessed a more gradual stepwise reduction in mortality, with the introduction of fibrinolytic and antiplatelet therapy (Fig. 6). However the number of patients needed to treat to show benefit, and hence the size of the clinical trials, has increased dramatically. Most recently, the COMMIT/CCS-2 trial (20) enrolled

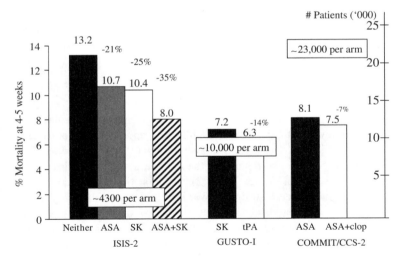

Figure 6 Mortality reduction over time with improved pharmacologic therapies in ST-elevation myocardial infarction. In the ISIS-2 trial (5), both ASA and SK each independently reduced mortality, while their combination showed additive benefits. Because the mortality rate in the comparator arm (placebo) was high by today's standards (13.2%) and the treatment effect was large (21–25%), only ~4300 patients per arm were required to demonstrate a statistical reduction in mortality. A mortality reduction was also seen in the GUSTO-1 trial (36) with tPA compared with SK. However, because the mortality in the comparator arm was now only 7.2% and the benefit of tPA over SK was more modest (14% RRR), nearly 10,000 patients per arm were required. In the COMMIT/CCS-2 trial (20), the most recent study of a new pharmacologic that reduced mortality in AMI, ~23,000 patients per arm were enrolled to demonstrate a 7% reduction in mortality with aspirin + clopidogrel compared with aspirin monotherapy. *Abbreviations*: tPA, tissue plasminogen activator; SK, streptokinase; ASA, aspirin; AMI, acute myocardial infarction.

45,852 patients with AMI to demonstrate a 7% relative (0.6% absolute, $p = 0.03$) reduction in mortality with the addition of clopidogrel. Alternatives to ever-increasing trial size (and extended study durations) include use of surrogate endpoints, composite endpoints, and noninferiority trial designs.

Surrogate Endpoints

A Surrogate endpoint ideally represents an alternative, intermediate endpoint that occurs more frequently or sooner than the clinical endpoint of interest and is closely predictive of that clinical event. In AMI studies, surrogate endpoints of interest have focused on measures of reperfusion, since early trials established a close link between early restoration of coronary perfusion and subsequent mortality reduction, known as the "Open Artery Theory" (21). However, complexities of large clinical trials (see above) make the link between a surrogate endpoint and clinical events observed in earlier smaller, homogenous trials less certain. For example, improved epicardial flow (22), myocardial flow (23), and ST segment resolution (24) each has been independently shown to correlate with lower mortality. However, in the INTEGRITI trial (25), combination therapy with eptifibatide + half-dose tenecteplase improved each of these three surrogates compared with tenecteplase monotherapy, but in the ADVANCE-MI trial (26), the rate of the primary clinical endpoint (death or severe congestive heart failure) tended to be higher with combination therapy (10.1% vs. 2.6%, $p = 0.09$). Similarly, while meta-analyses of facilitated PCI with pharmacologic therapy have demonstrated better epicardial flow with a variety of therapies (27), neither metanalyses of trials exploring the clinical benefit of such facilitated therapies (27,28) nor large-scale clinical endpoint trials have demonstrated the clinical benefit of facilitation with full-dose fibrinolytic (29), combination reduced-dose fibrinolytic + GP IIb/IIIa inhibitor (30), or GP IIb/IIIa monotherapy (30).

Composite Endpoints

A second alternative to a very large mortality trial is to use composite endpoints that combine death with other relevant clinical events. While this approach has been used successfully (e.g, enoxaparin, clopidogrel) to establish clinical benefits and achieve regulatory approval leading to commercial release on the market, a number of difficulties arise when combining multiple clinical events (Table 2). While at first glance combining death and nonfatal infarction might seem straightforward, to maintain uniformity across many hospitals and countries, clinical trials typically utilize a definition of MI that considers the clinical setting (spontaneous, post-revascularization), presence or absence of symptoms, type of cardiac biomarker available, and the relevant diagnostic threshold for the specific marker, presence of electrocardiogram (ECG) findings, and other

Table 2 Theoretical Difficulties with Composite Endpoints

1. Unequal importance (preventing one death $\neq$ one unstable angina episode)
2. Imbalanced frequency of events (nonfatal events typically occur more frequently than death)
3. Little or no effect on the most important endpoints
4. Arbitrary/varying definitions of nonfatal endpoints
5. Interpretation of composite endpoints when the individual components go in different directions (some are increased, others decreased) with the same treatment.

Table 3 Primary Composite Endpoint Results: Local Investigator Reporting Vs. Clinical Endpoint Committee (CEC) Adjudication in Four Landmark Trials

Trial Acronym	Experimental	Control	P-value
EPIC			
Investigator	9.0%	12.4%	0.12
CEC	8.3%	12.8%	0.009
IMPACT II			
Investigator	5.5%	7.8%	0.018
CEC	9.2%	11.4%	0.063
GUSTO Iib			
Investigator	8.4%	9.6%	0.016
CEC	8.9%	9.8%	0.058
PURSUIT			
Investigator	8.0%	10.0%	0.0007
CEC	14.2%	15.7%	0.04

supplemental data (e.g., new wall motion abnormalities on echocardiogram, postmortem findings). This results in a detailed definition that is long [564 words in one recent trial (31)], complicated, and most reliably applied by an independent group of experts, known as a clinical endpoint committee (CEC). The importance of CEC adjudication events should not be underestimated as research has shown that there can be considerable difference in the endpoints as assessed by the local investigator compared with those assessed by the CEC. In one such comparison (32), the CEC upgraded the primary endpoint from statistically nonsignificant (investigator determination) to highly statistically significant (CEC adjudication), and downgraded the primary events in three other trials that form statistically significant to borderline trends (Table 3). The changes in the frequency of the primary endpoint after CEC adjudication were substantial and in one trial (33) represented a 66% increase above what had been reported by the investigators.

Trials that combine efficacy and safety endpoints into a single primary composite endpoint are even more problematic and often face several challenges simultaneously. Consider the example of the REPLACE-2 trial (34), a randomized double-blind comparison of bivalirudin with standard therapy [unfractionated heparin (UFH) + GP IIb/IIIa antagonist] in 6010 patients undergoing urgent or elective PCI. The primary endpoint was a composite of death, MI, urgent revascularization, and inhospital major bleeding. Clearly, the relative importance of these endpoints is not the same, yet in most composite endpoint analyses no weighting of the individual components is performed. As expected, the frequency of death was much lower than the other endpoints, contributing only 0.3% (absolute) of the total primary composite event rate of 9.6%. The definition of bleeding was one that permitted less clinically severe manifestations of bleeding to count as "major," compared with other definitions, such as TIMI major (35) or GUSTO severe (36). In this study, the risks of bleeding and thrombosis tracked in opposition directions, as is typically the case when antithrombotic regimens of different potencies are compared. However, the relative contributions of bleeding and MI were highly dependent on the definitions employed (Figs. 7A and B). Furthermore, a similar trial [PROTECT-TIMI 30 (37)] in 857 patients with non-STE-ACS undergoing PCI demonstrated a directional different trade-off between bleeding and MI (0.4% net benefit in favor of standard therapy), in part explained by the higher-risk population, and in part due to different endpoint definitions.

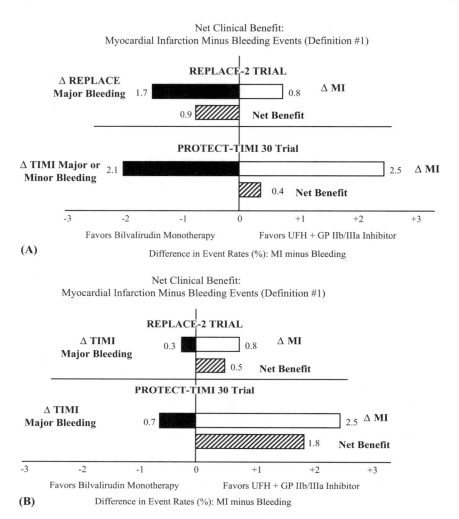

Figure 7 Assessment of the trade-off between bleeding and thrombosis is highly dependent upon the definitions used. Using lower threshold definitions of bleeding (**A**) in the REPLACE-2 (34) and PROTECT-TIMI 30 (37) trials, the former study favored bivalirudin monotherapy, while the latter favored UFH + GP IIb/IIIa inhibitor. However, when the more stringent definition of a TIMI major bleeding event was used (**B**), both studies demonstrated a more favorable balance of outcomes with UFH + GP IIb/IIIa inhibitor. *Abbreviations*: UFH, unfractionated heparin; GP, glycoprotein.

Indeed, difference of opinions regarding the relative merits of bleeding and prevention of ischemic complications are viewed differently by two authoritative guideline committees with respect to the early administration of clopidogrel in patients undergoing PCI and with fondaparinux in patients with non-STE-ACS. The reduction in early ischemic events that begins within the first 24 hours (38) after initiation of clopidogrel is counterbalanced by an increased risk in perioperative bleeding if a patient requires coronary artery bypass graft surgery within the next five days (39). The most recent PCI guideline from the European Society of Cardiology (ESC) (40) favors early treatment, recommending a 600-mg loading dose for patients undergoing immediate PCI or PCI within the next six hours, while 300 mg is considered an adequate clopidogrel load if PCI will not be performed until after six hours. Meanwhile, the North American PCI guideline (41) notes that the benefit and safety of a 600-mg clopidogrel loading dose is not well established and, thus, recommend 300 mg if the PCI is being performed six hours or more after a loading dose. Interestingly the positions of the European and North American experts in their respective 2007 UA/Non-STE-MI guidelines are switched with respect to the factor Xa inhibitor, fondaparinux, in patients with ACS. Fondaparinux was associated with a 48% ($p < 0.001$) reduction in bleeding in the OASIS-5 trial, but an excess of procedural-related thrombosis. In their respective guidelines, the ESC guidelines (42) give fondaparinux (then antithrombotic associated with less bleeding) the highest level of recommendation (Class IA) compared with the ACC/AHA guidelines (Class IB recommendation), which generally prefer UFH or enoxaparin (both Class IA) (43). Clearly, there is no consensus on how to balance these competing risks, particularly when these nonfatal endpoints are considered part of the same composite endpoint.

Noninferiority Design

An alternative to the use of a composite primary endpoint is a "noninferiority" trial design. In this type of study, rather than a null hypothesis that the two treatments are equal (with the hope of demonstrating the alternative hypothesis that the experimental arm is superior) as is the case in a typical superiority trial design, the null hypothesis becomes that the control arm is superior, and the (hoped for) alternative hypothesis is that the experimental arm is no worse than some small increment (i.e., not inferior more than some small arbitrary quantity). Noninferiority trials are especially susceptible to bias and must be carefully designed and conducted. A strong rationale for using a noninferiority design should be provided, as a superiority design would otherwise almost always be preferable. Trial participants should reflect those studies that were used to establish the selection of the active control. Blinding of the randomized treatments and endpoint assessment should be performed to minimize the chances that investigators could influence the results. The outcomes evaluated should use established definitions, as nonstandard definitions that increase the event rate tend to introduce "noise" and in general, reduce the chances of showing a difference between treatments. A critical variable for a noninferiority trial design is the definition of the noninferiority margin, as the larger the margin, the smaller the sample size required. However, trials with large margins (e.g., upper 95% CI of the RR = 1.50) run the risk of concluding that the experimental arm is "not inferior" to the control therapy when in fact it could be as much as 50% worse. Lastly, unlike a superiority trial, a poorly run noninferiority trial, with a high rate of crossover between treatment or premature dropouts, tends to *increase* the chances of a positive (i.e., noninferior) result. Despite these well-known guidelines, several recent noninferiority trials have been designed otherwise (44) and have had mixed acceptance in the clinical trial community (32) and the regulatory authorities.

Practical Issues

Several practical issues represent increasingly important challenges to clinical development of novel antithrombotics. The financial expenditures are enormous, with most large antithrombotic trials costing well in excess of $150 million, and total costs for the development program for a new drug exceeding $1 billion. Patents for drugs expire 20 years after filing, and exclusivity [exclusive marketing rights granted by the Food and Drug Administration (FDA) upon approval of a drug] run for only five (new chemical entity) or seven (orphan drug) years. Thus pharmaceutical companies often have only a few years to cover the costs of development for a new agent. Legal and regulatory requirements have been tightened in the wake of adverse experiences among patients during clinical development and after regulatory approval of new therapies. While many of these changes have improved study subject and patient safety, the addition of pages upon pages of required language into trial-informed consent documents is of questionable merit, particularly for patients with acute illnesses such as AMI when lifesaving therapies are time sensitive. Because of unfortunate severe adverse events that occasionally occur in clinical developments [and which may be highly publicized (45)], patients understandably become more hesitant to participate. Perhaps even more damaging are inaccurate reports in the lay press, such as those that followed the recent neutral results with ezetimibe in a trial of patients with heterozygous familial hypercholesterolemia (46). These widely read unscientific analyses only serve to frighten patients away from well-established therapies and ongoing trials. When these factors are added to the modest recognition and financial remuneration that clinical investigators and research coordinators receive for participation in a clinical study, it is not surprising that recent trials have extended timelines and required participation of less well-developed countries to achieve the enrollment goal.

POTENTIAL SOLUTIONS

While there are formidable challenges in evaluating new antithrombotic agents, there are a number of guiding principles that can help in the design of future trials. The principles can be derived by considering a large, simple, randomized controlled clinical trial comparing the clinical outcomes of two therapies (or new therapy vs. placebo).

Although mechanistic studies and trials exploring surrogate markers are helpful to fully understand a novel compound, there is no substitute for a well-designed clinical endpoint trial, as in the end, new therapies are sought to treat patients, not effect changes in intermediate markers. Since the number of available agents and targets can only increase, it is tempting to try to include multiple arms and treatments; however this is rarely successful. Unless the sample size or treatment effect is extremely large, studies with multiple comparisons are often underpowered (44); hence simpler trials that ask a single question, and compare to treatments head-to-head (such as the TARGET trial (47) that compared abciximab with tirofiban in patients undergoing PCI) are often much more informative. One exception is a 2×2 factorial randomization that can often answer two questions simultaneously without substantial loss of power (5). Because of the complexity of clinical practice, there has been a growing call for "real world trials" (48). Such studies are appealing since the rigid entry criteria and patient management in many studies do not reflect the richness and texture of clinical practice. However, an understated disadvantage of "real world trials" is that such a design can lead to unexpected complexity that precludes the ability to obtain a straightforward answer to a simple question. For example, the results of the SYNERGY trial (49) were difficult to interpret, in part due to the many degrees of freedom that were permitted regarding anticoagulant use prior to randomization and during or after catheterization, which resulted in 16 different combinations of enoxaparin and/or UFH that were administered to study patients before and after combination. While the trial mirrored the complexity of clinical practice, it is not clear that this study substantially added to our understanding of anticoagulant use in patients with non-STE-ACS. These confusing results stand in contrast to the unambiguous answer that came from the simply designed ISAR-REACT 2 study (15), which demonstrated that the benefit of abciximab in addition to 600 mg of clopidogrel in patients with non-STE-ACS was evident in patients with an elevated troponin at baseline.

An alternative to "messy" real-world trials are well-designed registries. Since the majority of patients treated in clinical practice do not qualify for most randomized trials, registries such as GRACE (50) and CRUSADE (51) can provide complementary information to the clinical trial database. These registries are also well suited to permit exploration of the generalizability of findings from the randomized trials. They serve as excellent sources of data for quality improvement efforts, and can identify important questions and generate hypotheses for testing in future RCTs [e.g., utility of early GP IIb/IIIa antagonists in non-STE-ACS (52)] Because registries have less restrictive entry criteria and a lower per patient cost, they are ideally suited to evaluate rare events in new therapies, such as subacute stent thrombosis (53).

Reporting of clinical trials in the medical literature could be improved if authors, reviewers, and editors used existing tools to improve quality. The CONSORT statement (54) identifies 22 items, covering key areas such as randomization, blinding, intention-to-treat, outcomes, sample size justification, and multiple endpoints, which should be described clearly in a clinical trial publication. Likewise, similar criteria exist for noninferiority trials (55), which recommend rigorous explanation and description of the rationale for noninferiority, study participants, interventions and outcomes, derivation of noninferiority margins, and justification for the analysis cohort (intention-to-treat vs. on-treatment). Equally important is education of the lay press, including print and media journalists, editors, and "authoritative experts" posting on the Internet, as these are the sources widely accessed by patients nowadays for medical information. Unfortunately, these sources, particularly the Internet, exhibit highly variable quality since there is essentially no regulation of content, and information that is incorrect and damaging often appears in high-profile publications (56).

The practical challenges to performing high-quality trials cannot be ignored since if they are left unaddressed, their impact will only increase. To ensure adequate financing of trials, streamlined data collection using electronic reporting with selective monitoring should reduce one of the most expensive line items in the trial budget. Legal and regulatory reforms should be pursued, which would permit greater centralized review of study documents, reduce duplicate reporting, and focus detailed collection of data for adverse events of interest (instead of the current comprehensive approach). Hospitals and communities should support subject recruitment in trials, rather than impeding the research team's efforts to identify potential study participants. Two potential incentives for such efforts could be recognition of trial participation as a hospital quality indicator, and more extensive and systematic feedback generated from trial data to participating hospitals regarding practice patterns and outcomes. Lastly, the hard work of the research team, which often occurs after hours and/or in addition to other responsibilities, must be recognized and rewarded. Academic credit (e.g., for continuing medical education), modest perks and benefits (e.g., favored parking for those who drive in off-hours to consent and randomize), and acknowledgment by hospital leadership of the service provided by the research team are small gestures that would help investigators feel that their efforts are valued.

SUMMARY

Testing of novel antithrombotics involves very complex systems and therapies. Whereas the choices for antithrombotic therapy during the 30-year period from 1950 to 1980 were limited to predominantly aspirin, heparin, warfarin, and streptokinase, the subsequent 30 years have witnessed an explosion in the number of classes and agents that are effective inhibitors of thrombosis. Fortunately, there are well-established methods to evaluate new therapies, and advances in study design and reporting have permitted higher quality evidence regarding the risks and benefits of these therapies to emerge. Nonetheless, owing to the complexity of modern clinical trials and the dissemination of their results, potential pitfalls abound. Rigorous attention to detail in trial design and reporting, along with greater efforts to address the many practical challenges faced by those involved in clinical studies is needed.

REFERENCES

1. Holy Bible. Nashville: Thomas Nelson Publishers, 1977.
2. Craven LL. Acetylasalicyclic acid, possible preventive of coronary thrombosis. Ann West Med Surg 1950; 4:95.
3. Elwood PC, Cochrane AL, Burr ML, et al. A randomized controlled trial of acetyl salicylic acid in the secondary prevention of mortality from myocardial infarction. Br Med J 1974; 1:436–440.
4. No authors listed. Effectiveness of intravenous thrombolytic treatment in acute myocardial infarction. Gruppo Italiano per lo Studio della Streptochinasi nell'Infarto Miocardico (GISSI). Lancet 1986; 1:397–402.
5. ISIS-2 (Second International Study of Infarct Survival) Collaborative group. randomized trial of intravenous streptokinase, oral aspirin, both, or neither among 17,187 cases of suspected acute myocardial infarction: ISIS-2. J Am Coll Cardiol 1988; 12:3A–13A.
6. Monroe DM, Hoffman M, Roberts HR. Platelets and thrombin generation. Arterioscler Thromb Vasc Biol 2002; 22:1381–1389.
7. Karvouni E, Katritsis DG, Ioannidis JP. Intravenous glycoprotein IIb/IIIa receptor antagonists reduce mortality after percutaneous coronary interventions. J Am Coll Cardiol 2003; 41:26–32.
8. Chew DP, Bhatt DL, Sapp S, et al. Increased mortality with oral platelet glycoprotein IIb/IIIa antagonists: a meta-analysis of phase III multicenter randomized trials. Circulation 2001; 103: 201–206.
9. Morrow DA, Murphy SA, McCabe CH, et al. Potent inhibition of thrombin with a monoclonal antibody against tissue factor (Sunol-cH36): results of the PROXIMATE-TIMI 27 trial. Eur Heart J 2005; 26:682–688.
10. Giugliano RP, Wiviott SD, Stone PH, et al. Recombinant nematode anticoagulant protein c2 (rNAPc2) in patients with non-ST-Elevation acute coronary syndrome – The ANTHEM (Anticoagulation with rNAPc2 To Help Eliminate MACE) - TIMI 32 Trial. J Am Coll Cardiol 2007, 49:2398–2407.
11. Wallentin L, Wilcox RG, Weaver WD, et al. Oral ximelagatran for secondary prophylaxis after myocardial infarction: the ESTEEM randomised controlled trial. Lancet 2003, 362:789–797.
12. Bhatt DL, Fox KA, Hacke W, et al. Clopidogrel and aspirin versus aspirin alone for the prevention of atherothrombotic events. N Engl J Med 2006; 354:1706–1717.
13. Antman EM, Cohen M, Bernink PJ, et al. The TIMI risk score for unstable angina/non-ST-elevation MI: A method for prognostication and therapeutic decision making. JAMA 2000; 284: 835–842.
14. Antman EM, McCabe CH, Gurfinkel EP, et al. Enoxaparin prevents death and cardiac ischemic events in unstable angina/non-Q-wave myocardial infarction. Results of the thrombolysis in myocardial infarction (TIMI) 11B trial [see comments]. Circulation 1999; 100:1593–1601.
15. Kastrati A, Mehilli J, Neumann FJ, et al. Abciximab in patients with acute coronary syndromes undergoing percutaneous coronary intervention after clopidogrel pretreatment: the ISAR-REACT 2 randomized trial. JAMA 2006; 295:1531–1538.
16. Gurbel PA, Bliden KP, Guyer K, et al. Platelet reactivity in patients and recurrent events post-stenting: results of the PREPARE POST-STENTING Study. J Am Coll Cardiol 2005; 46: 1820–1826.
17. Gurbel PA, Bliden KP, Hayes KM, et al. The relation of dosing to clopidogrel responsiveness and the incidence of high post-treatment platelet aggregation in patients undergoing coronary stenting. J Am Coll Cardiol 2005; 45:1392–1396.

18. Gurbel PA, Bliden KP, Samara W, et al. Clopidogrel effect on platelet reactivity in patients with stent thrombosis: results of the CREST Study. J Am Coll Cardiol 2005; 46:1827–1832.

19. Rieder MJ, Reiner AP, Gage BF, et al. Effect of VKORC1 haplotypes on transcriptional regulation and warfarin dose. N Engl J Med 2005; 352:2285–2293.

20. Chen ZM, Jiang LX, Chen YP, et al. Addition of clopidogrel to aspirin in 45,852 patients with acute myocardial infarction: randomised placebo-controlled trial. Lancet 2005; 366:1607–1621.

21. Braunwald E. The open-artery theory is alive and well—again. N Engl J Med 1993; 329:1650–1652.

22. Dalen JE, Gore JM, Braunwald E, et al. Six- and twelve-month follow-up of the phase I Thrombolysis in Myocardial Infarction (TIMI) trial. Am J Cardiol 1988; 62:179–185.

23. Gibson CM, Cannon CP, Murphy SA, et al. Relationship of TIMI myocardial perfusion grade to mortality after administration of thrombolytic drugs. Circulation 2000; 101:125–130.

24. Schroder R, Dissmann R, Bruggemann T, et al. Extent of early ST segment elevation resolution: a simple but strong predictor of outcome in patients with acute myocardial infarction. J Am Coll Cardiol 1994; 24:384–391.

25. Giugliano RP, Roe MT, Harrington RA, et al. Combination reperfusion therapy with eptifibatide and reduced-dose tenecteplase for ST-elevation myocardial infarction: results of the integrilin and tenecteplase in acute myocardial infarction (INTEGRITI) Phase II Angiographic Trial. J Am Coll Cardiol 2003; 41:1251–1260.

26. ADVANCE MI Investigators. Facilitated percutaneous coronary intervention for acute ST-segment elevation myocardial infarction: results from the prematurely terminated ADdressing the Value of facilitated ANgioplasty after Combination therapy or Eptifibatide monotherapy in acute Myocardial Infarction (ADVANCE MI trial). Am Heart J 2005; 150:116–122.

27. Keeley EC, Boura JA, Grines CL. Comparison of primary and facilitated percutaneous coronary interventions for ST-elevation myocardial infarction: quantitative review of randomised trials. Lancet 2006; 367:579–588.

28. Sinno MC, Khanal S, Al-Mallah MH, et al. The efficacy and safety of combination glycoprotein IIb/IIIa inhibitors and reduced-dose thrombolytic therapy-facilitated percutaneous coronary intervention for ST-elevation myocardial infarction: a meta-analysis of randomized clinical trials. Am Heart J 2007;153:579–586.

29. ASSENT-4 PCI Investigators. Primary versus tenecteplase-facilitated percutaneous coronary intervention in patients with ST-segment elevation acute myocardial infarction (ASSENT-4 PCI): randomised trial. Lancet 2006; 367:569–578.

30. Ellis SG, Tendera M, de Belder MA, et al. Facilitated PCI in patients with ST-elevation myocardial infarction. N Engl J Med 2008; 358:2205–2217.

31. Giugliano RP, Newby LK, Harrington RA, et al. The early glycoprotein IIb/IIIa inhibition in non-ST-segment elevation acute coronary syndrome (EARLY ACS) trial: a randomized placebo-controlled trial evaluating the clinical benefits of early front-loaded eptifibatide in the treatment of patients with non-ST-segment elevation acute coronary syndrome: study design and rationale. Am Heart J 2005; 149:994–1002.

32. Mahaffey KW, Harrington RA. Optimal timing for use of glycoprotein IIb/IIIa inhibitors in acute coronary syndromes: questions, answers, and more questions. JAMA 2007; 297:636–639.

33. The PURSUIT Trial Investigators. Inhibition of platelet glycoprotein IIb/IIIa with eptifibatide in patients with acute coronary syndromes. Platelet glycoprotein IIb/IIIa in unstable angina: receptor suppression using integrilin therapy (see comments). N Engl J Med 1998; 339:436–443.

34. Lincoff AM, Bittl JA, Harrington RA, et al. Bivalirudin and provisional glycoprotein IIb/IIIa blockade compared with heparin and planned glycoprotein IIb/IIIa blockade during percutaneous coronary intervention: REPLACE-2 randomized trial. JAMA 2003; 289:853–863.

35. Bovill EG, Terrin ML, Stump DC, et al. Hemorrhagic events during therapy with recombinant tissue-type plasminogen activator, heparin, and aspirin for acute myocardial infarction. Results of the Thrombolysis in Myocardial Infarction (TIMI), Phase II Trial. Ann Intern Med 1991; 115: 256–265.

36. The GUSTO investigators. An international randomized trial comparing four thrombolytic strategies for acute myocardial infarction. N Engl J Med 1993; 329:673–682.

37. Gibson CM, Morrow DA, Murphy SA, et al. A randomized trial to evaluate the relative protection against post-percutaneous coronary intervention microvascular dysfunction, ischemia, and inflammation among antiplatelet and antithrombotic agents: the PROTECT-TIMI-30 trial. J Am Coll Cardiol 2006; 47:2364–2373.

38. Yusuf S, Mehta SR, Zhao F, et al. Early and late effects of clopidogrel in patients with acute coronary syndromes. Circulation 2003; 107:966–972.

39. Fox KA, Mehta SR, Peters R, et al. Benefits and risks of the combination of clopidogrel and aspirin in patients undergoing surgical revascularization for non-ST-Elevation acute coronary syndrome: the Clopidogrel in Unstable angina to prevent Recurrent ischemic Events (CURE) trial. Circulation 2004; 110:1202–1208.

40. Silber S, Albertsson P, Aviles FF, et al. Guidelines for percutaneous coronary interventions: the task force for percutaneous coronary interventions of the European Society of Cardiology. Eur Heart J 2005; 26:804–847.

41. Smith SC Jr., Feldman TE, Hirshfeld JW Jr., et al. ACC/AHA/SCAI 2005 Guideline update for percutaneous coronary intervention—summary article. A report of the American College of Cardiology/American Heart Association Task Force on Practice Guidelines (ACC/AHA/SCAI Writing Committee to Update the 2001 Guidelines for Percutaneous Coronary Intervention). J Am Coll Cardiol 2006; 7:216–235.

42. Bassand JP, Hamm CW, Ardissino D, et al. Guidelines for the diagnosis and treatment of non-ST-segment elevation acute coronary syndromes. Eur Heart J 2007; 28:1598–1660.

43. Anderson JL, Adams CD, Antman EM, et al. ACC/AHA 2007 guidelines for the management of patients with unstable angina/non-ST-Elevation myocardial infarction: a report of the American College of Cardiology/American Heart Association Task Force on Practice Guidelines (Writing Committee to Revise the 2002 Guidelines for the Management of Patients With Unstable Angina/Non-ST-Elevation Myocardial Infarction) developed in collaboration with the American College of Emergency Physicians, the Society for Cardiovascular Angiography and Interventions, and the Society of Thoracic Surgeons endorsed by the American Association of Cardiovascular and Pulmonary Rehabilitation and the Society for Academic Emergency Medicine. J Am Coll Cardiol 2007, 50:e1-e157.

44. Stone GW, Bertrand M, Colombo A, et al. Acute Catheterization and Urgent Intervention Triage strategY (ACUITY) trial: study design and rationale. Am Heart J 2004, 148:764–775.

45. Suntharalingam G, Perry MR, Ward S, et al. Cytokine storm in a phase 1 trial of the anti-CD28 monoclonal antibody TGN1412. N Engl J Med 2006; 355:1018–1028.

46. Kastelein JJ, Akdim F, Stroes ES, et al. Simvastatin with or without ezetimibe in familial hypercholesterolemia. N Engl J Med 2008; 358:1431–1443.

47. Topol EJ, Moliterno DJ, Herrmann HC, et al. Comparison of two platelet glycoprotein IIb/IIIa inhibitors, tirofiban and abciximab, for the prevention of ischemic events with percutaneous coronary revascularization. N Engl J Med 2001; 344:1888–1894.

48. Freemantle N, Blonde L, Bolinder B, et al. Real-world trials to answer real-world questions. Pharmacoeconomics 2005; 23:747–754.

49. Ferguson JJ, Califf RM, Antman EM, et al. Enoxaparin vs. unfractionated heparin in high-risk patients with non-ST-segment elevation acute coronary syndromes managed with an intended early invasive strategy: primary results of the SYNERGY randomized trial. JAMA 2004; 292: 45–54.

50. GRACE Investigators. Rationale and design of the GRACE (Global Registry of Acute Coronary Events) Project: a multinational registry of patients hospitalized with acute coronary syndromes. Am Heart J 2001; 141:190–199.

51. Hoekstra JW, Pollack CV Jr., Roe MT, et al. Improving the care of patients with non-ST-Elevation acute coronary syndromes in the emergency department: the CRUSADE initiative. Acad Emerg Med 2002; 11:1146–1155.

52. Hoekstra JW, Menon V, Li Y, et al. Early use of GP IIb/IIIa inhibitors for non-ST-Elevation ACS is associated with lower mortality. Circulation 2003; 108, (suppl IV):580 (abstract).

53. Abbott JD, Voss MR, Nakamura M, et al. Unrestricted use of drug-eluting stents compared with bare-metal stents in routine clinical practice: findings from the National Heart, Lung, and Blood Institute Dynamic Registry. J Am Coll Cardiol 2007; 50:2029–2036.
54. Moher D, Schulz KF, Altman D. The CONSORT statement: revised recommendations for improving the quality of reports of parallel-group randomized trials. JAMA 2001; 285: 1987–1991.
55. Piaggio G, Elbourne DR, Altman DG, et al. Reporting of noninferiority and equivalence randomized trials: an extension of the CONSORT statement. JAMA 2006; 295:1152–1160.
56. Carey J. Do cholesterol drugs do any good?. BusinessWeek, 2008.

4

Pharmacogenomics and Warfarin Anticoagulation

Melkon Hacobian
Venous Thromboembolism Research Group, Cardiovascular Division, Brigham and Women's Hospital, Harvard Medical School, Boston, Massachusetts, U.S.A.

Samuel Z. Goldhaber
Cardiovascular Division, Department of Medicine, Brigham and Women's Hospital, Harvard Medical School, Boston, Massachusetts, U.S.A.

WARFARIN: PROBLEMS AND PROMISES

Warfarin has been commercially available since 1954 and is the sole oral anticoagulant available in the United States. The Food and Drug Administration (FDA) estimates that 2,000,000 patients in the United States start taking warfarin each year to prevent or treat thrombotic conditions.

Achieving safe and effective warfarin dosing is challenging, because a standard fixed dose is not available (Table 1). Doses must be titrated to the prothrombin time coagulation test, standardized and reported as the International Normalized Ratio (INR). The INR is a prothrombin time that is standardized according to the type of thromboplastin reagent used by the coagulation laboratory. Too high a warfarin dose predisposes to bleeding complications; too low a dose predisposes to thrombotic events such as stroke or pulmonary embolism. Dosing is further complicated by numerous drug-drug and drug-food interactions that affect the INR. Medical comorbidites, age, weight, and liver function affect the INR as well. Sometimes, the INR fluctuates markedly for unknown reasons. Optimal dosing of warfarin requires dose titration to achieve and maintain the desired target range INR.

The promise of pharmacogenomics is to personalize warfarin dosing with rapid turnaround genetic testing. Ideally, accurate-dosing nomograms can be devised to integrate genetic testing results with clinical variables such as age, gender, weight, nutrition, other medications, and medical comorbidites.

Warfarin is a combination of S and R enantiomers. The S enantiomer has three to five times greater anticoagulant activity (1). Warfarin has a half-life of 36 to 42 hours. Acenocoumarol and phenprocoumon are members of the coumarin family that are not

Table 1 Warfarin Advantages and Disadvantages

Advantages	Disadvantages
INR available to assess effectiveness	Narrow therapeutic index
INR available to optimize dosing	Wide interindividual difference
Available antidotes	Bleeding with excessive dose
Occasional missed dose is rarely important	Multiple drug-drug, drug-food interaction
Only available oral anticoagulant in the United States	Recurrent VTE or stroke with subtherapeutic dosing
Inexpensive	No standard dosing method
	Difficult to achieve a therapeutic INR
	Trial and error as the common practice
	Consistent laboratory monitoring required

Abbreviations: INR, International Normalized Ratio; VTE, venous thromboembolism.

available in the United States. Compared with warfarin, the half-life of acenocoumarol is shorter whereas the half-life of phenprocoumon is much longer (2).

Warfarin is almost completely absorbed through the gastrointestinal tract mucosa and primarily binds to albumin. The non-albumin-bound warfarin is the biologically active part. Therefore, any agent that binds to albumin and displaces warfarin may increase warfarin's biological activity (3). The increased sensitivity to warfarin in elderly patients may be related to lower albumin concentrations or slower warfarin clearance (4).

Cytochrome P450 is a group of enzymes responsible for hepatic metabolism of drugs and chemicals, including warfarin. The encoding genes for each enzyme differ in the sequence of amino acids. If they have more than 40% similarity in their sequences, then they are categorized to a family identified by a number. If the amino acid sequences have more than 55% similarity, they are assigned to a subfamily identified by a letter (5). Cytochrome P450 2C9 metabolizes the S enantiomer of warfarin in the liver (5).

γ-Carboxylation of prothrombotic vitamin K is an important step in the proper functioning of anticoagulation factors II, VII, IX, and X, as well as antithrombotic endogenous protein C and protein S. γ-Carboxylation of vitamin K allows these clotting proteins to bind calcium at phospholipid surfaces upon which coagulation occurs. As a vitamin K antagonist, warfarin blocks the recycling of vitamin K, inhibits the vitamin K–dependent γ-carboxylation of factors II, VII, IX, and X, and causes the liver to synthesize nonfunctional coagulation factors. Warfarin also inhibits the vitamin K–dependent γ-carboxylation of proteins C and S, the two antithrombotic proteins required to inhibit activated clotting factors VIII and V. Warfarin interferes with the vitamin K cycle by inhibiting the reduction of vitamin K to vitamin K hydroquinone. Warfarin also interferes with the reduction of vitamin K epoxide (KO) to vitamin K hydroquinone (K1H2) by blocking the vitamin K epoxide reductase complex (VKORC). VKORC is the most important enzyme in recycling of vitamin K (Fig. 1).

The most vulnerable period for bleeding and clotting complications occurs at the time warfarin is initiated. In 472 patients with atrial fibrillation newly started on warfarin therapy, the first 90 days of therapy were associated with a threefold increased risk of major bleeding (6). Advanced age was also associated with a higher rate of major hemorrhage. The rate of major bleeding was 13% in patients older than 80 years, compared with 4.8% in the group younger than 80 years. An INR greater than 4 was also a strong risk factor for bleeding. Unfortunately, the rates of major hemorrhage were higher in patients with more risk factors for developing embolic stroke (CHADS$_2$ scores of $\geq$3) (6).

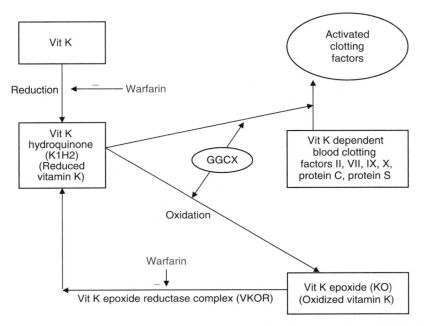

Figure 1 Vitamin K cycle and warfarin. Vitamin K reduced form (K1H2) is essential for γ-carboxylation of vitamin K–dependent blood-clotting factors II, VII, IX, and X, as well as antithrombotic proteins C and S. Warfarin interferes with the recycling of vitamin K and also blocks the γ-carboxylation of these clotting factors, resulting in nonfunctional coagulation factors. *Abbreviations*: Vit K, vitamin K; GGCX, γ-glutamyl carboxylase.

To determine the optimal INR range to prevent strokes, 13,559 patients with non-valvular atrial fibrillation were studied, and maintaining an INR between 2 and 4 maximized the efficacy and safety. The rate of intracranial hemorrhage increased when the INR exceeded 4 (7). Although the overall mortality rate from hemorrhagic events was low, intracranial bleeding was responsible for 90% of deaths and disabilities (8). In the same cohort population, the risk of major bleeding was higher in older patients, and the rate of intracranial hemorrhage was significantly higher in patients 80 years and older (9).

In a national survey of Emergency Department visits for adverse drug events, warfarin was the second most common problematic medication (after insulin). Patients older than 65 years of age were especially vulnerable (10).

In August 2006, the FDA added a warning "black box" to the labeling of warfarin, emphasizing the risk of bleeding with this medication. The warning states that bleeding is more likely to occur during the warfarin-initiation period and with a higher dose. Important risk factors include advanced age, prior history of gastrointestinal bleeding, hypertension, unstable INR values, cerebrovascular disease, heart disease, anemia, malignancy, trauma, chronic kidney disease, concomitant drugs, and long-term warfarin therapy. In patients with a higher risk for bleeding, regular monitoring of INR with greater frequency, careful dose adjustment, and shorter duration of therapy (if appropriate) with warfarin are the measures recommended by the FDA to minimize risk (11).

There is no standard dosing method for warfarin. Most dosing is empiric, with "educated guessing" based upon trial and error. Most patients receive an initial dose of 5 mg daily for about three days with subsequent doses titrated based on INR results. Some investigators propose warfarin 10 mg daily as a superior starting dose because it allows more rapid achievement of a therapeutic INR (12). Others found better INR control and less frequent excessive anticoagulation with a 5-mg rather than a 10-mg warfarin-initiating dose (13,14). In a randomized trial of 50 patients initiating warfarin, 5 mg compared with 10 mg warfarin-dosing nomograms were equally safe and effective (15). There are also data indicating that lower than 5 mg warfarin-dosing regimens tend to be more effective and safer in the elderly population (16). The Seventh ACCP Conference on Antithrombotic and Thrombolytic Therapy guidelines recommend initiation of oral anticoagulation with doses between 5 and 10 mg for one or two days and subsequent dose adjustment on the basis of INR results (17). There is also a specific recommendation for patients older than 60 years old to start warfarin with a dose not greater than 5 mg daily because of the reduced clearance of this medication in the elderly (17).

The wide range of INR responses to warfarin, especially during the warfarin initiation period, have been the focus of multiple investigations. Available dosing nomograms work poorly. In 1984, Fennerty proposed a 16-hour warfarin-dosing initiation nomogram for patients with venous thromboembolism (18). This nomogram never gained wide support because of the awkward dosing interval and because it was used in a patient population much younger than the average population of patients who take warfarin. The "modified Fennerty" nomogram was introduced with a dosing interval of 24 hours. While this nomogram was utilized in an older population, 35% of these patients had excessively high INRs that exceeded 4 within the first four days of warfarin therapy and this modified Fennerty nomogram was not found to be useful (4).

Thus, neither dosing by nomograms nor dosing empirically has resulted in consistent maintenance of patients within the therapeutic INR range. However, guidelines from ACC/AHA/ESC recommend at least once-a-week INR testing in elderly population during the initiation of oral anticoagulant therapy (19).

Many clinical factors predispose to an excessively high INR. These include advanced age, abnormal liver function, decreased vitamin K intake due to poor nutrition or poor appetite, diarrhea, many antibiotics, other concomitant medications, alcohol in binges, and changes in warfarin preparation (substituting one generic preparation for another or interchanging generic warfarin with brand name Coumadin®). The most common reason for abnormally low INRs is intake of high amounts of vitamin K, certain drug-warfarin interactions such as antithyroid agents, azathioprine, barbiturates, bosentan, carbamazepine, and most importantly, forgetting to take or deliberately omitting warfarin.

The availability of rapid turnaround genetic testing raises the issue of whether warfarin dosing should be personalized according to an individual's genetic profile (Table 2). The

Table 2 Possible Advantages and Disadvantages Associated with Genetic-Based Dosing

Possible advantages
Precise dosing
Less major bleeding
Less VTE recurrence
Better INR monitoring
Decreased laboratory costs
Patient convenience
Possible disadvantages
High cost
Slow turnaround
Lack of clinical trial evidence

Abbreviations: VTE, venous thromboembolism; INR, International Normalized Ratio.

alternative is to continue standard dosing with warfarin solely on the basis of clinical factors such as age, weight, comorbid illnesses, diet, concomitant medications, and clinical intuition or "gestalt."

In August 2007, the FDA added another cautionary note to warfarin labeling and stated that a "lower initiation dose should be considered for patients with certain genetic variations in CYP2C9 and VKORC1 enzymes" (20). The addition of this labeling generated controversy, because routine genetic testing has not been proven to maintain patients more frequently in the targeted therapeutic INR range when compared with standard dosing without genetic testing. Additional objections include the added cost of genetic testing, inconvenience, and slowing down the process of initiating warfarin dosing (Table 2). This new FDA labeling may also result in medicolegal complications that make physicians feel compelled to order genetic testing, even in the absence of evidence to support its routine use.

To estimate how personalized dosing of warfarin would affect health care costs, two renowned think tanks, the American Enterprise Institute and Brookings, worked together to conduct a theoretical study (21). They estimated that 2,000,000 patients initiate warfarin annually in the United States. They also estimated that one-third of these patients would carry a variant genotype. They relied upon the findings of Higashi et al., discussed later in this chapter, where 28% (16 of 58) of patients with one of the CYP2C9 variants developed hemorrhagic events, whereas only 13% (16 of 127) of patients with no variants had similar episodes (22). They hypothesized that routine rapid turnaround genetic testing would halve the rate of major bleeding. They also hypothesized that rapid turnaround genetic testing would halve the rate of embolic strokes due to atrial fibrillation. They further estimated the cost of genetic testing to be $350 per patient.

They concluded that with accurate warfarin dosing based on genotype information, approximately 85,000 major bleeding cases as well as about 17,000 ischemic strokes could be prevented annually. The calculations in this hypothetical exercise yielded a net savings of $ 1.1 billion in United States health care costs annually, even after accounting for the expense of rapid turnaround genetic testing (21). Thus, in this controversial think-tank paper, genotype-based dosing theoretically reduced both overall adverse event rates and medical costs.

Importantly, while it is easy to conceptualize how rapid turnaround genetic testing might help pinpoint the optimal initial dose of warfarin, it is difficult to understand how genetic testing will improve the maintenance dosing of warfarin over the long term.

Cytochrome P450 2C9 mutations are associated with impaired warfarin metabolism. The CYP2C9 genotype accounts for about 10% of warfarin-dose variance (23). Vitamin K receptor polymorphism testing can identify whether the patients require low, intermediate, or high doses of warfarin. Five common vitamin K receptor gene haplotypes account for about an additional 25% of warfarin-dose variance (24). These genotypes are discussed in detail below.

CYP2C9

The Cytochrome P450 2C9 family of enzymes is responsible for metabolism of the S-enantiomer of warfarin, which is the active enantiomer responsible for warfarin's anticoagulant effect (Table 3).

There are two known allelic variants, CYP2C9 *2 and CYP2C9 *3. Both are associated with low warfarin-dose requirements. These genetic mutations result in impaired hydroxylation of the S enantiomer of warfarin. These two variants differ from

Table 3 Cytochrome P2C9

Metabolism of S-enantiomer
Polymorphism with single amino acid substitution
PCR to detect two common variants
CYP2C9 *2 has 30% and *3 has 70% less activity
Lower warfarin doses required with these variants
Excess anticoagulation risk with the two variants

Abbreviations: PCR, polymerase chain reaction; CYP2C9, cytochrome P2C9.

the wild-type CYP2C9 *1 by a single amino acid substitution. The CYP2C9 *2 variant is a C to T substitution at codon 144, resulting the replacement of arginine by cysteine. The CYP2C9 *3 is an A to C substitution in codon 359, resulting the replacement of isoleucine with leucine (25).

There is a strong association between low warfarin-dose requirements and these polymorphisms. In one study, to evaluate the effect of CYP2C9 polymorphisms on warfarin-dose requirements, 29 of 36 (81%) patients requiring low warfarin doses had at least one of the variant alleles, compared to 40 of 100 patients (40%) in the control group. Subjects with low warfarin-dose requirements were six times more likely to have one or more of the variant alleles associated with impaired S-warfarin metabolism compared with the general population. The risk of major bleeding complications in patients requiring low-dose warfarin was four times higher than the control group (25).

The association between CYP2C9*2 and *3 polymorphisms and excessively high INRs has been established. A retrospective cohort study of 185 patients taking warfarin evaluated the association between the genetic variants and clinical outcomes (22). Patients with variant genotypes of CYP2C9 had an increased risk of above range INRs and longer time to achieve a stable INR. The rate of major bleeding was higher in patients with a genetic variant compared to the wild type (22).

One of the first attempts to combine genetic, clinical, and demographic factors to develop a warfarin-dosing algorithm was initiated at Washington University in St. Louis (23). Clinical information on 369 patients included age, gender, body surface area, race, renal function, serum albumin level, smoking status, dietary history, and concomitant medications. Each subject was screened for CYP2C9 polymorphisms. The warfarin maintenance dose was 19% lower in CYP2C9 *2 group and 29% lower in CYP2C9 *3 group. Overall, the investigators were able to explain 10% of warfarin-maintenance dose variability by considering these single nucleotide polymorphisms (23).

In a separate study (26), the genetic impact on warfarin dosing was examined exclusively, without including any demographic or clinical factors. In this study, 73 patients mostly with atrial fibrillation or venous thromboembolism were enrolled. These subjects were on a stable warfarin dose with a therapeutic INR for more than a month. They were divided into low-, moderate-, and high-dose warfarin groups requiring ≤ 2 mg, 4 to 6 mg, and ≥ 10 mg, respectively. After enrollment, the subjects were evaluated for CYP2C9 polymorphisms. Most of the subjects in the low-dose warfarin group had at least one CYP2C9 *2 or *3 polymorphism. The rate of excessive anticoagulation was two- to threefold higher in these patients compared with the group carrying the wild-type allele. Patients in high dose group mostly had the wild-type CYP2C9 allele (26).

The first prospective trial testing pharmacogenetic-based versus standard warfarin dosing was done in 48 orthopedic patients undergoing total hip or knee arthroplasty (27). The central hypothesis was that dosing by genetic testing would help achieve a stable INR. Before the study began, a combined genetics-clinical nomogram was developed on the basis of CYP2C9 genotypes. Clinical information factored into the nomogram included age, race, body surface area, and amiodarone or statin use (27). Unexpectedly, the time to achieve a stable therapeutic INR was similar in all patients regardless of CYP2C9 genotype. Paradoxically, despite the nomogram, patients receiving genotype-guided dosing with CYP2C9 *2 or *3 variants were more likely to have an excessively high INR (27).

In another randomized trial of 185 hospitalized warfarin-naïve patients, dosing was assigned to either a clinical algorithm or a CYP2C9 genotype-based algorithm (28). In this study, the genotype-based dosing group more rapidly achieved a therapeutic INR and had fewer bleeding events compared with the empiric group. Patients in the standard dosing group more often had excessively high INR levels. These findings supported CYP2C9 genotype-guided warfarin dosing (28).

VITAMIN K EPOXIDE REDUCTASE COMPLEX 1

Vitamin K epoxide reductase is the molecular target of warfarin. Vitamin K reductase complex 1 (VKORC1) is the gene encoding the warfarin-sensitive component of KO reductase. Warfarin resistance is associated with mutations in VKORC1. A single nucleotide polymorphism is responsible for the resistance (Table 4).

VKORC1, the key enzyme of the vitamin K cycle, recycles oxidized KO to the reduced form of vitamin K (K1H2) (Fig. 1). Vitamin K1H2 is essential for γ-carboxylation of the vitamin K–dependent clotting factors II, VII, IX, and X and proteins C and S. γ-Carboxylation is the rate-limiting step required to activate these coagulation proteins. During the vitamin K cycle, KO is reduced to K1H2, an essential cofactor for γ-carboxylation by γ-glutamyl carboxylase. Warfarin blocks γ-carboxylation, resulting in synthesis of nonfunctional coagulation factors.

VKORC1 haplotypes determine 25% to 40% of warfarin-dose variability. Therefore, VKORC1 is the most important genetic factor identified thus far to determine the variability in warfarin dose. Its effect on warfarin dosing is approximately three times greater than that of the CYP2C9 genotype (24).

In a landmark study to evaluate the effect of VKORC1 haplotypes on the warfarin dose, two haplotype groups, A and B, predicted low dose and high dose, respectively (24). VKORC1 was used to stratify patients in low-, intermediate-, and high-dose warfarin groups. Patients with A/A haplotypes required low-dose warfarin (on average 2.7 mg) as a maintenance dose, B/B haplotypes required high doses (on average 6.2 mg), and A/B haplotypes remained in the intermediate group (on average 4.9 mg). Group A haplotypes predicted the low warfarin-dose phenotype and were common in the Asian population, whereas group B haplotypes with higher dose requirements were more common among the African-American population (24).

VKORC1 haplotypes are more closely associated with initial INR variability than CYP2C9 variants (29). The effects of CYP2C9 genotypes and VKORC1 haplotypes were evaluated for the time necessary to achieve the first therapeutic INR and also the time until an excessively high INR (above 4). In a cohort study of 297 patients initiating

Table 4 Vitamin K Epoxide Reductase Complex 1

Warfarin-receptor gene encodes VKORC1
Important in vitamin K cycle
10 noncoding single nucleotide polymorphisms with five major haplotypes

Abbreviation: VKORC1, vitamin K epoxide reductase complex 1.

warfarin, those with group A haplotype had higher INR values during the first week of warfarin therapy compared with those with the non-A group (29).

GENETIC VS. CLINICAL FACTORS

Variants of CYP2C9 and VKORC1, combined with clinical factors, determine the individual patient's warfarin dose. Clinical considerations include age, gender, weight, diet, and medical comorbidites. This does not mean that genotyping will eliminate the necessity of monitoring INR values in guiding therapy; however, genotyping may help predict initial dosing, thereby reducing the risk of excessive anticoagulation or subtherapeutic anticoagulation in the period before dose stabilization is achieved. The association between genotyping and dose variance has been evaluated in multiple investigations, but prospective testing and development of combined genotype-based and clinical algorithms are required to test the potential superiority of this method over the traditional empirical dosing.

A prospective randomized trial of genotype-guided warfarin dosing versus standard dosing called Couma-Gen failed to demonstrate the primary end point: an increase in time within the therapeutic INR range (30). Patients were randomized into either a genotype-guided INR dosing group or a standard empirical dosing group. They used swabs from buccal mucosa to identify variants of CYP2C9 *2, *3 and VKORC1. Genotype-based group patients were placed on a dosing regimen based on a novel algorithm that took into account genetic variants, age, gender, and weight. Patients in empirical group were started on 10 mg initial dose of warfarin daily. Subsequent doses were adjusted on the basis of INR results. The algorithm, guided by pharmacogenetic and clinical factors, selected an initial dose more closely predictive of the eventual maintenance dose, necessitated fewer and smaller dose adjustments, and required fewer INR measurements. However, the time within the therapeutic INR range did not differ between the two groups (30).

Millican and colleagues (31) developed an algorithm for 92 orthopedic surgical patients combining genetic and clinical information. They found a close correlation between the warfarin dose predicted by their nomogram and the therapeutic dose that was eventually required to achieve the target INR (31). They also posted an algorithm on their Web site (www.WarfarinDosing.org) to provide clinicians with a starting point for estimating the warfarin dose based upon clinical as well as genetic information rather than reverting to the traditional trial and error method.

Other investigators have designed algorithms to encompass clinical factors such as weight, age, and gender, in addition to VKORC1 and CYP2C9 genotypes (32). In a prospective study of 213 outpatients, clinical factors such as age, gender, and weight described only 12% of warfarin-dose variability. However, genotype variations of CYP2C9 and VKORC1 contributed to 33% of interindividual dose differences. The majority of warfarin-dosing variability could not be explained by either clinical or genetic factors (32).

Controversy swirls around proposed routine genetic testing for warfarin dosing (33). For now, it is premature to initiate routine rapid turnaround genetic testing to dose warfarin.

NATIONAL HEART, LUNG, AND BLOOD INSTITUTE PROJECTS

To investigate the controversy surrounding the effectiveness of a genotype-based warfarin-dosing algorithm, the National Heart, Lung, and Blood Institute (NHLBI) is sponsoring a randomized trial of about 2,000 patients allocated to one of three groups:

trial and error empirical dosing (the control group), clinical algorithm dosing, and clinical plus genetic algorithm dosing. The primary end point is the percent of time that patients remain in the targeted therapeutic INR range.

OTHER GENETIC PROTEINS

Interindividual differences in warfarin-dose requirement are multifactorial. It is essential to consider all the genetic and nongenetic factors together to explain these differences.

In addition to relatively well-studied VKORC1 and CYP2C9 variants, γ-glutamyl carboxylase, microsomal epoxide hydrolase (EPHX1), and endoplasmic reticulum Ca^{2+} binding protein calumenin (CALU) have been studied for their rare mutations and their associations with warfarin-dose requirements (34).

Using a broader approach, a recent trial combined the effects of genetic polymorphisms in association with warfarin dosing (34). There was a significant difference in warfarin-dosing requirement, between the patients with mutant and wild-type CALU genotype in combination with other variants of CYP2C9 and VKORC1. Patients with the wild-type CYP2C9, and VKORC1, and mutant CALU genotype required the highest doses, whereas the patients with the mutant CYP2C9, VKORC1, and wild-type CALU genotype had the lowest dose requirements. Less VKORC1 inhibition in mutant CALU genotype and enhanced inhibition of VKORC1 in wild type CALU were thought to explain these differences. This trial showed that the combination of VKORC1, CYP2C9, and CALU genotyping might constitute the major determinants of warfarin doses.

In summary, the current data available for genetic testing and its effect on warfarin dosing are promising. Incorporating genetic information into warfarin-dosing algorithms may reduce the health care expenses, adverse bleeding, clotting events, and the time necessary to achieve and maintain a stable INR. However, for now, there is not enough evidence to support a change in the standard of care. The NHLBI trial should clarify the current controversy. Nevertheless, even with advances in the art and science of warfarin dosing, the clinical use of warfarin is likely to diminish because of the introduction of novel oral anticoagulants that do not necessitate laboratory coagulation monitoring.

REFERENCES

1. Takahashi H, Echizen H. Pharmacogenetics of warfarin elimination and its clinical implications. Clin Pharmacokinet 2001; 40(8):587–603.
2. Oldenburg J, Bevans CG, Fregin A, et al. Current pharmacogenetic developments in oral anticoagulation therapy: The influence of variant VKORC1 and CYP2C9 alleles. Thromb Haemost 2007; 98:570–578.
3. Sands CD, Chan ES, Welty TE. Revisiting the significance of warfarin protein-binding displacement interactions. Ann Pharmacother 2002; 36:1642–1644.
4. Cooper MW, Hendra TJ. Prospective evaluation of a modified Fennerty regimen for anticoagulating elderly people. Age Aging 1998; 27:655–656.
5. Nebert DW, Russell DW. Clinical importance of the cytochrome P450. Lancet 2002; 360:1155–1162.
6. Hylek EM, Evans-Mlolina C, Shea C, et al: Major hemorrhage and tolerability of warfarin in the first year of therapy among elderly patients with atrial fibrillation. Circulation 2007; 115:2689–2696.
7. Hylek EM, Go AS, Chang Y, et al. Effect of intensity of oral anticoagulation on stroke severity and mortality in atrial fibrillation. N Engl J Med 2003; 349(11):1019–1026.
8. Fang MC, Go AS, Chang Y, et al. Death and disability from warfarin-associated intracranial and extracranial hemorrhages. Am J Med 2007; 120:700–705.

9. Fang MC, Go As, Hylek EM, et al. Age and the risk of warfarin-associated hemorrhage: the anticoagulation and risk factors in atrial fibrillation study. J Am Geriatr Soc 2006; 54(8):1231–1236.
10. Budnitz DS, Pollock DA, Weidenbach KN, et al. National surveilance of emergency department visits for outpatient adverse drug events. JAMA 2006; 296(15):1858–1866.
11. Medication guide. Coumadin tablets. Available at: www.fda/gov/medwatch/safety/2006/coumadin_medguide.pdf. Accessed on April 9, 2008.
12. Kovacs MJ, Rodger M, Anderson D, et al. Comparison of 10 mg and 5 mg warfarin initiation nomograms together with low molecular weight heparin for outpatient treatment of acute venous thromboembolism: a randomized, double-blind, controlled trial. Ann Intern Med 20003; 138:714–719.
13. Crowther MA, Ginsberg JB, Kearon C, et al. A randomized trial comparing 5 mg and 10 mg warfarin loading doses. Arch Intern Med 1999; 159:46–48.
14. Harrison L, Johnston M, Massicotte MP, et al. Comparison of 5 mg and 10 mg loading doses in initiation of warfarin therapy. Ann Intern Med 1997; 126:133–136.
15. Quiroz R, Gerhard-Herman M, Kosowsky JM, et al. Comparison of a single end point to determine optimal initial warfarin dosing (5 mg versus 10 mg) for venous thromboembolism. Am J Cardiol 2006; 98(4):535–537.
16. Gedge J, Orme S, Hampton KK, et al. A comparison of a low-dose warfarin induction regimen with the modified Fennerty regimen in elderly in patients. Age Ageing 2000; 29:31–34.
17. Ansell J, Hirsh J, Poller L, et al. The pharmacology and management of the vitamin K antagonists. The seventh ACCP conference on antithrombotic and Thrombolytic therapy. Chest 2004; 126(3):204–233.
18. Fennerty A, Dolben J, Thomas P, et al. Flexible induction dose regimen for warfarin and prediction of maintenance dose. Br Med J 1984; 288:1268–1270.
19. Fuster V, Ryden LE, Asinger RW, et al. ACC/AHA/ESC Guidelines for the management of patients with atrial fibrillation: executive summary a report of the American college of cardiology/American heart association task force on practice guidelines and the European society of cardiology committee for practice guidelines and policy conferences (committee to develop guidelines for the management of patients with atrial fibrillation) developed in collaboration with the North American Society of Pacing and Electrophysiology. Circulation 2001; 104:2118–2150.
20. U.S. Food and Drug Administration. FDA approves updated warfarin (Coumadin) prescribing information. Available at: http://www.fda.gov/bbs/topics/NEWS/2007/NEW01684.html. Accessed on April 9, 2008.
21. McWilliam A, Lutter R, Nardinelli C. Health Care savings from personalizing medicine using genetic testing: The case of warfarin. 2006 AEI-Brookings Joint Center: 27 July 2007. Available at: http://aei-brookings.org/publications/abstract.php=1127. Accessed on April 9, 2008.
22. Higashi MK, Veenstra DL, Kondo LM, et al. Association between CYP2C9 genetic variants and anticoagulation-related outcomes during warfarin therapy. JAMA 2002; 287:1690–1698.
23. Gage BF, Eby C, Milligan PE, et al. Use of pharmacogenetics and clinical factors to predict the maintenance dose of warfarin. Thromb Haemost 2004; 91:87–94.
24. Reider MJ, Reiner AP, Gage BF, et al. Effect of VKORC1 haplotypes on transcriptional regulation and warfarin dose. N Engl J Med 2005; 352:2285–2293.
25. Aithal GP, Day CP, Kesteven PJL, et al. Association of polymorphisms in the cytochrome P450 CYP2C9 with warfarin dose requirement and risk of bleeding complications. Lancet 1998; 353: 717–719.
26. Joffe HV, Xu R, Johnson FB, et al. Warfarin dosing and cytochrome P450 2C9 polymorphisms. Thromb Haemost 2004; 91:1123–1128.
27. Voora D, Eby C, Linder MW, et al. Prospective dosing of warfarin based on cytochrome P450 2C9 genotype. Thromb Haemost 2005; 93:1–6.
28. Caraco Y, Blotnick S, Muszkat M. CYP2C9 genotype-guided warfarin prescribing enhances the efficacy and safety of anticoagulation: a prospective randomized controlled study. Clin Pharmacol Ther 2008; 83(3):460–470.

29. Schwarz UI, Ritchie MD, Bradford Y, et al. Genetic determinants of response to warfarin during anticoagulation. N Engl J Med 2008; 358:999–1008.
30. Anderson JL, Horne BD, Stevens SM, et al. Randomized trial of genotype-guided versus standard warfarin dosing in patients initiating oral anticoagulation. Circulation 2007; 116:1–8.
31. Millican EA, Lenzini PA, Milligan PE, et al. Genetic- based dosing in orthopedic patients beginning warfarin therapy. Blood 2007; 110:1511–1515.
32. Carlquist JF, Horne BD, Muhlestein JB, et al. Genotypes of the cytochrome P450 isoform, CYP2C9, and the vitamin K epoxide reductase complex subunit 1 conjointly determine stable warfarin dose: a prospective study. J Thromb Thrombolysis 2006; 22:191–197.
33. McClain MR, Palomki GE, Piper M, et al. A rapid-ACCE review of CYP2C9 and VKORC1 alleles testing to inform warfarin dosing in adults at elevated risk for thrombotic events to avoid serious bleeding. Genet Med 2008; 10(2):89–98.
34. Vescler M, Lobestein R, Almog S, et al. Combined genetic profiles of components and regulators of the vitamin K-dependent γ-carboxylation system affect individual sensitivity to warfarin. Thromb Haemost 2006; 95:205–211.

5

Pharmacogenomics of Platelet Inhibitors

Srikanth Nagalla
The Cardeza Foundation for Hematologic Research and the Department of Medicine, Jefferson Medical College, Philadelphia, Pennsylvania, U.S.A.

Suzanne M. Leal
Department of Human and Molecular Genetics, Baylor College of Medicine, Houston, Texas, U.S.A.

Paul F. Bray
The Cardeza Foundation for Hematologic Research and the Department of Medicine, Jefferson Medical College, Philadelphia, Pennsylvania, U.S.A.

INTRODUCTION

Formation of platelet thrombi at the sites of ruptured atherosclerotic plaques is responsible for the majority of acute ischemic events in coronary, cerebral, and peripheral arteries. Platelet activation with exposure of phosphotidyl serine is also believed to play a role in some venous thrombotic disorders. In vitro assays demonstrating reduced platelet function correlate with mild (e.g., platelet secretion defects) and severe (e.g., Glanzmann thrombasthenia) clinical bleeding. More recently, there has been an increasing awareness of the prothrombotic risk of platelet hyperreactivity in normal subjects and those with coronary artery disease (1). This hemostasis-thrombosis heterogeneity in the population may be linked to the well-known interindividual variation in *ex vivo* measures of platelet reactivity. Although there may be acquired and technical explanations for interindividual variation in platelet phenotypes, there is strong evidence that heritability contributes to this variation (2,3). These genetic effects are consistent with an increasing number of reports of platelet gene polymorphisms that show associations with clinical outcomes and laboratory assays of platelet function (4–14).

There is a well-established role for therapeutic platelet inhibition in the primary (15) or secondary (16) prevention of the complications of occlusions in coronary, cerebral, and peripheral arteries. For example, aspirin reduces the risk of recurrent myocardial infarction (MI), stroke, and death by 25% (15). Not all pharmacologic agents have equivalent efficacy for all individuals, and genetic variability contributes to this altered

Table 1 Table of Platelet Inhibitors Studied for Pharmacogenetic Regulation

Drug class	Drugs
(1) Cyclooxygenase inhibitors	Aspirin
(2) ADP receptor inhibitors	Clopidogrel, ticlopidine, prasugrel
(3) Glycoprotein IIb/IIIa receptor blockers	Abciximab, eptifibatide, tirofiban
(4) Phosphodiesterase inhibitors	Dipyridamole, cilostazol

efficacy (17). In addition, pharmacologic agents can have toxic effects in some individuals (17,18). Not surprisingly, there is a marked interindividual variation in both the clinical and in vitro responsiveness to antiplatelet agents, and there is a genetic contribution to this variation (19). There are currently available a substantial number of genetic biomarkers with high sensitivity and specificity to predict efficacy or toxicity of numerous drugs (17). Thus, pharmacogenetics and technology development can lead to the development of personalized medicine where genetic testing can identify subsets of individuals who (*i*) will benefit from a particular drug or (*ii*) could potentially suffer adverse events from a drug exposure. In the latter situation, depending on the drug, patients could be treated with a lower/safer drug dose or an alternative, safer therapy.

This chapter considers platelet pharmacogenetics; i.e., the field of pharmacology dealing with the interindividual variability in drug response based on genetic determinants. These genetic determinants could be at the level of (*i*) drug absorption, (*ii*) drug distribution, (*iii*) drug metabolism, (*iv*) drug elimination, and (*v*) mechanisms that regulate the drug-target interaction. Genetic variation could alter the quantity or structure of the proteins involved in these processes. Table 1 classifies the platelet inhibitors in current use as (*i*) cyclooxygenase (COX) inhibitors, (*ii*) inhibitors of ADP-induced platelet aggregation, (*iii*) integrin $\alpha_{IIb}\beta_3$ [glycoprotein (GP) IIb/IIIa] receptor blockers, and (*iv*) phosphodiesterase inhibitors. Many candidate platelet genes have been studied for their interaction with antiplatelet agents, and, in some cases, the same genetic variant has been investigated with different platelet inhibitors. This necessitates some repetition in the subheadings of any discussion of this topic, but we have elected to organize this chapter according to antiplatelet drug classes.

ASPIRIN

Production of thromboxane A_2 (TXA_2) is an important positive feedback mechanism for maximal platelet activation. There are several key enzymes involved in the biochemical pathway, resulting in TXA_2 (Fig. 1): (*i*) phospholipase, which triggers the release of arachidonic acid from membrane phospholipids; (*ii*) COX (prostaglandin H synthase), which converts arachidonic acid to prostaglandin H_2 (PGH_2); and (*iii*) thromboxane synthase, which transforms PGH_2 to TXA_2. COX has two isoforms, COX-1 and COX-2, which catalyze the same reactions. COX-1 is constitutively expressed in all tissues, including platelets. COX-2 is induced in many tissues under inflammatory conditions, but is expressed at low levels in newly formed platelets (20). Serum thromboxane B_2 (TXB_2) and urinary 11-dehydrothromboxane B_2 are the stable metabolites of TXA_2 that are routinely measured. Serum TXB_2, unlike urinary 11-dehydrothromboxane B_2, is largely produced from TXA_2 of the COX-1 pathway (21). Prostacyclin, a potent inhibitor of platelet activation, requires endothelial cell COX-2 for its biosynthesis.

The meta-analysis by the Antiplatelet Trialists' Collaboration established the benefit of aspirin in the secondary prevention of cardiovascular events, including MI, strokes, or vascular death (16). Aspirin is also recommended in the primary prevention of

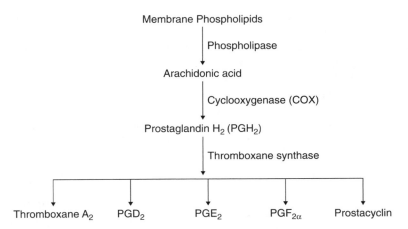

Figure 1 Biochemical pathway resulting in thromboxane A_2. Cyclooxygenase is also called prostaglandin H synthase. *Abbreviations*: PGD_2, prostaglandin D_2; PGE_2, prostaglandin E_2; $PGF_{2\alpha}$, prostaglandin $F_{2\alpha}$.

cardiovascular events in high-risk population with diabetes, peripheral arterial disease, carotid stenosis, and end-stage kidney disease requiring dialysis (15).

Individual response to aspirin can be assessed using either clinical outcomes or laboratory studies of platelet inhibition. Patients who have recurrent ischemic events on therapeutic doses of aspirin may be deemed clinically as aspirin nonresponders (see chap. 7). In addition, there are numerous *ex vivo* assays of platelet reactivity, many of which appear to predict clinical efficacy (1,22–24). And while it is beyond the scope of this chapter to discuss the issue of "aspirin resistance," suffice it to say that there is marked interindividual variability in the inhibitory effects of aspirin when platelets are tested functionally *ex vivo*. Although there are many causes for apparent inadequate responses to the inhibitory effects of aspirin, recent evidence indicates that heritable factors contribute to the variability in *ex vivo* tests of residual platelet responsiveness after aspirin administration (19).

Aspirin and Cyclooxygenase-1

Aspirin irreversibly acetylates COX-1 at serine residue 529 (25), preventing access of arachidonic acid to the catalytic site of COX-1 and thus inhibiting TXA_2 synthesis (26). Since the major antiplatelet effects of aspirin are mediated through the COX-1 pathway, it was natural for investigators to consider whether genetic variations in COX-1 might affect aspirin responsiveness. *COX1* is located on chromosome 9, is 22 kb in length, and consists of 11 exons (27). There are at least 24 single nucleotide polymorphisms (SNPs) that have been identified throughout *COX1* (27–29). Several studies have re-sequenced the exons and 5′ region of *COX1* using DNA samples from individuals from a limited number of ethnic groups (27–29). Ulrich et al. identified 18 *COX1* polymorphisms and found the allele frequencies of the nonsynonymous polymorphisms to be low. SNPs with a minor allele frequency (MAF) of $\geq$4% resulting in amino acid changes were C22T (R8W), C50T (P17L), and C714A (L237M) in European-Americans and C50T (P17L) in African-Americans. *COX1* polymorphisms A842G and C50T are very rare in the Chinese population (30). The most commonly studied SNPs in the pharmacogenetic studies of aspirin have been –842A→G (promoter region), C22T (exon 2, signal peptide region), C50T (exon 2, signal peptide region), G128A (exon 3), C644A (exon 6), and C714A (exon 7) (27,28,31,32).

All aspirin pharmacogenetic studies to date have utilized laboratory endpoints, not clinical endpoints. The initial study on the effects of *COX1* polymorphisms on response to aspirin utilized 38 healthy European-American volunteers (27) and assessed arachidonic acid–induced platelet aggregation and arachidonic acid–induced $PGF_{2\alpha}$ and TXB_2 production. The *COX1* SNP $-842A\rightarrow G$ was in complete linkage disequilibrium (LD) with C50T. Aspirin-treated platelets from $-842G/50T$ heterozygous subjects generated significantly less $PGF_{2\alpha}$ compared with the wild-type homozygous group ($-842A/50C$). However, there was no genotype effect on TXB_2 production and arachidonic acid–induced platelet aggregation after aspirin incubation. Two other *COX1* SNPs (C22T and C644A) showed no interaction with aspirin for any platelet phenotype. In contrast, two studies in patients with coronary artery disease found that the $-842G$ was associated with aspirin nonresponsiveness (31,32). A study by Maree et al. genotyped 5 *COX1* SNPs, inferred haplotypes, and found that *COX1* haplotypes were associated with aspirin inhibition of (*i*) arachidonic acid–induced platelet aggregation and (*ii*) serum TXB_2 levels. In some instances, haplotypes may provide more statistical power than individual SNPs because they can be more highly correlated with functional variants.

In summary, and specifically when considering the limitations of the pharmaco-genetic studies described below, there is no firm evidence for a pharmacogenetic interaction between aspirin and *COX1*. Currently, there is no clinical indication for *COX1* genotyping when using aspirin to prevent vascular thrombosis.

Aspirin and Cyclooxygenase-2

Aspirin irreversibly acetylates COX-2 at serine residue 516 (33). Aspirin is 170 times less potent against COX-2 than COX-1 (34). TXA_2 generated by COX-2 may be one mechanism contributing to aspirin insensitivity. A $-765G\rightarrow C$ SNP in the promoter of *COX2* causes lower promoter activity and gene expression (35). However, platelet *COX2* mRNA and protein levels do not appear to be different between subjects with platelets showing different responsiveness to aspirin (36). There are no studies of aspirin and COX-2 that consider clinical thrombosis endpoints. A single small study of healthy volunteers found that the $-765C$ *COX2* variant was associated with slightly greater aspirin-induced inhibition of urinary TXB_2 than the wild-type $-765G$ allele (37). Considering that the effects of aspirin on COX-2 may be more relevant in non-platelet tissues, additional studies are needed.

Aspirin and Platelet Membrane Glycoproteins

The initial platelet contact with exposed subendothelium is a tethering to subendothelial von Willebrand factor (vWF) via GP Ibα (see chap. 2) (38–40). Subendothelial collagen mediates platelet activation and stable platelet adhesion through GPVI and integrin $\alpha_2\beta_1$ (GP Ia/IIa), respectively. An expanding thrombus ensues when platelets aggregate via the intercellular bridging of fibrinogen and vWF to the activated conformation of integrin $\alpha_{IIb}\beta_3$ (GP IIb/IIIa) (41). There is a substantial body of literature assessing the main effect of candidate SNPs on coronary heart disease outcomes (42). Because many of these studies involved patients with arterial vascular disease, a few were able to consider the pharmacogenetics of aspirin and these adhesive platelet GPs.

Aspirin and the PI$^{A1/A2}$ Polymorphism of *INTB3* (Leu33Pro Substitution of Integrin β3)

The $\alpha_{IIb}\beta_3$ receptor is the most abundant receptor in the platelet membrane at about 80,000 copies per cell. Platelet $\alpha_{IIb}\beta_3$ (GP IIb/IIIa) is known as the "classic" fibrinogen receptor, although it binds other ligands, including vWF. A relatively common SNP of *INTB3* results in the substitution of proline (also called Pl^{A2}) for leucine (also called Pl^{A1}) at residue 33 of integrin β3. Perhaps because this SNP could potentially impact on the final common pathway of platelet aggregation, it has been studied extensively at genetic, clinical epidemiologic, and functional levels (43), although there is little support for a direct biochemical interaction between aspirin and α$_{IIb}$β$_3$.

There are no studies of aspirin and the Pl$^{A1/A2}$ polymorphism that consider clinical arterial thrombosis endpoints. Unfortunately, the Physician Health Study used a composite venous and arterial thrombosis endpoint in its analysis (44). Several studies have examined the relationship between aspirin and the Pl$^{A1/A2}$ polymorphism, with bleeding as an endpoint and observed that Pl^{A1} homozygotes are more sensitive to the effects of aspirin compared with Pl^{A2} heterozygotes (45,46). The remainder of work in this area—similar to the rest of platelet pharmacogenetics—is left with intermediate outcomes of platelet function studies. Compared with Pl^{A1} homozygotes, platelets from Pl$^{A1/A2}$ subjects have been associated with increased aspirin sensitivity in some studies (47–49), but with reduced sensitivity in others (50–52); these conflicting findings may be related to different methodology for assessing platelet reactivity or due to small sample size and random variability. Assays of blood from sites of bleeding-time wounds have shown that Pl^{A2}-positive subjects exhibit enhanced thrombin formation and an impaired antithrombotic response to aspirin compared with Pl^{A2}-negative subjects (53–55). It is possible that platelets with the Pl$^{A1/A2}$ genotype may be more resistant to aspirin suppression in subjects with established coronary artery disease, and/or that this relationship is only observed with some platelet agonists and not others (51). In summary, most (45–55), but not all (36,56–59), studies have shown that the Pl^A polymorphism is associated with significant variation in platelet inhibition by aspirin. Although it is difficult to compare studies of different design, the literature suggests that carriers of the Pl^{A2} allele are less sensitive to effects of aspirin than are Pl^{A1} homozygotes, particularly in response to collagen; furthermore, Pl^{A1} homozygotes may be at a higher risk of bleeding in some clinical situations.

Aspirin and the Polymorphisms of *GP1BA*

The GPIb-IX-V complex is the second-most abundant platelet receptor, with about 25,000 copies per platelet (60). The binding sites for vWF and α-thrombin are located in the N-terminal domain of the GPIbα subunit (61,62). The three most commonly studied polymorphisms in GPIbα are the Kozak polymorphism (–5T/C), the Thr/Met145 polymorphism (Br or HPA-2), and the variable tandem repeats (VNTR) polymorphism (42). A single study observed no association between the –5T/C SNP of *GP1BA* and platelet responsiveness to aspirin (48).

Aspirin and the Polymorphisms of *ITGA2*

Integrin α$_2$β$_1$ (also known as GP Ia/IIa) is one of the two primary collagen receptors on the surface of the platelets (63). The 807T SNP of *ITGA2* is strongly associated with a higher-level receptor expression than 807C (64,65). Three studies have shown no effect of this 807 T/C SNP on the platelet response to aspirin as assessed by the Platelet Function Analyzer (PFA)-100 (37,48,57).

Aspirin and the Polymorphisms of Platelet GPVI

GPVI is the major collagen-signaling receptor on platelets. C13254T is a *GP6* dimorphism that results in a serine to proline substitution at amino acid residue 219

(Ser219Pro) that has been associated with an increased risk of MI in men, but not women (66–68). A single study has suggested that the C13254T polymorphism of *GP6* is associated with aspirin nonresponse as defined by PFA-100 testing (31).

Aspirin and the Polymorphisms of P2 Purinergic Receptors

The purinergic receptors P2Y1 and P2Y12 are discussed in more detail in the next section ("Thienopyridines") but will be briefly introduced here. There are two major haplotypes of *P2Y12*, H1 and H2. Neither haplotype appears to influence platelet aspirin sensitivity or the occurrence of neurologic events in patients with peripheral arterial disease taking aspirin (56,69,70). No association was observed between an A1622G SNP in *P2Y1* and the platelet response to aspirin (56), whereas Jefferson et al. found that the C893T polymorphism of *P2Y1* was associated with responsiveness defined by arachidonic acid–induced platelet aggregation (71). A plausible biologic mechanism is elusive, and in the absence of good compliance information, aspirin insensitivity based on arachidonic acid–induced aggregation is suboptimal.

Aspirin and Coagulation Factor XIII

Upon activation by thrombin, activated Factor XIII catalyzes the cross-linking of α- and γ-fibrin chains (72). A G$\rightarrow$T transition in exon 2 of the Factor XIII gene results in the substitution of leucine for valine at amino acid 34 (73). Since this substitution takes place 3 amino acids away from the thrombin cleavage site, it has been suggested that the Val34Leu polymorphism might alter the Factor XIII activity. The hypothesis that treatment with aspirin alters the influence of the Val34Leu polymorphism on the Factor XIII activation was studied in 37 healthy volunteers (74). The rationale for this study was based on data that acetylation of fibrinogen by aspirin alters the coagulation properties of fibrinogen and thrombin-mediated Factor XIII activation is stimulated by fibrinogen and/or fibrin (72,75). Low-dose aspirin was shown to enhance the inhibition of Factor XIII activation in 34Leu carriers. These findings raise the possibility that low-dose aspirin might be more effective in 34Leu carriers compared with the Val34 homozygotes for reducing the risk of coronary artery events.

THIENOPYRIDINES

The activation of platelet P2 purinergic receptors initiates a complex signaling cascade leading to platelet activation and thrombus formation. P2Y1, P2Y12, and P2X1 are the P2 purinergic receptors present on the platelet surface. ADP acts as the agonist for two G protein–coupled receptors: G_q-coupled P2Y1 receptor and G_i-P2Y12 receptor, whereas ATP acts as the agonist for the ligand-gated channel P2X1 (76).

Ticlopidine and clopidogrel are the representative drugs of this class of platelet inhibitors, and their molecular target is the P2Y12 receptor on the platelet surface (77). Clopidogrel is absorbed in the gastrointestinal tract and metabolized via the cytochrome P_{450}-dependent pathway, ultimately resulting in the highly labile active metabolite that irreversibly modifies the P2Y12 receptor by forming a disulfide bridge between one or more cysteine residues of the receptor (Fig. 2) (78). This effect of the clopidogrel metabolite on the P2Y12 receptor blocks ADP binding and downstream platelet signaling and activation. As with aspirin, there is interindividual variability in the response to clopidogrel, and several studies have associated recurrent ischemic events with a suboptimal treatment response to clopidogrel (79). The major in vitro tests that have been

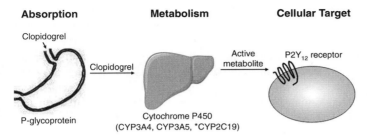

Figure 2 Pharmacokinetics of thienopyridines. Clopidogrel is metabolized by the CYP3A system that consists of the CYP3A4 and CYP3A5 isoenzymes, as well as CYP2C19. Ticlopidine is known to be metabolized via CYP2C19.

used to assess clopidogrel responsiveness include ADP-induced platelet aggregation, platelet P-selectin expression, integrin $\alpha_{IIb}\beta_3$ activation, and phosphorylated vasodilator-stimulated phosphoprotein (VASP) (79).

Clopidogrel and P-Glycoprotein

Variability in the absorption of clopidogrel in the intestine can lead to the interindividual differences in clopidogrel response. P-glycoprotein encoded by the multidrug resistance gene *MDR1* (*ABCB1*) is an adenosine triphosphate–binding cassette (ABC) efflux transporter (80). The oral bioavailability of thienopyridines is affected by luminal secretion by the ABC transporters present in the apical membrane of the intestinal mucosa. Some measures of clopidogrel absorption may be modified by a common C3435T polymorphism in exon 26 of *MDR1*, depending upon the loading dose (81).

Clopidogrel and Cytochrome P$_{450}$ Enzymes

Most drugs are metabolized in the liver by phase I and phase II reactions. Hydroxylation, reduction, and oxidation are phase I reactions performed by cytochrome P$_{450}$ (CYP) enzymes. The cytochrome P$_{450}$ enzyme families 1–3 carry out 80% of the phase I dependent metabolic reactions, and the most important enzymes are CYP1A2, CYP3A, CYP2C9, CYP2C19, CYP2D6, and CYP2E1 (82). Clopidogrel is predominantly metabolized by the CYP3A system that consists of the CYP3A4 and CYP3A5 isoenzymes (83). The other thienopyridines metabolized by the cytochrome P$_{450}$ system are ticlopidine (via CYP2C19), tienilic acid (via CYP2C9), and prasugrel (via CYP3A4 and 2B6) (84–86). Variability in the platelet inhibition may be caused by altered clopidogrel metabolism due to (*i*) other drugs that interact with cytochrome P450 enzymes and (*ii*) functional polymorphisms in these enzymes.

Clopidogrel and CYP3A4

The influence of *CYP3A4* polymorphisms on response to clopidogrel and platelet reactivity has been examined in three studies (1 large study with 1419 patients), but no effect was observed on ADP-induced platelet aggregation (87–89).

Clopidogrel and CYP3A5

CYP3A5 is the other isoenzyme in the CYP3A system that metabolizes clopidogrel to its active metabolite. A functional polymorphism in *CYP3A5* distinguishes an expresser genotype (*1/*1 or *1/*3 allele) from a non-expresser genotype (*3/*3 allele). The non-expresser genotype is caused by the introduction of an alternate splice site, giving rise to a truncated protein with reduced enzymatic activity (90,91). Korean patients with the non-expresser *CYP3A5* genotype had a lower extent of platelet inhibition by clopidogrel compared with the patients with the expresser genotype (92). Patients with the non-expresser genotype had worse six-month clinical outcomes after bare-metal stent placement for CAD. However, similar pharmacogenetic interactions were not confirmed in two additional studies (93,94)

Clopidogrel and CYP2C19

A 681G→A polymorphism of *CYP2C19* (the *2 "loss-of-function" allele) results in aberrant mRNA splicing and a truncated protein with nonfunctional enzyme activity. There has been uniformity in findings from three different groups of investigators that carriers of the *2 allele exhibit less platelet inhibition by clopidogrel than *1/*1 subjects. This reduction in clopidogrel effect by *CYP2C19* *1/*2 genotype was observed in both healthy young men and women of Northern European decent (88,94,95), as well as in a large population of high-risk coronary patients from Italy (89). An allele dose response was observed in the latter study. Brandt et al. showed that the loss-of-function allele of *CYP2C19* was associated with reduced generation of the active metabolite of clopidogrel, but not prasugrel (95). The consistent study findings with the *2 allele of *CYP2C19* seem to warrant clinical trials testing the utility of this polymorphism in patient management.

Clopidogrel and the Genes for P2 Purinergic Receptors

Fontana et al. demonstrated two major haplotypes, H1 and H2, for *P2Y12* that were associated with ADP-induced platelet aggregation in healthy subjects (10). Although it is biologically plausible to consider the pharmacogenetic interaction of variants of *P2Y12* with clopidogrel, no effect has been observed in either healthy subjects or patients with acute coronary syndromes, regardless of the clopidogrel dose used or the outcome measured (56,69,89,93,96–98). Limited data is available on the interaction between clopidogrel and the C34T SNP of *P2Y12*, but a single study found an increase in neurologic events in patients with the 34T allele compared with 34 C/C homozygotes (69).

   To date, no effect of the *P2Y1* A1622G polymorphism has been observed on clopidogrel inhibition of ADP-induced aggregation in patients with coronary artery disease (56,99).

Clopidogrel and Polymorphisms of *ITGB3* and *ITGA2*

Although the metabolite of clopidogrel is not believed to directly act on platelet-adhesive receptors, a number of studies have nevertheless tested the pharmacogenetic interaction of clopidogrel and platelet integrins utilizing laboratory endpoints. Most studies have not shown any association between the response to clopidogrel and this polymorphism (51,56,100). Single small studies have suggested enhanced (101) or reduced (102) clopidogrel effects in carriers of the Pl^{A2} polymorphism of *ITGB3* compared with subjects who do not express this variant.

   The 807C/T SNP of *ITGA2* does not appear to influence the effect of clopidogrel inhibition of platelet reactivity (103). Small studies suggest that carriers of the 807T allele have enhanced platelet responsiveness despite clopidogrel therapy (104,105).

INTEGRIN $\alpha_{IIb}\beta_3$ (GP IIb/IIIa) ANTAGONISTS

$\alpha_{IIb}\beta_3$ Antagonists block ligand (fibrinogen or vWF) binding. The first drug developed in this class for clinical use was the monoclonal antibody against $\alpha_{IIb}\beta_3$, abciximab. Subsequently, low molecular competitive antagonists of $\alpha_{IIb}\beta_3$ like eptifibatide and tirofiban were developed. Eptifibatide is a cyclic heptapeptide antagonist, whereas tirofiban is a non-peptide tyrosine derivative (106). Abciximab, eptifibatide, and tirofiban are parenteral compounds. Parenteral $\alpha_{IIb}\beta_3$ antagonists are used in patients with coronary artery disease undergoing percutaneous coronary intervention and in high-risk patients treated with medical therapy alone. Chronic administrations of oral $\alpha_{IIb}\beta_3$ antagonists like orbofiban and sibrafiban resulted in increased mortality and are currently not in clinical use (107,108).

$\alpha_{IIb}\beta_3$ Antagonists and the Pl^A Polymorphism of *ITGB3*

An obvious mechanism for a potential pharmacogenetic effect exists if a drug has different binding characteristics for its target depending on inherited variations in the target. Using stably transfect cell lines, Wheeler et al. showed reduced abciximab affinity for Pl^{A2}-positive platelets compared with Pl^{A1}-homozygous platelets (109), although this difference did not meet statistical significance ($p = 0.12$). These investigators also assessed *ex vivo* platelet reactivity in patients with coronary artery disease who had received abciximab intravenously, and found that compared with Pl^{A1}-homozygous platelets, Pl^{A2}-positive platelets were less well inhibited by $\alpha_{IIb}\beta_3$ antagonists (109). Some, but not all, studies have confirmed this pharmacogenetic effect in healthy subjects in whom platelets were treated *ex vivo* with abciximab (49,110). Probably the best evidence that the Pl^{A2} polymorphism interacts with $\alpha_{IIb}\beta_3$ antagonists comes from the OPUS-TIMI-16 (orbofiban in patients with unstable coronary syndromes–thrombolysis in MI 16) trial (111). These investigators found that compared with Pl^{A1} homozygotes, Pl^{A2}-positive patients had significantly less bleeding when receiving orbofiban.

MISCELLANEOUS PLATELET PHARMACOGENETIC INTERACTIONS

Postmenopausal hormone therapy and statins are commonly used in populations at risk for arterial vascular thrombosis. SNPs in the genes encoding platelet GPIbα and GPVI have been shown to interact with estrogen plus progesterone for recurrent coronary heart events in women participating in the Heart and Estrogen/progestin Replacement Study (HERS) (66). Certain combinations of *GP1BA* and *GP6* genotypes predicted risk for recurrent events with hormone use, while other combinations predicted benefit. Several studies have found that Pl^{A2}-positive patients with coronary artery disease received greater statin benefit for clinical endpoints than Pl^{A2}-negative patients (112,113). Other drugs like angiotensin-converting enzyme inhibitors, angiotensin receptor blockers, selective serotonin reuptake inhibitors and nitrates also have antiplatelet effects (114–117), but currently there is no platelet-pharmacogenetic data for these drugs.

LIMITATIONS OF THE CURRENT PHARMACOGENETICS OF PLATELET-INHIBITING AGENTS

Very few studies have utilized clinical endpoints, and the few that have are underpowered or less than optimally analyzed (15,45,46,69,92,111). The overwhelming majority of pharmacogenetic studies have utilized an intermediate phenotype for the outcome; i.e., an assay of platelet function. Among these, most studies examined *ex vivo* platelet reactivity in subjects who have ingested the platelet inhibitor, while some have tested platelet reactivity after the in vitro incubation of the drug. Both study designs may have value, but clearly the former may be affected by numerous variables, including compliance for taking the medication and variation (including genetic variation) in drug absorption, transportation, and metabolism. Only a minority of studies have made any effort to assess compliance. This may be especially important in platelet pharmacogenetics if, for example, aspirin resistance is defined as an unusually high extent of platelet aggregation to arachidonic acid. The only large study that formally considered compliance found that inhibition of aggregation to arachidonic acid was profound, with 94% of subjects demonstrating no measurable response after aspirin (118). And the use of an intermediate phenotype presents another somewhat unique problem: unlike simply measuring serum glucose, platelet biologists must choose between a multitude of assays, agonist concentrations, shear rates, specimen handling issues, etc., which makes comparisons between studies extremely difficult.

Most platelet pharmacogenetic studies are underpowered. Analyses that test for interactions between the two variables (drug use and gene variation) require a larger sample size. Power can be limited further when the minor allele frequency is low, such that a small fraction of the study population carries the genetic alteration of interest. Finally, because many variables affect platelet reactivity (age, gender, other drugs, comorbid condition, etc.), proper statistical analysis requires a large sample size, since an uneven distribution of these variables could have a profound effect on power. Many existing platelet pharmacogenetic studies do not consider these potential confounders or factor pre-drug platelet reactivity into the analysis. Regarding the latter, some studies considering clopidogrel use have shown that subjects with the 807T allele of *ITGA2* have increased platelet reactivity in response to collagen compared with subjects without this allele. However, if the 807T-positive subjects also display increased platelet reactivity in response to collagen before taking clopidogrel, should this be considered a pharmacogenetic effect? Several studies have shown that pre-aspirin platelet reactivity is a predictor of post-aspirin reactivity (19,37), but few consider this variable when conducting aspirin pharmacogenetic studies.

Most of the inconsistent findings in the above study can be explained by small sample sizes and different study designs. Additionally, the SNP that is being studied is often not functional but only in linkage disequilibrium (LD) with the causal variant. The strength of LD between the associated SNP and causal variant can vary between groups especially those from different ethnic backgrounds, thus leading to inconsistent findings. Furthermore, the minimal contribution of any one SNP to the overall phenotypic variance may be difficult to quantify, especially since multiple mechanisms and complex pathways lead to the development of vascular occlusion. For example, oxidative stress is involved in the complex pathophysiology of atherosclerosis and can induce thromboxane production independent of COX, leading to aspirin-resistant platelet aggregation (36).

LINKS BETWEEN DRUG TARGETS AND GENETIC VARIANTS

The biologic plausibility supporting many pharmacogenetic studies is extremely attractive, and is summarized in Figure 3. Knowing the precise targets of aspirin and the clopidogrel metabolite makes genetic variations in *COX1* and *P2Y12*, respectively, ideal candidates for pharmacogenetic interactions; likewise, for $\alpha_{IIb}\beta_3$ and its inhibitors. However, on the basis of our current understanding and as illustrated in Figure 3, some

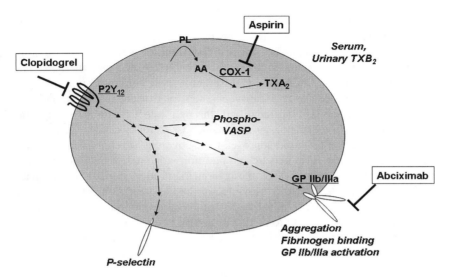

Figure 3 Platelet pharmacogenetic linkages. Drugs are in boxes; targets are underlined; commonly used platelet function read-outs are in italics. Arrows represent molecules involved in signaling pathways. *Abbreviations*: PL, phospholipase; AA, arachidonic acid; COX-1, cyclooxygenase-1; TXA$_2$, thromboxane A$_2$; TXB$_2$, thromboxane B$_2$; Phospho-VASP, phosphorylated vasodilator-stimulated phosphoprotein.

investigations make little sense, such as aspirin and *P2Y12* or clopidogrel and integrin genes. Since $\alpha_{IIb}\beta_3$ is the final common mediator of platelet aggregation, there may be more rationale for considering SNPs in *ITGA2B* or *ITGB3* as mediating effects of many drugs that target "upstream" aspects of platelet activation. However, Figure 3 is also meant to illustrate that the "further away" the drug target (such as P2Y12) is from the "read out" (such as VASP phosphorylation vs. fibrinogen binding) and the more alternative pathways that lead to the read-out, the more difficult it is likely to be to detect the effect.

Several other biologic factors may impact on results of pharmacogenetic studies. First, the drug may act on substrates that are not commonly considered. For example, aspirin acetylates fibrinogen as well as other plasma proteins. Such acetylation could be affected by amino acid–altering SNPs of fibrinogen or platelet adhesive GPs. Secondly, many SNPs affect protein expression or function in non-platelet tissue; therefore, a drug could directly affect non-platelet tissue to affect a clinical (or non-platelet) phenotype even though no pharmacogenetic effect was observed on an *ex vivo* measure of platelet function. This may explain the pharmacogenetic effects that have been observed between statins and *ITGB3* (112,113) and between estrogen and *GP1BA* and *GP6* (66).

CONCLUSION AND FUTURE DIRECTIONS

The pharmacogenetics of antiplatelet agents is in its infancy. As such, most of the studies are hypothesis-generating and none have been designed in a manner that permits incorporation into clinical practice. Nevertheless, there is strong data supporting a pharmacogenetic effect of the *2 allele of *CYP2C19* on platelet inhibition in response to clopidogrel. Future exploratory studies should be based on biologic plausibility (e.g., clopidogrel and variants in CYP enzymes), rather than testing for gene–drug interactions that have little rationale (e.g., clopidogrel and variants in *ITGB3*) and lead to "noise" in the literature. Large clinical trials using different ethnic groups must include pharmacogenetic analyses if we are to identify potential pharmacogenetic biomarkers. Pharmacogenetic biomarkers may be identified through genetic studies using the candidate gene approach. In addition, genome-wide association studies present an important opportunity to use an unbiased approach to discovering novel pharmacogenetic biomarkers. State-of-the-art statistical genetic and bioinformatic analyses are essential for either approach, and replication studies of these biomarkers are essential to eliminate false-positive results. Candidate biomarkers should also be validated in biochemical, cell biologic, and animal studies. Lastly, clinical trials would be needed to test whether these pharmacogenetic biomarkers are useful to predict drug benefit or adverse reactions. In the future the profile of an individual's pharmacogenetic biomarkers should aid in decisions pertaining to safer and more effective antiplatelet therapy for patients with arterial vascular disease.

REFERENCES

1. Bray PF. Platelet hyperreactivity: predictive and intrinsic properties. Hematol Oncol Clin North Am 2007; 21:633–645.
2. Bray PF, Mathias RA, Faraday N, et al. Heritability of platelet function in families with premature coronary artery disease. J Thromb Haemost 2007; 5:1617–1623.
3. O'Donnell CJ, Larson MG, Feng D, et al. Genetic and environmental contributions to platelet aggregation: the Framingham heart study. Circulation 2001; 103:3051–3056.
4. Boekholdt SM, Peters RJ, de Maat MP, et al. Interaction between a genetic variant of the platelet fibrinogen receptor and fibrinogen levels in determining the risk of cardiovascular events. Am Heart J 2004; 147:181–186.
5. Bojesen SE, Juul K, Schnohr P, et al. Platelet glycoprotein IIb/IIIa Pl(A2)/Pl(A2) homozygosity associated with risk of ischemic cardiovascular disease and myocardial infarction in young men: the Copenhagen City Heart Study. J Am Coll Cardiol 2003; 42:661–667.
6. Burr D, Doss H, Cooke GE, et al. A meta-analysis of studies on the association of the platelet PlA polymorphism of glycoprotein IIIa and risk of coronary heart disease. Stat Med 2003; 22:1741–1760.
7. Cavallari U, Trabetti E, Malerba G, et al. Gene sequence variations of the platelet P2Y12 receptor are associated with coronary artery disease. BMC Med Genet 2007; 8:59.
8. Di Castelnuovo A, de Gaetano G, Donati MB, et al. Platelet glycoprotein receptor IIIa polymorphism PLA1/PLA2 and coronary risk: a meta-analysis. Thromb Haemost 2001; 85:626–633.
9. Faraday N, Martinez EA, Scharpf RB, et al. Platelet gene polymorphisms and cardiac risk assessment in vascular surgical patients. Anesthesiology 2004; 101:1291–1297.
10. Fontana P, Dupont A, Gandrille S, et al. Adenosine diphosphate-induced platelet aggregation is associated with P2Y12 gene sequence variations in healthy subjects. Circulation 2003; 108:989–995.
11. Fontana P, Gaussem P, Aiach M, et al. P2Y12 H2 haplotype is associated with peripheral arterial disease: a case-control study. Circulation 2003; 108:2971–2973.
12. Hetherington SL, Singh RK, Lodwick D, et al. Dimorphism in the P2Y1 ADP receptor gene is associated with increased platelet activation response to ADP. Arterioscler Thromb Vasc Biol 2005; 25:252–257.
13. Wu AH, Tsongalis GJ. Correlation of polymorphisms to coagulation and biochemical risk factors for cardiovascular diseases. Am J Cardiol 2001; 87:1361–1366.

14. Yee DL, Bray PF. Clinical and functional consequences of platelet membrane glycoprotein polymorphisms. Semin Thromb Hemost 2004; 30:591–600.
15. Antithrombotic Trialists' Collaboration. Collaborative meta-analysis of randomised trials of antiplatelet therapy for prevention of death, myocardial infarction, and stroke in high risk patients. BMJ 2002; 324:71–86.
16. Antiplatelet Trialists' Collaboration. Collaborative overview of randomised trials of antiplatelet therapy–I: Prevention of death, myocardial infarction, and stroke by prolonged antiplatelet therapy in various categories of patients. BMJ 1994; 308:81–106.
17. Brockmoller J, Tzvetkov MV. Pharmacogenetics: data, concepts and tools to improve drug discovery and drug treatment. Eur J Clin Pharmacol 2008; 64:133–157.
18. Ingelman-Sundberg M. Pharmacogenomic biomarkers for prediction of severe adverse drug reactions. N Engl J Med 2008; 358:637–639.
19. Faraday N, Yanek LR, Mathias R, et al. Heritability of platelet responsiveness to aspirin in activation pathways directly and indirectly related to cyclooxygenase-1. Circulation 2007; 115:2490–2496.
20. Weber AA, Zimmermann KC, Meyer-Kirchrath J, et al. Cyclooxygenase-2 in human platelets as a possible factor in aspirin resistance. Lancet 1999; 353:900.
21. Hankey GJ, Eikelboom JW. Aspirin resistance. Lancet 2006; 367:606–617.
22. Gum PA, Kottke-Marchant K, Welsh PA, et al. A prospective, blinded determination of the natural history of aspirin resistance among stable patients with cardiovascular disease. J Am Coll Cardiol 2003; 41:961–965.
23. Eikelboom JW, Hirsh J, Weitz JI, et al. Aspirin-resistant thromboxane biosynthesis and the risk of myocardial infarction, stroke, or cardiovascular death in patients at high risk for cardiovascular events. Circulation 2002; 105:1650–1655.
24. Grotemeyer KH, Scharafinski HW, Husstedt IW. Two-year follow-up of aspirin responder and aspirin non responder. A pilot-study including 180 post-stroke patients. Thromb Res 1993; 71:397–403.
25. Roth GJ, Machuga ET, Ozols J. Isolation and covalent structure of the aspirin-modified, active-site region of prostaglandin synthetase. Biochemistry 1983; 22:4672–4675.
26. Roth GJ, Calverley DC. Aspirin, platelets, and thrombosis: theory and practice. Blood 1994; 83:885–898.
27. Halushka MK, Walker LP, Halushka PV. Genetic variation in cyclooxygenase 1: effects on response to aspirin. Clin Pharmacol Ther 2003; 73:122–130.
28. Hillarp A, Palmqvist B, Lethagen S, et al. Mutations within the cyclooxygenase-1 gene in aspirin non-responders with recurrence of stroke. Thromb Res 2003; 112:275–283.
29. Ulrich CM, Bigler J, Sibert J, et al. Cyclooxygenase 1 (COX1) polymorphisms in African-American and Caucasian populations. Hum Mutat 2002; 20:409–410.
30. Li Q, Chen BL, Ozdemir V, et al. Frequency of genetic polymorphisms of COX1, GPIIIa and P2Y1 in a Chinese population and association with attenuated response to aspirin. Pharmacogenomics 2007; 8:577–586.
31. Lepantalo A, Mikkelsson J, Resendiz JC, et al. Polymorphisms of COX-1 and GPVI associate with the antiplatelet effect of aspirin in coronary artery disease patients. Thromb Haemost 2006; 95:253–259.
32. Maree AO, Curtin RJ, Chubb A, et al. Cyclooxygenase-1 haplotype modulates platelet response to aspirin. J Thromb Haemost 2005; 3:2340–2345.
33. Lecomte M, Laneuville O, Ji C, et al. Acetylation of human prostaglandin endoperoxide synthase-2 (cyclooxygenase-2) by aspirin. J Biol Chem 1994; 269:13207–13215.
34. Vane JR, Bakhle YS, Botting RM. Cyclooxygenases 1 and 2. Annu Rev Pharmacol Toxicol 1998; 38:97–120.
35. Papafili A, Hill MR, Brull DJ, et al. Common promoter variant in cyclooxygenase-2 represses gene expression: evidence of role in acute-phase inflammatory response. Arterioscler Thromb Vasc Biol 2002; 22:1631–1636.
36. Kranzhofer R, Ruef J. Aspirin resistance in coronary artery disease is correlated to elevated markers for oxidative stress but not to the expression of cyclooxygenase (COX) 1/2, a novel COX-1 polymorphism or the PlA(1/2) polymorphism. Platelets 2006; 17:163–169.

37. Gonzalez-Conejero R, Rivera J, Corral J, et al. Biological assessment of aspirin efficacy on healthy individuals: heterogeneous response or aspirin failure? Stroke 2005; 36:276–280.

38. Bolhuis PA, Sakariassen KS, Sander HJ, et al. Binding of factor VIII-von Willebrand factor to human arterial subendothelium precedes increased platelet adhesion and enhances platelet spreading. J Lab Clin Med 1981; 97:568–576.

39. Fredrickson BJ, Dong JF, McIntire LV, et al. Shear-dependent rolling on von Willebrand factor of mammalian cells expressing the platelet glycoprotein Ib-IX-V complex. Blood 1998; 92:3684–3693.

40. Nieswandt B, Watson SP. Platelet-collagen interaction: is GPVI the central receptor? Blood 2003; 102:449–461.

41. Savage B, Almus-Jacobs F, Ruggeri ZM. Specific synergy of multiple substrate-receptor interactions in platelet thrombus formation under flow. Cell 1998; 94:657–666.

42. Afshar-Kharghan V, Vijayan KV, Bray PF. Platelet Polymorphisms. In: Michelson AD, eds. Platelets. San Diego: Academic Press, 2007:281–307.

43. Vijayan KV, Bray PF. Molecular mechanisms of prothrombotic risk due to genetic variations in platelet genes: Enhanced outside-in signaling through the Pro33 variant of integrin beta3. Exp Biol Med (Maywood) 2006; 231:505–513.

44. Ridker PM, Hennekens CH, Schmitz C, et al. PIA1/A2 polymorphism of platelet glycoprotein IIIa and risks of myocardial infarction, stroke, and venous thrombosis. Lancet 1997; 349:385–388.

45. Potapov EV, Ignatenko S, Nasseri BA, et al. Clinical significance of PlA polymorphism of platelet GP IIb/IIIa receptors during long-term VAD support. Ann Thorac Surg 2004; 77:869–874 (discussion 874).

46. Potapov EV, Hetzer R. Impact of PlA polymorphism of platelet GP IIb/IIIa receptors on clinical course during long-term LVAD support is independent of type of LVAD. Ann Thorac Surg 2006; 82:1167.

47. Cooke GE, Bray PF, Hamlington JD, et al. PlA2 polymorphism and efficacy of aspirin. Lancet 1998; 351:1253.

48. Macchi L, Christiaens L, Brabant S, et al. Resistance in vitro to low-dose aspirin is associated with platelet PlA1 (GP IIIa) polymorphism but not with C807T(GP Ia/IIa) and C-5T Kozak (GP Ibalpha) polymorphisms. J Am Coll Cardiol 2003; 42:1115–1119.

49. Michelson AD, Furman MI, Goldschmidt-Clermont P, et al. Platelet GP IIIa Pl(A) polymorphisms display different sensitivities to agonists. Circulation 2000; 101:1013–1018.

50. Lim E, Carballo S, Cornelissen J, et al. Dose-related efficacy of aspirin after coronary surgery in patients With Pl(A2) polymorphism (NCT00262275). Ann Thorac Surg 2007; 83:134–138.

51. Cooke GE, Liu-Stratton Y, Ferketich AK, et al. Effect of platelet antigen polymorphism on platelet inhibition by aspirin, clopidogrel, or their combination. J Am Coll Cardiol 2006; 47:541–546.

52. Szczeklik A, Undas A, Sanak M, et al. Relationship between bleeding time, aspirin and the PlA1/A2 polymorphism of platelet glycoprotein IIIa. Br J Haematol 2000; 110:965–967.

53. Dropinski J, Musial J, Sanak M, et al. Antithrombotic effects of aspirin based on PLA1/A2 glycoprotein IIIa polymorphism in patients with coronary artery disease. Thromb Res 2007; 119:301–303.

54. Undas A, Brummel K, Musial J, et al. Pl(A2) polymorphism of beta(3) integrins is associated with enhanced thrombin generation and impaired antithrombotic action of aspirin at the site of microvascular injury. Circulation 2001; 104:2666–2672.

55. Undas A, Sanak M, Musial J, et al. Platelet glycoprotein IIIa polymorphism, aspirin, and thrombin generation. Lancet 1999; 353:982–983.

56. Lev EI, Patel RT, Guthikonda S, et al. Genetic polymorphisms of the platelet receptors P2Y(12), P2Y(1) and GP IIIa and response to aspirin and clopidogrel. Thromb Res 2007; 119:355–360.

57. Bernardo E, Angiolillo DJ, Ramirez C, et al. Lack of association between gene sequence variations of platelet membrane receptors and aspirin responsiveness detected by the PFA-100 system in patients with coronary artery disease. Platelets 2006; 17:586–590.

58. Pamukcu B, Oflaz H, Nisanci Y. The role of platelet glycoprotein IIIa polymorphism in the high prevalence of in vitro aspirin resistance in patients with intracoronary stent restenosis. Am Heart J 2005; 149:675–680.

59. Papp E, Havasi V, Bene J, et al. Glycoprotein IIIA gene (PlA) polymorphism and aspirin resistance: is there any correlation? Ann Pharmacother 2005; 39:1013–1018.

60. Lopez JA, Dong JF. Structure and function of the glycoprotein Ib-IX-V complex. Curr Opin Hematol 1997; 4:323–329.

61. Coller BS, Peerschke EI, Scudder LE, et al. Studies with a murine monoclonal antibody that abolishes ristocetin-induced binding of von Willebrand factor to platelets: additional evidence in support of GPIb as a platelet receptor for von Willebrand factor. Blood 1983; 61:99–110.

62. Yamamoto N, Kitagawa H, Tanoue K, et al. Monoclonal antibody to glycoprotein Ib inhibits both thrombin- and ristocetin-induced platelet aggregations. Thromb Res 1985; 39:751–759.

63. Clemetson KJ, Clemetson JM. Platelet collagen receptors. Thromb Haemost 2001; 86:189–197.

64. Kritzik M, Savage B, Nugent DJ, et al. Nucleotide polymorphisms in the alpha2 gene define multiple alleles that are associated with differences in platelet alpha2 beta1 density. Blood 1998; 92:2382–2388.

65. Kunicki TJ, Kritzik M, Annis DS, et al. Hereditary variation in platelet integrin alpha 2 beta 1 density is associated with two silent polymorphisms in the alpha 2 gene coding sequence. Blood 1997; 89:1939–1943.

66. Bray PF, Howard TD, Vittinghoff E, et al. Effect of genetic variations in platelet glycoproteins Ibalpha and VI on the risk for coronary heart disease events in postmenopausal women taking hormone therapy. Blood 2007; 109:1862–1869.

67. Ollikainen E, Mikkelsson J, Perola M, et al. Platelet membrane collagen receptor glycoprotein VI polymorphism is associated with coronary thrombosis and fatal myocardial infarction in middle-aged men. Atherosclerosis 2004; 176:95–99.

68. Croft SA, Samani NJ, Teare MD, et al. Novel platelet membrane glycoprotein VI dimorphism is a risk factor for myocardial infarction. Circulation 2001; 104:1459–1463.

69. Ziegler S, Schillinger M, Funk M, et al. Association of a functional polymorphism in the clopidogrel target receptor gene, P2Y12, and the risk for ischemic cerebrovascular events in patients with peripheral artery disease. Stroke 2005; 36:1394–1399.

70. Bierend A, Rau T, Maas R, et al. P2Y(12) polymorphisms and antiplatelet effects of aspirin in patients with coronary artery disease. Br J Clin Pharmacol 2007.

71. Jefferson BK, Foster JH, McCarthy JJ, et al. Aspirin resistance and a single gene. Am J Cardiol 2005; 95:805–808.

72. Lorand L. Factor XIII: structure, activation, and interactions with fibrinogen and fibrin. Ann N Y Acad Sci 2001; 936:291–311.

73. Wells PS, Anderson JL, Scarvelis DK, et al. Factor XIII Val34Leu variant is protective against venous thromboembolism: a HuGE review and meta-analysis. Am J Epidemiol 2006; 164:101–109.

74. Undas A, Sydor WJ, Brummel K, et al. Aspirin alters the cardioprotective effects of the factor XIII Val34Leu polymorphism. Circulation 2003; 107:17–20.

75. He S, Blomback M, Yoo G, et al. Modified clotting properties of fibrinogen in the presence of acetylsalicylic acid in a purified system. Ann N Y Acad Sci 2001; 936:531–535.

76. Kahner BN, Shankar H, Murugappan S, et al. Nucleotide receptor signaling in platelets. J Thromb Haemost 2006; 4:2317–2326.

77. Hollopeter G, Jantzen HM, Vincent D, et al. Identification of the platelet ADP receptor targeted by antithrombotic drugs. Nature 2001; 409:202–207.

78. Nguyen T, Frishman WH, Nawarskas J, et al. Variability of response to clopidogrel: possible mechanisms and clinical implications. Cardiol Rev 2006; 14:136–142.

79. Maree AO, Fitzgerald DJ. Variable platelet response to aspirin and clopidogrel in atherothrombotic disease. Circulation 2007; 115:2196–2207.

80. Mizuno N, Niwa T, Yotsumoto Y, et al. Impact of drug transporter studies on drug discovery and development. Pharmacol Rev 2003; 55:425–461.

81. Taubert D, von Beckerath N, Grimberg G, et al. Impact of P-glycoprotein on clopidogrel absorption. Clin Pharmacol Ther 2006; 80:486–501.

82. Wijnen PA, Op den Buijsch RA, Drent M, et al. Review article: The prevalence and clinical relevance of cytochrome P450 polymorphisms. Aliment Pharmacol Ther 2007; 26(suppl 2): 211–219.

83. Clarke TA, Waskell LA. The metabolism of clopidogrel is catalyzed by human cytochrome P450 3A and is inhibited by atorvastatin. Drug Metab Dispos 2003; 31:53–59.

84. Ha-Duong NT, Dijols S, Macherey AC, et al. Ticlopidine as a selective mechanism-based inhibitor of human cytochrome P450 2C19. Biochemistry 2001; 40:12112–12122.

85. Lopez-Garcia MP, Dansette PM, Mansuy D. Thiophene derivatives as new mechanism-based inhibitors of cytochromes P-450: inactivation of yeast-expressed human liver cytochrome P-450 2C9 by tienilic acid. Biochemistry 1994; 33:166–175.

86. Rehmel JL, Eckstein JA, Farid NA, et al. Interactions of two major metabolites of prasugrel, a thienopyridine antiplatelet agent, with the cytochromes P450. Drug Metab Dispos 2006; 34:600–607.

87. Angiolillo DJ, Fernandez-Ortiz A, Bernardo E, et al. Contribution of gene sequence variations of the hepatic cytochrome P450 3A4 enzyme to variability in individual responsiveness to clopidogrel. Arterioscler Thromb Vasc Biol 2006; 26:1895–1900.

88. Fontana P, Hulot JS, De Moerloose P, et al. Influence of CYP2C19 and CYP3A4 gene polymorphisms on clopidogrel responsiveness in healthy subjects. J Thromb Haemost 2007; 5:2153–2155.

89. Giusti B, Gori AM, Marcucci R, et al. Cytochrome P450 2C19 loss-of-function polymorphism, but not CYP3A4 IVS10 + 12G/A and P2Y12 T744C polymorphisms, is associated with response variability to dual antiplatelet treatment in high-risk vascular patients. Pharmacogenet Genomics 2007; 17:1057–1064.

90. Hustert E, Haberl M, Burk O, et al. The genetic determinants of the CYP3A5 polymorphism. Pharmacogenetics 2001; 11:773–779.

91. Kuehl P, Zhang J, Lin Y, et al. Sequence diversity in CYP3A promoters and characterization of the genetic basis of polymorphic CYP3A5 expression. Nat Genet 2001; 27:383–391.

92. Suh JW, Koo BK, Zhang SY, et al. Increased risk of atherothrombotic events associated with cytochrome P450 3A5 polymorphism in patients taking clopidogrel. CMAJ 2006; 174:1715–1722.

93. Smith SM, Judge HM, Peters G, et al. Common sequence variations in the P2Y12 and CYP3A5 genes do not explain the variability in the inhibitory effects of clopidogrel therapy. Platelets 2006; 17:250–258.

94. Hulot JS, Bura A, Villard E, et al. Cytochrome P450 2C19 loss-of-function polymorphism is a major determinant of clopidogrel responsiveness in healthy subjects. Blood 2006; 108:2244–2247.

95. Brandt JT, Close SL, Iturria SJ, et al. Common polymorphisms of CYP2C19 and CYP2C9 affect the pharmacokinetic and pharmacodynamic response to clopidogrel but not prasugrel. J Thromb Haemost 2007; 5:2429–2436.

96. von Beckerath N, von Beckerath O, Koch W, et al. P2Y12 gene H2 haplotype is not associated with increased adenosine diphosphate-induced platelet aggregation after initiation of clopidogrel therapy with a high loading dose. Blood Coagul Fibrinolysis 2005; 16:199–204.

97. Cuisset T, Frere C, Quilici J, et al. Role of the T744C polymorphism of the P2Y12 gene on platelet response to a 600-mg loading dose of clopidogrel in 597 patients with non-ST-segment elevation acute coronary syndrome. Thromb Res 2007; 120:893–899.

98. Angiolillo DJ, Fernandez-Ortiz A, Bernardo E, et al. Lack of association between the P2Y12 receptor gene polymorphism and platelet response to clopidogrel in patients with coronary artery disease. Thromb Res 2005; 116:491–497.

99. Sibbing D, von Beckerath O, Schomig A, et al. P2Y1 gene A1622G dimorphism is not associated with adenosine diphosphate-induced platelet activation and aggregation after administration of a single high dose of clopidogrel. J Thromb Haemost 2006; 4:912–914.

100. Papp E, Havasi V, Bene J, et al. Does glycoprotein IIIa gene (Pl(A)) polymorphism influence clopidogrel resistance?: a study in older patients. Drugs Aging 2007; 24:345–350.

101. Dropinski J, Musial J, Jakiela B, et al. Anti-thrombotic action of clopidogrel and Pl(A1/A2) polymorphism of beta3 integrin in patients with coronary artery disease not being treated with aspirin. Thromb Haemost 2005; 94:1300–1305.

102. Angiolillo DJ, Fernandez-Ortiz A, Bernardo E, et al. PlA polymorphism and platelet reactivity following clopidogrel loading dose in patients undergoing coronary stent implantation. Blood Coagul Fibrinolysis 2004; 15:89–93.

103. Cuisset T, Frere C, Quilici J, et al. Lack of association between the 807 C/T polymorphism of glycoprotein Ia gene and post-treatment platelet reactivity after aspirin and clopidogrel in patients with acute coronary syndrome. Thromb Haemost 2007; 97:212–217.

104. Angiolillo DJ, Fernandez-Ortiz A, Bernardo E, et al. 807 C/T Polymorphism of the glycoprotein Ia gene and pharmacogenetic modulation of platelet response to dual antiplatelet treatment. Blood Coagul Fibrinolysis 2004; 15:427–433.

105. Angiolillo DJ, Fernandez-Ortiz A, Bernardo E, et al. Variability in platelet aggregation following sustained aspirin and clopidogrel treatment in patients with coronary heart disease and influence of the 807 C/T polymorphism of the glycoprotein Ia gene. Am J Cardiol 2005; 96:1095–1099.

106. Schror K, Weber AA. Comparative pharmacology of GP IIb/IIIa antagonists. J Thromb Thrombolysis 2003; 15:71–80.

107. Second SYMPHONY Investigators. Randomized trial of aspirin, sibrafiban, or both for secondary prevention after acute coronary syndromes. Circulation 2001; 103:1727–1733.

108. Cannon CP, McCabe CH, Wilcox RG, et al. Oral glycoprotein IIb/IIIa inhibition with orbofiban in patients with unstable coronary syndromes (OPUS-TIMI 16) trial. Circulation 2000; 102:149–156.

109. Wheeler GL, Braden GA, Bray PF, et al. Reduced inhibition by abciximab in platelets with the PlA2 polymorphism. Am Heart J 2002; 143:76–82.

110. Rozalski M, Watala C. Antagonists of platelet fibrinogen receptor are less effective in carriers of Pl(A2) polymorphism of beta(3) integrin. Eur J Pharmacol 2002; 454:1–8.

111. O'Connor FF, Shields DC, Fitzgerald A, et al. Genetic variation in glycoprotein IIb/IIIa (GPIIb/IIIa) as a determinant of the responses to an oral GPIIb/IIIa antagonist in patients with unstable coronary syndromes. Blood 2001; 98:3256–3260.

112. Bray PF, Cannon CP, Goldschmidt-Clermont P, et al. The platelet Pl(A2) and angiotensin-converting enzyme (ACE) D allele polymorphisms and the risk of recurrent events after acute myocardial infarction. Am J Cardiol 2001; 88:347–352.

113. Walter DH, Schachinger V, Elsner M, et al. Statin therapy is associated with reduced restenosis rates after coronary stent implantation in carriers of the Pl(A2)allele of the platelet glycoprotein IIIa gene. Eur Heart J 2001; 22:587–595.

114. Stamler JS, Loscalzo J. The antiplatelet effects of organic nitrates and related nitroso compounds in vitro and in vivo and their relevance to cardiovascular disorders. J Am Coll Cardiol 1991; 18:1529–1536.

115. Skowasch D, Lentini S, Andrie R, et al. Decreased platelet aggregation during angiotensin-converting enzyme inhibitor therapy. Results of a pilot study. Dtsch Med Wochenschr 2001; 126:707–711.

116. Bauriedel G, Skowasch D, Schneider M, et al. Antiplatelet effects of angiotensin-converting enzyme inhibitors compared with aspirin and clopidogrel: a pilot study with whole-blood aggregometry. Am Heart J 2003; 145:343–348.

117. Malinin AI, Ong S, Makarov LM, et al. Platelet inhibition beyond conventional antiplatelet agents: expanding role of angiotensin receptor blockers, statins and selective serotonin reuptake inhibitors. Int J Clin Pract 2006; 60:993–1002.

118. Faraday N, Becker DM, Yanek LR, et al. Relation between atherosclerosis risk factors and aspirin resistance in a primary prevention population. Am J Cardiol 2006; 98:774–779.

6

The Effects of Antiplatelet, Antithrombotic, and Thrombolytic Agents on Inflammation and Circulating Inflammatory Biomarkers

Erdal Cavusoglu
Division of Cardiology, Department of Medicine, SUNY Downstate Medical Center, Brooklyn, New York, U.S.A.

INTRODUCTION

This chapter will review the effects of the drugs used for the treatment of atherothrombotic disorders on inflammation and inflammatory biomarkers. While these medications were developed primarily to target components of the thrombotic process, many have been found to have unanticipated inhibitory effects on inflammation and inflammatory biomarkers. Such effects may have potential implications both for the selection of therapy (the choice of one agent vs. another of the same general class) as well as the duration and intensity of this therapy. An additional reason for the clinician to be aware of the anti-inflammatory properties of these agents is that they may provide insights into the mechanism of action of these drugs. While there have been no studies to date designed specifically to determine the clinical significance of such effects, given the growing recognition of the importance of inflammation in atherosclerotic disease, knowledge of the anti-inflammatory effects of such agents has the potential to lead to improved therapeutic strategies and drug development. Accordingly, the effects of such therapies on inflammation and on circulating markers form an important topic. This chapter will systematically examine the effects of the various antiplatelet, antithrombotic, and thrombolytic agents on both inflammation in general and the circulating biomarkers in particular. The review will be restricted to the FDA-approved commercially available agents in the United States. A summary of the relevant clinical studies are provided in Table 1.

(Text continues on page 77)

Table 1 Summary of the Clinical Studies Investigating the Effects of Antiplatelet, Antithrombotic, and Thrombolytic Agents on Inflammation and Circulating Inflammatory Biomarkers

Study	Drug dose and duration	Population	Design	Main findings
Feng et al. (1)	ASA 81–325 mg/day × 7 days	32 healthy men	Randomized, double blind, parallel study	No effect of ASA on CRP levels either at rest or post exercise.
Feldman et al. (2)	ASA 81 mg/day × 31 days	57 healthy male and female volunteers	Placebo-controlled trial	Low doses of ASA had no detectable effect on serum CRP levels in healthy men and women.
Azar et al. (3)	ASA 325 mg/day × 8 wks	37 healthy volunteers	Randomized, prospective, crossover study	No effect of ASA on serum levels of CRP, IL-6, s-ICAM, and monocyte expression of the CD11b/CD18 receptor.
Ikonomidis et al. (4)	ASA 300 mg/day × 3 wks	40 men with coronary artery disease	Placebo-controlled, randomized, double blind crossover trial	Serum CRP levels were significantly lower after ASA therapy compared with placebo.
Solheim et al. (5)	(i) ASA 160 mg/day or (ii) ASA 75 mg/day + warfarin or (iii) warfarin alone	310 patients who were 3 mos post-MI	Substudy of WARIS II trial, retrospective analysis	ASA 160 mg/day was associated with significantly lower levels of hs-CRP and TNF-α over 4 yr compared with warfarin alone.
Takeda et al. (6)	81–162 mg/day × 3 mos	1457 patients with and without ischemic heart disease referred for coronary angiography	Cross-sectional, not placebo-controlled	Treatment with ASA had no effect on CRP levels in either group.
Woodward et al. (7)	ASA 75 mg/day or Clopidogrel 75 mg/day, for 6 mos	184 patients who were 3–7 days post MI	Randomized, double blind multicenter trial (the CADET trial)	At 1 mo, fibrinogen, D-dimer, vWF, and CRP were significantly reduced from baseline values in both groups; at 6 mo, no difference between the 2 treatment groups.
Monakier et al. (8)	Rofecoxib 25 mg/day + ASA 100 mg/day or placebo + ASA 100 mg/day, for 3 mos	34 NSTEMI patients	Prospective, randomized, double blind, placebo-controlled study	Rofecoxib + ASA group had statistically significant reductions in CRP and IL-6 levels at 1 mo and lower CRP levels at 3 mos: ASA + placebo group had no change in CRP or IL-6 levels at any time point.

Reference	Treatment	Study type	Subjects	Findings
Rogowski et al. (9)	Chronic therapy with ASA ≤325 mg/day	Retrospective analysis of participants of a large registry	370 patients with low atherothrombotic risk profile	ASA at these doses was not associated with any significant effect on concentrations of CRP.
Dunzendorfer et al. (10)	Clopidogrel 75 mg/day or ASA 100 mg/day, for 8 days	Ex vivo	8 healthy volunteers	Clopidogrel reduced the plasma-dependent chemokinesis in monocytes and plasma-dependent cytokine-triggered neutrophil transendothelial migration in endothelial cells, as well as plasma levels of sICAM-1; these effects were not seen with ASA.
Hermann et al. (11)	Clopidogrel 75 mg/day × 7 days	Ex vivo	10 healthy male volunteers	ADP-induced expression of CD40L was completely abolished with clopidogrel treatment.
Nannizzi-Alaimo et al. (12)	ASA 325 mg/d × 7 days	Ex vivo	7 volunteer donors	Platelets from aspirin-treated patients were partially protected from sCD40L release, but only when the agonist was collagen (and not when platelets were stimulated with ADP or TRAP).
Klinkhardt et al. (13)	Clopidogrel 150 mg/day × 1 day, then 75 mg/day × 5 days	Ex vivo	10 healthy volunteers	Clopidogrel significantly reduced CD62 expression and formation of platelet-leukocyte aggregates induced by TRAP or ADP.
Vivekananthan et al. (14)	Clopidogrel 75 mg/day with no pretreatment or Clopidogrel 75 mg/day with pretreatment. Pretreatment with clopidogrel was defined as (i) a 300- to 600-mg loading dose on the day of (but before) the interventional procedure, or (ii) an initial 75-mg/day loading dose ≥ 1 day before the procedure.	Retrospective analysis of registry patients who had pre- and post-procedural levels of CRP drawn	833 patients undergoing percutaneous coronary intervention	Clopidogrel pretreatment was associated with an attenuation of the peri-procedural increase in CRP.

(Continued)

Table 1 Summary of the Clinical Studies Investigating the Effects of Antiplatelet, Antithrombotic, and Thrombolytic Agents on Inflammation and Circulating Inflammatory Biomarkers (*Continued*)

Study	Drug dose and duration	Population	Design	Main findings
Quinn et al. (15)	Clopidogrel pretreatment with varying doses (>24 hr before PCI) or No clopidogrel pretreatment (only procedural treatment with 300–450 mg load)	74 patients undergoing PCI	Prospective non-randomized study	Clopidogrel pretreatment was associated with lower ADP-activated platelet CD40L expression in baseline and post-procedural samples. Similarly, platelet P-selectin expression at all time points in ADP-activated and in baseline and post-procedural TRAP-activated samples was lower in patients pretreated with clopidogrel. Clopidogrel pretreatment did not affect serum IL-6 or CD40L levels.
Xiao and Theroux (16)	Clopidogrel 300 mg loading dose	23 NSTEMI patients within 24 hr of hospital admission; 20 normal individuals served as controls	Ex vivo	Loading dose of clopidogrel attenuated the formation of platelet-monocyte and platelet-neutrophil conjugates.
Cha et al. (17)	Clopidogrel (300 mg on day 1, then 75 mg/day) and ASA (100 mg/day) or IV heparin (aPTT-monitored) and ASA (100 mg/day), for 7 days	52 patients with acute stage of atherosclerotic ischemic stroke (<24 hr)	Randomized	Treatment with Clopidogrel + ASA was associated with a significant reduction in platelet P-selectin expression as well as CRP levels at the end of 7 days.
Klinkhardt et al. (18)	(*i*) Clopidogrel (75 mg/day) or (*ii*) Aspirin (100 mg/day) or (*iii*) Combination or (*iv*) No antiplatelet treatment	44 patients with generalized atherosclerosis and peripheral occlusions on an antiplatelet regimen	Cross-sectional study of patients with PVD, ex vivo	Patients receiving clopidogrel (either alone or in combination with ASA) exhibited significantly lower expression of CD62 and formation of platelet-leukocyte aggregates.

Reference	Intervention	Patients	Study type	Results
Harding et al. (19)	Clopidogrel 75 mg/day × 28 days	20 patients with type 2 diabetes mellitus without evidence of CV disease	Prospective	Compared with baseline values, 28 day of treatment with Clopidogrel reduced platelet-leukocyte interactions, monocyte activation, and plasma concentrations of RANTES; no effect on surface expression of CD40L or sCD40L.
Lincoff et al. (20)	Abciximab bolus plus 12-hr infusion (standard dose) or placebo	160 patients undergoing high-risk balloon angioplasty or directional atherectomy	Substudy of the EPIC trial, retrospective analysis	Treatment with abciximab was associated with reductions of 30–100% in the magnitude of rise in CRP, IL-6, and TNF-α.
James et al. (21)	(i) Abciximab bolus plus 24-hr infusion or (ii) Abciximab bolus plus 48-hr infusion or (iii) matching placebo (bolus plus 48-hr infusion) All patients received aspirin and subcutaneous dalteparin for 5–7 days or until either discharge or PCI	404 patients with NSTEMI	Substudy of the GUSTO IV trial, retrospective analysis	Prolonged treatment with abciximab had no influence on IL-6, CRP, fibrinogen, and PAI-1.
Gurbel et al. (22)	(i) Clopidogrel 300 mg or (ii) Clopidogrel 600 mg or (iii) Clopidogrel 300 mg plus eptifibatide (standard dose) or (iv) Clopidogrel 600 mg plus eptifibatide (standard dose)	120 consecutive patients undergoing elective coronary stenting	2 × 2 randomized investigation	Compared with clopidogrel alone, clopidogrel plus eptifibatide was associated with a significant decrease in CRP and TNF-α release.

(Continued)

Table 1 Summary of the Clinical Studies Investigating the Effects of Antiplatelet, Antithrombotic, and Thrombolytic Agents on Inflammation and Circulating Inflammatory Biomarkers (*Continued*)

Study	Drug dose and duration	Population	Design	Main findings
Welt et al. (23)	(*i*) Eptifibatide bolus plus 16-hr infusion or (*ii*) Abciximab bolus plus 12-hr infusion or (*iii*) No GP IIb/IIIa inhibitor	45 consecutive patients undergoing PCI (relatively low risk)	Prospective observational study, non-randomized	PCI in the absence of GP IIb/IIIa inhibitor was associated with a small but measurable rise in CD40L and the platelet-derived chemokine RANTES. In contrast, eptifibatide significantly lowered baseline sCD40L and RANTES levels, while abciximab had no such effect.
Aggarwal et al. (24)	Abciximab bolus plus 12-hr infusion or Eptifibatide double bolus plus 18-hr infusion	50 patients undergoing coronary stenting	Prospective, randomized comparison	Comparable suppression of CRP, IL-6, and IL-1 receptor antagonist during the first 24 hr after coronary stent implantation.
Furman et al. (25)	(*i*) Abciximab bolus plus 12-hr infusion or (*ii*) Eptifibatide double bolus plus 16-hr infusion or (*iii*) No GP IIb/IIIa antagonist	98 consecutive ACS patients undergoing PCI	Non-randomized, choice of agent at operator discretion	At almost all time points post-PCI (up to 24 hr), abciximab was superior to both control and eptifibatide in the reduction of soluble CD40L and formation of platelet-leukocyte aggregates.
Ercan et al. (26)	Tirofiban bolus plus 48-hr infusion + heparin or Heparin alone	57 patients with NSTEMI undergoing PCI	Prospective and randomized	Tirofiban attenuated the rise in CRP at 48- and 72-hr post baseline compared with the heparin alone group.
Akbulut et al. (27)	Tirofiban bolus plus 24-hr infusion or 24-hr saline infusion	107 patients with stable angina undergoing stent placement	Prospective but non-randomized	Tirofiban had no effect on the levels of fibrinogen, CRP, IL-1, IL-6, IL-8, and TNF-α at prespecified time points (up to 48 hr) after PCI.

Study	Treatment	Patients	Design	Results
Montalescot et al. (28)	Enoxaparin (100 anti-Xa units/kg subcutaneously every 12 hr) or UFH (bolus + infusion), for a minimum of 48 hr and up to a maximum of 8 days	68 patients hospitalized for unstable coronary artery disease	Substudy of the ESSENCE trial	The early increase of vWF (a protein of the acute-phase reaction) was more frequent and more severe with UFH than with enoxaparin.
Montalescot et al. (29)	(i) Enoxaparin (100 anti-Xa units/kg SC every 12 hr) or (ii) Dalteparin (120 anti-Xa units/kg SC every 12 hr) or (iii) UFH (bolus + infusion) or (iv) PEG-hirudin (bolus + infusion)	154 patients with unstable coronary artery disease	Non-randomized, patients were enrolled in different centers participating in various different trials	There was a significant rise in vWF levels over the initial 48 hr in those treated with UFH or dalteparin which was not seen in those treated with either PEG-hirudin or enoxaparin.
Montalescot et al. (30)	48–120 hr of either (i) enoxaparin (100 anti-factor Xa U/kg subcutaneously at 12-hr intervals), (ii) dalteparin (120 anti-factor Xa U/kg subcutaneously at 12-hr intervals), or (iii) UFH (bolus + infusion)	141 patients with unstable angina or NSTEMI	Multicenter, prospective, randomized, open-label study with 3 parallel treatment groups	Compared with UFH, both enoxaparin and dalteparin reduced the release of vWF and CRP after ≥ 48 hr of treatment.
Hodl et al. (31)	Dalteparin (120 IU/kg subcutaneously at 12-hr intervals) or enoxaparin 1 mg/kg subcutaneously at 12-hr intervals)	61 patients with unstable angina or NSTEMI	Prospective and randomized	No significant differences between the treatment groups at any time point with respect to vWF levels (up to 66 hr after initiation of low molecular weight heparin treatment).

(Continued)

Table 1 Summary of the Clinical Studies Investigating the Effects of Antiplatelet, Antithrombotic, and Thrombolytic Agents on Inflammation and Circulating Inflammatory Biomarkers (*Continued*)

Study	Drug dose and duration	Population	Design	Main findings
Oldgren et al. (32)	Dalteparin (5000–7500 IU subcutaneously twice daily) or placebo, for 3 mos	555 patients with unstable angina and NSTEMI	Substudy of the FRISC II trial (restricted to the noninvasive cohort), retrospective analysis	There was no beneficial effect of prolonged dalteparin treatment with respect to acute-phase proteins, with persistently elevated levels of vWF found throughout the course of treatment.
Keating et al. (33)	Bivalirudin 0.75 mg/kg bolus plus infusion at 1.75 mg/kg/hr or Eptifibatide double bolus plus 18-hr infusion + UFH	63 patients undergoing elective PCI	Randomized	The early effects on inflammation were similar between the 2 groups. Bivalirudin was associated with significantly lower CRP levels at 30 days.
Keating et al. (34)	Bivalirudin 0.75 mg/kg bolus plus infusion at 1.75 mg/kg/hr or Eptifibatide double bolus plus 18-hr infusion + UFH	60 patients undergoing PCI	Randomized	Compared with those treated with bivalirudin, patients treated with UFH plus eptifibatide exhibited a 2-fold increase in platelet surface expression of P-selectin in pre-procedural samples. Platelet-leukocyte aggregation in vivo was greater with UFH plus eptifibatide as was concentration of MPO. Patients treated with UFH + eptifibatide exhibited a decrease in the capacity of platelets to bind fibrinogen.
Anand et al. (35)	(i) Bivalirudin 0.75 mg/kg bolus plus infusion at 1.75 mg/kg/hr or (ii) Bivalirudin 0.75 mg/kg bolus plus infusion at 1.75 mg/kg/hr plus Clopidogrel 300 mg or (iii) UFH (40–50 U/kg bolus)	50 patients undergoing elective PCI	Prospective, non-randomized observational study	Bivalirudin significantly reduced plasma sCD40L, an effect not seen with UFH (5 min after administration of bivalirudin).

Li et al. (36)	Bivalirudin 0.75 mg/kg bolus plus infusion at 1.75 mg/kg/hr or Eptifibatide double bolus plus 18-hr infusion + UFH	24 patients undergoing nonurgent PCI	Randomized and prospective	Patients treated with UFH + eptifibatide experienced a 2.3 fold increase in MPO levels which was not seen in those treated with bivalirudin.
Gibson et al. (37)	(i) Eptifibatide double bolus plus 18-24-hr infusion + UFH or (ii) Eptifibatide double bolus plus 18-24-hr infusion + 0.5 mg/kg IV of enoxaparin or (iii) Bivalirudin 0.75 mg/kg bolus plus infusion at 1.75 mg/kg/hr	857 moderate-to-high risk patients with ACS undergoing PCI	Randomized, open-label multicenter study	The peak increase from baseline in biomarkers (CRP, sCD40L, RANTES, and IL-6) did not differ between treatment strategies (sampled up to 24 hr post PCI).
Merlini et al. (38)	Thrombolytic therapy (rt-PA) or Heparin alone	39 patients hospitalized with acute myocardial infarction within 12 hr of symptom onset	Prospective, but non-randomized observational study	Patients receiving thrombolytic therapy had early activation of inflammation (as reflected by increases in CRP and IL-6 at 24 hr) which paralleled the activation of the contact system and coagulation cascade.
Pietila et al. (39)	Thrombolytic therapy with SK (1.8 mµ over 1 hr) or no thrombolytic therapy	23 patients with acute STEMI	Prospective observational study	In patients treated with SK, CRP was useful in assessing the success of thrombolysis. In patients with successful reperfusion the CRP response was only approximately 20% of that in patients in whom reperfusion failed or who did not receive lytic therapy (matched for infarct size).
Andreotti et al. (40)	Thrombolytic therapy with rt-PA	24 patients with STEMI receiving rt-PA within 6 hr	Prospective observational study	Early coronary recanalization with successful thrombolytic therapy curtails the response of fast acting plasminogen activator inhibitor and vWF (two procoagulant acute-phase proteins) and CRP to myocardial infarction, most likely by reducing the extent of necrosis and consequent acute-phase reaction.

(Continued)

Table 1 Summary of the Clinical Studies Investigating the Effects of Antiplatelet, Antithrombotic, and Thrombolytic Agents on Inflammation and Circulating Inflammatory Biomarkers (*Continued*)

Study	Drug dose and duration	Population	Design	Main findings
Andreotti et al. (41)	Thrombolytic therapy with rt-PA	30 patients with acute STEMI receiving rt-PA	Prospective observational study	Patients with successful lysis and patent infarct-related artery had a significant fall in vWF, plasminogen activator inhibitor, and CRP (during the first 3 days of myocardial infarction).
Tsakiris et al. (42)	Thrombolytic therapy (with either tenecteplase or reteplase) or No thrombolytic therapy	36 patients with STEMI	Prospective observational study	Patients who were thrombolysed had lower CRP values on admission, at 24 hr and at 48 hr, compared with those without thrombolysis.
Audebert et al. (43)	Thrombolytic therapy (with rt-PA) or No thrombolytic therapy	346 patients with acute ischemic stroke (43 patients with thrombolysis)	Retrospective analysis	Successful thrombolysis was related to a significantly attenuated inflammatory response as reflected in a reduction of body temperature, CRP, and WBC.
Pietila et al. (44)	Thrombolytic therapy with either accelerated alteplase, streptokinase, or a combination of both	146 patients with STEMI	Substudy of the GUSTO I trial	Thrombolytic treatment with accelerated alteplase was associated with a smaller acute-phase reaction (as reflected by lower CRP values) than treatment with either SK or a combination of SK and alteplase. The low-peak serum CRP values were associated with complete reperfusion of the infarct-related coronary artery. More efficient reperfusion with alteplase compared with the other regimens may reduce the inflammatory reaction of acute MI.

ASPIRIN

Preclinical Data

One of the strongest pieces of evidence in support of the anti-inflammatory properties of aspirin comes from its established inhibitory effects on the activity of nuclear factor kB (NF-kB), a transcription factor that is required for the expression of genes encoding pro-inflammatory molecules such as monocyte chemoattractant protein-1 (MCP-1), interleukin (IL)-1, IL-6, and adhesion molecules (45–48). In a classic study using both human and mouse cell lines, Kopp and Ghosh demonstrated that sodium salicylate and aspirin (in relatively high doses) inhibited the activation of NF-kB (45). This inhibition prevented the degradation of the NF-kB inhibitor, which resulted in the retention of NF-kB in the cytosol. Thus, NF-kB was unable to be translocated to the nucleus where it binds to DNA and regulates transcription of specific genes in response to a variety of inflammatory triggers. In a subsequent study, Cyrus et al. sought to determine the effect of low-dose aspirin on vascular inflammation, plaque composition, and atherogenesis in low-density lipoprotein (LDL) receptor–deficient mice fed a high-fat diet (49). They found that in LDL receptor-deficient mice fed a high-fat diet, low-dose aspirin induced a significant decrease in circulating levels and vascular formation of various inflammatory cytokines (such as sICAM-1, MCP-1, and TNF-α), without affecting lipid levels. Importantly, these effects were associated with significant reduction of the NF-kB activity in the aorta as well as a reduction in the extent of atherosclerosis. Consistent with these observations, Muller et al. demonstrated that chronic aspirin treatment of transgenic rats over-expressing the human renin and angiotensionogen genes protected from angiotensin II induced end-organ damage by inhibiting NF-kB activation in vivo (50).

Clinical Data

Because of the strong basic science literature in support of the anti-inflammatory actions of aspirin, there has been much interest in measuring these effects clinically, and attempting to correlate them with the benefits seen with aspirin usage. To this end, almost all studies that have tried to do so have looked at C-reactive protein (CRP) as the surrogate circulating inflammatory marker, and have examined the effect of aspirin therapy on baseline CRP levels. In general, these studies have provided conflicting results, possibly reflecting the different populations studied, as well as differences in the dose and duration of treatment with aspirin. These studies can be classified into those conducted in healthy volunteers versus those performed in patients with established atherosclerosis.

Healthy Populations

Three prospective studies have examined the effect of low-dose aspirin treatment on serum CRP levels in healthy subjects. These three studies were done specifically with aspirin doses shown to be cardioprotective (81–325 mg/day). In the first of these studies, Feng et al. found no significant effect of seven days of aspirin therapy (81 or 325 mg/day) on CRP levels, either at rest or post exercise, in a randomized, double blind study involving 32 healthy men (1). Similarly, in a placebo-controlled trial in 57 healthy male and female volunteers, Feldman et al. found that 31 days of treatment with 81 mg of aspirin produced no significant reduction in serum levels of high-sensitivity CRP compared with baseline (2). This lack of effect occurred despite the demonstration that this low-dose therapy was associated with a marked inhibition of platelet COX-1 activity, as manifested by a profound decline in platelet-derived serum thromboxane B_2

concentrations. In the third study, Azar and colleagues studied the effects of eight weeks of aspirin therapy (325 mg/day) on the levels of CRP, cytokines, and adhesion molecules in 37 healthy volunteers without evidence of cardiovascular disease (3). This study was randomized and prospective, and had a crossover design. The investigators found that the levels of CRP, IL-6, s-ICAM, and CD11b/CD18 expression on monocytes measured at different time intervals were not reduced with aspirin therapy. Of note, the duration of therapy in this study was eight weeks, longer than that in the studies by Feng et al. and Feldman et al. Because the aspirin dosage used in all of these studies was relatively low, however, the possibility still remains that higher doses may in fact be associated with greater suppression of inflammatory markers. Although there are no clinical studies in apparently healthy individuals examining the effect of higher doses of aspirin on CRP, one study which looked at the effect of aspirin at a daily dose of 2400 mg for four days in healthy volunteers found no significant effect on α-1 acid glycoprotein (GP) levels, an acute-phase protein and marker of inflammation (51).

Ex vivo studies of the effects of aspirin on platelets have also been performed in healthy volunteers. In one such study, Dunzendorfer et al. investigated the role of aspirin in ex vivo endothelial activation for interactions with leukocytes in healthy volunteers (10). Administration of aspirin was not associated with a decrease in the levels of adhesion molecules and platelet-derived mediators. In another study, adenosine diphosphate (ADP)-induced CD40L expression was not inhibited by aspirin in washed human platelets obtained from healthy volunteers (11). Finally, Nannizzi-Alaimo et al. found that platelets from healthy volunteers treated with aspirin 325 mg/day for seven days were partially protected from soluble CD40 ligand (sCD40L) release, but only when the agonist was collagen (not ADP or TRAP) (12).

Patients with Established Atherosclerosis

Clinical studies in patients with established atherosclerosis have also been performed. Specifically, data in this regard are available for patients with non-ST-segment elevation myocardial infarction (NSTEMI), acute stroke, peripheral arterial disease, diabetes mellitus, as well as patients undergoing percutaneous coronary intervention (PCI). Ikonomidis et al. administered 300 mg aspirin/day for three weeks or placebo to 40 men with coronary artery disease (4). Serum CRP levels were significantly lower after aspirin therapy than they were after placebo. In a substudy of the WARIS II trial, Solheim and colleagues assessed the influence of aspirin on selected inflammatory markers in patients recovering from acute myocardial infarction (MI) (5). Patients participating in the WARIS II trial were randomized to either aspirin 160 mg/day or aspirin 75 mg/day plus warfarin, or warfarin alone after acute MI. In this setting, aspirin 160 mg/day was associated with significantly lower levels of high-sensitivity CRP and TNF-α than warfarin alone over four years. Of note, the investigators found reduced levels of high-sensitivity CRP and TNF-α after four years in all three groups, indicating reduced inflammatory activity irrespective of the study medication. The authors postulated that this may be related to the use of statins during follow-up, which are known to reduce inflammatory markers in patients with coronary artery disease.

In contrast to the studies by Ikonomidis et al. and Solheim et al., four other studies in patients with established coronary artery disease have provided negative results. In a large study of patients with ($n = 1231$) and without ($n = 226$) ischemic heart disease referred for coronary angiography, Takeda and colleagues examined CRP levels at baseline and after three months of therapy with aspirin at a dose of 81–162 mg/day (6). They found that, while CRP levels were higher in those with ischemic heart disease compared with those without disease, treatment with aspirin did not have any effect on the

CRP level in either group. This was in contrast to treatment with statins, which was associated with significant reductions in CRP in both groups, and in contrast to either angiotensin-converting enzyme inhibitors or angiotensin II receptor blockers, which were associated with significant reductions in CRP levels only in the group of patients with ischemic heart disease. In another study, Woodward and colleagues randomized 184 patients who had experienced an MI within the previous three to seven days to aspirin (75 mg/day) versus clopidogrel (75 mg/day) in order to compare the effects of these two antiplatelet agents on thrombotic variables and CRP over a six-month period of treatment (7). Blood samples were taken at baseline and then at clinic visits at 1, 3 and 6 months. By one month, fibrinogen, D-dimer, von Willebrand factor, and CRP were significantly reduced from baseline values in both treatment groups. In addition, tissue plasminogen activator antigen was reduced in the aspirin group at this time point. At six months, however, there were no differences between treatment groups for any of the variables. Similarly, there were no differences between treatments with respect to baseline and final values for any of the variables. The authors attributed the reduction in markers at one month to the resolution of the acute-phase protein response for patients with acute MI. Furthermore, there was no evidence that these decreases between baseline and one month were affected by the type of treatment received (aspirin vs. clopidogrel). In another study, Monakier and colleagues randomized 34 patients hospitalized with non-ST-segment elevation acute coronary syndrome to receive rofecoxib 25 mg/day plus aspirin 100 mg/day, or placebo plus aspirin 100 mg/day for a period of three months (8). Blood samples for CRP and IL-6 levels were drawn prior to randomization, and after one month and three months. In contrast to the group receiving rofecoxib, who experienced statistically significant reductions in CRP and IL-6 levels at one month and lower CRP levels at three months, patients in the placebo group (receiving only aspirin) had no significant change in either CRP or IL-6 levels at any time point. Finally, in a more recent analysis of 370 subjects with a low atherothrombotic risk profile, low dose of aspirin (defined as < 325 mg/day) was not associated with any significant effect on concentrations of CRP (9).

Summary

In conclusion, it appears that the totality of the evidence would suggest a lack of effect of aspirin therapy (at least in clinically relevant doses) on circulating markers of inflammation, specifically CRP. The data in this regard are most consistent in apparently healthy subjects, where all studies to date have failed to demonstrate any effect of such therapy on circulating CRP levels. The data in patients with established atherosclerosis are somewhat conflicting, although the majority are also negative. Because some of these studies were conducted in patients across a broad spectrum of risk, it is conceivable that there may be subgroups in whom aspirin therapy is associated with meaningful reductions in inflammatory markers. Along the same lines, it is also conceivable that the ability to detect statistically significant reductions in CRP concentrations in those subjects with low or even moderately elevated baseline levels would require substantially larger numbers of patients. Such large studies have not been performed to date.

CLOPIDOGREL

Preclinical Data

There is experimental evidence to suggest that clopidogrel has an inhibitory effect on the activation of the endothelium. In this regard, Savi and colleagues were among the first to study the effects of aspirin and clopidogrel on platelet-dependent tissue factor expression in endothelial cells (52). When rat platelets were incubated with cultured bovine aortic endothelial cells, a significant increase in tissue factor expression was observed, which was further enhanced by the addition of thrombin or 2-methylthio-ADP. When administered orally in this setting, clopidogrel was able to inhibit the increase in tissue factor expression, whereas aspirin was ineffective in this regard. In a subsequent study by the same group of investigators, clopidogrel significantly inhibited, in the presence of platelets, the ex vivo generation of thrombin triggered by low concentrations of tissue factor (53). Importantly, the dose of clopidogrel that inhibited thrombin generation in this study also strongly inhibited platelet aggregation. As the authors stated, this would suggest that antiplatelet agents such as clopidogrel likely make a major contribution to inhibition of thrombin generation by decreasing platelet deposition and/or decreasing platelet activation.

In a very recent animal study, clopidogrel was shown to have inhibitory effects on CRP. Using a porcine model of percutaneous transluminal coronary angioplasty plus brachytherapy, Ayral and colleagues studied the effect of prolonged clopidogrel treatment on CRP concentrations (54). All animals received a 300-mg loading dose of clopidogrel one day before intervention, followed by clopidogrel 75 mg/day, in addition to aspirin 325 mg/day. Angioplasty plus radiation treatment was associated with an increase in CRP concentration in the blood of pigs immediately post intervention. Treatment with clopidogrel for three months reduced CRP levels more than did clopidogrel therapy for one month. Plasma clotting was not affected by prolonged clopidogrel therapy.

Clinical Data

There have been a number of clinical studies that have examined the effect of clopidogrel on platelet-mediated inflammation in apparently healthy human subjects. These studies have all used changes in surrogate markers (such as platelet expression of CD40L or P-selectin) as evidence of a reduction in platelet-mediated inflammation. In general, and in contrast to the studies with aspirin, the results have been fairly consistent in demonstrating an inhibitory effect of clopidogrel on markers of inflammation.

Healthy Populations

Hermann and colleagues studied the effects of aspirin and clopidogrel on platelet CD40L expression (11). In ten healthy male volunteers who were treated with 75 mg/day of clopidogrel for seven days, ADP-induced expression of CD40L was completely abolished. In contrast, ADP-induced CD40L expression was not inhibited by aspirin. In another study examining the roles of clopidogrel and aspirin in ex vivo endothelial activation for interactions with leukocytes, Dunzendorfer and colleagues found that plasma obtained from healthy volunteers treated with 75 mg/day of clopidogrel for eight days reduced plasma-dependent chemokinesis in monocytes and plasma-dependent cytokine-triggered neutrophil transendothelial migration in endothelial cells, as well as plasma levels of sICAM-1 (10). In addition, the effect on neutrophil transmigration was reversed after clopidogrel treatment was discontinued, suggesting that a continued anti-inflammatory effect with clopidogrel requires prolonged treatment. Importantly, because plasma-dependent endothelial activation for endothelium-leukocyte interaction is considered an early stage in the development of atherosclerosis and its complications, inhibition of plasma-promoted endothelial activation by clopidogrel may indicate a novel role in the prevention of atherosclerosis (10). In another study performed in ten healthy male volunteers, Klinkhardt et al. demonstrated that clopidogrel significantly reduced CD62 expression and formation of platelet-leukocyte aggregates induced by thrombin receptor agonist peptide (TRAP) or ADP (13). In a more recent study, Evangelista and colleagues demonstrated that pretreatment of human platelets with the active metabolite of clopidogrel in vitro resulted in a profound inhibition of platelet P-selectin expression, platelet-polymorphonuclear leukocyte adhesion, and production of reactive oxygen species by polymorphonuclear leukocytes (55). In addition, the active metabolite of clopidogrel inhibited rapid tissue factor exposure on platelets as well as on leukocyte surfaces in whole blood. Thus, this study showed that clopidogrel reduced platelet-dependent upregulation of inflammatory and pro-atherothrombotic functions in leukocytes. In this way, clopidogrel may have a beneficial effect in reducing the inflammation that underlies the atherosclerotic process.

Patients with Established Atherosclerosis

Studies in patients with established atherosclerotic diseases have both confirmed and extended the observations derived from healthy cohorts with respect to the inhibitory effects of clopidogrel on markers of inflammation. Perhaps the best data in this regard come from the PCI literature. Persistent elevations of CRP following stent implantation have been suggested to reflect a prolonged inflammatory reaction to coronary stent implantation, which might be causally involved in the restenotic process (56,57). In addition, both pre- and post-procedural elevations of CRP have been associated with short- and long-term adverse outcomes following PCI (56). In one of the earliest studies of its kind, Chew and colleagues from the Cleveland Clinic demonstrated that, among patients with an elevated baseline CRP level undergoing coronary stenting, pretreatment with clopidogrel was associated with a substantial reduction in 30-day death or MI (58). In a follow-up study, Vivekananthan and colleagues from the same institution reported that clopidogrel pretreatment was associated with an attenuation of the peri-procedural increase of CRP (14). Notably, this reduction in CRP levels was on top of that seen with the concomitant use of GP IIb/IIIa inhibitors, which have also been shown to have a similar effect on CRP levels. The authors speculated as to whether the known clinical benefit of pretreatment with clopidogrel in patients undergoing PCI was related to the blunting of the procedure-related inflammatory response associated with clopidogrel use.

In a similar study, Quinn et al. examined the effect of clopidogrel pretreatment on platelet inflammatory marker expression in patients undergoing PCI in a non-randomized fashion (15). Clopidogrel pretreatment was associated with lower ADP-activated platelet CD40L expression in baseline and post-procedural samples. Similarly, platelet P-selectin expression at all time points in ADP-activated and in baseline and post-procedural TRAP-activated samples was lower in patients pretreated with clopidogrel. Clopidogrel pretreatment did not affect serum IL-6 or CD40L levels.

Xiao and Theroux extended the observations about the anti-inflammatory effects of clopidogrel to patients with non-ST-segment elevation acute coronary syndrome (16). They found that a 300-mg loading dose of clopidogrel attenuated the agonist effects of ADP and TRAP on platelet secretion, aggregation, and formation of platelet-monocyte and platelet-neutrophil conjugates in patients with acute coronary syndrome. The authors suggested that these effects may contribute to the clinical benefits of clopidogrel in these syndromes.

Similar studies have also been performed in patients with established atherosclerosis in other vascular beds. Cha and colleagues examined the effects of clopidogrel on P-selectin expression on platelets and the plasma concentration of CRP in the acute stage of atherosclerotic ischemic stroke (17). Patients with acute ischemic stroke (<24 hours) were randomized for seven days to a combined regimen of clopidogrel and aspirin ($n = 24$) or intravenous heparin with aspirin ($n = 28$). Treatment with the combination of clopidogrel and aspirin (but not heparin and aspirin) was associated with a significant reduction in platelet P-selectin expression as well as plasma concentrations of CRP at the end of seven days compared with the baseline values of these parameters. Importantly, the beneficial inflammatory effects seen in the aspirin and clopidogrel group correlated with clinical improvement as well, as assessed by the NIH stroke scale score. Klinkhardt and colleagues extended the observations about the anti-inflammatory effects of clopidogrel to patients with peripheral vascular disease (18). In a cross-sectional study of patients with peripheral vascular disease, they demonstrated that untreated patients and those receiving aspirin monotherapy exhibited significantly higher expression of CD62 and formation of platelet-leukocyte aggregates than patients receiving clopidogrel alone or in combination with aspirin. This was observed both in blood samples in vivo (unstimulated baseline) and after in vitro stimulation of platelets with ADP or TRAP. Expression of MAC-1 on stimulation was significantly reduced in patients receiving clopidogrel or combined treatment, as compared with untreated patients or those receiving aspirin. Thus, their findings suggest that antiplatelet therapy with clopidogrel or combined therapy with clopidogrel and aspirin may exert an indirect anti-inflammatory effect through reduction of leukocyte activation by adherent platelets.

Another population at risk for developing atherosclerosis are diabetics. This group of patients are characterized by increased platelet reactivity, vascular inflammation, and are at elevated risk for the development of atherothrombotic events. Harding and colleagues examined the effects of clopidogrel on systemic inflammatory markers and on platelet, monocyte and endothelial activation in patients with type 2 diabetes mellitus (19). Twenty patients with type 2 diabetes mellitus without clinical evidence of cardiovascular disease were treated with clopidogrel 75 mg daily for 28 days, and blood samples were obtained at baseline and at 28 days. Clopidogrel treatment in these patients not only reduced platelet activation but also reduced platelet-leukocyte interactions, monocyte activation, and plasma concentrations of the chemokine RANTES. In contrast to P-selectin and RANTES, neither platelet surface expression of CD40L nor sCD40L was reduced by clopidogrel. The authors contrasted their findings with respect to CD40L to those by Xiao and Theroux (16), who reported a 27% reduction in plasma concentrations of sCD40L in patients with acute coronary syndromes. Importantly, in the study by Harding et al., baseline platelet activation and sCD40L levels were substantially lower than in the acute coronary syndrome population studied by Xiao and Theroux. Thus, it may be that clopidogrel may not have the same effect on CD40L in patients with lower baseline levels of platelet activation and sCD40L (19).

Summary

In summary, there is strong and consistent data demonstrating that clopidogrel treatment is associated with a reduction in markers of inflammation, such as CD40L, CRP, P-selectin, and platelet-leukocyte aggregate formation. This effect of clopidogrel is seen in healthy populations, those at risk (such as diabetics), as well as in those with established atherosclerosis. Furthermore, the effect of clopidogrel in reducing inflammatory markers is consistent across the full spectrum of patients with established atherosclerosis, including those with cerebrovascular disease, coronary artery disease, and peripheral vascular disease. Notably, these consistent findings with clopidogrel are in contrast to the conflicting data on the effects of aspirin on inflammatory markers. This raises the possibility that the effects of clopidogrel on inflammatory markers may therefore be due to its unique mechanism of action of P2Y12 ADP-receptor antagonism, and not to the more general effect of inhibition of platelet activation (48). Whether the apparent clinical superiority of clopidogrel over aspirin in certain clinical settings (59) is in fact related to their differential effects on inflammatory markers remains unknown.

THE GLYCOPROTEIN IIb/IIIa ANTAGONISTS

There is evidence to suggest that all three of the commercially available GP IIb/IIIa inhibitors have attenuating effects on inflammatory markers. In a subset of patients from the EPIC trial, a placebo-controlled evaluation of abciximab in high-risk PCI patients, Lincoff et al. showed that the use of abciximab was associated with a significant suppression of the peri-procedural rise in markers of systemic inflammation (20). Specifically, treatment with abciximab was associated with reductions of 30% to 100% in the magnitude of rise in CRP, IL-6, and TNF-α. Because the influence of abciximab on inflammatory markers in this study seemed to occur independently of the inhibition of ischemic events by this agent, some of the immediate or long-term benefit of abciximab in the setting of coronary intervention may be related to the suppression of inflammation (20). However, more recently, James and colleagues did an analysis of the 404 patients with non-ST-elevation acute coronary syndromes who had been enrolled in the GUSTO IV substudy on markers of inflammation and coagulation to determine if there was any effect of prolonged abciximab treatment on markers of inflammation (IL-6, CRP, and fibrinogen), coagulation (thrombin/anithrombin complex and soluble fibrin), and fibrinolysis (PAI-1) (21). In addition to aspirin and dalteparin, all patients were randomized to receive abciximab infusion for 24 hours or 48 hours or corresponding placebo without early revascularization. Plasma samples were obtained at baseline and at 24, 48, and 72 hours. The authors found that in non-ST-elevation acute coronary syndrome, there was a simultaneous activation of inflammation, coagulation, and fibrinolysis systems despite aspirin and dalteparin treatment. Furthermore, prolonged treatment with abciximab had no influence on the activation of these systems. These findings are in contrast to those by Lincoff et al. (20). It has been suggested that these disparate findings may have been related to differences in the reduction of myocardial damage associated with abciximab use in the two studies (greater reduction in the study by Lincoff et al. due to a higher rate of coronary intervention), with greater suppression of inflammation associated with prevention of myocardial damage (21).

Gurbel and colleagues examined the effect of eptifibatide on early inflammation and cardiac marker release after elective stenting when used in conjunction with clopidogrel (22). Compared with a strategy of clopidogrel alone, clopidogrel plus eptifibatide reduced the release of cardiac markers. A marked reduction in platelet aggregation and active GP IIb/IIIa expression with clopidogrel plus eptifibatide was associated with a decrease in CRP and TNF-α release. The decrease in inflammatory response by GP IIb/IIIa blockade was accompanied by maximum inhibition of platelet aggregation and GP IIb/IIIa receptor expression, but not P-selectin expression. These data would suggest that the decrease in the inflammatory response may be independent of P-selectin expression (22). In another study, Welt and colleagues measured plasma sCD40L and inflammatory markers (at baseline and at various time intervals post PCI) in a cohort of patients receiving abciximab, eptifibatide, or no GP IIb/IIIa inhibitor (23). PCI in the absence of GP IIb/IIIa inhibitor was associated with a small but measurable rise in sCD40L and the platelet-derived chemokine RANTES. In contrast, eptifibatide significantly lowered baseline sCD40L and RANTES levels, while abciximab had no such effect. However, in another study comparing abciximab and eptifibatide, Aggarwal and colleagues found comparable suppression of inflammation by these two agents after coronary stenting (24). In yet a third study comparing the two agents by Furman and colleagues, abciximab was superior to both untreated and eptifibatide-treated ACS patients undergoing PCI (25). They measured the effects of abciximab, eptifibatide, and no GPIIb/IIIa (control) on sCD40L and the formation of platelet-leukocyte aggregates. At almost all time points post PCI, abciximab was superior to both control and eptifibatide in the reduction of these parameters.

Data for tirofiban are also available. Ercan and colleagues investigated the effect of tirofiban on CRP levels in patients with NSTEMI (26). In a small but prospective and randomized study of 57 patients with NSTEMI already receiving aspirin, clopidogrel, and unfractionated heparin, the addition of tirofiban was shown to attenuate the rise in CRP at 48- and 72-hours post baseline compared with those not receiving tirofiban. Importantly, this effect was seen on top of traditional therapy, consisting of both aspirin and clopidogrel. However, in another study by Akbulut et al. of 107 patients with stable angina undergoing stent placement, tirofiban treatment had no significant effect on the levels of a variety of inflammatory markers (including CRP) at prespecified time points after PCI (27). The discrepant findings in these two studies may again highlight the importance of the status of the underlying inflammatory state, as the baseline CRP levels in the study by Ercan (consisting of NSTEMI patients) were higher than those by Akbulut (consisting of stable angina patients).

In summary, the totality of the evidence seems to suggest that the GP IIb/IIIa inhibitors have beneficial effects on inflammation and inflammatory markers. In addition, in the highest-risk patients these beneficial effects seem to occur on top of those already achieved with standard antiplatelet therapy. Importantly, however, the vast majority of studies examining this issue have been performed in the highly select population of patients undergoing PCI. It is unclear if these classes of agents would have similar effects in healthy populations or in coronary artery disease patients not undergoing PCI. Finally, given the limited number of small studies, there are not enough data regarding the superiority of one agent over another in this regard.

THE LOW MOLECULAR WEIGHT HEPARINS

Several studies have examined the effects of the commercially available low molecular weight heparins, enoxaparin and dalteparin, on circulating markers of inflammation. In one of the first studies in this regard, Montalescot and colleagues performed an analysis of a subgroup of 68 patients who had participated in the ESSENCE study, which was a multicenter and randomized trial that had demonstrated the clinical superiority of enoxaparin compared with adjusted-dose intravenous unfractionated heparin in patients hospitalized for unstable coronary artery disease (28). In this substudy, the investigators measured the levels of CRP, fibrinogen, von Willebrand factor antigen, endothelin-1, and troponin-I on admission and after 48 hours. All acute-phase reactant proteins were elevated on admission and increased further at 48 hours. By multivariate analysis, the rise of von Willebrand factor over 48 hours was a significant and independent predictor of the composite endpoint (consisting of death, MI, recurrent angina, or revascularization) at both 14 days and at 30 days. Of note, the early increase of von Willebrand factor was more frequent and more severe with unfractionated heparin than with enoxaparin. Thus, the authors concluded that enoxaparin provided protection as evidenced by the reduced release of von Willebrand factor (a protein of the acute-phase reaction), which represented a favorable prognostic finding.

In a follow-up study to this, Montalescot and colleagues compared the effects of different anticoagulant treatments on von Willebrand factor release in 154 patients with unstable angina (29). Patients were treated for at least 48 hours with either intravenous unfractionated heparin, enoxaparin, dalteparin, or the direct thrombin inhibitor PEG-hirudin. As in their earlier study, the authors confirmed that von Willebrand factor was released acutely during the first 48 hours of unstable angina and that an early and important rise of von Willebrand factor was associated with an adverse outcome at one-month follow-up. Importantly, however, they also found that there was a differential effect of the various anticoagulant regimens on the release of von Willebrand factor in this setting. Namely, there was a significant rise in von Willebrand factor levels over the initial 48 hours in those who were treated with either unfractionated heparin or dalteparin, which was not seen in those treated with either PEG-hirudin or enoxaparin.

In another study of 141 patients with unstable angina or NSTEMI, Montalescot and colleagues aimed to identify markers of blood cell activation that were independent predictors of outcomes at one month and sought to compare the effects of enoxaparin, dalteparin, and unfractionated heparin on these markers (30). Patients were randomized to treatment for 48 to 120 hours with either enoxaparin, dalteparin, or unfractionated heparin. Blood samples were drawn at baseline (pre-randomization) and after 48 hours of treatment. By multivariate analysis, increased plasma levels of von Willebrand factor and decreased platelet levels of GP Ib/IX complexes were independent predictors of adverse outcomes at one month. Importantly, von Willebrand factor release was strongly related to inflammation as measured by CRP. Compared with unfractionated heparin, both enoxaparin and dalteparin reduced the release of von Willebrand factor and CRP in plasma. Enoxaparin had a more favorable effect on GP Ib/IX complexes than either dalteparin or unfractionated heparin. The incidence of the composite clinical efficacy endpoint was lowest with enoxaparin and highest with unfractionated heparin. The authors concluded that von Willebrand factor was linked to inflammation and, like GP Ib/IX, was affected more favorably by the low molecular weight heparins than by unfractionated heparin.

In contrast to the studies by Montalescot and colleagues, two other groups reported negative results with respect to the effects of the low molecular weight heparins on inflammatory markers. Hodl and colleagues prospectively randomized 61 consecutive patients with unstable angina or NSTEMI to either subcutaneous dalteparin or enoxaparin every 12 hours for 60 hours (31). Levels of von Willebrand factor exhibited a nonsignificant increase after 4 and 66 hours, but there were no significant differences between the two treatment groups at any time of blood sampling. In perhaps the largest study to date, Oldgren and colleagues performed an analysis on the effects of prolonged dalteparin therapy in a subgroup of patients who had participated in the FRISC II study, which was a large, randomized, double blind multicenter trial designed to determine the efficacy of long-term dalteparin administration in patients with unstable coronary artery disease (32). Patients were treated with subcutaneous dalteparin twice daily for five to seven days and randomized to placebo or gender and weight-adjusted doses of dalteparin twice daily for three months. In this particular analysis, serial blood samples were obtained from 555 of 2267 unstable coronary artery disease patients in the FRISC II study. There was no beneficial effect of prolonged dalteparin treatment with respect to acute-phase proteins, with persistently elevated levels of von Willebrand factor found throughout the course of treatment. Although von Willebrand factor levels decreased with time during prolonged dalteparin treatment, they were still significantly higher than in the placebo group at six months. In addition, and in contrast to other studies, IL-6, CRP, and fibrinogen levels were also unaffected by dalteparin treatment.

In summary, the data with respect to the low molecular weight heparins are limited and conflicting in nature. While one group of investigators has consistently reported a beneficial effect of these agents on inflammatory markers, two other groups have found negative results.

BIVALIRUDIN

Because of the well-characterized pro-inflammatory actions of thrombin (60), it has been logical to assume that thrombin inhibition (whether direct or indirect) would have salutary effects on inflammation. There have been only a limited number of studies looking at the effects of bivalirudin on inflammation in general and on inflammatory markers in particular. Most of these have used unfractionated heparin as the comparator, either alone or in combination with a GP IIb/IIIa inhibitor. Keating and colleagues were among the first to study the effects of bivalirudin in this regard. In one of their earlier studies, they compared the effects of bivalirudin with those of unfractionated heparin plus eptifibatide on inflammatory markers in patients treated with aspirin and clopidogrel undergoing elective PCI (33). They found that the early effects on inflammation were similar with both treatment strategies. However, treatment with bivalirudin was associated with a significantly lower concentration of CRP in blood 30 days after PCI compared with adjuvant treatment with unfractionated heparin plus eptifibatide. The authors speculated as to whether this greater attenuation of inflammation seen with bivalirudin may have contributed to the trend toward a lower mortality one year after PCI, associated with bivalirudin in the REPLACE-2 study (61). In another study, the same group of investigators again randomized patients undergoing PCI to either unfractionated heparin plus eptifibatide or bivalirudin. They measured platelet-monocyte aggregates and platelet-neutrophil aggregates with the use of flow cytometry, as well as elaboration of myeloperoxidase by ELISA (34). Compared with those treated with bivalirudin, patients treated with unfractionated heparin plus eptifibatide exhibited a twofold increase in platelet surface expression of P-selectin in pre-procedural samples. Furthermore, platelet-leukocyte aggregation in vivo was greater with unfractionated heparin plus eptifibatide as was the concentration in blood of myeloperoxidase. In contrast, patients treated with unfractionated heparin plus eptifibatide exhibited a 45% decrease in the capacity of platelets to bind fibrinogen compared with those treated with bivalirudin.

Other investigators have also reported beneficial effects of bivalirudin on inflammation. In one small study, Anand and colleagues found that bivalirudin, either alone or in combination with clopidogrel, significantly reduced plasma sCD40L in PCI patients; this effect was not seen in patients treated with unfractionated heparin alone (35). Li and colleagues studied the effects of unfractionated heparin and GP IIb/IIIa antagonists versus bivalirudin on myeloperoxidase release from neutrophils (36). Patients undergoing nonurgent PCI of a native coronary artery were randomized to receive adjunctive therapy with bivalirudin or unfractionated heparin plus eptifibatide. The use of unfractionated heparin plus eptifibatide was associated with a rapid rise in plasma myeloperoxidase levels immediately after percutaneous coronary revascularization that was attributed to a direct effect of heparin on neutrophils. This effect was not seen with the use of bivalirudin. Furthermore, in an in vitro assay, heparin, but not bivalirudin or eptifibatide, stimulated myeloperoxidase release from neutrophils and neutrophil activation. Since myeloperoxidase is generally viewed as a mediator of cardiovascular disease and as a marker of increased risk, these findings would suggest that adjuvant therapy in the form of unfractionated heparin during PCI may be associated with pro-inflammatory effects. Such effects do not seem to occur with bivalirudin. In another experimental study using a model of normothermic cardiopulmonary bypass in rats, Welsby and colleagues found that bivalirudin was superior to heparin alone in attenuating the inflammatory response (as judged by the levels of TNF-α, IL-1β, IL-6, and IL-10) (62).

In contrast to these positive studies, one recent study found no differential effect of bivalirudin on inflammatory biomarkers. In this study of moderate- to high-risk patients with acute coronary syndrome undergoing PCI randomly assigned to one of three different treatment strategies (eptifibatide plus reduced dose unfractionated heparin, eptifibatide plus reduced dose enoxaparin, or bivalirudin monotherapy), the peak increase from baseline in biomarkers (CRP, sCD40 ligand, RANTES, and IL-6) did not differ between treatment strategies (37).

In summary, most of the available literature with regard to the effects of bivalirudin on circulating inflammatory markers suggest that treatment with bivalirudin is associated with a significant reduction in a variety of such markers. Because bivalirudin is currently FDA-approved only for use during PCI, these studies have all been done in the select population of patients undergoing coronary intervention, and it is unclear if bivalirudin would have similar effects in other populations. Finally, whether the apparent superiority of bivalirudin over other antithrombotic agents seen in recent clinical trials is related to the anti-inflammatory actions of bivalirudin is unknown.

THROMBOLYTIC AGENTS

The effects of thrombolytic agents on systemic inflammation and circulating markers have been extensively studied. The relation between thrombolytic therapy and inflammation is complex, with thrombolysis having effects on inflammation and inflammation itself predicting (or perhaps even influencing) the efficacy of thrombolysis. Accordingly, both the baseline level of inflammation pre-thrombolytic therapy as well as the nature of the inflammatory response to thrombolytic therapy (magnitude and direction) have been suggested as appropriate gauges for predicting the success of such therapy.

Thrombolytic agents dissolve clot by stimulating the plasmin system. However, they also have the undesirable effects of activating the complement and kinin systems, and increasing thrombin generation (along with accompanying pro-inflammatory effects) (38,63,64). Merlini and colleagues have shown that thrombolytic therapy leads to the activation of factor XII, which was associated with the induction of an early proinflammatory state (38). Specifically, they demonstrated that thrombolytic therapy resulted in an early increase in cleaved kininogen levels, thrombin generation, and IL-6 levels. Because the early (i.e., 90 minutes) rise in IL-6 levels that occurred in patients treated with thrombolysis did not occur in those treated with heparin alone, the authors concluded that the rise in IL-6 levels was not related to tissue damage known to occur starting 14 hours after an MI.

There have been numerous clinical studies demonstrating that an elevated baseline level of inflammation pre-thrombolytic therapy is associated with subsequent thrombolytic failure. These studies are summarized in Table 2. Barron and colleagues showed that a heightened inflammatory state (as reflected by an elevation of WBC count pre-thrombolytic therapy) was associated with resistance to thrombolytic therapy as well as increased thrombus burden and impaired microvascular perfusion in patients treated for acute MI (65). Zairis and colleagues prospectively studied 318 consecutive patients who received intravenous thrombolysis because of ST-segment elevation acute MI and classified them according to tertiles of plasma CRP levels on admission (66). They found that patients at the top tertile had a significantly lower incidence of complete ST-segment

Table 2 Summary of Clinical Studies Investigating the Association Between the Baseline Inflammatory State and the Efficacy of Subsequent Thrombolytic Therapy

Study	Drug dose and duration	Population	Design	Main findings
Barron et al. (65)	Thrombolytic therapy with either tenecteplase or front-loaded rt-PA	975 patients with STEMI	Substudy of the TIMI 10A and 10B trials, retrospective analysis	Elevation in baseline WBC count was associated with reduced epicardial blood flow and myocardial perfusion, thromboresistance (arteries open later and have a greater thrombus burden), and a higher incidence of new congestive heart failure and death.
Zairis et al. (66)	Thrombolytic therapy (either streptokinase or t-PA) + UFH for 48 hr	318 consecutive patients who received IV thrombolysis because of STEMI	Prospective, observational	Patients in the top tertile of CRP values on admission had greater reperfusion failure and mortality.
Amasyali et al. (67)	Thrombolytic therapy with streptokinase + UFH for 24 hr	45 consecutive patients with first STEMI who underwent streptokinase therapy and subsequent coronary angiography	Prospective, observational	Higher CRP levels on admission were associated with lower TIMI flow grades and higher residual stenosis of the infarct-related artery after lysis.
Dibra et al. (68)	(i) Stenting plus abciximab or (ii) Thrombolysis alone (full-dose alteplase) or (iii) Thrombolysis (half-dose alteplase) plus abciximab	250 patients presenting with acute myocardial infarction treated with 3 different reperfusion strategies as part of trial	Substudy of STOP-AMI 1 and 2 trials	A high CRP on admission was associated with a significantly lower salvage index among patients treated with thrombolysis alone.
Foussas et al. (69)	Thrombolytic therapy with either streptokinase, alteplase, reteplase, or tenecteplase	786 patients with ST-segment elevation MI who received intravenous thrombolysis within 6 hr of index pain	Prospective, observational study	High circulating levels of both cTnI and CRP were related to an independent increased risk of thrombolytic failure and 30-day cardiac mortality.

Study	Intervention	Population	Study type	Findings
Murphy et al. (70)	Thrombolytic therapy with either streptokinase or accelerated t-PA	29 patients presenting with first STEMI	Prospective, observational study	Elevated levels of sVCAM-1 (endothelial activation) at presentation were associated with thrombolytic failure (as judged by vessel patency on day 5 post MI).
Bennermo et al. (71)	Thrombolytic therapy with either streptokinase or front-loaded alteplase	208 patients with STEMI	Prospective, observational study	Increased plasma concentrations of IL-6 at admission and at 48 hr after admission were associated with worse prognosis.
Mega et al. (72)	Thrombolytic therapy with full-dose tenecteplase or half-dose tenecteplase plus abciximab, with either UFH or enoxaparin	438 patients presenting within 6 hr of STEMI	Substudy of the ENTIRE-TIMI-23 study	An elevated BNP level before fibrinolysis was associated with a lower likelihood of successful epicardial and myocardial perfusion.
Cruden et al. (73)	Thrombolytic therapy with either SK or rt-PA in standard doses	110 patients with acute STEMI treated with thrombolytic therapy	Prospective, observational study	Plasma TAFI, CD40L, PAI-1, t-PA, CRP did not predict perfusion following thrombolysis.

resolution or thrombolysis in myocardial infarction (TIMI)-3 flow in the infarct-related artery, greater in-hospital mortality, and greater three-year cardiac mortality. They concluded that plasma levels of CRP on admission may be a predictor of reperfusion failure and of short- and long-term prognosis in patients with ST-segment elevation acute MI. These data would suggest a possible role of inflammation in the pathophysiologic mechanisms underlying response to thrombolysis. In another study with consistent findings, Amasyali and colleagues investigated the influence of CRP levels before thrombolytic therapy on infarct-related artery patency and the degree of residual stenosis in 45 consecutive patients with a first attack of acute MI, who underwent streptokinase therapy and subsequent coronary angiography (67). They found that high serum CRP levels on admission in patients within six hours after the start of acute ST-segment elevation MI were associated with lower TIMI flow grades and higher residual stenosis of the infarct-related artery after intravenous streptokinase. More recently, Dibra and colleagues evaluated whether CRP levels on admission were predictive of myocardial salvage (using technetium sestamibi scintigraphy) achieved with different reperfusion strategies (including thrombolytics) in patients with acute MI (68). They found that while basal CRP was not related to myocardial salvage in patients treated with stenting plus abciximab or thrombolysis plus abciximab, a high CRP on admission was associated with a significantly lower salvage index among patients treated with thrombolysis alone. Thus, they concluded that CRP levels on admission could potentially predict the efficacy of reperfusion in patients with acute MI treated with thrombolysis alone. Most recently, Foussas and colleagues confirmed and expanded the previous observations regarding the significance of elevated baseline CRP levels in predicting the efficacy of thrombolytic therapy in one of the largest studies of its kind to date (69). Using the method of ST-segment monitoring by continuous 12-lead ECG, they evaluated the significance of simultaneously assessed cTnI and high-sensitivity CRP in the prediction of intravenous thrombolysis outcome in 786 consecutive patients with ST-segment elevation myocardial infarction (STEMI). They found that high circulating levels of both cTnI and high-sensitivity CRP were related with an independent increased risk of intravenous thrombolysis failure and 30-day cardiac death in patients who received intravenous thrombolysis in the first six hours of STEMI.

There are data for biomarkers other than CRP for predicting response to thrombolytic therapy. Murphy and colleagues measured levels of soluble adhesion molecules, CRP, and MCP-1 prior to thrombolysis in patients presenting with their first acute MI (70). An angiogram on day 5 after admission was performed to establish patency of the index vessel. They found elevated levels of the adhesion molecule sVCAM-1 at presentation in patients with acute MI who did not respond to thrombolysis. They suggested that endothelial activation (as reflected by high sVCAM-1 levels) may be important in thrombolysis resistance. Bennermo and colleagues investigated the prognostic value of plasma IL-6 concentrations and promoter polymorphisms of the IL-6 gene in 208 patients with acute MI treated with thrombolysis, who were followed for two to five years (71). Patients who died of cardiovascular causes or suffered a new MI during follow-up had increased plasma concentrations of IL-6 at admission and at 48 hours after admission compared with patients who had an uneventful course. IL-6 levels above the median at admission were independently associated with a worse prognosis. No associations were found between IL-6 levels and the promoter polymorphisms. In a substudy of the ENTIRE-TIMI-23 study, Mega and colleagues obtained samples from 438 patients presenting within six hours of STEMI (72). After adjusting for a variety of clinically significant covariates (including CRP and cTnI), a BNP level greater than 80 pg/mL was associated with a sevenfold higher mortality risk at 30 days. Furthermore, and most germane to the present discussion, patients with BNP greater than 80 pg/mL were also more likely to have impaired coronary flow and incomplete resolution of ST-segment elevation. Thus, an elevated BNP level before fibrinolysis was associated with a lower likelihood of successful epicardial and myocardial reperfusion. In contrast to the studies discussed above, one recent study found that inflammatory markers were not useful in predicting thrombolytic efficacy. In this study by Cruden and colleagues, the authors investigated whether admission plasma concentrations of novel fibrinolytic and vascular inflammatory factors, thrombin-activatable fibrinolysis factor (TAFI) and sCD40L, predicted reperfusion following thrombolytic therapy in 110 patients with acute MI (73). Other markers studied included t-PA, PAI-1, and CRP. The investigators found that none of these biomarkers predicted reperfusion in patients receiving thrombolytic therapy for STEMI. Although plasma CRP concentrations appeared to be lower in patients who reperfused, this was not statistically significant.

In addition to the baseline pretreatment inflammatory state, the inflammatory *response* to thrombolytic therapy has also been suggested as a gauge for its efficacy. In one of the earliest studies in this regard, Pietila and colleagues proposed that in patients treated with streptokinase CRP concentrations may be used to assess the success of thrombolysis (39). To this end, they found that in patients with successful reperfusion the CRP response was only approximately 20% of that in patients in whom reperfusion failed or who received no thrombolytic treatment and who were matched by infarct size. In another early report, Andreotti and colleagues investigated the effects of early recanalization on the plasma levels of two procoagulant acute-phase proteins, the fast acting plasminogen activator inhibitor and von Willebrand factor, in 24 patients with MI receiving rt-PA within six hours of the onset of symptoms (40). The levels of these markers, along with CRP, were measured before rt-PA infusion, daily for the first three days and after 90 days. Coronary angiography was performed before and 90 minutes after the start of rt-PA infusion. In the 16 patients with a patent infarct-related artery at 90 minutes, peak CRP levels were reduced significantly by more than twofold compared with values in the eight patients with an occluded artery at 90 minutes. The patients with early recanalization also had lower plasminogen activator–inhibitor activity on day 2 and day 3 and lower 0 to 72 hour averaged von Willebrand factor. The authors therefore concluded that early coronary recanalization curtails the response of plasminogen activator inhibitor activity and von Willebrand factor to MI, most likely by reducing the extent of ischemia and necrosis and the consequent acute-phase reaction. In a similar subsequent study, the same investigators assessed plasma von Willebrand factor, plasminogen activator inhibitor activity, and CRP as markers of coronary recanalization in 30 patients with acute MI receiving rt-PA (41). Blood samples were taken before rt-PA (time 0), four hourly for 24 hours and daily up to 72 hours. Coronary arteriography was performed 90 minutes and 24 hours after the start of rt-PA. Patients with a patent infarct artery ($n = 17$), compared with those with occluded artery ($n = 13$), showed a fall in von Willebrand factor from 0 to 24 hours, a greater fall in plasminogen activator inhibitor from 24 to 48 hours, and a fall in CRP from 48 to 72 hours. All these reductions achieved statistical significance. Thus, changes in plasma von Willebrand factor, plasminogen activator inhibitor, and CRP during the first three days of MI were shown to be indicative of thrombolytic efficacy. One possible interpretation of these two studies by Andreotti and colleagues is that the response of the various biomarkers to lytic therapy may be related more to the status of the infarct-related artery and the extent of subsequent myonecrosis than to the effects of these agents on biomarkers per se. More recently, Tsakiris and colleagues studied 36 patients with STEMI (28 of whom received thrombolytic therapy) and measured concentrations of CRP in all patients on admission,

24 and 48 hours later (42). They found that patients who received thrombolysis had statistically significant lower CRP values on admission, at 24 hours and 48 hours, compared with those who did not receive such therapy. They concluded that thrombolytic therapy in patients with STEMI is associated with a less pronounced response of CRP during the first 48 hours. Audebert and colleagues from Germany found similar findings in patients with stroke treated with thrombolytic therapy (43). These investigators examined whether successful thrombolysis resulted in a reduction in poststroke inflammation. They studied a variety of inflammatory parameters (body temperature, CRP, and WBC) in 346 stroke patients (43 of whom received thrombolytic therapy) and found that successful thrombolysis was related to a significantly attenuated inflammatory response as reflected in a reduction in each of these parameters.

In perhaps the only comparative study of its kind, Pietila and colleagues investigated the infarct-related acute-phase reaction after treatment with accelerated alteplase, streptokinase, or a combination of both in a substudy of the GUSTO I trial (44). Blood samples were available from 146 patients, 48 of whom had been treated with alteplase, 66 with streptokinase, and 32 with the combination of streptokinase and alteplase. Blood samples for the study were drawn at the start of thrombolytic treatment and at numerous time points thereafter (up to 96 hours). They were analyzed for CRP and hydroxybutyrate dehydrogenase. The authors found that thrombolytic treatment of acute MI with accelerated alteplase was associated with a smaller acute-phase reaction (as reflected by lower peak serum CRP values) than treatment with either streptokinase or a combination of streptokinase and alteplase. The low-peak serum CRP values were associated with complete reperfusion of the infarct-related coronary artery. Thus, they concluded that the more efficient reperfusion with alteplase compared with the other regimens may reduce the inflammatory reaction of acute MI.

Thus, the data with respect to thrombolytic therapy and biomarkers are consistent in demonstrating that the efficacy of lysis seems to be diminished in patients with a heightened inflammatory state pretreatment. Furthermore, an attenuated acute-phase reaction following treatment appears to be associated with successful therapy. Whether thrombolytic therapy has effects on biomarkers independent of its effects on myonecrosis (with the associated inflammatory state) has not been firmly established.

CONCLUSION

As reviewed in this chapter, many of the commercially available antiplatelet, antithrombotic, and thrombolytic agents have effects on inflammation and circulating inflammatory biomarkers. However, there are substantial differences between the various agents in the extent to which they inhibit inflammation. The data for an inhibitory effect are strongest for clopidogrel and bivalirudin, although there are only limited data for bivalirudin. In the case of some agents, the potentially beneficial anti-inflammatory effects appear to be congruent with their established clinical superiority (e.g., bivalirudin vs. unfractionated heparin). Importantly, there have been no studies to date that have linked the favorable inflammatory profile associated with the use of a particular agent to superior clinical outcomes. Clearly, such a mechanistic study would require a large number of patients with the ability to control for numerous covariates known to affect clinical outcomes. Similarly, clinical studies using the inflammatory response to guide the type and duration of therapy have also not been performed. While it may indeed seem logical to assume that a beneficial effect on the inflammatory state would translate into improved clinical outcomes, the limited number of studies performed to date that have specifically targeted inflammation per se have not supported this assumption. For example, in a recent prospective phase 3 study examining the conjunctive use of intravenous pexelizumab (a humanized monoclonal antibody that binds the C5 component of complement) in patients undergoing primary PCI for STEMI, there was no benefit seen with the use of this agent (74). This was despite the fact that pexelizumab was convincingly demonstrated in an earlier study to have potent anti-inflammatory effects, significantly reducing CRP and IL-6 levels in patients undergoing PCI (75). Similarly, two clinical trials found no incremental benefit with the use of an intravenous monoclonal antibody to the components of the CD11/CD18 integrin receptor when added to a standard regimen of thrombolytic therapy in patients with acute MI (76,77). Inhibition of leukocyte adhesion with antibodies to this family of adhesion molecules had been demonstrated in earlier animal models to result in a reduction in ischemia-reperfusion injury related to inflammation in the setting of acute MI (76). Thus, it is not entirely clear whether inflammation itself represents an appropriate target or gauge of the effectiveness of any therapy.

Assuming that inflammation is an appropriate target for these drugs, an important question is: which circulating biomarker should serve as the ideal gauge for monitoring the inflammatory response to these drugs? The majority of the studies discussed in this chapter have used CRP as the surrogate marker. CRP is probably the most validated of all the biomarkers for general prognostic purposes, and it has been claimed to have the profile of the ideal analyte (78). An additional appeal for CRP as the biomarker of choice for monitoring pharmacologic intervention has to do with the fact that there are data to suggest that CRP itself may be involved in the pathogenesis of cardiovascular disease (79–82), although this notion remains controversial (83,84). Finally, there is precedent for using CRP to monitor the efficacy of therapy with an entirely different class of pharmacologic agents, the statins. Statins have not only been shown to reduce CRP, but the reduction associated with their use has been shown to decrease the risk of cardiovascular events (85,86). However, to date, there are no firm data that lowering CRP levels per se will lower vascular risk (87). In addition, there are a large number of emerging candidate biomarkers that have also been shown to predict adverse outcomes in patients with known or suspected coronary artery disease (88–95). It is conceivable that another biomarker may be more selectively affected by a particular antiplatelet or antithrombotic drug, and therefore, serve as a more appropriate gauge for the efficacy of a particular therapy.

In conclusion, antiplatelet, antithrombotic, and thrombolytic agents have well documented inhibitory effects on inflammation and inflammatory biomarkers to varying degrees. To date, the clinical significance of these effects remains unknown. Larger studies designed to target therapy as a function of an anti-inflammatory endpoint are needed to better understand the implications of these anti-inflammatory effects.

REFERENCES

1. Feng D, Tracy RP, Lipinska I, et al. Effect of short-term aspirin use on C-reactive protein. J Thromb Thrombolysis 2000; 9:37–41.
2. Feldman M, Jialal I, Devaraj S, et al. Effects of low-dose aspirin on serum C-reactive protein and thromboxane B2 concentrations: a placebo-controlled study using a highly sensitive C-reactive protein assay. J Am Coll Cardiol 2001; 37:2036–2041.
3. Azar RR, Klayme S, Germanos M, et al. Effects of aspirin (325 mg/day) on serum high-sensitivity C-reactive protein, cytokines, and adhesion molecules in healthy volunteers. Am J Cardiol 2003; 92:236–239.

4. Ikonomidis I, Andreotti F, Economou E, et al. Increased proinflammatory cytokines in patients with chronic stable angina and their reduction by aspirin. Circulation 1999; 100:793–798.
5. Solheim S, Arnesen H, Eikvar L, et al. Influence of aspirin on inflammatory markers in patients after acute myocardial infarction. Am J Cardiol 2003; 92:843–845.
6. Takeda T, Hoshida S, Nishino M, et al. Relationship between effects of statins, aspirin and angiotensin II modulators on high-sensitive C-reactive protein levels. Atherosclerosis 2003; 169: 155–158.
7. Woodward M, Lowe GD, Francis LM, et al. A randomized comparison of the effects of aspirin and clopidogrel on thrombotic risk factors and C-reactive protein following myocardial infarction: the CADET trial. J Thromb Haemost 2004; 2:1934–1940.
8. Monakier D, Mates M, Klutstein MW, et al. Rofecoxib, a COX-2 inhibitor, lowers C-reactive protein and interleukin-6 levels in patients with acute coronary syndromes. Chest 2004; 125:1610–1615.
9. Rogowski O, Shapira I, Ben Assayag E, et al. Lack of significant effect of low doses of aspirin on the concentrations of C-reactive protein in a group of individuals with atherothrombotic risk factors and vascular events. Blood Coagul Fibrinolysis 2006;17:19–22.
10. Dunzendorfer S, Reinisch CM, Kaneider NC, et al. Inhibition of plasma-dependent monocyte chemokinesis and cytokine-triggered endothelial activation for neutrophil transmigration by administration of clopidogrel in man. Acta Med Austriaca 2002; 29:100–106.
11. Hermann A, Rauch BH, Braun M, et al. Platelet CD40 ligand (CD40L)–subcellular localization, regulation of expression, and inhibition by clopidogrel. Platelets 2001; 12:74–82.
12. Nannizzi-Alaimo L, Alves VL, Phillips DR. Inhibitory effects of glycoprotein IIb/IIIa antagonists and aspirin on the release of soluble CD40 ligand during platelet stimulation. Circulation 2003; 107:1123–1128.
13. Klinkhardt U, Graff J, Harder S. Clopidogrel, but not abciximab, reduces platelet leukocyte conjugates and P-selectin expression in a human ex vivo in vitro model. Clin Pharmacol Ther 2002; 71:176–185.
14. Vivekananthan DP, Bhatt DL, Chew DP, et al. Effect of clopidogrel pretreatment on periprocedural rise in C-reactive protein after percutaneous coronary intervention. Am J Cardiol 2004; 94:358–360.
15. Quinn MJ, Bhatt DL, Zidar F, et al. Effect of clopidogrel pretreatment on inflammatory marker expression in patients undergoing percutaneous coronary intervention. Am J Cardiol 2004; 93:679–684.
16. Xiao Z, Theroux P. Clopidogrel inhibits platelet-leukocyte interactions and thrombin receptor agonist peptide-induced platelet activation in patients with an acute coronary syndrome. J Am Coll Cardiol 2004; 43:1982–1988.
17. Cha JK, Jeong MH, Lee KM, et al. Changes in platelet P-selectin and in plasma C-reactive protein in acute atherosclerotic ischemic stroke treated with a loading dose of clopidogrel. J Thromb Thrombolysis 2002; 14:145–150.
18. Klinkhardt U, Bauersachs R, Adams J, et al. Clopidogrel but not aspirin reduces P-selectin expression and formation of platelet-leukocyte aggregates in patients with atherosclerotic vascular disease. Clin Pharmacol Ther 2003; 73:232–241.
19. Harding SA, Sarma J, Din JN, et al. Clopidogrel reduces platelet-leucocyte aggregation, monocyte activation and RANTES secretion in type 2 diabetes mellitus. Heart 2006; 92:1335–1337.
20. Lincoff AM, Kereiakes DJ, Mascelli MA, et al. Abciximab suppresses the rise in levels of circulating inflammatory markers after percutaneous coronary revascularization. Circulation 2001; 104:163–167.
21. James SK, Siegbahn A, Armstrong P, et al. Activation of the inflammation, coagulation, and fibrinolysis systems, without influence of abciximab infusion in patients with non-ST-elevation acute coronary syndromes treated with dalteparin: a GUSTO IV substudy. Am Heart J 2004; 147: 267–274.
22. Gurbel PA, Bliden KP, Tantry US. Effect of clopidogrel with and without eptifibatide on tumor necrosis factor-alpha and C-reactive protein release after elective stenting: results from the CLEAR PLATELETS 1b study. J Am Coll Cardiol 2006; 48:2186–2191.

23. Welt FG, Rogers SD, Zhang X, et al. GP IIb/IIIa inhibition with eptifibatide lowers levels of soluble CD40L and RANTES after percutaneous coronary intervention. Catheter Cardiovasc Interv 2004; 61:185–189.
24. Aggarwal A, Schneider DJ, Terrien EF, et al. Comparison of effects of abciximab versus eptifibatide on C-reactive protein, interleukin-6, and interleukin-1 receptor antagonist after coronary arterial stenting. Am J Cardiol 2003; 91:1346–1349.
25. Furman MI, Krueger LA, Linden MD, et al. GPIIb-IIIa antagonists reduce thromboinflammatory processes in patients with acute coronary syndromes undergoing percutaneous coronary intervention. J Thromb Haemost 2005; 3:312–320.
26. Ercan E, Tengiz I, Duman C, et al. Effect of tirofiban on C-reactive protein in non-ST-elevation myocardial infarction. Am Heart J 2004; 147:E1.
27. Akbulut M, Ozbay Y, Gundogdu O, et al. Effects of tirofiban on acute systemic inflammatory response in elective percutaneous coronary interventions. Curr Med Res Opin 2004; 20:1759–1767.
28. Montalescot G, Philippe F, Ankri A, et al. Early increase of von Willebrand factor predicts adverse outcome in unstable coronary artery disease: beneficial effects of enoxaparin. French Investigators of the ESSENCE Trial. Circulation 1998; 98:294–299.
29. Montalescot G, Collet JP, Lison L, et al. Effects of various anticoagulant treatments on von Willebrand factor release in unstable angina. J Am Coll Cardiol 2000; 36:110–114.
30. Montalescot G, Bal-dit-Sollier C, Chibedi D, et al. Comparison of effects on markers of blood cell activation of enoxaparin, dalteparin, and unfractionated heparin in patients with unstable angina pectoris or non-ST-segment elevation acute myocardial infarction (the ARMADA study). Am J Cardiol 2003; 91:925–930.
31. Hodl R, Huber K, Kraxner W, et al. Comparison of effects of dalteparin and enoxaparin on hemostatic parameters and von Willebrand factor in patients with unstable angina pectoris or non–ST- segment elevation acute myocardial infarction. Am J Cardiol 2002; 89:589–592.
32. Oldgren J, Fellenius C, Boman K, et al. Influence of prolonged dalteparin treatment on coagulation, fibrinolysis and inflammation in unstable coronary artery disease. J Intern Med 2005; 258:420–427.
33. Keating FK, Dauerman HL, Whitaker DA, et al. The effects of bivalirudin compared with those of unfractionated heparin plus eptifibatide on inflammation and thrombin generation and activity during coronary intervention. Coron Artery Dis 2005; 16:401–415.
34. Keating FK, Dauerman HL, Whitaker DA, et al. Increased expression of platelet P-selectin and formation of platelet-leukocyte aggregates in blood from patients treated with unfractionated heparin plus eptifibatide compared with bivalirudin. Thromb Res 2006; 118:361–369.
35. Anand SX, Kim MC, Kamran M, et al. Comparison of platelet function and morphology in patients undergoing percutaneous coronary intervention receiving bivalirudin versus unfractionated heparin versus clopidogrel pretreatment and bivalirudin. Am J Cardiol 2007; 100:417–424.
36. Li G, Keenan AC, Young JC, et al. Effects of unfractionated heparin and glycoprotein IIb/IIIa antagonists versus bivalirdin on myeloperoxidase release from neutrophils. Arterioscler Thromb Vasc Biol 2007; 27:1850–1856.
37. Gibson CM, Morrow DA, Murphy SA, et al. A randomized trial to evaluate the relative protection against post-percutaneous coronary intervention microvascular dysfunction, ischemia, and inflammation among antiplatelet and antithrombotic agents: the PROTECT-TIMI-30 trial. J Am Coll Cardiol 2006; 47:2364–2373.
38. Merlini PA, Cugno M, Rossi ML, et al. Activation of the contact system and inflammation after thrombolytic therapy in patients with acute myocardial infarction. Am J Cardiol 2004; 93:822–825.
39. Pietila K, Harmoinen A, Poyhonen L, et al. Intravenous streptokinase treatment and serum C-reactive protein in patients with acute myocardial infarction. Br Heart J 1987; 58:225–229.
40. Andreotti F, Roncaglioni MC, et al. Early coronary reperfusion blunts the procoagulant response of plasminogen activator inhibitor-1 and von Willebrand factor in acute myocardial infarction. J Am Coll Cardiol 1990: 16:1553–1560.

41. Andreotti F, Hackett DR, Haider AW, et al. Von Willebrand factor, plasminogen activator inhibitor-1 and C-reactive protein are markers of thrombolytic efficacy in acute myocardial infarction. Thromb Haemost 1992; 68:678–682.
42. Tsakiris AK, Marnelos PG, Nearchou NS, et al. The influence of thrombolytic therapy on C-reactive protein in ST-segment elevation acute myocardial infarction. Hellenic J Cardiol 2006; 47:218–222.
43. Audebert HJ, Rott MM, Eck T, et al. Systemic inflammatory response depends on initial stroke severity but is attenuated by successful thrombolysis. Stroke 2004; 35:2128–2133.
44. Pietila K, Hermens WT, Harmoinen A, et al. Comparison of peak serum C-reactive protein and hydroxybutyrate dehydrogenase levels in patients with acute myocardial infarction treated with alteplase and streptokinase. Am J Cardiol 1997; 80:1075–1077.
45. Kopp E, Ghosh S. Inhibition of NF-kappa B by sodium salicylate and aspirin. Science 1994; 265:956–959.
46. Weyrich AS, McIntyre TM, McEver RP, et al. Monocyte tethering by P-selectin regulates monocyte chemotactic protein-1 and tumor necrosis factor-alpha secretion. Signal integration and NF-kappa B translocation. J Clin Invest 1995; 95:2297–2303.
47. Martin T, Cardarelli PM, Parry GC, et al. Cytokine induction of monocyte chemoattractant protein-1 gene expression in human endothelial cells depends on the cooperative action of NF-kappa B and AP-1. Eur J Immunol 1997; 27:1091–1097.
48. Steinhubl SR, Badimon JJ, Bhatt DL, et al. Clinical evidence for anti-inflammatory effects of antiplatelet therapy in patients with atherothrombotic disease. Vasc Med 2007; 12:113–122.
49. Cyrus T, Sung S, Zhao L, et al. Effect of low-dose aspirin on vascular inflammation, plaque stability, and atherogenesis in low-density lipoprotein receptor-deficient mice. Circulation 2002; 106:1282–1287.
50. Muller DN, Heissmeyer V, Dechend R, et al. Aspirin inhibits NF-kappaB and protects from angiotensin II-induced organ damage. FASEB J 2001; 15:1822–1824.
51. Prichard PJ, Poniatowska TJ, Willars JE, et al. Effect in man of aspirin, standard indomethacin, and sustained release indomethacin preparations on gastric bleeding. Br J Clin Pharmacol 1988; 26:167–172.
52. Savi P, Bernat A, Dumas A, et al. Effect of aspirin and clopidogrel on platelet-dependent tissue factor expression in endothelial cells. Thromb Res 1994; 73:117–124.
53. Herault JP, Dol F, Gaich C, et al. Effect of clopidogrel on thrombin generation in platelet-rich plasma in the rat. Thromb Haemost 1999; 81:957–960.
54. Ayral Y, Rauch U, Goldin-Lang P, et al. Prolonged application of clopidogrel reduces inflammation after percutaneous coronary intervention in the porcine model. Cardiovasc Revasc Med 2007; 8:183–188.
55. Evangelista V, Manarini S, Dell'Elba G, et al. Clopidogrel inhibits platelet-leukocyte adhesion and platelet-dependent leukocyte activation. Thromb Haemost 2005: 94:568–577.
56. Kereiakes DJ. Inflammation as a therapeutic target: a unique role for abciximab. Am Heart J 2003; 146:S1–S4.
57. Versaci F, Gaspardone A, Tomai F, et al. Immunosuppressive therapy for the prevention of restenosis after coronary artery stent implantation (IMPRESS Study). J Am Coll Cardiol 2002; 40:1935–1942.
58. Chew DP, Bhatt DL, Robbins MA, et al. Effect of clopidogrel added to aspirin before percutaneous coronary intervention on the risk associated with C-reactive protein. Am J Cardiol 2001; 88:672–674.
59. A randomised, blinded, trial of clopidogrel versus aspirin in patients at risk of ischaemic events (CAPRIE). CAPRIE Steering Committee. Lancet 1996; 348:1329–1339.
60. Vergnolle N, Hollenberg MD, Wallace JL. Pro- and anti-inflammatory actions of thrombin: a distinct role for proteinase-activated receptor-1 (PAR1). Br J Pharmacol 1999; 126:1262–1268.
61. Lincoff AM, Kleiman NS, Kereiakes DJ, et al. Long-term efficacy of bivalirudin and provisional glycoprotein IIb/IIIa blockade vs heparin and planned glycoprotein IIb/IIIa blockade during percutaneous coronary revascularization: REPLACE-2 randomized trial. JAMA 2004; 292:696–703.

62. Welsby IJ, Jones WL, Arepally G, et al. Effect of combined anticoagulation using heparin and bivalirudin on the hemostatic and inflammatory responses to cardiopulmonary bypass in the rat. Anesthesiology 2007; 106:295–301.

63. Eisenberg PR, Sherman LA, Jaffe AS. Paradoxic elevation of fibrinopeptide A after streptokinase: evidence for continued thrombosis despite intense fibrinolysis. J Am Coll Cardiol 1987; 10: 527–529.

64. Agostoni A, Gardinali M, Frangi D, et al. Activation of complement and kinin systems after thrombolytic therapy in patients with acute myocardial infarction. A comparison between streptokinase and recombinant tissue-type plasminogen activator. Circulation 1994; 90: 2666–2670.

65. Barron HV, Cannon CP, Murphy SA, et al. Association between white blood cell count, epicardial blood flow, myocardial perfusion, and clinical outcomes in the setting of acute myocardial infarction: a thrombolysis in myocardial infarction 10 substudy. Circulation 2000; 102:2329–2334.

66. Zairis MN, Manousakis SJ, Stefanidis AS, et al. C-reactive protein levels on admission are associated with response to thrombolysis and prognosis after ST-segment elevation acute myocardial infarction. Am Heart J 2002; 144:782–789.

67. Amasyali B, Kose S, Kilic A, et al. C-reactive protein on admission and the success of thrombolytic therapy with streptokinase: is there any relation? Int J Cardiol 2003; 92:27–33.

68. Dibra A, Mehilli J, Schwaiger M, et al. Predictive value of basal C-reactive protein levels for myocardial salvage in patients with acute myocardial infarction is dependent on the type of reperfusion treatment. Eur Heart J 2003; 24:1128–1133.

69. Foussas SG, Zairis MN, Makrygiannis SS, et al. The significance of circulating levels of both cardiac troponin I and high-sensitivity C reactive protein for the prediction of intravenous thrombolysis outcome in patients with ST-segment elevation myocardial infarction. Heart 2007; 93:952–956.

70. Murphy RT, Foley JB, Mulvihill N, et al. Endothelial inflammation and thrombolysis resistance in acute myocardial infarction. Int J Cardiol 2002; 83:227–231.

71. Bennermo M, Held C, Green F, et al. Prognostic value of plasma interleukin-6 concentrations and the -174 G > C and -572 G > C promoter polymorphisms of the interleukin-6 gene in patients with acute myocardial infarction treated with thrombolysis. Atherosclerosis 2004; 174:157–163.

72. Mega JL, Morrow DA, De Lemos JA, et al. B-type natriuretic peptide at presentation and prognosis in patients with ST-segment elevation myocardial infarction: an ENTIRE-TIMI-23 substudy. J Am Coll Cardiol 2004; 44:335–339.

73. Cruden NL, Graham C, Harding SA, et al. Plasma TAFI and soluble CD40 ligand do not predict reperfusion following thrombolysis for acute myocardial infarction. Thromb Res 2006; 118: 189–197.

74. APEX AMI Investigators. Pexelizumab for acute ST-segment elevation myocardial infarction in patients undergoing primary percutaneous coronary intervention. JAMA 2007; 297:43–51.

75. Theroux P, Armstrong PW, Mahaffey KW, et al. Prognostic significance of blood markers of inflammation in patients with ST-segment elevation myocardial infarction undergoing primary angioplasty and effects of pexelizumab, a C5 inhibitor: a substudy of the COMMA trial. Eur Heart J 2005; 26:1964–1670.

76. Baran KW, Nguyen M, McKendall GR, et al. Double-blind, randomized trial of an anti-CD18 antibody in conjunction with recombinant tissue plasminogen activator for acute myocardial infarction: limitation of myocardial infarction following thrombolysis in acute myocardial infarction (LIMIT AMI) study. Circulation 2001; 104:2778–2783.

77. Faxon DP, Gibbons RJ, Chronos NA, et al. The effect of blockade of the CD11/CD18 integrin receptor on infarct size in patients with acute myocardial infarction treated with direct angioplasty: the results of the HALT-MI study. J Am Coll Cardiol 2002; 40:1199–1204.

78. Pearson TA, Mensah GA, Alexander RW, et al. Markers of inflammation and cardiovascular disease: application to clinical and public health practice: A statement for healthcare

professionals from the Centers for Disease Control and Prevention and the American Heart Association. Circulation 2003; 107:499–511.

79. Pasceri V, Willerson JT, Yeh ET. Direct proinflammatory effect of C-reactive protein on human endothelial cells. Circulation 2000; 102:2165–2168.

80. Zwaka TP, Hombach V, Torzewski J. C-reactive protein-mediated low density lipoprotein uptake by macrophages: implications for atherosclerosis. Circulation 2001; 103:1194–1197.

81. Venugopal SK, Devaraj S, Yuhanna I, et al. Demonstration that C-reactive protein decreases eNOS expression and bioactivity in human aortic endothelial cells. Circulation 2002; 106: 1439–1441.

82. Devaraj S, Xu DY, Jialal I. C-reactive protein increases plasminogen activator inhibitor-1 expression and activity in human aortic endothelial cells: implications for the metabolic syndrome and atherothrombosis. Circulation 2003; 107:398–404.

83. Hirschfield GM, Gallimore JR, Kahan MC, et al. Transgenic human C-reactive protein is not proatherogenic in apolipoprotein E-deficient mice. Proc Natl Acad Sci USA 2005; 102:8309–8314.

84. Tennent GA, Hutchinson WL, Kahan MC, et al. Transgenic human CRP is not pro-atherogenic, pro-atherothrombotic or pro-inflammatory in apoE−/− mice. Atherosclerosis 2008; 196: 248–255.

85. Ridker PM, Rifai N, Clearfield M, et al. Measurement of C-reactive protein for the targeting of statin therapy in the primary prevention of acute coronary events. N Engl J Med 2001; 344: 1959–1965.

86. Ridker PM, Cannon CP, Morrow D, et al. C-reactive protein levels and outcomes after statin therapy. N Engl J Med 2005; 352: 20–28.

87. Tsimikas S, Willerson JT, Ridker PM. C-reactive protein and other emerging blood biomarkers to optimize risk stratification of vulnerable patients. J Am Coll Cardiol 2006; 47:C19–C31.

88. Vasan RS. Biomarkers of cardiovascular disease: molecular basis and practical considerations. Circulation 2006; 113: 2335–2362.

89. Cavusoglu E, Chhabra S, Jiang XC, et al. Relation of baseline plasma phospholipid levels to cardiovascular outcomes at two years in men with acute coronary syndrome referred for coronary angiography. Am J Cardiol 2007; 100:1739–1743.

90. Cavusoglu E, Eng C, Chopra V, et al. Low plasma RANTES levels are an independent predictor of cardiac mortality in patients referred for coronary angiography. Arterioscler Thromb Vasc Biol 2007; 27:929–935.

91. Cavusoglu E, Eng C, Chopra V, et al. Usefulness of the serum complement component C4 as a predictor of stroke in patients with known or suspected coronary artery disease referred for coronary angiography. Am J Cardiol 2007; 100:164–168.

92. Cavusoglu E, Kornecki E, Sobocka MB, et al. Association of plasma levels of F11 receptor/ junctional adhesion molecule-A (F11R/JAM-A) with human atherosclerosis. J Am Coll Cardiol 2007; 50:1768–1776.

93. Cavusoglu E, Ruwende C, Chopra V, et al. Adiponectin is an independent predictor of all-cause mortality, cardiac mortality, and myocardial infarction in patients presenting with chest pain. Eur Heart J 2006; 27:2300–2309.

94. Cavusoglu E, Ruwende C, Chopra V, et al. Tissue inhibitor of metalloproteinase-1 (TIMP-1) is an independent predictor of all-cause mortality, cardiac mortality, and myocardial infarction. Am Heart J 2006; 151:1101, e1–e8.

95. Cavusoglu E, Ruwende C, Eng C, et al. Usefulness of baseline plasma myeloperoxidase levels as an independent predictor of myocardial infarction at two years in patients presenting with acute coronary syndrome. Am J Cardiol 2007; 99:1364–1368.

7

The Role of Platelet Function Testing in the Development of Platelet Inhibitors

Alan D. Michelson
Center for Platelet Function Studies, Departments of Pediatrics, Medicine, and Pathology, University of Massachusetts Medical School, Worcester, Massachusetts, U.S.A.

INTRODUCTION

This chapter is divided into two sections. First, the advantages and disadvantages of the many available platelet function tests for measuring the effects of platelet inhibitors are discussed. Second, the following four roles of platelet function testing in the development of platelet inhibitors are discussed: (*i*) elucidation of mechanisms of action, (*ii*) determination of optimal dose and frequency of administration, (*iii*) comparison of different platelet inhibitors, and (*iv*) monitoring of "resistance" or hyporesponsiveness to platelet inhibitors.

PLATELET FUNCTION TESTS FOR MONITORING PLATELET INHIBITORS

The mechanisms of action of antiplatelet drugs are well known. Aspirin irreversibly acetylates serine 529 of cyclooxygenase 1 (COX-1), resulting in inhibition of the generation of thromboxane A_2 from platelets (1). Thienopyridines (including ticlopidine and clopidogrel) irreversibly inhibit platelet $P2Y_{12}$ adenosine diphosphate (ADP) receptors (2) and glycoprotein (GP) IIb-IIIa antagonists (including abciximab, integrilin, and tirofiban) inhibit the final common pathway of platelet-to-platelet aggregation (3).

Platelets circulate in a resting discoid form. Platelet activation results in the formation of filopodia and lamellipodia and then in platelet aggregation. The goal of antiplatelet drug therapy is to prevent, or reverse, this process. Tests of platelet function attempt to measure at what point in this activation process are the platelets of an individual patient. The effects of platelet inhibitors on platelet function can be assessed by many different tests, each of which has advantages and disadvantages (Table 1).

Table 1 Methods for the Measurement of Platelet Function in Patients

Test	Basis	Advantages	Disadvantages
Turbidometric aggregometry	Platelet aggregation	Historical gold standard	High sample volume Sample preparation Time consuming
Impedance aggregometry	Platelet aggregation	Whole blood assay	High sample volume Sample preparation Time consuming
VerifyNow®	Platelet aggregation	Simple, rapid Point-of-care (no pipetting required) Low sample volume Whole blood assay	Limited hematocrit and platelet count range
Plateletworks®	Platelet aggregation	Minimal sample prep. Whole blood assay	Not well studied
Platelet surface P-selectin, activated GPIIb-IIIa, leukocyte-platelet aggregates	Activation-dependent changes in platelet surface	Low sample volume Whole blood assays Fixed samples can be mailed to core lab	Sample preparation Requires flow cytometer and experienced technician Not commercially available
TEG® PlateletMapping™ system	Platelet contribution to clot strength	Whole blood assay Clot information	Limited studies Requires pipetting
Impact® cone-and-plate(let) analyzer	Shear induced platelet adhesion	Simple, rapid Point-of-care Low sample volume No sample prep. Whole blood assay Shear	Requires pipetting Instrument not widely used
PFA-100®	In vitro cessation of high shear blood flow by platelet plug	Simple, rapid Point-of-care Low sample volume No sample prep. Whole blood assay Shear	Dependent on VWF & hematocrit Requires pipetting Does not correlate well with clopidogrel therapy
VASP	Activation-dependent signaling	Dependent on clopidogrel target, $P2Y_{12}$ Low sample volume Whole blood assay Blood samples can be mailed at RT to core lab	Sample preparation Requires flow cytometer and experienced technician
Serum thromboxane B_2	Activation-dependent release from platelets	Directly dependent on aspirin target, COX-1	Indirect measure Not platelet-specific
Urinary 11-dehydro thromboxane B_2/ creatinine ratio	Stable urinary metabolite of thromboxane B_2	Directly dependent on aspirin target, COX-1	Indirect measure Not platelet-specific

Abbreviations: COX, cyclooxygenase; GP, glycoprotein; VASP, vasodilator-stimulated phosphoprotein; PFA, platelet function analyzer.
Source: Modified from Ref. 4.

Specific Tests of Platelet Function

Platelet Aggregometry

Turbidometric platelet aggregometry in platelet-rich plasma was originally described by Gustav Born (5) and John O'Brien (6). The end point of this assay is change in light transmission as a result of integrin αIIbβ3 (GPIIb-IIIa)-dependent platelet-to-platelet aggregation in response to an agonist (7). The main advantage of platelet aggregometry is that it is the historical gold standard, although Born and O'Brien designed the test as a measure of defective platelet function, not as a predictor of thrombosis. The disadvantages of platelet aggregometry are that platelet-rich plasma needs to be prepared, and the test is therefore time-consuming and a high sample volume is required.

Impedance Aggregometry

Platelet aggregation can be measured in anticoagulated whole blood by the use of impedance rather than turbidometry (7,8). Impedance is the same method that is used in a Coulter counter. Although impedance aggregometry and turbidometric aggregometry conceptually measure the same thing—integrin αIIbβ3 (GPIIb-IIIa)-dependent platelet-to-platelet aggregation—the size of the platelet aggregates measured by impedance aggregometry is smaller than the platelet aggregates measured by turbidometric aggregometry. The major advantage of impedance aggregometry is that it is more physiologic in that it is a whole blood assay that does not require the separation of platelet-rich plasma. However, impedance aggregometry still requires a fairly high sample volume and the assay is still time consuming and expensive because a technician needs to monitor the agonist-induced aggregation over a number of minutes.

VerifyNow®

VerifyNow® (Accumetrics, San Diego, California, U.S.) formerly known as the Ultegra rapid platelet function analyzer (RPFA) is a point-of-care device that, like turbidometric aggregation and impedance aggregation, is based on integrin αIIbβ3 (GPIIb-IIIa) - dependent platelet aggregation (9). However, platelet aggregation is augmented by the presence of fibrinogen-coated beads. Unlike turbidometric aggregation, but like impedance aggregation, the VerifyNow assay is performed in anticoagulated whole blood. Other advantages of the VerifyNow assay are that it is simple, rapid, and requires only a small sample volume. Furthermore, it is a true point-of-care device in that no pipetting is required. Although the VerifyNow assay has a limited hematocrit and platelet count range, this applies to many tests of platelet function.

Plateletworks®

Plateletworks® (Helena Laboratories, Beaumont, Texas, U.S.) is another device that is based on integrin αIIbβ3 (GPIIb-IIIa)-dependent platelet aggregation (8). It is a conceptually simple method in which the platelet count is compared in samples with and without agonists. Minimal sample preparation is required and it is a whole blood assay. The main disadvantage of Plateletworks is that it is not well studied.

Platelet Surface P-selectin, Activated GPIIb-IIIa, and Leukocyte Platelet Aggregates

Platelet surface P-selectin, activated integrin αIIbβ3 (GPIIb-IIIa), and leukocyte platelet aggregates can be measured by flow cytometry (10). Integrin αIIbβ3 is normally present on the platelet surface, but it is in a resting confirmation. With platelet activation, the confirmation of the integrin αIIbβ3 changes and a specific monoclonal antibody, PAC-1, only binds to integrin αIIbβ3 when it is in this activated confirmation (11). So a PAC-1-negative platelet is a resting platelet and a PAC-1-positive platelet is an activated platelet.

When platelets are activated, they degranulate and P-selectin, which is normally present on the α-granule membrane not the platelet plasma membrane, becomes exteriorized on the platelet surface (12). So a P-selectin-negative platelet is a resting platelet and a P-selectin-positive platelet is an activated platelet. In addition, P-selectin-positive platelets very rapidly bind to leukocytes via their constitutively expressed counter receptor, P-selectin glycoprotein ligand 1 (PSGL-1) (12,13). Therefore, circulating leukocyte-platelet aggregates (especially monocyte-platelet aggregates) are a more sensitive marker of in vivo platelet activation than circulating P-selectin-positive platelets (13).

The advantages of the flow cytometric measurement of platelet function by platelet surface P-selectin, activated integrin αIIbβ3, and/or leukocyte platelet aggregates are that these assays require a very low sample volume and they are whole blood assays. Furthermore, we have standardized these assays such that fixed samples can be mailed to a core laboratory; this is particularly useful in multicenter clinical trials (14). The disadvantages of these assays are that sample preparations are needed, and they require an expensive machine (a flow cytometer) and an experienced technician. These assays are therefore currently mainly research tools.

TEG® PlateletMapping™ System

Although the thromboelastogram was invented more than 50 years ago, it has recently been updated to a more platelet-specific test in the form of the TEG® PlateletMapping™ System (Haemoscope, Niles, Illinois, U.S.) (8). The particular advantage of the TEG PlateletMapping System is that in addition to measuring platelet function, it specifically measures the platelet contribution to clot strength. Although platelet function and coagulation are often considered separately, they are of course completely interrelated processes (15). So it may be advantageous to measure the two processes in the one assay (16). An additional advantage of the TEG PlateletMapping System is that it is a whole blood assay. Its disadvantages are that it is not a true point-of-care instrument in that it requires pipetting and there are a limited number of published studies (16).

Impact® Cone and Plate(let) Analyzer

The Impact® cone and plate(let) analyzer (Diamed, Cressier, Switzerland) was originally developed in Israel by David Varon and Naphtali Savion. The end point of this assay is shear-induced platelet adhesion. This is potentially very advantageous because shear is very important for platelet function (17), particularly in the setting of coronary artery disease (18). Although turbidometric aggregometry and impedance aggregometry are performed in stirred samples, the shear rate in these assays is an order of magnitude below the shear rate that is relevant to coronary artery disease. The research version of the Impact has an adjustable shear rate, and in the clinical version of the Impact, the shear rate is directly relevant to that in coronary artery disease (19). Additional advantages of the Impact are simplicity, rapid readout, low sample volume, no sample preparation, and its being a whole blood assay. The disadvantages of the Impact are that it is not a true point-of-care instrument in that it requires pipetting, and, although there are a number of published studies (19), the instrument is not widely used.

Platelet Function Analyzer -100®

The platelet function analyzer (PFA)-100® also has the advantage of including a physiologically relevant shear rate (20). This device has been referred to as an "in vitro bleeding time"—not an ideal term—but the concept is of an in vitro method to look at cessation of blood flow in a high shear environment, as determined by the closure time of an aperture by the formation of a platelet plug. In addition to shear, the advantages of the PFA-100 (Siemens Healthcare Diagnostics, Newark, Delaware) are its simplicity, rapid readout, low sample volume, no sample preparation and its being a whole blood assay The disadvantages of the PFA-100 are that the closure time is very dependent on von Willebrand factor levels and hematocrit. Although initial pipetting of the blood sample is necessary, one then just inserts the sample into a cassette, presses a button and gets a rapid readout. The PFA-100 has two available cartridges: a collagen-epinephrine cartridge and a collagen-ADP cartridge. The PFA-100 has been widely used to study aspirin response (8,21). Surprisingly however, the PFA-100, even with the collagen-ADP cartridge, is not sensitive to clopidogrel therapy.

Phosphorylation of Vasodilator-Stimulated Phosphoprotein

Phosphorylation of vasodilator-stimulated phosphoprotein (VASP) for the measurement of $P2Y_{12}$ antagonism is available commercially as a flow cytometry kit (BioCytex, Marseilles, France) (10). Prostaglandin E_1 (PGE_1) binds to its IP receptor on the platelet surface and signals through a G stimulatory (G_s) protein and adenylyl cyclase (AC) to convert ATP to cyclic AMP (cAMP), and then through protein kinase A (PKA) to convert VASP to phosphorylated VASP (VASP-P) (Fig. 1). ADP binds to its $P2Y_{12}$ receptor on the platelet surface and signals through a G inhibitory (G_i) protein to inhibit

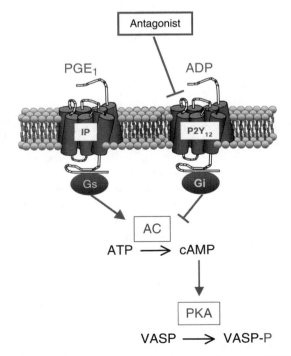

Figure 1 VASP assay for the measurement of $P2Y_{12}$ antagonism. See text for explanation. *Source*: Modified from Ref. 22. *Abbreviations*: VASP, vasodilator-stimulated phosphoprotein.

PGE$_1$-induced signaling through AC. P2Y$_{12}$ antagonists, e.g., the active metabolite of clopidogrel, inhibit this ADP-induced effect. Therefore, in the presence of both PGE$_1$ and ADP, VASP-P is directly proportional to the degree of P2Y$_{12}$ antagonism (Fig. 1). VASP-P is measured by whole blood flow cytometry, using permeabilization and a monoclonal antibody specific for the phosphorylated form of VASP.

The advantages of the VASP assay are that it is dependent on clopidogrel's target (P2Y$_{12}$), low sample volume, and whole blood assays. In addition, quite remarkably, citrated blood samples can be mailed at room temperature to a core laboratory; this is particularly useful in multicenter clinical trials (14). The disadvantages of the VASP assay are sample preparation, and the requirement for a flow cytometer and an experienced technician.

Serum Thromboxane B$_2$

Thromboxane A$_2$ is released from platelets in an activation-dependent manner, and then rapidly converted to its stable metabolite thromboxane B$_2$ (23). The advantage of measuring serum thromboxane B$_2$ is that it is directly dependent on aspirin's target, COX-1. The disadvantages of measuring serum thromboxane B$_2$ are that it is an indirect measure in the sense that platelets are not directly assayed and that it may not be entirely platelet-specific (24).

Urinary 11-dehydro thromboxane B$_2$

Urinary 11-dehydro thromboxane B$_2$ is a stable urinary metabolite of thromboxane A$_2$ (23). The advantage of measuring urinary 11-dehydro thromboxane B$_2$ is that it is directly dependent on aspirin's target, COX-1. The disadvantages of measuring urinary 11-dehydro thromboxane B$_2$ are that it is an indirect measure in the sense that platelets are not directly assayed and that it may not be entirely platelet specific (24). The potential effects of renal function are obviated by measuring the urinary 11-dehydro thromboxane B$_2$/creatinine ratio (25).

Approach to Monitoring Antiplatelet Therapy

Platelet Function Tests for Monitoring Aspirin
Considering this cornucopia of available platelet function tests (Table 1), how should the effects of aspirin be monitored? There are three categories of available tests (Table 2).

First, thromboxane could be used as the end point, with an assay of either serum thromboxane B$_2$ or urinary 11-dehydro thromboxane B$_2$. The advantage of this approach is that aspirin specifically inhibits platelet COX-1 and, therefore, thromboxane generation. A possible disadvantage is that nearly all patients who are compliant with taking aspirin are inhibited as judged by serum thromboxane B$_2$ or urinary 11-dehydro thromboxane B$_2$ assays—but not necessarily as judged by other assays (27,28).

Second, arachidonic acid can be used as the stimulus. The advantage of this approach is that arachidonic acid results in specific signaling through COX-1, the point of inhibition by aspirin. Again, the assumption is that all of aspirin's effects result from its inhibition of COX-1, which might not be entirely so (27,28). With arachidonic acid as the stimulus, one of a number of end points could be chosen, including turbidometric platelet aggregometry, impedance platelet aggregometry, the VerifyNow aspirin assay, Plateletworks, platelet surface activated GPIIb-IIIa, platelet surface P-selectin, leukocyte-platelet aggregates, TEG PlateletMapping System, and the Impact cone and plate(let) analyzer. However, older studies of the VerifyNow (Ultegra rapid platelet function assay),

Table 2 Platelet Function Tests for Monitoring Aspirin, Clopidogrel, and GPIIb-IIIa Antagonists

Aspirin
Thromboxane as the end point
Serum thromboxane B_2
Urinary 11-dehydro thromboxane B_2
Arachidonic acid as the stimulus
Platelet aggregometry (turbidometric)
Platelet aggregometry (impedance)
VerifyNow aspirin assay
Plateletworks
Platelet surface–activated GPIIb-IIIa, platelet surface P-selectin, leukocyte-platelet aggregates
(flow cytometry)
TEG platelet mapping system
Impact cone and plate(let) analyzer
Other
PFA-100
Clopidogrel
$P2Y_{12}$ specific
VASP phosphorylation (flow cytometry)
ADP stimulated
Platelet aggregometry (turbidometric)
Platelet aggregometry (impedance)
VerifyNow $P2Y_{12}$ assay
Plateletworks
Platelet surface activated GPIIb-IIIa, platelet surface P-selectin, leukocyte-platelet aggregates
(flow cytometry)
TEG platelet mapping system
Impact cone and plate(let) analyzer
GPIIb-IIIa antagonists
Platelet aggregation
Platelet aggregometry (turbidometric)
Platelet aggregometry (impedance)
VerifyNow TRAP assay
Plateletworks
Activation-dependent conformational change in GPIIb-IIIa by flow cytometry
Platelet surface–activated GPIIb-IIIa (PAC-1)
LIBS

Abbreviations: LIBS, Ligand-induced binding site; GP, glycoprotein.
Source: Modified from Ref. 26.

including the widely quoted study by Chen et al. (29), used propyl gallate, not arachidonic acid, as the stimulus.

Third, the PFA-100 has been widely used to study the response of platelets to aspirin (30). Unlike the first two categories in Table 2, the PFA-100 is not COX-1 specific. Is that a disadvantage, or could it be an advantage if aspirin also has non-COX-1-mediated inhibitory effects (27,28) on platelets?

Platelet Function Tests for Monitoring Clopidogrel

How should the effects of clopidogrel be monitored? There are two categories of available tests (Table 2). First, only the VASP phosphorylation assay is specific with regard to signaling through $P2Y_{12}$, and therefore the platelet-inhibitory effects of clopidogrel (Fig. 1).

Second, ADP can be used as the stimulus. The alternative approach is to add ADP and look at one of a number of end points. However, it is important to consider that ADP binds to its platelet surface $P2Y_1$ receptor as well as its platelet surface $P2Y_{12}$ receptor (31)—and that the active metabolite of clopidogrel only inhibits at $P2Y_{12}$ not $P2Y_1$ (2). Therefore, the effects of ADP on platelet function reflect not only the inhibitory effects of clopidogrel on $P2Y_{12}$, but also the unblocked effect of ADP-induced signaling through $P2Y_1$. With ADP as the stimulus, one of a number of end points could be chosen, including turbidometric platelet aggregometry, impedance platelet aggregometry, the VerifyNow $P2Y_{12}$ assay, Plateletworks, platelet surface activated GPIIb-IIIa, platelet surface P-selectin, leukocyte-platelet aggregates, TEG PlateletMapping System, and the Impact cone and plate(let) analyzer.

Platelet Function Tests for Monitoring GPIIb-IIIa Antagonists

GPIIb-IIIa antagonists can be monitored by two categories of tests (Table 2). First, because GPIIb-IIIa antagonists block the final common pathway of platelet aggregation (3), inhibition of platelet aggregation can be assessed by one of a number of end points, turbidometric platelet aggregometry, impedance aggregometry, VerifyNow TRAP assay, or Plateletworks. Second, because platelet aggregation cannot occur without a conformational change in integrin $\alpha IIb\beta 3$, flow cytometry can be used to measure a conformational change in platelet surface activated GPIIb-IIIa[reported by monoclonal antibody PAC-1 (10,11)] or a ligand-induced binding site (LIBS) (32,33).

Point-of-Care Assays

Point-of-care assays (also referred to as point-of-service assays) have potentially great advantages, for example, to help immediate decision-making about the type and dose of antiplatelet therapy in the interventional cardiology suite. A rigorous definition of a point-of-care assay is one that meets all of the following criteria: Use at or near the patient bedside, easy to use without special skills, no sample processing, no pipetting, and rapid readout. The only currently available device that fits these criteria is VerifyNow (9). However, at least two other devices are in development: T-Guide (ThromboVision, Houston,Texas, U.S.), based on agonist-induced laser light scattering, and PRT (PlaCor, Plymouth, Minnesota, U.S.), based on a fingerstick capillary blood sample with no exogenously added agonist.

POTENTIAL ROLES OF PLATELET FUNCTION TESTING IN THE DEVELOPMENT OF PLATELET INHIBITORS

Elucidation of Mechanisms of Action

Remarkably, the two most widely used platelet inhibitors in clinical medicine, aspirin and clopidogrel, were both shown to have a beneficial antithrombotic effect long before their mechanism of action as inhibitors of platelet function was elucidated. Subsequently, aspirin was demonstrated to irreversibly acetylate serine 529 of COX-1, thereby inhibiting generation of the potent endogenous platelet activator thromboxane A_2 (34). More recently, the active metabolite of clopidogrel was demonstrated to inhibit the ADP platelet receptor $P2Y_{12}$ (35)—a receptor whose existence was unknown when clopidogrel, and its similarly acting predecessor ticlopidine, were already widely used in patients.

Nevertheless, additional mechanisms of action of these well-established antiplatelet drugs continue to be investigated. For example, in a recent 700-patient study of aspirin-treated patients, we demonstrated that there is residual arachidonic acid-induced platelet activation via an ADP-dependent but COX-1- and COX-2-independent pathway (27).

Turbidometric platelet aggregation may be used to study congenital platelet disorders and, in response to all agonists except Ristocetin is defective in Glanzmann thrombasthenia (36). Glanzmann thrombasthenia was subsequently determined to be a defect in GPIIb-IIIa (integrin $\alpha IIb\beta 3$) (36). This finding eventually resulted in the development of the first rationally designed antiplatelet agents: GPIIb-IIIa antagonists (37).

In the development of novel platelet inhibitors, in vitro platelet function tests are initially used to demonstrate that an agent is in fact a platelet inhibitor. Further development of novel platelet inhibitors involves the use of platelet function tests in animal studies and then human phase I, II, and III studies—as described in detail in subsequent chapters in this book.

Determination of Optimal Dose and Frequency of Administration

The determination of the optimal dose and frequency of administration of platelet inhibitors is largely dependent on platelet function tests (38). Furthermore, platelet function tests have been used to determine the optimal dose of platelet inhibitors in different age groups. For example, we recently performed a prospective, multicenter, randomized, placebo-controlled trial to demonstrate that clopidogrel 0.2 mg/kg/day in children 0 to 24 months of age achieves a platelet-inhibition level similar to that in adults taking the standard clopidogrel maintenance dose of 75 mg/day (39).

Comparison of Different Platelet Inhibitors

Although the optimal comparison between different platelet inhibitors is a phase III clinical outcomes study, platelet function tests can be very useful and are, of course, much less expensive. For example, we recently compared the relative antiplatelet effects of prasugrel (a novel $P2Y_{12}$ antagonist) versus high-dose clopidogrel in percutaneous coronary intervention patients in the prasugrel in comparison to clopidogrel for inhibition of platelet activation and aggregation–thrombolysis in myocardial infarction 44 (PRINCIPLE-TIMI 44) trial (14). This study compared prasugrel 60-mg loading dose followed by 10 mg/day versus clopidogrel 600-mg loading dose followed by 150 mg/day in 201 patients undergoing cardiac catheterization for planned percutaneous coronary intervention. Greater inhibition of platelet aggregation at all time points measured from 30 minutes to 24 hours was observed with patients receiving prasugrel compared with high-loading-dose clopidogrel. During the maintenance-dose phase, greater inhibition of platelet aggregation was also seen in subjects receiving prasugrel compared with high-maintenance-dose clopidogrel. The trial was not powered for clinical end points. Bleeding tended to be more frequent with prasugrel, although no significant differences were observed. Prasugrel has been compared with standard-dose clopidogrel in a large-scale clinical events trial [trial to assess improvement in therapeutic outcomes by optimizing platelet inhibition with prasugrel thrombolysis in myocardial infarction 38 (TRITON-TIMI 38)] (40), and, along with the data from PRINCIPLE-TIMI 44, demonstrate that greater inhibition of platelet aggregation is seen with prasugrel compared with high-loading-dose and high-maintenance-dose clopidogrel (14).

Monitoring of "Resistance" or Hyporesponsiveness to Platelet Inhibitors

Antiplatelet drugs are beneficial in the treatment of coronary artery disease, ischemic stroke, and peripheral arterial disease (38). Platelet function tests have been studied in cardiovascular diseases as a means to predict clinical outcomes and monitor antiplatelet drugs (4). There is a well-documented variability between patients (and normal volunteers) with regard to laboratory test responses to antiplatelet drugs (25,29,41–48). Evidence from small clinical studies suggests that decreased response, or "resistance", to antiplatelet drugs is associated with subsequent major adverse clinical events (MACE) (25,29,41–44,46,48–52). However, it remains unknown whether altering therapy based on platelet function tests is beneficial to patients.

Aspirin "Resistance"

Aspirin reduces the odds of a serious arterial thrombotic event in high-risk patients by $\sim 25\%$ (53). Despite aspirin's clearly demonstrated clinical antithrombotic effect (38,53) and excellent cost effectiveness profile (54), 10% to 20% of patients with an arterial thrombotic event who are treated with aspirin have a recurrent arterial thrombotic event during long-term follow up (53). In some studies, the occurrence of an arterial thrombotic event despite aspirin therapy has been termed (clinical) "aspirin resistance." However, because arterial thrombosis is multifactorial, an arterial thrombotic event in a patient may reflect treatment failure rather than resistance to aspirin (55,56). Furthermore, patient noncompliance with aspirin administration is a confounding problem (57,58). Nevertheless, there is a well-documented variability between patients (and normal volunteers) with regard to laboratory test responses to aspirin (25,29,41–44). Less-than-expected inhibition of platelet function by aspirin has been termed (laboratory) "aspirin resistance" or "aspirin nonresponsiveness" (4,55,56,59–61). In this chapter, the term "aspirin resistance" will be used to refer to a less than expected inhibition of platelet function by aspirin, as determined by a laboratory test. Depending on the assay used, aspirin resistance occurs in 5% to 60% of aspirin-treated patients (4,55,56,59–61). Assays for the measurement of aspirin resistance are listed in Table 2. Possible mechanisms of aspirin resistance are listed in Table 3.

A key question is whether laboratory tests of aspirin resistance (Table 2) predict clinical aspirin resistance, i.e., MACE. A clinically meaningful definition of aspirin resistance can only be based on data linking aspirin-dependent laboratory tests to relevant clinical outcomes (4,55). There is evidence that future MACE in the settings of acute coronary syndromes, stroke/transient ischemic attacks, and peripheral arterial disease can be predicted by the following in vitro tests of aspirin resistance: arachidonic acid–and ADP-induced platelet aggregation (turbidometric), ADP- and collagen-induced platelet aggregation (impedance), VerifyNow aspirin assay, PFA-100, and urinary 11-dehydro thromboxane B_2 (25,29,41–44,51,52).

However, there are three important disclaimers: (*i*) The number of MACE was low in all these studies (25,29,41–44,51,52). (*ii*) The reported incidence of aspirin resistance varies greatly depending on the platelet function assay used (25,29,41–44,51,52,62), but it is not known which is the optimal platelet function test for determining aspirin resistance. (*iii*) It remains unknown which, if any, of the platelet function tests shown in Table 2 provides the best criterion for changing aspirin therapy based on a finding of aspirin resistance (4,55).

Aspirin resistance is an issue with potentially important public health implications because of the very high prevalence of coronary artery disease and concomitant use of aspirin therapy. It is estimated that in the United States alone, approximately 30 million individuals take aspirin daily for cardioprotection (63). Identification of a more optimal

Table 3 Possible Mechanisms of Aspirin and Clopidogrel "Resistance" or Response Variability

Bioavailability
   Noncompliance
   Underdosing
   Poor absorption (enteric-coated aspirin)
   Interference (NSAIDs/aspirin, atorvastatin/clopidogrel)
Platelet function
   Incomplete suppression of thromboxane A_2 generation (aspirin)
   Accelerated platelet turnover, with introduction into bloodstream of newly formed,
     drug-unaffected platelets
   Stress-induced COX-2 in platelets (aspirin)
   Increased platelet sensitivity to ADP and collagen
Single-nucleotide polymorphisms
   Receptors: GPIIb-IIIa, $P2Y_1$, $P2Y_{12}$, thromboxane receptor, etc.
   Enzymes: COX-1, COX-2, TxA_2 synthase, etc. (aspirin), cytochrome P450 (clopidogrel)
Bioavailability
   Noncompliance
   Underdosing
   Poor absorption (enteric-coated aspirin)
   Interference (NSAIDs/aspirin, atorvastatin/clopidogrel)
Platelet function
   Incomplete suppression of thromboxane A_2 generation (aspirin)
   Accelerated platelet turnover, with introduction into bloodstream of newly formed,
     drug-unaffected platelets
   Stress-induced COX-2 in platelets (aspirin)
   Increased platelet sensitivity to ADP and collagen
Single-nucleotide polymorphisms
   Receptors: GPIIb-IIIa, $P2Y_1$, $P2Y_{12}$, thromboxane receptor, etc.
   Enzymes: COX-1, COX-2, TxA_2 synthase, etc. (aspirin), cytochrome P450 (clopidogrel)
Platelet interactions with other blood cells
   Endothelial cells and monocytes make thromboxane A_2 and the TXA_2 intermediate, PGH_2, both
     of which may be taken up by platelets (bypassing COX-1) (aspirin)
Other factors
   Smoking, hypercholesterolemia, etc.
Rather than resistance, is it
   treatment failure (because arterial thrombosis is multifactorial)?
   aspirin or clopidogrel response variability?
   platelet response variability?

Abbreviations: COX, cyclooxygenase; ADP, adenosine diphosphate; GP, glycoprotein.
Source: Modified from Ref. 4.

dosing of aspirin could therefore have a much larger impact on death and disability than many newer treatments (64). However, it is not certain that increasing the dose of aspirin based on laboratory evidence of aspirin resistance will be clinically beneficial. Meta-analysis of published studies has not demonstrated a difference between the benefit of low dose (e.g., 81 mg) and higher dose (e.g., ≥ 325 mg) aspirin (53)—although the accompanying editorial to this article pointed out that such overviews are "reductionist, blunt instruments" that "are unlikely to elucidate aspirin resistance" in subpopulations of patients (65). Because arterial thrombosis is multifactorial, an adverse arterial thrombotic outcome in a patient may reflect treatment failure rather than aspirin resistance.

Furthermore, patient noncompliance with aspirin (57,58) may have been a (hard to detect) confounding factor in studies that report MACE can be predicted by laboratory tests of aspirin resistance (25,29,41–44,51,52). Finally, hemorrhagic side effects (especially gastrointestinal bleeding) are increased with higher doses of aspirin (38,66).

Many clinicians increase the dose of aspirin based on laboratory evidence of aspirin resistance (67,68). However, no published studies address the clinical effectiveness of altering therapy based on a laboratory finding of aspirin resistance. The correct treatment, if any, of aspirin resistance therefore remains unknown. The International Society on Thrombosis and Haemostasis (ISTH) *Working Group on Aspirin Resistance* concluded that "other than in research trials, it is not currently appropriate to test for aspirin resistance in patients or to change therapy based on such tests" (55). Similar conclusions have been published by both the American College of Chest Physicians 7th Consensus Conference on Antithrombotic Therapy (38) and the Consensus Task Force on the Use of Antiplatelet Agents in Patients with Atherosclerotic Cardiovascular Disease of the European Society of Cardiology (ESC) (66).

Clopidogrel "Resistance"

There is variability between patients with regard to clopidogrel-induced inhibition of platelet function assays (4,–45–47,61,69). A relative lack of clopidogrel-induced inhibition of platelet function assays has been termed clopidogrel "resistance" (4,45–47,61). Assays for the measurement of clopidogrel resistance are listed in Table 2.

A number of possible mechanisms for clopidogrel resistance have been proposed (Table 3), including poor bioavailability [noncompliance, underdosing, poor absorption, interference by atorvastatin with cytochrome P450–mediated metabolism of clopidogrel (47)], accelerated platelet turnover (with the introduction into the blood stream of newly formed, drug-unaffected platelets) and SNPs [e.g., the $P2Y_{12}$ H2 haplotype (69)]. However, in the absence of clopidogrel, it is well known that there is a wide inter-individual variation in platelet response to ADP, the causes of which may include SNPs in the $P2Y_1$(70) and/or $P2Y_{12}$ (69). ADP receptors and variations in the platelet surface density of the $P2Y_1$ receptor (71). Indeed, we have provided evidence that clopidogrel resistance is, at least in part, the result of preexistent platelet response variability that is not increased by clopidogrel administration (72).

Some (46,49,50), but not all (73), studies suggest that patients with higher residual platelet reactivity after the initiation of clopidogrel therapy have more subsequent MACE. However, as for aspirin resistance (see above): (*i*) The number of MACE was low in all these studies (46,49,50,73). (*ii*) The reported incidence of clopidogrel resistance varies greatly depending on the platelet function assay used, but it is not known which is the optimal platelet function test for determining clopidogrel resistance. (*iii*) It remains unknown which, if any, of the platelet function tests shown in Table 2 provides the best criterion for changing clopidogrel therapy based on a finding of clopidogrel resistance.

The correct treatment of clopidogrel resistance is unknown. Higher doses of clopidogrel (74–77) or other antiplatelet therapy may be beneficial. However, definitive evidence for the benefit of guided antiplatelet therapy based on the degree of platelet reactivity will have to await the results of prospective clinical outcomes studies (4). The first report of such a guided therapy study concluded that in a small number of patients with clopidogrel resistance according to measurement of phosphorylated VASP (Fig. 1), adjusting the loading dose of clopidogrel significantly improves clinical outcomes (78). The 2006 American College of Cardiology/American Heart Association guidelines for PCI provided a class IIB recommendation (based on level C evidence) that, in patients in whom subacute stent thrombosis may be catastrophic or lethal, platelet aggregation studies may be considered and the maintenance dose of clopidogrel increased from 75 mg to 150 mg per day if less than 50% inhibition of platelet aggregation is demonstrated (79). In addition, novel thienopyridines may provide a therapeutic advantage over clopidogrel. For example, prasugrel results in more rapid and more potent inhibition of $P2Y_{12}$ receptors, with much less inter-individual variability in platelet response to ADP (14,40,80,81).

GPIIb-IIIa Antagonist Resistance

The GPIIb-IIIa antagonists [abciximab (ReoPro®), eptifibatide (Integrilin®), tirofiban (Aggrastat®)] inhibit fibrinogen binding to platelet surface GPIIb-IIIa (integrin αIIbβ3), the final common pathway of platelet aggregation (82). The term "GPIIb-IIIa antagonist resistance" could be used (4), because there is substantial patient-to-patient variability in the degree of inhibition of platelet function by GPIIb-IIIa antagonists (48) and there is evidence that an in vitro test of abciximab "resistance" (VerifyNow) predicts MACE (48). However, no published studies address the clinical effectiveness of altering therapy based on a laboratory finding of GPIIb-IIIa antagonist resistance.

REFERENCES

1. Awtry EH, Loscalzo J. Aspirin. In: Michelson AD, ed. Platelets. 2nd ed. San Diego, CA: Elsevier/Academic Press, 2007:1099–1125.
2. Cattaneo M. ADP receptor antagonists. In: Michelson AD, ed. Platelets. 2nd ed. San Diego, CA: Elsevier/Academic Press, 2007:1127–1144.
3. Agah R, Plow EF, Topol EJ. aIIbb3 (GPIIb-IIIa) antagonists. In: Michelson AD, ed. Platelets. 2nd ed. San Diego, CA: Elsevier/Academic Press, 2007:1145–1163.
4. Michelson AD. Platelet function testing in cardiovascular diseases. Circulation 2004; 110: e489–e493.
5. Born GVR. Aggregation of blood platelets by adenosine diphosphate and its reversal. Nature 1962; 194:927–929.
6. O'Brien JR. Platelet aggregation. Part II: Some results of a new method. J Clin Pathol 1962; 15:452–455.
7. Jennings LK, White MM. Platelet aggregation. In: Michelson AD, ed. Platelets. 2nd ed. San Diego, CA: Elsevier/Academic Press, 2007:495–508.
8. Harrison P, Keeling D. Clinical tests of platelet function. In: Michelson AD, ed. Platelets. 2nd ed. San Diego, CA: Elsevier/Academic Press, 2007:445–474.
9. Steinhubl SR. The VerifyNow system. In: Michelson AD, ed. Platelets. 2nd ed. San Diego, CA: Elsevier/Academic Press, 2007:509–518.
10. Michelson AD, Linden MD, Barnard MR, et al. Flow cytometry. In: Michelson AD, ed. Platelets, 2nd ed. San Diego, CA: Elsevier/Academic Press, 2007:545–564.
11. Shattil SJ, Hoxie JA, Cunningham M, et al. Changes in the platelet membrane glycoprotein IIb-IIIa complex during platelet activation. J Biol Chem 1985; 260:11107–11114.
12. McEver RP. P-Selectin/PSGL-1 and other interactions between platelets, leukocytes, and endothelium. In: Michelson AD, ed. Platelets. 2nd ed. San Diego, CA: Elsevier/Academic Press, 2007:231–249.
13. Michelson AD, Barnard MR, Krueger LA, et al. Circulating monocyte-platelet aggregates are a more sensitive marker of in vivo platelet activation than platelet surface P-selectin: studies in baboons, human coronary intervention, and human acute myocardial infarction. Circulation 2001; 104:1533–1537.
14. Wiviott SD, Trenk D, Frelinger AL, et al. Prasugrel compared with high loading- and maintenance-dose clopidogrel in patients with planned percutaneous coronary intervention: the

Prasugrel in Comparison to Clopidogrel for Inhibition of Platelet Activation and Aggregation-Thrombolysis in Myocardial Infarction 44 trial. Circulation 2007; 116:2923–2932.

15. Bouchard BA, Butenas S, Mann KG, et al. Interactions between platelets and the coagulation system. In: Michelson AD, ed. Platelets. 2nd ed., San Diego, CA: Elsevier/Academic Press, 2007:377–402.

16. Tantry US, Bliden KP, Gurbel PA. Overestimation of platelet aspirin resistance detection by thrombelastograph platelet mapping and validation by conventional aggregometry using arachidonic acid stimulation. J Am Coll Cardiol 2005; 46:1705–1709.

17. Savage B, Ruggeri ZM. Platelet thrombus formation in flowing blood. In: Michelson AD, ed. Platelets. 2nd ed. San Diego, CA: Elsevier/Academic Press, 2007:359–376.

18. Ruggeri ZM. Platelets in atherothrombosis. Nature Med 2002; 8:1227–1234.

19. Varon D, Savion N. Impact cone and plate(let) analyzer. In: Michelson AD, ed. Platelets. 2nd ed. San Diego, CA: Elsevier/Academic Press, 2007:535–544.

20. Francis JL. The platelet function analyzer (PFA)-100. In: Michelson AD, ed. Platelets. 2nd ed. San Diego, CA: Elsevier/Academic Press, 2007:519–534.

21. Harrison P, Frelinger AL, III, Furman MI, et al. Measuring antiplatelet drug effects in the laboratory. Thrombos Res 2007; 120:323–336.

22. Cattaneo M. In: Michelson AD, ed. Platelets, 2nd ed. Elsevier/Academic Press, 2007:325.

23. Grosser T, Fries S, FitzGerald GA. Thromboxane generation. In: Michelson AD, ed. Platelets. 2nd ed. San Diego, CA: Elsevier/Academic Press, 2007:565–574.

24. Catella F, FitzGerald GA. Paired analysis of urinary thromboxane B2 metabolites in humans. Thromb Res 1987; 47:647–656.

25. Eikelboom JW, Hirsh J, Weitz JI, et al. Aspirin-resistant thromboxane biosynthesis and the risk of myocardial infarction, stroke, or cardiovascular death in patients at high risk for cardiovascular events. Circulation 2002; 105:1650–1655.

26. Michelson AD, Frelinger AL, III, Furman MI, et al. Resistance to antiplatelet drugs. Eur Heart J 2006; (8):G53–G58.

27. Frelinger AL, III, Furman MI, Linden MD, et al. Residual arachidonic acid-induced platelet activation via an adenosine diphosphate-dependent but cyclooxygenase-1- and cyclooxygenase-2-independent pathway: a 700-patient study of aspirin resistance. Circulation 2006; 113:2888–2296.

28. Gurbel PA, Bliden KP, DiChiara J, et al. Evaluation of dose-related effects of aspirin on platelet function: results from the Aspirin-Induced Platelet Effect (ASPECT) study. Circulation 2007; 115:3156–3164.

29. Chen WH, Lee PY, Ng W, et al. Aspirin resistance is associated with a high incidence of myonecrosis after non-urgent percutaneous coronary intervention despite clopidogrel pretreatment. J Am Coll Cardiol 2004; 43:1122–1126.

30. Crescente M, Di Castelnuovo A, Iacoviello L, et al. Response variabilty to aspirin as assessed by the platelet function analyzer (PFA)-100: a systematic review. Thromb Haemost 2008; 99:14–26.

31. Cattaneo M. The platelet P2 receptors. In: Michelson AD, ed. Platelets 2nd ed. San Diego, CA: Elsevier/Academic Press, 2007:201–220.

32. Frelinger AL, Cohen I, Plow EF, et al. Selective inhibition of integrin function by antibodies specific for ligand-occupied receptor conformers. J Biol Chem 1990; 265:6346–6352.

33. Jennings LK, White MM. Expression of ligand-induced binding sites on glycoprotein IIb-IIIa complexes and the effect of various inhibitors. Am Heart J 1998; 35:S179–S183.

34. Roth GJ, Stanford N, Majerus PW. Acetylation of prostaglandin synthase by aspirin. Proc Natl Acad Sci USA 1975; 72:3073–3076.

35. Hollopeter G, Jantzen HM, Vincent D, et al. Identification of the platelet ADP receptor targeted by antithrombotic drugs. Nature 2001; 409:202–207.

36. Nurden AT, Nurden P. Inherited disorders of platelet function. In: Michelson AD, ed. Platelets. 2nd ed. San Diego, CA: Elsevier/Academic Press, 2007:1029–1050.

37. Coller BS. Platelet GPIIb-IIIa antagonists: the first anti-integrin receptor therapeutics. J Clin Invest 1997; 99:1467–1471.

38. Patrono C, Coller B, FitzGerald GA, et al. Platelet-active drugs: the relationships among dose, effectiveness, and side effects. Chest 2004; 126:234S–264S.
39. Li JS, Yow E, Berezny KY, et al. Dosing of Clopidogrel for Platelet Inhibition in Infants and Young Children: Primary Results of the Platelet Inhibition in Children On cLOpidogrel (PICOLO) Trial. Circulation 2008; 117:553–559.
40. Wiviott SD, Braunwald E, McCabe CH, et al. Prasugrel versus clopidogrel in patients with acute coronary syndromes. N Engl J Med 2007; 357:2001–2015.
41. Mueller MR, Salat A, Stangl P, et al. Variable platelet response to low-dose ASA and the risk of limb deterioration in patients submitted to peripheral arterial angioplasty. Thromb Haemost 1997; 78:1003–1007.
42. Grotemeyer KH, Scharafinski HW, Husstedt IW. Two-year follow-up of aspirin responder and aspirin non-responder. A pilot-study including 180 poststroke patients. Thromb Res 1993; 71:397–403.
43. Gum PA, Kottke-Marchant K, Welsh PA, et al. A prospective, blinded determination of the natural history of aspirin resistance among stable patients with cardiovascular disease. J Am Coll Cardiol 2003; 41:961–965.
44. Grundmann K, Jaschonek K, Kleine B, et al. Aspirin non-responder status in patients with recurrent cerebral ischemic attacks. J Neurol 2003; 250:63–66.
45. Gurbel PA, Bliden KP, Hiatt BL, et al. Clopidogrel for coronary stenting: response variability, drug resistance, and the effect of pretreatment platelet reactivity. Circulation 2003; 107:2908–2913.
46. Matetzky S, Shenkman B, Guetta V, et al. Clopidogrel resistance is associated with increased risk of recurrent atherothrombotic events in patients with acute myocardial infarction. Circulation 2004; 109:3171–3175.
47. Lau WC, Gurbel PA, Watkins PB, et al. Contribution of hepatic cytochrome P450 3A4 metabolic activity to the phenomenon of clopidogrel resistance. Circulation 2004; 109:166–171.
48. Steinhubl SR, Talley JD, Braden GA, et al. Point-of-care measured platelet inhibition correlates with a reduced risk of an adverse cardiac event after percutaneous coronary intervention: results of the GOLD (AU-Assessing Ultegra) multicenter study. Circulation 2001; 103:2572–2578.
49. Gurbel PA, Bliden KP, Samara W, et al. Clopidogrel effect on platelet reactivity in patients with stent thrombosis: results of the CREST study. J Am Coll Cardiol 2005; 46:1827–1832.
50. Cuisset T, Frere C, Quilici J, et al. High post-treatment platelet reactivity identified low responders to dual antiplatelet therapy at increased risk of recurrent cardiovascular events after stenting for acute coronary syndrome. J Thromb Haemost 2006; 4:542–549.
51. Snoep JD, Hovens MM, Eikenboom JC, et al. Association of laboratory-defined aspirin resistance with a higher risk of recurrent cardiovascular events: a systematic review and meta-analysis. Arch Intern Med 2007; 167:1593–1599.
52. Krasopoulos G, Brister SJ, Beattie WS, et al. Aspirin "resistance" and risk of cardiovascular morbidity: systematic review and meta-analysis. Br Med J 2008; 336:195–203.
53. Antithrombotic Trialists' Collaboration. Collaborative meta-analysis of randomised trials of antiplatelet therapy for prevention of death, myocardial infarction, and stroke in high risk patients. Br Med J 2002; 324:71–86.
54. Gaspoz JM, Coxson PG, Goldman PA, et al. Cost-effectiveness of aspirin, clopidogrel, or both for secondary prevention of coronary heart disease. N Engl J Med 2002; 346:1800–1806.
55. Michelson AD, Cattaneo M, Eikelboom JW, et al. Aspirin resistance: position paper of the Working Group on Aspirin Resistance. J Thromb Haemost 2005; 3:1309–1311.
56. Patrono C. Aspirin resistance: definition, mechanisms, and clinical read-outs. J Thromb Haemost 2003; 1:1710–1713.
57. Cotter G, Shemesh E, Zehavi M, et al. Lack of aspirin effect: aspirin resistance or resistance to taking aspirin? Am Heart J 2004; 147:293–300.
58. Schwartz KA, Schwartz DE, Ghosheh K, et al. Compliance as a critical consideration in patients who appear to be resistant to aspirin after healing of myocardial infarction. Am J Cardiol 2005; 95:(973–975).
59. Hankey GJ, Eikelboom JW. Aspirin resistance. Br Med J 2004; 328:477–479.

60. Bhatt DL. Aspirin resistance: more than just a laboratory curiosity. J Am Coll Cardiol 2004; 43:1127–1129.

61. Cattaneo M. Aspirin and clopidogrel: efficacy, safety, and the issue of drug resistance. Arterioscler Thromb Vasc Biol 2004; 24:1980–1987.

62. Harrison P, Segal H, Blasbery K, et al. Screening for aspirin responsiveness after transient ischemic attack and stroke: comparison of 2 point-of-care platelet function tests with optical aggregometry. Stroke 2005; 36:1001–1005.

63. Steinhubl SR, Charnigo R, Moliterno DJ. Resistance to antiplatelet resistance. Is it justified? J Am Coll Cardiol 2005; 45:1757–1758.

64. Quinn MJ, Aronow HD, Califf RM, et al. Aspirin dose and six-month outcome after an acute coronary syndrome. J Am Coll Cardiol 2004; 43:972–978.

65. Reilly M, FitzGerald GA. Gathering intelligence on antiplatelet drugs: the view from 30,000 feet. When combined with other information, overviews lead to conviction. Br Med J 2002; 324:59–60.

66. Patrono C, Bachmann F, Baigent C, et al. Expert consensus document on the use of antiplatelet agents. The task force on the use of antiplatelet agents in patients with atherosclerotic cardiovascular disease of the European Society of Cardiology. Eur Heart J 2004; 25:166–181.

67. Pollack A. For some, aspirin may not help hearts. New York Times, 2004 Jul 20, F1.

68. Poulsen TS, Kristensen SR, Atar D, et al. A critical appraisal of the phenomenon of aspirin resistance. Cardiology 2005; 104:83–91.

69. Fontana P, Dupont A, Gandrille S, et al. Adenosine diphosphate-induced platelet aggregation is associated with P2Y12 gene sequence variations in healthy subjects. Circulation 2003; 108:989–995.

70. Hetherington SL, Singh RK, Lodwick D, et al. Dimorphism in the P2Y1 ADP receptor gene is associated with increased platelet activation response to ADP. Arterioscler Thromb Vasc Biol 2005; 25:252–257.

71. Hechler B, Zhang Y, Eckly A, et al. Lineage-specific overexpression of the P2Y1 receptor induces platelet hyper-reactivity in transgenic mice. J Thromb Haemost 2003; 1:155–163.

72. Michelson AD, Linden MD, Furman MI, et al. Evidence that pre-existent variability in platelet response to ADP accounts for "clopidogrel resistance". J Thromb Haemost 2007; 5:75–81.

73. Mobley JE, Bresee SJ, Wortham DC, et al. Frequency of nonresponse antiplatelet activity of clopidogrel during pretreatment for cardiac catheterization. Am J Cardiol 2004; 93:456–458.

74. Gurbel PA, Bliden KP, Zaman KA, et al. Clopidogrel loading with eptifibatide to arrest the reactivity of platelets. Results of the clopidogrel loading with eptifibatide to arrest the reactivity of platelets (CLEAR PLATELETS) study. Circulation 2005; 111:1153–1159.

75. Gurbel PA, Bliden KP, Hayes KM, et al. The relation of dosing to clopidogrel responsiveness and the incidence of high posttreatment platelet aggregation in patients undergoing coronary stenting. J Am Coll Cardiol 2005; 45:1392–1396.

76. Patti G, Colonna G, Pasceri V, et al. Randomized trial of high loading dose of clopidogrel for reduction of periprocedural myocardial infarction in patients undergoing coronary intervention. Results from the ARMYDA-2 (Antiplatelet therapy for Reduction of MYocardial Damage during Angioplasty) study. Circulation 2005; 111:2099–2106.

77. Hochholzer W, Trenk D, Frundi D, et al. Time dependence of platelet inhibition after a 600-mg loading dose of clopidogrel in a large, unselected cohort of candidates for percutaneous coronary intervention. Circulation 2005; 111:2560–2564.

78. Bonello L, Camoin L, Arques S, et al. Adjusted clopidogrel loading doses according to VASP phosphorylation index decrease rate of major adverse cardiovascular events in patients with clopidogrel resistance: a multicentre randomized prospective study. J Am Coll Cardiol 2008; 51:A258.

79. Smith SC, Feldman TE, Hirshfeld JW, et al. ACC/AHA/SCAI 2005 guideline update for percutaneous coronary intervention—summary article: a report of the American College of Cardiology/American Heart Association Task Force on Practice Guidelines (ACC/AHA/SCAI 2005 Writing Committee to Update the 2001 Guidelines for Percutaneous Coronary Intervention). Circulation 2006; 113:156–175.

80. Jernberg T, Payne CD, Winters KJ, et al. Prasugrel achieves greater inhibition of platelet aggregation and a lower rate of non- responders compared with clopidogrel in aspirin-treated patients with stable coronary artery disease. Eur Heart J 2006; 27:1166–1173.

81. Wiviott SD, Antman EM, Winters KJ, et al. Randomized comparison of prasugrel (CS-747, LY640315), a novel thienopyridine P2Y12 antagonist, with clopidogrel in percutaneous coronary intervention: results of the Joint Utilization of Medications to Block Platelets Optimally (JUMBO)-TIMI 26 trial. Circulation 2005; 28:111, 3366–3373.

82. Plow EF, Pesho MM, Ma Y-Q. Integrin αIIbβ3. In: Michelson AD, ed. Platelets. 2nd ed. San Diego, CA: Elsevier/Academic Press, 2007:165–178.

8

The Role of Proteomics and Transcriptomics in the Development of Antithrombotics

Lisa Senzel
Department of Pathology, State University of New York, Stony Brook, New York, U.S.A.

Dmitri V. Gnatenko and Wadie F. Bahou
Department of Medicine, State University of New York, Stony Brook, New York, U.S.A.

INTRODUCTION

The transcriptome is the mRNA pool found within a cell. Transcriptomic discovery approaches include microarray-based technologies as well as sequencing-based technologies. Transcriptomic experiments provide dynamic information about gene expression at the tissue level. Complementing the transcriptome, the proteome is the pool of proteins expressed in a cell, tissue, or fluid at a given time and circumstance. The word "proteomics" summarizes several technologies for visualization, quantitation, and identification of these proteins. Unlike transcriptomic studies, proteomic studies can give information about localization, interactions, posttranslational modifications, and activation states of gene products. Protein separation can be accomplished using two-dimensional electrophoresis (2-DE), protein chips with an affinity matrix, or by a variety of advanced chromatographic methods. Then mass spectrometry (MS) is used to identify separated proteins using bioinformatics approaches linked to protein sequence databases. In another approach, peptide libraries are being used to identify molecules, which bind to platelets and to enzymatic components of the coagulation cascade. This chapter will discuss how transcriptomic and proteomic techniques are being used to study thrombosis in model systems and in patients with atherosclerotic disease and hypercoagulable conditions. The drive to discover new antithrombotic drugs using these techniques has met with several limitations and, while holding promise, has not yet reached the bedside. This chapter will explore these challenges and enumerate strategies for moving forward.

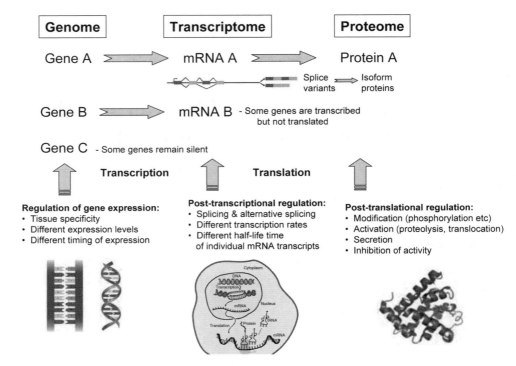

Figure 1 Types of information generated by transcriptomic and proteomic experiments. While the genome is static, the transcriptome represents the dynamic mRNA pool at the tissue level. Transcriptomic profiles capture physiological fluctuations in gene expression, but cannot show whether a gene product is translated. Proteomic experiments can delineate localization, interactions, posttranslational modifications, and activation states of gene products.

EXPRESSION GENOMICS: THE INTERROGATION OF THE TRANSCRIPTOME

Genomics includes the analysis of genetic mutations and polymorphisms, which represent static information. Expression profiles are dynamic, take place at the tissue level, and can capture physiological fluctuations (Fig. 1). The utility of expression genomics is in the simultaneous measurement of thousands of genes and the ability to assess many samples for comparison. The resultant expression footprints are akin to signatures of cellular states and can be used to distinguish between subtle differences. Thus, cell lineage makes a greater impact than biochemical pathways, and in turn, greater than individual gene effects (1). The transcriptome can be studied using microarrays as well as sequencing-based approaches. Microarrays can discern disease classes that standard clinical assays and assessments cannot. Serial analysis of gene expression (SAGE) and massively parallel signature sequencing (MPSS) can assess the expression of unknown or unexpected genes and can be useful for gene discovery.

PRINCIPLES OF MICROARRAY EXPERIMENTS

In microarrays, thousands of probes are fixed to a surface, and RNA samples (the targets) are labeled with fluorescent dyes for hybridization to the microarray. After hybridization, laser light is used to excite the fluorescent dye. The hybridization intensity is represented by the amount of fluorescent emission, which gives an estimate of the relative amounts of the different transcripts that are represented. There are many microarray platforms that differ in array fabrication and dye selection.

In cDNA microarrays, mRNA from biological samples is reverse transcribed and simultaneously labeled with Cy3 and Cy5. After hybridization, Cy3 and Cy5 fluorescence is measured separately, and captured in two images, which are merged to produce a composite image. Long-oligonucleotide microarrays [typically 75 base pair (bp)] are similar to cDNA microarrays, but the probes are derived from genomic or EST sequences. High-density oligonucleotide microarrays involving shorter probe sequences (typically 25 bp) use only a single fluorescence color, because the mRNA sample is converted to biotinylated cRNA and only one target is hybridized to each array (2).

Microarray experiments generate lists of differentially expressed genes. Genes of interest are those that appear to be upregulated or downregulated in disease states or other conditions. When selecting genes for further study, statistical criteria such as the p value can be considered along with the fold change (3). Differences in gene expression must still be confirmed using PCR-based or other hybridization assays, and must also be confirmed at the protein level to assess functional significance.

THROMBOTIC DISEASE STATES STUDIED BY TRANSCRIPTOMIC PROFILING: HUMAN PATIENTS

Microarray experiments using human patients have profiled several thrombotic disease states, as shown in Table 1. Two groups studied gene expression changes after ischemic stroke and identified different gene lists in spite of using similar Affymetrix platforms. The studies differed in that Moore et al. (4) profiled peripheral blood mononuclear cells (PBMCs), which include lymphocytes and monocytes, whereas Tang et al. (5) profiled neutrophils as well as PBMCs. Tang et al. (5) found that neutrophils expressed the genes that best predicted stroke. Thus far, gene lists could not differentiate between ischemic

Table 1 Thrombosis Models and Disease States Studied by Transcriptomic Profiling

Context	Ref.
Human patients	
Stroke	4,5
Coronary artery disease	6–9
Acute myocardial infarction	10
Antiphospholipid syndrome	11
Cardiopulmonary bypass	12,13
Essential thrombocythemia	14
Animal models and cell lines	
HUVEC stimulated by thrombin	15
HUVEC incubated with patient-derived antiphospholipid antibodies	16
Human microvascular endothelial cells stimulated by thrombin	17
Human coronary artery smooth muscle cells stimulated by prostaglandins	18
Human coronary artery endothelial cells activated by cytokines/APC	19
HUVEC treated with antithrombin	20
HUVEC stimulated by cytokines/APC/thrombin	21
Zebrafish hemostatic mutants	22,23
Buffy coat cells from mice with hyperhomocysteinemia	24

Abbreviations: HUVEC, human umbilical vein endothelial cells; APC, activated protein C.

and hemorrhagic stroke. Ma et al. (6) identified 108 differentially expressed genes in leukocytes among subjects with coronary heart disease versus healthy control subjects. These studies were extended when other groups found gene expression patterns which correlated well between animal and human studies during atherosclerotic lesion progression (7–9,25). In contrast, cross-species patterns in acute stroke correlated poorly between rats and humans (5). Cardiopulmonary bypass produced a "primed" phenotype of circulating PBMCs in which adhesion and signaling factors were overexpressed (12). Another study demonstrated that the coating on the cardiopulmonary bypass circuit affected leukocyte gene patterns. Heparin coating resulted in a more profound alteration in leukocyte gene expression when compared with protein coating (13).

In antiphospholipid syndrome, gene expression patterns from PBMCs predicted an individual's predisposition to developing thrombosis (11). This study was retrospective, and some of the differences could have been secondary to thrombosis. No attempt was made to subfractionate the starting mononuclear cell population, which also included platelets. Still, the study represents a paradigm for a genomic approach that could be applied to other populations of patients with thrombosis. Platelet profiling, as performed in human patients, is described later in this chapter.

TRANSCRIPTOMIC PROFILING IN ANIMAL STUDIES AND MODEL SYSTEMS OF THROMBOSIS

In endothelial cells, transcriptomic studies have facilitated the discovery of signaling pathways involving thrombin, cytokines, adhesion molecules, and other mediators of coagulation and inflammation (Table 1). Microarray experiments have identified changes in human umbilical vein (15) and microvascular (17) endothelial cells after thrombin stimulation. In the second study, thrombin increased thrombospondin-1 expression via activation of a signaling cascade, which included the G-protein coupled protease-activated receptor-1 (PAR-1) (17). Hamid et al. (16) incubated human umbilical vein endothelial cells with anti-β2-glycoprotein I antibodies derived from patients with antiphospholipid syndrome and uncovered genes, which may contribute to the vasculopathy associated with the disease. In microarray studies, the prostacyclin mimetic iloprost caused upregulation of thrombomodulin in human coronary artery smooth muscle cells (18). This finding led to the identification of a novel platelet-independent mechanism to explain the prothrombotic effects of cyclooxygenase-2 inhibitors (26). Franscini et al. (19) exposed human coronary artery endothelial cells to proinflammatory cytokines and performed microarray studies that uncovered a novel antiinflammatory mechanism of gene regulation, in which activated protein C (APC) caused c-Fos-dependent induction of monocyte chemotactic protein-1 (MCP-1) and intercellular adhesion molecule-1 (ICAM-1). Riewald and Ruf (21) identified differences in gene patterns in cytokine-stimulated mouse endothelial cells, which explained how APC and thrombin could exert distinct effects by signaling through the same receptor PAR-1. Zhang et al. (20) treated endothelial cells with antithrombin and discovered the importance of the proangiogenic heparan sulfate proteoglycan, perlecan in mediating the antiangiogenic effects of antithrombin. In another endothelial cell microarray study, C-reactive protein augmented the expression of matrix metalloproteinase (MMP)-1 and MMP-10 (27). The MMPs are participants in plaque disruption and thrombosis, and as such represent potential therapeutic drug targets (25).

In animal studies, microarray technology has been used to study atherosclerosis (described above), hyperhomocysteinemia, and other conditions related to thrombosis. Ebbesen et al. (24) found that hyperhomocysteinemia induced changes in the expression of genes involved in platelet activation, fibrinolysis, and contact activation in folate-deficient rats. Zebrafish have been used as a model system for hemostasis and thrombosis and have been studied by expression profiling (28). High throughput screens with chemicals using laser-induced thrombosis methods in zebrafish may lead to the discovery of novel antithrombotic compounds (22,23).

PLATELET TRANSCRIPTOME: THE APPLICATION OF MICROARRAY ANALYSIS TO PLATELETS

Platelets are particularly well suited to transcriptomic studies as they lack nuclear DNA and their genome consists of a small subset of megakaryocyte-derived mRNA transcripts. This complete pool of platelet RNAs is significantly smaller than that of nucleated cells. The study of the platelet transcriptome has been called "genomics without a genome" (29). Platelet RNAs have been studied by microarray approaches and by SAGE. SAGE represents an open transcript profiling system, which relies on the observation that short sequences (tags) within 3-mRNAs can stringently discriminate among genes. Differentially expressed genes can be identified in a quantitative manner, and genes expressed at very low levels can be identified by SAGE. The overrepresentation of mitochondrial transcripts in the platelet transcriptome limits the applicability of SAGE in platelet diseases, but the technique is useful for gene discovery (30).

Microarray studies using platelet-derived mRNAs are in general agreement on platelet transcript quantitation and gene expression patterns (31–35). Microarray analysis has been used to identify genes that are differentially expressed in several platelet-related diseases, including essential thrombocythemia. These studies demonstrate the feasibility of platelet transcript profiling in identifying differentially expressed genes, characterizing novel platelet-expressed genes, and elucidating the molecular signature of a disease (essential thrombocythemia) with potential application for platelet diagnostics (10,14,36). Transcriptomic data represented the basis for the discovery of novel molecules in platelets such as the transporters for GABA, glutamate, and dopamine (35,37,38).

Recently, platelet transcriptomes were analyzed from patients with acute myocardial infarction (MI) and stable coronary artery disease (CAD) to identify candidate genes with differential expression. The strongest discriminators of ST-segment-elevation MI were CD69 and myeloid-related protein-14 (MRP-14). Plasma levels of MRP-8/14 heterodimer were elevated in STEMI patients. A validation study found that MRP-8/14 levels could independently predict the risk of any vascular event in apparently healthy women (10). This study was criticized for non-agreement with microarray and proteomic studies by others and for possible contamination of the platelet fraction by leukocyte microparticles (39). The authors countered that they demonstrated MRP-14 expression in both megakaryocytes and in platelets, which lacked antibody staining for leukocyte markers. Irrespective, this study clearly used platelet expression profiling to identify a novel determinant of cardiovascular events, and this determinant was validated in one clinical study.

LIMITATIONS OF MICROARRAY EXPERIMENTS

When microarrays were developed in the early 1990s, their reliability was highly questioned. Cross-experimental, cross-platform and cross-laboratory variability made it difficult to compare experiments. Several multi-institutional projects are now under way to develop more reliable experimental protocols and controls, and progress has already been made (40). For example, the MicroArray Quality Control project gauged the performance of seven microarray platforms and queried the abundance of more than 12,000 genes in the same two RNA samples. The results confirmed that the distinct platforms and test sites performed comparably, reaffirming the robust nature of the technology. However, the starting samples were mixtures from cell lines and from brain tissue. Often, investigators begin with biological samples that have a smaller signal-to-noise ratio. The development of control RNAs that can be "spiked in" to any sample should help with standardization and sharing of microarray data (3). The Microarray Gene Expression Data (MGED) Society put forward a proposal in 2001 for experimental annotation standards known as "minimum information about a microarray experiment" (MIAME), designed to record key details about factors such as sample preparation and experimental design. These standards were particularly stringent, and simpler formats have been proposed (40).

Limitations of modern transcript profiling approaches include reliable and reproducible detection of low-abundant transcripts, feasibility of truly quantitative transcript profiling, and bulky and complex data processing. The transcriptome is complex and dynamically controlled at different levels, including regulation by microRNAs (miRNAs), signal-dependent pre-mRNA splicing, and translational control pathways. Despite significant progress in microarray chip design, accurate transcript profiling still requires validation by quantitative polymerase chain reaction (Q-PCR) or other techniques, followed by protein antigenic and functional correlational analyses. Efficient mRNA amplification, development of more sensitive whole genome microarrays (which detect alternatively spliced transcripts), and enhancements to bioinformatics software should obviate some of these restrictions. In the case of the platelet, accurate transcript profiling requires stringent attention to purification methodologies because a single nucleated cell (i.e., leukocyte) contains considerably more mRNA than a platelet.

The expense of global transcript and profiling precludes investigators from performing larger disease cohort studies. The development of cost-effective and reliable tools for transcript profiling would facilitate such experimentation. We have fabricated a first-generation custom platelet microarray that can be used in conjunction with proteomic analyses to study normal and diseased platelets. The final transcript list contains 432 genes, which clearly cosegregate by cell type (platelet vs. leukocyte) (30). The development of platelet-specific gene (and protein) chips should lead to more widespread applicability of this technology to dissect mechanisms of platelet-related thrombotic disorders.

FROM TRANSCRIPTOMICS TO PROTEOMICS

Transcriptomic studies give information about gene expression but not about certain aspects of gene function (Fig. 1). Proteomic approaches can yield data about localization, interactions, posttranslational modifications, and activation states of gene products. While the human genome encodes some 22,000 genes (41), the number of functional proteins that can be generated through alternative splicing and posttranslational modifications is estimated to be at least one million (42).

PROTEOMIC TECHNIQUES: PROTEIN/PEPTIDE SEPARATION OPTIONS

Proteomic experiments begin with a protein mixture, which is digested to a peptide mixture, either in a gel or in solution. 2-DE has been available since the 1970s. Newer protein separation methods, which use in-solution proteolytic digestion, can detect proteins not well represented by 2-DE, such as transmembrane and basic proteins (43,44).

Peptide mixtures can be directly analyzed by MS, or separated by high-pressure liquid chromatography (HPLC) before mass-spectrometric analysis. The use of liquid chromatography-mass spectrometry (LC-MS) not only adds a time-consuming step, but also results in a dramatically higher number of detected peptides and facilitates automation (45). Multidimensional protein identification technology (MudPIT) employs ion-exchange and reverse-phase LC for peptide separation (46).

PROTEIN IDENTIFICATION: MASS-SPECTROMETRIC OPTIONS

MS has the capacity to identify proteins in a high throughput manner. The two main mass-spectroscopic options are electrospray ionization (ESI) and matrix-assisted laser desorption/ionization (MALDI). ESI is usually performed with tandem mass spectrometry (MS/MS) capability. MALDI is usually performed with time-of-flight (TOF) instruments recording only the mass spectrum of the peptide ions; no fragmentation information is collected. MALDI-TOF analysis can be performed rapidly but generates less statistical information than MS/MS data. For experiments with high sample complexity and a wide dynamic range, LC-MS/MS is the method now chosen by most proteomics researchers, and peptides are ionized via ESI (45).

PLASMA/SERUM PROTEOME

Plasma contains proteins whose concentrations vary over at least 15 orders of magnitude (47). Most abundant are albumin (50% of plasma protein content), immunoglobulins, fibrinogen, transferrin, haptoglobin, and lipoproteins. Removal of fibrinogen by clotting induces the disappearance of many other proteins involved in coagulation, such as prothrombin, which is absent in serum. Conversely, many peptides absent in plasma but detectable in serum are identified after coagulation.

"PEPTIDOMICS" AND "METABOLOMICS"

Peptides often have specific functions as mediators and indicators of biological processes. They play important roles as messengers, e.g., as hormones, growth factors, and cytokines, and also serve as indicators of protease activity. For analysis of circulating peptides and small proteins less than 20 kDa, also known as the "peptidome," use of platelet-depleted EDTA or citrate plasma is recommended. When serum is used, many peptides are generated from cellular components including platelets, enzymatic activities of coagulation cascades, and other proteases. These peptides impede discovery efforts because they mimic and obscure the desired "message from tissue" and cause false-positive results. Heparin alters the elution behavior of peptides (48). Protein modifications resulting in particular peptide patterns may reflect disease-specific protease activity in vivo, which produce useful biomarkers. The application of surface-enhanced laser desorption ionization (SELDI) to delineate low-molecular-weight proteomic profiles in patient-groups is discussed later in this chapter.

Metabolomics seeks to quantify small molecules that serve as physiological indicators within plasma or particular cells and tissues. The potential list of small molecules includes carbohydrates, peptides, lipids and metabolic intermediates such as amino acids, organic acids, and drug metabolites. Quantification is generally based on various methods of spectroscopy or chromatography. One of the challenges in this field is simultaneously detecting myriad compounds across a broad concentration range (25).

COAGULATION "SUBPROTEOME" IN HUMAN PLASMA

The pilot phase of the Plasma Proteome Project, organized by the Human Proteome Organization (HUPO), identified 34 coagulation-related proteins in human plasma (49). These included coagulation factors and their cofactors, natural anticoagulants, and regulators of fibrinolysis. However, several well-known coagulation factors escaped identification in this pilot phase, including factor VII, tissue factor, and thrombomodulin.

THE PLATELET PROTEOME: ACTIVATION-DEPENDENT CHANGES

Quiescent platelets display minimal translational activity. Platelet activation leads to the rapid translation of preexisting mRNA, with the release or derivation of platelet-secreted proteins, cytokines, exosomes, and microparticles. Using thrombin-stimulated platelets, a combination of MALDI-TOF and MudPIT identified more than 300 released proteins (50). Several of the secreted proteins have been identified in atherosclerotic lesions but are absent in normal vasculature; these include secretogranin III (a monocyte chemo-attractant precursor), cyclophilin A, and calumenin. These and other proteins released from platelets may contribute to atherosclerosis and to the thrombosis that complicates the disease. In another study, the use of 2-DE, MALDI-TOF, and LC-ESI MS/MS to study platelet dense granules led to the identification of an extracellular role for 14-3-3 zeta protein in atherosclerosis (51). Such secreted proteins are potential targets for future drug development, given their extracellular localization, without the risk of bleeding that complicates direct inhibition of platelet activation (43).

Maguire et al. (43) used LC-MS/MS to profile platelet proteins associated with detergent-resistant membrane lipid rafts. These lipid rafts may act as concentrating platforms that co-cluster receptors and signaling molecules, thus coordinating platelet activation and secretion. Proteins recruited upon vWF activation included GPIbα, glucose transporter 14 and C-terminal LIM protein 36. Targeting of such proteins may represent a novel therapeutic strategy in the prevention of thrombosis.

Novel membrane proteins that signal during platelet aggregation have been identified using LC-MS/MS, combined fractional diagonal chromatography, and micro-array techniques (52–54). Some of these proteins become phosphorylated on tyrosine or serine residues on platelet aggregation. Garcia et al. identified 41 proteins, which were differentially phosphorylated following stimulation by thrombin receptor activating peptide (TRAP) (55). Several of the proteins had not been previously reported in platelets, including the adapter downstream of tyrosine kinase 2 (Dok-2). Functional studies revealed the implication of Dok-2 in other signaling cascades, with a potentially important role in thrombus formation (56).

PROTEOME OF PROCOAGULANT MICROPARTICLES

Microparticles (MP) are small membrane vesicles that are released from cells upon activation or during apoptosis. Hardly detectable in the peripheral blood of healthy individuals, procoagulant MPs circulating at elevated levels are often associated with thrombotic propensity (57). MPs are thought to support coagulation by exposure of tissue factor as well as anionic phospholipids, and also stimulate cells to produce cytokines, cell-adhesion molecules, growth factors and TF (58). Thus, pharmacologic approaches could theoretically target the prothrombotic potential associated with MPs with respect to quantitative or qualitative endpoints.

Endothelial cell-derived procoagulant MPs have been studied by proteomic methods using human umbilical cord endothelial cells (HUVEC) (58). Endothelial dysfunction is associated with pre-eclampsia, thrombotic thrombocytopenic purpura (TTP), diabetes, systemic lupus erythematosis (SLE), antiphospholipid syndrome (APLS), and CAD. The platelet microparticle proteome has been characterized (59), and appears to have a composition distinct from the plasma proteome (60). This could be significant because while plasma-derived MPs imply cellular activation and possible damage, platelet-derived MPs appear to be present in healthy individuals. Smalley et al. (60) compared the proteomic profiles of plasma-derived and platelet-derived MPs using two methods, spectral count analysis and isotope-coded affinity tag (ICAT) labeling of proteins. Proteins present only in the plasma MPs included several associated with apoptosis, iron transport, complement components, and the coagulation process (protein S and factor VIII). Von Willebrand factor was enriched in plasma MPs, supporting the idea that plasma MPs are a procoagulant surface and associate with nascent thrombi.

FINDING BIOMARKERS FOR THROMBOTIC DISEASE STATES USING PROTEOMICS

SELDI-TOF MS has been used to study low-molecular-weight (1–20 kDa) proteomic profiles in patient groups. SELDI uses protein chips with an affinity matrix (charge, hydrophobicity, or other) and various wash buffers to allow the differential binding of proteins to the surface of the chip based on the stringency of their binding under various conditions. Marshall et al. (61) found that in MI a spectral pattern originated from the cleavage of complement C3-α chain to release the C3f peptide and cleavage of fibrinogen to release peptide A. However, ex vivo aminopeptidase activity can confound such findings (62). Svensson et al. reported that the proteomic analysis of plasma samples from a large family with type I protein C deficiency was able to discriminate those members who presented with deep vein thrombosis before the age of 40 from those who did not (63). They hypothesized that the approach may assist with discovery of a gene, which modifies the type I protein C deficiency phenotype of the early onset patients or their unaffected kindred. While they could not identify the individual peaks using SELDI, they noted that higher resolution instruments are becoming available, such as orthogonal MALDI (prOTOF). Their approach may have the power to produce a fingerprint profile indicative of thrombotic risk (64).

The use of proteomic techniques has led to the identification of potentially useful clinical markers for several disease states (Table 2). These include clusterin for preeclampsia (65), serum amyloid A for HELLP syndrome (66), ApoC-I and ApoC-III for stroke (67), fatty acid binding protein for stroke (68), α-1-antitrypsin isoform1 for acute coronary syndrome (69), and vitamin D binding protein for aspirin resistance in coronary ischemia (70).

PROTEOMIC DATA RESOURCES FOR BLOOD CELLS, THEIR DERIVATIVES, AND PLASMA/SERUM

Proteomic data about blood cells and components have become increasingly available in various databases. The Reactome Web site (http://www.reactome.org) includes continuously updated information for the complex biochemical networks that comprise hemostasis. Reactome, an online curated resource for human pathway data, provides an

Table 2 Plasma/Serum Biomarkers for Thrombotic Disease States Identified Using Proteomics

Context	Methods	Protein(s) identified	Ref.
Human patients			
Preeclampsia	2-DE	Clusterin	65
HELLP	2-DE	Serum amyloid A	66
Stroke	SELDI	Abnormal protein profile	67,68
Heart infarction	2-DE	α-1-antitrypsin isoform 1	69
Aspirin resistant coronary disease	2-DE	Vitamin D–binding protein	70
Congenital protein C deficiency with and without deep venous thrombosis	SELDI	Distinct protein profiles	63
Animal models			
Rat pulmonary embolism	2-DE	Abnormal protein profile	71

Abbreviations: 2-DE, two-dimensional electrophoresis; SELDI, surface-enhanced laser desorption ionization.

infrastructure for the interpretation of large-scale datasets including microarray data (72). The HUPO Proteomics Standards Initiative has produced a document, known as the "minimum information about a proteomics experiment" (MIAPE), which enumerates several integrated databases (73). Proteomic data for serum and plasma can be accessed through web sites of HUPO (http://www.hupo.org) and the Plasma Proteome Institute (http://www.plasmaproteome.org). Proteomic data have been published for platelets (reviewed in (29,30,56,74)), platelet-α granules (75), platelet dense granules (51), red blood cells (76,77), neutrophils (78), plasma and platelet-derived microparticles (59,60), and endothelial cell-derived microparticles (58).

INTEGRATING TRANSCRIPTOMIC AND PROTEOMIC STUDIES

Although studies in platelets have shown relatively good correlation between proteomic and transcriptomic data in the endpoints of detection and identification, there is sometimes discordance between the two. Microarray studies have shown that receptors, integrins, and glycoproteins are over-represented in platelets, and proteomic studies have supported these findings (35). The lack of detailed quantitative correlations limits the ability to compare platelet gene and protein levels with those of nucleated cells. Some studies have found that about one third of platelet proteins identified by proteomic methods are not reflected in the transcriptome (33,79–81). The discordance may be due to (*i*) the limited mRNA stability of these genes, (*ii*) failure of microarray analysis to detect very low levels of RNA, (*iii*) the occurrence of proteins which may be synthesized in megakaryocytes, after which mRNA is degraded, and (*iv*) the fact that some proteins may be taken up from plasma or from other cells rather than synthesized in megakaryocytes or platelets (81). Conversely, mRNA transcripts identified by transcriptomic methods are sometimes not detected by proteomic techniques; the frequency of this problem is unclear. When proteins are not identified, this may be due to the failure of current proteomic methods to identify proteins with certain structural or biochemical characteristics, and/or due to lack of translation of mRNA (81). Using suppressive-subtractive hybridization PCR, one group found gender differences in platelet transcripts, which were consistently reflected in protein levels (82).

There is no clear relationship between mRNA (or protein) levels and the importance of the resulting protein to cellular function. Dynamic changes in levels of rare transcripts can have more relevance to cellular function than absolute levels of common transcripts. For some genes and their corresponding proteins, substantial fluctuations in levels may be normal, whereas for others, small changes may carry a large impact on platelet function. The level of redundancy of transcripts and the amplification of small signals by downstream transduction pathways are factors that contribute to the unequal relationship between abundance and functional significance.

PEPTIDE LIBRARIES, PEPTIDE MICROARRAYS, AND ACTIVITY-BASED PROTEIN PROFILING

New methods for mapping protease specificity are being used as strategies for the design of enzyme inhibitors of the coagulation cascade (83). Competitive activity-based protein profiling (ABPP) uses active site-directed probes to identify enzyme inhibitors (84,85). Peptide libraries that include fluorogenic and binding tags are generated by solid-phase synthesis and screened for protease substrate recognition. When these peptide libraries are very large, microarrays have advantages over well plates. Gosalia et al. (86) used peptide microarrays to examine the specificities of human blood serine proteases including thrombin, factor Xa, plasmin, and urokinase plasminogen activator. The arrays provided complete maps of protease specificity for the substrates tested and allowed for detection of cooperative interactions between substrate subsites. Peptide-peptide nucleic acid libraries have been subjected to thrombin, plasmin, and human plasma (normal or warfarin-treated) (87). Raffler et al. identified a novel class of small peptides that inhibit thrombin using mRNA display (88). Dickopf et al. identified 60 ligands for factor VIIa using surface plasmon resonance detection of arrays presenting a variety of compound fragments. Phage display has been applied to factor Xa, urokinase plasminogen activator, and other proteases, leading to generation of peptide inhibitors (83). Blue et al. (89) used high throughput screening to identify a novel small molecule inhibitor of αIIbβ3-mediated platelet interaction with fibrinogen.

CONCLUSIONS AND FUTURE PERSPECTIVES

High throughput technologies have facilitated the understanding of dynamic changes in gene and protein expression in platelets, endothelial cells, and other players in thrombogenesis. Microarray data identified differentially expressed genes that comprise molecular signatures for several thrombotic diseases (Table 1). Transcriptome data constituted the basis for the discovery of novel molecules in platelets, such as the transporters for GABA, glutamate, and dopamine, as well as receptors involved in signaling. Proteomic approaches have identified biomarkers for thrombotic disease states (Table 2) as well as a wealth of data about blood cells and their derivatives. Proteomic experiments have uncovered proteins, previously not known to be secreted by activated platelets, which represent potential therapeutic targets in atherothrombosis. Figure 2 illustrates how transcriptomics and proteomics can direct the search for new therapeutic drugs. Both transcriptomic and proteomic approaches still face challenges in the areas of sample processing, separating signal from noise, and obtaining statistical power. Advances in technology make it more likely that these approaches will reach the bedside in the form of new antithrombotic agents.

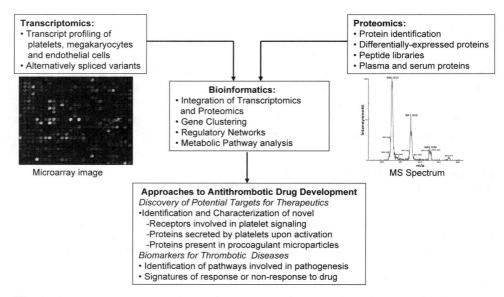

Microarray image   MS Spectrum

Figure 2 A model outlining the application of transcriptomic and proteomic data for the development of new antithrombotic agents.

REFERENCES

1. Liu ET. Expression genomics and drug development: towards predictive pharmacology. Brief Funct Genomic Proteomic 2005; 3(4):303–321.
2. Allison DB, Cui X, Page GP, et al. Microarray data analysis: from disarray to consolidation and consensus. Nat Rev Genet 2006; 7(1):55–65.
3. Strauss E. Arrays of hope. Cell 2006; 127(4):657–659.
4. Moore DF, Li H, Jeffries N, et al. Using peripheral blood mononuclear cells to determine a gene expression profile of acute ischemic stroke: a pilot investigation. Circulation 2005; 111(2):212–221.
5. Tang Y, Xu H, Du X, et al. Gene expression in blood changes rapidly in neutrophils and monocytes after ischemic stroke in humans: a microarray study. J Cereb Blood Flow Metab 2006; 26(8):1089–1102.
6. Ma J, Liew CC. Gene profiling identifies secreted protein transcripts from peripheral blood cells in coronary artery disease. J Mol Cell Cardiol 2003; 35(8):993–998.
7. Tabibiazar R, Wagner RA, Ashley EA, et al. Signature patterns of gene expression in mouse atherosclerosis and their correlation to human coronary disease. Physiol Genomics 2005; 22(2):213–226.
8. Karra R, Vemullapalli S, Dong C, et al. Molecular evidence for arterial repair in atherosclerosis. Proc Natl Acad Sci U S A 2005; 102(46):16789–16794.
9. Seo D, Wang T, Dressman H, et al. Gene expression phenotypes of atherosclerosis. Arterioscler Thromb Vasc Biol 2004; 24(10):1922–1927.
10. Healy AM, Pickard MD, Pradhan AD, et al. Platelet expression profiling and clinical validation of myeloid-related protein-14 as a novel determinant of cardiovascular events. Circulation 2006; 113(19):2278–2284.
11. Potti A, Bild A, Dressman HK, et al. Gene-expression patterns predict phenotypes of immune-mediated thrombosis. Blood 2006; 107(4):1391–1396.
12. Tomic V, Russwurm S, Moller E, et al. Transcriptomic and proteomic patterns of systemic inflammation in on-pump and off-pump coronary artery bypass grafting. Circulation 2005; 112(19):2912–2920.

13. Seeburger J, Hoffmann J, Wendel HP, et al. Gene expression changes in leukocytes during cardiopulmonary bypass are dependent on circuit coating. Circulation 2005; 112 (9 suppl):I224–I228.
14. Gnatenko DV, Cupit LD, Huang EC, et al. Platelets express steroidogenic 17beta-hydroxysteroid dehydrogenases. Distinct profiles predict the essential thrombocythemic phenotype. Thromb Haemost 2005; 94(2):412–421.
15. Okada M, Suzuki K, Takada K, et al. Detection of up-regulated genes in thrombin-stimulated human umbilical vein endothelial cells. Thromb Res 2006; 118(6):715–721.
16. Hamid C, Norgate K, D'Cruz DP, et al. Anti-beta2GPI-antibody-induced endothelial cell gene expression profiling reveals induction of novel pro-inflammatory genes potentially involved in primary antiphospholipid syndrome. Ann Rheum Dis 2007; 66(8):1000–1007.
17. McLaughlin JN, Mazzoni MR, Cleator JH, et al. Thrombin modulates the expression of a set of genes including thrombospondin-1 in human microvascular endothelial cells. J Biol Chem 2005; 280(23):22172–22180.
18. Meyer-Kirchrath J, Debey S, Glandorff C, et al. Gene expression profile of the Gs-coupled prostacyclin receptor in human vascular smooth muscle cells. Biochem Pharmacol 2004; 67(4):757–765.
19. Franscini N, Bachli EB, Blau N, et al. Gene expression profiling of inflamed human endothelial cells and influence of activated protein C. Circulation 2004; 110(18):2903–2909.
20. Zhang W, Chuang YJ, Swanson R, et al. Antiangiogenic antithrombin down-regulates the expression of the proangiogenic heparan sulfate proteoglycan, perlecan, in endothelial cells. Blood 2004; 103(4):1185–1191.
21. Riewald M, Ruf W. Protease-activated receptor-1 signaling by activated protein C in cytokine-perturbed endothelial cells is distinct from thrombin signaling. J Biol Chem 2005; 280(20):19808–19814.
22. Jagadeeswaran P, Kulkarni V, Carrillo M, et al. Zebrafish: from hematology to hydrology. J Thromb Haemost 2007; 5(suppl 1):300–304.
23. Rubinstein AL. Zebrafish: from disease modeling to drug discovery. Curr Opin Drug Discov Devel 2003; 6(2):218–223.
24. Ebbesen LS, Olesen SH, Kruhoffer M, et al. Folate deficiency induced hyperhomocysteinemia changes the expression of thrombosis-related genes. Blood Coagul Fibrinolysis 2006; 17(4):293–301.
25. Miller DT, Ridker PM, Libby P, et al. Atherosclerosis: the path from genomics to therapeutics. J Am Coll Cardiol 2007; 49(15):1589–1599.
26. Rabausch K, Bretschneider E, Sarbia M, et al. Regulation of thrombomodulin expression in human vascular smooth muscle cells by COX-2-derived prostaglandins. Circ Res 2005; 96(1):e1–e6.
27. Montero I, Orbe J, Varo N, et al. C-reactive protein induces matrix metalloproteinase-1 and -10 in human endothelial cells: implications for clinical and subclinical atherosclerosis. J Am Coll Cardiol 2006; 47(7):1369–1378.
28. Zon LI, Peterson RT. In vivo drug discovery in the zebrafish. Nat Rev Drug Discov 2005; 4(1):35–44.
29. Macaulay IC, Carr P, Gusnanto A, et al. Platelet genomics and proteomics in human health and disease. J Clin Invest 2005; 115(12):3370–3377.
30. Gnatenko DV, Perrotta PL, Bahou WF. Proteomic approaches to dissect platelet function: half the story. Blood 2006; 108(13):3983–3991.
31. Gnatenko DV, Dunn JJ, McCorkle SR, et al. Transcript profiling of human platelets using microarray and serial analysis of gene expression. Blood 2003; 101(6):2285–2293.
32. Rox JM, Bugert P, Muller J, et al. Gene expression analysis in platelets from a single donor: evaluation of a PCR-based amplification technique. Clin Chem 2004; 50(12):2271–2278.
33. McRedmond JP, Park SD, Reilly DF, et al. Integration of proteomics and genomics in platelets: a profile of platelet proteins and platelet-specific genes. Mol Cell Proteomics 2004; 3(2):133–144.
34. Bugert P, Dugrillon A, Gunaydin A, et al. Messenger RNA profiling of human platelets by microarray hybridization. Thromb Haemost 2003; 90(4):738–748.
35. Bugert P, Kluter H. Profiling of gene transcripts in human platelets: an update of the platelet transcriptome. Platelets 2006; 17(7):503–504.

36. Raghavachari N, Xu X, Harris A, et al. Amplified expression profiling of platelet transcriptome reveals changes in arginine metabolic pathways in patients with sickle cell disease. Circulation 2007; 115(12):1551–1562.
37. Frankhauser P, Grimmer Y, Bugert P, et al. Characterization of the neuronal dopamine transporter DAT in human blood platelets. Neurosci Lett 2006; 399(3):197–201.
38. Rainesalo S, Keranen T, Saransaari P, et al. GABA and glutamate transporters are expressed in human platelets. Brain Res Mol Brain Res 2005; 141(2):161–165.
39. Krishnan U, Goodall AH, Bugert P. Letter by Krishnan et al regarding article, "Platelet expression profiling and clinical validation of myeloid-related protein-14 as a novel determinant of cardiovascular events". Circulation 2007; 115(6):e186.
40. Eisenstein M. Microarrays: quality control. Nature 2006; 442(7106):1067–1070.
41. Finishing the euchromatic sequence of the human genome Nature 2004; 431(7011):931–945.
42. Hochstrasser DF, Sanchez JC, Appel RD. Proteomics and its trends facing nature's complexity. Proteomics 2002; 2(7):807–812.
43. Maguire PB, Foy M, Fitzgerald DJ. Using proteomics to identify potential therapeutic targets in platelets. Biochem Soc Trans 2005; 33(Pt 2):409–412.
44. de Hoog CL, Mann M. Proteomics. Annu Rev Genomics Hum Genet 2004; 5:267–293.
45. Kocher T, Superti-Furga G. Mass spectrometry-based functional proteomics: from molecular machines to protein networks. Nat Methods 2007; 4(10):807–815.
46. Delahunty CM, Yates JR III. MudPIT: multidimensional protein identification technology. Biotechniques 2007; 43(5):563, 565, 567.
47. Thadikkaran L, Siegenthaler MA, Crettaz D, et al. Recent advances in blood-related proteomics. Proteomics 2005; 5(12):3019–3034.
48. Tammen H, Schulte I, Hess R, et al. Peptidomic analysis of human blood specimens: comparison between plasma specimens and serum by differential peptide display. Proteomics 2005; 5(13):3414–3422.
49. Ping P, Vondriska TM, Creighton CJ, et al. A functional annotation of subproteomes in human plasma. Proteomics 2005; 5(13):3506–3519.
50. Coppinger JA, Cagney G, Toomey S, et al. Characterization of the proteins released from activated platelets leads to localization of novel platelet proteins in human atherosclerotic lesions. Blood 2004; 103(6):2096–2104.
51. Hernandez-Ruiz L, Valverde F, Jimenez-Nunez MD, et al. Organellar proteomics of human platelet dense granules reveals that 14-3-3zeta is a granule protein related to atherosclerosis. J Proteome Res 2007; 6(11):4449–4457.
52. Martens L, Van DP, Van DJ, et al. The human platelet proteome mapped by peptide-centric proteomics: a functional protein profile. Proteomics 2005; 5(12):3193–3204.
53. Moebius J, Zahedi RP, Lewandrowski U, et al. The human platelet membrane proteome reveals several new potential membrane proteins. Mol Cell Proteomics 2005; 4(11):1754–1761.
54. Nanda N, Bao M, Lin H, et al. Platelet endothelial aggregation receptor 1 (PEAR1), a novel epidermal growth factor repeat-containing transmembrane receptor, participates in platelet contact-induced activation. J Biol Chem 2005; 280(26):24680–24689.
55. Garcia A, Prabhakar S, Hughan S, et al. Differential proteome analysis of TRAP-activated platelets: involvement of DOK-2 and phosphorylation of RGS proteins. Blood 2004; 103(6):2088–2095.
56. Garcia A. Proteome analysis of signaling cascades in human platelets. Blood Cells Mol Dis 2006; 36(2):152–156.
57. Morel O, Toti F, Hugel B, et al. Procoagulant microparticles: disrupting the vascular homeostasis equation? Arterioscler Thromb Vasc Biol 2006; 26(12):2594–2604.
58. Banfi C, Brioschi M, Wait R, et al. Proteome of endothelial cell-derived procoagulant microparticles. Proteomics 2005; 5(17):4443–4455.
59. Garcia BA, Smalley DM, Cho H, et al. The platelet microparticle proteome. J Proteome Res 2005; 4(5):1516–1521.
60. Smalley DM, Root KE, Cho H, et al. Proteomic discovery of 21 proteins expressed in human plasma-derived but not platelet-derived microparticles. Thromb Haemost 2007; 97(1):67–80.

61. Marshall J, Kupchak P, Zhu W, et al. Processing of serum proteins underlies the mass spectral fingerprinting of myocardial infarction. J Proteome Res 2003; 2(4):361–372.
62. Misek DE, Kuick R, Wang H, et al. A wide range of protein isoforms in serum and plasma uncovered by a quantitative intact protein analysis system. Proteomics 2005; 5(13):3343–3352.
63. Svensson AM, Whiteley GR, Callas PW, et al. SELDI-TOF plasma profiles distinguish individuals in a protein C-deficient family with thrombotic episodes occurring before age 40. Thromb Haemost 2006; 96(6):725–730.
64. Scully MF. Plasma peptidome: A new approach for assessing thrombotic risk? Thromb Haemost 2006; 96(6):697.
65. Watanabe H, Hamada H, Yamada N, et al. Proteome analysis reveals elevated serum levels of clusterin in patients with preeclampsia. Proteomics 2004; 4(2):537–543.
66. Heitner JC, Koy C, Kreutzer M, et al. Differentiation of HELLP patients from healthy pregnant women by proteome analysis—on the way towards a clinical marker set. J Chromatogr B Analyt Technol Biomed Life Sci 2006; 840(1):10–19.
67. Allard L, Lescuyer P, Burgess J, et al. ApoC-I and ApoC-III as potential plasmatic markers to distinguish between ischemic and hemorrhagic stroke. Proteomics 2004; 4(8):2242–2251.
68. Zimmermann-Ivol CG, Burkhard PR, Le Floch-Rohr J, et al. Fatty acid binding protein as a serum marker for the early diagnosis of stroke: a pilot study. Mol Cell Proteomics 2004; 3(1):66–72.
69. Mateos-Caceres PJ, Garcia-Mendez A, Lopez FA, et al. Proteomic analysis of plasma from patients during an acute coronary syndrome. J Am Coll Cardiol 2004; 44(8):1578–1583.
70. Lopez-Farre AJ, Mateos-Caceres PJ, Sacristan D, et al. Relationship between vitamin D binding protein and aspirin resistance in coronary ischemic patients: a proteomic study. J Proteome Res 2007; 6(7):2481–2487.
71. Li SQ, Qi HW, Wu CG, et al. Comparative proteomic study of acute pulmonary embolism in a rat model. Proteomics 2007; 7(13):2287–2299.
72. Vastrik I, D'Eustachio P, Schmidt E, et al. Reactome: a knowledge base of biologic pathways and processes. Genome Biol 2007; 8(3):R39.
73. Taylor CF, Paton NW, Lilley KS, et al. The minimum information about a proteomics experiment (MIAPE). Nat Biotechnol 2007; 25(8):887–893.
74. Dittrich M, Birschmann I, Stuhlfelder C, et al. Understanding platelets. Lessons from proteomics, genomics and promises from network analysis. Thromb Haemost 2005; 94(5):916–925.
75. Maynard DM, Heijnen HF, Horne MK, et al. Proteomic analysis of platelet alpha-granules using mass spectrometry. J Thromb Haemost 2007; 5(9):1945–1955.
76. Zhang Y, Zhang Y, Adachi J, et al. MAPU: Max-Planck Unified database of organellar, cellular, tissue and body fluid proteomes. Nucleic Acids Res 2007; 35(Database issue):D771–D779.
77. Pasini EM, Kirkegaard M, Mortensen P, et al. In-depth analysis of the membrane and cytosolic proteome of red blood cells. Blood 2006; 108(3):791–801.
78. Lominadze G, Powell DW, Luerman GC, et al. Proteomic analysis of human neutrophil granules. Mol Cell Proteomics 2005; 4(10):1503–1521.
79. Marcus K, Immler D, Sternberger J, et al. Identification of platelet proteins separated by two-dimensional gel electrophoresis and analyzed by matrix assisted laser desorption/ionization-time of flight-mass spectrometry and detection of tyrosine-phosphorylated proteins. Electrophoresis 2000; 21(13):2622–2636.
80. O'Neill EE, Brock CJ, von Kriegsheim AF, et al. Towards complete analysis of the platelet proteome. Proteomics 2002; 2(3):288–305.
81. Bugert P, Ficht M, Kluter H. Towards the identification of novel platelet receptors: Comparing RNA and proteome approaches. Transfus Med Hemother 2006; 33:236–243.
82. Hillmann AG, Harmon S, Park SD, et al. Comparative RNA expression analyses from small-scale, single-donor platelet samples. J Thromb Haemost 2006; 4(2):349–356.
83. Diamond SL. Methods for mapping protease specificity. Curr Opin Chem Biol 2007; 11(1):46–51.
84. Jessani N, Cravatt BF. The development and application of methods for activity-based protein profiling. Curr Opin Chem Biol 2004; 8(1):54–59.

85. Hagenstein MC, Sewald N. Chemical tools for activity-based proteomics. J Biotechnol 2006; 124(1):56–73.
86. Gosalia DN, Salisbury CM, Maly DJ, et al. Profiling serine protease substrate specificity with solution phase fluorogenic peptide microarrays. Proteomics 2005; 5(5):1292–1298.
87. Winssinger N, Damoiseaux R, Tully DC, et al. PNA-encoded protease substrate microarrays. Chem Biol 2004; 11(10):1351–1360.
88. Raffler NA, Schneider-Mergener J, Famulok M. A novel class of small functional peptides that bind and inhibit human alpha-thrombin isolated by mRNA display. Chem Biol 2003; 10(1):69–79.
89. Blue R, Murcia M, Karan C, et al. Application of high throughput screening to identify a novel {alpha}IIb-specific small molecule inhibitor of {alpha}IIb{beta}3-mediated platelet interaction with fibrinogen. Blood 2008; 111(3):1248–1256.

9

Overview of New Anticoagulant Drugs

Nahid Qushmaq and Jeffrey I. Weitz
Department of Medicine, Henderson Research Centre and McMaster University, Hamilton, Ontario, Canada

INTRODUCTION

Arterial and venous thromboses are major causes of morbidity and mortality. Whereas arterial thrombosis is the most common cause of myocardial infarction (MI), stroke, and limb gangrene, venous thrombosis can be complicated by potentially fatal pulmonary embolism (PE) and post-phlebitic syndrome. Arterial thrombi, which form under high-shear conditions, consist of platelet aggregates held together by small amounts of fibrin. Because of the preponderance of platelets, strategies to inhibit arterial thrombogenesis focus mainly on drugs that block platelet function. However, such strategies often include anticoagulants to prevent fibrin deposition, and these are also the drugs of choice for prevention of cardioembolic events. In contrast to arterial thrombi, venous thrombi are predominantly composed of fibrin and trapped red blood cells and contain relatively few platelets. Consequently, anticoagulants are the mainstay for prevention and treatment of venous thrombosis. Focusing on new anticoagulant drugs for the prevention and treatment of arterial and venous thrombosis, this chapter (*i*) reviews arterial and venous thrombogenesis, (*ii*) outlines new anticoagulant strategies, and (*iii*) provides clinical perspective as to which new strategies have the greatest chance of success.

THROMBOGENESIS

Arterial thrombosis is typically initiated by spontaneous or mechanical rupture of atherosclerotic plaque, a process that exposes thrombogenic material found in the lipid-rich core of the plaque to the blood (1). Intraluminal thrombus superimposed on disrupted atherosclerotic plaque impairs blood flow. Higher shear promotes platelet and fibrin deposition, resulting in the formation of an occlusive thrombus that can obstruct blood flow to organs, including the heart, brain, or extremities.

Venous thrombi, which consist mainly of fibrin and red blood cells, develop under low-flow conditions. Often originating in the muscular veins of the calf or in the valve cusp pockets of the deep calf veins, coagulation in these sites is likely initiated by activation of the vascular endothelium and is augmented by venous stasis. Damage to the vessel wall may also contribute to venous thrombosis after major hip or knee surgery.

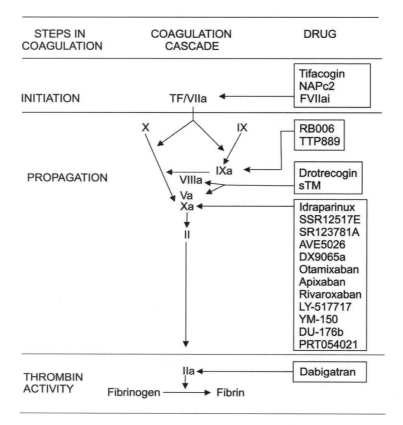

Figure 1 Steps in blood coagulation and sites of action of new anticoagulants. Initiation of coagulation is triggered by the factor VIIa/tissue factor complex (VIIa/TF), which activates factor IX (IX) and X (X). Activated factor IX (IXa) propagates coagulation by activating X in a reaction that utilizes activated factor VIII (VIIIa) as a cofactor. Activated factor X (Xa), with activated factor V (Va) as a cofactor, converts prothrombin to thrombin (IIa). Thrombin then converts fibrinogen to fibrin. Tifacogin, a recombinant form of TFPI, NAPc2, and active site–blocked factor VIIa (VIIai), target VIIa/TF. RB006 and TTP889 inhibit IXa. Drotrecogin, a recombinant form of activated protein C, inhibits propagation of coagulation by inactivating Va and VIIIa. By catalyzing thrombin-mediated activation of protein C, sTM also promotes the inactivation of Va and VIIIa. Idraparinux, SSR12517E, SR123781A, and AVE5026 are indirect inhibitors of Xa, whereas DX9065a, otamixaban, apixaban, rivaroxaban, LY-517717, YM-150, DU-176b, and PRT054021 are direct Xa inhibitors. Dabigatran etexilate is a direct inhibitor of IIa. *Abbreviations*: TFPI, tissue factor pathway inhibitor; NaPc2, nematode anticoagulant peptide; sTM, soluble thrombomodulin.

Initiation of coagulation in veins or arteries is triggered by tissue factor (Fig. 1), a cellular receptor for activated factor VII (factor VIIa) and factor VII (2). Most nonvascular cells express tissue factor in a constitutive fashion, whereas de novo tissue factor synthesis can be induced in monocytes (3,4). Injury to the arterial or venous wall exposes nonvascular tissue factor–expressing cells to blood (2). Lipid-laden macrophages in the core of atherosclerotic plaques are particularly rich in tissue factor (1), thereby explaining the propensity for thrombus formation at sites of plaque disruption. Factor VIIa, found in small amounts in normal plasma, binds to exposed tissue factor, as does factor VII. Bound factor VII can undergo autoactivation and, thereby, augment the local concentration of factor VIIa (5). The factor VIIa/tissue factor complex then activates factors IX and X, leading to the generation of factors IXa and Xa, respectively. Factor IXa binds to factor VIIIa on membrane surfaces to form intrinsic tenase, a complex that amplifies coagulation by promoting additional factor X activation (2).

Factor Xa propagates coagulation by binding to factor Va on membrane surfaces to form the prothrombinase complex, which converts prothrombin to thrombin. Once it dissociates from the membrane surface, thrombin converts fibrinogen to fibrin monomer. Fibrin monomers polymerize to form the fibrin mesh, which is stabilized and cross-linked by factor XIIIa, a thrombin-activated transglutaminase. Thrombin amplifies its own generation by feedback activation of factor V and factor VIII, cofactors in the prothrombinase and intrinsic tenase complexes, respectively. Thrombin also serves as a potent platelet agonist, thereby triggering platelet activation and aggregation at sites of vascular injury (6).

NEW ANTICOAGULANT STRATEGIES

Anticoagulant strategies to inhibit thrombogenesis have focused on blocking initiation of coagulation, preventing the propagation of coagulation, or inhibiting thrombin (Fig. 1). Initiation of coagulation can be inhibited by agents that target the factor VIIa/tissue factor complex. Propagation of coagulation can be blocked by drugs that target factor IXa or factor Xa, or by inactivation of factors Va and VIIIa, key cofactors in coagulation. Finally, thrombin inhibitors prevent fibrin formation and block thrombin-mediated feedback activation of factors V and VIII. Drugs that target each of these steps will be discussed in turn.

INHIBITORS OF INITIATION OF COAGULATION

Drugs that target the factor VIIa/tissue factor complex inhibit the initiation of coagulation. Only parenteral agents in this category have reached phase II or III clinical testing (Table 1). These include tifacogin, a recombinant form of tissue factor pathway inhibitor, recombinant nematode anticoagulant peptide (NAPc2), and active site–inhibited factor VIIa (factor VIIai).

Tifacogin

A recombinant form of tissue factor pathway inhibitor expressed in *Saccharomyces cerevisae*, tifacogin has been evaluated in patients with sepsis. The drug has a half-life of minutes, which necessitates intravenous infusion, and is cleared by the liver. In a phase II

Table 1 Inhibitors of the Factor VIIa/Tissue Factor Complex

Drug	Route of administration	Mechanism of action	Stage of development as of 2008
Tifacogin	Intravenous	Inhibits factor VIIa in a factor Xa-dependent fashion	Phase III
NAPc2	Subcutaneous	Inhibits factor VIIa in a factor X or Xa-dependent fashion	Phase II
Factor VIIai	Intravenous	Competes with factor VIIa for tissue factor	Halted

Abbreviation: NaPc2, nematode anticoagulant peptide.

trial (7), 210 sepsis patients were randomized to receive one of two doses of tifacogin (25 or 50 g/kg/hr) by continuous infusion or placebo for four days. Compared with placebo, tifacogin produced a 20% relative reduction in 28-day mortality. Major bleeding occurred in 9% of patients treated with tifacogin and in 6% of those given placebo, a difference that was not statistically significant. Building on these results, a phase III trial compared tifacogin with placebo in 1754 severe sepsis patients (8). The primary endpoint, 28-day mortality, was similar with tifacogin and placebo (34.2% and 33.9%, respectively), while the rate of bleeding was significantly higher with tifacogin (6.5% and 4.8%, respectively). An ongoing phase III clinical trial is comparing two doses of tifacogin with placebo in patients with severe community-acquired pneumonia (www .clinicaltrials.gov).

NAPc2

An 85-amino acid polypeptide originally isolated from the canine hookworm *Ancylostoma caninum* (9), recombinant NAPc2 is expressed in yeast. NAPc2 binds to a noncatalytic site on factor X or factor Xa (10). Once bound to factor Xa, the NAPc2/factor Xa complex inhibits tissue factor–bound factor VIIa. Because it binds factor X with high affinity, NAPc2 has a half-life of approximately 50 hours after subcutaneous injection (11). Consequently, the drug can be given on alternate days.

Initial clinical trials with NAPc2 focused on venous thromboprophylaxis. In a phase II dose-finding study (12), 293 patients undergoing elective knee arthroplasty were given subcutaneous NAPc2 on the day of surgery, and every second day thereafter to a maximum of four doses. Best results were observed with a NAPc2 dose of 3.0 g/kg administered one hour after surgery. With this dose, the rate of venographically detected DVT in the operated leg was 12%, while the rate of proximal DVT was 1%. Major bleeding occurred in 2% of patients. Compared with historical controls, NAPc2 appears to have efficacy and safety similar to those of low-molecular-weight heparin (LMWH). However, prospective randomized trials are needed to confirm these findings.

More recent studies with NAPc2 have focused on arterial thrombosis. In a series of phase II clinical trials, NAPc2 was evaluated in patients with unstable angina or non-ST-elevation MI and in those undergoing percutaneous coronary interventions (PCIs). Addition of NAPc2 to usual antithrombotic therapy in 203 patients with acute coronary syndromes (ACS) reduced levels of prothrombin fragment 1.2 in a dose-dependent fashion without increasing the risk of bleeding (13). In a second trial, adjunctive NAPc2 (in doses ranging from 3.5 to 10 μg/kg) suppressed levels of prothrombin fragment 1.2 in patients undergoing elective PCI (14). An ongoing trial is evaluating NAPc2 as a substitute for heparin in the setting of PCI.

Factor VIIai

Recombinant factor VIIa that has its active site irreversibly blocked competes with factor VIIa for tissue factor binding, thereby attenuating the initiation of coagulation by the factor VIIa/tissue factor complex. On the basis of promising results in animal models of thrombosis (15,16), factor VIIai, given in doses ranging from 50 to 400 g/kg with or without adjunctive heparin, was compared with heparin alone in 491 patients undergoing elective PCI (17). Factor VIIai, with or without adjunctive heparin, produced no significant reduction in the primary endpoint, a composite of death, MI, need for urgent revascularization, abrupt vessel closure, or bailout use of glycoprotein IIb/IIIa antagonists or heparin at day 7 or at hospital discharge. Rates of major bleeding were similar with factor VIIai and heparin. Because of these disappointing results, factor VIIai has not been developed further for treatment of arterial thrombosis.

INHIBITORS OF PROPAGATION OF COAGULATION

Propagation of coagulation can be inhibited by drugs that target factor IXa or factor Xa or by agents that inactivate their respective cofactors, factor VIIIa and factor Va, respectively.

Factor IXa Inhibitors

Both parenteral and oral factor IXa inhibitors have been developed (Table 2). The parenteral factor IXa inhibitor is an RNA aptamer (designated RB006) that binds factor IXa with high affinity (18). In phase I studies (19), this aptamer produced rapid anticoagulation, as evidenced by a dose-dependent prolongation of the activated partial thromboplastin time. A unique aspect of RB006 is its potential for rapid neutralization by a complementary oligonucleotide (designated RB007). This drug-antidote pair is being explored for use in cardiopulmonary bypass surgery or in other indications where rapid anticoagulant reversal may be beneficial (20).

An orally active direct factor IXa inhibitor also has been evaluated. Designated TTP889, this agent completed a phase IIa clinical trial that was negative (21). On the basis of these results, further development of TTP880 has been halted.

Factor Xa Inhibitors

New factor Xa inhibitors include agents that block factor Xa indirectly or directly. Indirect inhibitors act by catalyzing factor Xa inhibition by antithrombin. In contrast, direct factor Xa inhibitors bind directly to the active site of factor Xa, thereby blocking its interaction with its substrates. Unlike the heparin/antithrombin complex, which has limited capacity to inhibit factor Xa incorporated into the prothrombinase complex (22,23), direct factor Xa inhibitors inhibit both free and platelet-bound factor Xa (24,25). This property may endow direct factor Xa inhibitors with an advantage over indirect inhibitors.

Indirect Factor Xa Inhibitors

The prototype of the new indirect factor Xa inhibitors is fondaparinux, a first-generation synthetic analog of the antithrombin-binding pentasaccharide found in heparin or LMWH (26). On the basis of the results of well-designed randomized clinical trials, fondaparinux is already licensed for prevention of venous thromboembolism (VTE) in patients

Table 2 Factor IXa Inhibitors

Drug	Route of administration	Mechanism of action	Stage of development as of 2008
RB006	Intravenous	Factor IXa-directed inhibitory RNA aptamer	Phase I
TTP889	Oral	Inhibits factor IXa incorporation into intrinsic tenase	Halted

Table 3 Indirect Factor Xa Inhibitors

Drug	Route of administration	Mechanism of action	Stage of development as of 2008
Idraparinux	Subcutaneous	Inhibits factor Xa in an antithrombin-dependent fashion	Completed phase III
SSR12517E	Subcutaneous	Biotinylated form of idraparinux	Phase III
SR123781A	Subcutaneous	Synthetic hexadecasaccharide that inhibits factor Xa and thrombin in an antithrombin-dependent fashion	Phase II
AVE5026	Subcutaneous	Ultra LMWH with an anti-Xa:anti-IIa ratio of 30:1	Phase III

Abbreviation: LMWH, low-molecular-weight heparin.

undergoing high-risk orthopedic surgery (27,28) and, in some countries, for VTE prevention in general surgical (29) or medical patients (30). Fondaparinux is also approved as an alternative to heparin or LMWH for initial treatment of VTE (31,32). Fondaparinux has been evaluated in patients with non-ST-segment elevation and with ST-segment elevation MI (33,34). In patients with non-ST-segment elevation ACS, fondaparinux is as effective as enoxaparin but causes less bleeding (33). However, catheter thrombosis can occur if fondaparinux-treated patients undergo PCI (33,34). Adjunctive heparin appears to reduce the risk of catheter thrombosis in this setting, but additional studies are needed to determine the safety of this approach.

Newer indirect factor Xa inhibitors are second and third-generation variants of fondaparinux, which include idraparinux, SSR126517E and SR123781A, as well as AVE5026, an ultra-LMWH (Table 3).

Idraparinux A hypermethylated derivative of fondaparinux, idraparinux binds antithrombin with such high affinity that its plasma half-life of 80 hours is similar to that of antithrombin (35). Because of its long half-life, idraparinux can be given subcutaneously on a once-weekly basis. In a phase II dose-finding trial, idraparinux was compared with warfarin in 659 patients with proximal deep vein thrombosis (DVT) (36). After a five- to seven-day course of enoxaparin, patients were randomized to receive once-weekly subcutaneous idraparinux (2.5, 5.0, 7.5, or 10 mg) or warfarin for 12 weeks. The primary endpoint, thrombus burden, as assessed by measuring changes in compression ultrasound and perfusion lung scan findings, was similar in all idraparinux groups and did not differ from that in the warfarin group. There was a clear dose response for major bleeding in patients given idraparinux with an unacceptably high frequency in those given the 10-mg dose. Two patients, both of whom received 5 mg of idraparinux once weekly, suffered a fatal bleed. Patients given the lowest dose of idraparinux had less bleeding than those randomized to warfarin ($p = 0.029$). On the basis of these results, a once-weekly 2.5-mg dose of idraparinux was chosen for further trials.

The phase III Van Gogh DVT and PE trials (37) randomized 2904 patients with acute symptomatic DVT and 2215 patients with PE to either a three- to six-month course of once-weekly subcutaneous idraparinux (at a dose of 2.5 mg) or a conventional therapy with LMWH or heparin followed by a vitamin K antagonist with dose adjusted to achieve a target international normalized ratio (INR) between 2 and 3. In the DVT patients, the rate of recurrent VTE at three months was similar in the idraparinux and conventionally treated groups (2.9% and 3.0%, respectively). Clinically relevant bleeds were less common with idraparinux than with conventional treatment (4.5% and 7.0%, respectively; $p = 0.004$). In the PE patients, idraparinux was less effective than conventional therapy at three months. Thus, recurrent VTE occurred in 3.4% of patients given idraparinux and in 1.6% of those receiving conventional therapy. Clinically relevant bleeding occurred in 5.8% of those given idraparinux and in 8.2% of those treated with heparin or LMWH followed by a vitamin K antagonist. On the basis of the results of these trials, idraparinux appears to have an acceptable safety profile compared with that of warfarin. The discordant results in the DVT and PE trials highlight the importance of adequate levels of anticoagulation for initial PE treatment because the majority of the recurrences occurred early. These findings suggest that PE patients require higher initial doses of idraparinux than DVT patients.

The efficacy of long-term idraparinux was evaluated in the van Gogh extension study (38). In this trial, 1215 patients who had completed six months of initial treatment of DVT or PE with either idraparinux or a vitamin K antagonist were randomized to an additional six months of treatment with either once-weekly subcutaneous idraparinux or with placebo. Compared with placebo, idraparinux produced a 72.9% relative reduction in the risk of recurrent VTE ($p = 0.002$), reducing recurrent events from 3.7% to 1%. Major bleeding occurred in 3.7% of those given idraparinux and included three fatal intracranial bleeds. In contrast, there were no major bleeds in the placebo group. These findings suggest that although effective compared with placebo, idraparinux causes excessive bleeding.

The AMADEUS trial randomized patients with atrial fibrillation to once-weekly subcutaneous idraparinux (at a dose of 2.5 mg) or to a vitamin K antagonist with the dose adjusted to achieve a target INR of 2 to 3 (39). The trial was stopped after 4576 patients were enrolled because of an excess in the rate of clinically relevant bleeds with idraparinux compared with that of vitamin K antagonists (19.7% and 11.3%, respectively; $p < 0.001$). Intracranial bleeding was also more frequent with idraparinux than with vitamin K antagonists (1.1% and 0.4%, respectively; $p = 0.014$). Elderly patients and those with renal insufficiency appeared to have the highest risk of bleeding. Rates of thromboembolism were lower with idraparinux than with vitamin K antagonists (hazard ratio 0.71; 95% confidence interval, 0.39–1.30). These findings raise the possibility that the dose of idraparinux was too high, particularly in older individuals or in those with renal impairment.

Based on the results of the van Gogh and AMADEUS trials, it is unlikely that idraparinux will be developed further. Instead, attention has shifted to SSR12517E.

SSR12517E A biotinylated form of idraparinux, SSR12517E exhibits the same pharmacokinetic and pharmacodynamic profile as idraparinux. Like idraparinux, SSR12517E is given subcutaneously on a once-weekly basis. The only difference is that the anticoagulant activity of SSR12517E can be rapidly neutralized by intravenous administration of avidin. A large tetrameric protein derived from egg white, avidin, binds biotin with high affinity to form a 1:1 stoichiometric complex, which is then cleared via the kidneys.

SSR12517E is now undergoing phase III evaluation in patients with symptomatic PE with or without evidence of DVT. Patients are given at least five days of heparin or LMWH before being randomized to SSR12517E or to a vitamin K antagonist.

SR123781A A synthetic hexadecasaccharide, SR123781A is composed of the antithrombin-binding synthetic pentasaccharide plus a thrombin-binding sulfated tetrasaccharide joined together by a central nonsulfated heptasaccharide. SR123781A binds antithrombin with high affinity (40). In addition to catalyzing factor Xa inhibition by antithrombin, SR123781A is long enough to bridge antithrombin to thrombin, thereby enhancing thrombin inhibition. Like heparin, therefore, SR123781A catalyzes the inhibition of both factor Xa and thrombin (40). Unlike heparin, SR123781A does not bind platelet factor 4 (PF4) or fibrin. Because it does not bind PF4, heparin-induced thrombocytopenia is unlikely to occur with SR123781A. Without affinity for fibrin, SR123781A does not promote the formation of the ternary heparin/thrombin/fibrin complex that protects fibrin-bound thrombin from inhibition by the antithrombin/heparin complex (41). In contrast to heparin, therefore, SR123781A appears capable of inhibiting fibrin-bound thrombin (42).

SR123781A is administered subcutaneously. It exhibits almost complete bioavailability after subcutaneous administration and produces a dose proportional increase in the activated partial thromboplastin time and anti-factor Xa activity. The drug is primarily cleared by the kidneys where it is excreted intact. SR123781A has completed phase II evaluation for prophylaxis in patients undergoing knee arthroplasty. Although the results have not been reported, further development of SR123781A has been halted.

AVE5026 An ultra-LMWH, AVE5026 has a mean molecular weight less than 3000. Like fondaparinux, AVE5026 exhibits almost complete bioavailability after subcutaneous injection and has a half-life of 17 hours. Therefore, AVE5026 is given subcutaneously on a once-daily basis. Unlike fondaparinux, which only catalyzes factor Xa inhibition by antithrombin, AVE5026 retains residual activity against thrombin and has an anti-Xa to anti-IIa ratio of 30 to 1. AVE5026 also induces TFPI release, which is not a feature of fondaparinux.

In the phase II TREK trial, once-daily subcutaneous AVE5026 (at doses of 5, 10, 20, or 40 mg) was compared with enoxaparin (40 mg) for prophylaxis in 678 patients undergoing elective knee-replacement surgery. AVE5026 produced a dose-dependent reduction in total VTE from 40% to 5.3%, and at doses of 20, 40, and 60 mg, AVE5026 appeared to be more efficacious than enoxaparin (VTE rates of 15.6%, 13.6%, and 5.3%, respectively, compared with 35.8% with enoxaparin). There was also a dose-dependent increase in major plus minor bleeding with AVE5026 (from 0% to 3.4%), and rates of bleeding were higher with AVE5026 than with enoxaparin at doses of 40 mg/day or higher (43). AVE5026 is now undergoing phase III evaluation for prevention of VTE in a variety of medical and surgical settings.

Direct Factor Xa Inhibitors

Direct factor Xa inhibitors include parenteral agents, such as DX9065a and otamixaban, as well as several orally active drugs. All the direct factor Xa inhibitors are small molecules that reversibly block the active site of factor Xa (Table 4). The large number of oral factor Xa inhibitors under development highlight the continued focus on identifying new oral anticoagulants that can replace the vitamin K antagonists, such as warfarin.

DX-9065a A synthetic nonpeptidic direct factor Xa inhibitor, DX9065a is administered parentally, has a dose-dependent half-life that ranges from 40 minutes to 5 hours, and is cleared by the kidneys (44–46). DX9065a was evaluated in patients with non-ST-elevation ACS and in patients undergoing PCI. In the ACS trial, 402 patients were randomized to weight-adjusted heparin or to low- or high-dose DX-9065a (47). The primary efficacy endpoint, a composite of death, MI, urgent revascularization, or ischemia, occurred in 33.6%, 34.3%, and 31.3% of patients, respectively. Major bleeding

Table 4 Direct Factor Xa Inhibitors

Drug	Route of administration	Stage of development as of 2007
DX-9065a	Intravenous	Stopped at phase II
Otamixaban	Intravenous	Phase II
Razaxaban	Oral	Halted
Rivaroxaban	Oral	Phase III
Apixaban	Oral	Phase III
LY-517717	Oral	Phase II
YM-150	Oral	Phase II
DU-176b	Oral	Phase II
PRT054021	Oral	Phase II

occurred in 3.3% of those randomized to heparin and in less than 1% of those who received DX-9065a. In the PCI trial, 175 patients were randomized to open-label DX-9065a or to heparin in one of four sequential phases (48). Although thrombotic events were rare in all phases of the study, enrollment in the phase evaluating the lowest dose of DX-9065 was stopped because of catheter thrombosis. Major bleeding events were uncommon, and there was no apparent dose response. Although promising, DX9065a has not undergone further clinical evaluation.

Otamixaban A noncompetitive inhibitor of factor Xa, this agent is administered intravenously and has a half-life of two to three hours (49). It is excreted unchanged in the urine, whereas metabolites appear in the feces. A phase IIa study compared a 24-hour otamixaban infusion with placebo in patients with stable coronary artery disease. The addition of otamixaban to usual medications did not cause bleeding, and otamixaban produced a rapid and sustained increase in anti-factor Xa activity (50). A phase II trial comparing otamixaban with heparin in patients undergoing nonurgent PCI demonstrated greater reductions in the levels of prothrombin fragment 1.2 with otamixaban than with heparin and no difference in the rate of major bleeding (51). An ongoing phase II trial is comparing otamixaban with heparin plus eptifibatide in patients undergoing PCI (clinical trials.gov).

Razaxaban Razaxaban, a nonpeptidic oral factor Xa inhibitor, underwent phase II evaluation for thromboprophylaxis after knee arthroplasty (52). The primary endpoint, a composite of venographically detected DVT and symptomatic VTE, occurred in 8.6% of patients randomized to the lowest dose of razaxaban and in 15.9% of those given enoxaparin. Major bleeding occurred in 0.7% of patients given the lowest dose of razaxaban and in none of those treated with enoxaparin. The three higher dose razaxaban arms were stopped prematurely because of increased rates of major bleeding. Because of the narrow therapeutic index and pharmacological limitations, further development of razaxaban was halted in favor of apixaban.

Apixaban A variant of razaxaban that has superior pharmacological properties, apixaban has high oral bioavailability and a half-life of about 12 hours (53). Food has no effect on its absorption, and the drug produces a predictable anticoagulant effect. Apixaban is cleared through both the fecal and renal route with renal elimination accounting for about 25% of drug clearance (53).

In a phase II trial in 1238 patients undergoing knee-replacement surgery, apixaban was compared with enoxaparin or with warfarin (54). Apixaban was given in total daily doses of 5, 10, or 20 mg using a once-daily or twice-daily regimen. The primary endpoint, a composite of total VTE and all-cause mortality, was lower with all doses of apixaban than with enoxaparin or warfarin. At daily doses of 10 or 20 mg, the efficacy of apixaban appeared to be better with twice-daily as compared with that of once-daily dosing. Total bleeding was less frequent with 5-mg apixaban once daily or with 2.5-mg twice daily than it was with enoxaparin or warfarin. With higher doses of apixaban, there was more bleeding than with enoxaparin or warfarin. On the basis of these data, a dose of 2.5-mg apixaban twice daily will be compared with that of enoxaparin in two phase III trials in patients undergoing knee-replacement surgery and in one trial in patients undergoing hip-replacement surgery. This dose will also be evaluated for thromboprophylaxis in medical patients. In a phase II trial, 520 patients with proximal DVT were randomized to a three-month course of treatment with apixaban (at doses of 5- or 10-mg twice daily or 20-mg once daily) or to conventional anticoagulant therapy with LMWH or fondaparinux followed by a vitamin K antagonist. The primary efficacy endpoint, a composite of recurrent VTE and increased thrombus burden (as detected by repeated ultrasound and perfusion lung scanning), occurred in 6.0%, 5.6%, and 2.6% of patients given apixaban at doses of 5- or 10-mg twice daily or 20-mg once daily, respectively, and in 4.2% of those treated with conventional therapy. Rates of major plus clinically relevant nonmajor bleeding were 8.6%, 4.5%, and 7.3%, respectively, in the apixaban arms and 7.9% in those given conventional treatment. On the basis of these results, phase III trials will evaluate a 2.5- and a 5-mg twice-daily regimen of apixaban for initial and extended treatment of VTE.

Apixaban also is being compared with warfarin or with aspirin in two separate phase III trials in patients with atrial fibrillation. Phase II dose-finding studies are examining the utility of apixaban for thromboprophylaxis in cancer patients and for prevention of recurrent ischemia in ACS patients.

Rivaroxaban An oxazolidone derivative, rivaroxaban has oral bioavailability of 80%, inhibits factor Xa with a K_i of 0.4 nM, and has a half-life of about nine hours. It is cleared by the kidneys and the gut (55). Rivaroxaban has been evaluated for thromboprophylaxis in patients undergoing knee or hip arthroplasty in four phase II trials. Proof of principle was established in a series of dose-finding studies in patients undergoing elective hip or knee arthroplasty (56–60). These phase II trials compared once- or twice-daily oral rivaroxaban dosing regimens, in total daily doses ranging from 5 to 60 mg, with those of enoxaparin. There was no clear dose-response relationship for efficacy, and once-daily dosing appeared to be as effective as the twice-daily regimens. Compared with enoxaparin, the point estimates for major bleeding were higher with rivaroxaban at daily doses higher than 10 mg. On the basis of these results, a 10-mg once-daily dose was evaluated in the phase III program.

The REgulation of Coagulation in major Orthopedic surgery reducing the Risk of DVT and PE (RECORD)-3 trial compared oral rivaroxaban (10-mg once daily, started 6–8 hours after surgery) with subcutaneous enoxaparin (40-mg once daily, started the evening before surgery) in 2531 patients undergoing knee-replacement surgery (61). Both regimens were continued for 10 to 14 days. The primary efficacy endpoint, a composite of DVT, nonfatal PE, and all-cause mortality, occurred in 9.6% of patients receiving rivaroxaban and in 18.9% of those given enoxaparin. Thus, rivaroxaban was associated with a 49% reduction in relative risk, a difference that was statistically significant ($p < 0.001$). Major VTE, a composite of proximal DVT, nonfatal PE, and VTE-related mortality, occurred in 1.0% of patients given rivaroxaban and in 2.6% of those treated with enoxaparin; a difference that was statistically significant ($p = 0.01$). Symptomatic VTE occurred in 1.0% and 2.7% of those given rivaroxaban or enoxaparin, respectively. Major bleeding rates were 0.6% and 0.5% in the rivaroxaban and enoxaparin-treated groups, respectively, whereas any bleeding occurred in 4.9% and 4.8%, respectively. Three other phase III orthopedic trials have been conducted with rivaroxaban. Two are completed and the third is underway.

The RECORD 1 and 2 trials evaluated rivaroxaban in patients undergoing hip arthroplasty. In the RECORD 1 trial (62), 4541 such patients were randomized to either oral rivaroxaban (10-mg once daily) or to subcutaneous enoxaparin (40-mg once daily). Both drugs were given for five weeks. Compared with enoxaparin, rivaroxaban reduced the rate of total VTE from 3.7% to 1.1% ($p < 0.001$) and the rate of major VTE from 2.0% to 0.2% ($p < 0.001$). Rates of major bleeding with rivaroxaban and enoxaparin were similar (0.3% and 0.1%, respectively) as were the rates of nonmajor bleeding (5.8% and 5.8%, respectively).

In the RECORD 2 trial (63), 2509 patients undergoing hip arthroplasty were randomized to receive either oral rivaroxaban (10-mg once daily for 5 weeks) or subcutaneous enoxaparin (40-mg once daily for 2 weeks). At five weeks, the rate of total VTE was lower with extended rivaroxaban treatment than it was with enoxaparin (2.0% and 9.3%, respectively; $p < 0.001$) as was the rate of major VTE (0.6% and 5.1%, respectively; $p < 0.001$). Rates of major bleeding were similar with rivaroxaban and enoxaparin (0.1% and 0.1%, respectively; $p = 0.98$) as were the rates of nonmajor bleeding (6.5% and 5.5%, respectively; $p = 0.25$).

A fourth study in patients undergoing knee arthroplasty compared the 10-mg once-daily dose of oral rivaroxaban with that of subcutaneous enoxaparin. In this trial, enoxaparin was started postoperatively at a dose of 30-mg twice daily, the enoxaparin regimen that is often used in North America. The trial has been completed, but the results have not yet been published.

Rivaroxaban also has been evaluated for treatment of proximal DVT in two dose-ranging studies. The first trial randomized 613 patients to a three-month course of rivaroxaban (at doses of 10, 20, or 30-mg twice daily or 40-mg once daily) or to LMWH followed by a vitamin K antagonist (64). The primary efficacy outcome, reduced thrombus burden based on repeated ultrasound evaluation at 21 days without evidence of recurrent VTE, was achieved in 43.8% to 59.2% of patients given rivaroxaban and in 45.9% of those treated with LMWH followed by a vitamin K antagonist.

In the second study, 543 patients with proximal DVT were randomized to a three-month course of once-daily rivaroxaban (at doses of 20, 30, or 40 mg) or to heparin or LMWH followed by a vitamin K antagonist (65). The primary endpoint, a composite of symptomatic events (VTE-related death, DVT, or PE) plus an increase in thrombus burden (as detected by repeated ultrasound and ventilation-perfusion lung scanning), occurred in 6% of those given rivaroxaban and in 9.9% of those receiving conventional therapy. There was no apparent dose response with rivaroxaban. In both trials, rates of major bleeding were low with rivaroxaban and with conventional therapy. Phase III studies evaluating rivaroxaban for treatment of VTE and for stroke prevention in atrial fibrillation are underway. A 20-mg once-daily dose of rivaroxaban is being evaluated for these indications.

LY-517717 With oral bioavailability of 25% to 82%, LY-517717 inhibits factor Xa with a K_i of 5 to 7 nM. LY-517717 has a half-life of about 25 hours and is given once daily. LY-517717 was evaluated in a phase II noninferiority study that randomized 511 patients undergoing hip or knee arthroplasty to one of six doses of LY-517717 (25, 50, 75, 100,

125, or 150 mg started 6–8 hours after wound closure) or to once-daily subcutaneous enoxaparin (40 mg started the evening before surgery) (66). Both treatments were administered for a total of 6 to 10 doses. Randomization to the three lower doses of LY-517717 was stopped early due to lack of efficacy. The three higher doses of LY-517717 had efficacy similar to that of enoxaparin (17.1–24.0% and 22.2%, respectively). Adjudicated major bleeding events were uncommon in all study arms. Additional studies are needed to determine the efficacy and safety of this agent.

YM 150 An oral agent that inhibits factor Xa with a K_i of 31 nM, YM 150 is given once daily. YM 150 was evaluated in 174 patients undergoing elective hip arthroplasty (67). YM 150 at once-daily doses of 3, 10, 30, or 60 mg produced a statistically significant dose response for efficacy. No major bleeds were reported, and there was no dose-response trend for clinically relevant nonmajor bleeding. Although the point estimates for DVT appeared to favor the two highest doses of YM 150 over enoxaparin, the small study sample size precludes any firm conclusions. Ongoing phase II trials are evaluating YM150 in patients undergoing hip or knee arthroplasty and in patients with atrial fibrillation. A second phase II trial in patients undergoing elective hip arthroplasty is ongoing.

DU-176b An oral factor Xa inhibitor, DU-176b inhibits factor Xa with a K_i of 0.56 nM (68). Building on preclinical evidence of antithrombotic efficacy in animal models, DU-176b has completed phase II evaluation in hip arthroplasty patients and is now being compared with warfarin for stroke prevention patients with atrial fibrillation.

PRT 054021 With oral bioavailability of 47% and a half-life of 19 hours, PRT 054021 inhibits factor Xa with a K_i of 0.12 nM. PRT 054021 exhibited antithrombotic activity in animal models and was well tolerated in humans in a phase I trial that included 64 subjects. In the phase II EXPERT trial, oral PRT 054021 at doses of 15- or 40-mg twice daily was compared with that of subcutaneous enoxaparin (30-mg twice daily) for postoperative thromboprophylaxis in 215 patients undergoing elective knee arthroplasty. Randomization was done in a 2:2:1 fashion, and treatment was given for 10 to 14 days. DVT and nonfatal PE occurred in 20% and 15% of patients given 15 or 40 mg of PRT 054021, respectively, and in 10% of those given enoxaparin. There were no major bleeds in the 171 patients given PRT 054021, and there was one major bleed in the 43 patients given enoxaparin (69).

FACTOR Va INHIBITORS

Factor Va is the major target of activated protein C. Activated protein C acts as an anticoagulant by proteolytically degrading and inactivating factor Va, a key cofactor in thrombin generation. Factor Va is directly inhibited by drotrecogin-α (activated), a recombinant form of activated protein C. ART-123, a recombinant analog of the extracellular domain of thrombomodulin, binds thrombin and enhances its capacity to activate protein C (Table 5). Although drotrecogin-α (activated) and ART-123 have anticoagulant properties, both are being used in sepsis.

Drotrecogin-α (Activated)

A recombinant form of activated protein C, drotrecogin is licensed for treatment of severe sepsis. Approval for this indication was based on a trial comparing drotrecogin with placebo in 1690 severely septic patients (70). When given as an infusion of 24 µg/kg/hr

Table 5 Inhibitors of Factor Va

Drug	Route of administration	Mechanism of action	Stage of development as of 2007
Drotrecogin	Intravenous	Proteolytically degrades and inactivates factor Va	Licensed for severe sepsis
ART-123	Subcutaneous	Binds thrombin and promotes its activation of protein C	Phase II

over 96 hours, drotrecogin C produced a 19% reduction in mortality at 28 days (from 30.8% to 24.7%; $p = 0.005$). The rate of major bleeding was higher with drotrecogin than with placebo (3.5% and 2%, respectively; $p = 0.06$). Since approval, two additional clinical trials, one in adults with sepsis and a low risk of death and the other in children with sepsis, were stopped prematurely due to lack of efficacy and the potential to cause harm because of bleeding (71).

ART-123

A recombinant analog of the extracellular domain of thrombomodulin (72), ART-123 binds thrombin and converts it from a procoagulant enzyme into a potent activator of protein C. ART-123 has nearly 100% bioavailability after subcutaneous administration and a half-life of two to three days. In a phase IIa dose-ranging study in patients undergoing elective hip arthroplasty, the primary endpoint (a composite of venographically detected DVT and symptomatic PE) occurred in 4.3% of the 94 patients given lower-dose ART-123 and in none of the 99 patients receiving the higher dose (73). Major bleeding occurred in 1.6% and 5.7% of patients receiving low- or high-dose ART-123, respectively. ART-123 is currently being evaluated in patients with sepsis.

INHIBITORS OF FIBRIN FORMATION

Thrombin, the enzyme that converts fibrinogen to fibrin, can be inhibited indirectly or directly. Indirect inhibitors that are specific for thrombin act by catalyzing heparin cofactor II. In contrast, direct inhibitors bind to thrombin and block its interaction with substrates. Three parenteral direct thrombin inhibitors (lepirudin, argatroban, and bivalirudin) have been licensed in North America for limited indications. Lepirudin, a recombinant form of hirudin, and argatroban are approved for treatment of patients with heparin-induced thrombocytopenia, whereas bivalirudin is licensed as an alternative to heparin in PCI patients with or without heparin-induced thrombocytopenia. These will not be discussed. The new agents are oral thrombin inhibitors. Three such drugs have been developed: odiparcil is an indirect inhibitor, whereas ximelagatran and dabigatran etexilate are direct thrombin inhibitors (Table 6).

Odiparcil

An oral β-D-xyloside, odiparcil, primes the synthesis of circulating dermatan sulfate-like glycosaminoglycans (74). These glycosaminoglycans indirectly inhibit thrombin by catalyzing heparin cofactor II. Steady-state levels of glycosaminoglycans are achieved after two to three days of odiparcil administration. Like warfarin, therefore, odiparcil has a delayed onset of action. The anticoagulant activity of odiparcil can be partially reversed

Table 6 Thrombin Inhibitors

Drug	Route of administration	Mechanism of action	Stage of development as of 2007
Odiparcil	Oral	Primes the synthesis of dermatan sulfate-like glycosaminoglycans	Halted
Ximelagatran	Oral	Prodrug of melagatran, a reversible inhibitor of the active site of thrombin	Briefly licensed in Europe and now withdrawn worldwide
Dabigatran etexilate	Oral	Prodrug of dabigatran, a reversible inhibitor of the active site of thrombin	Phase III

with protamine sulfate. In a phase II dose-finding trial, three different doses of oral odiparcil were compared with warfarin for thromboprophylaxis in patients undergoing knee arthroplasty (75). Because of lack of efficacy, further development of odiparcil has been halted.

Ximelagatran

A prodrug of melagatran, ximelagatran is absorbed from the gastrointestinal tract with a bioavailability of 20%. Once absorbed, ximelagatran undergoes rapid biotransformation to melagatran via two intermediate metabolites, H338/57 and H415/04 (76). Melagatran has a half-life of four to five hours and is administered twice daily.

Ximelagatran does not interact with food, has a low potential for drug interactions, and produces a predictable anticoagulant response. Ximelagatran underwent extensive evaluation for prevention and treatment of VTE, prevention of cardioembolic events in patients with nonvalvular atrial fibrillation, and prevention of recurrent ischemia in patients with recent MI (77). Initial studies led to its temporary licensing in Europe for thromboprophylaxis in patients undergoing major orthopedic surgery. However, the drug was not approved in North America and was eventually withdrawn from the world market because of potential hepatic toxicity. Thus, in a total of 6948 patients randomized to ximelagatran, there was one death from hepatorenal failure and two other deaths from hepatic failure (78). Added to this was a patient who developed severe hepatic injury several weeks after receiving a four-week course of ximelagatran for thromboprophylaxis after orthopedic surgery. AZD0837, a follow-up compound to ximelagatran that appears to have a lower risk of hepatic toxicity, has completed phase II evaluation (79) and will likely move forward into phase III testing.

Dabigatran Etexilate

A double prodrug, dabigatran etexilate is absorbed from the gastrointestinal tract with a bioavailability of 5% to 6% (79–81). Absorption requires an acid microenvironment and is reduced by acid suppression therapy. Once absorbed, dabigatran etexilate is converted by esterases into its active metabolite, dabigatran (BIBR 953). Plasma levels of dabigatran peak at two hours, and dabigatran has a half-life of eight hours after single-dose administration and up to 17 hours after multiple doses. Consequently, it is possible to administer dabigatran etexilate once daily for some indications. At least 80% of dabigatran is excreted unchanged via the kidneys; therefore, the drug is contraindicated in patients with renal failure.

Dabigatran etexilate has been evaluated for thromboprophylaxis in patients undergoing hip or knee arthroplasty in phase II and III trials and for prevention of stroke in patients with atrial fibrillation in phase II trials. In the phase II arthroplasty trial, 1973 patients were randomized to receive one of four doses of dabigatran etexilate for 6 to 10 days after surgery (with the first dose administered 1–4 hours postoperatively) or enoxaparin 40-mg once daily started 12 hours prior to surgery (82). The primary efficacy outcome was a composite of venographically detected DVT or symptomatic VTE. The three highest dabigatran etexilate dose regimens produced a statistically significant reduction in the incidence of VTE compared with enoxaparin. However, this was balanced by a trend for more major bleeding with higher dabigatran doses than with enoxaparin.

In the phase III RE-MODEL trial (83), 2076 patients undergoing knee arthroplasty were randomized to receive either dabigatran etexilate (at doses of 150- or 220-mg once daily, starting with a half dose given 1–4 hours after surgery) or enoxaparin (given subcutaneously once daily at a dose of 40 mg, starting 12 hours prior to surgery). The primary endpoint, a composite of VTE and all-cause mortality, occurred in 40.5% and 36.4% of patients given 150 and 220 mg of dabigatran etexilate, respectively, and in 37.7% of those randomized to enoxaparin. Major bleeding occurred in 1.3%, 1.5%, and 1.3% of those given 150-mg dabigatran etexilate, 220-mg dabigatran etexilate, and enoxaparin, respectively, while rates of major bleeding plus clinically relevant, nonmajor bleeding were 7.1%, 7.4%, and 6.6%, respectively. None of these differences was statistically significant. Levels of alanine aminotransferase greater than three times the upper limit of normal were observed in 3.7% and 2.8% of patients receiving 150 and 220 mg of dabigatran etexilate, respectively, compared with 4.0% of those given enoxaparin.

Dabigatran etexilate has been evaluated in two other phase III orthopedic trials. The RE-NOVATE trial randomized 3494 patients undergoing hip-replacement surgery to oral dabigatran etexilate (150- or 220-mg once –daily, starting with a half dose given 1–4 hours after surgery) or subcutaneous enoxaparin (40-mg once –daily, starting 12 hours prior to surgery) for an average of 33 days (84). The primary efficacy endpoint, a composite of DVT, nonfatal PE, and all-cause mortality, occurred in 8.6% and 6.0% of patients given dabigatran etexilate 150 or 220 mg, respectively, and in 6.7% of those treated with enoxaparin. Major bleeding occurred in 1.3% and 2.0% of patients treated with dabigatran etexilate 150 and 220 mg, respectively, and in 1.6% of those given enoxaparin. None of these differences was statistically significant.

In the North American RE-MOBILIZE trial, patients undergoing knee-replacement surgery were randomized to oral dabigatran etexilate (150- or 220-mg once daily, starting with a half dose given 8–12 hours after surgery) or subcutaneous enoxaparin (30-mg twice daily, starting 12–24 hours after surgery) for 10 to 14 days (85). The primary efficacy endpoint, a composite of DVT, nonfatal PE, and all-cause mortality, occurred in 33.7% and 31.1% of patients treated with dabigatran 150 or 220 mg, respectively, and in 25.3% of those given enoxaparin. Major bleeding occurred in 0.6% of patients treated with either dose of dabigatran and in 1.4% of those given enoxaparin, differences that were not statistically significant. Unlike the other two phase III trials, dabigatran was inferior to enoxaparin in this trial. This difference may reflect the higher-dose enoxaparin regimen used as a comparator and/or the delayed start of dabigatran etexilate.

A phase II trial in 502 patients with atrial fibrillation compared a three-month course of treatment with three different doses of dabigatran etexilate (50-, 150-, or 300-mg twice daily) or with warfarin (with doses adjusted to achieve a target INR of

2 to 3) (86). Using a factorial design, patients were also randomized to aspirin (81 or 325 mg daily) or to placebo. Recruitment into the high-dose dabigatran etexilate plus aspirin arm was stopped early because of four gastrointestinal bleeds in 63 patients. Addition of aspirin in the other groups did not appear to increase the risk of bleeding. In the low-dose dabigatran etexilate arm, 2 of 105 patients suffered a thromboembolic event. Building on these data, 361 of the 432 patients randomized to dabigatran etexilate continued open-label treatment at doses of 50-, 100-, or 300-mg twice daily or 150- or 300-mg once daily for at least 16 months. The two lowest doses of dabigatran etexilate (50 twice daily or 150 once daily) were discontinued early because of annual stroke rates of 8.4% and 8.1%, respectively. The annual stroke rate with the 300-mg once-daily dose was 9.5%, whereas rates were lower with the other doses. The cumulative frequency of elevations in alanine aminotransferase of greater than three times the upper limit of normal was 2% in patients receiving dabigatran etexilate for at least 12 months compared with 1% in those given warfarin. On the basis of these data, the ongoing phase III RELY trial is comparing dabigatran etexilate doses of 110- or 150-mg twice daily with dose-adjusted warfarin for stroke prevention in over 18,000 patients with nonvalvular atrial fibrillation. In addition, dabigatran etexilate also is undergoing phase III evaluation for initial and extended treatment of VTE, while a phase II trial is examining its utility for prevention of recurrent ischemia in ACS patients.

CONCLUSIONS AND FUTURE DIRECTIONS

New anticoagulants have the potential to streamline the prevention and treatment of venous and arterial thrombosis. The introduction of LMWH and fondaparinux has largely shifted the treatment of VTE from the hospital to the outpatient setting. In addition to reducing health care costs, this approach also has increased patient satisfaction.

Where do we go from here? Most of the excitement is centered on new oral anticoagulants, which have the potential to replace warfarin and simplify long-term therapy. Emerging data suggest that factor Xa and thrombin are both good targets for new anticoagulants. Regardless of whether thrombin generation is attenuated or thrombin activity is suppressed, the relative efficacy and safety appear to be similar. Since head-to-head trials comparing factor Xa inhibitors with thrombin inhibitors are unlikely to be conducted in the near future, we will see parallel development of the two classes of drugs over the next few years.

The first new oral anticoagulant to market may gain a competitive edge. However, such advantage is likely to be small because the initial indication will be restricted to VTE prevention, a limited market. More important will be the first drug to yield favorable clinical results when compared with warfarin for stroke prevention in patients with atrial fibrillation. This is the area of greatest need because the burden of atrial fibrillation continues to increase as the population ages. The availability of an oral anticoagulant that can be given in fixed doses without monitoring will simplify stroke prevention in these patients, thereby enhancing uptake of preventive therapy.

Will the new oral anticoagulants be more effective or safer than warfarin? This is a definite possibility because the novel agents have been designed to produce a predictable anticoagulant response. However, demonstrating superiority requires innovative clinical trial design. In patients with atrial fibrillation, the focus should be on incident cases because the risk of bleeding with warfarin therapy is "front loaded." The high initial risk reflects a combination of patient factors plus the difficulty identifying the therapeutic dose of warfarin, which varies from patient to patient. The latter problem will be circumvented by the new oral anticoagulants because these drugs yield stable anticoagulation from the initiation of therapy. Therefore, clinical trials that focus mainly on warfarin-naïve patients should demonstrate superiority of the new oral anticoagulants over warfarin. In contrast, trials that enter a preponderance of warfarin-experienced patients are unlikely to demonstrate superiority because such patients are at lower risk of bleeding or suffering embolic events.

Why is it important to demonstrate superiority? New oral anticoagulants will be more expensive than warfarin. Rationalizing this added cost solely on the basis of convenience is difficult. In contrast, if these new drugs prove superior to warfarin, the added cost can be justified.

What are the potential challenges associated with these new anticoagulants? Management of bleeding episodes will be difficult. There are no antidotes for these new agents, and the utility of procoagulants, such as activated factor VII, to arrest such bleeding has not been established. Furthermore, the thrombotic risks of procoagulants in patients with underlying thrombotic diseases are unknown. Coagulation monitoring also will be problematic. Thus, the novel agents have variable effects on routine tests of coagulation. How will we monitor them, should a patient present with a hemorrhagic or thrombotic event? Even if we can monitor them, how will we know the target therapeutic range if monitoring has not been part of their clinical development program? These issues will need to be addressed.

Finally, compliance may be more important with the new oral anticoagulants than with warfarin. With shorter half-lives than warfarin, missed doses may have a more profound effect on outcomes with the new drugs. Although inconvenient, INR monitoring provides ongoing assessment of compliance with warfarin. How will compliance be assessed with the new agents?

Finally, we will need to watch for off-target side effects. Hepatic toxicity was the downfall of ximelagatran. Will this or other side effects, such as rebound activation of coagulation, plague the new drugs? Results from large clinical trials and postmarketing surveillance exclude these possibilities.

We are in exciting times. Never has there been such an extensive array of new antithrombotic agents. With so many drugs in development, some are likely to succeed. Expanding our armamentarium of agents will help to reduce the burden of thrombotic disease, the number one cause of death and morbidity worldwide.

REFERENCES

1. Fuster V, Badimon L, Badimon JJ, et al. The pathogenesis of coronary artery disease and the acute coronary syndromes. N Engl J Med 1992; 326:310–318.
2. Furie B, Furie BC. Molecular and cellular biology of blood coagulation. N Engl J Med 1992; 326:800–806.
3. van den Eijnden MM, Steenhauer SI, Reitsma PH, et al. Tissue factor expression during monocyte-macrophage differentiation. Thromb Haemost 1997; 7:1129–1136.
4. Neumann FJ, Ott I, Marx N, et al. Effect of human recombinant interleukin-6 and interleukin-8 on monocyte procoagulant activity. Arterioscler Thromb Vasc Biol 1997; 17:3399–3405.
5. Yamamoto M, Nakagaki T, Kisiel W. Tissue factor-dependent autoactivation of human blood coagulation factor. J Biol Chem 1992; 267:19089–19094.
6. Broze GJ Jr. Tissue factor pathway inhibitor. Thromb Haemost 1995; 74:90–93.
7. Abraham E, Reinhart K, Svoboda P, et al. Assessment of the safety of recombinant tissue factor pathway inhibitor in patients with severe sepsis: a multicenter, randomized, placebo-controlled, single-blind, dose escalation study. Crit Care Med 2001; 29(11):2081–2089.

8. Abraham E, Reinhart K, Opal S, et al. Efficacy and safety of tifacogin (recombinant tissue factor pathway inhibitor) in severe sepsis: a randomized controlled trial. JAMA 2003; 290(2): 238–247.

9. Cappello M, Vlasuk GP, Bergum PW, et al. *Ancylostoma caninum* anticoagulant peptide: a hookworm-derived inhibitor of human coagulation factor Xa. Proc Natl Acad Sci USA 1995; 92: 6152–6156.

10. Bergum PW, Cruikshank A, Maki S, et al. Role of zymogen and activated factor X as scaffolds for the inhibition of the blood coagulation factor VIIa-tissue factor complex by recombinant nematode anticoagulant protein c2. J Biol Chem 2001; 276(13):10063–10071.

11. Vlasuk GP, Bradbury A, Lopez-Kinniger L, et al. Pharmacokinetics and anticoagulant properties of the factor VIIa-tissue factor inhibitor recombinant Nematode Anticoagulant Protein c2 following subcutaneous administration in man. Dependence on the stoichiometric binding to circulating factor X. Thromb Haemost 2003; 90(5):803–812.

12. Lee A, Agnelli G, Buller H, et al. Dose-response study of recombinant factor VIIa/tissue factor inhibitor recombinant nematode anticoagulant protein c2 in prevention of postoperative venous thromboembolism in patients undergoing total knee replacement. Circulation 2001; 104(1):74–78.

13. Giugliano RP, Wiviott SD, Morrow DA, et al. Addition of a tissue-factor/factor VIIa inhibitor to standard treatments in NSTE-ACS managed with an early invasive strategy: results of the Phase II ANTHEM-TIMI 32 double-blind randomized clinical trial. In: Program and Abstracts of the American Heart Association Meeting; 2005, November; Dallas Texas (TX) (abstr 2095/C16).

14. Moons AH, Peters RJ, Bijsterveld NR, et al. Recombinant nematode anticoagulant protein c2, an inhibitor of the tissue factor/factor VIIa complex, in patients undergoing elective coronary angioplasty. J Am Coll Cardiol 2003; 41:2147–2153.

15. Taylor FB Jr. Role of tissue factor and factor VIIa in the coagulant and inflammatory response to LD100 *Escherichia coli* in the baboon. Haemostasis 1996; 26:83–91.

16. Jang Y, Guzman LA, Lincoff AM, et al. Influence of blockade at specific levels of the coagulant cascade on restenosis in a rabbit atherosclerotic femoral artery injury model. Circulation 1995; 92: 3041–3050.

17. Lincoff AM. First clinical investigation of a tissue-factor inhibitor administered during percutaneous coronary revascularization: a randomized, double-blind, dose-escalation trial assessing safety and efficacy of FFR-FVIIa in percutaneous transluminal coronary angioplasty (ASIS) trial. J Am Coll Cardiol 2000; 36:312 (abstract).

18. Rusconi CP, Scardino E, Layzer J, et al. RNA aptamers as reversible antagonists of coagulation factor IXa. Nature 2002; 419(6902):90–94.

19. Dyke CK, Steinhubl SR, Kleiman NS, et al. First-in-human experience of an antidote-controlled anticoagulant using RNA aptamer technology: a phase 1a pharmacodynamic evaluation of a drug-antidote pair for the controlled regulation of factor IXa activity. Circulation 2006; 114(23): 2490–2497.

20. Nimjee SM, Keys JR, Pitoc GA, et al. A novel antidote-controlled anticoagulant reduces thrombin generation and inflammation and improves cardiac function in cardiopulmonary bypass surgery. Mol Ther 2006; 14(3):408–415.

21. Eriksson BI, Dahl OE, Lassen MR, et al. Partial factor IXa inhibition with TTP889 for prevention of venous thromboembolism; an exploratory study. J Thromb Haemost 2008; 6:457–463.

22. Rezaie AR. Prothrombin protects factor Xa in the prothrombinase complex from inhibition by the heparin-antithrombin complex. Blood 2001; 97:2308–2313.

23. Brufatto N, Nesheim ME. The use of prothrombin (S525C) labeled with fluorescein to directly study the inhibition of prothrombinase by antithrombin during prothrombin activation. J Biol Chem 2001; 276:17663–17671.

24. Krishnaswamy S, Vlasuk GP, Bergum PW. Assembly of the prothrombinase complex enhances the inhibition of bovine factor Xa by tick anticoagulant peptide. Biochemistry 1994; 33(25): 7897–7907.

25. Herault JP, Bernat A, Pflieger AM, et al. Comparative effects of two direct and indirect factor Xa inhibitors on free and clot-bound prothrombinase. J Pharmacol Exp Ther 1997; 283(1):16–22.

26. Boneu B, Necciari J, Cariou R, et al. Pharmacokinetics and tolerance of the natural pentasaccharide (SR90107/ORG31540) with high affinity to antithrombin III in man. Thromb Haemost 1995; 74:1468–1473.

27. Turpie AG, Bauer KA, Eriksson BI, et al. Fondaparinux vs enoxaparin for the prevention of venous thromboembolism in major orthopedic surgery: a meta-analysis of 4 randomized double-blind studies. Arch Intern Med 2002; 162(16):1833–1840.

28. Turpie AG, Bauer KA, Eriksson BI, et al. Superiority of fondaparinux over enoxaparin in preventing venous thromboembolism in major orthopedic surgery using different efficacy end points. Chest 2004; 126(2):501–508.

29. Agnelli G, Bergqvist D, Cohen AT, et al. Randomized clinical trial of postoperative fondaparinux versus perioperative dalteparin for prevention of venous thromboembolism in high-risk abdominal surgery. Br J Surg 2005; 92(10):1212–1220.

30. Cohen AT, Davidson BL, Gallus AS, et al. Efficacy and safety of fondaparinux for the prevention of venous thromboembolism in older acute medical patients: randomised placebo controlled trial. Br Med J 2006; 332(7537):325–329.

31. Buller HR, Davidson BL, Decousus H, et al. Fondaparinux or enoxaparin for the initial treatment of symptomatic deep venous thrombosis: a randomized trial. Ann Intern Med 2004; 140(11):867–873.

32. Buller HR, Davidson BL, Decousus H, et al. Subcutaneous fondaparinux versus intravenous unfractionated heparin in the initial treatment of pulmonary embolism. N Engl J Med 2003; 349(18): 1695–1702.

33. Fifth Organization to Assess Strategies in Acute Ischemic Syndromes Investigators; Yusuf, S, Mehta SR, Chrolavicius S, et al. Comparison of fondaparinux and enoxaparin in acute coronary syndromes. N Engl J Med 2006; 354(14):1461–1476.

34. Yusuf S, Mehta SR, Chrolavicius S, et al. Effects of fondaparinux on mortality and reinfarction in patients with acute ST-segment elevation myocardial infarction: the OASIS-6 randomized trial. JAMA 2006; 295(13):1519–1530.

35. Herbert JM, Herault JP, Bernat A, et al. Biochemical and pharmacological properties of SANORG 34006, a potent and long-acting synthetic pentasaccharide. Blood 1998; 91: 4197–4205.

36. The Persist Investigators. A novel long-acting synthetic factor Xa inhibitor (SanOrg34006) to replace warfarin for secondary prevention in deep vein thrombosis. A phase II evaluation. J Thromb Haemost 2004; 2(1):47–53.

37. van Gogh Investigators, Buller HR, Cohen AT, et al. Idraparinux versus standard therapy for venous thromboembolic disease. N Engl J Med 2007; 357(11):1094–1104.

38. van Gogh Investigators, Buller HR, Cohen AT, et al. Extended prophylaxis of venous thromboembolism with idraparinux. N Engl J Med 2007; 357(11):1105–1112.

39. The Amadeus Investigators. Comparison of idraparinux with vitamin K antagonists for prevention of thromboembolism in patients with atrial fibrillation: a randomized, open-label, non-inferiority trial. Lancet 2008; 371:315–321.

40. Herbert JM, Herault JP, Bernat A, et al. SR123781A, a synthetic heparin mimetic. Thromb Haemost 2001; 85(5):852–860.

41. Becker DL, Fredenburgh JC, Stafford AR, et al. Exosites 1 and 2 are essential for protection of fibrin-bound thrombin from heparin-catalyzed inhibition by antithrombin and heparin cofactor II. J Biol Chem 1999; 274(10):6226–6233.

42. Herault JP, Cappelle M, Bernat A, et al. Effect of SanOrg123781A, a synthetic hexadecasaccharide, on clot-bound thrombin and factor Xa in vitro and in vivo. J Thromb Haemost 2003; 1(9):1959–1965.

43. Lassen MR, Dahl OE, Mirmetti P, et al. AVE5026, a new anticoagulant for the prevention of venous thromboembolism in total knee replacement surgery—TREK: a dose ranging study. Blood 2007; 110(11):98a (abstract #311).

44. Herbert JM, Bernat A, Dol F, et al. DX-9065a, a novel synthetic, selective and orally active inhibitor of Factor Xa: in vitro and in vivo studies. J Pharmacol Exp Ther 1996; 276:1030–1038.

45. Maruyama I, Tanaka M, Kunitada S, et al. Tolerability, pharmacokinetics and pharmacodynamics of DX-9065a, a new synthetic potent anticoagulant and specific Factor Xa inhibitor, in healthy male volunteers. Clin Pharmacol Ther 1996; 66:258–264.

46. Becker RC, Alexander JH, Dyke C, et al. Effect of the novel direct Factor Xa inhibitor DX-9065a on thrombin generation and inhibition among patients with stable atherosclerotic coronary artery disease. Thromb Res 2006; 117:439–446.

47. Alexander JH, Yang H, Becker RC, et al. First experience with direct, selective Factor Xa inhibition in patients with non-ST-elevation acute coronary syndromes: results of the XaNADU-ACS Trial. J Thromb Haemost 2005; 3:436–438.

48. Alexander JH, Dyke CK, Yang H, et al. Initial experience with factor Xa inhibition in percutaneous coronary intervention: the XaNADU-PCI pilot. J Thromb Haemost 2004; 2:234–241.

49. Paccaly A, Ozooux ML, Chu V, et al. Pharmacodynamic markers in the early clinical assessment of otamixaban, a direct Factor Xa inhibitor. Thromb Haemost 2005; 94:1156–1163.

50. Hinder M, Frick A, Jordaan P, et al. Direct and rapid inhibition of factor Xa by otamixaban: a pharmacokinetic and pharmacodynamic investigation in patients with coronary artery disease. Clin Pharmacol Ther 2006; 80(6):691–702.

51. Cohen M, Bhatt DL, Alexander JH, et al. Randomized, double-blind, dose-ranging study of otamixaban, a novel, paternal, short-acting direct factor Xa inhibitor, in percutaneous coronary intervention: the SEPIA-PCI trial. Circulation 2007; 115(20):2642–2651.

52. Lassen MR, Davidson BL, Gallus A, et al. A phase II randomized, double blind, five-arm, parallel group, dose-response study of a new oral directly acting Factor Xa inhibitor, razaxaban, for the prevention of deep vein thrombosis in knee replacement surgery. Blood 2003; 102:15a (abstract 41).

53. Kan H, Bing H, Grace JE, et al. Preclinical pharmacokinetic and metabolism of apixaban, a potent and selective factor Xa inhibitor. Blood 2006; 108(11):(abstr 910).

54. Lassen MR, Davidson BL, Gallus A, et al. The efficacy and safety of apixaban, an oral, direct factor Xa inhibitor, as thromboprophylaxis in patients following total knee replacement. J Thromb Haemost 2007 Sept 15; [epub ahead of print].

55. Kubitza D, Becka M, Wensing G, et al. Safety, pharmacodynamics of BAY 59-7939—an oral, direct Factor Xa inhibitor—after multiple dosing in healthy male subjects. Eur J Clin Pharmcol 2005; 61(12):873–880.

56. Eriksson BI, Borris LC, Dahl OE, et al. Dose-escalation study of rivaroxaban (BAY 59-7939)—an oral, direct Factor Xa inhibitor—for the prevention of venous thromboembolism in patients undergoing total hip replacement. Thromb Res 2007; 120(5):685–693.

57. Eriksson BI, Borris L, Dahl OE, et al. Oral, direct Factor Xa inhibition with BAY 59-7939 for the prevention of venous thromboembolism after total hip replacement. J Thromb Haemost 2006; 4(1):121–128.

58. Turpie AG, Fisher WD, Bauer KA, et al. BAY 59-7939: an oral, direct factor Xa inhibitor for the prevention of venous thromboembolism in patients after total knee replacement. A phase II dose-ranging study. J Thromb Haemos 2005; 3(11):2479–2486.

59. Fisher WD, Eriksson BI, Bauer KA, et al. Rivaroxaban for thromboprophylaxis after orthopedic surgery: pooled analysis of two studies. Thromb Haemost 2007; 97(6):931–937.

60. Eriksson BI, Borris LC, Dahl OE, et al. A once daily, oral, direct Factor Xa inhibitor, rivaroxaban (BAY 59-7939), for thromboprophylaxis after total hip replacement. Circulation 2006; 114(22):2374–2381.

61. Lassen MR, Turpie AG, Rosencher N, et al. Late breaking clinical trial: Rivaroxaban—an oral, direct factor Xa inhibitor—for the prevention of venous thromboembolism in total knee replacement surgery: results of the RECORD-3 study. J Thromb Haemost 2007; 5(suppl 2): (abstr #O-S-006B).

62. Eriksson BI, Borris LC, Friedman RJ, et al. Oral rivaroxaban compared with subcutaneous enoxaparin for extended thromboprophylaxis after total hip arthroplasty: the RECORD 1 trial. Blood 2007; 110:9a (abstr 6).

63. Kakkar AK, Brenner B, Dahl OE, et al. Extended thromboprophylaxis with rivaroxaban compared with enoxaparin after total hip arthroplasty: the RECORD 2 trial. Blood 2007; 110:97a (abstr 307).

64. Agnelli G, Gallus A, Goldhaber SZ, et al. Treatment of proximal deep-vein thrombosis with the oral direct factor Xa inhibitor rivaroxaban (BAY 59-7939): The ODIXa-DVT (Oral Direct Factor Xa Inhibitor BAY 59-7939 in Patients with Acute Symptomatic Deep-Vein Thrombosis) study. Circulation 2007; 116(2):180–187.

65. Buller HR, on behalf of the EINSTEIN-DVT study group. Once-daily treatment with an oral, direct factor Xa inhibitor—rivaroxaban (BAY 59-7939)—in patients with acute, symptomatic deep vein thrombosis. The EINSTEIN-DVT dose-finding study. Eur Heart J 2006; 27 (suppl):761 (abstr P4568).

66. Agnelli G, Haas S, Ginsberg JS, et al. A phase II study of the oral factor Xa inhibitor LY517717 for the prevention of venous thromboembolism after hip or knee replacement. J Thromb Haemost 2007; 5(4):746–753.

67. Eriksson BI, Turpie AG, Lassen MR, et al. A dose escalation study of YM150, an oral direct factor Xa inhibitor, in the prevention of venous thromboembolism in elective primary hip replacement surgery. J Thromb Haemost 2007; 5(8):1660–1665.

68. Turpie AG. Oral direct factor Xa inhibitors in development for the prevention and treatment of thromboembolic diseases. Arterioscler Thromb Vasc Biol 2007; Mar 22 (epub ahead of print).

69. Turpie AG, Gent M, Bauer K, et al. Evaluation of the factor Xa (FXa) inhibitor, PRT054021 (PRT021), against enoxaparin in a randomized trial for the prevention of venous thromboembolic events after total knee replacement (EXPERT). J Thromb Haemost 2007; 5(suppl 2):(abstr #P-T-652).

70. Bernard GR, Vincent JL, Laterre PF, et al. Efficacy and safety of recombinant human activated protein C for severe sepsis. N Engl J Med 2001; 344:699–709.

71. Abraham E, Laterre PF, Garg R, et al. Drotrecogin alfa (activated) for adults with severe sepsis and a low risk of death. N Engl J Med 2005; 353:1332–1341.

72. Parkinson JF, Grinnell BW, Moore RE, et al. Stable expression of a secretable deletion mutation of recombinant human thrombomodulin in mammalian cells. J Biol Chem 1990; 265: 12602–12610.

73. Kearon C, Comp P, Douketis JD, et al. Dose-response study of recombinant human soluble thrombomodulin (ART-123) in the prevention of venous thromboembolism after total hip replacement. J Thromb Haemost 2005; 3:962–968.

74. Tommey JR, Abboud MA, Valocik RE, et al. A comparison of the β-D-xyloside, odiparcil, to warfarin in a rat model of venous thrombosis. J Thromb Haemost 2006; 4:1989–1996.

75. Bates SM, Buller H, Lassen MR, et al. A phase II double-blind placebo-controlled parallel-group randomized study of extended prophylaxis with odiparcil following total hip arthroplasty (THA). J Thromb Haemost 2007; 5(suppl 2):(abstr #P-M-653).

76. Gustafsson D, Nystrom J, Carlsson S, et al. The direct thrombin inhibitor melagatran and its oral prodrug H376/95: intestinal absorption properties, biochemical and pharmacodynamic effects. Thromb Res 2001; 101:171–181.

77. Testa L, Andreotti F, Biondi Zoccai GG, et al. Ximelagatran/melagatran against conventional anticoagulation: A meta-analysis based on 22,639 patients. Int J Cardiol 2007; Jan 11 (epub ahead of print).

78. Lee WM, Larrey D, Olsson R, et al. Hepatic findings in long-term clinical trials of ximelagatran. Drug Saf 2005; 28(4):351–370.

79. Gustafsson D. Oral direct thrombin inhibitors in clinical development. J Int Med 2003; 254: 322–334.

80. Weitz JI. Emerging anticoagulants for the treatment of venous thromboembolism. Thromb Haemost 2006; 96(3):274–284.

81. Stangier J, Rathgen K, Stahle H, et al. The pharmacokinetics, pharmacodynamics and tolerability of dabigatran etexilate, a new oral direct thrombin inhibitor, in healthy male subjects. Br J Clin Pharmacol 2007; 64(3):292–303.

82. Eriksson BI, Dahl OE, Buller HR, et al. A new oral direct thrombin inhibitor, dabigatran etexilate, compared with enoxaparin for prevention of thromboembolic events following total hip or knee replacement: the BISTRO II randomized trial. J Thromb Haemost 2005; 3: 103–111.

83. Eriksson BI, Dahl OE, Rosencher N, et al. Dabigatran etexilate versus enoxaparin for the prevention of venous thromboembolism after total knee replacement: the RE-MODEL randomized trial. J Thromb Haemost 2007; Aug 24 (epub ahead of print).
84. Eriksson BI, Dahl OE, Rosencher N, et al. Dabigatran etexilate versus enoxaparin for prevention of venous thromboembolism after total hip replacement: a randomized, double-blind, non-inferiority trial. Lancet 2007; 370(9591):949–956.
85. Caprini JA, Hwang E, Hantel S, et al. The oral direct thrombin inhibitor, dabigatran etexilate, is effective and safe for prevention of major venous thromboembolism following major orthopedic surgery. J Thromb Haemost 2007; 5(suppl 2) (abstr #O-W-050).
86. Wallentin L, Ezekowitz M, Simmers TA, et al. Safety and efficacy of a new oral direct thrombin inhibitor dabigatran in atrial fibrillation: a dose finding trial with comparison to warfarin. Eur Heart J 2005; 26: (abstr 482).

10

Anticoagulants for the Treatment of Venous Thromboembolism

Sam Schulman
Department of Medicine, McMaster University, Hamilton, Ontario, Canada

INTRODUCTION

The medical treatment of venous thromboembolism dates back to the 1940s, when unfractionated heparin (UFH) and vitamin K antagonists (VKAs) were first used for this indication. The treatment changed little until low–molecular weight heparin (LMWH) was introduced about 20 years ago. The introduction of LMWH allowed outpatient treatment of most patients with deep-vein thrombosis (DVT) and, more recently, a substantial proportion of patients with pulmonary embolism (PE). A pentasaccharide is the smallest entity of heparin that can bind to and change the conformation of antithrombin for selective inhibition of factor Xa. One such pentasaccharide, fondaparinux, has recently been approved for several indications requiring anticoagulation. Several orally available, selective coagulation factor inhibitors are presently in advanced phase of clinical trials. This chapter reviews the above-mentioned anticoagulant agents and their profile in established venous thromboembolism.

UNFRACTIONATED HEPARIN

Characteristics

Both UFH and LMWH are sulfated glycosaminoglycans extracted from animal sources, most commonly, porcine intestinal mucosa. The molecular range of UFH is 3000 to 30,000 Da. UFH serves as a catalyst to antithrombin by binding to lysine residues on the serine protease inhibitor and inducing a conformational change in its reactive center loop. This increases the inhibiting capacity of antithrombin by several orders of magnitude, and it binds covalently to the serine residue in the active center of coagulation factors XIIa, XIa, IXa, Xa, and thrombin. Subsequently, heparin dissociates from antithrombin and is then available to bind to additional antithrombin molecules (1).

The half-life of UFH increases from 0.5 hour at prophylactic doses to 2.5 hours at full therapeutic doses. Elimination occurs via the endothelium and macrophages, which internalize and depolymerize the mucopolysaccharides, and also via the kidneys. The

Table 1   Treatment Regimens for Anticoagulation in Acute Venous Thromboembolism

Agent	Route	Initial bolus	Maintenance dose	Monitoring	Indication	Reference
UFH	i.v.	80 U/kg	18 U/kg/hr	APTT	DVT, PE	2
UFH	i.v.	5000 U	1300 U/hr	APTT	DVT, PE	3
UFH	s.c.	5000 U **i.v.**	250 U/kg s.c. every 12 hr	APTT	DVT, PE	4
UFH	s.c.	333 U/kg s.c.	250 U/kg s.c. every 12 hr	None	DVT, PE	5
Low–molecular weight heparin						
Dalteparin	s.c.	–	200 IU/kg once daily	None	DVT, PE	6
Or		–	120 IU/kg every 12 hr	None	PE	7
Enoxaparin	s.c.	–	1.5 mg/kg once daily	None	DVT, PE	8
Or		–	1 mg/kg every 12 hr	None	PE	8
Nadroparin	s.c.	–	171 IU/kg once daily	None	DVT	
Or		–	85 IU/kg every 12 hr	None	PE	4
Tinzaparin	s.c.	–	175 IU/kg once daily	None	DVT, PE	9
Pentasaccharide Fondaparinux	s.c.		5/7.5/10 mg once daily	none	DVT, PE	10, 11

Abbreviations: UFH, unfractionated heparin; i.v., intravenous; s.c., subcutaneous; APTT, activated partial thromboplastin time; DVT, deep-vein thrombosis; PE, pulmonary embolism.

anticoagulant effect of UFH is variably reduced by binding to plasma proteins, such as von Willebrand factor and platelet factor 4, as well as to different cells (1).

For treatment of venous thromboembolism, UFH is given by intravenous (i.v.) infusion or subcutaneous (s.c.) injection (Table 1). The former is initiated with an i.v. bolus dose of 5000 U or 80 U/kg and then continued with infusion of 18 U/kg/hr. Weight-based dosing improves the effect of UFH as measured by achievement of a therapeutic activated partial thromboplastin time (APTT), defined as >1.5 times the control, and reduces the incidence of recurrent thrombosis (2). The s.c. regimens are either an initial i.v. bolus of 5000 U followed by 250 U/kg subcutaneously every 12 hours (4) or an initial s.c. dose of 333 U/kg and then 250 U/kg every 12 hours (5).

Monitoring of UFH treatment is most commonly done using the APTT. It is recommended that the dose be adjusted according to a local nomogram, based on the sensitivity of the APTT reagent and the coagulometer (1). The treatment is typically targeted at an APTT range of 1.5 to 2.5 times control, which should correspond to an anti-Xa activity of 0.3 to 0.7 IU/mL (1). With a weight-based subcutaneous injection regimen, it appears possible to manage patients without coagulation monitoring and thus without hospitalization (5).

Clinical Data

In the classical study by Barritt and Jordan, which compared UFH with control in 35 patients with clinically diagnosed PE, UFH produced an absolute risk reduction for death and fatal and nonfatal PE of 22%, 26%, and 26%, respectively (12). In two placebo-controlled studies that each included more than a hundred patients with venous thromboembolism, the absolute risk reduction for recurrence was 15% [95% confidence interval (CI) 3–27] (13) and 13% (95% CI 2–24) (14) during 3 and 24 weeks of follow-up, respectively.

In a meta-analysis of six randomized controlled trials (RCTs) that compared s.c. injection versus i.v. infusion of UFH, progression of venous thromboembolism was demonstrated in 7.4% and 10.3%, respectively (odds ratio 0.62, 95% CI 0.39–0.98) (15). The bioavailability of UFH is lower with s.c. administration, and therefore, identical doses to the i.v. regimen result in a subtherapeutic APTT for many of the patients treated with the former and a higher risk of recurrence—19.3% versus 5.2% in an RCT by Hull et al. (16).

When UFH is given intravenously, careful anticoagulation monitoring is essential to ensure that a therapeutic level is achieved. The i.v. infusion can be stopped in case of bleeding or need for invasive procedures. Once stopped, UFH is quickly cleared from the circulation. However, if more rapid reversal is needed, protamine sulfate can be administered. The dose is 1 mg for neutralization of 100 U of heparin.

UFH is recommended for patients with PE and hemodynamic instability, after thrombolysis in massive PE, in case of recurrence or progression during treatment with LMWH, and in ill patients, particularly those with severe renal failure or those with a recent hemorrhage.

Adverse reactions to UFH include heparin-induced thrombocytopenia (chap. 17) with or without thrombotic complications, nonspecific mild thrombocytopenia, elevation of liver transaminases, allergic skin reactions, and, with long-term exposure, osteoporosis.

LOW–MOLECULAR WEIGHT HEPARIN

Characteristics

Low molecular weight heparins contain glycosaminoglycan chains of 2000 to 9000 Da, which are obtained by fragmentation or depolymerization of UFH. These shorter chains are not long enough to bridge thrombin to antithrombin. Consequently, inhibition of factor Xa becomes the dominant effect. Because of differences in the methods for production of LMWHs, there are differences in their mean molecular weight, pharmacokinetic characteristics, and biological effects. The ratio of inhibition of factor Xa relative to thrombin varies from 2:1 to 4:1. LMWHs exhibit less binding to cells and plasma proteins than UFH, and therefore, LMWHs have more predictable pharmacokinetics and almost 100% bioavailability after s.c. injection. The peak concentration is reached three to five hours after injection, half-life is three to six hours, and elimination occurs mainly via the kidneys.

The administration of LMWHs is invariably via the s.c. route, and the dose is adjusted according to body weight. Once-daily injection is sufficient, because of its longer half-life than that of UFH. A meta-analysis of five RCTs that compared once- versus twice-daily LMWH regimens did not show any difference in clinical endpoints (17). The LMWH dose should be increased linearly in obese patients, at least to a body weight of 190 kg (18). Dose regimens for commonly used LMWHs are shown in Table 1.

Accumulation of LMWH occurs in patients with renal failure, and the risk of bleeding is higher in patients with a creatinine clearance <30 mL/min than it is in those with a high creatinine clearance (odds ratio 2.25, 95% CI 1.19–4.27) (19). Thus, LMWH should not be used for treatment of venous thromboembolism in patients with a creatinine clearance <30 mL/min, except for tinzaparin, which may be given down to a creatinine clearance of 20 mL/min (19).

There is no need for laboratory monitoring of LMWH when it is used for the initial treatment of venous thromboembolism because there is no clear relationship between high anti-Xa levels and bleeding. In case of moderate renal failure or morbid obesity, there is uncertainty regarding the optimal dose, and anti-factor Xa monitoring at peak drug

Table 2 Outcomes in a Meta-Analysis of 22 Trials Comparing Fixed-Dose Low–Molecular Weight Heparin with Adjusted-Dose Unfractionated Heparin for the Treatment of VTE

Outcome	Studies	Odds ratio (95% confidence interval)
VTE overall		
Recurrence		
During initial treatment period	15	0.68 (0.48–0.97)
At 3 mo	13	0.68 (0.53–0.88)
At 6 mo	6	0.68 (0.48–0.96)
At end of follow-up	18	0.68 (0.55–0.84)
Major hemorrhage	19	0.57 (0.39–0.83)
Death at end of follow-up	18	0.76 (0.62–0.92)
Proximal deep-vein thrombosis alone		
Recurrence at end of follow-up	9	0.57 (0.44–0.75)
Major hemorrhage	8	0.50 (0.29–0.85)
Death	8	0.62 (0.46–0.84)
Pulmonary embolism alone		
Recurrence at end of follow-up	4	0.88 (0.48–1.63)

Source: From Ref. 21.

levels is recommended. The target anti-Xa level is 0.6 to 1.2 IU/mL. During pregnancy, when LMWH is used for many months and the pharmacokinetics may change, monitoring once a month is also advisable (20).

Clinical Data

A meta-analysis of 22 RCTs demonstrated that LMWH is more effective and safer than UFH for initial treatment of venous thromboembolism in general and of DVT alone (Table 2) (21). Four RCTs compared LMWH with UFH for treatment of patients with PE, and no statistically significant differences were seen regarding rates of recurrence, major bleeding, or death (21). The once-daily s.c. regimen with LMWH makes it suitable for outpatient treatment. In a systematic review, two RCTs that compared treatment in hospital with the same treatment at home yielded no differences in clinical endpoints (22). However, outpatient treatment is estimated to reduce costs by 56%.

The adverse reactions seen with UFH are also observed with LMWH, but heparin-induced thrombocytopenia (HIT) is less frequent and the risk of osteoporosis during long-term treatment in pregnancy appears to be minimal (23).

Protamine sulfate only reverses the anti-IIa effect of LMWH. Recombinant factor VIIa has been reported as an alternative antidote, and future options may be heparinase I, platelet factor 4, or concatameric peptides (24).

PENTASACCHARIDES

Fondaparinux

The shortest mucopolysaccharide chain that binds to antithrombin consists of five saccharide units and was first synthesized in 1983 by the group of Choay (25). Like UFH and LMWH, the pentasaccharide, which is designated as fondaparinux, is an indirect inhibitor of coagulation, but it lacks any effect on thrombin. Pentasaccharides are not derived from animal sources, and there is batch-to-batch consistency. Fondaparinux has been modified from the native pentasaccharide by the addition of four specific sulfate groups, which optimize the binding to antithrombin. It catalyzes the inhibition of pure factor Xa without any effect on platelets or tissue factor pathway inhibitor (26). The bioavailability after s.c. injection is almost 100%, and binding in plasma is almost exclusively to antithrombin. The half-life in plasma is 14 hours, increasing to 21 hours in the elderly, and elimination is via the kidneys without any prior metabolism.

The dose used for treatment of venous thromboembolism is a once-daily s.c. injection with 5, 7.5, or 10 mg for body weight <50 kg, 50 to 100 kg, and >100 kg, respectively (Table 1). There is no need for monitoring, and standard tests such as prothrombin time or APTT are insensitive. The anti-Xa assay with a fondaparinux standard appears to correlate with antithrombotic activity (26).

Clinical Data

In a dose-finding study, 5, 7.5, and 10 mg of fondaparinux once daily were compared with dalteparin for the initial treatment of 453 patients with symptomatic proximal DVT (27). There were no significant differences between the groups regarding thromboembolic or bleeding complications.

Two phase III trials in patients with venous thromboembolism have been performed, and primary endpoints were clinical outcome after three months. In the phase III PE trial, 2213 patients with PE were randomized to treatment with fondaparinux once daily subcutaneously or UFH by continuous i.v. infusion for at least five days and until treatment with a VKA had reached a therapeutic level (10). Recurrence of venous thromboembolism, major bleeding, and death did not differ significantly between the groups. In the fondaparinux group, 14% were treated as outpatients (10).

In the phase III DVT trial, 2205 patients with acute DVT were randomized to receive the same fondaparinux regimen or enoxaparin (1 mg/kg subcutaneously twice daily). There were no statistically significant differences in clinical outcome between the two groups (11).

Since most LMWHs have a similar once-daily dosing regimen, there is no convenience advantage for fondaparinux. Because of the absence of animal proteins, the risk of allergic reactions is very small. Initially, it was believed that fondaparinux would not cause heparin-induced thrombocytopenia. However, fondaparinux induces HIT antibody formation to the same extent as LMWH (28), and there has been a case report of clinical HIT with fondaparinux (29).

For indications other than treatment of venous thromboembolism, the risk-benefit ratio of bleeding with a lower dose of fondaparinux (2.5 mg) has been somewhat contradictory. When used for prophylaxis against DVT after major orthopedic surgery, this dose of fondaparinux was associated with more surgical bleeding, measured as bleeding index, and major bleeding, but improved efficacy compared with a prophylactic dose of enoxaparin (11). Conversely, in acute coronary syndromes, there was less bleeding (hazard ratio, 0.52; $p < 0.001$) and similar efficacy as compared with a therapeutic dose of enoxaparin (30).

Protamine sulfate does not reverse the anticoagulant effect of fondaparinux. Hemodialysis only reduces fondaparinux plasma levels by approximately 20%. Although recombinant factor VIIa reverses the effect of fondaparinux on thrombin generation in vitro and in human volunteers (24), the ability of recombinant factor VIIa to stop bleeding is limited to single case reports (31).

Idraparinux

Addition of seven methyl groups to fondaparinux produces a pentasaccharide with high affinity for antithrombin and a half-life of 80 hours. Indeed, only when antithrombin is metabolized does idraparinux dissociate from it and bind to another antithrombin molecule. The pharmacokinetics are linear, and there is low inter-and intraindividual variability. Elimination is dependent on renal function.

In a dose-finding study in 659 patients with proximal DVT, idraparinux (at doses of 2.5, 5, 7.5, and 10 mg once weekly) was compared with warfarin (32). During the course of the study, but after complete recruitment, the 10-mg arm was stopped because of a high incidence of bleeding. There was a dose response for bleeding but not for efficacy. On the basis of these results, the 2.5-mg dose was carried forward into the phase III program.

The results of the phase III program in venous thromboembolism (van Gogh studies) are summarized in Table 3. In the two studies, treatment was either with once-weekly idraparinux or with UFH/LMWH followed by a VKA, and the treatment duration was three or six months (33). In the extended treatment trial, all patients received six months of study drug (34). In summary, idraparinux was effective for DVT but not for PE, where both fatal and nonfatal recurrence and all-cause mortality were increased compared with conventional therapy. The incidence of fatal and nonfatal venous thromboembolism in the standard therapy group with PE was at 92 days, however, only 1.6% and 1.9%, respectively, depended on stratification. In the MATISSE PE trial, it was 5.0% during the corresponding period (10) without any difference in quality of oral anticoagulant therapy, measured as "time in therapeutic range," between these studies. Conversely, the incidence

Table 3 Results of the Phase III Clinical Trials with Idraparinux in Venous Thromboembolism (van Gogh Program)

Variable Treatment	van Gogh DVT		van Gogh PE		van Gogh extension	
	Idraparinux	Standard	Idraparinux	Standard	Idraparinux	Placebo
N (%)	1452	1452	1095	1120	594	621
3-mo stratum at 3 mo						
Recurrent VTE	4 (1.2)	5 (1.6)	2 (2.0)	2 (1.9)	NA	NA
Fatal PE	0	0	2	2	NA	NA
Nonfatal PE	3	3	0	0	NA	NA
DVT only	1	2	0	0	NA	NA
6-mo stratum at 6 mo						
Recurrent VTE	42 (3.7)	42 (3.7)	40 (4.0)[a]	20 (2.0)[a]	6 (1.0)[b]	23 (3.7)[b]
Fatal PE	5	6	11	4	2	1
Nonfatal PE	19	18	16	4	1	11
DVT only	18	18	13	12	3	11
Death any cause	55 (4.9)	44 (3.9)	64 (6.4)[c]	45 (4.4)[c]	9 (1.5)	4 (0.6)
Major bleeding	21 (1.9)	17 (1.5)	14 (1.4)[c]	28 (2.8)[c]	11 (1.9)[d]	0[d]
Clinically relevant nonmajor	73 (6.5)	75 (6.6)	62 (6.2)	71 (7.0)	27 (4.5)[b]	9 (1.5)[b]

NA = not applicable
All other differences are nonsignificant.
[a] $p = 0.007$
[b] $p = 0.002$
[c] $p = 0.04$
[d] $p < 0.001$
Abbreviations: DVT, deep-vein thrombosis; PE, pulmonary embolism.
Source: From Refs. 33, 34.

Table 4 Treatment Regimens for Selective Anticoagulants Currently in Clinical Phase III Studies of Treatment for Established Venous Thromboembolism

Agent	Target	Initial phase	Secondary prophylaxis	Route
Ximelagatran[a]	Thrombin	36 mg twice daily for 6 mo	24 mg twice daily for 7–24 mo	Oral
Dabigatran	Thrombin	Unfractionated heparin or LMWH for 5–7 days	150 mg every 12 hr for 6–24 mo	Oral
SSR126517E	Factor Xa	LMWH for 5 days	3 mg once weekly for 3 or 6 mo	Subcutaneous
Rivaroxaban	Factor Xa	15 mg every 12 hr × 3 wk	20 mg once daily for 3–24 mo	Oral

[a]Withdrawn from the market and development.
Abbreviation: LMWH, low–molecular weight heparin.

in the idraparinux group of 2.0% to 3.5% was similar to previous reports on the efficacy of fondaparinux and of UFH-VKA in the MATISSE PE trial (3.8% and 5.0%, respectively) (10) and LMWH-VKA or UFH-VKA in a meta-analysis (3.0% and 4.4%, respectively) (35). The incidence of major bleeding was, on the other hand, lower in the idraparinux than in the conventional therapy group in the PE study. It is unclear whether patients with PE should therefore be treated with a higher dose of idraparinux than those with DVT. In the extended therapy study, idraparinux was more effective than placebo but caused more major as well as nonmajor clinically relevant bleeding and thus did not produce a net clinical benefit. This is in contrast with a similar study on an oral thrombin inhibitor that has been withdrawn from the market (ximelagatran), which was effective without a difference in bleeding compared with placebo (36). Finally, if the three studies with idraparinux are pooled for the six-month treatment duration, there was a higher all-cause mortality than in the comparator groups (4.7% versus 3.4%, $p = 0.01$) due to a combination of more deaths in PE and in cancer.

In a large RCT that compared idraparinux with warfarin for stroke prevention in atrial fibrillation, idraparinux was associated with an increase in intracranial hemorrhage (1.1 versus 0.4 per 100 patient-years, $p = 0.014$) and clinically relevant bleeding (19.7 versus 11.3 per 100 patient-years, $p < 0.0001$). Because of these findings, the trial study was stopped prematurely (37).

The development of the clinical program with a long-acting pentasaccharide has now been focused on a biotinylated form of idraparinux, SSR126517E, which can be neutralized with i.v. avidin in case of bleeding. This product is being evaluated for equipotency with idraparinux in a study with 700 patients and in phase III in a trial with 3200 patients with PE as well as in a study in atrial fibrillation.

Recombinant factor VIIa has a similar reversing effect on idraparinux as described above for fondaparinux (24).

VITAMIN K ANTAGONISTS

Characteristics

VKAs are derivatives of either coumarin or indanedione. They inhibit vitamin K epoxide reductase (VKOR) or vitamin K reductase, thereby blocking regeneration of vitamin KH_2 from vitamin K epoxide. Depletion of vitamin K results in deficient posttranslational

γ-carboxylation of approximately 10 glutamic acid residues located in the Gla domain of coagulation factors II, VII, IX, and X and also in the corresponding domains of the anticoagulants, protein C, protein S, and protein Z, as well as nonhemostatic proteins such as osteocalcin, proline-rich Gla protein 2, matrix γ-glutamic acid protein, and the protein encoded by growth arrest-specific gene (GAS6). The hypo-γ-carboxylated coagulation factors bind calcium poorly and fail to localize the coagulation process to phospholipid surfaces (38).

The VKAs generally have good absorption, about 99% binding to plasma proteins, mainly albumin, and are metabolized by the cytochrome P450 (CYP) system. The half-life varies from 10 hours (acenocoumarol) to three to five days (phenprocoumon). Warfarin, the most widely used VKA, has a half-life of 35 to 45 hours (38). The VKAs are susceptible to a large number of drug and food interactions through a variety of mechanisms. In addition, polymorphisms in complex 1 of VKOR (VKORC1), in the hydroxylating enzyme CYP2C9, which is mainly responsible for the metabolism of warfarin, and to a lesser extent, in γ-carboxylase, microsomal epoxide hydrolase, and calumenin contribute to the 40-fold range in daily dose requirement in individuals (38).

The full anticoagulant effect occurs only after about five days of VKA treatment. Therefore, VKA therapy should be initiated concomitantly with UFH or LMWH and overlapped for at least five days (39). The dose of VKA is adjusted to maintain a target international normalized ratio (INR) of 2.5 (range 2.0–3.0). The duration of treatment depends on a large number of factors, including presence of reversible risk factors, localization and extent of the thrombus, number of episodes of venous thromboembolism, presence of thrombophilic abnormalities or cancer, history of bleeding, patient age, and compliance. It can thus vary from six weeks to indefinitely, as recently reviewed elsewhere (40).

Clinical Data

Secondary prophylaxis against venous thromboembolism is necessary, since UFH without subsequent VKA treatment is associated with a 20% risk of early recurrence, as shown in a RCT with 51 patients suffering from calf vein thrombosis (41). Moreover, in RCTs where the short-duration arm was only four to six weeks, the rate of recurrence was significantly higher than when the duration was at least three months (42,43). Properly managed anticoagulation virtually eliminates the risk of recurrence (44,45), with the exceptions usually explained by active cancer. Optimal management of treatment with VKA is, however, challenging (38,46).

The most common complication of treatment is bleeding. In a meta-analysis of 33 trials, major bleeding occurred in 2.1% of the patients within the first three months of therapy, with fatal bleeding occurring in 0.37% (47). The case fatality of major bleeding was 13%, and in cases of intracranial bleeding, it was 46% (47). In patients with active cancer, LMWH should be used for secondary prophylaxis for three to six months instead of VKA, because of a favorable risk-benefit profile and possibly better survival (39). A lower risk of bleeding with LMWH than with VKA has also been shown for patients in general according to a meta-analysis of seven trials (odds ratio 0.45, 95% CI 0.2–1.1) (48). Therefore, LMWH is an attractive alternative when the planned duration is six weeks or less.

Infrequent side effects of VKA are skin necrosis, limb gangrene, purple toes, skin allergy, eosinophilic pleurisy, vasculitis, alopecia, diarrhea, osteoporosis, toxic hepatitis, and intrahepatic jaundice. In addition, VKAs are teratogenic if given during pregnancy weeks 6 to 12, with an incidence of embryopathy of approximately 6% (49).

Major bleeding requires reversal of VKA with vitamin K, usually in combination with prothrombin complex concentrate or recombinant factor VIIa, whereas plasma in adequate doses cannot be transfused fast enough and often causes volume overload (24).

ORAL DIRECT THROMBIN INHIBITORS

In the quest for orally available alternatives to VKA, the main requirements were simplified dosing regimens, elimination of the need for laboratory monitoring, and rapid onset and offset of action. The development has focused mainly on highly selective inhibitors, which reversibly bind to the active site of factor Xa or thrombin. However, drugs against other targets, such as factor IXa and factor VIIa, also have been explored. The first candidate to reach approval, albeit short lived, was ximelagatran, a prodrug of melagatran. This orally available thrombin inhibitor was withdrawn from the market in February 2006 because of potential liver toxicity. However, a 36-mg twice-daily dose of unmonitored ximelagatran was as effective as warfarin for the treatment of patients with venous thromboembolism (50). In another study with 1233 patients, ximelagatran (at a dose of 24 mg twice daily) was compared with placebo for secondary prophylaxis extending from 6 to 24 months (36). Recurrent venous thromboembolism was effectively reduced (hazard ratio 0.16, 95% CI 0.09–0.30, $p < 0.001$) without an increase in major bleeding or any bleeding.

Dabigatran

The second orally available direct thrombin inhibitor is dabigatran etexilate. Conversion of the prodrug to dabigatran occurs in two steps via ubiquitous esterases. Bioavailability is low (4–6%), plasma protein binding is only 30% to 38%, and peak concentration is seen two hours after ingestion. About 30% of dabigatran is glucuronidated, although still active, and the drug is eliminated via the kidneys. The half-life is eight hours, increasing to 14 to 17 hours after repeated dosing, and steady state is achieved after three days. No drug interactions have been identified (51). Prothrombin time, thrombin time, and ecarin clotting time have a linear correlation, and APTT has a curvilinear correlation with the plasma concentration of dabigatran. The slope is quite flat for the prothrombin time, which renders it less useful for assessing overdose. At high plasma concentrations, the bleeding time becomes prolonged.

Dabigatran should be considered contraindicated in pregnancy. With the exception of bleeding, there have not been any reports of drug-specific adverse events in humans. In particular, there is no evidence that dabigatran produces liver toxicity as was seen with ximelagatran.

Dabigatran has proven effective in comparison with enoxaparin (40 mg once daily) as primary thromboprophylaxis after major orthopedic surgery (52,53), and in 2008 the drug was approved for marketing on this indication in Europe and in several countries in other parts of the world. The clinical trial program has, at this point, already involved 34,000 patients. For established venous thromboembolism, no phase II studies were performed. Instead, data from the dose-finding study in atrial fibrillation were used to determine the dose. There are currently four ongoing phase III trials evaluating a dose of dabigatran etexilate of 150 mg twice daily (Table 4). Each one will include >2000 patients. Two trials focus on patients with acute DVT or PE, who are randomized to dabigatran etexilate or warfarin for six months after initial treatment with UFH or LMWH. The design is double blind, double dummy, with sham INR results and non-inferiority analysis. A third trial recruits patients at low risk of recurrence and randomizes them to dabigatran etexilate or placebo, whereas a fourth trial aiming at patients with a high risk of recurrence, randomizes patients to dabigatran or warfarin. Both trials use a double-blind, double-dummy design, and patients receive 18 months of extended therapy.

There is no antidote for dabigatran. In animal models, bleeding after a dose of ximelagatran could be attenuated with activated prothrombin complex concentrate (54).

ORAL DIRECT FACTOR Xa INHIBITORS

Factor Xa is currently the most popular target for new oral anticoagulants. Its strategic location at the intersection of the intrinsic and extrinsic pathways of coagulation is often claimed as ideal for inhibition. It is however impossible to objectively rate one target as better than the other at this point in time. Favorable pharmacokinetics and successful selection of the appropriate dose for the clinical trials may play a greater role for obtaining superior results.

Rivaroxaban

Rivaroxaban is a small, non-peptidic molecule, which binds with high selectivity to the active site of factor Xa. Maximum plasma concentration is reached 2.5 to 4 hours after ingestion with oral bioavailability of about 80%. The half-life is 5.8 to 9.2 hours, and elimination occurs mainly without prior metabolism by fecal/biliary and renal excretion. The enzymes involved in the metabolism include CYP3A4 and CYP2J2. In addition, rivaroxaban is a substrate for the transporter proteins P-glycoprotein (P-gp) and breast cancer resistance protein (Bcrp). CYP3A4 and P-gp are strongly inhibited by ketoconazole and ritonavir, which may cause a clinically significant enhancement of the anticoagulant effect, whereas the CYP3A4 and P-gp inducers rifampicin and probably also phenytoin, carbamazepine, phenobarbitone, and St John's wort may reduce the effect. There is an additive effect on inhibition of factor Xa with concomitant administration of rivaroxaban and enoxaparin. Rivaroxaban does not affect the bleeding time, but there is a linear correlation between prothrombin time and rivaroxaban concentration. Factor Xa inhibition and parameters of thrombin generation are also inhibited dose dependently (55). Concomitant ingestion of food delays the time to maximum plasma concentration by 1.25 hours and increases the peak concentration and area under the curve (56), but this is probably of minimal clinical significance. The dose brought forward to phase III in major orthopedic surgery is 10 mg once daily. For treatment of venous thromboembolism, an initial dose of 15 mg twice daily followed by 20 mg once daily has been selected (Table 4). Rivaroxaban crosses the placenta and is contraindicated in pregnancy.

For prevention of venous thromboembolism after total knee arthroplasty, rivaroxaban was compared with enoxaparin (40 mg once daily) in 2531 patients in a non-inferiority study that actually showed superiority (57). The rate of any thromboembolism and all-cause death was 9.6% versus 18.9% ($p < 0.001$), of proximal DVT 1.1% versus 2.2%, of symptomatic venous thromboembolism 1.0% versus 2.7% ($p = 0.006$) and of major bleeding 0.6% versus 0.5% for rivaroxaban and enoxaparin, respectively (57). Rivaroxaban was approved in 2008 for marketing in Europe and Canada on the indication thromboprophylaxis in major orthopedic surgery.

Two dose-finding studies in patients treated for venous thromboembolism have been performed. In the first study, 604 patients were randomized to rivaroxaban (10, 20, or 30 mg twice daily or 40 mg once daily) or enoxaparin plus VKA for three months (58). The primary efficacy endpoint, reduced thrombus burden on day 21, was achieved in

43.8% to 59.2% of the rivaroxaban-treated patients, without any relationship to dose, and in 45.9% in the conventional therapy group. Major bleeding occurred in 1.7% to 3.3% in the rivaroxaban groups versus none in the standard therapy group, but this difference was not statistically significant (58). In the second study, 542 patients were randomized to rivaroxaban (20, 30, or 40 mg once daily) versus UFH/LMWH and VKA for 12 weeks (59). The primary efficacy endpoint was the composite of symptomatic recurrent venous thromboembolism and increased thrombotic burden, which was observed in 5.4% to 6.6% versus 9.9% in the rivaroxaban groups and standard group, respectively, whereas the rate of major bleeding was 0% to 1.5% and 1.5%, respectively. There was no dose response for any of the variables in either study.

Currently, a phase III program is being conducted with treatment for 6 or 12 months after acute DVT ($n = 2900$) or PE ($n = 3300$). Rivaroxaban is started immediately after diagnosis (Table 4) and compared in an open-label, non-inferiority design with enoxaparin and VKA. Moreover, in a study on extended treatment, 1300 patients, who have already received 6 or 12 months of anticoagulation therapy, are randomized to another 6 or 12 months of rivaroxaban (20 mg daily) or placebo in a double-blind, superiority design.

There is no known antidote to rivaroxaban, and hemorrhagic complications should be treated symptomatically with transfusions of red cells and plasma as needed.

Apixaban

In a dose-finding study in total knee replacement, the oral, direct factor Xa inhibitor razaxaban was effective but caused an increased rate of major bleeding compared with enoxaparin. The program was halted, and several modifications were made to the substance, resulting in the compound apixaban (60). The pharmacokinetic profile was thereby improved, and the oral bioavailability is high without influence from food. Peak plasma concentration is achieved after 3 hours, the half-life is 12 hours, and elimination is combined renal (25%) and fecal (61).

In a phase II study in total knee replacement, apixaban (5, 10 or 20 mg once daily or the same dose divided and given twice daily) was compared with enoxaparin (30 mg twice daily) or warfarin in 1217 patients (62). All apixaban groups experienced a lower rate of venous thromboembolism and all-cause mortality than the comparators, but there was also a higher rate of major bleeding in most apixaban groups versus the comparators. The preferred regimen appeared to be 2.5 mg twice daily, which has been brought forward to currently recruiting phase III studies in major orthopedic surgery and in medically ill patients (n ≈ 6500).

Patients with established venous thromboembolism ($n = 520$) were included in a phase II trial with apixaban 5 or 10 mg twice daily, 20 mg once daily, or standard therapy, which was either LMWH or fondaparinux, followed by VKA for three months (63). The primary efficacy endpoint, recurrent symptomatic venous thromboembolism, or increased thrombotic burden occurred in 6.0%, 5.6% and 2.6% in the apixaban groups without a clear dose response and in 4.2% with standard therapy. Major bleeding was low, 0% to 0.8%. At the moment of writing this chapter, the dose selected for phase III on this indication is unknown.

CONCLUSION

The treatment of venous thromboembolism is effective and safe today and rarely requires hospitalization. Now the major unmet need is convenient secondary prophylaxis. Indefinite duration of anticoagulation is justified in a large number of patients with risk factors for recurrence but is often avoided because of the aversion from both patients and physicians. The development of new, orally available anticoagulants, which do not require routine monitoring and dose adjustments, is well under way. A few agents can be expected to reach marketing approval in two to three years on the indication established venous thromboembolism. It remains to be seen if efficacy can be maintained without routine monitoring and associated feedback mechanisms when clinical practice patients, less compliant than the ideal study patients, are involved. Another potential concern is that the treatment will be simplified to the extent that objective diagnosis may not be pursued and many patients may be treated *ex juvantibus*. Good clinical training in the diagnosis and appropriate treatment of venous thromboembolism will continue to be important.

REFERENCES

1. Hirsh J, Raschke R. Heparin and low-molecular-weight heparin. Chest 2004; 126:188S–203S.
2. Raschke RA, Reilly BM, Guidry JR, et al. The weight-based heparin dosing nomogram compared with a "standard care" nomogram. A randomized controlled trial. Ann Intern Med 1993; 119:874–881.
3. Kearon C, Kahn SR, Agnelli G, et al. Antithrombotic therapy for venous thromboembolic disease. Chest 2008; 133(Suppl):454S–545S.
4. Prandoni P, Carnovali M, Marchiori A, et al. Subcutaneous adjusted-dose unfractionated heparin vs. fixed-dose low-molecular-weight heparin in the initial treatment of venous thromboembolism. Arch Intern Med 2004; 164:1077–1083.
5. Kearon C, Ginsberg JS, Julian JA, et al. Comparison of fixed-dose weight-adjusted unfractionated heparin and low-molecular-weight heparin for acute treatment of venous thromboembolism. JAMA 2006; 296:935–942.
6. Fiessinger JN, Lopez-Fernandez M, Gatterer E, et al. Once-daily subcutaneous dalteparin, a low molecular weight heparin, for the initial treatment of acute deep vein thrombosis. Thromb Haemost 1996; 76:195–199.
7. Meyer G, Brenot F, Pacouret G, et al. Subcutaneous low-molecular-weight heparin fragmin versus intravenous unfractionated heparin in the treatment of acute non massive pulmonary embolism: an open randomized pilot study. Thromb Haemost 1995; 74:1432–1435.
8. Merli G, Spiro TE, Olsson CG, et al. Subcutaneous enoxaparin once or twice daily compared with intravenous unfractionated heparin for treatment of venous thromboembolic disease. Ann Intern Med 2001; 134:191–202.
9. Hull RD, Raskob GE, Pineo GF, et al. Subcutaneous low-molecular-weight heparin compared with continuous intravenous heparin in the treatment of proximal-vein thrombosis. N Engl J Med 1992; 326:975–982.
10. Büller HR, Davidson BL, Decousus H, et al. Subcutaneous fondaparinux versus intravenous unfractionated heparin in the initial treatment of pulmonary embolism. N Engl J Med 2003; 349:1695–1702.
11. Büller HR, Davidson BL, Decousus H, et al. Fondaparinux or enoxaparin for the initial treatment of symptomatic deep venous thrombosis: a randomized trial. Ann Intern Med 2004; 140:867–873.
12. Barritt DW, Jordan SC. Anticoagulant drugs in the treatment of pulmonary embolism. Lancet 1960; 1:1309–1312.
13. Rosenbeck-Hansen JV, Valdorf-Hansen F, Dige-Petersen H, et al. En kontrolleret undersøgelse af antikoagulationsbehandlingens effekt ved dyb venetrombose og lungeemboli. Nord Med 1968; 80:1305–1306.
14. Brandjes DP, Heijboer H, Buller HR, et al. Acenocoumarol and heparin compared with acenocoumarol alone in the initial treatment of proximal-vein thrombosis. N Engl J Med 1992; 327:1485–1489.

15. Hommes DW, Bura A, Mazzolai L, et al. Subcutaneous heparin compared with continuous intravenous heparin administration in the initial treatment of deep vein thrombosis. A meta-analysis. Ann Intern Med 1992; 116:279–284.

16. Hull RD, Raskob GE, Hirsh J, et al. Continuous intravenous heparin compared with intermittent subcutaneous heparin in the initial treatment of proximal-vein thrombosis. N Engl J Med 1986; 315:1109–1114.

17. Couturaud F, Julian JA, Kearon C. Low molecular weight heparin administered once versus twice daily in patients with venous thromboembolism: a meta-analysis. Thromb Haemost 2001; 86:980–984.

18. Spinler SA, Inverso SM, Cohen M, et al. Safety and efficacy of unfractionated heparin versus enoxaparin in patients who are obese and patients with severe renal impairment: analysis from the ESSENCE and TIMI 11B studies. Am Heart J 2003; 146:33–41.

19. Lim W, Dentali F, Eikelboom JW, et al. Meta-analysis: low-molecular-weight heparin and bleeding in patients with severe renal insufficiency. Ann Intern Med 2006; 144:673–684.

20. Laposata M, Green K, Elizabeth MVC, et al. College of American Pathologists Conference XXXI on Laboratory Monitoring of Anticoagulant Therapy. The clinical use and laboratory monitoring of low-molecular-weight heparin, danaparoid, hirudin and related compounds, and argatroban. Arch Pathol Lab Med 1998; 122:799–807.

21. van Dongen CJJ, van der Belt AGM, Prins MH, et al. Fixed-dose subcutaneous low molecular weight heparins versus adjusted dose unfractionated heparin for venous thromboembolism. Cochrane Database Syst Rev 2004; (4):CD001100.

22. Schraibman IG, Milne AA, Royle EM. Home versus in-patient treatment for deep vein thrombosis. Cochrane Database Syst Rev 2001; (2):CD003076.

23. Pettilä V, Leinonen P, Markkola A, et al. Postpartum bone mineral density in women treated for thromboprophylaxis with unfractionated heparin or LMW heparin. Thromb Haemost 2002; 87:182–186.

24. Schulman S, Bijsterveld NR. Anticoagulants and their reversal. Transfus Med Rev 2007; 21:37–48.

25. Torri G, Casu B, Gatti G, et al. Mono- and bidimensional 500 MHZ proton NMR spectra of a synthetic pentasaccharide corresponding to the binding sequence of heparin to antithrombin-III: evidence for conformational peculiarity of the sulphated iduronate residue. Biochem Biophys Res Commun 1985; 128:134–140.

26. Walenga JM, Jeske WP, Samama MM, et al. Fondaparinux: a synthetic heparin pentasaccharide as a new antithrombotic agent. Expert Opin Investig Drugs 2002; 11:397–407.

27. The Rembrandt Investigators. Treatment of proximal deep vein thrombosis with a novel synthetic compound (SR90107A/ORG31540) with pure anti-factor Xa activity. Circulation 2000; 102:2726–2731.

28. Greinacher A, Gopinadhan M, Gunther JU, et al. Close approximation of two platelet factor 4 tetramers by charge neutralization forms the antigens recognized by HIT antibodies. Arterioscler Thromb Vasc Biol 2006; 26:2386–2393.

29. Warkentin TE, Maurer BT, Aster RH. Heparin-induced thrombocytopenia associated with fondaparinux. N Engl J Med 2007; 356:2653–2655.

30. Yusuf S, Mehta SR, Chrolavicius S, et al. Comparison of fondaparinux and enoxaparin in acute coronary syndromes. N Engl J Med 2006; 354:1464–1476.

31. Huvers F, Slappendel R, Benraad B, et al. Treatment of postoperative bleeding after fondaparinux with rFVIIa and tranexamic acid. Neth J Med 2005; 63:184–186.

32. PERSIST investigators. A novel long-acting synthetic factor Xa inhibitor (SanOrg34006) to replace warfarin for secondary prevention in deep vein thrombosis. A phase II evaluation. J Thromb Haemost 2004; 2:47–53.

33. Büller HR, Cohen AT, Davidson B, et al. Idraparinux versus standard therapy for venous thromboembolic disease. N Engl J Med 2007; 357:1094–1104.

34. Büller HR, Cohen AT, Davidson B, et al. Extended prophylaxis of venous thromboembolism with idraparinux. N Engl J Med 2007; 357:1105–1112.

35. Quinlan DJ, McQuillan A, Eikelboom JW. Low-molecular-weight heparin compared with intravenous unfractionated heparin for treatment of pulmonary embolism: a meta-analysis of randomized, controlled trials. Ann Intern Med 2004; 140:175–183.

36. Schulman S, Wahlander K, Lundstrom T, et al. Secondary prevention of venous thromboembolism with the oral direct thrombin inhibitor ximelagatran. N Engl J Med 2003; 349:1713–1721.

37. The Amadeus Investigators. Comparison of idraparinux with vitamin K antagonists for prevention of thromboembolism in patients with atrial fibrillation; a randomised, open-label, non-inferiority trial. Lancet 2008; 371:315–321.

38. Ansell J, Hirsh J, Poller L, et al. The pharmacology and management of the vitamin K antagonists. Chest 2004; 126(suppl):204S–233S.

39. Büller HR, Agnelli G, Hull RD, et al. Antithrombotic therapy for venous thromboembolic disease. Chest 2004; 126(suppl):401S–428S.

40. Schulman S, Ogren M. New concepts in optimal management of anticoagulant therapy for extended treatment of venous thromboembolism. Thromb Haemost 2006; 96:258–266.

41. Lagerstedt CI, Olsson CG, Fagher BO, et al. Need for long-term anticoagulant treatment in symptomatic calf-vein thrombosis. Lancet 1985; 2:515–518.

42. Research Committee of the British Thoracic Society. Optimum duration of anticoagulation for deep-vein thrombosis and pulmonary embolism. Lancet 1992; 340:873–876.

43. Schulman S, Rhedin AS, Lindmarker P, et al. A comparison of six weeks with six months of oral anticoagulant therapy after a first episode of venous thromboembolism. Duration of Anticoagulation Trial Study Group. N Engl J Med 1995; 332:1661–1665.

44. Kearon C, Gent M, Hirsh J, et al. A comparison of three months of anticoagulation with extended anticoagulation for a first episode of idiopathic venous thromboembolism. N Engl J Med 1999; 340:901–907.

45. Schulman S, Granqvist S, Holmström M, et al. The duration of oral anticoagulant therapy after a second episode of venous thromboembolism. The Duration of Anticoagulation Trial Study Group. N Engl J Med 1997; 336:393–398.

46. Schulman S. Care of patients receiving long-term anticoagulant therapy. N Engl J Med 2003; 349:675–683.

47. Linkins LA, Choi PT, Douketis JD. Clinical impact of bleeding in patients taking oral anticoagulant therapy for venous thromboembolism: a meta-analysis. Ann Intern Med 2003; 139:893–900.

48. Iorio A, Guercini F, Pini M. Low-molecular-weight heparin for the long-term treatment of symptomatic venous thromboembolism: meta-analysis of the randomized comparisons with oral anticoagulants. J Thromb Haemost 2003; 1:1906–1913.

49. Chan WS, Anand S, Ginsberg JS. Anticoagulation of pregnant women with mechanical heart valves: a systematic review of the literature. Arch Intern Med 2000; 160:191–196.

50. Fiessinger JN, Huisman MV, Davidson BL, et al. Ximelagatran vs. low-molecular-weight heparin and warfarin for the treatment of deep vein thrombosis: a randomized trial. JAMA 2005; 293:681–689.

51. Ieko M. Dabigatran etexilate, a thrombin inhibitor for the prevention of venous thromboembolism and stroke. Curr Opin Investig Drugs 2007; 8:758–768.

52. Eriksson BI, Dahl OE, Rosencher N, et al. Oral dabigatran etexilate vs. subcutaneous enoxaparin for the prevention of venous thromboembolism after total knee replacement: the RE-MODEL randomized trial. J Thromb Haemost 2007; 5:2178–2185.

53. Eriksson BI, Dahl OE, Rosencher N, et al. Dabigatran etexilate versus enoxaparin for prevention of venous thromboembolism after total hip replacement: a randomised, double-blind, non-inferiority trial. Lancet 2007; 370:949–956.

54. Elg M, Carlsson S, Gustafsson D. Effects of activated prothrombin complex concentrate or recombinant Factor VIIa on bleeding time and thrombus formation during anticoagulation with a direct thrombin inhibitor. Thromb Res 2001; 101:145–157.

55. Kubitza D, Haas S. Novel factor Xa inhibitors for prevention and treatment of thromboembolic disease. Expert Opin Investig Drugs 2006; 15:843–855.

56. Kubitza D, Becka M, Zuehlsdorf M, et al. Effect of food, an antacid, and the H2 antagonist ranitidine on the absorption of BAY 59-7939 (rivaroxaban), an oral, direct factor Xa inhibitor, in healthy subjects. J Clin Pharmacol 2006; 46:549–558.

57. Lassen MR, Ageno W, Borris LC, et al. Rivaroxaban versus enoxaparin for thromboprophylaxis after total knee arthroplasty. N Engl J Med 2008; Jun 26; 358:2776–2786.

58. Agnelli G, Gallus A, Goldhaber SZ, et al. Treatment of proximal deep-vein thrombosis with the oral direct factor Xa inhibitor rivaroxaban (BAY 59-7939): the ODIXa-DVT (oral direct factor Xa inhibitor BAY 59-7939 in patients with acute symptomatic deep-vein thrombosis) study. Circulation 2007; 116:180–187.

59. Büller HR, Lensing AW, Prins MH, et al. A dose-ranging study evaluating once-daily oral administration of the factor Xa inhibitor rivaroxaban in the treatment of patients with acute symptomatic deep vein thrombosis: the Einstein-DVT Dose-Ranging Study. Blood 2008; 112:2242–2247.

60. Pinto DJ, Orwat MJ, Koch S, et al. Discovery of 1-(4-methoxyphenyl)-7-oxo-6-(4-(2-oxopiperidin-1-yl)phenyl)-4,5,6,7-tetrahydro-1H-pyrazolo[3,4-c]pyridine-3-carboxamide (apixaban, BMS-562247), a highly potent, selective, efficacious, and orally bioavailable inhibitor of blood coagulation factor Xa. J Med Chem 2007; 50:5339–5356.

61. Turpie AG. New oral anticoagulants in atrial fibrillation. Eur Heart J 2008; 29:155–165.

62. Lassen MR, Davidson BL, Gallus A, et al. The efficacy and safety of apixaban, an oral, direct factor Xa inhibitor, as thromboprophylaxis in patients following total knee replacement. J Thromb Haemost 2007; 5:2368–2375.

63. Büller HR. A dose finding study of the oral direct factor Xa inhibitor apixaban in the treatment of patients with acute symptomatic deep vein thrombosis—the Botticelli investigators. J Thromb Haemost 2007; 5(suppl 2):O-S-003.

11

Anticoagulation in Acute Coronary Syndromes

Simon J. McRae
Institute of Medical and Veterinary Science, The Queen Elizabeth Hospital, South Australia, Australia

John W. Eikelboom
Department of Medicine, McMaster University, Thrombosis Service, Hamilton General Hospital, Hamilton, Ontario, Canada

INTRODUCTION

Cardiovascular disease is the leading cause of death in the industrialized world and is expected to become the single most common cause of morbidity and mortality in the developing world by 2020 (1). Acute coronary syndrome (ACS) refers to a spectrum of clinical presentations in patients with acute myocardial ischemia, most often caused by a complication of atherosclerotic coronary artery disease (CAD) (2). In 2005, there were over 1.5 million hospital admissions for either a primary or secondary diagnosis of ACS in the United States (3). Patients with ACS are at high risk for both short- and long-term morbidity and mortality (4,5). Therefore, prompt diagnosis and appropriate management are essential. This chapter critically examines the evidence for the efficacy and safety of anticoagulant therapy in the immediate management of patients with ACS.

Pathogenesis of ACSs and Definitions

Atherosclerosis is a chronic immuno-inflammatory fibroproliferative disease that results in lipid accumulation within the intimal layer of medium-sized and large arteries (6). Uncomplicated, the disease typically progresses over many years, resulting in luminal narrowing and manifesting clinically as stable angina. Atherosclerotic plaques may also progress through episodes of instability characterized by activation of T cells and macrophages (7), metalloproteinase expression, and plaque thinning (8). Plaque fissuring or rupture exposes collagen and von Willebrand factor to the circulating blood, leading to platelet adhesion and activation (9). Exposure of tissue factor activates coagulation, and assembly of clotting factor complexes results in thrombin generation. Thrombin promotes further platelet recruitment and activation and triggers the formation of a platelet-rich thrombus within the coronary artery (7). The central role of thrombus formation in the development of ACS has been demonstrated in autopsy series (10,11) and by angiographic and angioscopic detection of intra-coronary thrombi in symptomatic patients (12).

The location and extent of coronary artery thrombos are major determinants of the clinical presentation of patients with ACS, which can be subdivided into two major categories:

1. Non-ST-elevation ACS (NSTE-ACS): Patients presenting with symptoms of ACS who do not have persistent ST elevation on their electrocardiogram (ECG) typically have incomplete or transient thrombotic occlusion of a coronary artery (13). Patients with NSTE-ACS can be further categorized as having either non-ST-elevation myocardial infarction (NSTEMI), if biochemical evidence of myocardial necrosis is present (14), or unstable angina (UA), if there is no evidence of myocardial necrosis (15). The immediate therapeutic objective in patients with NSTE-ACS is to prevent the development of complete thrombotic occlusion of the culprit coronary artery, and commonly involves the use of an early invasive management strategy in combination with aggressive antithrombotic therapy.

2. ST-elevation myocardial infarction (STEMI): Patients presenting with symptoms of ACS who have persistent ST elevation on their ECG typically have complete thrombotic occlusion of a coronary artery and most will develop biochemical evidence of myocardial infarction (MI) (6). The immediate therapeutic objective in patients with STEMI is to restore coronary perfusion. This can be achieved mechanically via primary angioplasty or pharmacologically through the use of fibrinolytic therapy. With either approach, aggressive antithrombotic therapy also is employed (2,15).

ANTITHROMBOTIC THERAPY IN PATIENTS WITH NSTE-ACS

Antithrombotic therapy has been used for the management of unstable angina for more than 50 years (16). Aspirin was the only antiplatelet treatment used in the early trials, but more recent trials have used increasingly aggressive combinations of antiplatelet drugs, anticoagulants, and early revascularization procedures, complicating their comparison with earlier trials (15). We will consider separately the results of trials in which a predominantly conservative management strategy was used and the results of trials in which the majority of patients underwent an early invasive management strategy.

Anticoagulation in a Conservative Strategy for NSTE-ACS

Unfractionated Heparin
Unfractionated heparin (UFH) is a sulfated glycosaminoglycan that exerts its anticoagulant effect by binding to antithrombin (AT) via a unique pentasaccharide sequence. Once bound to AT, heparin induces a conformational change that accelerates the rate at which AT inhibits thrombin (factor IIa) and factor Xa (17). UFH catalyzes the inhibition of thrombin by acting as a binding template for both AT and thrombin in a reaction that requires a heparin chain length of at least 18 saccharide units. By contrast, binding of heparin to AT via the critical pentasaccharide sequence is all that is required to inhibit factor Xa (18). UFH also inhibits coagulation factors IXa and XIa. Commercial UFH is a heterogeneous mixture of carbohydrate chains ranging in molecular weight from 3000 to 30,000 d (19), but only one-third of heparin chains contain the unique pentasaccharide

sequence required for binding to AT (20). The molecular heterogeneity and nonspecific binding of heparin to plasma proteins and cells are responsible for its unpredictable anticoagulant effect and major side effects (discussed below).

The first placebo-controlled trial of UFH reported a significant reduction in the incidence of MI (21). The results of subsequent trials directly comparing UFH with aspirin were conflicting (22–26), but aspirin was later shown to be effective for preventing death or MI (26–28). Thus, the relevant clinical question was whether the addition of UFH to aspirin was more effective than aspirin alone.

Trials of UFH vs. placebo (or no UFH) Six randomized controlled trials (RCTs) involving a combined total of 1353 patients have compared UFH plus aspirin with aspirin alone in conservatively managed patients with NSTE-ACS (Table 1) (26,29–32). A meta-analysis of these trials reported a borderline significant 33% reduction in the combined endpoint of death or MI in patients receiving UFH for up to one week (OR 0.67; 95% CI, 0.45–0.99; $p = 0.045$) (38), predominantly due to a reduction in nonfatal MI with no reduction in death. The duration of anticoagulation therapy in the trials ranged from 48 hours to 7 days. UFH did not reduce recurrent angina (OR 0.94; 95% CI, 0.58–1.54; $p = 0.81$) or need for revascularization procedures (OR 1.25; 95% CI, 0.76–2.06; $p = 0.37$), but increased major bleeding (OR 1.88; 95% CI, 0.60–5.87; $p = 0.28$) (38). There is evidence of rebound activation of coagulation during the first few hours after discontinuation of UFH. Rebound activation of coagulation is associated with an increased risk of reinfarction (39,40).

Increasing the intensity of anticoagulation with UFH [as reflected by an activated partial thromboplastin time (aPTT) > 80 seconds] does not appear to offer any efficacy advantage compared with moderate intensity anticoagulation (aPTT 45–60 seconds) (41,42). For patients with ACS, a weight-adjusted UFH protocol involving an initial bolus of 60 U/kg (maximum 4000 U) followed by an infusion of 12 U/kg/hr (maximum 1000 U/hr) appears to be the most effective regimen for achieving an aPTT within the target range of 45 to 70 seconds at 6 hours (43).

Low-Molecular-Weight Heparin

Low-molecular-weight heparin (LWMH) is produced by controlled enzymatic or chemical depolymerization of UFH and has a mean molecular weight of approximately 5000 d (18). Compared with UFH, LMWH has fewer carbohydrate chains that exceed 18 saccharide units, and it is, therefore, a less effective inhibitor of thrombin. The molecular weights and chain lengths of different LMWH preparations vary depending on their method of production. Consequently, the ratio of anti-factor Xa to anti-factor IIa activity of commercially available LMWH preparations ranges from 1.9 to 3.8 (18).

The lower molecular size and charge of LMWH compared with UFH result in less nonspecific binding to endothelium, macrophages, and heparin-binding plasma proteins (44). Consequently, LMWH has a higher bioavailability and longer half-life than UFH and produces a more predictable anticoagulant dose-response, allowing it to be administered subcutaneously in a fixed, weight-adjusted dose without laboratory monitoring. LMWH is cleared primarily via the kidneys (18), and a reduced dose is recommended when the creatinine clearance is < 30 mL/min. LMWH is contraindicated in patients with severe renal impairment.

Trials of LMWH vs. placebo (or no LMWH) Two trials have compared LMWH plus aspirin with aspirin alone for short-term treatment (up to 6 days) of patients with NSTE-ACS (Table 1) (32,33). Pooled data from the two trials reveal a 66% reduction in death or

Table 1 Trials of UFH and LMWH in Patients with NSTE-ACS Managed Conservatively

Study	Year	n	Active treatment	Control treatment	Duration (day)	Death or myocardial infarction		
						Active arm	Control arm	Odds ratio OR (95% CI)
UFH vs. placebo or untreated control								
Theroux et al. (22)	1988	243	UFH bolus + infusion	Placebo bolus + infusion	5–6	2/122 (1.6%)	4/121 (3.3%)	0.50 (0.10–2.53)
Cohen et al. (29)	1990	69	UFH bolus + infusion	Untreated control	3–4	0/37 (0.0%)	1/32 (3.1%)	0.12 (0.01–5.89)
RISC (26)	1990	399	UFH bolus 6 hourly	Placebo bolus 6 hourly	4	3/210 (1.4%)	7/189 (3.7%)	0.40 (0.11–1.39)
Cohen et al. (30)	1994	214	UFH bolus + infusion	Untreated control	3–4	4/105 (3.8%)	9/109 (8.2%)	0.46 (0.15–1.41)
Holdright et al. (31)	1994	285	UFH bolus + infusion	Untreated control	2	42/154 (27.3%)	40/131 (30.5%)	0.85 (0.51–1.43)
Gurfinkel et al. (32)	1995	143	UFH bolus + infusion	Placebo bolus + infusion	5–7	4/70 (5.7%)	7/73 (9.6%)	0.58 (0.17–1.98)
Pooled data for UFH vs. placebo/control						55/698 (7.9%)	68/655 (10.4%)	0.67 (0.45–0.99)
LMWH vs. placebo or untreated control								
Gurfinkel et al. (32)	1995	141	Nadroparin 214 ICU b.i.d	Untreated control	5–7	0/68 (0.0%)	7/73 (9.6%)	0.13 (0.03–0.60)
FRISC I (33)	1996	1506	Dalteparin 120 IU/kg b.i.d	Placebo b.i.d	6	4/70 (5.7%)	36/757 (4.8%)	0.39 (0.22–0.68)
Pooled data for LMWH vs. placebo/control						13/809 (1.6%)	43/830 (5.2%)	0.34 (0.20–0.58)
Pooled data for UFH + LMWH vs. placebo/control						68/1507 (4.5%)	104/1412 (7.4%)	0.53 (0.38–0.73)
LMWH vs. UFH								
Gurfinkel et al. (32)	1995	138	Nadroparin 214 ICU b.i.d	UFH bolus + infusion	5–7	0/68	4/70	0.13 (0.02–0.97)
FRIC (34)	1997	1482	Dalteparin 120 IU/kg b.i.d	UFH bolus + infusion	6	29/751 (3.9%)	26/731 (3.6%)	1.09 (0.64–1.87)
ESSENCE (35)	1997	3171	Enoxaparin 1 mg/kg b.i.d	UFH bolus + infusion	2–8	17/1607 (1.1%)	20/1564 (1.3%)	0.83 (0.43–1.58)
TIMI IIB (36)	1999	3910	Enoxaparin 30 mg bolus, 1 mg/kg b.i.d	UFH bolus + infusion	3–8	33/1953 (1.7%)	42/1959 (2.1%)	0.79 (0.50–1.24)
FRAXIS (37)	1999	3468	Nadroparin 87 IU/kg b.i.d	UFH bolus + infusion	6	69/2317 (3.0%)	36/1151 (3.1%)	0.95 (0.63–1.44)
Pooled data for LMWH vs. UFH						148/6696 (2.2%)	128/5475 (2.3%)	0.88 (0.69–1.12)

Abbreviations: UFH, unfractionated heparin; LMWH, low-molecular-weight heparin.

MI during treatment (OR 0.34; 95% CI, 0.20–0.58; $p < 0.0001$), with no reduction in death and a nonsignificant increase in major bleeding (OR 1.48; 95% CI, 0.45–4·84; $p = 0.51$) (38).

A meta-analysis of all trials comparing either UFH or LMWH with placebo (or untreated control) for the initial treatment of patients with NSTE-ACS reported a 47% reduction in death or MI (OR 0.53; 95% CI, 0.38–0.73; $p = 0.0001$) with no statistical evidence of heterogeneity among the trial results (38). In absolute terms, this translates to 29 events (death or MI) prevented for every 1000 patients treated. There was no reduction in death, and there was a numerical excess of major bleeding that was not statistically significant (OR 1.41; 95% CI, 0.62–3·23).

Trials of short-term LMWH vs. UFH RCTs have compared short-term LMWH with UFH for the management of NSTE-ACS in more than 25,000 patients. The first five trials were conducted prior to the year 2000 and primarily involved patients who were conservatively managed and did not receive a glycoprotein (GP) IIb/IIIa inhibitor (Table 1). Two of these trials evaluated enoxaparin (35,36), two nadroparin (32), and one dalteparin (34).

Enoxaparin vs. UFH The ESSENCE and TIMI-IIB trials compared subcutaneous (SC) enoxaparin (1 mg/kg twice daily) with intravenous (IV) UFH in patients with UA/NSTEMI (35). In the ESSENCE trial, the duration of anticoagulation was two to eight days (45). In the TIMI-B trial, the first dose of enoxaparin was given IV (30 mg bolus), and treatment was continued for three to eight days (36). The median duration of treatment was significantly longer in patients randomized to receive enoxaparin compared with UFH. Treatment of patients completing the initial treatment period without complications was continued in an extended phase, with those patients who were initially assigned to UFH receiving SC placebo injections twice daily and those originally assigned to enoxaparin receiving enoxaparin 40 mg SC twice daily until day 43. The results of the extended treatment phase of the trial are considered later in this chapter.

A prospectively planned meta-analysis of data from ESSENCE and TIMI-B reported a significant reduction in death or MI at day 8 with enoxaparin in comparison with UFH (OR 0.77; 95% CI, 0.62–0.95; $p = 0.02$), primarily due to a reduction in nonfatal MI with no reduction in death, no increase in major bleeding (1.3% vs. 1.1%, OR 1.23; 95% CI, 0.80–1.89; $p = 0.35$), and an increase in minor bleeding, primarily at injection sites (10.0% vs. 4.3%, $p = 0.0001$) (45). There was no significant reduction in death or MI at one year (12.7% vs. 13.7%, $p = 0.19$) (46).

Thus enoxaparin, as administered in the ESSENCE and TIMI 11B trials, is superior to UFH for preventing death or MI in the short term in conservatively managed patients with NSTE-ACS, at the expense of an increase in minor bleeding. Compared with UFH, enoxaparin also appears to be cost effective (47,48).

Nadroparin vs. UFH Although an initial small randomized trial reported improved outcomes in NTSE-ACS patients treated with nadroparin compared with UFH (32), the substantially larger FRAXIS (Fraxiparine during Ischaemic Syndromes) trial found no benefit of either 6 or 14 days of treatment with SC nadroparin compared with 6 days of IV UFH (37). The combined endpoint of cardiac death, MI, refractory angina, or recurrence of angina by day 14 occurred in 18·1%, 17·8%, and 20.0% of the patients receiving UFH, 6 days of nadroparin, and 14 days of nadroparin, respectively. The incidence of major hemorrhage was higher in patients receiving 14 days of nadroparin than it was in those receiving UFH (3·5% vs. 1.6%; $p = 0.0035$).

Dalteparin vs. UFH The FRIC (Fragmin in Unstable Coronary Artery Disease) study randomized 1482 patients with NSTE-ACS to receive twice daily weight-adjusted SC dalteparin (120 IU/kg) or IV UFH for five days (34). Patients were then re-randomized to a prolonged (days 6–45) treatment phase with either dalteparin (7500 IU once daily) or placebo. The results of the prolonged treatment phase of the trial are considered below. There was no significant difference between dalteparin and UFH during the first five days in the composite endpoint, death, MI, or recurrence of angina (UFH 7.6% vs. 9.3% dalteparin; RR 1.18; 95% CI, 0.84–1.66) or the composite endpoint, death, or MI (UFH 3.6% vs. dalteparin 3.9%; RR 1.07; 95% CI, 0.63–1.80). During the same period, the incidence of major bleeding with UFH treatment was 1.0% in comparison with 1.1% with dalteparin. Thus dalteparin appears to be as effective and safe as UFH for the initial treatment of NSTE-ACS.

Pooled analysis of short term LMWH vs. UFH A meta-analysis of the first five trials comparing LMWH with UFH during the acute phase in conservatively managed patients with NSTE-ACS demonstrated no significant reduction in death or MI (OR 0.88; 95% CI, 0.69–1.12; $p = 0.34$), a borderline significant reduction in recurrent angina (OR 0.84; 95% CI, 0.71–1.00; $p = 0.05$), and no increase in major bleeding (OR 1.00; 95% CI, 0.64–1.57; $p = 0.99$) (38).

Trials of extended duration LMWH vs. UFH Five trials have compared extended LMWH therapy with placebo in NSTE-ACS (33,34,36,37,49). A meta-analysis of these trials showed no reduction in death or MI (OR 0.98; 95% CI, 0.81–1.17; $p = 0.80$), recurrent angina (OR 1.12; 95% CI, 0.85–1.49; $p = 0.42$) or need for revascularization (OR 0.89; 95% CI 0.75–1.05; $p = 0.16$) during/up to 90 days of therapy (38). Extended treatment with LMWH significantly increased major bleeding (OR 2.26; 95% CI, 1.6–3.1; $p < 0.001$), equating to an excess of 12 major bleeds per 1000 patients treated.

Pharmacokinetics and dosing of LMWH An analysis of pharmacokinetic data from patients with NSTE-ACS treated with a single 30-mg IV bolus of enoxaparin followed by 1.0 or 1.25 mg/kg SC twice daily revealed an average enoxaparin clearance of 0.733 L/hr and an elimination half-life of 5 hours (50). Enoxaparin clearance was related to patients' weight and creatinine clearance and was a predictor of bleeding events. A creatinine clearance of <40 mL/min was associated with a 22% decrease in enoxaparin clearance compared with that in patients with normal (creatinine clearance ≥ 88 mL/min) renal function.

Adherence to the recommended LMWH dosing schedule is an independent determinant of patient outcome. In a study of 803 unselected UA patients treated with SC enoxaparin, patients with low anti-Xa levels (<0.5 IU/mL), mostly due to suboptimal dosing, had a threefold increase in the risk of 30-day mortality compared with patients who had anti-Xa levels in the target range of 0.5 to 1.2 IU/mL ($p = 0.004$) (51). The CRUSADE National Quality Improvement Initiative showed that up to half of the patients treated with enoxaparin for ACS did not receive the recommended dose (52). Elderly patients, those with lower body weights, and females were more likely to receive excessive doses (>10 mg above the recommended dose), and those who received excessive doses had an increased risk of major bleeding (OR 1.43; 95% CI, 1.18–1.75) and death (OR 1.35; 95% CI, 1.03–1.77). Inadequate dosing (>10 mg below the recommended dose) was associated with a trend toward higher mortality (OR 1.25; 95% CI, 0.93–1.68). There is no evidence to support dose capping in obese patients (53,54).

Accumulation of LMWH in patients with impaired renal function is associated with an increased risk of major bleeding (53). Pharmacokinetic simulation and clinical data suggest that after an initial loading enoxaparin dose of 1 mg/kg, a 12 hourly dose of

0.6 mg/kg is likely to maintain peak levels between 0.5 and 1.2 anti-Xa units/mL (55,56). The enoxaparin drug package insert recommends 1 mg/kg once daily in patients with severe renal impairment (<30 mL/min). It may be prudent to monitor anti-Xa levels in patients with severe renal impairment who require more than a brief period of treatment.

Anticoagulation in Patients Receiving a GP IIB/IIIA Inhibitor

GP IIb/IIIa inhibitors are effective for the treatment of ACS (57), particularly in patients undergoing percutaneous coronary intervention (PCI) (58), and are often administered to patients with NSTE-ACS managed with an early invasive strategy. In most of the early GP IIb/IIIa inhibitor trials, patients received concurrent anticoagulant therapy with IV UFH (59–63). Three RCTs, in which the majority of patients did not undergo an early invasive procedure, compared enoxaparin with UFH in patients with NSTE-ACS treated with a GP IIb/IIIa inhibitor (64–67). The INTERACT (Integrilin and Enoxaparin Randomized Assessment of Acute Coronary Syndrome Treatment) and ACUTE-II (Antithrombotic Combination Using Tirofiban and Enoxaparin-II) trials, which were primarily designed to evaluate safety, compared with IV UFH, showed that SC enoxaparin (1 mg/kg twice daily) either reduced major bleeding (1.8% vs. 4.6%, $p = 0.03$) or did not alter the risk of major bleeding (0.3% vs. 1.0%, $p = 0.57$), respectively. The larger follow-up, that is, A to Z trial randomized 3987 patients with NSTE-ACS who were treated with tirofiban to receive either open-label SC enoxaparin or weight-adjusted UFH and was designed as a non-inferiority study (66). The primary composite endpoint of death, MI, or refractory ischemia at seven days occurred in 8.4% of patients randomized to enoxaparin compared with 9.4% in patients receiving UFH (HR 0.88; 95% CI, 0.71–1.08), which met the prespecified criterion for non-inferiority. Compared with IV UFH, enoxaparin significantly increased TIMI major bleeding (0.9% vs. 0.4%, $p = 0.05$). In each of these three studies, about 60% of patients underwent diagnostic catheterization and about 30% underwent early PCI (68).

Anticoagulation in an Invasive Strategy

The American College of Cardiology/American Heart Association (ACC/AHA) and European Society of Cardiology guidelines recommend that patients with NSTE-ACS who have refractory symptoms, clinical instability or high-risk features, should undergo early diagnostic catheterization with the intent to perform revascularization as appropriate (6,15,69).

Anticoagulation in Patients Undergoing PCI

UFH remains the most widely used anticoagulant for patients undergoing PCI, although it has never been evaluated in RCTs. In patients not receiving a GP IIb/IIIa inhibitor, UFH is usually given IV in a dose of 70 to 100 IU/kg to achieve a target activated clotting time (ACT) of 250 to 350 seconds. The dose of UFH should be reduced to 50 to 60 IU/kg in patients receiving a GP IIb/IIIa inhibitor, aiming for a target ACT of 200 to 250 seconds (70).

Several small trials have reported favourable results with the use of LMWH instead of UFH during PCI (71–75). The largest study to date is the Superior Yield of New strategy with Enoxaparin, Revascularization and Glycoprotein IIb/IIIa inhibitors (SYNERGY) trial, which compared the safety and efficacy of enoxaparin with UFH in patients with NSTE-ACS planned for an early invasive strategy (catheterization within 48 hours of admission) (67). The use of GP IIb/IIIa inhibitors was at the discretion of the treating physician and was administered to approximately 60% of patients in both randomized treatment groups. The primary endpoint of death or nonfatal MI at 30 days occurred in 14.0% of patients assigned to enoxaparin and 14.5% of patients assigned to UFH (HR 0.96; 95% CI, 0.86–1.06). There was no difference in the rate of abrupt vessel closure (1.3% vs. 1.7%, $p = 0.32$), but enoxaparin significantly increased TIMI major bleeding (9.1% vs. 7.6%, $p = 0.008$). Excess bleeding with enoxaparin in the SYNERGY trial has been attributed to a high rate of switching between anticoagulants, but this hypothesis has yet to be confirmed.

Data from the SYNERGY trial were combined with the results of the earlier A to Z, INTERACT, ACUTE-II, ESSENCE, and TIMI-IIB trials in a meta-analysis of the enoxaparin trials (68). The percentage of patients undergoing early PCI ranged from 15% in ESSENCE to 47% in SYNERGY. In the approximately 22,000 patients included in this meta-analysis compared with IV UFH, enoxaparin did not reduce death at 30 days (3.0% vs. 3.0%; OR 1.00; 95% CI, 0.85–1.17), but reduced death or nonfatal MI (10.1% vs. 11.0%; OR 0.91; 95% CI, 0.83–0.99) (Fig. 1). There was no difference in major bleeding (OR 1.04; 95% CI, 0.83–1.30).

The enoxaparin meta-analysis data indicate that enoxaparin is superior to IV UFH for preventing MI in patients with NSTE-ACS. The benefits were primarily evident in the early trials (ESSENCE and TIMI-IIB), but the results were consistent in later trials, where a greater proportion of patients were managed invasively. However, only one of these trials (i.e., SYNERGY) involved patients who were routinely managed using an invasive strategy, and this study showed a significant excess of major bleeding and no efficacy advantage of enoxaparin compared with UFH.

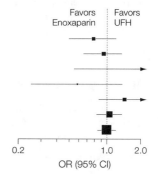

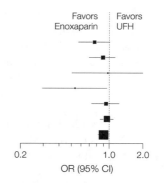

Figure 1 Pooled analysis of enoxaparin versus UFH for treatment of NSTE-ACS. *Abbreviations*: UFH, unfractionated heparin; NSTE-ACS, non-ST-elevation ACS. *Source*: From Ref. 68.

Table 2 Properties of Anticoagulants Used for Treatment of ACS

Anticoagulant	Mechanism of action	Half-life	Route of administration	Metabolism	Reversal agent
UFH	Indirect inhibition FIIa, FIXa, FXa, FXIa	60–90 min	IV or SC	Reticulo-endothelial	Yes
LMWH	Indirect inhibition Fxa > FIIa	~4 hr	SC	Renal	Partial
Fondaparinux	Indirect FXa inhibitor	15–20 hr	SC	Renal	No
Bivalirudin	Direct thrombin inhibitor	25 min	IV	Renal	No

Abbreviations: UFH, unfractionated heparin; LMWH, low-molecular-weight heparin; IV, intravenous; SC, subcutaneous.

Limitations of UFH and LMWH

The non-pharmacokinetic limitations of UFH appear to be related to its nonspecific binding to cells. UFH binding to osteoblasts and osteoclasts causes heparin-induced osteoporosis, and UFH interaction with platelet factor 4 and platelets can cause immune-mediated platelet activation and heparin-induced thrombocytopenia (HIT) (76). LMWH is less likely than UFH to cause osteoporosis and HIT, presumably because it is less negatively charged. However, LMWH is primarily cleared by the kidneys, which renders it problematic in patients with renal insufficiency, and the anticoagulant effect of LMWH is only partially reversed with protamine sulfate.

Recognition of the limitations of UFH and LMWH has prompted active research into the development of alternative anticoagulants for the management of ACS and other indications. Two newer anticoagulants, the indirect factor Xa inhibitor fondaparinux, and the direct thrombin inhibitor, bivalirudin, have been extensively evaluated and are increasingly used for the treatment of ACS. The pharmacological characteristics of these agents are summarized in Table 2.

Newer Anticoagulants

Fondaparinux
Fondaparinux is an indirect factor Xa inhibitor and is a synthetic analogue of the unique pentasaccharide sequence responsible for the binding of heparin to AT. The binding of fondaparinux to AT catalyses AT-mediated irreversible inhibition of free factor Xa. Fondaparinux has excellent bioavailability after SC injection and its plasma half-life of 17 hours permits once-daily administration. Fondaparinux is contraindicated in patients with severe renal insufficiency (77).

The OASIS (Organization to Assess Strategies for Ischemic Syndromes)-5 study randomized over 20,000 patients with NSTE-ACS to receive either fondaparinux (2.5 mg SC once daily) or enoxaparin (1 mg/kg SC twice daily) for up to eight days (78). At week 1, there was no difference between fondaparinux and enoxaparin in the proportion of patients developing the primary outcome of death, MI, or refractory ischemia (5.8% vs. 5.7%, $p = 0.007$ for non-inferiority) (Fig. 2). However, fondaparinux reduced the incidence of major bleeding by approximately 50% (2.2% vs. 4.1%, $p = 0.001$), and was associated with a 17% reduction in death at 30 days (2.9% vs. 3.5%, $p = 0.02$). More than 90% of the excess deaths in the enoxaparin arm occurred in patients who experienced bleeding. Among the 12,715 patients in OASIS-5 who underwent cardiac catheterization

(A) Death, Myocardial Infarction, or Refractory Ischemia through Day 9

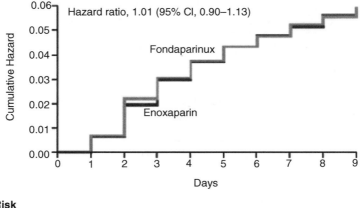

No. at Risk
Enoxaparin   10,021 9954 9824 9724 9652 9593 9550 9515 9470
Fondaparinux   10,057 9986 9836 9752 9684 9628 9589 9541 9510

(B) Major Bleeding through Day 9

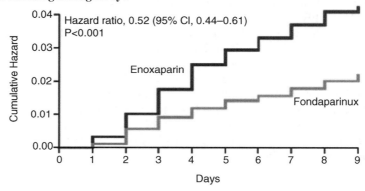

No. at Risk
Enoxaparin   10,021 9,979 9871 9774 9682 9625 9575 9527 9478
Fondaparinux   10,057 10,028 9951 9884 9838 9796 9773 9738 9709

Figure 2 Primary results of the OASIS-5 trial. Hazard ratios are for the fondaparinux group in comparison to the enoxaparin group. *Source*: From Ref. 78.

(including 6238 patients who underwent PCI) (79), fondaparinux compared with enoxaparin reduced major bleeding by more than 50% at day 9 (2.4% vs. 5.1%, HR 0.46, $p = 0.00001$) with no difference in ischemic events. Fondaparinux significantly increased catheter-related thrombosis in patients undergoing PCI (0.9% vs. 0.4%, $p = 0.001$), but this did not appear to translate into an excess of ischemic cardiovascular events and was largely avoided by the use of UFH during PCI. These data suggest that selective factor Xa inhibition is inadequate to prevent contact activation caused by exposure of the artificial surface of the catheter to the circulating blood.

Thus, fondaparinux, at a dose of 2.5 mg once daily, appears to be at least as effective as and substantially safer than enoxaparin 1 mg/kg twice daily for the management of patients with NSTE-ACS. The increased risk of catheter thrombosis renders fondaparinux unsuitable for use as the sole anticoagulant during PCI, and additional anticoagulation with UFH at the time of the procedure is recommended.

Bivalirudin for Treatment of NSTE-ACS

Bivalirudin is a 20–amino acid synthetic polypeptide analogue of the direct thrombin inhibitor hirudin. Bivalirudin has a plasma half-life of 25 minutes after IV injection (80). Five randomized trials have compared bivalirudin with heparin in patients with ACS, predominantly in patients undergoing PCI (81–85).

In the initial large double-blind randomized trial performed prior to the routine use of GP IIb/IIIa inhibitors and clopidogrel, patients undergoing angioplasty for either unstable or post-infarct angina were randomized to either bivalirudin (bolus 1.0 mg/kg bolus followed by 2.5 mg/kg for 4 hours, then 0.2 mg/kg for 14–20 hours) or IV UFH (83). Bivalirudin did not reduce the primary combined endpoint of in-hospital death, MI, abrupt vessel closure, or rapid clinical deterioration of cardiac origin, but was associated with a lower incidence of major bleeding (3.8% vs. 9.8%, $p < 0.001$).

Subsequently, two smaller trials comparing bivalirudin with heparin in patients undergoing elective and/or urgent angioplasty in conjunction with GP IIb/IIIa inhibition demonstrated that bivalirudin was as effective as UFH (84,85).

The REPLACE-II (Randomized Evaluation in PCI Linking Angiomax to Reduced Clinical Events-II) trial randomized patients undergoing urgent or elective PCI to receive bivalirudin (0.75 mg/kg bolus followed by a 1.75 mg/kg/hr infusion during the procedure) and provisional GP IIb/IIIa therapy in the event of complications, or UFH therapy (65 U/kg bolus up to 7000 U at the time of the procedure) and routine GP IIb/IIIa inhibition (82). Approximately 35% of the patients enrolled in the trial had NSTE-ACS, and only 7% of patients randomized to bivalirudin received a GP IIb/IIIa inhibitor. Bivalirudin compared with UFH plus a GPIIb/IIIa inhibitor did not reduce the primary composite endpoint of death, MI, or urgent repeat revascularization at 30 days or in-hospital major bleeding (9.2% vs. 10.0%, OR 0.92; 95% CI 0.77–1.09; $p = 0.32$), but significantly reduced in-hospital major bleeding (2.4% vs. 4.1%; $p < 0.001$).

The largest study examining bivalirudin in the treatment of NSTE-ACS was the ACUITY (The Acute Catheterization and Urgent Intervention Triage Strategy) trial, in which 13,819 patients with NSTE-ACS were randomized to receive one of three antithrombotic regimens: bivalirudin alone, bivalirudin plus a GP IIb/IIIa inhibitor, or intravenous UFH or enoxaparin plus a GP IIb/IIIa inhibitor (81). Bivalirudin was started before angiography and given as a bolus of 0.1 mg/kg followed by an infusion of 0.25 mg/kg/hr; before PCI an additional bolus of 05 mg/kg was given, followed by an infusion of 1.75 mg/kg/hr during the procedure; 57% of patients underwent PCI during study drug administration. Bivalirudin plus a GP IIb/IIIa inhibitor compared with UFH (or LMWH) plus a GP IIb/IIIa inhibitor was associated with non-inferior 30-day rate of the primary composite ischemia endpoint (7.7% vs. 7.3%; RR 1.07; 95% CI, 0.92–1.23, $p = 0.39$) and major bleeding (5.3% vs. 5.7%, RR 0.93; 95% CI, 0.78–1.10, $p = 0.38$). Bivalirudin was non-inferior to UFH or enoxaparin plus GP IIb/IIIa inhibition for preventing the composite of death, MI, or unplanned revascularization at 30 days (7.8% vs. 7.3%, RR 1.08; 95% CI, 0.93–1.24; $p = 0.32$) (Fig. 3), and was associated with a lower rate of clinically important bleeding (3.0% vs. 5.7%, RR 0.53; 95% CI, 0.43–0.65; $p = 0.001$). In the 3304 patients who did not receive a thienopyridine before angiography or PCI, the composite ischemic event rate was higher in the group who received bivalirudin alone than it was in those who received heparin plus GP IIb/IIIa inhibition (9.1% vs. 7.1%, RR 1.29; 95% CI, 1.03–1.63). One-year follow-up of the ACUITY trial reported no difference between the three arms in the incidence of the composite ischemia endpoint or death (86).

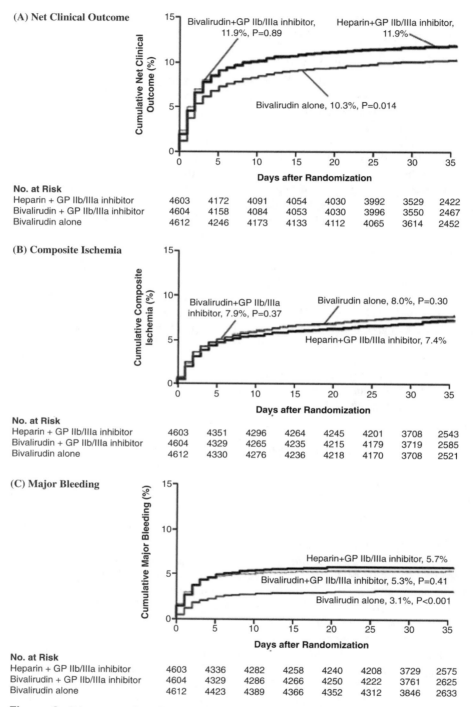

Figure 3 Primary results of the ACUITY trial. Net clinical outcome = occurrence of the composite ischemia end point or major bleeding. Composite ischemia endpoint = death from any cause, myocardial infarction, or unplanned revascularization for ischemia. *Source*: From Ref. 81.

Overall, bivalirudin monotherapy appears to be as effective as heparin plus GP IIb/IIIa inhibition in the treatment of patients with NSTE-ACS undergoing PCI, and causes less bleeding. It is unclear, however, whether bivalirudin monotherapy is as effective as the combination of heparin plus a GPIIb/IIIa inhibitor in very high-risk patients who may have been underrepresented in the ACUITY trial. Bivalirudin appears to be less effective in patients who have not received a thienopyridine.

Summary of Evidence and Current Guidelines

1. Short-term anticoagulation with UFH or LMWH in patients with NSTE-ACS results in a 40% to 50% reduction in risk of death or recurrent MI. Thus, in the absence of contraindications, all patients with NSTE-ACS should receive anticoagulant therapy.
2. In patients with NSTE-ACS managed by a conservative strategy, anticoagulant regimens using UFH, LMWH, or fondaparinux have been shown to be effective. Enoxaparin is more effective than UFH, while fondaparinux is at least as effective as enoxaparin and reduces bleeding.
3. In patients with NSTE-ACS managed by an invasive strategy, regimens using UFH, LMWH, fondaparinux, or bivalirudin are effective. Enoxaparin is no more effective than UFH and increases the risk of bleeding. Fondaparinux is at least as effective as enoxaparin and is associated with a lower bleeding risk. Fondaparinux should not be used as the sole anticoagulant in patients undergoing PCI because of the risk of catheter thrombosis. Monotherapy with bivalirudin appears to be as effective as the combination of UFH and a GPIIb/IIIa inhibitor and causes less bleeding.

The ACC/AHA and European Society of Cardiology guidelines for the anticoagulant management of patients with NSTE-ACS are summarized in Table 3.

Anticoagulation in Patients with STEMI

Aspirin and fibrinolytic therapy reduce the rate of re-infarction and death in patients with STEMI (87). Until recently, however, the role of adjunctive therapy with anticoagulant agents has been uncertain.

Unfractionated Heparin

Trials of UFH vs. placebo Four small trials involving a combined total of 1239 STEMI patients treated with aspirin and fibrinolytic therapy have compared IV UFH with placebo [two studies used streptokinase (88,89), one alteplase (90), and one anistreplase (91)] (Table 4) (101). The duration of UFH treatment was between one and five days. A meta-analysis of the four trials showed no significant reduction in re-infarction or death with UFH compared with control (OR re-infarction 1.08; 95% CI, 0.58–1.99, OR death 1.04, 95% CI, 0.62–1.78), and UFH did not significantly increase major bleeding or stroke. However the meta-analysis was unpowered to exclude a 30% or smaller reduction in re-infarction or death with UFH.

Despite the lack of evidence of efficacy from randomized trials, UFH is commonly administered to patients receiving fibrinolytic therapy for STEMI. This practice is based on the results of the large fibrinolytic trials in which UFH was routinely used. A lower-dose UFH regimen given with accelerated tissue plasminogen activator (tPA) has been shown to be associated with lower rates of intracerebral hemorrhage than higher-dose

Table 3 Summarized Existing Guidelines on Anticoagulant Therapy in NSTE-ACS

ACC/AHA Guidelines for the management of patients with UA/NSTEMI (Ref. 2)
1. Anticoagulant therapy should be added to antiplatelet therapy in UA/NSTEMI patients as soon as possible after presentation.
2. For patients in whom an invasive strategy is selected, regimens with established efficacy include enoxaparin, UFH, bivalirudin, and fondaparinux.
3. For patients in whom a conservative strategy is selected, regimens using either enoxaparin, UFH, or fondaparinux have established efficacy.
4. In patients in whom a conservative strategy is selected and who have an increased risk of bleeding, fondaparinux is preferable.
5. For UA/NSTEMI patients in whom an initial conservative strategy is selected, enoxaparin or fondaparinux is preferable to UFH as anticoagulant therapy, unless CABG is planned within 24 hr.[a]

European Society of Cardiology Guidelines for the diagnosis and treatment of NSTEMI-ACS (Ref. 6)
1. Anticoagulation is recommended for all patients in addition to antiplatelet therapy.
2. The choice of anticoagulant depends on the initial strategy (urgent invasive vs. early invasive vs. conservative strategy).
3. In an urgent invasive strategy, UFH, enoxaparin,[a] or bivalirudin should be immediately started.
4. In a nonurgent situation, as long as a decision between an early invasive and conservative strategy is pending.

   a) Fondaparinux is recommended on the basis of the most favorable efficacy/safety profile.
   b) Enoxaparin due to a less favorable safety profile than fondaparinux should be used only if the bleeding risk is low.[a]
   c) As the efficacy/safety profile of LMWH (other than enoxaparin) or UFH relative to fondaparinux is unknown, these anticoagulants cannot be recommended over fondaparinux.[a]

5. At PCI procedures, the initial anticoagulant should also be maintained during the procedure, apart from fondaparinux, where an additional dose of UFH (50–100 IU/kg bolus) is necessary.

[a]Class II recommendation (all other recommendations are class I).
Abbreviations: ACC/AHA, American College of Cardiology/American Heart Association; UA/NSTEMI, unstable angina/non-ST elevation myocardial infarction; UFH, unfractionated heparin; CABG, coronary artery bypass grafting; LMWH, low-molecular-weight heparin; ACS, acute coronary syndrome; PCI, percutaneous coronary intervention.

regimens (102). The ACC/AHA guidelines recommend that in STEMI patients treated with fibrin-specific lytic agents, UFH should be administered as a weight-adjusted bolus of 60 U/kg (maximum 4000 U), followed by an infusion of 12 U/kg (maximum 1000 U/hr) with a target aPTT of 50 to 70 seconds (87).

Low-Molecular-Weight Heparin

Trials of LMWH vs. placebo Four randomized trials have compared LMWH with placebo in patients with STEMI receiving fibrinolytic therapy [three trials used streptokinase (92,93,103) and one trial used either streptokinase or urokinase (94)] and aspirin (Table 4) (101). The duration of LMWH therapy was between 1 and 11 days. Treatment with LMWH resulted in an approximately 25% reduction in the risk of re-infarction (1.6% vs. 2.2%; OR, 0.72; 95% CI, 0.58–0.90) and a 10% reduction in death (7.8% vs. 8.7%; OR, 0.90; 95% CI, 0.80–0.99), with a nonsignificant increase in the risk of stroke (primarily intracerebral hemorrhage) and a significant increase in the risk of major bleeding (101). Most of the data in this comparison came from the large CREATE (The Clinical Trial of Reviparin and Metabolic Modulation in Acute Myocardial Infarction Treatment Evaluation) trial, which evaluated the LMWH, reviparin (94).

Table 4 Trials of UFH or LMWH for the Treatment of STEMI

Study	Year	n	Active treatment	Control treatment	Thrombolytic agent	Odds ratios	
						Death at 7 day	Re-infarction at 7 day
UFH vs. placebo or untreated control							
ISIS-2 Pilot (89)	1987	209	1000 IU/hr for 48 hr	Untreated control	SK 1.5 MU/1 hr	1.32 (0.44–3.95)	0.19 (0.02–1.63)
ECSG (90)	1992	652	Bolus + 1000 IU/hr for 48–120 hr	Placebo	tPA 100 MG/3 hr	0.80 (0.58–1.96)	0.99 (0.40–2.40)
OSIRIS (88)	1992	128	Bolus + 1000 IU/hr for 24 hr	Placebo bolus	SK 1.5 MU over 1 hr	0.32 (0.03–3.19)	2.03 (0.18–22.99)
DUCCS (91)	1994	250	15 IU/kg/hr 96 hr, aPTT 60–90 sec	Untreated control	APSAC 30 U over 2–5 min	1.47 (0.58–3.74)	2.23 (0.70–7.44)
Pooled data for UFH vs. placebo/ control						*1.08 (0.58–1.99)*	*1.04 (0.62–1.78)*
LMWH vs. placebo or untreated control							
FRAMI (92)	1997	776	Dalteparin 150 mg/kg b.i.d for 7–11 day	Placebo	SK 1.5 MU/1 hr	1.00 (0.55–1.82)	0.75 (0.26–2.17)
AMI-SK (93)	2002	496	Enoxaparin 30 mg bolus then 1 mg/kg for 3–8 day	Placebo	SK 1.5 MU/1 hr	1.26 (0.55–1.82)	0.33 (0.12–0.93)
CREATE (94)	2005	15570	Reviparin 3436–6871 IU b.i.d for 7 day	Placebo	SK or UK	0.89 (0.79–0.99)	0.76 (0.60–0.96)
Pooled data for LMWH vs. placebo/ control						*0.90 (0.80–0.99)*	*0.72 (0.58–0.90)*
LMWH vs. UFH							
ASSENT 3 (95)	2001	4078	Enoxaparin 1 mg/kg b.i.d for 7 day	Bolus then 12 IU/kg/hr for 7 day	TNK 30–50 mg	0.80 (0.60–1.07)	0.61 (0.43–0.86)
HART II (96)	2001	400	Enoxaparin 1 mg/kg b.i.d for 3 day	Bolus then 15 IU/kg/hr for 3 day	tPA weight adjusted	0.88 (0.33–2.34)	0.83 (0.25–2.76)

(continued)

Table 4 Trials of UFH or LMWH for the Treatment of STEMI (*Continues*)

Study	Year	n	Active treatment	Control treatment	Thrombolytic agent	Odds ratios	
						Death at 7 day	Re-infarction at 7 day
Baird et al. (97)	2002	300	Enoxaparin 40 mg t.i.d for 4 day	Bolus then 30 IU/day for 4 day	SK 1.5 MU or APSAC 30 IU or tPA 100 mg	0.75 (0.25–2.22)	0.71 (0.35–1.40)
ENTIRE-TIMI (98)	2002	242	Enoxaparin 1 mg/kg b.i.d for 7 day	Bolus then 12 IU/kg/hr for 3 day	TNK 0.53 mg/kg	0.50 (0.10–2.55)	0.14 (0.03–0.67)
ASSENT-PLUS (99)	2003	439	Dalteparin 90 IU/kg then 120 IU/kg b.i.d for 4–7 day	UFH Bolus then 800–1000 IU/hr for 48 hr	tPA 100 mg	0.59 (0.19–1.84)	0.25 (0.07–0.92)
ASSENT-3 PLUS (100)	2003	1639	Enoxaparin 1 mg/kg b.i.d for 7 day	Bolus then 12 IU/kg/hr for 3 day	TNK 30–50 mg	1.34 (0.90–2.00)	0.58 (0.36–0.93)
Pooled data for LMWH vs. UFH				148/6696 (2.2%)	6	0.92 (0.74–1.13)	0.57 (0.45–0.73)

Abbreviations: UFH, unfractionated heparin; LMWH, low-molecular-weight heparin.

Trials of LMWH vs. UFH Pooled data from six trials comparing LMWH (5 trials used enoxaparin) with UFH in patients with STEMI treated with fibrinolytic therapy found a significant reduction in the risk of re-infarction during hospitalization (3.0% vs. 5.2%; OR 0.57; 95% CI, 0.45–0.73), but no reduction in death (4.8% vs. 5.3%; OR, 0.92; 95% CI, 0.74–1.13) (95–101) (Table 4). Five of the six trials used a fibrin-specific fibrinolytic agent, and the duration of LMWH or UFH treatment was between 48 hours and 8 days. Patients randomized to LMWH generally received a longer duration of treatment than those receiving UFH. There was a nonsignificant increase in the risk of stroke and major bleeding with LMWH.

Subsequent to the above analyses, the large EXTRACT-TIMI 25 (Enoxaparin and Thrombolysis Reperfusion for Acute Myocardial Infarction Treatment—Thrombolysis in Myocardial Infarction 25) was completed (104). This trial compared enoxaparin (initial 30 mg IV bolus followed by 1.0 mg/kg SC twice daily up to 8 days) with IV UFH for 48 hours in 20,506 STEMI patients who received fibrinolytic therapy and aspirin with or without the addition of clopidogrel. In patients 75 years or older, no initial IV enoxaparin bolus was given and the dose of enoxaparin was reduced to 0.75 mg/kg twice daily. Patients with severe renal impairment received 1.0 mg/kg enoxaparin every 24 hours. Compared with IV UFH, enoxaparin reduced death or MI by 17% at 30 days (9.9% vs. 12%; $p < 0.001$; RR 0.83; 95% CI, 0.77–0.90), but increased TIMI major bleeding (2.1% vs. 1.4%; $p < 0.001$; RR 1.53; 95% CI, 1.23–1.89) and fatal bleeding (0.55% vs. 0.33%). If the rates of death, MI, or major bleeding are combined, there was a net clinical benefit of enoxaparin over UFH (11.0% vs. 12.8%; $p < 0.001$; RR 0.86; 95% CI, 0.80–0.93). A consistent benefit of enoxaparin was evident in patients undergoing non-primary PCI during study drug administration (15).

Thus, LMWH is superior to UFH in patients receiving aspirin and fibrinolytic therapy for STEMI. The data in patients undergoing primary PCI for STEMI are limited, and further trials are required to address this issue (44).

Fondaparinux

The OASIS-6 study randomized 12,092 patients with STEMI to either 2.5 mg fondaparinux SC once daily for up to eight days or to "standard care," either with placebo in patients in whom UFH was not thought to be indicated (stratum 1) or IV UFH for 48 hours in patients in whom anticoagulation was considered warranted (stratum 2) (105). Compared with standard care, fondaparinux reduced the risk of death or MI at day 8 by 17% (7.4% vs. 8.9%; RR 0.83; 95% CI, 0.73–0.94; $p = 0.003$) and at day 30 (9.7% vs. 11.2%; RR 0.86; 95% CI, 0.77–0.96; $p < 0.001$) (Fig. 4). While the apparent effect size of fondaparinux on the composite outcome of death or reinfarction was initially larger in stratum 1 (comparator placebo), by the end of 180 days of follow-up, the effect sizes in the two strata were almost identical (HRs of 0.87 in stratum 1 and 0.88 in stratum 2). Overall, the rate of bleeding was not increased with fondaparinux compared with the control group (1.8% vs. 2.1%, $p = 0.14$).

Nearly 4000 patients in the OASIS-6 trial underwent primary PCI. All patients in the control group who underwent primary PCI received UFH during the procedure compared with 21% in the fondaparinux group who received UFH. Compared with standard care, fondaparinux was associated with a trend toward a higher rate of re-infarction in patients (2.0% vs. 1.6%; RR 1.25; 95% CI, 0.77–2.05; $p = 0.360$) and a higher rate of guiding catheter thrombosis (0% vs. 22%, $p = 0.001$) and coronary complications (abrupt coronary artery closure, new angiographic thrombus, catheter thrombus, no reflow, dissection, or perforation; 225% vs. 270%; $p = 0.04$). In the

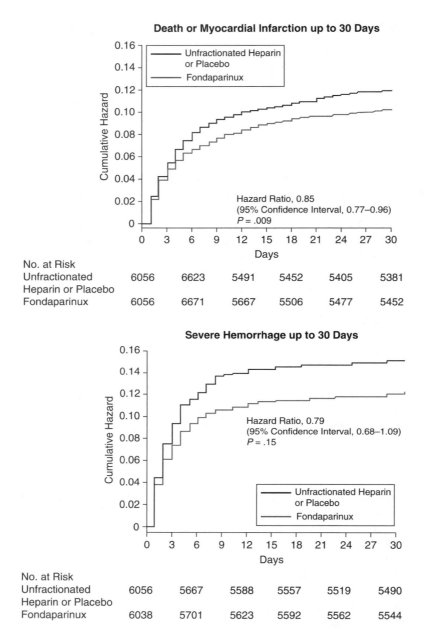

Figure 4 Primary results of the OASIS-6 trial. In both graphs, the UFH/placebo group is the upper line. *Abbreviation*: UFH, unfractionated heparin. *Source*: From Ref. 105.

496 patients who received UFH prior to primary PCI, the rate of catheter thrombosis was low in both arms (0 in controls vs. 2 with fondaparinux).

In summary, fondaparinux appears to be more effective than standard care (no anticoagulation or UFH) for preventing death and recurrent ischemic events in patients with STEMI, but is associated with a higher rate of catheter thrombosis in patients undergoing primary PCI. Similar to OASIS-5, the use of additional UFH with fondaparinux during PCI largely avoided catheter thrombosis.

Bivalirudin

The HERO-2 (The Hirulog and Early Reperfusion or Occlusion) trial randomized 17,073 patients with STEMI to either a 48-hour infusion of fixed-dose bivalirudin after an initial IV bolus or adjusted-dose UFH. Both were given in conjunction with streptokinase (106). Less than 2% of patients in each treatment arm underwent early PCI. Compared with UFH, bivalirudin did not reduce the incidence of death (10.8% vs. 10.9%, respectively; $p = 0.85$) or the composite of death or MI at 30 days (12.6% vs. 13.6%; RR 0.92; 95% CI, 0.83–1.01; $p = 0.07$), but increased major bleeding (0.7% vs. 0.5%, $p = 0.07$).

Additional support for the effectiveness and safety of bivalirudin in STEMI comes from the recently presented, but as yet unpublished, HORIZONS AMI trial in which 3600 STEMI patients were randomized within 12 hours of symptom onset to receive UFH [60 U/kg IV (with subsequent boluses titrated to achieve a target ACT of 200–250 seconds] plus a GP IIb/IIIa inhibitor or bivalirudin monotherapy (0.75 mg/kg bolus; infusion 1.75 mg/kg/hr) plus provisional GP IIb/IIIa inhibitor for large thrombi or refractory no-flow. All patients were treated with primary PCI, and 7.2% of patients in the bivalirudin-treated group received a GP IIb/IIIa inhibitor. Compared with UFH plus a GPIIb/IIIa inhibitor, bivalirudin did not reduce the primary endpoint of all-cause death, reinfarction, ischemic target vessel revascularization (TVR), or stroke, but reduced major bleeding by 40% (4.9% vs. 8.3%, $p < 0.0001$). Bivalirudin also significantly reduced the risk of cardiac death (1.8% vs. 2.9%, $p = 0.035$).

Thus, monotherapy with bivalirudin appears to be a reasonable alternative to UFH as an anticoagulant for the treatment of STEMI, particularly in patients undergoing primary PCI.

Summary of Evidence and Current Guidelines

1. There is little evidence to demonstrate the efficacy of short-term IV. UFH in patients with STEMI who are treated with fibrinolytic therapy, but UFH was widely used in the trials that evaluated the efficacy and safety of fibrin-specific lytic agents.
2. LMWH is superior to placebo for preventing death and re-infarction and is superior to UFH for preventing re-infarction in patients with STEMI who are treated with fibrinolytic therapy, but increases major bleeding. There are limited data for the effectiveness of LMWH in patients undergoing primary PCI for STEMI.
3. Fondaparinux is superior to UFH or placebo for preventing the combined endpoint of death and recurrent MI in patients with STEMI and does not increase the risk of bleeding. Additional UFH is required in patients treated with fondaparinux who undergo PCI to prevent catheter thrombosis.
4. Bivalirudin is as effective as UFH in patients with STEMI, including patients undergoing primary PCI. Compared with the combination of heparin plus a GPIIb/IIIa inhibitor, bivalirudin causes less bleeding.

The ACC/AHA and European Society of Cardiology guidelines for the anti-coagulant management of patients with STEMI are summarized in Table 5.

FUTURE DIRECTIONS

There is a very large body of evidence demonstrating the efficacy of UFH, LMWH, fondaparinux, or bivalirudin in patients with ACS. The advantages of UFH are that (*i*) its anticoagulant effect can be readily reversed and (*ii*) it can be used in patients with severe renal impairment. The disadvantages of UFH include (*i*) the need for monitoring because

Table 5 Summarized Existing Guidelines on Anticoagulant Therapy in STEMI

ACC/AHA Guidelines for the management of patients with STEMI (Ref. 13)
1. Patients receiving fibrinolytic therapy should also receive anticoagulant therapy for a minimum of 48 hr, and preferably for the duration of hospitalization, up to 8 day (regimens other than UFH are recommended if anticoagulant therapy is given for more than 48 hr because of the risk of HIT with prolonged UFH treatment).
2. Anticoagulant regimens with established efficacy include:

    i. UFH [IV bolus 60 U/kg (maximum 4000 U)] followed by an IV infusion of 12 U/kg/hr (maximum 1000 U/hr) initially, adjusted to maintain the aPTT 1.5–2.0 times control (approximately 50–70 sec).

    ii. Enoxaparin: for patients < 75 yr, an initial 30-mg IV bolus, followed by 1.0 mg/kg SC 12 hourly; for patients ≥ 75 yr, no bolus and reduce dose to 0.75 mg/kg 12 hourly. If the CrCl < 30 mL/min reduce dose to 1.0 mg/kg every 24 hr.

    iii. Fondaparinux (provided the serum creatinine < mg/Dl): initial dose 2.5 mg IV; subsequently 2.5 mg SC daily.

3. For patients undergoing PCI after receiving an anticoagulant regimen, the following recommendations are made:

    i. If prior treatment with UFH, administer additional boluses of UFH as needed to support the procedure, taking into account whether GP IIb/IIIa receptor antagonists have been administered. Bivalirudin may also be used in patients.

    ii. If prior treatment with enoxaparin, if the last SC dose was within the prior 8 hr, no additional enoxaparin should be given; if the last SC dose was 8–12 hr earlier, an IV dose of 0.3 mg/kg of enoxaparin should be given.

    iii. For prior treatment with fondaparinux, administer additional IV treatment with an anticoagulant possessing anti-IIa activity, taking into account whether GP IIb/IIIa receptor antagonists have been administered.[a]

European Society of Cardiology Guidelines for the diagnosis and treatment of NSTEMI-ACS (Ref. 107).
1. For patients receiving fibrinolytic therapy, concurrent therapy with UFH is suggested; dosing IV bolus: 60 U/kg (maximum 4000 U) followed by IV infusion 12 U/kg/hr (maximum 1000 U/hr) for 24–48 hr. Target aPTT: 50–70 sec.

[a]Class II recommendation.
Abbreviations: ACC/AHA, American College of Cardiology/American Heart Association; UFH, unfractionated heparin; STEMI, ST-elevation myocardial infarction; ACS, acute coronary syndrome; PCI, percutaneous coronary intervention; HIT, heparin induced thrombocytopenia; apt, activated partial thromboplastin time; CrCl, creatinine clearance.

of its unpredictable anticoagulant effects and (*ii*) the risk of HIT and osteoporosis. LMWH has a more predictable anticoagulant effect than UFH, is less likely to cause HIT or osteoporosis, and is more effective than UFH for preventing nonfatal MI. Recently introduced anticoagulants include fondaparinux and bivalirudin. Fondaparinux is superior to LMWH in patients with NSTE-ACS and is superior to UFH or placebo in patients with STEMI treated with fibrinolytics, but is not suitable as the sole anticoagulant in patients undergoing PCI. Bivalirudin is an attractive alternative to the combination of UFH and a GPIIb/IIIa inhibitor in patients undergoing PCI. All of the currently available anticoagulants for the initial management of patients with ACS must be given parenterally and apart from UFH, and to a lesser extent bivalirudin, are renally cleared. Several new oral direct factor Xa and thrombin inhibitors are currently being evaluated in ACS patients.

REFERENCES

1. Murray CJ, Lopez AD. Alternative projections of mortality and disability by cause 1990–2020: global burden of disease study. Lancet 1997; 349(9064):1498–1504.
2. Anderson JL, Adams CD, Antman EM, et al. ACC/AHA 2007 guidelines for the management of patients with unstable angina/non ST-elevation myocardial infarction: a report of the American College of Cardiology/American Heart Association Task Force on Practice Guidelines (Writing Committee to Revise the 2002 Guidelines for the Management of Patients With Unstable Angina/Non ST-Elevation Myocardial Infarction): developed in collaboration with the American College of Emergency Physicians, the Society for Cardiovascular Angiography and Interventions, and the Society of Thoracic Surgeons: endorsed by the American Association of Cardiovascular and Pulmonary Rehabilitation and the Society for Academic Emergency Medicine. Circulation 2007; 116(7):e148–e304.
3. Rosamond W, Flegal K, Furie K, et al. Heart disease and stroke statistics—2008 update: a report from the American Heart Association Statistics Committee and Stroke Statistics Subcommittee. Circulation 2008; 117(4):e25–e146.
4. Volmink JA, Newton JN, Hicks NR, et al. Coronary event and case fatality rates in an English population: results of the Oxford myocardial infarction incidence study. The Oxford Myocardial infarction incidence study group. Heart 1998; 80(1):40–44.
5. Savonitto S, Ardissino D, Granger CB, et al. Prognostic value of the admission electrocardiogram in acute coronary syndromes. JAMA 1999; 281(8):707–713.
6. Bassand JP, Hamm CW, Ardissino D, et al. Guidelines for the diagnosis and treatment of non-ST-segment elevation acute coronary syndromes. Eur Heart J 2007; 28(13):1598–1660.
7. Libby P, Theroux P. Pathophysiology of coronary artery disease. Circulation 2005; 111(25): 3481–3488.
8. Hansson GK, Libby P, Schonbeck U, et al. Innate and adaptive immunity in the pathogenesis of atherosclerosis. Circ Res 2002; 91(4):281–291.
9. Davi G, Patrono C. Platelet activation and atherothrombosis. N Engl J Med 2007; 357(24): 2482–2494.
10. Falk E. Unstable angina with fatal outcome: dynamic coronary thrombosis leading to infarction and/or sudden death. Autopsy evidence of recurrent mural thrombosis with peripheral embolization culminating in total vascular occlusion. Circulation 1985; 71(4):699–708.
11. Davies MJ, Thomas AC, Knapman PA, et al. Intramyocardial platelet aggregation in patients with unstable angina suffering sudden ischemic cardiac death. Circulation 1986; 73(3):418–427.
12. Mizuno K, Satomura K, Miyamoto A, et al. Angioscopic evaluation of coronary-artery thrombi in acute coronary syndromes. N Engl J Med 1992; 326(5):287–291.
13. Braunwald E. Unstable angina. A classification. Circulation 1989; 80(2):410–414.
14. Wu AH, Apple FS, Gibler WB, et al. National Academy of Clinical Biochemistry Standards of Laboratory Practice: recommendations for the use of cardiac markers in coronary artery diseases. Clin Chem 1999; 45(7):1104–1121.
15. Antman EM, Hand M, Armstrong PW, et al. 2007 Focused Update of the ACC/AHA 2004 Guidelines for the Management of Patients With ST-Elevation Myocardial Infarction: a report of the American College of Cardiology/American Heart Association Task Force on Practice Guidelines: developed in collaboration With the Canadian Cardiovascular Society endorsed by the American Academy of Family Physicians: 2007 Writing Group to Review New Evidence and Update the ACC/AHA 2004 Guidelines for the Management of Patients With ST-Elevation Myocardial Infarction, Writing on Behalf of the 2004 Writing Committee. Circulation 2008; 117(2):296–329.
16. Brown KW, Rykert HE. Heparin in the treatment of angina pectoris. Can Med Assoc J 1954; 70(6):617–620.
17. Rosenberg RD, Lam L. Correlation between structure and function of heparin. Proc Natl Acad Sci U S A 1979; 76(3):1218–1222.
18. Weitz JI. Low-molecular-weight heparins. N Engl J Med 1997; 337(10):688–698.

19. Hirsh J, Warkentin TE, Shaughnessy SG, et al. Heparin and low-molecular-weight heparin: mechanisms of action, pharmacokinetics, dosing, monitoring, efficacy, and safety. Chest 2001; 119(1 suppl):64S–94S.
20. Choay J, Lormeau JC, Petitou M, et al. Structural studies on a biologically active hexasaccharide obtained from heparin. Ann N Y Acad Sci 1981; 370:644–649.
21. Telford AM, Wilson C. Trial of heparin versus atenolol in prevention of myocardial infarction in intermediate coronary syndrome. Lancet 1981; 1(8232):1225–1228.
22. Theroux P, Ouimet H, McCans J, et al. Aspirin, heparin, or both to treat acute unstable angina. N Engl J Med 1988; 319(17):1105–1111.
23. Williams DO, Kirby MG, McPherson K, et al. Anticoagulant treatment of unstable angina. Br J Clin Pract 1986; 40(3):114–116.
24. Neri Serneri GG, Modesti PA, Gensini GF, et al. Randomised comparison of subcutaneous heparin, intravenous heparin, and aspirin in unstable angina. Studio Epoorine Sottocutanea nell'Angina Instobile (SESAIR) Refrattorie Group. Lancet 1995; 45(8959):1201–1204.
25. Theroux P, Waters D, Qiu S, et al. Aspirin versus heparin to prevent myocardial infarction during the acute phase of unstable angina. Circulation 1993; 88(5 pt 1):2045–2048.
26. The RISC Group. Risk of myocardial infarction and death during treatment with low dose aspirin and intravenous heparin in men with unstable coronary artery disease. Lancet 1990; 336(8719):827–830.
27. Lewis HD Jr., Davis JW, Archibald DG, et al. Protective effects of aspirin against acute myocardial infarction and death in men with unstable angina. Results of a Veterans Administration Cooperative Study. N Engl J Med 1983; 309(7):396–403.
28. Cairns JA, Gent M, Singer J, et al. Aspirin, sulfinpyrazone, or both in unstable angina. Results of a Canadian multicenter trial. N Engl J Med 1985; 313(22):1369–1375.
29. Cohen M, Adams PC, Hawkins L, et al. Usefulness of antithrombotic therapy in resting angina pectoris or non-Q-wave myocardial infarction in preventing death and myocardial infarction (a pilot study from the Antithrombotic Therapy in Acute Coronary Syndromes Study Group). Am J Cardiol 1990; 66(19):1287–1292.
30. Cohen M, Adams PC, Parry G, et al. Combination antithrombotic therapy in unstable rest angina and non-Q-wave infarction in nonprior aspirin users. Primary end points analysis from the ATACS trial. Antithrombotic Therapy in Acute Coronary Syndromes Research Group. Circulation 1994; 89(1):81–88.
31. Holdright D, Patel D, Cunningham D, et al. Comparison of the effect of heparin and aspirin versus aspirin alone on transient myocardial ischemia and in-hospital prognosis in patients with unstable angina. J Am Coll Cardiol 1994; 24(1):39–45.
32. Gurfinkel EP, Manos EJ, Mejail RI, et al. Low molecular weight heparin versus regular heparin or aspirin in the treatment of unstable angina and silent ischemia. J Am Coll Cardiol 1995; 26(2):313–318.
33. Fragmin during Instability in Coronary Artery Disease (FRISC) study group. Low-molecular-weight heparin during instability in coronary artery disease. Lancet 1996; 347(9001):561–568.
34. Klein W, Buchwald A, Hillis WS, et al. Fragmin in unstable angina pectoris or in non-Q-wave acute myocardial infarction (the FRIC study). Fragmin in unstable coronary artery disease. Am J Cardiol 1997; 80(5A):30E–304E.
35. Cohen M, Demers C, Gurfinkel EP, et al. A comparison of low-molecular-weight heparin with unfractionated heparin for unstable coronary artery disease. Efficacy and Safety of Subcutaneous Enoxaparin in Non-Q-Wave Coronary Events Study Group. N Engl J Med 1997; 337(7):447–452.
36. Antman EM, McCabe CH, Gurfinkel EP, et al. Enoxaparin prevents death and cardiac ischemic events in unstable angina/non-Q-wave myocardial infarction. Results of the thrombolysis in myocardial infarction (TIMI) 11B trial. Circulation 1999; 100(15):1593–1601.
37. (No authors listed).Comparison of two treatment durations (6 days and 14 days) of a low molecular weight heparin with a 6-day treatment of unfractionated heparin in the initial management of unstable angina or non-Q wave myocardial infarction: FRAX.I.S. (FRAxiparine in Ischaemic Syndrome). Eur Heart J 1999; 20(21):1553–1562.

38. Eikelboom JW, Anand SS, Malmberg K, et al. Unfractionated heparin and low-molecular-weight heparin in acute coronary syndrome without ST elevation: a meta-analysis. Lancet 2000; 355(9219):1936–1942.

39. Theroux P, Waters D, Lam J, et al. Reactivation of unstable angina after the discontinuation of heparin. N Engl J Med 1992; 327(3):141–145.

40. Granger C, Armstrong P. Reinfarction following discontinuation of intravenous heparin or hirudin for unstable angina and acute myocardial infarction. Circulation 1995; 92(8I):460.

41. Becker RC, Cannon CP, Tracy RP, et al. Relation between systemic anticoagulation as determined by activated partial thromboplastin time and heparin measurements and in-hospital clinical events in unstable angina and non-Q wave myocardial infarction. Thrombolysis in Myocardial Ischemia III B Investigators. Am Heart J 1996; 131(3):421–433.

42. Lee MS, Wali AU, Menon V, et al. The determinants of activated partial thromboplastin time, relation of activated partial thromboplastin time to clinical outcomes, and optimal dosing regimens for heparin treated patients with acute coronary syndromes: a review of GUSTO-IIb. J Thromb Thrombolysis 2002; 14(2):91–101.

43. Hochman JS, Wali AU, Gavrila D, et al. A new regimen for heparin use in acute coronary syndromes. Am Heart J 1999: 138(2 pt 1):313–318.

44. Hirsh J, Raschke R. Heparin and low-molecular-weight heparin: the Seventh ACCP Conference on Antithrombotic and Thrombolytic Therapy. Chest 2004: 126(3 suppl):188S–203S.

45. Antman EM, Cohen M, Radley D, et al. Assessment of the treatment effect of enoxaparin for unstable angina/non-Q-wave myocardial infarction. TIMI 11B-ESSENCE meta-analysis. Circulation 1999; 100(15):1602–1608.

46. Antman EM, Cohen M, McCabe C, et al. Enoxaparin is superior to unfractionated heparin for preventing clinical events at 1-year follow-up of TIMI 11B and ESSENCE. Eur Heart J 2002; 23(4):308–314.

47. O'Brien BJ, Willan A, Blackhouse G, et al. Will the use of low-molecular-weight heparin (enoxaparin) in patients with acute coronary syndrome save costs in Canada? Am Heart J 2000; 139(3):423–429.

48. Mark DB, Cowper PA, Berkowitz SD, et al. Economic assessment of low-molecular-weight heparin (enoxaparin) versus unfractionated heparin in acute coronary syndrome patients: results from the ESSENCE randomized trial. Efficacy and Safety of Subcutaneous Enoxaparin in Non-Q wave Coronary Events [unstable angina or non-Q-wave myocardial infarction]. Circulation 1998; 97(1 7):1702–1707.

49. FRagmin and Fast Revascularisation during InStability in Coronary artery disease Investigators. Long-term low-molecular-mass heparin in unstable coronary-artery disease: FRISC II prospective randomised multicentre study. Lancet 1999; 354(9180):701–707.

50. Becker RC, Spencer FA, Gibson M, et al. Influence of patient characteristics and renal function on factor Xa inhibition pharmacokinetics and pharmacodynamics after enoxaparin administration in non-ST-segment elevation acute coronary syndromes. Am Heart J 2002; 143(5):753–759.

51. Montalescot G, Collet JP, Tanguy ML, et al. Anti-Xa activity relates to survival and efficacy in unselected acute coronary syndrome patients treated with enoxaparin. Circulation 2004; 110 (4):392–398.

52. LaPointe NM, Chen AY, Alexander KP, et al. Enoxaparin dosing and associated risk of in-hospital bleeding and death in patients with non ST-segment elevation acute coronary syndromes. Arch Intern Med 2007; 167(14):1539–1544.

53. Spinler SA, Inverso SM, Cohen M, et al. Safety and efficacy of unfractionated heparin versus enoxaparin in patients who are obese and patients with severe renal impairment: analysis from the ESSENCE and TIMI 11B studies. Am Heart J 2003; 146(1):33–41.

54. Spinler SA, Dobesh P. Dose capping enoxaparin is unjustified and denies patients with acute coronary syndromes a potentially effective treatment. Chest 2005; 127(6):2288–2289; author reply 9–90.

55. Hulot JS, Montalescot G, Lechat P, et al. Dosing strategy in patients with renal failure receiving enoxaparin for the treatment of non-ST-segment elevation acute coronary syndrome. Clin Pharmacol Ther 2005; 77(6):542–552.

56. Collet JP, Montalescot G, Choussat R, et al. Enoxaparin in unstable angina patients with renal failure. Int J Cardiol 2001; 80(1):81–82.

57. Boersma E, Harrington RA, Moliterno DJ, et al. Platelet glycoprotein IIb/IIIa inhibitors in acute coronary syndromes: a meta-analysis of all major randomised clinical trials. Lancet 2002; 359(9302):189–198.

58. Roffi M, Chew DP, Mukherjee D, et al. Platelet glycoprotein IIb/IIIa inhibition in acute coronary syndromes. Gradient of benefit related to the revascularization strategy. Eur Heart J 2002; 23(18):1441–1448.

59. Global Organization of Network (PARAGON-B) Investigators. Randomized, placebo-controlled trial of titrated intravenous lamifiban for acute coronary syndromes. Circulation 2002; 105(3):316–321.

60. Simoons ML. Effect of glycoprotein IIb/IIIa receptor blocker abciximab on outcome in patients with acute coronary syndromes without early coronary revascularisation: the GUSTO IV-ACS randomised trial. Lancet 2001; 357(9272):1915–1924.

61. The PURSUIT Trial Investigators. Inhibition of platelet glycoprotein IIb/IIIa with eptifibatide in patients with acute coronary syndromes. Platelet Glycoprotein IIb/IIIa in Unstable Angina: Receptor Suppression Using Integrilin Therapy. N Engl J Med 1998; 339(7):436–443.

62. The PARAGON Investigators. International, randomized, controlled trial of lamifiban (a platelet glycoprotein IIb/IIIa inhibitor), heparin, or both in unstable angina. Platelet IIb/IIIa Antagonism for the Reduction of Acute coronary syndrome events in a Global Organization Network. Circulation 1998; 97(24):2386–2395.

63. Platelet Receptor Inhibition in Ischemic Syndrome Management in Patients Limited by Unstable Signs and Symptoms (PRISM-PLUS) Study Investigators. Inhibition of the platelet glycoprotein IIb/IIIa receptor with tirofiban in unstable angina and non-Q-wave myocardial infarction. N Engl J Med 1998; 338(21):1488–1497.

64. Cohen M, Theroux P, Borzak S, et al. Randomized double-blind safety study of enoxaparin versus unfractionated heparin in patients with non-ST-segment elevation acute coronary syndromes treated with tirofiban and aspirin: the ACUTE II study. The Antithrombotic Combination Using Tirofiban and Enoxaparin. Am Heart J 2002; 144(3):470–477.

65. Goodman SG, Fitchett D, Armstrong PW, et al. Randomized evaluation of the safety and efficacy of enoxaparin versus unfractionated heparin in high-risk patients with non-ST-segment elevation acute coronary syndromes receiving the glycoprotein IIb/IIIa inhibitor eptifibatide. Circulation 2003; 107(2):238–244.

66. Blazing MA, de Lemos JA, White HD, et al. Safety and efficacy of enoxaparin vs unfractionated heparin in patients with non-ST-segment elevation acute coronary syndromes who receive tirofiban and aspirin: a randomized controlled trial. JAMA 2004; 292(1):55–64.

67. Ferguson JJ, Califf RM, Antman EM, et al. Enoxaparin vs unfractionated heparin in high-risk patients with non-ST-segment elevation acute coronary syndromes managed with an intended early invasive strategy: primary results of the SYNERGY randomized trial. JAMA 2004; 292(1):45–54.

68. Petersen JL, Mahaffey KW, Hasselblad V, et al. Efficacy and bleeding complications among patients randomized to enoxaparin or unfractionated heparin for antithrombin therapy in non-ST-Segment elevation acute coronary syndromes: a systematic overview. JAMA 2004; 292(1):89–96.

69. Bavry AA, Kumbhani DJ, Rassi AN, et al. Benefit of early invasive therapy in acute coronary syndromes: a meta-analysis of contemporary randomized clinical trials. J Am Coll Cardiol 2006; 48(7):1319–1325.

70. Silber S, Albertsson P, Aviles FF, et al. Guidelines for percutaneous coronary interventions. The task force for percutaneous coronary interventions of the European society of cardiology. Eur Heart J 2005; 26(8):804–847.

71. Collet JP, Montalescot G, Golmard JL, et al. Subcutaneous enoxaparin with early invasive strategy in patients with acute coronary syndromes. Am Heart J 2004; 147(4):655–661.

72. Moser LR, Kalus JS. Role of low-molecular-weight heparin in invasive management of non-ST-elevation acute coronary syndromes. Ann Pharmacother 2004; 38(12):2094–2104.

73. Denardo SJ, Davis KE, Tcheng JE. Effectiveness and safety of reduced-dose enoxaparin in non-ST-segment elevation acute coronary syndrome followed by antiplatelet therapy alone for percutaneous coronary intervention. Am J Cardiol 2007; 100(9):1376–1382.

74. Wolak A, Ayzenberg Y, Cafri C, et al. Can enoxaparin safely replace unfractionated heparin during coronary intervention in acute coronary syndromes? Int J Cardiol 2004; 96(2):151–155.

75. Montalescot G, Ongen Z, Guindy R, et al. Predictors of outcome in patients undergoing PCI. Results of the RIVIERA study.Int J Cardiol 2007; [Epub ahead of print].

76. Warkentin TE, Greinacher A. Heparin-induced thrombocytopenia: recognition, treatment, and prevention: the seventh ACCP conference on antithrombotic and thrombolytic therapy. Chest 2004; 126(3 suppl):311S–37S.

77. Bates SM, Weitz JI. The status of new anticoagulants. Br J Haematol 2006; 134(1):3–19.

78. Yusuf S, Mehta SR, Chrolavicius S, et al. Comparison of fondaparinux and enoxaparin in acute coronary syndromes. N Engl J Med 2006; 354(14):1464–1476.

79. Mehta SR, Granger CB, Eikelboom JW, et al. Efficacy and safety of fondaparinux versus enoxaparin in patients with acute coronary syndromes undergoing percutaneous coronary intervention: results from the OASIS-5 trial. J Am Coll Cardiol 2007; 50(18):1742–1751.

80. Weitz JI, Crowther M. Direct thrombin inhibitors. Thromb Res 2002; 106(3):V275–V284.

81. Stone GW, McLaurin BT, Cox DA, et al. Bivalirudin for patients with acute coronary syndromes. N Engl J Med 2006; 355(21):2203–2216.

82. Lincoff AM, Bittl JA, Harrington RA, et al. Bivalirudin and provisional glycoprotein IIb/IIIa blockade compared with heparin and planned glycoprotein IIb/IIIa blockade during percutaneous coronary intervention: REPLACE-2 randomized trial. JAMA 2003; 89(7):853–863.

83. Bittl JA, Strony J, Brinker JA, et al. Treatment with bivalirudin (Hirulog) as compared with heparin during coronary angioplasty for unstable or postinfarction angina. Hirulog Angioplasty Study Investigators. N Engl J Med 1995; 333(12):764–769.

84. Lincoff AM, Kleiman NS, Kottke-Marchant K, et al. Bivalirudin with planned or provisional abciximab versus low-dose heparin and abciximab during percutaneous coronary revascularization: results of the Comparison of Abciximab Complications with Hirulog for Ischemic Events Trial (CACHET). Am Heart J 2002; 143(5):847–853.

85. Lincoff AM, Bittl JA, Kleiman NS, et al. Comparison of bivalirudin versus heparin during percutaneous coronary intervention (the Randomized Evaluation of PCI Linking Angiomax to Reduced Clinical Events [REPLACE]-1 trial). Am J Cardiol 2004; 93(9):1092–1096.

86. Stone GW, Ware JH, Bertrand ME, et al. Antithrombotic strategies in patients with acute coronary syndromes undergoing early invasive management: one-year results from the ACUITY trial. JAMA 2007; 298(21):2497–2506.

87. Antman EM, Anbe DT, Armstrong PW, et al. ACC/AHA guidelines for the management of patients with ST-elevation myocardial infarction—executive summary: a report of the American College of Cardiology/American Heart Association Task Force on Practice Guidelines (Writing Committee to Revise the 1999 Guidelines for the Management of Patients With Acute Myocardial Infarction). Circulation 2004; 110(5):588–636.

88. Col J, Decoster O, Hanique G, et al. Infusion of heparin conjunct to streptokinase accelerates reperfusion of acute myocardial infarction: results of a double blind randomized study (OSIRIS). Circulation 1992; 86(suppl 1):259a.

89. (No authors listed). Randomized factorial trial of high-dose intravenous streptokinase, of oral aspirin and of intravenous heparin in acute myocardial infarction. ISIS (International Studies of Infarct Survival) pilot study. Eur Heart J 1987; 8(6):634–642.

90. de Bono DP, Simoons ML, Tijssen J, et al. Effect of early intravenous heparin on coronary patency, infarct size, and bleeding complications after alteplase thrombolysis: results of a randomised double blind European Cooperative Study Group trial. Br Heart J 1992; 67(2):122–128.

91. O'Connor CM, Meese R, Carney R, et al. A randomized trial of intravenous heparin in conjunction with anistreplase (anisoylated plasminogen streptokinase activator complex) in acute myocardial infarction: the Duke University Clinical Cardiology Study (DUCCS) 1. J Am Coll Cardiol 1994; 23(1):11–18.

92. Kontny F, Dale J, Abildgaard U, et al. Randomized trial of low molecular weight heparin (dalteparin) in prevention of left ventricular thrombus formation and arterial embolism after acute anterior myocardial infarction: the Fragmin in Acute Myocardial Infarction (FRAMI) Study. J Am Coll Cardiol 1997; 30(4):962–969.

93. Simoons M, Krzeminska-Pakula M, Alonso A, et al. Improved reperfusion and clinical outcome with enoxaparin as an adjunct to streptokinase thrombolysis in acute myocardial infarction. The AMI-SK study. Eur Heart J 2002; 23(16):1282–1290.

94. Yusuf S, Mehta SR, Xie C, et al. Effects of reviparin, a low-molecular-weight heparin, on mortality, reinfarction, and strokes in patients with acute myocardial infarction presenting with ST-segment elevation. JAMA 2005; 293(4):427–435.

95. Assessment of the Safety and Efficacy of a New Thrombolytic Regimen (ASSENT)-3 Investigators. Efficacy and safety of tenecteplase in combination with enoxaparin, abciximab, or unfractionated heparin: the ASSENT-3 randomised trial in acute myocardial infarction. Lancet 2001; 358(9282):605–613.

96. Ross AM, Molhoek P, Lundergan C, et al. Randomized comparison of enoxaparin, a low-molecular-weight heparin, with unfractionated heparin adjunctive to recombinant tissue plasminogen activator thrombolysis and aspirin: second trial of Heparin and Aspirin Reperfusion Therapy (HART II). Circulation 2001; 104(6):648–652.

97. Baird SH, Menown IB, McBride SJ, et al. Randomized comparison of enoxaparin with unfractionated heparin following fibrinolytic therapy for acute myocardial infarction. Eur Heart J 2002; 23(8):627–632.

98. Antman EM, Louwerenburg HW, Baars HF, et al. Enoxaparin as adjunctive antithrombin therapy for ST-elevation myocardial infarction: results of the ENTIRE-Thrombolysis in Myocardial Infarction (TIMI) 23 Trial. Circulation 2002; 105(14):1642–1649.

99. Wallentin L, Bergstrand L, Dellborg M, et al. Low molecular weight heparin (dalteparin) compared to unfractionated heparin as an adjunct to rt-PA (alteplase) for improvement of coronary artery patency in acute myocardial infarction-the ASSENT Plus study. Eur Heart J 2003; 24(10):897–908.

100. Wallentin L, Goldstein P, Armstrong PW, et al. Efficacy and safety of tenecteplase in combination with the low-molecular-weight heparin enoxaparin or unfractionated heparin in the prehospital setting: the Assessment of the Safety and Efficacy of a New Thrombolytic Regimen (ASSENT)-3 PLUS randomized trial in acute myocardial infarction. Circulation 2003; 108(2):135–142.

101. Eikelboom JW, Quinlan DJ, Mehta SR, et al. Unfractionated and low-molecular-weight heparin as adjuncts to thrombolysis in aspirin-treated patients with ST-elevation acute myocardial infarction: a meta-analysis of the randomized trials. Circulation 2005; 112(25):3855–3867.

102. Giugliano RP, McCabe CH, Antman EM, et al. Lower-dose heparin with fibrinolysis is associated with lower rates of intracranial hemorrhage. Am Heart J 2001; 141(5):742–750.

103. Frostfeldt G, Ahlberg G, Gustafsson G, et al. Low molecular weight heparin (dalteparin) as adjuvant treatment of thrombolysis in acute myocardial infarction—a pilot study: biochemical markers in acute coronary syndromes (BIOMACS II). J Am Coll Cardiol 1999; 33(3):627–633.

104. Antman EM, Morrow DA, McCabe CH, et al. Enoxaparin versus unfractionated heparin with fibrinolysis for ST-elevation myocardial infarction. N Engl J Med 2006; 354(14):1477–1488.

105. Yusuf S, Mehta SR, Chrolavicius S, et al. Effects of fondaparinux on mortality and reinfarction in patients with acute ST-segment elevation myocardial infarction: the OASIS-6 randomized trial. JAMA 2006; 295(13):1519–1530.

106. White H. Thrombin-specific anticoagulation with bivalirudin versus heparin in patients receiving fibrinolytic therapy for acute myocardial infarction: the HERO-2 randomised trial. Lancet 2001; 358(9296):1855–1863.

107. Van de Werf F, Ardissino D, Betriu A, Management of acute myocardial infarction in patients presenting with ST-segment elevation. Eur Heart J 2003; 24:28–66.

12

Anticoagulation in Pregnancy

Shannon M. Bates
Department of Medicine, McMaster University and Henderson Research Centre, Hamilton, Ontario, Canada

INTRODUCTION

Anticoagulants are indicated during pregnancy for the prevention and treatment of venous thromboembolism (VTE), in patients with mechanical heart valves, as well as for the prevention of pregnancy loss in women with antiphospholipid antibodies (APLA). Anticoagulant therapy is also increasingly being employed for prevention of pregnancy complications in women with hereditary thrombophilia. Anticoagulant use during pregnancy is challenging because of the potential for fetal, as well as maternal, complications and because there is a paucity of high-quality clinical trials in this patient population upon which to make management decisions. This chapter will review the use of anticoagulants during pregnancy and in breast-feeding women and provide recommendations for the treatment and prevention of VTE, anticoagulant management in women with prosthetic mechanical valves, and prevention of pregnancy complications in women with thrombophilias.

FETAL COMPLICATIONS OF ANTICOAGULANT USE DURING PREGNANCY

Potential fetal complications of maternal anticoagulant therapy include teratogenicity, loss, and bleeding. Given their potential for deleterious effects on the fetus, vitamin K antagonists should only be used during pregnancy when potential maternal benefits justify potential fetal risks. Although unfractionated heparin (UFH) and low-molecular-weight heparin (LMWH) are as effective as vitamin K antagonists in the management of VTE, vitamin K antagonists may be more effective than these agents in patients with mechanical prosthetic valves.

Vitamin K Antagonist Exposure In Utero

Vitamin K antagonists readily cross the placenta and have the potential to cause fetal wastage, teratogenicity, and bleeding (1–3). In a systematic review examining outcomes in pregnant women with prosthetic valves (3), congenital anomalies were reported in 6.4% of live births (95% CI, 4.6–8.9%) when vitamin K antagonists were continued throughout pregnancy. The most common fetal anomaly was characteristic coumarin embryopathy, which typically consists of nasal hypoplasia and/or stippled epiphyses, although hypoplasia of the limbs and/or phalanges has been reported in up to one-third of cases (4). The severity of embropathy is variable and, in one literature review, one-half of affected infants had no severe disability (2). However, in severe cases true choanal stenosis and upper airway obstruction have been reported. In the systematic review described above, the substitution of heparin for vitamin K antagonists at or prior to six weeks appeared to eliminate the risk of embryopathy (0%; 95% CI, 0–3.4%) (3), raising the possibility that vitamin K antagonists are safe with regard to this complication during the first six weeks of gestation.

Although there is a definite risk of embryopathy if coumarin derivatives are taken between six and 12 weeks of gestation (2), the true incidence of embryopathy is difficult to determine because of the likelihood of case-reporting bias and a lack of uniform reporting of the trimester of exposure to anticoagulants. Therefore, it is not surprising that reported estimates of the risk of this anomaly vary widely, ranging from 0% (5–10) up to 29.6% (11). The latter is likely to represent an overestimate; however, as only two infants (5.7%) were described as having classic features of warfarin embryopathy, while the others had minor facial defects or facial bone features suggestive of embryopathy. Other research also supports a lower risk estimate. When the pregnancies of 666 European women who contacted Teratology Information Services seeking advice about gestational exposure to vitamin K antagonists were prospectively followed, there were only two cases of embryopathy among 356 live births (0.6%) (12). Both of these cases involved exposure to phenprocoumon until at least the end of the first trimester. In this study, there were no cases of embryopathy among children born to women who discontinued vitamin K antagonists before the eighth week after the first day of the last menstrual period (12).

Central nervous system abnormalities have been reported after exposure to vitamin K antagonists during any trimester (2). Two patterns of central nervous system damage have been described: dorsal midline dysplasia (agenesis of the corpus callosum, Dandy-Walker malformation, and midline cerebellar atrophy) and ventral midline dysplasia leading to optic atrophy (2). The incidence of these anomalies appears to be less than 5% (1,2,11); however, the sequelae appear more debilitating than those of warfarin embryopathy (2,3). In one review, all live-born affected infants had cognitive impairment, half were blind, one-third had spasticity, and seizures were found in one-quarter (2).

One cohort study that examined the long-term effects of prenatal vitamin K antagonist exposure in 274 school-aged children described an increased risk of minor neurodevelopmental problems (OR 1.9; 95% CI, 1.1–3.4) in children exposed to coumarins in the second and third trimester of pregnancy, compared with age-matched nonexposed controls (13). However, the significance of these problems is uncertain because there were no differences in mean intelligence quotient or performance on tests for reading, spelling, and arithmetic between exposed and nonexposed children (14).

Vitamin K antagonists have been associated with fetal wastage (3,15) and can cause fetal hemorrhagic complications, likely because the fetal liver is immature and produces lower levels of vitamin K dependent coagulation factors. Fetal coagulopathy is of particular concern at the time of delivery, when the combination of the anticoagulant effect and trauma of delivery can lead to neonatal bleeding. The risk of delivering an anticoagulated infant can be reduced by substituting UFH or LMWH for vitamin K antagonists approximately three weeks prior to planned delivery (15) and discontinuing these medications shortly before delivery. Others have advocated the use of planned cesarean section at 38 weeks with only a two- to three-day interruption of vitamin K antagonist therapy (16). Although this strategy appeared to result in good neonatal and maternal outcomes, only 30 babies were delivered using this regimen. Further, it should be noted that caesarean section is not without risk and is not routinely recommended for other conditions associated with an increased risk of neonatal intracranial hemorrhage at the time of delivery (e.g., immune thrombocytopenic purpura).

Physicians should counsel women receiving vitamin K antagonist therapy who are contemplating pregnancy about the risks of these medications before pregnancy occurs. If pregnancy is still desired, there are two options to reduce the risk of warfarin embryopathy. The first is performance of frequent pregnancy tests and substitution of adjusted-dose UFH or LMWH for warfarin when pregnancy is achieved (and before the sixth week of gestation), while the second is the replacement of vitamin K antagonists with UFH or LMWH before conception is attempted. Both approaches have limitations. The first option (*i*) assumes that vitamin K antagonists are safe during the first four to six weeks of gestation and (*ii*) places a higher value on avoiding the risks, inconvenience and costs of UFH or LMWH therapy while awaiting pregnancy than it does on minimizing the risks of early miscarriage associated with vitamin K antagonist therapy. The second option increases the duration of exposure to heparin and, therefore, is costly and exposes the patient to a higher risk of complications related to the use of UFH or LMWH.

UFH and LMWH Exposure In Utero

UFH does not cross the placenta (17) and, therefore, does not have the potential to cause fetal bleeding or teratogenicity; although bleeding at the uteroplacental junction is possible. Several studies strongly suggest that UFH therapy is safe for the fetus (1,18) and should be used as necessary for maternal indications.

LMWH is also a safe anticoagulant choice for the fetus because it also does not cross the placenta (19,20). There is no evidence of an increased risk of teratogenicity or fetal bleeding associated with maternal LMWH use (21).

Danaparoid Exposure In Utero

Danaparoid is a glycosaminoglycan that is often used as an alternative anticoagulant in patients with heparin-induced thrombocytopenia (HIT). Although the available literature suggests that there is no demonstrable fetal toxicity with maternal danaparoid use, the quality of evidence available to support that claim is limited and consists of one investigation demonstrating negligible movement across guinea pig placenta (22) and two case reports in which clinicians using danaparoid detected no anti-Xa activity in fetal cord plasma (23,24). In a review of 51 pregnancies in 49 danaparoid-treated patients, three fetal deaths were reported but all were associated with maternal complications antedating danaparoid use (25).

Direct Thrombin Inhibitor Exposure In Utero

Investigations have documented placental transfer of hirudin in rabbits and rats (26,27). Although small numbers of case reports of successful outcomes with hirudin use in pregnancy have been published (26,28,29), there are insufficient data to confirm its safety in this setting.

Pentasaccharide Exposure In Utero

Although no placental passage of fondaparinux was demonstrated in an in vitro human cotyledon model (30), anti-factor Xa activity at approximately one-tenth of that detected in maternal plasma was found in the umbilical cord plasma in newborns of five mothers treated with fondaparinux (31). Although there have been reports of the successful use of this agent in pregnant woman (32,33), potential deleterious effects on the fetus cannot be excluded.

Fibrinolytic Agent Exposure During Pregnancy

Concerns about the use of fibrinolytic therapy during pregnancy center on its effects on the placenta (i.e., premature labor, placental abruption, fetal demise) and the safety of fibrinolytic agents in this setting are unclear. Investigations have demonstrated minimal transplacental passage of ^{131}I-labeled streptokinase (34) and placental transfer of tissue plasminogen activator is unlikely because of its molecular size. Although there have been several reports of successful fibrinolysis in pregnancy with no harm to the fetus (35,36), the use of fibrinolytic therapy in pregnancy is best reserved for life-threatening maternal thromboembolism.

Aspirin Exposure In Utero

In a meta-analysis of 14 randomized studies including a total of 12,416 women (37), low-dose (50 to 150 mg/day) aspirin administered during the second and third trimesters of pregnancy to women at risk for pre eclampsia was safe for the mother and the fetus. However, the safety of aspirin ingestion during the first trimester remains uncertain. A meta-analysis of eight studies that evaluated the risk of congenital anomalies with aspirin exposure during the first trimester found no evidence of an increase in the overall risk of congenital malformations associated with aspirin use but there may have been a twofold increase in the risk for gastroschisis (OR, 2.37; 95% CI, 1.44–3.88) (38), a rare anomaly that occurs in three to six of every 100,000 births in which the intestines herniate through a congenital defect in the abdominal wall on one side of the umbilical cord. However, the reliability of this risk estimate is questionable because the use of other drugs, the type of control subjects selected, and failure to definitively confirm the diagnosis in all patients could have biased these results. Thus, although the safety of aspirin ingestion during the first trimester remains uncertain, there is no clear evidence of harm to the fetus, and, if fetal anomalies are caused by early aspirin exposure, they are very rare.

ANTICOAGULANT USE IN NURSING WOMEN

Risks to the neonate must be also considered when prescribing anticoagulants to breast-feeding women. In order for a drug to pose a risk to the breast-fed infant, not only must it be transferred and excreted into breast milk, it must also be absorbed by the infant's gut. Drugs that are poorly absorbed orally are unlikely to affect the neonate. Lipid soluble drugs with a low molecular weight that are not highly protein bound are more likely to be transferred into breast milk (39).

Many obstetricians remain reluctant to prescribe warfarin to lactating women. These concerns likely represent extrapolations from warfarin's fetopathic effects (40). There have been two reports demonstrating that nursing mothers can safely breast-feed their infants while taking warfarin. In the first, 13 nursing mothers with detectable plasma warfarin activity were studied and in each instance, less than 0.08 μmol of warfarin per liter of breast milk was found. Warfarin was not found in the plasma of any of the seven infants being breast-fed by their mothers (41). In the second study, the plasma and breast milk of two nursing mothers who had received warfarin for at least eight weeks were studied (42). Although the prothrombin times and levels of vitamin K–dependent clotting factors were altered in the mothers' plasma, the prothrombin times and factor levels of their infants' plasma showed 100% of control activity. Again, no warfarin was detected in the breast milk.

UFH's high molecular weight and strong negative charge prevent it from passing into breast milk, and it can be safely given to nursing mothers (43). Although a case series demonstrated excretion of small amounts of LMWH into the breast milk in 11 of 15 women receiving 2500 IU of LMWH (44), orally ingested heparin has a very low bioavailability, and there is unlikely to be any clinically relevant effect on the nursing infant. It is not known whether or to what extent fondaparinux is excreted in breast milk.

A small number of case reports have reported no or very low anti-Xa activity in the breast milk of danaparoid-treated women (26). Because danaparoid is not absorbed after oral intake, it is unlikely that any anticoagulant effect would appear in breast-fed infants.

In a single case report, no hirudin was detected in the breast milk of a nursing mother with a therapeutic plasma hirudin level (45). Enteral absorption of hirudin appears to be low (27) and, therefore, it is unlikely that exposed infants would experience a significant anticoagulant effect, even if small amounts of hirudin were to appear in breast milk.

MATERNAL COMPLICATIONS OF ANTICOAGULANT THERAPY

Maternal complications of anticoagulant therapy are similar to those seen in nonpregnant patients and include bleeding (for all anticoagulants), as well as HIT, heparin-associated osteoporosis, and pain at injection sites for heparin-related compounds.

UFH Therapy

In a study of 100 pregnant women treated with various doses of UFH, the rate of major bleeding was 2% (18), which is consistent with reported rates of bleeding associated with heparin therapy for the treatment of deep vein thrombosis (DVT) in nonpregnant patients (46). A persistent anticoagulant effect seen with therapeutic doses of subcutaneous UFH can complicate its use around the time of delivery because of increased risks of bleeding and hematoma with epidural anesthesia. In a cohort of 11 patients, prolongation of the activated partial thromboplastin time (aPTT) persisted for up to 28 hours after the last injection of adjusted-dose subcutaneous heparin given at 12-hour intervals (47). The mechanism responsible for this prolonged effect is unclear.

Approximately 3% of nonpregnant patients receiving UFH develop HIT (48). There are insufficient data to derive an estimate of the risk of HIT in pregnant and postpartum women, although it is reasonable to expect that the frequency would be similar. In the pregnant population, HIT should be differentiated from incidental thrombocytopenia of pregnancy (49) and HELLP (hemolysis, elevated liver enzymes and low platelets) syndrome, as well as from the early, benign, transient thrombocytopenia that can occur with initiation of UFH.

Long-term treatment with UFH has been reported to cause osteoporosis in both laboratory animals and humans because of decreased rates of bone formation, accompanied by increased bone resorption (50–58). Symptomatic vertebral fractures have been reported to occur in approximately 2% to 3% of the patient population and significant reductions of bone density have been reported in up to 30% of pregnant patients receiving UFH for prolonged periods (50,51).

LMWH Therapy

LMWH is now commonly used for prophylaxis and treatment of maternal thromboembolism. Although there is a paucity of supportive data from controlled trials or large prospective observational studies in the pregnant population, large trials in nonpregnant patients have demonstrated that LMWHs are at least as safe and effective as UFH for the treatment of VTE (59,60) and acute coronary syndromes (61,62), as well as for prophylaxis in high-risk patients (63). LMWH's better bioavailability, longer plasma-half-life, a more predictable dose response, and an improved safety profile also render it preferable to UFH (63–65).

Retrospective analyses and systematic reviews suggest that the incidence of bleeding in pregnant women receiving LMWH is low (21,64,65). An early review of LMWH use in 486 pregnancies identified a frequency of minor bleeding of 2.7% and no major hemorrhagic events (64). In a more recent systematic review of 64 studies reporting 2777 pregnancies, the frequencies of significant bleeding were 0.43% (95% CI, 0.22–0.75%) for antepartum hemorrhage, 0.94% (95% CI, 0.61–1.37%) for postpartum hemorrhage, and 0.61% (95% CI, 0.36%–0.98%) for wound hematoma; giving an overall frequency of 1.98% (95% CI, 1.50–2.57%) (65). Although HIT can occur with LMWH therapy, the risk appears lower with LMWH than with UFH (48), and no confirmed cases were identified in the two reviews described above (64,65).

Studies in both animals (57) and humans suggest that the risk of osteoporosis is lower with LMWHs than with UFH. In a study in which 80 men and women with a mean age of 68 years were treated with either subcutaneous dalteparin (5000 units twice daily) or UFH (10,000 units twice daily) for a period of three to six months, the risk of vertebral fractures was higher in those receiving UFH [15%, (95% CI, 6–30%)] than in those receiving dalteparin [3% (95% CI 0–11%)] (54). In another randomized trial in which pregnant women were allocated to prophylactic doses of dalteparin ($n = 21$) or UFH ($n = 23$), lumbar spine bone density following delivery did not differ between women receiving dalteparin and untreated patients but was significantly lower in those receiving UFH (55). On multiple logistic regression analysis, the type of heparin used was the only independent factor associated with reduced bone mass. Finally, in a prospective observational study in which preconception and postdelivery lumbar spine dual energy X-ray absorptiometry scans were performed in 55 pregnant women treated with prophylactic LMWH and aspirin and 20 other pregnant women who were not treated with antithrombotic agents, the loss in lumbar spine bone mineral density was similar in both groups. These results suggest that bone loss associated with prophylactic LMWH therapy is similar to normal physiologic losses during pregnancy (66).

TREATMENT RECOMMENDATIONS

There are no large well-conducted randomized trials or prospective cohort studies in the pregnant population to provide guidance for prevention and treatment of VTE or for the prevention of systemic embolism in patients with valvular heart disease. As a result, recommendations are usually based on extrapolations from nonpregnant patients, in addition to case reports and case series of pregnant patients (67).

Table 1 Subcutaneous LMWH Dosing Regimens for the Initial Treatment of VTE

LMWH	Twice-daily regimen	Once-daily regimen
Dalteparin	100 U/kg	200 U/kg
Tinzaparin	Not applicable	175 U/kg
Enoxparin	1 mg/kg	1.5 mg/kg

Abbreviation: LMWH, low-molecular-weight heparin.

VTE During Pregnancy

It has been recognized for many years that pregnant women are at increased risk of developing VTE and pulmonary embolism (PE) remains the leading cause of maternal mortality in the western world (68,69). VTE complicates between 0.6 and 1.3 per 1000 deliveries (70–75). Although these rates are low, they represent a 5- to 10-fold increase in risk compared with those reported for nonpregnant women of comparable age (76,77). Approximately two-thirds of pregnancy-related DVT occur antepartum, with these events distributed relatively equally throughout all three trimesters (78). In contrast, 43 to 60% of pregnancy-related episodes of PE appear to occur in the four to six weeks after delivery (71,75). Since the antepartum period is much longer than the six-week postpartum period, the daily risk of PE, as well as DVT, is considerably higher after delivery than antepartum.

Despite a paucity of supportive data from randomized trials or large prospective observation studies, LMWH is now commonly used for the treatment of maternal VTE. If LMWH is used for the treatment of pregnancy-related VTE, a weight-adjusted dose is recommended (Table 1). Optimal dosing regimens for LMWH in this setting are unknown because pregnant women are routinely excluded from clinical trials and pharmacologic studies. LMWH requirements may be influenced by physiologic changes that occur during pregnancy, such as maternal weight gain, alterations in volume of distribution of LMWH, and increases in glomerular filtration rate in the second trimester. The need for dose adjustments over the course of pregnancy remains controversial. On the basis of small studies showing the need for dose escalation to maintain "therapeutic" anti-Xa LMWH levels (79,80), some suggest that periodic (e.g., every one to three months) anti-factor Xa LMWH levels should be performed four hours after injection with dose adjustment to maintain anti-Xa levels of 0.6 to 1.0 U/mL if a twice-daily regimen is used and approximately 1.0 to 2.0 U/mL if a once-daily regimen is chosen. It has also been suggested that the LMWH dose should be increased in proportion to changes in weight (81). However, other researchers have demonstrated that few women require dose-adjustment when therapeutic doses of LMWH are used (82). In the absence of large studies using clinical endpoints demonstrating that there is an optimal "therapeutic anti-Xa LMWH range" or that dose-adjustments increase the safety or efficacy of therapy, any of these approaches is reasonable.

There have been no randomized trials evaluating routes of administration or dosages of UFH therapy during pregnancy. Clinicians selecting UFH can use either initial intravenous therapy followed by subcutaneous UFH administered every 12 hours in doses adjusted to prolong the mid-interval (six hour postinjection) aPTT into the therapeutic range or twice-daily adjusted-dose subcutaneous UFH for both initial and long-term treatment. When given subcutaneously, a starting regimen of at least 17,500 units every 12 hours is recommended. Because UFH requirements vary as pregnancy progresses, the mid-interval aPTT should be monitored every one to two weeks and the heparin dose adjusted to obtain a result within the therapeutic range.

Regimens in which the intensity of LMWH is reduced later during the course of therapy to an intermediate dose regimen (54) or 75% of a full treatment dose (83) have been used successfully in the nonpregnant population. There have been no studies directly comparing full-dose LMWH with one of these modified dosing strategies in pregnant women and it remains unclear whether the dose of UFH or LMWH can be reduced after an initial phase of therapeutic anticoagulation in these patients. However, a modified dosing regimen may be useful in pregnant women at increased risk of bleeding or heparin-associated osteoporosis.

Prevention of VTE in Pregnant Women

Women with thrombophilia and those with a history of VTE appear to have an increased risk of DVT or PE in subsequent pregnancies. Thromboprophylaxis during pregnancy involves long-term parenteral UFH or LMWH, both of which are expensive, inconvenient and painful to administer, and associated with risks of bleeding, osteoporosis, and HIT. Rational administration of prophylaxis depends on quantifying the risk of thrombosis and identifying those women whose risk is sufficiently high to merit intervention. The threshold for recommending postpartum prophylaxis is lower than that for antepartum prophylaxis because the length of required treatment is shorter (i.e., six weeks), the average daily risk of VTE is higher in the postpartum period (71,75,78), and warfarin is safe during this time period, even if the mother is breast-feeding (41,42).

Prevention of VTE in Pregnant Women with Thrombophilia and No Prior VTE

Thrombophilic defects predisposing to VTE vary in prevalence and in the magnitude of the associated increase in risk of VTE. Approximately 50% of gestational VTE are associated with heritable thrombophilia (84,85). Although inherited thrombophilias are common and affect approximately 15% of Western populations, only approximately 1 in 1000 pregnancies is complicated by DVT or PE. Therefore, the presence of thrombophilia alone does not consistently result in VTE.

In a systematic review of nine studies that assessed the risk of VTE in pregnant women with heritable thrombophilias, all congenital thrombophilias with the exception of homozygosity for the thermolabile methylene tetrahydrofolate reductase variant (MTHFR C677T) were found to be associated with a statistically significant increase in the risk of pregnancy-related VTE (Table 2) (86). The highest risks were associated with homozygosity for the factor V Leiden mutation or the prothrombin G20210A variant. The most common inherited thrombophilias, heterozygosity for the factor V Leiden mutation or for the prothrombin G20210A variant, were associated with lower risks. Given a background incidence of VTE during pregnancy of approximately 1 of 1000 deliveries, it is clear that the absolute risk of VTE in women without a prior event remains modest for those who have the common inherited thrombophilias. These results are supported by those of observational studies. In a recent report, there were no venous thromboembolic events among members of a prospectively followed cohort of 134 carriers of the heterozygous form of the factor V Leiden mutation with a singleton pregnancy and no prior history of VTE (0%, 95% CI, 0–2.7%) (87). On the other hand, in other cohort studies, the absolute risk of pregnancy-associated VTE has been reported to range from 9 to 16% in those homozygous for the factor V Leiden mutation (88–93). Double heterozygosity for factor V Leiden and prothrombin G20210A mutation has been reported to have an absolute risk of pregnancy-associated VTE of 4.0% (95% C1, 1.4 to 16.9%) (90). The reported risks of pregnancy-related VTE in the systematic review

Table 2 Risk of VTE and Pregnancy Complications in Women with Inherited Thrombophilia

	VTE	Recurrent early loss	Late loss	Preeclampsia	Placental abruption	IUGR
			Odds ratio (95% CI)			
Antithrombin deficiency	4.7 (1.3–17.0)	0.9 (0.2–4.5)	7.6 (0.3–196)	3.9 (0.2–97.2)	1.1 (0.1–18.1)	NA
Protein C deficiency	4.8 (2.1–10.6)	2.3 (0.2–26.4)	3.0 (0.2–38.5)	5.1 (0.3–102)	5.9 (0.2–152)	NA
Protein S deficiency	3.2 (1.5–6.9)	3.6 (0.3–35.7)	20.1 (3.7–109)	2.83 (0.8–10.6)	2.1 (0.5–9.3)	NA
Factor V Leiden (+/−)	8.3 (5.4–12.7)	1.7 (1.1–2.6)	2.1 (1.1–3.9)	2.2 (1.5–3.3)	4.7 (1.1–19.6)	2.7 (0.6–12.1)
Factor V Leiden (+/+)	34.4 (9.9–120)	2.7 (1.3–5.6)	2.0 (0.4–9.7)	1.9 (0.4–7.9)	8.4 (0.4–171)	4.64 (0.2–116)
Prothombin gene variant (+/−)	6.8 (2.5–18.8)	2.5 (1.2–5.0)	2.7 (1.3–5.5)	2.5 (1.5–4.2)	7.7 (3.0–19.8)	2.7 (0.6–12.1)
Prothombin gene variant (+/+)	26.4 (1.2–559)					
MTHFR C667T (+/+)	0.7 (0.2–2.5)	1.4 (0.8–2.6)	1.3 (0.9–1.9)	1.4 (1.1–1.8)	1.5 (0.4–5.3)	1.2 (0.8–1.8)

Note: Shaded areas contain statistically significant odds ratios.

Abbreviations: VTE, venous thromboembolism.

Source: From Ref. 86.

described above were lower for women with deficiencies of the endogenous anti-coagulants (antithrombin, protein C, and protein S) than traditionally described in older small retrospective studies of selected patients (94–96), which may have overestimated the risks of VTE. In more recent methodologically sound retrospective and case-control studies not included in the systematic review, estimates of the incidence of pregnancy-related VTE have ranged from 0.2% to 0.9% in those with protein C deficiency and from 0.2% to 36% in those deficient in antithrombin (97,98). Taken together, these data suggest that women with antithrombin deficiency or homozygous for the factor V Leiden mutation, as well as double heterozygotes, should be managed more aggressively than those with other heritable thrombophilias, especially in symptomatic kindreds.

Acquired thrombophilias have been less well studied but persistent APLA [lupus anticoagulants (nonspecific inhibitors) or anticardiolipin antibodies] are likely associated with an increased risk of pregnancy-related VTE (99).

The management of pregnant women with known thrombophilia and no prior VTE remains controversial because of our limited knowledge of the natural histories of various thrombophilias and the paucity of high-quality data measuring the effectiveness and safety of antithrombotic agents in preventing VTE in pregnant women with thrombophilia and no prior history of DVT or PE. Postpartum prophylaxis for approximately six weeks is generally recommended, even in the absence of prior VTE. Either prophylactic doses of LMWH or UFH or vitamin K antagonists targeted to an INR of 2.0 to 3.0 with a short initial course of prophylactic UFH or LMWH are typically used. In general, either careful clinical surveillance or pharmacologic prophylaxis is acceptable antepartum management options, depending on patient and physician preference. The indication for active antipasto prophylaxis appears stronger for women with high-risk thrombophilias as described above. Commonly used prophylactic regimens are outlined in Table 3.

Prevention of VTE in Pregnant Women with Prior Disease

The extent to which pregnancy influences the risk of recurrent VTE remains somewhat uncertain; however, in a retrospective study of 109 women who had at least one pregnancy without receiving thrombosis prophylaxis after an episode of VTE, recurrence rates per 100 patient-years were 10.9% during and 3.7% outside of pregnancy (RR during

Table 3 Subcutaneous LMWH Dosing Regimens for Prevention of VTE

LMWH	Prophylactic	Intermediate-dose
• Dalteparin	5000 units daily	5000 units every 12 hr or once-daily dosing adjusted to anti-Xa level of 0.2–0.6 U/mL
• Tinzaparin	4500 units daily OR 75 U/kg daily	Once-daily dosing adjusted to anti-Xa level of 0.2–0.6 U/mL
• Enoxaparin	40 mg daily	40 mg every 12 hr or Once-daily dosing adjusted to anti-Xa level of 0.2–0.6 U/mL
UFH	5000 units every 12 hr	5000 units every 12 hr in doses adjusted to target anti-Xa level of 0.1–0.3 U/mL

Abbreviations: LMWH, low-molecular-weight heparin; VTE, venous thromboembolism; UFH, unfractionated heparin.

Table 4 Risk of Pregnancy-Related Recurrent VTE

Study	Design	N	Antepartum VTE % (95% CI)
Brill-Edwards (101)	Prospective	125	2.4 (0.2–6.9)
Pabinger (102)	Retrospective	159	6.2 (1.6–10.9)
De Stefano (103)	Retrospective	88	5.8 (3.0–10.6)

Abbreviation: VTE, venous thromboembolism.

pregnancy 3.5; 95% CI, 1.6–7.8) (100). The most reliable data regarding the risk of recurrent VTE come from a prospective study of 125 pregnant women with a single previous episode of objectively diagnosed VTE in which antepartum heparin was withheld and anticoagulants (usually warfarin with a target INR of 2.0 to 3.0 with an initial short course of UFH or LMWH) were given in the postpartum period for four to six weeks. In this study, the overall frequency of antepartum recurrence was 2.4% (95% CI, 0.2–6.9%) (101). A post hoc subgroup analysis identified women without thrombophilia who had a temporary risk factor (including pregnancy and oral contraceptive therapy) at the time of their prior event as being at low risk of recurrence (0%, 95% CI, 0.0–8.0%) compared with those women with abnormal results on thrombophilia testing and/or a previous episode of thrombosis that was unprovoked (5.9%; 95% CI, 1.2–16.0%). Some have suggested that the above prospective study may have underestimated the risk of recurrence because women with known thrombophilia were excluded and the median gestational age at enrollment was relatively advanced (approximately 15 weeks) and two subsequent retrospective cohort studies suggested that the risk of antepartum recurrence might be slightly higher (Table 4) (102,103). Moreover, in these studies, the presence or absence of temporary risk factors or of a definable thrombophilia did not appear to influence the risk of recurrent VTE associated with pregnancy. The retrospective nature of these studies, differences in study population (including the inclusion of women with more than one prior episode of VTE) and failure to independently adjudicate recurrent events might account for the higher reported risk of recurrence. However, in both studies, the overall risk of antepartum recurrent VTE was less than 10% and CIs around the risk estimates are overlapping.

There have been no large clinical trials assessing the role of prophylaxis in pregnant women with previous VTE. As a result, the optimal approach to thrombosis prophylaxis in pregnant women with prior VTE is uncertain. However, on the basis of risk estimates reported in the single prospective study (101), antepartum prophylaxis appears unwarranted in women without thrombophilia whose previous episode of thrombosis was associated with a temporary risk factor. However, this decision should be considered on an individual basis, taking all the woman's risk factors for VTE and patient preference into account. Although pregnancy and oral contraceptive therapy were included as transient risk factors in the prospective study, the number of women whose prior event occurred in the setting of increased estrogen was small and many experts believe that these women have sufficiently high risk of antepartum recurrence to merit prophylaxis prior to delivery, as well as postpartum. At present, either antepartum clinical surveillance or pharmacologic prophylaxis can be justified in pregnant women with a prior history of unprovoked VTE or VTE associated with thrombophilia. Antepartum prophylaxis is easier to justify in women with higher risk thrombophilias and in women with more than one VTE event.

Common antepartum prophylactic regimens are outlined in Table 3. Until comparative studies are performed, it is not possible to make definitive recommendations about which prophylactic regimen is preferable. As with therapeutic LMWH, the need to adjust prophylactic LMWH dosing according to anti-Xa levels remains controversial. However, the appropriate "therapeutic range" for prophylaxis is uncertain and it has not been shown that dose adjustment to attain a specific anti-Xa level increases safety or efficacy of prophylaxis. Moreover, routine monitoring of anti-Xa levels is expensive and inconvenient and its reliability is compromised by inter-assay and instrument variability of anti-Xa results (104,105). Although supportive data from clinical trials are lacking, postpartum prophylaxis with either vitamin K antagonists targeted to an INR of 2.0 to 3.0 or prophylactic LMWH is suggested for pregnant women with prior VTE.

Prevention of Pregnancy Complications in Patients with Thrombophilia

Recent data suggests that there is a link between thrombophilia and adverse pregnancy outcomes, including fetal loss, placental abruption, and preeclampsia. There is convincing evidence from clinical studies that the presence of APLAs is associated with an increased risk of pregnancy loss (86,106–109). However, there is less agreement on the association between the presence of APLA and the occurrence of other pregnancy complications, including preeclampsia, placental abruption, and intrauterine growth restriction (110–127).

Many studies have examined the association between heritable thrombophilia and pregnancy complications, often with differing results (86), likely reflecting heterogeneity of study design, sample size, inclusion criteria, population studied, outcome definition, and thrombophilias studied. However, the results of a recent systematic review that examined 25 studies in 7167 women confirms the associations between some thrombophilias and early (recurrent) fetal loss, late fetal loss, preeclampsia, and placental abruption (Table 2) (86). Although there was a trend toward an increased risk of intrauterine growth restriction (IUGR) in women with congenital thrombophilia, no statistically significant associations were found (86).

The combination of UFH and low-dose aspirin has been shown to be effective in reducing miscarriage rates in women with APLA syndrome with prior recurrent fetal loss (109). On its own, aspirin has demonstrated no significant reduction in pregnancy loss compared with usual care or placebo (109). Although the results of one systematic review suggest that the combination of LMWH and aspirin had no statistically significant effect on pregnancy loss when compared with aspirin alone, the point estimate was in the direction of benefit (109). If UFH's effect on prevention of recurrent loss is mediated by its antithrombotic properties, then LMWH should be equally effective. Consistent with this, the results of two subsequently published pilot studies suggest that the combination of LMWH and aspirin might be equivalent to UFH and aspirin in preventing recurrent pregnancy loss (128,129).

The data surrounding the use of antithrombotic therapy in women with hereditable thrombophilia and pregnancy loss are less convincing and predominantly consist of small uncontrolled trials or observational studies (130–132). In the LIVE-ENOX trial, in which women with hereditary thrombophilia and recurrent pregnancy loss were randomized to one of two doses of enoxaparin (40 mg per day or 80 mg per day), there was no significant difference in pregnancy outcomes between the two groups; however, the rate of live birth was higher than might have been expected given the patients' prior histories (133,134). However, this trial has significant limitations (135,136), including heterogeneous entry criteria, absence of an untreated control group to establish efficacy, and the risk of regression toward the mean. More recently, Gris et al. reported that treatment with 40 mg enoxaparin daily in women with a thrombophilia (factor V Leiden mutation, prothrombin gene variant, or protein S deficiency) and one previous pregnancy loss after 10 weeks gestation, resulted in a significantly higher live birth rate (86%) compared with low-dose aspirin alone (29%) (137). This trial also has limitations including small sample size, absence of an untreated control group, and inadequate concealment of allocation. Further, given that the success rate of subsequent pregnancies is relatively high after a single miscarriage, it is difficult to assess the implications of these results.

Although there is circumstantial evidence that LMWH may improve the pregnancy outcome in women with heritable thrombophilia and recurrent pregnancy loss or loss after 10 weeks, available studies have important methodologic limitations and firm recommendations cannot be provided regarding the use of antithrombotic therapy in this patient population. Decisions should be made after reviewing with the patient the limitations of the available data, along with the potential benefits, harms and costs of any intervention. It is also important to note that treatment that prevents fetal loss may not prevent other complications and, at present, there are insufficient data on the effect of antithrombotic interventions on other adverse pregnant outcomes.

Prevention of Systemic Embolism in Pregnant Women with Valvular Heart Disease

The management of pregnant women with mechanical heart valves is a challenge. The use of vitamin K antagonists during pregnancy carries the potential for serious risks to the fetus, especially if these drugs are administered during the first trimester or at term. Although LMWH or UFH can be substituted for vitamin K antagonists, doubt has been raised about their effectiveness for prevention of systemic embolism.

In a systematic review of the literature examining outcomes in pregnant women with prosthetic valves (Table 5), the overall pooled of maternal mortality rate was 2.9%, while major bleeding occurred in 2.5% of all pregnancies, mostly at the time of delivery (3). The regimen associated with the lowest risk of valve thrombosis/systemic embolism was the use of vitamin K antagonists throughout pregnancy. Using UFH only between six

Table 5 Frequency of Maternal Complications Reported with Various Anticoagulation Regimens in Pregnant Women with Prosthetic Valves

Anticoagulant regimen	Thromboembolic complications	Deaths (all causes)
	n/N (%)	
Vitamin K antagonists throughout with/without UFH near term	31/788 (3.9%)[a]	10/56 (1.8%)
UFH starting at/before 6 wk and throughout 1st trimester, then vitamin K antagonists with/without UFH near term	21/229 (9.2%)[b]	7/167 (4.2%)
UFH throughout	7/21 (33.3%)	3/20 (15.0%)
• Adjusted dose	• 4/16 (25.0%)	• 1/15 (6.7%)
• Low dose	• 3/5 (60.0%)	• 2/5 (40.0%)

[a]8 cases occurred on UFH.
[b]All 21 cases occurred on UFH.
Abbreviation: UFH, unfractioned heparin.
Source: From Ref. 3.

and 12 weeks of gestation was associated with an increased risk of valve thrombosis. The risk of thromboembolic complications was highest when heparin was used throughout pregnancy and events occurred in women receiving intravenous or adjusted-dose subcutaneous heparin, as well as in those treated with low-dose heparin. Additional studies have been published subsequent to this analysis that also reported fewer thromboembolic events in women receiving warfarin than in those treated with heparin (10,138); however, other authors report conflicting findings (139). Although these data suggest that vitamin K antagonists are more efficacious than UFH for thromboembolic prophylaxis in pregnant women with mechanical heart valves, some events in women treated with UFH might be explained by inadequate dosing or use of an inappropriate target aPTT range. Therefore, if UFH is used, it should be initiated at doses at 17,500 to 20,000 units every 12 hours and adjusted to prolong the mid-interval aPTT into the therapeutic range. Careful monitoring is essential because UFH requirements fluctuate over time.

Treatment failures have also been reported with LMWH (140–144) and the safety of LMWH for this indication has been questioned in a warning from one manufacturer (145). This warning is based on postmarketing reports of valve thrombosis in an undisclosed number of patients receiving this LMWH, as well as by clinical outcomes in an open-label randomized study comparing LMWH (enoxaparin) with warfarin and UFH in pregnant women with prosthetic heart valves. The study was terminated after 12 of planned 110 patients were enrolled because of two deaths in the enoxaparin arm. On the basis of the small numbers in the trial and the inability to determine accurate incidence rates from postmarketing data, the true incidence of valve thrombosis in enoxaparin-treated pregnant women with mechanical valves is unknown. It also is uncertain whether thrombosis rates are higher in such women than in warfarin-treated nonpregnant patients. A comprehensive literature review of outcomes in pregnant women with mechanical heart valves treated with LMWH reported that valve thrombosis occurred in 7 of 81 pregnancies (8.64%; 95% CI, 2.52–14.76%) and the overall thromboembolic rate was 12.35% (10/81; 95% CI, 5.19%-19.51%) (146). However, 9 of the 10 patients with thromboembolic complications had received fixed dose LMWH (including 2 patients in whom a fixed low dose was utilized). Among 51 pregnancies in which anti-factor Xa LMWH levels were monitored and LMWH doses were adjusted according to these results, only one patient was reported to have suffered a thromboembolic complication. Thus, LMWH may provide adequate protection provided the drug is given twice daily, therapy is closely monitored, and the dose is adjusted to maintain a target anti-Xa levels of about 1.0 U/mL measured four hours after injection.

Given the above data, there is no single accepted treatment option for physicians managing pregnant women with mechanical heart valves. Several approaches remain acceptable: (*i*) vitamin K antagonists throughout pregnancy (despite medicolegal concerns) with LMWH or UFH substitution close to term, (*ii*) either LMWH or UFH between 6 and 12 weeks and close to term only and vitamin K antagonists at other times, (*iii*) aggressive adjusted-dose UFH throughout pregnancy, or (*iv*) aggressive adjusted-dose LMWH throughout pregnancy. The decision as to which regimen to use should be made after full discussion with the patient. Additional risk factors for thromboembolism such as valve type, position, and prior history of thromboembolism, as well as patient preference, should be taken into consideration. The option of vitamin K antagonist use throughout pregnancy until close to term might be a reasonable option in a very high-risk patient (e.g., first-generation mechanical valve in the mitral position, history of thromboembolism, or associated atrial fibrillation). Extrapolating from data in non-pregnant patients with mechanical valves receiving vitamin K antagonists (147); for the same high-risk women, the addition of aspirin, 75 to 100 mg/day can be considered in an attempt to reduce the risk of thrombosis, recognizing that it increases the risk of bleeding.

MANAGEMENT OF ANTICOAGULANTS AROUND THE TIME OF DELIVERY

In order to avoid an unwanted anticoagulant effect during delivery (especially with neuroaxial anesthesia) in women receiving adjusted-dose subcutaneous UFH (47) or LMWH, these agents should be discontinued 24 to 36 hours before elective induction of labor or cesarean section. If spontaneous labor occurs in fully anticoagulated women, neuroaxial anesthesia should not be employed. In women receiving subcutaneous UFH, careful monitoring of the aPTT is required and, if it is prolonged, protamine sulfate may be required to reduce the risk of bleeding. If available, anti-Xa LMWH levels should be checked in women treated with LMWH. If bleeding occurs, protamine sulfate may provide partial neutralization (148). Although recombinant activated factor VII has been used successfully to reduce LMWH-induced bleeding in the nonpregnant population (149), experience with this strategy is limited and there continue to be concerns about the thrombogenicity of this agent. Therefore, the use of recombinant activated factor VII should be reserved for cases where there is major bleeding unresponsive to conventional therapy (150).

In order to shorten the duration of time without therapeutic anticoagulation in women with a very high risk for recurrent VTE or with mechanical valves, therapeutic intravenous UFH can be substituted for LMWH or subcutaneous UFH and then discontinued four to six hours prior to the expected time of epidural insertion or delivery. Retrievable inferior vena caval filters that can be removed postpartum have been successfully used in women diagnosed with proximal DVT or PE shortly before delivery (151).

Postpartum, anticoagulants can be reintroduced as soon as adequate hemostasis is achieved after delivery, usually within 12 to 24 hours of delivery. Postpartum heparin and vitamin K antagonists can be started at the same time and heparin discontinued once a therapeutic INR is reached. There are no appropriately designed trials to guide the duration of postpartum anticoagulation for women diagnosed with VTE during pregnancy. In general, at least six months of anticoagulant therapy is suggested with treatment continued until at least six weeks postpartum.

SUMMARY

Evidence-based recommendations for the use of anticoagulant therapy in pregnancy have been published (67); however, given the paucity of available data, these guidelines are based largely upon extrapolations from data in nonpregnant patients, in addition to case reports and case series of pregnant patients. Consequently, the clinician is often left to make management decisions in the absence of sufficient information regarding the safety and efficacy of various therapeutic options.

Although LMWH, UFH, and danaparoid are safe for the fetus, it is clear that vitamin K antagonists are fetopathic. However, the true risks of warfarin embryopathy and CNS abnormalities remain unknown. There is still debate about the safety of aspirin during the first trimester and only limited data are available about the safety of newer anticoagulants, like fondaparinux and the direct thrombin inhibitors, during pregnancy. Although doubt has been raised about the effectiveness of UFH or LMWH for the prevention of systemic embolism in pregnant women with mechanical heart valves, observed failures could have been caused by inadequate dosing. Finally, the optimum management of pregnant women with thrombophilia, either asymptomatic or with prior pregnancy complications and/or prior VTE, is unknown. Accordingly, although clinical trials involving pregnant women are difficult to perform, the need for methodologically rigorous studies in this patient population cannot be overemphasized.

REFERENCES

1. Ginsberg JS, Hirsh J, Turner DC, et al. Risks to the fetus of anticoagulant therapy during pregnancy. Thromb Haemost 1989; 61(2):197–203.
2. Hall JAG, Paul RM, Wilson KM. Maternal and fetal sequelae of anticoagulation during pregnancy Am J Med 1980; 68(1):122–140.
3. Chan WS, Anand S, Ginsberg JS. Anticoagulation of pregnant women with mechanical heart valves: A systematic review of the literature. Arch Intern Med 2000; 160(2):191–196.
4. Shaul WL, Hall JG. Multiple congenital anomalies associated with oral anticoagulants. Am J Obstet Gynecol 1977; 12(2):191–198.
5. Ben Ismail M, Abid F, Trabelsi S, et al. Cardiac valve prostheses, anticoagulation and pregnancy.Br Heart J 1986, 55(1):101–105.
6. Sareli P, England MJ, Berk MR, et al. Maternal and fetal sequelae of anticoagulation during pregnancy in patients with mechanical heart valve prostheses.Am J Cardiol 1989; l63(20): 1462–1465.
7. Born D, Martinez EE, Almeida PA, et al. Pregnancy in patients with prosthetic heart valves. The effect of anticoagulation on mother, fetus, and neonate. Am Heart J 1992; 124(2): 413–417.
8. Pavankumar P, Venugopal P, Kaul U, et al. Pregnancy in patients with prosthetic cardiac valves. A 10 years experience. Scan J Thorac Cardiovasc Surg 1988; 22(1):19–22.
9. Larrea JL, Nunez L, Reque JA, et al. Pregnancy and mechanical valves prostheses: a high risk situation for the mother and the fetus. Ann Thorac Surg 1983; 36(4):459–463.
10. Al-Lawati AA, Venkitraman M, Al-Delaime T, et al. Pregnancy and mechanical heart valves replacement; dilemma of anticoagulation. Eur J Cardiothorac Surg 2002; 22(2):223–227.
11. Iturbe Alessio J, Fonseca MC, Mutchinik O, et al. Risks of anticoagulant therapy in pregnant women with artificial heart valves. N Engl J Med 1986; 315(22):1390–1393.
12. Schaefer C, Hannemann D, Meister R, et al. Vitamin K antagonists and pregnancy outcome. A multi-centre prospective study. Thromb Haemost 2006; 95(6):949–957.
13. Wesseling J, van Driel D, Heymans HS, et al. Coumarins during pregnancy: long term effects on growth and development in school age children. Thromb Haemost 2001; 85(4):609–613.
14. van Driel D, Wesseling J, Sauer PJ, et al. In utero exposure to coumarins and cognition at 8 to 14 years old. Pediatr 2001;107(1):123–129.
15. Hirsh J, Cade JF, O'Sullivan EF. Clinical experience with anticoagulant therapy during pregnancy. Br Med J 1970; 1:270–273.
16. Vitale N, De Feo M, De Santo LS, et al. Dose-dependent fetal complications of warfarin in pregnant women with mechanical heart valves. J Am Coll Cardiol 1999; 33(6):1637–1641.
17. Flessa HC, Kapstrom AB, Glueck HI, et al. Placental transport of heparin. Am J Obstet Gynecol 1965; 93(4):570–573.
18. Ginsberg JS, Kowalchuk G, Hirsh J, et al. Heparin therapy during pregnancy: Risks to the fetus and mother. Arch Intern Med 1989; 149(10):2233–2236.
19. Forestier F, Daffos F, Capella-Pavlovsky M. Low molecular weight heparin (PK 10169) does not cross the placenta during the second trimester of pregnancy: study by direct fetal blood sampling under ultrasound. Thromb Res 1984; 34(6):557–560.
20. Forestier F, Daffos F, Rainaut M, et al. Low molecular weight heparin (CY 216) does not cross the placenta during the third trimester of pregnancy. Thromb Haemost 1987; 57(2):234.

21. Lepercq J, Conard J, Borel-Derlon A et al. Venous thromboembolism during pregnancy: a retrospective study of enoxaparin safety in 624 pregnancies. Br J Obstet Gynaecol 2001; 108(11): 1134–1140.

22. Peeters LL, Hobbelen PM, Verkeste CM, et al. Placental transfer of Org 10172, a low-molecular-weight heparinoid in the awake late-pregnant guinea pig. Thromb Res 1986; 44(3):277–283.

23. Henny CP, ten Cate H, ten Cate JW, et al. Thrombosis prophylaxis in an AT III deficient pregnant woman: application of a low molecular-weight heparinoid.Thromb Haemost 1986; 55(2):301 (letter).

24. Greinacher A, Eckhardt T, Mussmann J, et al. Pregnancy-complicated by heparin associated thrombocytopenia: management by a prospectively in vitro selected heparinoid (Org 10172). Thromb Res 1993; 71(2):123–126.

25. Lindhoff-Last E, Kreutzenbeck H-J, Magnani HN. Treatment of 51 pregnancies with danaparoid because of heparin intolerance. Thromb Haemost 2005; 93(1):63–69.

26. Lindhoff-Last E, Bauersachs R. Heparin-induced thrombocytopenia – alternative anti-coagulation in pregnancy and lactation. Semin Thromb Hemost 2002; 28(5):439–445.

27. Markwardt F, Fink G, Kaiser B, et al. Pharmacological survey of recombinant hirudin. Pharmazie 1988; 43(3):202–207.

28. Mehta R, Golichowski A. Treatment of heparin induced thrombocytopenia and thrombosis during first trimester of pregnancy.J Thromb Haemost 2004; 2(9):1665–1666 (letter).

29. Furlan A, Vianello F, Clementi M, et al. Heparin-induced thrombocytopenia occurring in the first trimester of pregnancy: successful treatment with lepirudin. A case-report.Haematologica 2006; 91(suppl 8):19–20 (letter).

30. Lagrange F, Vergnes C, Brun JL, et al. Absence of placental transfer of pentasaccharide (fondaparinux, Arixtra) in the dually perfused human cotyledon in vitro. Thromb Haemost 2002; 87(5):831–835.

31. Dempfle CE. Minor transplacental passage of fondaparinux in vivo.N Engl J Med 2004; 350(18): 1914–1915 (letter).

32. Harenberg J. Treatment of a woman with lupus and thromboembolism and cutaneous intolerance of heparins using fondaparinux during pregnancy. Thromb Res 2007; 119(3):385–388.

33. Mazzolai L, Hohfeld P, Spertini F, et al. Fondaparinux is a safe alternative in case of heparin intolerance during pregnancy. Blood 2006; 108(5):1569–1570.

34. Pfeifer GW. Distribution studies and placental transfer of 131 I streptokinase. Australas Ann Med 1970; 19(suppl 1):17–18.

35. Leonhardt G, Gaul C, Nietsch HH, et al. Thrombolytic therapy in pregnancy. J Thromb Thrombolysis 2006; 21(3):271–276.

36. Ahearn GS, Hadjilaiadis D, Govert JA, et al. Massive pulmonary embolism during pregnancy treated with recombinant tissue plasminogen activator. A case report and review of treatment options. Arch Intern Med 2002; 162(11):1221–1226.

37. Coomarasamy A, Honest H, Papaioannou S, et al. Aspirin for prevention of preeclampsia in women with historical risk factors: a systematic review. Obstet Gynecol 2003; 101(6):1319–1332.

38. Kozer E, Nikfar S, Costei A, et al. Aspirin consumption during the first trimester of pregnancy and congenital anomalies: a meta-analysis. Am J Obstet Gynecol 2002; 187(6):1623–1630.

39. Berlin CM, Briggs GG. Drugs and chemicals in human milk. Semin Fetal Neonatal Med 2005; 10(2):149–159.

40. Clark SL, Porter TF, West FG. Coumarin derivatives and breast-feeding. Obstet Gynecol 2000; 95(6 part 1):938–940.

41. Orme ML, Lewis PJ, de Swiet M, et al. May mothers given warfarin breast-feed their infants? Br Med J 1977; 1:1564–1565.

42. McKenna R, Cole ER, Vasan V. Is warfarin sodium contraindicated in the lactating mother? J Pediatr 1983; 103(2):325–327.

43. O'Reilly R. Anticoagulant, antithrombotic and thrombolytic drugs. In: Gilman AG, Goodman LS, Gilman A, eds. The Pharmacologic Basis of Therapeutics, 6th ed. New York: Macmillan, 1980:1347.

44. Richter C, Sitzmann J, Lang P, et al. Excretion of low-molecular-weight heparin in human milk. Br J Clin Pharmacol 2001; 52(6):708–710.
45. Lindhoff-Last E, Willeke A, Thalhammer C, et al. Hirudin treatment in a breastfeeding woman.Lancet 2000; 355:467–468 (letter).
46. Hull R, Delmore T, Carter CJ, et al. Adjusted subcutaneous heparin versus warfarin sodium in the long-term treatment of venous thromboembolism. N Engl J Med 1982; 306(4):189–194.
47. Anderson DR, Ginsberg JS, Burrows R, et al. Subcutaneous heparin therapy during pregnancy: a need for concern at the time of delivery. Thromb Haemost 1991; 65(3):248–250.
48. Warkentin TE, Levine MN, Hirsh J, et al. Heparin induced thrombocytopenia in patients treated with low molecular weight heparin or unfractionated heparin. N Engl J Med 1994; 332(20): 1330–1335.
49. Burrow RF, Kelton JG. Incidentally detected thrombocytopenia in healthy mothers and their infants. N Engl J Med 1988; 319(3):142–145.
50. Douketis JD, Ginsberg JS, Burrows RF, et al. The effects of long-term heparin therapy during pregnancy on bone density. Thromb Haemost 1996; 75(2):254–257.
51. Dahlman TC. Osteoporotic fractures and the recurrence of thromboembolism during pregnancy and the puerperium in 184 women undergoing thromboprophylaxis with heparin. Am J Obstet Gynecol 1993; 168(4):1265–1270.
52. Ginsberg JS, Kowalchuk G, Hirsh J, et al. Heparin effect on bone density. Thromb Haemost 1990; 64(2):286–289.
53. Dahlman T, Lindvall N, Hellgren M. Osteopenia in pregnancy during long-term heparin treatment: a radiological study post-partum. Br J Obstet Gynecol 1990; 7(3):221–228.
54. Montreal M, Lafoz E, Olive A, et al. Comparison of subcutaneous unfractionated heparin with low molecular weight heparin (Fragmin) in patients with venous thromboembolism and contraindications to coumarin. Thromb Haemost 1994; 71(1):7–11.
55. Pettila V, Leinonen P, Markkola A, et al. Postpartum bone mineral density in women treated with thromboprophylaxis with unfractionated heparin or LMW heparin. Thromb Haemost 2002; 87(2):182–186.
56. Muir J, Andrew M, Hirsh J, et al. Histomorphometric analysis of the effect of standard heparin on trabecular bone in vivo. Blood 1996; 88(4):1314–1320.
57. Muir JM, Hirsh J, Weitz JI, et al. A histomorphometric comparison of the effects of heparin and low-molecular-weight heparin on cancellous bone in rats. Blood 1997; 89(9):3236–3242.
58. Shaughnessy SG, Hirsh J, Bhandari M, et al. A histomorphometric evaluation of heparin-induced bone loss after discontinuation of heparin-treatment in rats. Blood 1999; 93(4): 1231–1236.
59. Gould MK, Dembitzer AD, Doyle RL, et al. Low-molecular-weight heparins compared with unfractionated heparin for treatment of acute venous thrombosis: a meta-analysis of randomized, controlled trials. Ann Intern Med 1999; 130(10):800–809.
60. Quinlan DJ, McQuillan A, Eikelboom JW. Low-molecular-weight heparin compared with intravenous unfractionated heparin for treatment of pulmonary embolism. A meta-analysis of randomized controlled trials. Ann Intern Med 2004; 140(3):175–183.
61. Eikelboom JW, Quinlan DJ, Mehta SR, et al. Unfractionated heparin and low-molecular-weight heparin as adjuncts to thrombolysis in aspirin-treated patients with ST-elevation myocardial infarction: a meta-analysis of the randomized trials. Circulation 2005; 112(25): 3855–3867.
62. Eikelboom JW, Anand SS, Malmberg K, et al. Unfractionated heparin and low-molecular-weight heparin in acute coronary syndrome without ST elevation: a meta-analysis. Lancet 2000; 355:1936–1942.
63. Weitz JI. Low-molecular-weight heparin. N Engl J Med 1997; 337(10):688–698.
64. Sanson BJ, Lensing AWA, Prins MH, et al. Safety of low-molecular-weight heparin in pregnancy: a systematic review. Thromb Haemost 1999; 81(5):668–672.
65. Greer IA, Nelson-Piercy C. Low molecular weight heparins for thromboprophylaxis and treatment of venous thromboembolism in pregnancy: a systematic review of safety and efficacy. Blood 2005; 106(2):401–407.

66. Carlin AJ, Farquharson RG, Quenby SM, et al. Prospective observational study of bone mineral density during pregnancy: low molecular-weight heparin versus control. Hum Reprod 2004; 19(5):1211–1214.

67. Bates SM, Greer IA, Hirsh J, et al. Use of antithrombotic agents during pregnancy: the Seventh ACCP Conference on Antithrombotic and Thrombolytic Therapy. Chest 2004; 126 (suppl 3):627S–644S.

68. Confidential Enquiries into Maternal and Child Health. "Why Mothers Die: 2000-02". The Sixth Report of the UK Confidential Enquiries into Maternal Deaths. London: The Royal College of Obstetricians and Gynaecologists Press, 2004. Available at: www.cemach.org.uk.

69. Chang J, Elam-Evans LD, Berg CJ, et al. Pregnancy-related mortality surveillance: United States, 1991-1999. MMWR Surveill Summ 2003; 52(2):1–8.

70. Macklon NS, Greer IA. Venous thromboembolic disease in obstetrics and gynaecology: the Scottish experience. Scott Med J 1996; 41(3):83–86.

71. Gherman RB, Goodwin TM, et al. Incidence, clinical characteristics, and timing of objectively diagnosed venous thromboembolism during pregnancy. Obstet Gynecol 1999; 94(5 part 1): 730–734.

72. McColl MD, Ellison J, Greer IA, et al. Prevention of the post-thrombotic syndrome in young women with previous venous thromboembolism. Br J Haematol 2000; 108(2):272–274.

73. Lindqvist P, Dahlback B, Marsal K. Thrombotic risk during pregnancy: a population study. Obstet Gynecol 1999; 94(4):595–599.

74. Andersen BS, Steffensen FH, Sorensen HT, et al. The cumulative incidence of venous thromboembolism during pregnancy and puerperium: an 11 year Danish population-based study of 63,300 pregnancies. Acta Obstet Gynecol Scand 1998; 77(2):170–173.

75. Simpson EL, Lawrenson RA, Nightingale AL, et al. Venous thromboembolism in pregnancy and the puerperium: incidence and additional risk factors from a London perinatal database. BJOG 2001; 108(1):56–60.

76. Anderson FA Jr, Wheeler HB, Goldberg RJ, et al. A population-based perspective of the hospital incidence and case-fatality rates of deep vein thrombosis and pulmonary embolism. The Worcester DVT Study. Arch Intern Med 1991; 151(5):933–938.

77. Nordstrom M, Lindblad B, Bergqvist D, et al. A prospective study of the incidence of deep vein thrombosis within a defined urban population. J Intern Med 1992; 232(2):155–160.

78. Ray JG, Chan WS. Deep vein thrombosis during pregnancy and the puerperium: a meta-analysis of the period of risk and leg of presentation. Obstet Gynecol Surv 1999; 54(4): 254–271.

79. Barbour LA, Oja JL, Schultz LK. A prospective trial that demonstrates that dalteparin requirements increase in pregnancy to maintain therapeutic levels of anticoagulation. Am J Obstet Gynecol 2004; 191(3):1024–1029.

80. Jacobsen AF, Qvisgstad E, Sandset PM. Low molecular weight heparin (dalteparin) for treatment of venous thromboembolism in pregnancy. BJOG 2002; 110(2):139–144.

81. Crowther MA, Spitzer K, Julian J, et al. Pharmacokinetic profile of a low-molecular weight heparin (Reviparin) in pregnant patients: a prospective cohort study. Thromb Res 2000; 98(2): 133–138.

82. Rodie VA, Thomson AJ, Stewart FM, et al. Low molecular weight heparin for the treatment of venous thromboembolism in pregnancy: case series. Br J Obstet Gynaecol 2002; 109(9): 1020–1024.

83. Lee AY, Levine MN, Baker RI, et al. Low-molecular-weight heparin versus a coumarin for the prevention of recurrent venous thromboembolism in patients with cancer. N Engl J Med 2003; 349(2):146–153.

84. De Stefano V, Rossi E, Za T, et al. Prophylaxis and treatment of venous thromboembolism in individuals with inherited thrombophilia. Semin Thromb Hemost. 2006; 32(8):767–780.

85. Greer IA. Thrombosis in pregnancy: maternal and fetal issues. Lancet 1999; 353:1258–1265.

86. Robertson L, Wu O, Langhorne P, et al. for The Thrombosis Risk and Economic Assessment of Thrombophilia Screening (Treats) Study. Thrombophilia in pregnancy: a systematic review. Br J Haematol 2005; 132(2):171–196.

87. Dizon-Townson D, Miller C, Sibai B, et al. for the National Institute of Child Health and Human Development Maternal-Fetal Medicine Units Network. The relationship of the factor V Leiden mutation and pregnancy outcomes for mother and fetus. Obstet Gynecol 2005; 106(3): 517–524.

88. Middledorp S, Van der Meer J, Hamulyak K, et al. Counseling women with factor V Leiden homozygosity: use absolute instead of relative risks. Thromb Haemost 2001; 87(2):360–361.

89. Middledorp S, Libourel EJ, Hamulyak K, et al. The risk of pregnancy-related venous thromboembolism in women who are homozygous for factor V Leiden. Br J Haematol 2001; 113(2):553–555.

90. Martinelli I, Legnani C, Bucciarelli P, et al. Risk of pregnancy-related venous thrombosis in carriers of severe inherited thrombophilia. Thromb Haemost 2001; 86(3):800–803.

91. Pabinger I, Nemes L, Rintelen C, et al. Pregnancy-associated risk for venous thromboembolism and pregnancy outcome in women homozygous for factor V Leiden. Hematol J 2000; 1(1): 37–41.

92. Tormene D, Simioni P, Prandoni P, et al. Factor V Leiden mutation and the risk of venous thromboembolism in pregnant women. Haematologica 2001; 86(12):1305–1309.

93. Procare Group. Risk of venous thromboembolism during pregnancy in homozygous carriers of the factor V Leiden mutation: are there any predictive factors? J Thromb Haemost 2004; 2(2): 359–360.

94. Conard J, Horellou MH, Van Dreden P, et al. Thrombosis and pregnancy in congenital deficiencies in AT III, protein C or protein S: study of 78 women. Thromb Haemost 1990; 63(2): 319–320.

95. De Stefano V, Leone G, Mastrangelo S, et al. Thrombosis during pregnancy and surgery in patients with congenital deficiency of antithrombin III, protein C, protein S.Thromb Haemost 1994; 71(6):799–800 (letter).

96. Pabinger I, Schneider B for the Gessellscaft fur Thrombose-und Hamostaseforschung (GTH) Study Group on Natural Inhibitors. Thrombotic Risk in Hereditary Antithrombin III, Protein C, or Protein S Deficiency. Arterioscler Thromb Vasc Biol 1996; 16(6):742–748.

97. McColl M, Ramsay JE, Tait RC, et al. Risk factors for pregnancy associated venous thromboembolism. Thromb Haemost 1997; 78(4):1183–1188.

98. Zotz RB, Gerhardt A, Scharf RE. Prediction, prevention, and treatment of venous thromboembolic disease in pregnancy. Semin Thromb Hemostas. 2003; 29(2):143–154.

99. Long AA, Ginsberg JS, Brill-Edwards P, et al. The relationship of antiphospholipid antibodies to thromboembolic disease in systemic lupus erythematosus: A cross-sectional study. Thromb Haemost 1991; 66(5):520–524.

100. Pabinger I, Grafenhofer H, Kyrle PA, et al. Temporary increase in the risk for recurrence during pregnancy in women with a history of venous thromboembolism. Blood 2002; 100(3): 1060–1062.

101. Brill-Edwards P, Ginsberg JS, Gent M, et al. for the Recurrence Of Clot In This Pregnancy (ROCIT) Study Group. Safety of withholding antepartum heparin in women with a previous episode of venous thromboembolism. N Engl J Med 2000; 343(20):1439–1444.

102. Pabinger I, Grafenhofer H, Kaider A, et al. Risk of pregnancy-associated venous thromboembolism in women with a history of venous thrombosis. J Thromb Haemost 2005; 3(5):949–954.

103. De Stefano V, Martinelli I, Rossi E, et al. The risk of recurrent venous thromboembolism in pregnancy and puerperium without antithrombotic prophylaxis. Br J Haematol 2006; 135(3): 386–391.

104. Kovacs MJ, Keeney M. Inter-assay and instrument variability of anti-Xa results. Thromb Haemost 2000; 85(1):138.

105. Kitchen S, Iampietro R, Woolley AM, et al. Anti-Xa monitoring during treatment with low-molecular-weight heparin or danaparoid: inter-assay variability. Thromb Haemost 1999; 82(4): 1289–1293.

106. Ginsberg JS, Brill-Edwards P, Johnston M, et al. Relationship of antiphosopholipid antibodies to pregnancy loss in patients with systemic lupus erythematosis: a cross-sectional study. Blood 1992; 80(4):975–980.

107. Laskin CA, Bombardier C, Hannah ME, et al. Prednisone and aspirin in women with autoantibodies and unexplained recurrent fetal loss. N Engl J Med 1997; 337(3):148–153.

108. Rai RS, Clifford K, Cohen H, et al. High prospective fetal loss rate in untreated pregnancies of women with recurrent miscarriage and antiphospholipid antibodies. Hum Reprod 1995; 10(12): 3301–3304.

109. Empson M, Lassere M, Craig J, et al. Prevention of recurrent miscarriage for women with antiphospholipid antibody or lupus anticoagulant.Cochrane Database Syst Rev 2005; (2): CD002859.

110. Branch DW, Andres R, Digre KB, et al. The association of antiphospholipid antibodies with severe preeclampsia. Obstet Gynecol 1989; 73(4):541–545.

111. Yasuda M, Takakuwa K, Tokunaga A, et al. Prospective studies of the association between anticardiolipin antibody and outcome of pregnancy. Obstet Gynecol 1995; 86(4 part 1):555–559.

112. Polzin WJ, Kopelman JN, Robinson RD, et al. The association of antiphospholipid antibodies with pregnancies complicated by fetal growth restriction. Obstet Gynecol 1991; 78(6): 1108–1111.

113. Lockwood CJ, Romero R, Feinberg RF, et al. The prevalence and biologic significance of lupus anticoagulant and anticardiolipin antibodies in a general obstetric population. Am J Obstet Gynecol 1989; 161(2):369–373.

114. Lockshin MD, Druzin ML, Goei S, et al. Antibody to anticardiolipin as a predictor of fetal distress or death in pregnant women with systemic lupus erythematosus. N Engl J Med 1985; 313(3):152–156.

115. Reece EA, Gabrielli S, Cullen MT, et al. Recurrent adverse pregnancy outcome and antiphospholipid antibodies. Am J Obstet Gynecol 1990; 163(1 part 1):162–169.

116. Milliez J, Lelong F, Bayani N, et al. The prevalence of autoantibodies during third-trimester pregnancy complicated by hypertension or idiopathic fetal growth retardation. Am J Obstet Gynecol 1991; 165(1):51–56.

117. El-Roeiy A, Myers SA, Gleicher N. The relationship between autoantibodies and intrauterine growth retardation in hypertensive disorders of pregnancy. Am J Obstet Gynecol 1991; 164(5 pt 1): 1253–1261.

118. Allen JY, Tapia-Santiago C, Kutteh WH. Antiphospholipid antibodies in patients with preeclampsia. Am J Reprod Immunol 1996; 36(2):81–85.

119. von Tempelhoff G-F, Heilmann L, Spanuth E, et al. Incidence of the factor V Leiden mutation, coagulation inhibitor deficiencies and elevated antiphospholipid antibodies in patients with preeclampsia or HELLP syndrome (letter to the editors in chief). Thromb Res 2000; 100(4): 363–365.

120. Sletnes KE, Wisloff F, Moe N, et al. Antiphospholipid antibodies in pre-eclamptic women: relation to growth retardation and neonatal outcome. Acta Obstet Gynecol Scand 1992; 71(2): 112–117.

121. Lynch A, Marlar R, Murphy J, et al. Antiphospholipid antibodies in predicting adverse pregnancy outcome: a prospective study. Ann Intern Med 1994; 120(6):470–475.

122. Harris EN, Sinnato JA. Should anticardiolipin tests be performed in otherwise healthy pregnant women? Am J Obstet Gynecol 1991; 165(5 pt 1):1272–1277.

123. Branch DW, Porter TF, Rittenhouse L, et al for the National Institute of Child Health and Human Development Maternal-Fetal Medicine Units Network. Antiphospholipid antibodies in women at risk for preeclampsia. Am J Obstet Gynecol 2001; 184(5):825–835.

124. Out HJ, Bruinse HW, Christiaens GC, et al. A prospective, controlled multicentre study on the obstetric risks of pregnant women with antiphospholipid antibodies. Am J Obstet Gynecol 1992; 167(1):26–32.

125. Faux JA, Byron MA, Chapel HM. Clinical relevance of specific IgG antibodies to cardiolipin. Lancet 1989; 2:1457–1458.

126. Taylor PV, Skerrow SM, Redman CW. Pre-eclampsia and antiphospholipid antibody. Br J Obstet Gynecol 1991; 98(6):604–606.

127. Scott RA. Anti-cardiolipin antibodies and pre-eclampsia. Br J Obstet Gynaecol 1987; 94(6): 604–605.

128. Noble LS, Kutteh WH, Lashey N, et al. Antiphospholipid antibodies associated with recurrent pregnancy loss: prospective, multicenter, controlled pilot study comparing treatment with low-molecular-weight heparin versus unfractionated heparin. Fertil Steril 2005; 83(3): 684–690.

129. Stephenson MD, Ballem PJ, Tsang P, et al. Treatment of antiphospholipid antibody syndrome (APS) in pregnancy: a randomized pilot trial comparing low molecular weight heparin to unfractionated heparin. J Obstet Gynaecol Can 2004; 26(8):729–734.

130. Brenner B, Hoffman R, Blumenfeld Z, et al. Gestational outcome in thrombophilic women with recurrent pregnancy loss treated by enoxaparin. Thromb Haemost 2000; 83(5):693–697.

131. Carp H, Dolitzky M, Inbal A. Thromboprophylaxis improves the live birth rate in women with consecutive recurrent miscarriages and hereditary thrombophilia. J Thromb Haemost 2003; 1(3): 433–438.

132. Kupferminc MJ, Fait G, Many A, et al. Low-molecular-weight heparin for the prevention of obstetric complications in women with thrombophilias. Hypertens Pregnancy 2001; 20(1):35–44.

133. Brenner B, Bar J, Ellis M, et al. Effects of enoxaparin on late pregnancy complications and neonatal outcome in women with recurrent pregnancy loss and thrombophilia: results from the Live-Enox study. Fertil Steril 2005; 84(3):770–773.

134. Brenner B, Hoffman R, Carp H, et al. Efficacy and safety of two doses of enoxaparin in women with thrombophilia and recurrent pregnancy loss: the LIVE-ENOX study. J Thromb Haemost 2005; 3(4):227–229.

135. Walker ID, Kujovich JL, Greer IA, et al. The use of LMWH in pregnancies at risk: new evidence or perception? J Thromb Haemost 2005; 3(4):778–793.

136. Lindqvist PG, Merlo J. Low molecular weight heparin for repeated pregnancy loss: is it based on solid evidence? J Thromb Haemost 2005; 3(2):221–223.

137. Gris JC, Mercier E, Quere I, et al. Low-molecular-weight heparin versus low-dose aspirin in women with one fetal loss and a constitutional thrombophilic disorder. Blood 2004; 103(10): 3695–3699.

138. Geelani MA, Singh S, Verma A, et al. Anticoagulation in patients with mechanical valves during pregnancy. Asian Cardiovasc Thorac Ann 2005; 13(1):30–33.

139. Nassar AH, Hobeika EM, Abd Essamad HM, et al. Pregnancy outcome in women with prosthetic heart valves. Am J Obstet Gynecol 2004; 191(3):1009–1013.

140. Roberts N, Ross D, Flint SK, et al. Thromboembolism in pregnant women with mechanical prosthetic heart valves anticoagulated with low molecular weight heparin. Br J Obstet Gynaecol 2001; 108(3):327–329.

141. Leyh RG, Fischer S, Ruhparwar A, et al. Anticoagulation for prosthetic heart valves during pregnancy: is low-molecular-weight heparin an alternative. Eur J Cardiothorac Surg 2002; 21(3): 577–579.

142. Mahesh B, Evans S, Bryan AJ. Failure of low molecular weight heparin in the prevention of prosthetic mitral valve thrombosis during pregnancy: case report and review of options for anticoagulation. J Heart Valve Dis 2002; 11(5):745–750.

143. Lev-Ran O, Kramer A, Gurevitch J, et al. Low-molecular-weight heparin for prosthetic heart valves: treatment failure. Ann Thorac Surg 2000; 69(1):264–265.

144. Shapira Y, Sagie A, Battler A. Low-molecular-weight heparin for the treatment of patients with mechanical heart valves. Clin Cardiol 2002; 25(7):323–327.

145. Lovenox Injection (package insert). Bridgewater, NJ: Aventis Pharmaceuticals, 2004.

146. Oran B, Lee-Parritz A, Ansell J. Low molecular weight heparin for the prophylaxis of thromboembolism in women with prosthetic mechanical heart valves during pregnancy. Thromb Haemost 2004; 92(4):747–751.

147. Turpie AGG, Gent M, Laupacis A, et al. A comparison of aspirin with placebo in patients treated with warfarin after heart-valve replacement. N Engl J Med 1993; 329(8):524–529.

148. Massonnet-Castel S, Pelissier E, Bara L, et al. Partial reversal of low molecular-weight heparin (PK 101699) anti-Xa activity by protamine sulfate: in vitro and in vivo study during cardiac surgery with extracorporeal circulation. Haemostasis 1986; 16(2):139–146.

149. Firozvi K, Deveras RA, Kessler CM. Reversal of low-molecular-weight heparin-induced bleeding in patients with pre-existing hypercoagulable states with recombinant activated factor VII concentrate. Am J Hematol 2006; 81(8):582–589.
150. Franchini M, Lippi G, Franchi M. The use of recombinant activated factor VII in obstetric and gynecologic haemorrhage. BJOG 2007; 114(1):8–15.
151. Cheung MC, Asch MR, Gandhi S, et al. Temporary inferior vena caval filter use in pregnancy. J Thromb Haemost. 2005; 3(5):1096–1097.

13

Anticoagulants in Cancer

Edward N. Libby
Division of Hematology/Oncology, University of New Mexico Cancer Center,
Albuquerque, New Mexico, U.S.A.

Agnes Y. Lee
Department of Medicine, McMaster University and Hamilton Health Sciences,
Henderson Hospital, Hamilton, Ontario; and Department of Medicine, University of
British Columbia and Vancouver Coastal Health, Vancouver, British Columbia, Canada

INTRODUCTION

Venous thromboembolism (VTE) is an important cause of morbidity and mortality in cancer patients. Safe and efficacious prophylaxis and treatment of deep venous thrombosis (DVT) and pulmonary embolism (PE) are more difficult to achieve in cancer patients because of drug interactions, anemia, thrombocytopenia, frequent gastrointestinal disturbances, and other comorbid conditions. Consequently, the incidence of VTE in cancer patients is high, and complications of anticoagulant use are common. Furthermore, pharmacological agents currently available for prevention and treatment are troublesome to administer and have significant rates of breakthrough thrombosis and hemorrhage.

The most notable advance in thrombosis therapy in the past decade is the introduction of low-molecular-weight heparin (LMWH). Shown to be comparable to unfractionated heparin (UFH) for primary prevention and initial treatment of venous thromboembolism, LMWHs have also been shown to be tolerable, safe, and more effective than warfarin for the long-term, secondary prevention of recurrent VTE in cancer patients. More recently, a new class of anticoagulants, activated factor X (fXa) inhibitors, represented currently by the parenteral pentasaccharide fondaparinux, has been introduced, but has yet to be studied in a systematic fashion in oncology patients. A multitude of novel anticoagulants are also in development, ranging from direct oral thrombin (factor IIa) inhibitors to tissue factor (TF) pathway antagonists. On the basis of preliminary data, the mechanisms of action and safety profiles of these new agents hold promise for improved convenience and, possibly, better efficacy and safety in cancer patients.

In addition to their role in inhibition of coagulation, anticoagulants may have anticancer properties. Recently, laboratory studies and results from clinical trials have raised the possibility that LMWHs may retard tumor progression and improve patient survival. Further work is needed to elucidate the mechanisms by which LMWHs may exert their antitumor effects and to determine whether these translate into a benefit for cancer patients.

THROMBOSIS IN CANCER PATIENTS

Background

The association between cancer and thrombosis was recognized by Armand Trousseau in 1865 (1), when he noted that unexplained thrombosis may be a sign of underlying malignancy. This observation has been examined more carefully in recent years, using large population databases, registries, and small prospective studies. Several large trials have shown that approximately 10% of patients with apparent idiopathic DVT have an underlying malignancy (2). Hence there are ongoing debates regarding the need for cancer screening in patients with idiopathic DVT. In addition, the development of DVT has been shown to be a poor prognostic sign for cancer patients (3). Patients who have cancer and thrombosis are significantly more likely to die within a year after development of VTE (4). Although the majority of these patients are reported to die from advanced cancer, some die prematurely of fatal PE. Depending on tumor type, up to 40% of cancer patients have evidence of PE at autopsy (5,6).

Many factors can contribute to the development of thrombosis in oncology patients, and many of these are iatrogenic. For example, chemotherapeutic drugs, hormonal agents, and multiagent regimens significantly increase the risk of thrombosis. The increased incidence of thrombosis varies from a twofold higher risk for tamoxifen use to a 10-fold higher incidence of DVT reported with the combination of thalidomide and doxorubicin (7). Surgery, which plays an important role in the diagnosis and treatment of cancer, is also an important contributor to thrombosis. Common malignancies that often require extensive surgical procedures for diagnosis and treatment include colon, prostate, and non–small cell lung cancer. The debulking procedures that are often necessary in gynecologic malignancies (ovarian, cervical, and endometrial) are usually long and extensive and impart a very high risk for postoperative venous thromboembolism. Whether radiation therapy contributes to DVT is uncertain. Recently, growth factors, such as erythopoetin and darbepoetin, have been shown to increase the risk of DVT (8). This finding is worrying given the widespread and routine usage of these agents in the supportive care of cancer patients. Finally, thrombosis is also a well-known complication of the indwelling central venous catheters that are widely utilized to improve the delivery of chemotherapy and facilitate laboratory monitoring in cancer patients. The incidence of symptomatic catheter-related thrombosis is approximately 4% (9). At present, there is no clearly effective method for prevention of central venous catheter thrombosis (10).

Pathophysiology and Mechanisms

The list of potential mechanisms that contribute to development of venous thrombosis in oncology patients is extensive. Many distinct thrombophilic mechanisms are represented and the pathogenesis of thrombosis in an individual patient is multifactorial (11). Some of the best-described pathogenic mechanisms are discussed below.

Venous Stasis

Many solid cancers can grow to significant sizes within the chest, pelvis, or abdominal cavity. Compression of vessels by tumor masses or bulky adenopathy can cause stasis and abnormal blood flow and promote thrombus formation. Although the exact mechanisms have yet to be clarified, it is proposed that stasis leads to activation of coagulation via induction of hypoxia (12). Injury to the endothelial lining from vessel wall compression can also initiate the extrinsic pathway of coagulation through TF exposure.

Tissue Factor

TF is the physiological activator of coagulation in the normal state and is a critical procoagulant for thrombosis in malignancy. In the healthy state, TF is only expressed on the surface of stromal cells below the endothelial lining. In the event of vessel or endothelial injury, which can occur as a result of surgery or chemotherapy, TF in the subendothelial matrix is exposed and initiates clotting. In patients with malignancies, TF expression is often upregulated on tumor cells, monocytes, and endothelial cells (13). Thus, TF expression is significantly enhanced in a number of malignancies, including glioblastoma, pancreas, lung, and colon cancer. This upregulation may be partly responsible for the elevated levels of circulating TF-bearing microparticles in cancer patients, which, in turn, likely contribute to the systemic coagulopathy noted in a variety of tumor types. In addition to activating coagulation, the TF-activated factor VII (TF-fVIIa) complex is thought to enhance tumor growth via both *clotting-dependent* and *clotting-independent* mechanisms (14). Clotting-dependent augmentation of cancer occurs via TF-fVIIa activation of the coagulation cascade with subsequent thrombin generation, fibrin formation, and deposition of cellular matrix in the vicinity of tumor invasion. Furthermore, thrombin has a multitude of downstream signaling functions, including many that encourage tumor growth and metastasis. Clotting-independent enhancement of tumor growth is produced through activation of the cytoplasmic tail of TF, which causes activation of protease-activated receptors (PARS), leading to upregulation of vascular endothelial growth factor (VEGF) and activation of other pathways involved in angiogenesis, cell growth, and differentiation (Fig. 1).

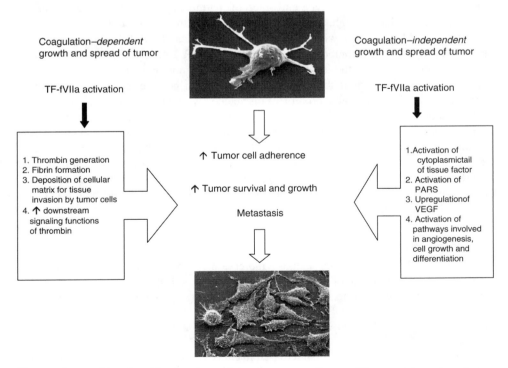

Figure 1 Possible effect(s) of anticoagulants on cancer. *Source*: Electron microscopy images courtesy of Getty Images, Inc, Seattle Washington, U.S.

Cancer Procoagulant

Cancer procoagulant is a cysteine protease expressed primarily on malignant cells. This enzyme, which directly activates factor X in the absence of fVII, represents an additional mechanism for activation of coagulation in cancer patients (15). There is also evidence that cancer procoagulant can induce dose-dependent platelet activation by a mechanism that appears to be similar to that of thrombin. The expression of cancer procoagulant in acute promyelocytic leukemia blasts parallels the degree of malignant transformation and response to all-trans retinoic acid (16). However, the specific protease has yet to be isolated and characterized.

Host Inflammatory Response

Host inflammatory response is an important component contributing to the hyper-coagulable state in cancer patients. Chemotherapy and radiation can produce cellular and tissue damage that induces an inflammatory response involving monocytes and other immune regulatory cells that further fuel the prothrombotic process (17). Tumor cells also release inflammatory cytokines and chemokines, such as tissue necrosis factor (TNF), interleukin-1 (IL-1), and VEGF, which act on leukocytes and endothelial cells to further enhance procoagulant activity (18). Release of potent inflammatory mediators such as TNF and IL-1 can elicit downstream responses that can promote thrombin generation.

Hereditary Thrombophilia

The contribution of inherited thrombophilia to thrombotic complications in cancer is incompletely studied (19). On the basis of the concept that individual thrombotic risk factors contribute in a stepwise fashion to the overall thrombotic risk, it is reasonable to surmise that for a given tumor type and stage of malignancy, patients with an inherited thrombophilia will have a higher risk for thrombosis than those without the defect (20). A large study of 3220 patients with DVT in the Netherlands showed that among patients with cancer, the risk of thrombosis is twofold higher (OR 2.2; 95% CI 0.3–17.8) among those who were carriers of the factor V Leiden or prothrombin gene mutation than cancer patients without these mutations (21). However, this increase was not statistically significant. Acquired activated protein C resistance (without the presence of factor V Leiden mutation) is frequently seen in cancer patients and may contribute to the prothrombotic state (22,23). Some authors have suggested that screening cancer patients for inherited thrombophilia is warranted to help assess the individual's risk for thrombosis and the need for prophylactic anticoagulation. This strategy has not been studied and should not be incorporated into routine practice until further information is available. Patients with known inherited thrombophilia who develop cancer should be individually considered for thromboprophylaxis.

Other Mechanisms

Less well-described mechanisms such as suppression of fibrinolysis (24,25), shedding of endothelial protein C receptor (26), and platelet-tumor cell aggregation (27) have also been reported to contribute to thrombosis risk in oncology patients.

Risk and Prognosis

In general, the risk of thrombosis is increased in cancer patients by four- to sevenfold over the general population. The exact risk in individual patients is dependent on a number of factors (Table 1) (28–38). Tumor histology and the stage are likely the strongest cancer-related determinants of the absolute risk of thrombosis. For example, it has been consistently shown in a number of population-based studies and registries that the solid tumors associated with the highest incidence of thrombosis are those of the pancreas, brain, stomach, kidneys, and ovary (Table 2) (39–44). The presence of metastasis further increases the risk by 20-fold as compared with early stage or limited disease (21). The risk of thrombosis is especially high (up to 53-fold increased) in the first few months after the cancer diagnosis.

The prognosis of cancer patients with thrombosis is far worse than that in patients without thrombotic complications. Only 12% of patients who receive a concurrent

Table 1 Determinants of the Risk of Thrombosis in Cancer Patients

Cancer-related
    Histology
    Stage or extent
    Time since cancer diagnosis

Noncancer-related factors
    Chemotherapy (e.g., asparaginase)
    Hormonal agents (e.g., tamoxifen)
    Antiangiogenic or imids agents (e.g., thalidomide)
    Growth factors (recombinant erythropoietin)
    Major surgery
    Long-term central venous catheterization
    Previous history of thrombosis
    Comorbid conditions (e.g., immobility, hereditary thrombophilia)

Abbreviation: imids, immunomodulatory.
Source: From Refs. 28–38.

Table 2 Incidence of VTE Among Some Solid Tumors

Tumor sites	VTE/100 pt-yr during 1st yr (39,44) (N = 235,149)	VTE/1000 pt during 1st 6 m (40) (N = 66,329)	VTE/10,000 pt-yr (41) (N = 1,211,944)	VTE/100 hospitalizations (42) (N = 40, 487,000)	VTE/100 neutropenic hosp pts (43) (N = 66,106)
Pancreas	20.0	22.7	110	4.3	12.10
Brain	11.1	32.1	117	3.5	9.50
Stomach	10.7	15.4	85	2.7	7.41
Bladder	7.9	12.9	22	1.0	6.60
Uterine	6.4	10.5	44	2.2	—
Kidney	6.0	12.6	84	2.0	7.55
Lung	5.0	13.8	61	2.1	7.00
Melanoma	4.4	2.7	—	—	—
Colon	4.3	13.4	76	1.9	6.75
Ovary	3.6	32.6	120	1.9	6.50
Breast	2.8	8.0	22	1.7	3.93
NHL	2.5	19.8	98	—	5.01
Prostate	0.9	9.5	55	2.0	7.29

Source: From Refs. 39–44.
Abbreviation: VTE, venous thromboembolism; NHL, non Hodgkin's lymphoma

diagnosis of cancer and thrombosis survive for more than one year, as compared with 36% of matched controls diagnosed with cancer but not with thrombosis (4). Among cancer patients, the inpatient mortality is also twofold higher when a venous thrombotic event occurs during hospitalization (43). Consequently, ensuring adequate provision of primary prophylaxis in hospitalized cancer patients could lead to a significant improvement in their survival (45,46).

ANTITHROMBOTIC AGENTS FOR PREVENTION AND TREATMENT OF THROMBOSIS

Acetylsalicylic Acid (Aspirin)

An irreversible inhibitor of cyclooxygenase-1, aspirin blocks thromboxane A_2 synthesis, which plays an important role in platelet aggregation. Hence, aspirin is effective for primary and secondary prevention of arterial thrombosis but is not considered an effective agent for prevention or treatment of venous thrombosis (28). Nonetheless, it is currently utilized for the prevention of arterial or venous thrombotic complications in patients with multiple myeloma and in patients with polycythemia vera.

The immunomodulatory (imids) drugs thalidomide and lenalidomide are two relatively new but highly effective therapies for multiple myeloma. These drugs are often combined with high doses of steroids to improve efficacy. Reported incidences of thrombosis for the combination of thalidomide and dexamethasone have ranged from 15% to 25%. These rates are approximately eightfold higher than expected (35). When the imids are combined with cytotoxic therapies, such as the anthracyclines, up to 58% of patients have developed thromboembolism (47,48). The high incidence of thrombotic complications observed in early studies of imid-cytotoxic drug combinations have led some investigators to recommend the routine use of aspirin for thromboprophylaxis. Several small, nonrandomized, uncontrolled trials have suggested that aspirin might be of benefit (49), but randomized trials evaluating the efficacy of aspirin for primary prevention of venous thrombosis in myeloma patients have not been performed (50). Such trials are critical because most patients with myeloma are elderly and have other comorbidities that confer a high risk of bleeding, even with low doses of aspirin (51).

Aspirin has also been recommended in patients with polycythemia vera. The risk of venous and arterial thrombosis is high in patients with this myeloproliferative disease. In a placebo-controlled trial, daily aspirin decreased the incidence of a composite outcome of arterial and venous thrombotic events, including deaths from cardiovascular causes (3.2% vs. 7.9%; $p = 0.03$) (52). However, the reduction in venous thromboembolic events was not significant (1.6% vs. 3.8%; $p = 0.28$).

Warfarin

Vitamin K antagonists, such as warfarin, have long been utilized as the long-term anticoagulant of choice in patients with thrombosis. These agents act as competitive antagonists of vitamin K by blocking enzymatic recycling of the reduced and oxidized forms of vitamin K. Vitamin K is essential for carboxylation of the procoagulant proteins factors II, VII, IX, and X. Such carboxylation is necessary for the effective participation of these clotting proteins in the assembly of the tenase and prothrombinase complexes. Vitamin K antagonists have a slow onset of action and a prolonged duration of the anticoagulant effect. This reflects the half-lives of clearance and production of the vitamin K–dependent coagulant factors (53).

Although vitamin K antagonists are highly effective in inhibiting thrombin generation, they are difficult to use because of their metabolism by the P450 system. As a result, the anticoagulant activity of these drugs is highly affected by vitamin K content in the diet, endogenous vitamin K production by bowel flora, and interactions with other drugs. Common genetic polymorphisms also produce wide-ranging dose responses. In addition, because vitamin K antagonists have a narrow therapeutic window, frequent monitoring of the international normalized ratio (INR) is required to ensure that a therapeutic anticoagulant effect is achieved. In cancer patients, these limitations are particularly problematic because nausea, vomiting, and cachexia are common but difficult to control, and the burden of frequent laboratory visits and dose modifications is high. There is also evidence that, despite a therapeutic INR, warfarin is less effective in preventing recurrent VTE in cancer patients than in patients without cancer (54).

Heparin

UFH accelerates inhibition of thrombin and factor Xa by antithrombin. In addition to binding to antithrombin, UFH also binds nonspecifically to plasma proteins, the levels of which vary between patients. This results in an unpredictable anticoagulant response. Consequently, UFH requires laboratory monitoring to ensure that a therapeutic anticoagulant effect has been achieved.

In the past decade, UFH has largely been replaced by LMWH. Nonetheless, UFH is still utilized for primary thromboprophylaxis and for treatment of acute VTE in patients with renal insufficiency or massive PE or in those at high risk for bleeding. A recent randomized controlled trial demonstrated that UFH can be given subcutaneously in an outpatient setting without laboratory monitoring (55). However, large volumes of drug and twice-daily injections are required.

Low-Molecular-Weight Heparins

LMWHs are fragments of UFH. Like UFH, LMWHs bind to antithrombin via a unique pentasaccharide sequence and accelerate the inactivation of thrombin and factor Xa. LMWHs exhibit less binding to plasma proteins than UFH and, subsequently, produce a more predictable anticoagulant response. Many studies have demonstrated that the efficacy and safety of LMWHs are comparable to those of UFH for primary prevention of thrombosis in the surgical setting, and placebo-controlled studies have shown a reduction in thrombotic complications in complex medical patients admitted to the hospital (56).

By allowing outpatient treatment and eliminating routine coagulation monitoring, LMWHs have simplified the treatment paradigm for all patients with thrombotic disease. There is also evidence that LMWHs are more efficacious and safer than UFH for initial treatment of VTE and that short-term administration is associated with an improvement in overall survival, particularly in patients with malignancy (57).

More recently, the CLOT trial showed that LMWH is more efficacious than warfarin therapy for long-term secondary prevention of recurrent VTE in patients with cancer (58). The CLOT trial randomized 772 cancer patients with acute VTE to receive long-term dalteparin (200U/kg subcutaneously once daily for the first month followed by approximately 150 IU/kg once daily for an additional 5 months) or dalteparin 200 IU/kg once daily for five to seven days followed by a vitamin K antagonist for six months (58). Superior results were seen with dalteparin, where 27/336 (8%) of patients had a recurrent VTE compared with 53/336 (15.8%) of patients in the control group, corresponding to a hazard ratio of 0.48 ($p = 0.002$) in favor of long-term dalteparin. Bleeding and mortality were similar in both groups.

Three other trials also studied the use of LMWH for extended secondary prophylaxis of VTE in cancer patients. The CANTHANOX trial randomized 146 cancer patients with VTE to treatment with either LMWH (enoxaparin 1.5 mg/kg/d) or warfarin (target INR 2–3) for months. Using a combined outcome of major bleeding and recurrent VTE, there were fewer major outcome events in the LMWH group; 7/71 (10.5%), as compared to the warfarin group 15/75 (21.1%), but the difference was not statistically significant (59). No difference was seen in cancer mortality between the two groups. The ONCENOX pilot study also studied enoxaparin for long-term use. This study enrolled 102 cancer patients with acute VTE for long-term treatment with enoxaparin (either 1.0 mg/kg/d or 1.5 mg/kg/d) or for routine care with a VKA (60). Treatment was continued for a total of 180 days. The primary outcome event was feasibility, while the secondary outcomes were safety (bleeding) and efficacy (VTE). The study was closed prematurely after only 122 patients were enrolled. Rates of recurrent VTE and hemorrhage were similar in all three groups. A substudy of the LITE trial (Long-term Innovations in TreatmEnt program) included 200 cancer patients randomized to either once daily tinzaparin or to conventional VKA therapy for long-term (3 months) secondary prevention of VTE. At 12 months, the routine care group had more than twice the rate of recurrent VTE [16/100 (16%) vs. 7/100 (7%) receiving tinzaparin]. However, this difference was not statistically significant at three months, when the study drugs were stopped (61).

Because of its size and design, the CLOT trial provides a benchmark, which documents that recurrent VTE in oncology patients is more effectively prevented with LMWH than with warfarin. Monotherapy with LMWH is now considered the first line treatment by national and international bodies, including the American Society of Clinical Oncology (62), the National Comprehensive Cancer Network (63), the 2004 American College of Chest Physicians Consensus Guidelines (64), and the British Society of Haematology (65).

Fondaparinux

Fondaparinux is a synthetic pentasaccharide that binds directly to antithrombin and catalyzes the inhibition of fXa. Unlike UFH and LMWHs, fondaparinux has no activity against thrombin. Fondaparinux is cleared entirely by the kidneys. Fondaparinux is administered by once daily subcutaneous injection and is given in a weight-based fashion. Coagulation monitoring is unnecessary. The major advantage of fondaparinux is its lower risk of heparin-induced thrombocytopenia. Fondaparinux has been studied for the prevention of VTE in medical, surgical, and orthopedic patients; treatment of DVT and PE; and for treatment of patients with acute coronary syndromes (66–70). Fondaparinux has yet to be studied in a systematic fashion in cancer patients.

CHALLENGES IN PROPHYLAXIS AND TREATMENT OF THROMBOSIS IN CANCER PATIENTS

Variability and Control of the Anticoagulant Effect

Cancer patients experience greater instability in anticoagulant control than noncancer patients. This likely contributes to higher rates of recurrent VTE and hemorrhage (71,72). The mechanisms contributing to unpredictable anticoagulant responses for warfarin include greater nonspecific binding of the heparins, drug-drug interactions, and vitamin K competition. Maintaining therapeutic anticoagulant levels is critical, but it is especially difficult in cancer patients because of their comorbid conditions and multiple concurrent medications. Warfarin dose reduction is usually required in patients with significant gastrointestinal effects from their chemotherapy and in those who are receiving broad-spectrum antibiotics. Conversely, dose escalation of warfarin is necessary in patients receiving enteral feeding or total parenteral nutrition, as many of these products contain high concentrations of vitamin K.

Recurrence of VTE on Anticoagulant Therapy

Rates of recurrent VTE are higher in cancer patients than they are in patients without a malignancy. Higher rates of recurrence are observed despite adequate anticoagulation with warfarin (54,72,73). In a study examining the outcomes of recurrent VTE and major bleeding, according to the INRs achieved in randomized controlled trials, the rate of recurrent VTE was 18.9 events per 100 pt-yrs in cancer patients, as compared with 7.2 events per 100 pt-yrs in those without cancer, during treatment periods with therapeutic INRs (54). In the CLOT study, cancer patients treated with a vitamin K antagonist had a recurrent VTE risk of 17% over six months, despite having INR levels above 2.0 for 70% of the total treatment time. The risk with dalteparin was 9% over the 6-month treatment period, despite maintaining 75% to 100% of the full therapeutic dose during that time (58).

To date, very little information is available on the treatment of recurrent VTE or cases of "anticoagulant failure." It has been recommended that patients who develop recurrent VTE on warfarin should be switched to LMWH at therapeutic doses. Higher doses of LMWH might be effective in patients who experience recurrent VTE while receiving weight-adjusted doses of LMWH.

Hemorrhagic Complications of Anticoagulants

Hemorrhagic complications of anticoagulation are clearly increased in cancer patients. A large Italian trial comparing cancer patients with controls reported annual rates of bleeding of 12.4% and 4.9%, respectively (72). Dutch investigators reported similar results of 13.1% and 2.1% in cancer and control patients, respectively (54). The higher bleeding rates are explained, at least in part, by the multiple risk factors for bleeding that exist in cancer patients, including the presence of friable, tumor tissue on mucosal surfaces, tumor invasion of vascular structures, the advanced age of most of the patients, the need for invasive procedures, and the prevalence of thrombocytopenia due to chemotherapy, radiation, or tumor invasion of bone marrow.

Thrombocytopenia

Thrombocytopenia is common and sometimes unpredictable in cancer patients. Causes of thrombocytopenia include myelosuppression due to chemotherapy and/or radiation, immune thrombocytopenic purpura, disseminated intravascular coagulation, and bone marrow invasion by tumor. Heparin-induced thrombocytopenia can also occur and it should be ruled out as the cause of a precipitous, unexpected drop in the platelet count in patients receiving UFH or LMWH.

The risk of bleeding from anticoagulants in cancer patients with thrombocytopenia has not been carefully studied. However, dose reduction or discontinuation of the anticoagulant should be considered when the platelet count is less than 50×10^9/L, and most clinicians stop anticoagulant therapy if the platelet count is less than 20×10^9/L. Alternatively, if the risk of thrombus extension or recurrence is deemed to be high, full dose anticoagulation may be continued if the platelet count can be maintained above

Table 3 New Anticoagulants

Xa inhibitors	Administration	Clearance	Stage of development
Apixaban	PO	Renal and GI	Phase III-VTE and AF
Betrixaban (PRT-054021)	PO	Hepatic	Phase II- VTE prevention
DU-176b	PO	unavailable	Phase II-orthopedic surgery
LY517717	PO	GI	Phase IIb- VTE completed
Otamixaban	IV	GI/hepatic	Phase II
Rivaroxaban[a]	PO	Hepatic 2/3, renal 1/3	Phase III- AF and VTE
YM150	PO	unavailable	Phase II-VTE and AF
YM-60828	PO	unavailable	Phase II-orthopedic surgery
Idraparinux	SQ	Renal	Phase III- VTE and AF
Biotinylated idraparinux	SQ	Renal	Phase III-VTE and AF
Thrombin inhibitors			
Dabigatran etexilate[a]	PO	Renal	Phase III-VTE and AF
FVIIa-Tissue factor inhibitors			
rNAPc2	SQ	Hepatic	Phase II

[a]Agent is now approved for use for prophylaxis in patients undergoing major joint replacement.
Abbreviations: PO, oral; SQ, subcutaneous; IV, intravenous; VTE, venous thromboembolism; GI, gastrointestinal; AF, atrial fibrillation.

$50 \times 10^9/L$ with platelet transfusions. Careful consideration should be given to the presence of a bleeding source and the overall goals of therapy in such patients.

NEW ANTICOAGULANTS

Several new anticoagulants are now in advanced stages of development. The majority of these agents are oral inhibitors of thrombin or factor Xa (Table 3). All can be given in fixed doses without routine laboratory monitoring, rendering them more convenient than warfarin. Although oncology patients may benefit from new anticoagulants with these properties, there are several issues of concern, including compliance, monitoring, reversal of the anticoagulant effect when needed, and safety in patients with impaired renal or hepatic function. None of the novel antithrombotic agents in development have been studied carefully in cancer patients. In fact, most cancer patients are excluded from clinical trials with these new anticoagulants. Given the potential for drug-drug interactions with chemotherapeutic agents that could result in altered dose responses and enhanced organ toxicity, it is prudent that such outcomes are examined carefully before new agents are accepted for general use in this highly vulnerable population.

EFFECT(S) OF ANTICOAGULANTS ON CANCER

For decades, anticoagulants have been reputed to have positive effects on the outcomes of cancer patients. Interestingly, improved overall survival has been described in patients with only a brief exposure to anticoagulant therapy (57,74). The mechanisms are not established and the clinical evidence is inconsistent. Nonetheless, given the critical interplays between TF, thrombin, vasculogenesis, and tumor growth, it is reasonable to propose that interference with coagulation activation, TF activity, or thrombin generation can impair the necessary or permissive pathways for tumor progression, and result in improved survival in patients with selected malignancies (14,75–78). Reduced fibrin formation by anticoagulants may also directly impair angiogenesis in the tumor environment that is necessary for tumor growth.

Potential Antitumor Effects

Biologic actions of anticoagulants on tumor biology have been examined in various in vitro or animal models. Most of the data appear to indicate that anticoagulants, particularly heparin and LMWH, inhibit metastasis as one of the key mechanisms. In rodents, administration of UFH or LMWH prior to intravenous injection of cancer cells results in a significant reduction in the number and size of metastatic pulmonary deposits (79,80). Potential mechanisms that have been reported include: (1) attenuation of the coagulation cascade, causing reduction in thrombin generation, (2) increased TF pathway inhibitor (TFPI) release, (3) inhibition of platelet and leukocyte adhesion to endothelial cells, (4) inhibition of adherence of tumor cells to vascular endothelium, and (5) heparanase binding and inhibition. Modified heparins, which possess little anticoagulant activity but are otherwise intact can inhibit tumor cell metastasis, suggesting that the antitumor effect of heparin is independent of the pentasaccharide sequence (27).

In numerous animal studies, TFPI has been shown to inhibit metastasis. The mechanism is uncertain but it has been suggested that TFPI acts through coagulation-dependent and coagulation-independent pathways to arrest tumor spread. Coagulation-*dependent* suppression of tumor spread takes place via direct inhibition of the TF/VIIa complex (81,82). This leads to attenuation of the coagulation cascade and less fibrin formation, thus reducing the cellular matrix that tumor cells can utilize for tissue invasion and growth and a decrease in the production of thrombin, which has major signaling roles in the enhancement of tumor growth and spread. Coagulation-*independent* arrest of tumor growth and metastasis occurs through arrest of TF intracellular downstream signaling pathways (83–85).

Clinical Evidence

Warfarin has been suggested to inhibit metastasis and to improve survival in cancer patients (86). A retrospective analysis of a study evaluating optimal duration of anticoagulation following an episode of unprovoked VTE showed that the incidence of new cancers was higher in patients who received a six-weeks course of warfarin, as compared to six months of therapy [OR 1.6; 95% CI 1.3–5.0 (74)]. A survival benefit for warfarin in cancer patients, however, has been inconsistently reported in prospective clinical trials (87).

Heparin was the first anticoagulant reported to have antitumor effects (88). Since that time, a number of clinical studies have provided conflicting data. The most promising results came from a trial in patients with small cell lung cancer (89), in which patients were randomized to chemoradiation or chemoradiation with adjusted doses of UFH to maintain the activated partial thromboplastin time between two and three times the control value. Statistically significant improvements in complete remission, median, and two-year overall survival were observed in the UFH group. Further studies have not been conducted to confirm these findings.

LMWH has also been reported to prolong overall survival of cancer patients in several trials but the effect was not detected in all studies. Improved survival was also reported in patients with small cell lung cancer in one trial (90), while another positive study included patients with a variety of advanced solid malignancies (91). Similar results were not observed in two other trials in patients with advanced cancers (92,93). Whether the discrepancy is due to heterogeneity of the patient populations, different dose and drug regimens used, or chance effect remains uncertain. The notable consistent findings among all of these studies are that patients with early stage or limited disease experienced greater benefit in survival when given an LMWH and that the survival benefit was observed following the discontinuation of the LMWH, indicating that a reduction in fatal PE is not the contributing mechanism.

IMPORTANT AREAS FOR FUTURE RESEARCH

Much work is needed to improve the safety, efficacy, and tolerability of anticoagulants for use in oncology patients. Major improvements in reducing drug and food interactions, minimizing or eliminating the need for monitoring, and the development of fast-acting oral drugs that can be utilized for rapid anticoagulation and long term for outpatient treatment would dramatically improve the lives of oncology patients. Better anticoagulants would be easier to incorporate into therapeutic plans for cancer patients and would likely improve compliance with primary prophylaxis.

The potential of treating cancer by inhibition of the coagulation cascade is tantalizing. Even if anticoagulants have only limited effects on cancer growth and metastasis, they could be combined with other agents to achieve a positive therapeutic benefit. To understand the effects of anticoagulants on cancer biology, future clinical trials should focus carefully on specific tumor settings rather than studying cancer as a single-disease entity. Carefully designed studies of cancer patients with similar histology, well-defined stages of disease, and standardized anticoagulant dosing regimens need to be performed. Whether all anticoagulants have similar effects on tumor progression remains uncertain. It is possible that drugs that target specific enzymes in the coagulation cascade may have less antitumor activity than nonspecific anticoagulants, such as LMWH.

Lastly, the oncology community and others who provide health care to patients with cancer need to be better educated regarding the negative impact that thrombosis has on the quality of life and life expectancy of these patients. Although developing new agents is exciting and potentially more beneficial in the long term, improving physician compliance with primary prophylaxis and proper treatment of established thrombosis could have a tremendous impact on the burden of disease and should be identified as research priorities.

REFERENCES

1. Varki A. Trousseau's syndrome: Multiple definitions and multiple mechanisms. Blood 2007; 110:1723–1729.
2. Sorensen HT, Mellemkjaer L, Steffensen FH, et al. The risk of a diagnosis of cancer after primary deep venous thrombosis or pulmonary embolism. N Engl J Med 1998; 338:1169–1173.
3. Mandala M, Reni M, Cascinu S, et al. Venous thromboembolism predicts poor prognosis in irresectable pancreatic cancer patients. Ann Oncol 2007; 18:1660–1665.
4. Sorensen HT, Mellemkjaer L, Olsen JH, et al. Prognosis of cancers associated with venous thromboembolism. N Engl J Med 2000; 343:1846–1850.
5. Ambrus JL, Ambrus CM, Pickern J, et al. Hematologic changes and thromboembolic complications in neoplastic disease and their relationship to metastasis. J Med 1975; 6:433–458.
6. Ogren M, Bergqvist D, Wahlander K, et al. Trousseau's syndrome—what is the evidence? A population-based autopsy study. Thromb Haemost 2006; 95:541–545.
7. Zangari M, Anaissie E, Barlogie B, et al. Increased risk of deep-vein thrombosis in patients with multiple myeloma receiving thalidomide and chemotherapy. Blood 2001; 98:1614–1615.
8. Rizzo JD, Somerfield MR, Hagerty KL, et al. Use of epoetin and darbepoetin in patients with cancer: 2007 American Society of Clinical Oncology/American Society of Hematology clinical practice guideline update. J Clin Oncol 2008; 26:132–149.

9. Verso M, Agnelli G. Venous thromboembolism associated with long-term use of central venous catheters in cancer patients. J Clin Oncol 2003; 21:3665–3675.
10. Akl EA, Karmath G, Yosuico V, et al. Anticoagulation for thrombosis prophylaxis in cancer patients with central venous catheters.Cochrane Database Syst Rev 2007:CD006468.
11. Franchini M, Montagnana M, Targher G, et al. Pathogenesis, clinical, and laboratory aspects of thrombosis in cancer. J Thromb Thrombolysis 2007; 24:29–38.
12. Lopez JA, Kearon C, Lee AY. Deep venous thrombosis.Hematol Am Soc Hematol Educ Program 2004:439–456.
13. Rauch U, Antoniak S, Boots M, et al. Association of tissue-factor upregulation in squamous-cell carcinoma of the lung with increased tissue factor in circulating blood. Lancet Oncol 2005; 6:254.
14. Rickles FR, Patierno S, Fernandez PM. Tissue factor, thrombin, and cancer. Chest 2003; 124:58S–68S.
15. Gordon SG, Mielicki WP. Cancer procoagulant: a factor x activator, tumor marker, and growth factor from malignant tissue. Blood Coagul Fibrinolysis 1997; 8:73–86.
16. Falanga A, Consonni R, Marchetti M, et al. Cancer procoagulant and tissue factor are differently modulated by all-trans-retinoic acid in acute promyelocytic leukemia cells. Blood 1998; 92:143–151.
17. Falanga A. Mechanisms of hypercoagulation in malignancy and during chemotherapy. Haemostasis 1998; 28(suppl 3):50–60.
18. Gale AJ, Gordon SG. Update on tumor cell procoagulant factors. Acta Haematol 2001; 106:25–32.
19. Decousus H, Moulin N, Quenet S, et al. Thrombophilia and risk of venous thrombosis in patients with cancer. Thromb Res 2007; 120(suppl 2):S51–S61.
20. Rosendaal FR. Venous thrombosis: a multicausal disease. Lancet 1999; 353:1167–1173.
21. Blom JW, Doggen CJ, Osanto S, et al. Malignancies, prothrombotic mutations, and the risk of venous thrombosis. JAMA 2005; 293:715–722.
22. Green D, Maliekel K, Sushko E, et al. Activated-Protein-C resistance in cancer patients. Haemostasis 1997; 27:112–118.
23. Elice F, Fink L, Tricot G, et al. Acquired resistance to activated protein c (aapcr) in multiple myeloma is a transitory abnormality associated with an increased risk of venous thromboembolism. Br J Haematol 2006; 134:399–405.
24. van Marion AM, Auwerda JJ, Minnema MC, et al. Hypofibrinolysis during induction treatment of multiple myeloma may increase the risk of venous thrombosis. Thromb Haemost 2005; 94:1341–1343.
25. Yagci M, Sucak GT, Haznedar R. Fibrinolytic activity in multiple myeloma. Am J Hematol 2003; 74:231–237.
26. Woodley-Cook J, Shin LY, Swystun L, et al. Effects of the chemotherapeutic agent doxorubicin on the protein c anticoagulant pathway. Mol Cancer Ther 2006; 5:3303–3311.
27. Borsig L, Wong R, Feramisco J, et al. Heparin and cancer revisited: mechanistic connections involving platelets, p-selectin, carcinoma mucins, and tumor metastasis. Proc Natl Acad Sci U S A 2001; 98:3352–3357.
28. Geerts WH, Pineo GF, Heit JA, et al. Prevention of venous thromboembolism: The Seventh ACCP Conference on Antithrombotic and Thrombolytic Therapy. Chest 2004; 126:338S–400S.
29. Leonardi MJ, McGory ML, Ko CY. A systematic review of deep venous thrombosis prophylaxis in cancer patients: implications for improving quality. Ann Surg Oncol 2007; 14:929–936.
30. Chan AT, Atiemo A, Diran LK, et al. Venous thromboembolism occurs frequently in patients undergoing brain tumor surgery despite prophylaxis. J Thromb Thrombolysis 1999; 8:139–142.
31. Grady D, Ettinger B, Moscarelli E, et al. Safety and adverse effects associated with raloxifene: multiple outcomes of raloxifene evaluation. Obstet Gynecol 2004; 104:837–844.
32. Shapiro AD, Clarke SL, Christian JM, et al. Thrombosis in children receiving l-asparaginase. Determining patients at risk. Am J Pediatr Hematol Oncol 1993; 15:400–405.
33. Payne JH, Vora AJ. Thrombosis and acute lymphoblastic leukaemia. Br J Haematol 2007; 138:430–445.
34. Vaitkus PT, Leizorovicz A, Cohen AT, et al. Mortality rates and risk factors for asymptomatic deep vein thrombosis in medical patients. Thromb Haemost 2005; 93:76–79.

35. El Accaoui RN, Shamseddeen WA, Taher AT. Thalidomide and thrombosis. A meta-analysis. Thromb Haemost 2007; 97:1031–1036.
36. Bennett CL, Angelotta C, Yarnold PR, et al. Thalidomide- and lenalidomide-associated thromboembolism among patients with cancer. JAMA 2006; 296:2558–2560.
37. Press MF, Lenz HJ. EGFR, HER2 and VEGF pathways: validated targets for cancer treatment. Drugs 2007; 67:2045–2075.
38. Shah MA, Ilson D, Kelsen DP. Thromboembolic events in gastric cancer: high incidence in patients receiving irinotecan- and bevacizumab-based therapy. J Clin Oncol 2005; 23:2574–2576.
39. Chew HK, Wun T, Harvey D, et al. Incidence of venous thromboembolism and its effect on survival among patients with common cancers. Arch Intern Med 2006; 166:458–464.
40. Blom JW, Vanderschoot JP, Oostindier MJ, et al. Incidence of venous thrombosis in a large cohort of 66,329 cancer patients: results of a record linkage study. J Thromb Haemost 2006; 4:529–535.
41. Levitan N, Dowlati A, Remick SC, et al. Rates of initial and recurrent thromboembolic disease among patients with malignancy versus those without malignancy. Risk analysis using medicare claims data. Medicine (Baltimore) 1999; 78:285–291.
42. Stein PD, Beemath A, Meyers FA, et al. Incidence of venous thromboembolism in patients hospitalized with cancer. Am J Med 2006; 119:60–68.
43. Khorana AA, Francis CW, Culakova E, et al. Thromboembolism in hospitalized neutropenic cancer patients. J Clin Oncol 2006; 24:484–490.
44. Semrad TJ, O'Donnell R, Wun T, et al. Epidemiology of venous thromboembolism in 9,489 patients with malignant glioma. J Neurosurg 2007; 106:601–608.
45. Cohen AT, Tapson VF, Bergmann JF, et al. Venous thromboembolism risk and prophylaxis in the acute hospital care setting (ENDORSE study): a multinational cross-sectional study. Lancet 2008; 371:387–394.
46. Kucher N, Koo S, Quiroz R, et al. Electronic alerts to prevent venous thromboembolism among hospitalized patients. N Engl J Med 2005; 352:969–977.
47. Oakervee H, Brownell A, Cervi P, et al. A study of the safety and efficacy of thalidomide combined with vincristine, adriamycin, and dexamethasone (T-VAD) in the treatment of younger patients with multiple myeloma: A UK Myeloma Forum study. Br J Haematol 2002; 117:65.
48. Baz R, Li L, Kottke-Marchant K, et al. The role of aspirin in the prevention of thrombotic complications of thalidomide and anthracycline-based chemotherapy for multiple myeloma. Mayo Clin Proc 2005; 80:1568–1574.
49. Niesvizky R, Martinez-Banos D, Jalbrzikowski J, et al. Prophylactic low-dose aspirin is effective antithrombotic therapy for combination treatments of thalidomide or lenalidomide in myeloma. Leuk Lymphoma 2007; 48:2330–2337.
50. Hirsh J. Risk of thrombosis with lenalidomide and its prevention with aspirin. Chest 2007; 131:275–277.
51. Palumbo A, Rajkumar SV, Dimopoulos MA, et al. Prevention of thalidomide- and lenalidomide-associated thrombosis in myeloma. Leukemia 2008; 22(2):414–423.
52. Landolfi R, Marchioli R, Kutti J, et al. Efficacy and safety of low-dose aspirin in polycythemia vera. N Engl J Med 2004; 350:114–124.
53. Ansell J, Hirsh J, Poller L, et al. The pharmacology and management of the vitamin K antagonists: The Seventh ACCP Conference on Antithrombotic and Thrombolytic Therapy. Chest 2004; 126:204S–233S.
54. Hutten BA, Prins MH, Gent M, et al. Incidence of recurrent thromboembolic and bleeding complications among patients with venous thromboembolism in relation to both malignancy and achieved international normalized ratio: a retrospective analysis. J Clin Oncol 2000; 18:3078–3083.
55. Kearon C, Ginsberg JS, Julian JA, et al. Comparison of fixed-dose weight-adjusted unfractionated heparin and low-molecular-weight heparin for acute treatment of venous thromboembolism. JAMA 2006; 296:935–942.

56. Francis CW. Clinical practice. Prophylaxis for thromboembolism in hospitalized medical patients. N Engl J Med 2007; 356:1438–1444.

57. van Dongen CJ, van den Belt AG, Prins MH, et al. Fixed dose subcutaneous low molecular weight heparins versus adjusted dose unfractionated heparin for venous thromboembolism. Cochrane Database Syst Rev 2004:CD001100.

58. Lee AY, Levine MN, Baker RI, et al. Low-molecular-weight heparin versus a coumarin for the prevention of recurrent venous thromboembolism in patients with cancer. N Engl J Med 2003; 349:146–153.

59. Meyer G, Marjanovic Z, Valcke J, et al. Comparison of low-molecular-weight heparin and warfarin for the secondary prevention of venous thromboembolism in patients with cancer: a randomized controlled study. Arch Intern Med 2002; 162:1729–1735.

60. Deitcher SR, Kessler CM, Merli G, et al. Secondary prevention of venous thromboembolic events in patients with active cancer: enoxaparin alone versus initial enoxaparin followed by warfarin for a 180-day period. Clin Appl Thromb Hemost 2006; 12:389–396.

61. Hull RD, Pineo GF, Brant RF, et al. Long-term low-molecular-weight heparin versus usual care in proximal-vein thrombosis patients with cancer. Am J Med 2006; 119:1062–1072.

62. Lyman GH, Khorana AA, Falanga A, et al. American Society of Clinical Oncology guideline: recommendations for venous thromboembolism prophylaxis and treatment in patients with cancer. J Clin Oncol 2007; 25:5490–5505.

63. http://www.nccn.org/professionals/physician_gls/PDF/vte.pdf (accessed April 2008).

64. Kearon C, Kahn SR, Agnelli G, et al. Antithrombotic therapy for venous thromboembolic disease: American College of Chest Physicians Evidence-Based Clinical Practice Guidelines (8th Edition). Chest 2008; 133(6 Suppl):454S–545S.

65. Baglin T, Barrowcliffe TW, Cohen A, et al. Guidelines on the use and monitoring of heparin. Br J Haematol 2006; 133:19–34.

66. Cohen AT, Davidson BL, Gallus AS, et al. Efficacy and safety of fondaparinux for the prevention of venous thromboembolism in older acute medical patients: randomised placebo controlled trial. BMJ 2006; 332:325–329.

67. Agnelli G, Bergqvist D, Cohen AT, et al. Randomized clinical trial of postoperative fondaparinux versus perioperative dalteparin for prevention of venous thromboembolism in high-risk abdominal surgery. Br J Surg 2005; 92:1212–1220.

68. Buller HR, Davidson BL, Decousus H, et al. Fondaparinux or enoxaparin for the initial treatment of symptomatic deep venous thrombosis: a randomized trial. Ann Intern Med 2004; 140:867–873.

69. Turpie AG, Bauer KA, Eriksson BI, et al. Fondaparinux vs. enoxaparin for the prevention of venous thromboembolism in major orthopedic surgery: a meta-analysis of 4 randomized double-blind studies. Arch Intern Med 2002; 162:1833–1840.

70. Yusuf S, Mehta SR, Chrolavicius S, et al. Comparison of fondaparinux and enoxaparin in acute coronary syndromes. N Engl J Med 2006; 354:1464–1476.

71. Palareti G, Legnani C, Lee A, et al. A comparison of the safety and efficacy of oral anticoagulation for the treatment of venous thromboembolic disease in patients with or without malignancy. Thromb Haemost 2000; 84:805–810.

72. Prandoni P, Lensing AW, Piccioli A, et al. Recurrent venous thromboembolism and bleeding complications during anticoagulant treatment in patients with cancer and venous thrombosis. Blood 2002; 100:3484–3488.

73. Gitter MJ, Jaeger TM, Petterson TM, et al. Bleeding and thromboembolism during anticoagulant therapy: a population-based study in Rochester, Minnesota. Mayo Clin Proc 1995; 70:725–733.

74. Schulman S, Lindmarker P. Incidence of cancer after prophylaxis with warfarin against recurrent venous thromboembolism. Duration of anticoagulation trial. N Engl J Med 2000; 342:1953–1958.

75. Ruf W. Tissue factor and par signaling in tumor progression. Thromb Res 2007; 120(suppl 2): S7–S12.

76. Ramachandran R, Hollenberg MD. Proteinases and signaling: pathophysiological and therapeutic implications via pars and more. Br J Pharmacol 2008; 153:S263–S282.

77. Nierodzik ML, Karpatkin S. Thrombin induces tumor growth, metastasis, and angiogenesis: evidence for a thrombin-regulated dormant tumor phenotype. Cancer Cell 2006; 10:355–362.
78. Wojtukiewicz MZ, Sierko E, Rak J. Contribution of the hemostatic system to angiogenesis in cancer. Semin Thromb Hemost 2004; 30:5–20.
79. Stevenson JL, Choi SH, Varki A. Differential metastasis inhibition by clinically relevant levels of heparins-correlation with selectin inhibition, not antithrombotic activity. Clin Cancer Res 2005; 11:7003–7011.
80. Hu L, Lee M, Campbell W, et al. Role of endogenous thrombin in tumor implantation, seeding, and spontaneous metastasis. Blood 2004; 104:2746–2751.
81. Amirkhosravi A, Meyer T, Amaya M, et al. The role of tissue factor pathway inhibitor in tumor growth and metastasis. Semin Thromb Hemost 2007; 33:643–652.
82. Niers TM, Klerk CP, DiNisio M, et al. Mechanisms of heparin induced anti-cancer activity in experimental cancer models. Crit Rev Oncol Hematol 2007; 61:195–207.
83. Versteeg HH, Schaffner F, Kerver M, et al. Inhibition of tissue factor signaling suppresses tumor growth. Blood 2008; 111:190–199.
84. Mackman N. Role of tissue factor in hemostasis, thrombosis, and vascular development. Arterioscler Thromb Vasc Biol 2004; 24:1015–1022.
85. Bromberg ME, Bailly MA, Konigsberg WH. Role of protease-activated receptor 1 in tumor metastasis promoted by tissue factor. Thromb Haemost 2001; 86:1210–1214.
86. Zacharski LR, Henderson WG, Rickles FR, et al. Effect of warfarin on survival in small cell carcinoma of the lung. Veterans administration study no. 75. JAMA 1981; 245:831–835.
87. Weitz IC, Liebman HA. The role of oral anticoagulants in tumor biology. Semin Thromb Hemost 2007; 33:695–698.
88. Goerner A. The influence of anticlotting agents on transplantation and growth of tumour tissue. J Lab Clin Med 1930; 16:369–372.
89. Lebeau B, Chastang C, Brechot JM, et al. Subcutaneous heparin treatment increases survival in small cell lung cancer. "Petites cellules" Group. Cancer 1994; 74:38–45.
90. Altinbas M, Coskun HS, Er O, et al. A randomized clinical trial of combination chemotherapy with and without low-molecular-weight heparin in small cell lung cancer. J Thromb Haemost 2004; 2:1266–1271.
91. Klerk CP, Smorenburg SM, Otten HM, et al. The effect of low molecular weight heparin on survival in patients with advanced malignancy. J Clin Oncol 2005; 23:2130–2135.
92. Kakkar AK, Levine MN, Kadziola Z, et al. Low molecular weight heparin, therapy with dalteparin, and survival in advanced cancer: The Fragmin Advanced Malignancy Outcome Study (FAMOUS). J Clin Oncol 2004; 22:1944–1948.
93. Sideras K, Schaefer PL, Okuno SH, et al. Low-molecular-weight heparin in patients with advanced cancer: a phase 3 clinical trial. Mayo Clin Proc 2006; 81:758–767.

14

Anticoagulation in Children

Paul T. Monagle
Department of Pediatrics, University of Melbourne, and Department of Hematology, Royal Children's Hospital, Melbourne, Victoria, Australia

Anthony K.C. Chan
Department of Pediatrics, McMaster University, Hamilton; Career Investigator Heart and Stroke Foundation of Canada, Coagulation Laboratory, The Hospital for Sick Children, Toronto, Ontario, Canada

INTRODUCTION

Thromboembolic disease in children and the use of anticoagulant drugs for its prevention and treatment have increased dramatically over recent years. There are many reasons for this increase. First, improved survival of children, who previously would have died of primary illness, has created a population at risk for thromboembolic disease. In addition, increased use of central venous, and arterial access, devices has dramatically increased the frequency of iatrogenic thromboembolic disease. Finally, improved imaging techniques have enabled more accurate diagnosis of thromboembolic diseases in specific circumstances.

With more occurrences of thromboembolic disease in children, there is a greater need for better drugs for its prevention and treatment. Experience with the use of anticoagulant drugs in the pediatric population is limited, with most of the focused research occurring within the last 10 to 15 years. This has coincided with the introduction of numerous new anticoagulants for use in adults. However, all anticoagulants must be considered as being relatively new in children. Drugs such as unfractionated heparin (UFH) and warfarin, which have undergone approximately 50 years of research and clinical experience in adults, remain unlicensed in all countries for pediatric use. Despite a wealth of information about adults, accurate pharmacokinetic analyses, validated therapeutic ranges, and proven risk-to-benefit profiles are not available about children. The lessons we are learning about the use of so-called established anticoagulant drugs in children must serve as a guide for the appropriate introduction of newer drugs for which data in adults remain limited.

There are important variables that render the use of anticoagulant drugs in pediatric patients different from that in adults. After highlighting these issues, this chapter will review our current knowledge about the use of individual anticoagulants in children.

Discussion of the current indications for anticoagulant therapy in children and management of specific thromboembolic conditions are beyond the scope of this chapter, and readers are referred to the most recent edition of the *American College of Chest Physicians Antithrombotic Guidelines* for this information.

VARIABLES THAT AFFECT THE USE OF ANTICOAGULANT DRUGS IN PEDIATRICS

Epidemiology of Thromboembolic Disease in Pediatric Patients

The epidemiology of thrombosis in pediatric patients has changed dramatically over recent years. Over the past 10 years, numerous national and international registries have published their findings on neonates and children (1–8). While some data are conflicting, there is agreement about the high proportion of secondary thrombosis in children with major underlying diseases, the overwhelming role of central venous access devices in the etiology of thrombosis, and the biphasic age dependence with neonates and adolescents being at highest risk for thrombosis. This last fact probably reflects, at least in part, the age distribution of major illnesses that necessitate insertion of central venous access devices, such as congenital heart disease and cancer, the influence of smaller caliber blood vessels in neonates, and the progressive maturation of the coagulation system in adolescents. The epidemiological differences between adult and pediatric patients with thromboembolism almost certainly influence the risk-to-benefit ratio of anticoagulation therapy.

Developmental Hemostasis

The hemostatic system is a dynamic evolving entity, which not only influences the frequency and natural history of thromboembolic disease in children but also the response to therapeutic agents (9–14). The concept of developmental hemostasis was first coined in the late 1980s and is now uniformly accepted. Not only are the plasma levels of many individual coagulation proteins different in pediatric patients than they are in adults, but the global functioning of the coagulation system also appears to be different. In addition to the well-documented quantitative differences, there is evidence, primarily from animal models, of qualitative differences in many coagulation proteins, especially in neonates (15,16). Data from animal studies also suggest that there are age-related differences in the antithrombotic properties of the blood vessel wall, reflecting altered concentrations of surface glycosaminoglycans (17). These differences not only impact on the risk of thrombosis but also may influence the response to certain anticoagulants. For example, plasma concentrations of antithrombin (AT) are physiologically low at birth (~0.50 U/mL) and do not increase to adult values until the age of three months. Sick, premature neonates frequently have plasma levels of AT of less than 0.30 U/mL. Fetal reference ranges indicate that AT levels range from 0.20 to 0.37 U/mL at gestational ages of 19 to 38 weeks. These low AT levels are likely to influence the response to heparin whose antithrombotic activity is dependent on catalysis of AT. AT inactivates a variety of coagulation enzymes, including thrombin. Even without heparin, thrombin generation in neonatal plasma is both delayed and decreased compared with adult plasma. In fact, endogenous thrombin generation in neonatal plasma resembles that in plasma from adults receiving therapeutic amounts of heparin (18). After infancy, the capacity for thrombin generation increases, but remains approximately 25% less than that in adult plasma throughout childhood (19). Both in vitro sensitivity and resistance to the anticoagulant effect of UFH have been reported in neonatal plasma. Increased sensitivity to UFH is observed when assays dependent on thrombin generation are used, such as the activated partial thromboplastin time (APTT). For example, a recent comparison of the in vitro effect of 0.25-U/mL UFH in plasma from neonates, children, or adults demonstrated delayed and reduced thrombin generation in plasma from children to relative plasma from adults. Thrombin generation was virtually absent in neonatal plasma (20). Resistance to UFH is observed when assays that measure the inhibition of exogenously added factor Xa or thrombin are used, because such assays are dependent on the plasma AT concentrations.

With low-molecular-weight heparin (LMWH) in vitro, thrombin generation is similar in plasma from adults and children. However, thrombin generation is delayed and reduced by approximately half in newborn plasma. These differences parallel reductions in the rates of prothrombin consumption (20).

The vitamin K-dependent coagulation factors have been extensively studied in infants. Physiologically low levels of factors (prothrombin) II, VII, IX, and X are found in infants who received vitamin K prophylaxis at birth. The levels of the vitamin K-dependent factors and the contact factors (factor XI, factor XII, prekallikrein, and high-molecular-weight kininogen) gradually increase to near adult values by six months of life. Thrombin generation in plasma from children receiving vitamin K antagonists is delayed and decreased by 25% compared with that in plasma from adults with a similar international normalized ratio (INR) (21).

Whether the overall activity of the protein C/protein S system varies with age is unknown. At birth, however, plasma concentrations of protein C are very low, and they remain low throughout the first six months of life. Although the total concentrations of protein S are decreased at birth, functional protein S activity is similar to that in adults, because all of the protein S at birth is in the free form, reflecting the absence of C4-binding protein (22,23). Furthermore, the interaction of protein S with activated protein C in newborn plasma may be influenced by the increased levels of α_2-macroglobulin. α_2-Macroglobulin has been shown to bind APC, hence reducing the capacity for protein S to form a complex with protein C, and thus reducing the inhibition of thrombin (24). Plasma concentrations of soluble thrombomodulin are increased in early childhood and decreased to adult values by late teenage years. However, the influence of age on endothelial cell thrombomodulin expression has not been determined (25).

Tissue factor pathway inhibitor (TFPI) levels in newborns are reported to be similar to those in older children or adults. However, the levels of free TFPI are significantly lower in newborns (9). The explanation for the age-related differences in free TFPI, not observed in total TFPI, are as yet not understood. One explanation could be differential binding, but further research is required to clarify this aspect (9).

Distribution, Binding, and Clearance of Antithrombotic Drugs

The distribution, binding, and clearance of antithrombotic drugs are age dependent. Although studies with UFH in newborns are limited, such studies indicate more rapid clearance in newborns compared with older children, reflecting the larger volume of distribution (26). The dose of UFH required to achieve a therapeutic APTT is higher in newborns than in older children (27). Pharmacokinetic studies in pigs show more rapid clearance of UFH in piglets than in adult pigs because of the larger volume of distribution (28). Heparin binding to endothelium and plasma proteins may also be different, although this has yet to be proven. These factors presumably contribute to the noted age-related differences in heparin dosing. Bolus doses of 75 to 100 U/kg result in therapeutic

APTT values in 90% of children. Maintenance heparin doses are age-dependent, with infants (up to 2 months corrected for gestational age) having the highest requirements (average 28 U/kg/hr) and children older than one year having lower requirements (average 22 U/kg/hr). The doses of heparin required for older children are similar to the weight-adjusted requirements in adults (18 U/kg/hr) (29).

The doses for LMWH are also age-dependent and exhibit far more patient-to-patient variability in neonates and children than in adults (30–33). Weight-adjusted doses required to achieve a target anti-factor Xa level in children may vary up to fourfold. In general, anti-factor Xa levels peak two to six hours after a subcutaneous LMWH injection. Infants aged two to three months or less than 5 kg require a higher per kg dose of LMWH, likely reflecting their larger volume of distribution. Alternative explanations for higher LMWH doses in young children include altered LMWH pharmacokinetics and/or reduced anticoagulant activity because of the low AT concentrations.

The published age-specific, weight-adjusted doses of warfarin for children vary, reflecting different study designs, patient populations, and possibly the small number of children studied. The largest cohort study ($n = 263$) reported that infants require an average of 0.33-mg/kg warfarin, whereas teenagers need 0.09-mg/kg warfarin to maintain a target INR of 2 to 3 (34). For adults, weight-adjusted doses are not precisely known, but are in the range of 0.04 to 0.08 mg/kg to achieve an INR in the 2 to 3 range. The mechanisms responsible for the age dependency of vitamin K antagonist dosing are not well understood.

Drug formulations

There are no specific pediatric formulations of anticoagulant drugs, making accurate, reproducible weight-adjusted dosing difficult. This is especially true for vitamin K antagonists where suspension or liquid preparations are lacking. Although the tablets can be dissolved in water for administration to newborns, there are no stability data, nor has this practice been critically evaluated. LMWH are conveniently provided in prefilled syringes. However, these syringes are geared to the adult population, and parents can have problems adjusting the doses for their infants or children.

Dietary Differences

Vitamin K antagonists are problematic in infants because breast milk and infant formulas contain different levels of vitamin K (35). Infant formula is supplemented with vitamin K to prevent hemorrhagic disease of the newborn. This renders formula-fed infants resistant to vitamin K antagonists. Such infants may require as much as 15 mg of warfarin per day to achieve a therapeutic INR. This dosing can increase the risk of bleeding should the infant have an intercurrent illness that transiently reduces formula intake. In contrast, breast milk contains little vitamin K. Consequently, breast-fed infants are sensitive to vitamin K antagonists. This can be overcome by giving them 30 to 60 mL of formula each day.

Other Patient-Related Differences

Diagnostic testing for thromboembolic disease in pediatric patients often requires general anesthesia to ensure that the patient remains still. Therefore, the threshold for testing tends to be higher in newborns and infants than it is in older children or adults. Vascular access also can be problematic in infants and children. Frequently, the choice of anticoagulant is influenced by the ease of administration. Often, vascular access devices are needed for drug delivery. These devices themselves increase the risk of thrombosis and complicate monitoring. With respect to warfarin, the frequency and types of intercurrent illnesses and concomitant medications vary with age. In particular, small infants have frequent viral infections, which often render warfarin management more difficult. Finally, compliance issues are vastly different in, for example, small infants who cannot understand the need for therapy, adolescents who intellectually comprehend but are unable to cooperate, and children in dysfunctional families who suffer the effects of inadequate parenting. The social, ethical, and legal implications of these issues cannot be underestimated and can interfere with the ability to provide the "best" individualized treatment.

Lack of Quality Evidence for Development of Treatment Guidelines

Recommendations for anticoagulant therapy in pediatrics have been extrapolated from adults because pediatric thromboembolic events were previously rare enough to hinder testing of specific therapeutic modalities, yet common enough to present significant management dilemmas that required therapeutic intervention.

The most widely used guidelines for anticoagulation therapy in neonates and children are those of the American College of Chest Physicians (ACCP) Consensus Conference (36–38). Since the first publication of pediatric guidelines in 1995, fewer than 10 multinational randomized controlled intervention trials assessing specific aspects of anticoagulant therapy in children have been initiated, and most of these have failed to enrol a sufficient number of patients to address the primary study question. This is in stark contrast to the large number of trials in adults. Most of the literature available to support the pediatric recommendations is in the form of uncontrolled studies, case reports, or in vitro experiments. Consequently, high-level recommendations cannot be made.

SPECIFIC ANTICOAGULANTS IN CHILDREN

Unfractionated Heparin

UFH remains one of the most commonly used anticoagulants in pediatric patients. In tertiary pediatric hospitals, approximately 15% of inpatients are exposed to UFH each day (39). Despite this fact, few general pediatricians have experience managing UFH in neonates and children. Thus, even though the use of UFH has increased, most children who require such therapy are treated in tertiary pediatric hospitals where they are managed by subspecialist teams.

The mechanism of action of UFH has been described.

Perhaps the most vexing issue related to UFH therapy in children is the question of the ideal therapeutic range. For adults, the recommended therapeutic range for treatment of venous thromboembolism is a UFH dose that results in an APTT that reflects a heparin level by protamine titration of 0.2 to 0.4 U/mL, or an anti-factor Xa level of 0.35 to 0.7 U/mL (40). The APTT therapeutic ranges are universally calculated using adult plasma. A number of studies suggest that extrapolating the APTT range from adults to pediatric patients is unlikely to be valid. For example, baseline APTT values in pediatric patients, especially neonates, are often higher than those in adults. Therefore, the therapeutic range represents a reduced relative increment in APTT values in pediatric patients than in adults (9). Recent in vitro and in vivo data suggest that the APTT range that correlates to an anti-factor Xa level of 0.35 to 0.70 U/mL varies significantly with age and may be significantly higher in children (41,42). Furthermore, there is considerable interpatient variability and correlation between the APTT, and anti-factor Xa levels is often poor. Not infrequently, children younger than one year receiving UFH have APTT values that are unrecordable in the clinical laboratory, yet their anti-factor Xa level is therapeutic. The lack of correlation between monitoring assays contributes to the uncertainty regarding therapeutic levels for UFH in children. While there are no published data to support the practice, many clinicians preferentially use anti-factor Xa assays to monitor UFH in children younger than one year or in those in the pediatric intensive care unit (PICU).

Anti-factor Xa assays also have problems. Different results can be obtained depending on the commercial kit used for the test. In a patient population that is relatively AT deficient compared with adults, kits that include exogenous AT likely introduce in vitro artifact. Alternatively, kits that contain dextran sulfate, which is known to displace UFH from plasma proteins, also may yield spurious results. The effect of these interfering substances appears to vary depending on the dose of UFH the patient is receiving, further confounding the interpretation of the results. This has implications not only for the use of anti-factor Xa assays to monitor UFH therapy but also for the determination of the therapeutic APTT ranges (43). However, as yet, there are no clinical outcome data to support changing clinical practice on the basis of variation in the anti-factor Xa assays. Likewise, there is no evidence to support one particular anti-factor Xa assay over another. With the information available, we still need to extrapolate from adult data. If one accepts that the therapeutic range in adults is appropriate for children, then one prospective cohort study used a weight-based normogram to identify the dose of UFH required to achieve therapeutic APTT values in pediatric patients (29). Bolus doses of 75 to 100 U/kg result in therapeutic APTT values in 90% of children four to six hours post bolus. Maintenance UFH doses are age-dependent, and infants (up to 2 months corrected for gestational age) have the highest requirements (average 28 U/kg/hr), while children older than one year have lower requirements (average 20 U/kg/hr). The doses of UFH required for older children are similar to the weight-adjusted requirements in adults (18 U/kg/hr) (44). There are little or no data to define optimal prophylactic doses of UFH. Clinicians commonly use a dose of 10 U/kg/hr administered as a continuous intravenous infusion (45).

Further studies examining dosing strategies in children are needed. In addition, specific data about the pharmacokinetics and pharmacodynamics of UFH in children of different ages are required (46,47). The reported adverse event profile for UFH in children is variable. One cohort study reported bleeding in 1.5% [95% confidence interval (CI), 0.0–8.3%] of children treated with UFH for deep-venous thrombosis (DVT)/pulmonary embolism (PE) (29). However, many children were treated with subtherapeutic doses of UFH (based on the target APTT) in this study (29). A more recent single center cohort study reported a major bleeding rate of 24% in children in the PICU receiving UFH therapy (48). Further studies are required to determine the true frequency of UFH-induced bleeding in optimally treated children.

As in adults, if anticoagulation with UFH needs to be discontinued for clinical reasons, termination of the UFH infusion will usually suffice because of the rapid clearance of UFH. If an immediate effect is required, protamine sulfate rapidly neutralizes UFH activity. The required dose of protamine sulfate is based on the amount of UFH received in the previous two hours. Protamine sulfate can be administered in a concentration of 10 mg/mL at a rate not to exceed 5 mg/min. Patients with known hypersensitivity reactions to fish and those who have received protamine-containing insulin or previous protamine therapy may be at risk for hypersensitivity reactions to protamine sulfate.

There are only three reported cases of UFH-induced osteoporosis in children. In two of these, the patient received concurrent steroid therapy (49–51). The third received high-dose intravenous UFH therapy for a prolonged period (52). However, given the convincing relationship between UFH and osteoporosis in adults, clinicians should avoid long-term use of UFH in children when alternative anticoagulants are available.

A number of case reports of pediatric heparin-induced thrombocytopenia (HIT) have described patients ranging in age from 3 months to 15 years (53–57). UFH exposure in these cases ranged from low-dose exposure through heparin flushes used to maintain patency of venous access devices to high doses of UFH given during cardiopulmonary bypass or hemodialysis. Studies specifically examining the frequency of HIT in children have yielded variable results, likely related to differences in patient selection and the laboratory tests used for diagnosis of HIT (39,58–62). Reported rates vary from almost nonexistent in unselected heparinized children (39) up to 2.3% in children in the PICU (59). A high index of suspicion is required to diagnose HIT in children, because many patients in the PICU who are exposed to UFH have multiple potential reasons for thrombocytopenia and/or thrombosis. Danaparoid, hirudin, and argatroban are alternatives to UFH in children with HIT (53,54,56,63–66).

LMWH

Despite their unproven efficacy, LMWHs have rapidly become the anticoagulant of choice in pediatric patients, both for primary prophylaxis and for treatment. The majority of all clinical data with respect to LMWH use in pediatric patients is from studies that used enoxaparin (33,67–74). The potential advantages of LMWH for pediatric patients include minimal monitoring requirements, which is helpful for pediatric patients with poor venous access, absence of drug-drug or dietary interactions, and lower risk of HIT and osteoporosis compared with UFH. However, the anticoagulant response to weight-adjusted doses of LMWH appears to be less predictable in the pediatric population than it is in adults.

The mechanism of action of LMWH is described elsewhere (20,75).

As for UFH, the therapeutic range for LMWH is extrapolated from data in adults and is based on anti-factor Xa levels. Anti-factor Xa levels between 0.50 and 1.0 U/mL measured four to six hours after dosing are considered therapeutic. Therapeutic ranges for once-daily LMWH in children are not reported in detail. Target anti-factor Xa levels for prophylactic LMWH are again extrapolated from adult data, although the PROTEKT trial used a range of 0.1 to 0.3 U/mL (76).

In pediatric patients, the doses of LMWH required to achieve therapeutic anti-factor Xa levels have been reported for enoxaparin, reviparin, dalteparin, and tinzaparin (Table 1) (31,32,77). In general, peak anti-factor Xa levels are achieved two to six hours after dosing. Although the reported doses are those most likely to yield therapeutic anti-factor Xa levels, there is considerable patient variability, suggesting that monitoring of anti-factor Xa levels is necessary in children and neonates. Infants younger than two to three months or less than 5 kg require larger doses of LMWH reflecting their larger volume of distribution, altered heparin pharmacokinetics (30), and/or lower plasma concentration of AT.

More work is needed to better define the optimal doses of LMWH. For example, the initial study recommending an enoxaparin dose of 1.5 mg/kg twice daily for children younger than two months was based on results in nine children and ignored their gestational age. A subsequent review of clinical experience with enoxaparin suggests that higher doses are needed. From 1996 to 2007, primary data have been published on 240 neonates receiving enoxaparin (78). The mean maintenance dose of enoxaparin ranged from 1.48 to 2.27 mg/kg twice daily, but doses of 1.9 to 2.27 mg/kg were needed for

Table 1 Recommended Starting Subcutaneous Doses of LMWH Required to Achieve Therapeutic Range in Children

Age of patient	<2 mo or 5 kg	2–12 mo	1–5 yr	5–10 yr	10 yr plus
Enoxaparin	1.75 mg/kg/dose q 12 hr	1.0 mg/kg/dose q 12 hr			
Tinzaparine	275 U/kg/dose q 24 hr	250 U/kg/dose q 24 hr	240 U/kg/dose q 24 hr	200 U/kg/dose q 24 hr	175 U/kg/dose q 24 hr
Dalteparin	129+/−43 U/kg/ dose q 24 hr				
Reviparin[a]	150 U/kg/dose q 12 hr	100 U/kg/dose q 12 hr			

[a]Doses for reviparin were studied according to weight range, i.e., <5 kg or >5 kg, as distinct from age.
Abbreviation: LMWH, low-molecular-weight heparin.

preterm neonates. These findings suggest that enoxaparin should be started at a dose of 1.75 mg/kg twice daily in term neonates and 2.0 mg/kg twice daily in preterm neonates, provided that the bleeding risk is low. However, further prospective studies are needed to validate this approach.

Intravenous enoxaparin has been used in one neonate; an eight-hourly dose of 1 mg/kg achieved therapeutic levels (67). In a nonrandomized prospective cohort study, a once-daily enoxaparin dose of 1.5 mg/kg was reported to be as effective as a twice-daily dose of 1 mg/kg in children with DVT after an initial 7 to 14 days of twice-daily treatment (69). However, the study was small, and the results cannot be considered definitive.

The recommended prophylactic doses of enoxaparin, reviparin, and dalteparin are listed in Table 2, but these doses have not been prospectively validated (31,32,77).

The risk of major bleeding in neonates is uncertain, but some information can be gleaned from studies that included neonates as part of larger patient populations. One pilot study reported no bleeding in seven infants younger than two months (0%, 95% CI, 0–47%) (30). In a larger series, 4 of 37 infants had major bleeding (10.8%, 95% CI, 3–25.4%) (33). Bleeding occurred locally (at the site of subcutaneous catheters in 2 newborns with little subcutaneous tissue) and into preexisting abnormalities in the central nervous system in two more newborns. On the basis of this limited information, subcutaneous catheters should likely be used with caution in newborns with little subcutaneous tissue. In a single institution cohort study of 146 courses of therapeutic enoxaparin given to children, major bleeds occurred in 4.8% (95% CI, 2–9.6%) of patients (33). In a randomized trial ($n = 37$) of reviparin, major bleeding occurred in 8.1% of patients (95% CI, 1.7–21.9%) (76). A recent review, which summarized the experience with enoxaparin in 240 neonates, reported a major bleeding rate of 12 % (95% CI, 0–19%) (78).

Table 2 Recommended Subcutaneous Doses for Prophylactic LMWH in Children

Age of patient	<2 mo or 5 kg	2–12 mo	1–5 yr	5–10 yr	10 yr plus
Enoxaparin	0.75 mg/kg/dose q 12 hr	0.5 mg/kg/dose q 12 hr			
Dalteparin	92 +/−52 U/kg/dose q 24 hr				
Reviparin[a]	50 U/kg/dose q 12 hr	30 U/kg/dose q 12 hr			

[a]Doses for reviparin were studied according to weight range, i.e., <5 kg or >5 kg, as distinct from age.
Abbreviation: LMWH, low-molecular-weight heparin.

The risk of osteoporosis, HIT, or other hypersensitivity reactions to LMWH in children is unknown.

Concerns about the reversibility of LMWH remain an important factor in patient selection. Protamine sulfate neutralizes the anti-factor IIa activity of LMWH but incompletely neutralizes its anti-factor Xa activity (79). In animal models, however, LMWH-induced bleeding is attenuated with protamine sulfate (80–83). Protocols for protamine sulfate reversal of LMWH have been published (80).

Vitamin K Antagonists

Vitamin K antagonists act as anticoagulants by reducing the functional plasma concentration of the vitamin K-dependent coagulation factors (II, VII, IX, and X). Vitamin K antagonists are problematic in newborns for several reasons that have been discussed previously. These include reduced plasma levels of the vitamin K-dependent coagulation factors, dietary implications of breast versus formula feeding, lack of pediatric-specific preparations, and blood-monitoring difficulties (35,84,85). Finally, although there is substantial information on the use of vitamin K antagonists in children older than three months, there is essentially no efficacy or safety information specific to their use in neonates.

Current therapeutic ranges for children are directly extrapolated from recommendations for adults because no pediatric trials have been done. Thus, for most indications, the target INR is 2.5 (range 2.0–3.0), and the low-dose prophylactic target INR is 1.7 (range 1.5–1.9). These targets are used despite ex vivo evidence that thrombin generation is delayed and decreased by 25% in plasma from children receiving vitamin K antagonists compared with adult plasma with a similar INR (21). On the basis of the ex vivo data, the therapeutic INR for children should be lower than that for adults. This hypothesis is supported by the observation that plasma concentrations of a marker of endogenous thrombin generation, prothrombin fragment 1.2, is significantly lower in children compared with that in adults at similar INR values (21). Outcome studies are needed to test this hypothesis.

An initial dose of 0.2 mg/kg, with subsequent dose adjustments made according to an INR nomogram, was evaluated in a prospective cohort study with warfarin (86). The published age-specific weight-adjusted doses of warfarin for children vary, reflecting different study designs, patient populations, and possibly the small numbers of children studied. The largest cohort study ($n = 319$) found infants required mean warfarin doses of 0.33 mg/kg, whereas teenagers needed 0.09 mg/kg to achieve an INR of 2 to 3 (87). For adults, weight-adjusted doses for vitamin K antagonists are not precisely known but are in the range of 0.04 to 0.08 mg/kg for an INR of 2 to 3 (88). The mechanisms responsible for the age dependency of vitamin K antagonist doses are not completely clear.

Warfarin therapy in children is problematic, and close supervision and frequent INR monitoring and dose adjustments are needed (86,87,89). Only 10% to 20% of children can be safely monitored on a once-monthly basis (86). Because venous access is often limited in children, point-of-care or capillary whole blood monitoring is gaining popularity. Whole blood INR monitors use various techniques to measure the time from application of fresh samples of capillary whole blood to clotting of the sample. The monitors include a batch-specific calibration code, which converts the result into an INR. Two point-of-care devices have been evaluated in the pediatric population: the CoaguChek S (Boehringer Mannheim, Germany) and the ProTime® Microcoagulation System (International Technidyne Corp., Edison, New Jersey, U.S.). Results with both monitors correlated well with INR values derived from venous blood samples analyzed in a coagulometer regardless of whether the monitors were used in an outpatient laboratory or in the home settings. Parents and patients received a formal education program prior to using the monitors. The major advantages identified by families included reduced trauma of venipuncture, minimal interruption of school and work, ease of operation, and portability (90–93). However, the cost per test with whole blood INR monitors is substantially higher. The recently released CoaguChek XS has yet to be validated in the pediatric population.

Bleeding is the main complication of vitamin K antagonist therapy. The risk of serious bleeding in children receiving vitamin K antagonists for mechanical prosthetic valves is less than 3.2% per patient year (13 case series) (36). In one large cohort study (391 warfarin years, variable target INR range), the bleeding rate was 0.5 % per patient year (87). In a randomized trial ($n = 41$, target INR range 2–3 for 3 months), bleeding occurred in 12.2% (95% CI, 4.1–26.2) of patients (78). A more recent single center study with a nurse-coordinated anticoagulant service reported a bleeding rate of 0.05% per patient year (94).

Treatment of vitamin K antagonist-induced bleeding is also based on experience in adults. If the INR is excessively prolonged (usually >8), and there is no significant bleeding, vitamin K can be given. Although data are limited, intravenous vitamin K in doses of 30 μg/kg have been used (95). If bleeding necessitates more rapid reversal, fresh-frozen plasma (FFP), prothrombin complex concentrates, or recombinant factor VIIa can be used.

Non-hemorrhagic complications of vitamin K antagonists, such as tracheal calcification or hair loss, have been described in young children, but are rare (96). Two cohort studies have described reduced bone density in children on warfarin for more than one year. However, these were uncontrolled studies, and the role of the underlying disorders in reducing bone density remains unclear (97,98).

Alternative Thrombin Inhibitors

A small number of case reports have documented the use of danaparoid, hirudin, or argatroban in pediatric patients (53,55,63,64,99), most commonly children with HIT. A protocol for danaparoid dosing in children is available (36).

A recent study reported in vitro comparisons of danaparoid, fondaparinux, and lepirudin in children and adults (100). Plasma samples from healthy children or adults were batched into age-specific pools. Varying concentrations of danaparoid, fondaparinux, or lepirudin were added to each age-specific pool, and anticoagulant response was measured. Danaparoid and fondaparinux, drugs with predominant anti-factor Xa activity, had similar effects in plasma from children as they did in adult plasma. In contrast, lepirudin, a thrombin inhibitor, had different effects on thrombin potential and APTT depending on the age of the patients from which the plasma was derived.

Lepirudin is usually monitored using the APTT, the activated clotting time (ACT), or ecarin clotting time (ECT). For both these tests, the study reported age-related differences in response for the same dose of the drug. Further, the impact on endogenous thrombin potential (ETP) was significantly increased in younger children for the same dose of lepirudin. This suggests that the response to lepirudin in children is different to that in adults and that the safety and effectiveness data from adults cannot be extrapolated to children. A previous study reported that increased doses of hirudin were required to achieve the same level of anticoagulation in cord plasma compared with adult plasma (101). However, cord plasma is known to be a different system to plasma from children.

In terms of fondaparinux, the results of the study indicated that in vitro there are no age-related differences in response to this drug. Similarly, as for danaparoid, this is probably related to the fact that this drug functions by inhibiting factor Xa and that the critical age-related factor appears to be thrombin (IIa).

CONCLUSIONS

Anticoagulation therapy in children remains in its infancy in terms of our understanding of the pharmacology of the various drugs in the setting of a dynamically evolving hemostatic system. Although we need to treat thromboembolic disease to reduce morbidity and mortality, even drugs such as UFH, LMWH, and warfarin, which are the mainstay of anticoagulant therapy in adults, are problematic in children. As studies with these drugs are done in children and infants, even the most basic premises on which these therapies are based are beginning to be questioned. Only through ongoing research will we gain a better understanding of anticoagulation therapy in children. Therapeutic ranges, drug-dosing strategies, and optimal-monitoring tests and protocols will likely need to be age-specific. In the interim, clinicians are left with no choice but to continue to extrapolate from adult practices as best they can, modifying therapy on the basis of first principles and experience.

REFERENCES

1. Nowak-Gottl U, Von Kries R, Gobel U. Neonatal symptomatic thromboembolism in Germany: two year survey. Arch Dis Child Fetal Neonatal Ed 1997; 76:F163–F167.
2. Schmidt B, Andrew M. Neonatal thrombosis: report of a prospective Canadian and international registry. Pediatrics 1995; 96:939–943.
3. Andrew M, David M, Adams M, et al. Venous thromboembolic complications (VTE) in children: first analyses of the Canadian registry of VTE. Blood 1994; 83:1251–1257.
4. Monagle P, Adams M, Mahoney M, et al. Outcome of pediatric thromboembolic disease: a report from the Canadian childhood thrombophilia registry. Pediatr Res 2000; 47:763–766.
5. Massicotte MP, Dix D, Monagle P, et al. Central venous catheter related thrombosis in children: analysis of the Canadian Registry of Venous Thromboembolic Complications. J Pediatr 1998; 133:770–776.
6. van Ommen C, Heijboer H, Buller HR, et al. Venous thromboembolism in childhood: a prospective two year registry in the Netherlands. J Pediatr 2001; 139:676–681.
7. Monagle P, Newall F, Barnes C, et al. Arterial thromboembolic disease: a single-centre case series study. J Paediatr Child Health 2007; 44:28–32.
8. Newall F, Wallace T, Crock C, et al. Venous thromboembolic disease: a single-centre case series study. J Paediatr Child Health 2006; 42:803–807.
9. Monagle P, Barnes C, Ignjatovic V, et al. Developmental haemostasis: impact for clinical haemostasis laboratories. Thromb Haemost 2006; 95:362–372.
10. Andrew M, Paes B, Milner R, et al. Development of the human coagulation system in the full-term infant. Blood 1987; 70:165–172.
11. Andrew M, Paes B, Johnston M. Development of the hemostatic system in the neonate and young infant. Am J Pediatr Hematol Oncol 1990; 12:95–104.
12. Andrew M, Paes B, Milner R, et al. Development of the human coagulation system in the healthy premature infant. Blood 1988; 72:1651–1657.
13. Reverdiau-Moalic P, Delahousse B, Body G, et al. Evolution of blood coagulation activators and inhibitors in the healthy human fetus. Blood 1996; 88:900–906.
14. Andrew M, Vegh P, Johnston M, et al. Maturation of the hemostatic system during childhood. Blood 1992; 80:1998–2005.
15. Greffe BS, Marlar RA, Manco-Johnson MJ. Neonatal protein C: molecular composition and distribution in normal term infants. Thromb Res 1989; 56:91–98.

16. Manco-Johnson MJ, Spedale S, Peters M, et al. Identification of a unique form of protein C in the ovine fetus: developmentally linked transition to the adult form. Pediatr Res 1995; 37:365–372.

17. Nitschmann E, Berry L, Bridge S, et al. Morphological and biochemical features affecting the antithrombotic properties of the aorta in adult rabbits and rabbit pups. Thromb Haemost 1998; 79:1034–1040.

18. Andrew M, Schmidt B, Mitchell L, et al. Thrombin generation in newborn plasma is critically dependent on the concentration of prothrombin. Thromb Haemost 1990; 63:27–30.

19. Andrew M, Mitchell L, Vegh P, et al. Thrombin regulation in children differs from adults in the absence and presence of heparin. Thromb Haemost 1994; 72:836–842.

20. Chan AK, Berry L, Monagle P, et al. Decreased concentrations of heparinoids are required to inhibit thrombin generation in plasma from newborns and children compared to plasma from adults due to reduced thrombin potential. Thromb Haemost 2002; 87:606–613.

21. Massicotte P, Leaker M, Marzinotto V, et al. Enhanced thrombin regulation during warfarin therapy in children compared to adults. Thromb Haemost 1998; 80:570–574.

22. Moalic P, Gruel Y, Body G, et al. Levels and plasma distribution of free and C4b-BP-bound protein S in human fetuses and full-term newborns. Thromb Res 1988; 49:471–480.

23. Schwarz HP, Muntean W, Watzke H, et al. Low total protein S antigen but high protein S activity due to decreased C4b-binding protein in neonates. Blood 1988; 71:562–565.

24. Cvirn G, Gallistl S, Koestenberger M, et al. α_2-macroglobulin enhances prothrombin activation and thrombin potential by inhibiting the anticoagulant protein C/protein S system in cord and adult plasma. Thromb Res 2002; 105:433–439.

25. Nako Y, Ohki Y, Harigaya A, et al. Plasma thrombomodulin level in very low birthweight infants at birth. Acta Paediatr 1997; 86:1105–1109.

26. Vieira A, Berry L, Ofosu F, et al. Heparin sensitivity and resistance in the neonate: an explanation. Thromb Res 1991; 63:85–98.

27. Andrew M, Schmidt B. The use of heparin in newborn infants. Semin Thromb Haemost 1988; 14:28–32.

28. Andrew M, Ofosu F, Schmidt B, et al. Heparin clearance and ex vivo recovery in newborn piglets and adult pigs. Thromb Res 1988; 52:517–527.

29. Andrew M, Marzinotto V, Massicotte P, et al. Heparin therapy in pediatric patients: a prospective cohort study. Pediatr Res 1994; 35:78–83.

30. Massicotte P, Adams M, Marzinotto V, et al. Low-molecular-weight heparin in pediatric patients with thrombotic disease: a dose finding study. J Pediatr 1996; 128:313–318.

31. Massicotte MP, Adams M, Leaker M, et al. A nomogram to establish therapeutic levels of the low molecular weight heparin (LMWH), clivarine in children requiring treatment for venous thromboembolism (VTE). Thromb Haemost 1997; 78:(suppl 282) (abstr).

32. Kuhle S, Massicotte MP, Andrew M, et al. A dose-finding study of tinzaparin in pediatric patients. Blood 2002; 100:279a (abstr).

33. Dix D, Andrew M, Marzinotto V, et al. The use of low molecular weight heparin in pediatric patients: a prospective cohort study. J Pediatr 2000; 136:439–445.

34. Streif W, Andrew M, Marzinotto V, et al. Analysis of warfarin therapy in pediatric patients: a prospective cohort study of 319 patients. Blood 1999; 94:3007–3014.

35. Haroon Y, Shearer MJ, Rahim S, et al. The content of phylloquinone (vitamin K1) in human milk, cows' milk and infant formula foods determined by high-performance liquid chromatography. J Nutr 1982; 112:1105–1117.

36. Michelson A, Bovill E, Andrew M. Antithrombotic therapy in children. Chest 1995; 108:506S–522S.

37. Monagle P, Michelson AD, Bovill E, et al. Antithrombotic therapy in children. Chest 2001; 119:344S–370S.

38. Monagle P, Michelson AD, Chan A, et al. Antithrombotic therapy in children: the seventh ACCP conference on antithrombotic and thrombolytic therapy. Chest 2004; 126:645S–687S.

39. Newall F, Barnes C, Ignjatovic V, et al. Heparin-induced thrombocytopenia in children. J Paediatr Child Health 2003; 39:289–292.

40. Hirsh J. Heparin. N Engl J Med 1991; 324:1565–1574.
41. Ignjatovic V, Furmedge J, Newall F, et al. Age-related differences in heparin response. Thromb Res 2006; 118:741–745.
42. Ignjatovic V, Summerhayes R, Than J, et al. Therapeutic range for unfractionated heparin therapy: age-related differences in response in children. J Thromb Haemost 2006; 4:2280–2282.
43. Ignjatovic V, Summerhayes R, Gan A, et al. Monitoring unfractionated heparin (UFH) therapy: which anti-factor Xa assay is appropriate? Thromb Res 2007; 120:347–351.
44. Raschke RA, Reilly BM, Guidry JR, et al. The weight-based heparin dosing nomogram compared with a "standard care" nomogram. A randomized controlled trial. Ann Intern Med 1993; 119:874–881.
45. Andrew M, de Veber G. Pediatric Thromboembolism and Stroke Protocols. 1st ed. Hamilton, Canada B.C.: Decker Inc., 1997:1–7.
46. McDonald MM, Jacobson LJ, Hay WW Jr., et al. Heparin clearance in the newborn. Pediatr Res 1981; 15:1015–1018.
47. Turner Gomes S, Nitschmann E, Benson L, et al. Heparin is cleared faster in children with congenital heart disease than adults. J Am Coll Cardiol 1993; 21:59a (abstr).
48. Kuhle S, Eulmesekian P, Kavanagh B, et al. A clinically significant incidence of bleeding in critically ill children receiving therapeutic doses of unfractionated heparin: a prospective cohort study. Haematologica 2007: 92:244–247.
49. Avioli LV. Heparin-induced osteopenia: an appraisal. Adv Exp Med Biol 1975; 52:375–387.
50. Schuster J, Meier-Ruge W, Egli F. [Pathology of osteopathy following heparin therapy]. Dtsch Med Wochenschr 1969; 94:2334–2338.
51. Murphy MS, John PR, Mayer AD, et al. Heparin therapy and bone fractures. Lancet 1992; 340:1098.
52. Sackler JP, Liu L. Heparin-induced osteoporosis. Br J Radiol 1973; 46:548–550.
53. Severin T, Sutor AH. Heparin-induced thrombocytopenia in pediatrics. Semin Thromb Hemost 2001; 27:293–299.
54. Potter C, Gill JC, Scott JP, et al. Heparin-induced thrombocytopenia in a child. J Pediatr 1992; 121:135–138.
55. Klement D, Rammos S, V Kries R, et al. Heparin as a cause of thrombus progression. Heparin-associated thrombocytopenia is an important differential diagnosis in paediatric patients even with normal platelet counts. Eur J Pediatr 1996; 155:11–14.
56. Murdoch IA, Beattie RM, Silver DM. Heparin-induced thrombocytopenia in children. Acta Paediatr 1993; 82:495–497.
57. Magnani HN. Heparin-induced thrombocytopenia (HIT): an overview of 230 patients treated with orgaran (Org 10172). Thromb Haemost 1993; 70:554–561.
58. Spadone D. Heparin induced thrombocytopenia in the newborn. J Vasc Surg 1996; 15:306–312.
59. Schmugge M, Risch L, Huber AR, et al. Heparin-induced thrombocytopenia-associated thrombosis in pediatric intensive care patients. Pediatrics 2002; 109:E10.
60. Boshkov L, Ibsen L, Kirby A, et al. Heparin-induced thrombocytopenia (HIT) in neonates and very young children undergoing congenital cardiac surgery: a likely under-recognized complication with significant morbidity and mortality: report of 4 sequential cases. J Thromb Haemost 2003; 1(suppl 1):1494a.
61. Etches W, Stang L, Conradi A. Incidence of heparin-induced thrombocytopenia in a pediatric intensive care population. Blood 2003; 102(suppl):536a.
62. Klenner AF, Fusch C, Rakow A, et al. Benefit and risk of heparin for maintaining peripheral venous catheters in neonates: a placebo-controlled trial. J Pediatr 2003; 143:741–745.
63. Saxon BR, Black MD, Edgell D, et al. Pediatric heparin-induced thrombocytopenia: management with Danaparoid (organan). Ann Thorac Surg 1999; 68:1076–1078.
64. Severin T, Zieger B, Sutor AH. Anticoagulation with recombinant hirudin and danaparoid sodium in pediatric patients. Semin Thromb Hemost 2002; 28:447–454.
65. Risch L, Fischer JE, Herklotz R, et al. Heparin-induced thrombocytopenia in paediatrics: clinical characteristics, therapy and outcomes. Intensive Care Med 2004; 30:1615–1624.

66. Klenner A. Heparin-induced thrombocytopenia in children. In: Warkentin T, Greinacher A, eds. Heparin-Induced Thrombocytopenia. 3rd ed. New York, NY: Marcel Dekker Inc., 2004:553–571.
67. Dunaway KK, Gal P, Ransom JL. Use of enoxaparin in a preterm infant. Ann Pharmacother 2000; 34:1410–1413.
68. Streif W, Goebel G, Chan AK, et al. Use of low molecular mass heparin (enoxaparin) in newborn infants: a prospective cohort study of 62 patients. Arch Dis Child Fetal Neonatal Ed 2003; 88:F365–F370.
69. Schobess R, During C, Bidlingmaier C, et al. Long-term safety and efficacy data on childhood venous thrombosis treated with a low molecular weight heparin: an open-label pilot study of once-daily versus twice-daily enoxaparin administration. Haematologica 2006; 91:1701–1704.
70. Burak CR, Bowen MD, Barron TF. The use of enoxaparin in children with acute, nonhemorrhagic ischemic stroke. Pediatr Neurol 2003; 29:295–298.
71. Elhasid R, Lanir N, Sharon R, et al. Prophylactic therapy with enoxaparin during L-asparaginase treatment in children with acute lymphoblastic leukemia. Blood Coagul Fibrinolysis 2001; 12:367–370.
72. Bontadelli J, Moeller A, Schmugge M, et al. Use of enoxaparin in the treatment of catheter-related arterial thrombosis in infants with congenital heart disease. Cardiol Young 2006; 16:27.
73. Dix D, Charpentier K, Sparling C, et al. Determination of trough anti-factor Xa levels in pediatric patients on low molecular weight heparin (LMWH). J Pediatr Hematol Oncol 1998; 20:398 (abstr 667).
74. Revel-Vilk S, Sharathkumar A, Massicotte P, et al. Natural history of arterial and venous thrombosis in children treated with low molecular weight heparin: a longitudinal study by ultrasound. J Thromb Haemost 2004; 2:42–46.
75. Hirsh J, Warkentin TE, Raschke R, et al. Heparin and low-molecular-weight heparin: mechanisms of action, pharmacokinetics, dosing considerations, monitoring, efficacy, and safety. Chest 1998; 114:489S–510S.
76. Massicotte P, Julian JA, Gent M, et al. An open-label randomized controlled trial of low molecular weight heparin for the prevention of central venous line-related thrombotic complications in children: the PROTEKT trial. Thromb Res 2003; 109:101–108.
77. Nohe N, Flemmer A, Rumler R, et al. The low molecular weight heparin dalteparin for prophylaxis and therapy of thrombosis in childhood: a report on 48 cases. Eur J Pediatr 1999; 158:S134–S139.
78. Malowany J, Monagle P, Knoppert D, et al. For the Canadian paediatric thrombosis and hemostasis network. Enoxaparin for neonatal thrombosis: a call for a higher dose for neonates. Thromb Res 2008; 122(6): 826–830.
79. Crowther MA, Berry LR, Monagle PT, et al. Mechanisms responsible for the failure of protamine to inactivate low-molecular-weight heparin. Br J Haematol 2002; 116:178–186.
80. Massonnet-Castel S, Pelissier E, Bara L, et al. Partial reversal of low molecular weight heparin (PK 10169) anti-Xa activity by protamine sulfate: in vitro and in vivo study during cardiac surgery with extracorporeal circulation. Haemostasis 1986; 16:139–146.
81. Harenberg J, Wurzner B, Zimmermann R, et al. Bioavailability and antagonization of the low molecular weight heparin CY 216 in man. Thromb Res 1986; 44:549–554.
82. Van Ryn-McKenna J, Cai L, Ofosu FA, et al. Neutralization of enoxaparine-induced bleeding by protamine sulfate. Thromb Haemost 1990; 63:271–274.
83. Thomas DP. Does low molecular weight heparin cause less bleeding? Thromb Haemost 1997; 78:1422–1425.
84. von Kries R, Shearer M, McCarthy PT, et al. Vitamin K1 content of maternal milk: influence of the stage of lactation, lipid composition, and vitamin K1 supplements given to the mother. Pediatr Res 1987; 22:513–517.
85. Bonduel MM. Oral anticoagulation therapy in children. Thromb Res 2006; 118:85–94.
86. Andrew M, Marzinotto V, Brooker LA, et al. Oral anticoagulation therapy in pediatric patients: a prospective study. Thromb Haemost 1994; 71:265–269.

87. Streif W, Andrew M, Marzinotto V, et al. Analysis of warfarin therapy in pediatric patients: A prospective cohort study of 319 patients. Blood 1999; 94:3007–3014.

88. Hirsh J, Dalen JE, Anderson DR, et al. Oral anticoagulants: mechanism of action, clinical effectiveness, and optimal therapeutic range. Chest 1998; 114:445S–469S.

89. Newall F, Savoia H, Campbell J, et al. Anticoagulation clinics for children achieve improved warfarin management. Thromb Res 2004; 114:5–9.

90. Massicotte P, Marzinotto V, Vegh P, et al. Home monitoring of warfarin therapy in children with a whole blood prothrombin time monitor. J Pediatr 1995; 127:389–394.

91. Nowatzke WL, Landt M, Smith C, et al. Whole blood international normalization ratio measurements in children using near-patient monitors. J Pediatr Hematol Oncol 2003; 25:33–37.

92. Marzinotto V, Monagle P, Chan A, et al. Capillary whole blood monitoring of oral anticoagulants in children in outpatient clinics and the home setting. Pediatr Cardiol 2000; 21:347–352.

93. Newall F, Monagle P, Johnston L. Home INR monitoring of oral anticoagulant therapy in children using the CoaguChek S point-of-care monitor and a robust education program. Thromb Res 2006; 118:587–593.

94. Newall F, Campbell J, Savoia H, et al. Incidence of major bleeding in a large paediatric cohort of patients requiring warfarin therapy. J Thromb Haemost 2005; 3:OR357 (abstr).

95. Bolton-Maggs P, Brook L. The use of vitamin K for reversal of over-warfarinization in children. Br J Haematol 2002; 118:924.

96. Taybi H, Capitanio MA. Tracheobronchial calcification: an observation in three children after mitral valve replacement and warfarin sodium therapy. Radiology 1990; 176:728–730.

97. Massicotte P, Julian J, Webber C, et al. Osteoporosis: a potential complication of long term warfarin therapy. Thromb Haemost 1999; (suppl):1333a (abstr).

98. Barnes C, Newall F, Ignjatovic V, et al. Reduced bone density in children on long-term warfarin. Pediatr Res 2005; 57:578–581.

99. Wilhelm MJ, Schmid C, Kececioglu D, et al. Cardiopulmonary bypass in patients with heparin-induced thrombocytopenia using Org 10172. Ann Thorac Surg 1996; 61:920–924.

100. Ignjatovic V, Summerhayes R, Yip YY, et al. The in vitro anticoagulant effects of Danaparoid, Fondaparinux, and Lepirudin in children compared to adults. Thromb Res 2008; 122(5): 709–714.

101. Baier K, Cvirn G, Fritsch P, et al. Higher concentrations of heparin and hirudin are required to inhibit thrombin generation in tissue factor-activated cord plasma than in adult plasma. Paediatr Res 2005; 57:685–689.

15

New Heparins: Synthetic Pentasaccharides

Pieter W. Kamphuisen and Harry R. Büller
*Department of Vascular Medicine, Academic Medical Center, Amsterdam,
The Netherlands*

INTRODUCTION

The efficacy of anticoagulant treatment for the prevention and treatment of thrombotic disorders has been well established. For decades, the anticoagulant compounds used most often for venous thromboembolism (VTE) were unfractionated heparin (UFH) and low-molecular-weight heparin (LMWH) for the initial treatment, and vitamin K antagonists (VKA) for long-term treatment (1). All these agents have disadvantages. In particular, VKA and UFH have unpredictable pharmacokinetics, and, as a consequence, they produced a highly variable anticoagulant response that necessitates frequent monitoring to prevent both under- or overdosing. In addition, heparins are derived from animal tissue and can cause heparin-induced thrombocytopenia (HIT). These features prompted the development of new synthetic, more selective, anticoagulant compounds. Currently, numerous new molecules are being evaluated for efficacy and safety in the treatment of thrombosis.

One of the most promising targets for new anticoagulant agents is activated factor X (factor Xa). Factor Xa is centrally located in the coagulation cascade, at the convergence point of the extrinsic and intrinsic pathways, and upstream to thrombin. Furthermore, because the concentration of serine protease is amplified at each step of the coagulation cascade, anticoagulants with targets higher up in the cascade, such as factor Xa, are attractive. Synthetic pentasaccharides that selectively block factor Xa are the first of a new class of anticoagulants and have been extensively evaluated for the prevention and treatment of thrombosis.

PHARMACOLOGY AND PHARMACOKINETICS OF PENTASACCHARIDES

Fondaparinux

Pentasaccharides contain structural features that allow tight binding to antithrombin. A methyl group stabilizes the anomeric end of the molecule and avoids nonspecific binding to plasma proteins (2). Figure 1 shows the molecular structure of fondaparinux (Arixtra®,

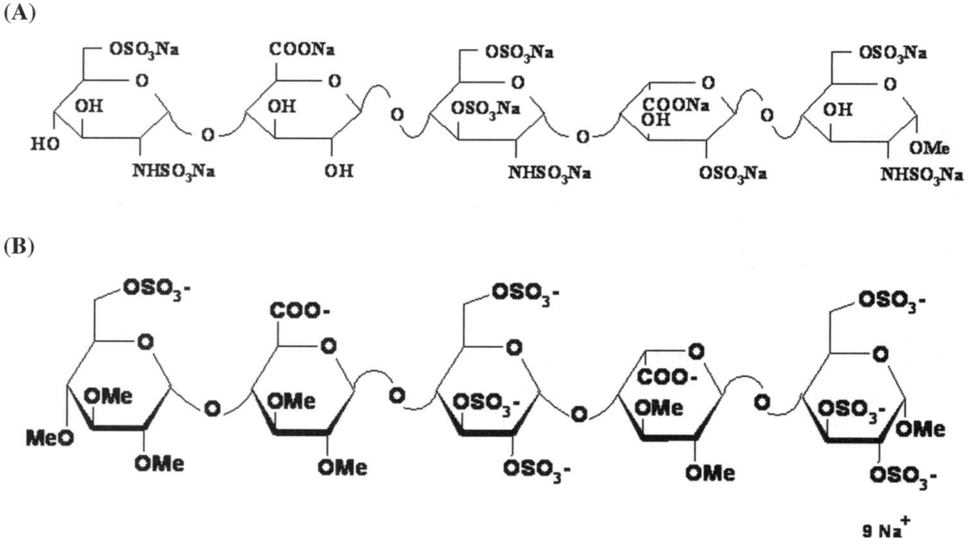

(A)

(B)

9 Na$^+$

Figure 1 (A) Structure of fondaparinux and (B) idraparinux.

GlaxoSmithKline, Brentford, Middlesex, U.K.; former Sanofi-Synthélabo, Paris, France), which is composed of three D-glucosamine units separated by one D-glucuronic acid unit and one L-iduronic acid unit. Fondaparinux bears several sulfonate groups in crucial positions. It directly binds to the heparin site of antithrombin with high affinity (dissociation constant Kd = 36 ± 11 nM) in a 1:1 stoichiometric fashion (3,4). This reversible binding induces a conformational change in the antithrombin molecule that results in a 300-fold increase in the rate of factor Xa inhibition by antithrombin. The mechanism is catalytic, because the binding of antithrombin to factor Xa releases the fondaparinux molecule, enabling the process to start again. Fondaparinux does not appear to inhibit platelet function.

The differences in pharmacokinetics between fondaparinux and UFH or LMWH are depicted in Table 1. The molecular weight of fondaparinux is lower (1728 Da) than those of LMWH (1000–10,000 Da) and UFH (3000–30,000 Da). After subcutaneous injection of fondapariunx in young healthy subjects, the peak plasma level (C_{max}) was achieved at two hours, and half this level ($C_{max}/2$) was obtained within 25 minutes, indicating a rapid onset of anticoagulant activity (5). The C_{max} for LMWH is three to four hours after subcutaneous injection. The elimination half-life of fondaparinux is 17 hours, much longer than that of subcutaneous LMWH or intravenous UFH. This renders fondaparinux suitable for once-daily injection. After injection of up to 20 mg intravenously, the peak plasma level and the area under the curve (AUC) were linearly related to the dose administered.

With repeated subcutaneous injection of increasing doses of fondaparinux (4 or 10 mg), steady-state plasma concentrations were reached after three to four days (5). Bioavailability after subcutaneous administration is 100%, and elimination is primarily via the kidneys. After fondaparinux injection, between 64% and 77% of the unchanged drug can be recovered in the urine (5). Fondaparinux does not undergo hepatic metabolism and does not interact with agents metabolized by the liver (6). Importantly, the pharmacokinetic profile of fondaparinux in the elderly is comparable to that in younger subjects (5). Finally, there was no interaction between fondaparinux and warfarin or aspirin when these agents were coadministered to healthy volunteers (7,8). Since the anticoagulant effect of fondaparinux

Table 1 Comparison of the Main Properties of Fondaparinux, Idraparinux, and Heparins

Property	UFH	LMWH	Fondaparinux	Idraparinux
Molecular weight (Da)	3000–30,000	1000–10,000	1728	1728
Source	Animal tissue	Animal tissue	Chemically synthesized	Chemically synthesized
Target	Factors IIa, IXa, Xa	Factors IIa, IXa, Xa	Factor Xa	Factor Xa
Route of administration	IV/SC	SC	SC	SC
Bioavailability	20–30%	85–95%	100%	100%
Half-life (hr)	1.30	4.0	17.0	80.0
Frequency of administration	Continuous IV or 2–3 times daily SC	Once to twice daily	Once daily	Once weekly
Monitoring	Yes	No	No	No
Elimination	Mainly kidneys	Mainly kidneys	Kidneys	Kidneys

Abbreviations: UFH, unfractionated heparin; LMWH, low-molecular-weight heparin; IV, intravenous; SC, subcutaneous.

is very predictable and stable, it does not require anticoagulation monitoring. There is no specific antidote for fondaparinux (see below).

Idraparinux

Although fondaparinux has advantages as a new treatment option for VTE, the need for once-daily subcutaneous injection may be problematic for some patients. Idraparinux is a second-generation pentasaccharide with the same anticoagulant target as fondaparinux, but with a much longer half-life (Fig. 1) (9). This hypermethylated derivative of fondaparinux binds to antithrombin with such a high affinity that is has a half-life of about 80 hours, which makes it suitable for once-weekly subcutaneous injection (10,11) (Table 1). Like fondapariunx, idraparinux has complete bioavailability after injection, binds specifically to antithrombin, and has a predictable anticoagulant response (11). Consequently, idraparinux does not need monitoring during treatment. There is no specific antidote for idraparinux. Idraparinux is also excreted by the kidneys; consequently, the dose must be downward adjusted in patients with renal insufficiency.

CLINICAL STUDIES

Clinical Trials with Fondaparinux

The efficacy and safety of fondaparinux have been extensively evaluated, first for the prevention of VTE in orthopedic surgery, followed by trials assessing its effects in the treatment for VTE and in acute coronary syndromes. The most important clinical trials are described below.

Prevention of Venous Thromboembolism

Orthopedic surgery The efficacy of fondaparinux for the prevention of VTE in patients undergoing orthopedic surgery was evaluated in five studies: one phase II dose-finding study (12) and four phase III trials (13–16). In all these studies, subcutaneous enoxaparin, an LMWH, was chosen as the reference antithrombotic agent. In two studies, enoxaparin was given in a dose of 40 mg once daily, 12 ± 2 hours preoperatively (13,16), while in the other trials enoxaparin was started 12 to 24 hours postoperatively and was given at a dose of 30 mg twice daily (12,14,15). In all these studies, fondaparinux was initiated 6 ± 2 hours postoperatively and was administered subcutaneously once daily.

In the first large dose-finding trial, 933 patients undergoing total hip replacement received subcutaneous fondaparinux in doses of 0.75, 1.5, 3.0, 6.0, or 8.0 mg once daily, or subcutaneous enoxaparin, 30-mg twice daily (12). Both treatments were given for up to 10 days. The rate of VTE was low with all fondaparinux doses with a clear dose-response effect: 11.8%, 6.7%, 1.7%, 4.4%, and 0%, respectively, compared with 9.4% in the enoxaparin group. At a dose of 3 mg, fondaparinux reduced VTE by 82% ($p = 0.01$) compared with enoxaparin. The fondaparinux 6- and 8-mg groups were stopped prematurely because of excess bleeding. Analysis of the results suggested that 2.5 mg of fondaparinux once daily was optimal for thromboprophylaxis in the phase III program.

In the phase III studies, the primary efficacy outcome was VTE up to 11 days after surgery. Mandatory bilateral contrast venography of the legs was done to detect deep vein thrombosis (DVT). The primary safety outcome was major bleeding. Two phase III trials, Ephesus and Pentathlon 2000, were performed in patients undergoing elective total hip surgery (13,14). In the European Ephesus trial, fondaparinux significantly reduced the incidence of VTE (4.1%, 37/908) compared with enoxaparin (9.2%, 85/919), with a relative risk reduction of 55.9% (95% confidence interval (CI), 33.1–72.8%) (13). In this study, enoxaparin was used at a dose of 40-mg once daily starting 12 ± 2 hours preoperatively. There was no difference in bleeding between the two groups. Pentathlon 2000, a study done in North America and Australia, showed a nonsignificant relative reduction of 26.3% (95% CI, 10.8–52.8%) in favor of fondaparinux, again without a difference in bleeding (14). This time enoxaparin was started 12 to 24 hours postoperatively and was given at a dose of 30 mg twice daily.

The efficacy of fondaparinux was further assessed in patients undergoing elective knee replacement (Pentamaks), where it was compared with enoxaparin (30 mg twice daily, starting 12–24 hours postoperatively) (15). In 724 patients, the incidence of VTE was significantly lower in the fondaparinux group compared with enoxaparin (12.5% vs. 27.8%, relative risk reduction 55.2%). Fondaparinux was associated with more major bleeding ($p = 0.006$). Finally, in the Penthifra study, fondaparinux was compared with 40 mg enoxaparin once daily, started 12 ± 2 hours preoperatively in 1250 patients undergoing surgery for hip fracture (16). The incidence of VTE was 8.3% in patients randomized to fondaparinux and 19.1% in those given enoxaparin. Therefore, fondaparinux was associated with a relative risk reduction of 56.4% (95% CI, 39.0–70.3%), without a difference in bleeding.

The results of a meta-analysis of the four phase III trials are illustrated in Figure 2 (17). In 5385 patients, the pooled odds ratio yielded a relative risk reduction of 55.2% in favor of fondaparinux, without heterogeneity among the studies. This benefit was also present for proximal DVT. There was no difference between fondaparinux and enoxaparin in the rates of nonfatal or fatal pulmonary embolism, fatal bleeding, bleeding in a critical organ, or bleeding leading to reoperation. However, fondaparinux caused more bleeding in the category of a "bleeding index >2," a combination of transfused packed cells and hemoglobin level. Importantly, the efficacy of fondaparinux was the same in patients who received the first dose either more than six hours after skin closure or before this period. However, the bleeding risk was decreased when fondaparinux was started at least six hours postoperatively. On the basis of these studies, fondaparinux was approved for thromboprophylaxis in patients undergoing orthopedic surgery in the

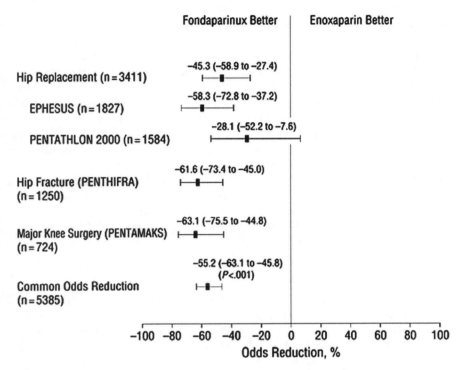

Figure 2 Meta-analysis of thromboprophylaxis studies with fondaparinux in orthopedic surgery. Incidence of venous thromboembolism up to day 11 (primary efficacy). Odds reduction per type of surgery and per study and estimated common odds reduction (exact 95% confidence interval) with fondaparinux relative to enoxaparin. *Source*: From Ref. 17.

United States and Europe. The approved dose is 2.5 mg once daily, starting six hours postoperatively.

To assess the optimal duration of prophylaxis, the Penthifra-plus trial randomized 428 patients who had all received one week of thromboprophylaxis with fondaparinux after surgery for hip fracture to an additional three weeks of fondaparinux (2.5 mg once daily) or placebo (18). During the three additional weeks of treatment, fondaparinux reduced the total incidence of VTE from 35% in the placebo group to 1.4% (relative risk reduction 95.5%); the incidence of symptomatic VTE was also reduced from 2.7% to 0.3% ($p = 0.021$). The incidence of major bleeding was higher in the fondaparinux group (2.4%) compared with placebo (0.6%), but this difference was of borderline significance ($p = 0.06$). There were no significant differences in clinically relevant bleeding or in mortality.

Abdominal surgery Fondaparinux (2.5 mg once daily) was also evaluated in 2927 patients undergoing abdominal surgery in the Pegasus trial (19). In this study, dalteparin was used for comparison. Dalteparin was started two hours before surgery and then continued once daily postoperatively. The first two doses consisted of 2500 units followed by 5000 units once daily. Ten days after surgery, the incidence of bilateral venographically detected VTE was 4.6% in the fondaparinux group and 6.1% in the dalteparin group, a nonsignificant relative risk reduction of 25%. The incidence of symptomatic VTE was 0.4% in both groups, and there was no difference in major bleeding.

Acute medical patients The efficacy of fondaparinux for the prevention of VTE in older acute medical patients was evaluated in the Artemis trial (20). Patients in this study were all over 60 years of age, acutely ill with congestive heart failure (class III/IV according to the New York Heart Association classification), acute respiratory illness in the presence of chronic lung disease, or clinically diagnosed acute infections or inflammatory disorders (such as arthritis or connective tissue disease). Patients were expected to stay in bed for at least four days. The primary outcome was the incidence of asymptomatic or symptomatic VTE up to day 15. Patients received either subcutaneous fondaparinux (2.5 mg once daily) or placebo for a median of seven days. The incidence of all VTE was 5.6% in the fondaparinux group, which was significantly lower than that in patients given placebo (10.5%, relative risk reduction 46.7%, 95% CI, 7.7–69.3%). No symptomatic thromboembolic events occurred in either group. During therapy, the incidence of major bleeding was similar in both arms. On the basis of this study, fondaparinux was approved for use in Europe and the United States for the prevention of VTE in medical patients who are immobilized because of acute illness.

Treatment of Venous Thromboembolism

Phases II and III trials with fondaparinux were conducted in patients with DVT and pulmonary embolism. In the Rembrandt phase IIb trial, the efficacy and safety of subcutaneous fondaparinux 5, 7.5, and 10 mg once daily were compared with those with subcutaneous dalteparin (100 IU/kg twice daily) in patients with acute DVT (21). These treatment regimens were administered for 5 to 10 days, after which the patients were treated with VKAs for three months. The primary outcome measure was the change in thrombus mass assessed by repeat ultrasonography of the leg veins and perfusion lung scintigraphy. The three fondaparinux dosages were comparable to the dalteparin treatment, with a low incidence of bleeding. The once-daily 7.5-mg dose was chosen for further evaluation in the phase III non-inferiority trials.

The randomized double-blind Matisse-DVT study compared subcutaneous fondaparinux 7.5 mg once daily with subcutaneous enoxaparin 1 mg/kg twice daily in patients with symptomatic DVT (22). This initial treatment was continued for at least five days and until VKA treatment produced an international normalized ratio (INR) greater than 2. In patients <50 kg, fondaparinux 5.0 mg was given, whereas those >100 kg received 10 mg. A total of 2205 patients were included, and the primary outcome measure was symptomatic VTE during three months of follow-up. Recurrent VTE occurred in 43 (3.9%) of the fondaparinux patients, while 45 (4.1%) of the enoxaparin group had recurrent VTE—a nonsignificant difference of –0.15% (95% CI, –1.8–1.5%) (Table 2). Major bleeding during initial treatment occurred in 1.1% of the patients given fondaparinux and in 1.2% of those treated with enoxaparin. Clinically relevant nonmajor bleeding or mortality was virtually the same in the two groups.

In the Matisse-PE trial, 2213 patients with acute pulmonary embolism were randomized to either fondaparinux (same regimen as in the Matisse-DVT study) or adjusted-dose intravenous UFH followed by VKA treatment (23). At three months, 42 (3.8%) of the fondaparinux patients and 56 (5.0%) of the patients who received UFH had recurrent VTE, a nonsignificant difference of –1.2% (95% CI, –3.0–0.5%) (Table 2). Major bleeding during initial treatment, clinically relevant nonmajor bleeding, and mortality were similar between the two groups. These two large studies showed that once-daily subcutaneous administration of fondaparinux 7.5 mg was effective and safe in patients with either acute DVT or acute pulmonary embolism. Thereafter, fondaparinux was approved in the United States and Europe for the initial treatment of acute VTE.

Table 2 The Efficacy and Safety of Fondaparinux in Phase III Trials for Venous Thromboembolism and Acute Coronary Syndrome

| Indication | Study | No. of subjects | Intervention | | | Outcome | |
			Fondaparinux	Control	Primary outcome	Efficacy	Major bleeding
DVT (22)	Matisse-DVT	2205	7.5 mg once daily	Enoxaparin 1 mg/kg twice daily and VKA	Recurrent VTE at 3 mo	Fondaparinux 3.9% Enoxaparin 4.1%	Fondaparinux 1.1% Enoxaparin 1.2%
PE (23)	Matisse-PE	2213	7.5 mg once daily	UFH and VKA	Recurrent VTE at 3 mo	Fondaparinux 3.8% UFH 5.0%	Fondaparinux 1.3% UFH 1.1%
NSTACS (24)	OASIS-5	20,078	2.5 mg once daily	Enoxaparin 1 mg/kg twice daily	Death, MI, or RI at 9 days	Fondaparinux 5.8% Enoxaparin 5.7%	Fondaparinux 2.2% Enoxaparin 4.1%
STEMI (25)	OASIS-6	12,092	2.5 mg once daily	Placebo or UFH	Death or MI at 30 days	Fondaparinux 9.7% Control 11.2%	Fondaparinux 1.8% Control 2.1%

Abbreviations: DVT, deep-vein thrombosis; PE, pulmonary embolism; NSTACS, non-ST-elevation acute coronary syndrome; NSTEMI, non-ST-elevation myocardial infarction; UFH, unfractionated heparin; VKA, Vitamin K antagonists; RI, reinfarction.

Acute coronary syndrome The role of fondaparinux in patients with acute coronary syndrome was assessed in several studies. In these studies, LMWH or UFH was used as the comparator. First, in the Pentua trial, four doses of fondaparinux (2.5, 4.0, 8.0, or 12.0 mg once daily) were compared with enoxaparin 1 mg/kg twice daily in 1147 patients with unstable angina or non-Q-wave myocardial infarction (26). At a dose of 2.5 mg, fondaparinux showed the best efficacy for the prevention of the composite endpoint of death, acute myocardial infarction, and recurrent ischemia. The Pentalyse study evaluated the combination of either intravenous UFH or low (4–6 mg), medium (6–10 mg), or high (10–12 mg) doses of fondaparinux and thrombolysis in 333 patients with ST-elevation myocardial infarction (STEMI) (27). All patients were treated with alteplase and aspirin. Thrombolysis in myocardial infarction (TIMI) flow grade 3 rates were comparable among the groups at 90 minutes, as was the incidence of major bleeding.

The large OASIS-5 (Organization to Assess Strategies for Ischemic Syndromes-5) study randomized 20,078 patients with acute coronary syndrome without ST-segment elevation to subcutaneous fondaparinux (2.5 mg once daily) or enoxaparin (1 mg/kg twice daily) (26). Patients were treated for up to eight days with a mean treatment duration of six days. The primary efficacy outcome was the composite of death, myocardial infarction, or refractory ischemia, and the trial was intended to show non-inferiority of fondaparinux compared with enoxaparin. The primary outcome was similar (5.8% vs. 5.7%) in the fondaparinux and enoxaparin groups, but at nine days the rate of major bleeding was 2.2% with fondaparinux versus 4.1% with enoxaparin ($p < 0.001$) (Table 2). At 30 days, fondaparinux also reduced mortality by 17% (2.9% vs. 3.5%), including fatal bleeding (7% vs. 22%) at 30 days. This study showed an important relationship between major bleeding and fatality: 13.2% of the patients who had a major bleeding episode during hospitalization died compared with 2.8% of those without major bleeding. Likewise the risk of reinfarction was also increased in patients with major bleeding. Finally, there was a higher rate of catheter-related thrombosis in the fondaparinux group (0.9% vs. 0.4% in the enoxaparin patients, $p = 0.001$), but only when patients were not additionally treated with UFH. The most remarkable result of this study was the reduction in bleeding associated with fondaparinux, which may be due to the difference in the intensity of anticoagulant effect between the prophylactic dose of fondaparinux and the therapeutic dose of enoxaparin (28). In the previous prevention trials in orthopedic patients, fondaparinux 2.5 mg was compared with enoxaparin 40 mg once daily or 30 mg twice daily. Nevertheless, the OASIS-5 study demonstrates clearly that fondaparinux 2.5 mg daily is effective and safe in patients with acute coronary syndrome.

The efficacy and safety of fondaparinux were also evaluated in patients with STEMI in the OASIS-6 study (28). This trial randomized 12,092 patients to either subcutaneous fondaparinux (2.5 mg once daily) for up to eight days or usual care. Patients were additionally treated with either placebo or intravenous therapeutic dose UFH followed by eight days of placebo. The decision as to whether patients were treated with UFH was based on the judgment of the treating physician. At 30 days, the number of deaths and reinfarction was 11.2% in the control group and 9.7% in the fondaparinux group (absolute risk reduction 1.5%, 95% CI, 0.4–2.6%) (Table 2). This difference was already present at nine days. The frequency of severe bleeding was not increased with fondaparinux compared with the control group (1.8% vs. 2.1%, $p = 0.13$). Fondaparinux did not benefit patients who underwent primary percutaneous coronary intervention. In addition, patients treated with fondaparinux had a higher rate of guiding catheter thrombosis unless adjunctive UFH was given. The results of this large trial indicate that fondaparinux 2.5 mg once daily is effective and safe in patients with STEMI. In patients with primary PCI, however, fondaparinux is not of benefit.

Catheter thrombosis is problematic but appears to be preventable with adjunctive UFH treatment at the time of PCI.

Clinical Trials with Idraparinux

Treatment of Venous Thromboembolism

The efficacy and safety of idraparinux for the treatment of VTE were evaluated in phases II and III trials. Idraparinux also was evaluated in patients with atrial fibrillation. In the phase II persist trial, consecutive patients aged between 18 and 85 years with acute symptomatic proximal DVT were treated with enoxaparin (1 mg/kg subcutaneously twice daily) for five to seven days, after which a bilateral ultrasound of the leg veins and perfusion scintigraphy of the lungs were performed to assess the thrombotic burden (29). Patients were randomized to warfarin or four doses of once-weekly subcutaneous administration of idraparinux: 2.5 mg, 5.0 mg, 7.5 mg, and 10 mg. Treatment duration was 12 weeks, and at the end of the treatment period, bilateral ultrasound of the leg veins and perfusion scintigraphy of the lungs were repeated. The primary efficacy outcome, change in thrombotic burden, was similar in all groups. Normalization of the affected veins occurred in 25% in all groups after three months. There was a statistically significant dose-response effect in both major and clinically relevant bleeds ($p = 0.003$ and $p = 0.001$, respectively). The incidence of major bleeding in the 10-mg idraparinux group was higher than that in patients treated with warfarin ($p = 0.01$). The incidence of any bleeding was lower in the 2.5-mg idraparinux group compared with that in the warfarin group. On the basis of this study, the 2.5-mg dose was selected for the phase III studies.

The phase III van Gogh non-inferiority trials compared 2.5-mg idraparinux once weekly with standard treatment for acute DVT or PE, i.e., LMWH or UFH followed by VKA dose adjusted to achieve an INR of 2 to 3 (30). Both studies were randomized open-label trials, with stratification according to the center and intended treatment duration (3 or 6 months as assessed by the treating physician). The primary efficacy outcome in both studies was symptomatic recurrent VTE at day 92. In the DVT study, 2904 patients were randomized, of whom 2.9% in the idraparinux group and 3.0% in the standard therapy group developed recurrent VTE (odds ratio 0.98, 95% CI, 0.63–1.50) (Fig. 3) (30). At three months, the incidence of clinically relevant bleeding was lower in the idraparinux group (4.5%) compared with that of standard treatment group (7.0%, $p = 0.004$). In the 2215 patients with acute pulmonary embolism, idraparinux treatment was less effective than conventional treatment (Fig. 3) (30); 3.4% of the patients treated with idraparinux and 1.6% given standard treatment developed a recurrent event in the first three months (odds ratio 2.14, 95% CI, 1.21–3.78) (Fig. 3). Like in the DVT study, the incidence of clinically relevant bleedings was lower in the idraparinux group (5.8%) than in the standard treatment group (8.2%, $p = 0.02$). In conclusion, idraparinux treatment was non-inferior to standard therapy in patients with acute DVT, but was inferior in the pulmonary embolism study. The exact reason for this discrepancy is unclear, but may be partially explained by the lower-than-expected recurrence rate of pulmonary embolism in the standard treatment group (1.6% after 3 months; see Fig. 3).

The extended use of idraparinux for prophylaxis against that for VTE was assessed in the van Gogh extension trial (31). In 1215 patients, most of whom had participated in the van Gogh DVT and PE trials and completed six months of treatment with either idraparinux or VKA were randomized to another six months of idraparinux (2.5 mg once weekly) or to placebo. Compared with placebo, idraparinux reduced the rate of

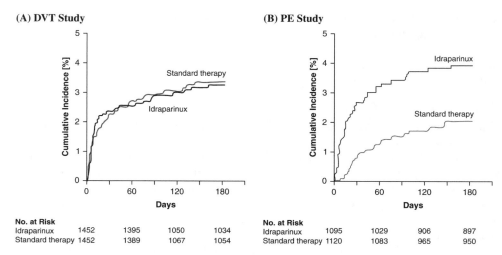

Figure 3 van Gogh study showing the cumulative incidence of venous thromboembolic events in patients (**A**) with DVT and (**B**) pulmonary embolism randomized to either idraparinux treatment or standard treatment. *Source*: From Ref. 30.

symptomatic VTE from 3.7% to 1.0% (odds ratio 0.27, 95% CI, 0.11–0.66). Major bleeding occurred in 1.9% of the idraparinux-treated patients and in none of the placebo patients ($p < 0.001$). Interestingly, both the incidences of thrombosis and bleeding were influenced by the use of idraparinux before randomization. In patients who had received idraparinux and who used placebo, the six-month recurrent thrombosis rate was only 0.7%, compared with 5.9% in the patients that had received VKAs before randomization to placebo. Vice versa, clinically relevant bleeding episodes occurred in 2.2% of the placebo patients who had received idraparinux before, compared with 0.9% of the patients who had received prior VKA therapy. These results suggest a prolonged antithrombotic effect after stopping the drug.

Atrial fibrillation Idraparinux has also been investigated in patients with non-valvular atrial fibrillation. This is an important group as patients with atrial fibrillation often have a lifelong indication for anticoagulant treatment and could benefit from once-weekly treatment with idraparinux. The Amadeus study was a non-inferiority trial that compared idraparinux 2.5 mg subcutaneous once weekly with VKA dose adjusted to achieve a target INR of 2 to 3 (32). The primary efficacy outcome was stroke and systemic embolism. Because of an excess of clinically relevant bleeding in the idraparinux group, the study was prematurely terminated after randomization of 4576 patients. Clinically relevant bleeding occurred in 19.7% of the idraparinux patients and in 11.3% of the patients given VKA (odds ratio 1.74, 95% CI, 1.47–2.06). Elderly patients and patients with renal insufficiency were at highest risk for bleeding. Idraparinux was non-inferior to VKA for stroke and systemic embolism prevention.

Biotinylated idraparinux The aforementioned excess of bleeding with idraparinux and the absence of a specific antidote prompted the development of biotinylated idraparinux. This compound has the same anticoagulant properties as idraparinux, but because of an additional biotin moiety, rapid reversal can be achieved after intravenous injection of avidin (11,33). Avidin is an egg white–derived protein that binds biotin with high affinity to form a stable complex that is cleared within minutes via the kidneys.

Two phase III trials with biotinylated idraparinux were initiated in 2006. The Equinox study, which has recently been completed, is a bioequipotency study between biotinylated idraparinux and idraparinux in 700 patients with acute DVT (see www.ClinicalTrials.gov; identifier NCT00311090). In a subset of patients, the effect of intravenous avidin on the biotinylated idraparinux-induced anti-Xa levels was analyzed. In the Cassiopeia study, 3200 patients with acute PE will be randomized after one-week treatment with LMWH to either biotinylated idraparinux (3 mg subcutaneously once weekly) and conventional treatment with LMWH or heparin followed by VKA (see www .ClinicalTrials.gov; identifier NCT00345618). Primary efficacy outcome will be recurrent VTE at three months. Finally, the very large Borealis-AF study will assess the efficacy and safety of biotinylated idraparinux 3 mg subcutaneously once weekly versus VKA in patients with non-valvular atrial fibrillation. This study started recruitment in December 2007 (see www.ClinicalTrials.gov; identifier NCT00580216).

Special Categories

Heparin-Induced Thrombocytopenia

Although uncommon, HIT is a potential life-threatening disorder that is caused by complex formation between heparin and platelet factor 4, which leads to platelet activation and aggregation (34). The risk of development of HIT is highest with therapeutic dose of UFH but can also occur with LMWH treatment (34). Fondaparinux is a potential alternative for prevention and treatment of HIT. In vitro, it has a very low cross reactivity with HIT antibodies (35). In addition, prophylactic treatment with 2.5 mg of fondaparinux in over 2700 orthopedic patients resulted in less than 3% of PF4 antibodies without the development of clinical HIT (36). The clinical experience with fondaparinux for the treatment of HIT is however scarce, and cases of HIT associated with fondaparinux have been reported (37). Recently, a study in patients with acute HIT has started that compares the efficacy and safety of fondaparinux 7.5 mg once daily with argatroban or lepirudin (see www.ClinicalTrials.gov; identifier NCT00603824).

Renal Insufficiency

Pentasaccharides are excreted via the kidneys without prior metabolism and therefore have the potential to accumulate inpatients with impaired renal function, which could lead to an increased risk of bleeding. Importantly, in the prophylaxis studies with fondaparinux, patients with a serum creatinine concentration above 2.04 mg/dL (180 µmol/L) were excluded, nearly the same criterion as in the therapeutic Matisse-VTE studies. In the OASIS trials in patients with acute coronary syndrome, patients were excluded when they had a serum creatinine concentration above 3 mg/dL (265 µmol/L). A subanalysis of the OASIS-5 trial examined the effect of renal dysfunction of fondaparinux 2.5 mg once daily in patients with acute coronary syndrome (38). After nine days of treatment, 2.8% of the patients with a glomerular filtration rate <58 mL/min per $1.73\ m^2$ and fondaparinux 2.5 mg once daily had a major bleeding event, compared with 6.4% of the patients assigned to enoxaparin, dose adjusted for severe renal impairment or 1 mg/kg twice daily (odds ratio 0.42, 95% CI, 0.32–0.56). In comparison, 1.6% of the patients with a normal renal function experienced a major bleeding event during treatment with fondaparinux.

In a recent pharmacokinetic and simulation study, fondaparinux concentrations in patients with severe renal impairment who received fondaparinux 2.5 mg every other day were predicted to be similar to those in patients with mild renal impairment with fondaparinux 2.5 mg once daily (39,40). Therefore, increasing the dosing interval for fondaparinux may be a reasonable strategy for dose adjustment in carefully selected patients with severe renal impairment. However, this first requires careful clinical investigation.

In patients with renal impairment (creatinine clearance <30 mL/min), the guidelines of the FDA and EMEA are somewhat conflicting. According to the FDA, fondaparinux is contraindicated in these patients, whereas the EMEA has recently approved fondaparinux 1.5 mg once daily in patients with a creatinine clearance of 20 to 50 mL/min (see www.emea.europa.eu/humandocs/PDFs/EPAR/arixtra/H-403-PI-en.pdf). In general, no adjustment in the fondaparinux dosage is required in patients with mild-to-moderate renal insufficiency (40). However, as with LMWH, fondaparinux should be used with caution in patients with moderate renal impairment (creatinine clearance 30–50 mL/min). In addition, as in all patients with renal impairment who are receiving new anticoagulants, renal function should be assessed periodically.

Although synthetic pentasaccharides have been developed for use without the need for anticoagulant monitoring, periodic monitoring could be helpful in special patient categories. The effect of LMWH treatment in patients with renal impairment can be monitored with anti-Xa levels, and dose adjustments can be made accordingly. The effect of pentasaccharides can also be monitored with anti-factor Xa assays, but it is important that these assays are pentasaccharides specific (11). In addition, knowledge of the optimal therapeutic range in terms of anti-Xa activity is a prerequisite.

Antidote For fondaparinux and idraparinux, as for nearly all new anticoagulants, no specific antidote is available. In cases of severe bleeding, recombinant factor VIIa can be administered, which normalizes the clotting tests and thrombin generation (41). The anticoagulant effect of biotinylated idraparinux can be directly reversed with an intravenous injection with avidin.

Pregnancy

In clinical trials with pentasaccharides, pregnant women were excluded. In vitro, in placentas obtained immediately following delivery, fondaparinux did not transfer the placental barrier at plasma concentrations corresponding to therapeutic levels (42). Fondaparinux, however, may cross the placental barrier in vivo. Low anti-factor Xa activity has been measured in umbilical cord blood after maternal treatment (43). Further evaluation of fondaparinux in this indication is therefore warranted.

CONCLUSIONS

Synthetic pentasaccharides form a new class of heparins that specifically target factor Xa through activation of antithrombin. Several large-scale trials have established that subcutaneous fondaparinux 2.5 mg once daily is effective in preventing VTE in orthopedic and abdominal surgery and in medical patients with acute illnesses. This dose is also effective and safe in patients with acute coronary syndrome. Fondaparinux 7.5 mg once daily has been shown to adequately prevent recurrent VTE in patients with either acute DVT or pulmonary embolism, without an excess in major bleeding complications. Idraparinux, the longer-acting pentasaccharide that can be administered once weekly, was halted from further development, since it caused more bleeding. Biotinylated idraparinux, of which the anticoagulant effect can directly be reversed with avidin, is currently being evaluated.

REFERENCES

1. Büller HR, Agnelli G, Hull RD, et al. Antithrombotic therapy for venous thromboembolic disease: the seventh ACCP conference on Antithrombotic and Thrombolytic Therapy. Chest 2004; 126(3 suppl):401S–428S.
2. Petitou M, Duchaussoy P, Lederman I. Synthesis of heparin fragments: a alpha-methyl pentaoside with high affinity for antithrombin III. Carbohydr Res 1987; 167:67–75.
3. Jin J, Abrahams JP, Skinner R. The anticoagulant activation of antithrombin by heparin. Proc Natl Acad Sci USA 1997; 94:14683–14688.
4. Olson ST, Björk I, Sheffer R. Role of the antithrombin-binding pentasaccharide in heparin acceleration of antithrombin-proteinase reactions. Resolution of the antithrombin conformational change contribution to heparin rate enhancement. J Biol Chem 1992; 267:12528–12538.
5. Donat F, Duret JP, Santoni R. The pharmacokinetics of fondaparinux sodium in healthy volunteers. Clin Pharmacokinet 2002; 41(suppl 2):1–9.
6. Lieu C, Shi J, Donat F. Fondaparinux sodium is not metabolised in mammalian liver fractions and does not inhibit cytochrome P450-mediated metabolism of concomitant drugs. Clin Pharmacokinet 2002; 41(suppl 2):19–26.
7. Faaij RA, Burggraaf J, Schoemaker RC, et al. Absence of an interaction between the synthetic pentasaccharide fondaparinux and oral warfarin. Br J Clin Pharmacol 2002; 54:304–308.
8. Ollier C, Faaij RA, Santoni A, et al. Absence of interaction of fondaparinux sodium with aspirin and piroxicam in healthy male volunteers. Clin Pharmacokinet 2002; 41(suppl 2):31–37.
9. Herbert JM, Herault JP, Bernat A, et al. Biochemical and pharmacological properties of SANORG 34006, a potent and long-acting synthetic pentasaccharide. Blood 1998; 91: 4197–4205.
10. Walenga JM, Jeske WP, Fareed J. Short- and long-acting synthetic pentasaccharides as antithrombotic agents. Expert Opin Investig Drugs 2005; 14:847–858.
11. Gross PL, Weitz JI. New anticoagulants for treatment of venous thromboembolism. Arterioscler Thromb Vasc Biol 2008; 28:380–386.
12. Turpie AGG, Gallus AS, Hoek JA. For the pentasaccharide investigators. A synthetic pentasaccharide for the prevention of deep-vein thrombosis after total hip replacement. N Engl J Med 2001; 344:619–625.
13. Lassen MR, Bauer KA, Eriksson BI, et al. Fondaparinux versus enoxaparin for the prevention of venous thromboembolism in elective hip replacement surgery. A randomized double-blind comparison. Lancet 2002; 359:1715–1720.
14. Turpie AGG, Bauer KA, Eriksson BI. A randomized double-blind comparison of fondaparinux with enoxaparin for the prevention of venous thromboembolism after elective hip replacement surgery. Lancet 2002; 359:1721–1726.
15. Eriksson BI, Bauer KA, Lassen MR, et al. Fondaparinux compared with enoxaparin for the prevention of venous thromboembolism after hip-fracture surgery. N Engl J Med 2001; 345: 1298–1300.
16. Bauer KA, Eriksson BI, Lassen MR, et al. Fondaparinux compared with enoxaparin for the prevention of venous thromboembolism after elective major knee surgery. N Engl J Med 2001; 345:1305–1310.
17. Turpie AGG, Bauer KA, Eriksson BI, et al. Fondaparinux vs enoxaparin for the prevention of venous thromboembolism in major orthopedic surgery. A meta-analysis of 4 randomized double-blind studies. Arch Intern Med 2002; 162:1833–1840.
18. Eriksson BI, Lassen MR. PENTasaccharide in HIp-fracture surgery plus investigators. duration of prophylaxis against venous thromboembolism with fondaparinux after hip fracture surgery: a multicenter, randomized, placebo-controlled, double-blind study. Arch Intern Med 2003; 163: 1337–1342.
19. Agnelli G, Bergqvist D, Cohen AT, et al. For the PEGASUS investigators. Randomized clinical trial of postoperative fondaparinux versus perioperative dalteparin for prevention of venous thromboembolism in high-risk abdominal surgery. Br J Surg 2005; 92:1212–1220.

20. Cohen AT, Davidson BL, Gallus AS, et al. Efficacy and safety of fondaparinux for the prevention of venous thromboembolism in older acute medical patients: randomised placebo controlled trial. Br Med J 2006; 332:325–329.

21. Büller HR, Cariou R, Gallus A, et al. Treatment of proximal deep vein thrombosis with a novel synthetic compound (SR90107A/ORG31540) with pure anti-factor Xa activity. Circulation 2000; 102:2726–2731.

22. Büller HR, Davidson BL, Decousus H, et al. Fondaparinux or enoxaparin for the initial treatment of symptomatic deep venous thrombosis: a randomized trial. Ann Intern Med 2004; 140:867–873.

23. Büller HR, Davidson BL, Decousus H, et al. Subcutaneous fondaparinux versus intravenous unfractionated heparin in the initial treatment of pulmonary embolism. N Engl J Med 2003; 349:1695–1702.

24. Yusuf S, Mehta SR, Chrolavicius S, et al. Comparison of fondaparinux and enoxaparin in acute coronary syndromes. N Engl J Med 2006; 354:1464–1476.

25. Yusuf S, Mehta SR, Chrolavicius S, et al. Effects of fondaparinux on mortality and reinfarction in patients with acute ST-segment elevation myocardial infarction: the OASIS-6 randomized trial. JAMA 2006; 295:1519–1530.

26. Simoons ML, Bobbink IW, Boland J, et al. A dose-finding study of fondaparinux in patients with non-ST-segment elevation acute coronary syndromes: the Pentasaccharide in Unstable Angina (PENTUA) Study. J Am Coll Cardiol 2004; 43:2183–2190.

27. Coussement PK, Bassand J-P, Convens C, et al. A synthetic factor-Xa inhibitor (ORG31540/SR90107A) as an adjunct to fibrinolysis in acute myocardial infraction. The PENTALYSE study. Eur Heart J 2001; 22:1716–1724.

28. Hirsh J, O'Donnell M, Eikelboom JW. Beyond unfractionated heparin and warfarin: current and future advances. Circulation 2007; 116:552–560.

29. PERSIST Investigators. A novel long-acting synthetic factor Xa inhibitor (SanOrg34006) to replace warfarin for secondary prevention in deep vein thrombosis: a phase II evaluation. J Thromb Haemost 2004; 2:47–53.

30. van Gogh investigators, Büller HR, Cohen AT, et al. Idraparinux versus standard therapy for venous thromboembolic disease. N Engl J Med 2007; 357:1094–1104.

31. van Gogh investigators, Büller HR, Cohen AT, et al. Extended prophylaxis of venous thromboembolism with idraparinux. N Engl J Med 2007; 357:1105–1112.

32. Amadeus investigators, Bousser MG, Bouthier J, et al. Comparison of idraparinux with vitamin K antagonists for prevention of thromboembolism in patients with atrial fibrillation: a randomised, open-label, non-inferiority trial. Lancet 2008; 371:315–321.

33. Spyropoulos AC. Investigational treatments of venous thromboembolism. Expert Opin Investig Drugs 2007; 16:431–440.

34. Warkentin TE, Greinacher A. Heparin-induced thrombocytopenia: recognition, treatment, and prevention: the seventh ACCP conference on Antithrombotic and Thrombolytic therapy. Chest 2004; 126:311S–375S.

35. Savi P, Chong BH, Greinacher A, et al. Effect of fondaparinux on platelet activation in the presence of heparin-dependent antibodies: a blinded comparative multicenter study with unfractionated heparin. Blood 2005; 105:139–144.

36. Warkentin TE, Cook RJ, Marder VJ, et al. Anti-platelet factor 4/heparin antibodies in orthopedic surgery patients receiving antithrombotic prophylaxis with fondaparinux or enoxaparin. Blood 2005; 106:3791–3796.

37. Warkentin TE, Maurer BT, Aster RH. Heparin-induced thrombocytopenia associated with fondaparinux. N Engl J Med 2007; 356:2653–2655.

38. Fox KAA, Bassand JP, Mehta SR, et al. Influence of renal function on the efficacy and safety of fondaparinux relative to enoxaparin in non–ST-segment elevation acute coronary syndromes. Ann Intern Med 2007; 147:304–310.

39. GlaxoSmithKline. Use of Arixtra in Patients with Renal Impairment. Medical information letter. Philadelphia, PA; 2006 May.

40. Lobo BL. Use of newer anticoagulants in patients with chronic kidney disease. Am J Health Syst Pharm 2007; 64:2017–2026.

41. Bijsterveld NR, Moons AH, Boekholdt SM, et al. Ability of recombinant factor VIIa to reverse the anticoagulant effect of the pentasaccharide fondaparinux in healthy volunteers. Circulation 2002; 106:2550–2554.

42. Lagrange F, Vergnes C, Paolucci F, et al. Absence of placental transfer of pentasaccharide (fondaparinux, Arixtra) in the dually perfused human cotyledon in vitro. Thromb Haemost 2002; 87:831–835.

43. Dempfle CE. Minor transplacental passage of fondaparinux in vivo. N Engl J Med 2004; 350: 1914–1915.

16

Treatment of Heparin-Induced Thrombocytopenia

Theodore E. Warkentin

Department of Pathology and Molecular Medicine, and Department of Medicine, Michael G. DeGroote School of Medicine, McMaster University, Transfusion Medicine, Hamilton Regional Laboratory Medicine Program, Hamilton Health Sciences, Hamilton General Site, Hamilton, Ontario, Canada

INTRODUCTION

The topic, "Treatment of Heparin-Induced Thrombocytopenia," befits a book entitled *New Therapeutic Agents in Thrombosis and Thrombolysis*. This is because the two most widely used anticoagulant classes—heparins and coumarins—are usually considered to be *contraindicated* for use during the acute (thrombocytopenic) phase of immune heparin-induced thrombocytopenia (HIT) (1). Furthermore, HIT confers an exceptionally high risk of venous and/or arterial thrombosis (odds ratio for thrombosis, 20 to 40) (2,3), even if the inciting agent—heparin—is stopped (4). Thus, most patients with HIT require treatment with an alternative, non-heparin anticoagulant with rapid onset of action. Indeed, two direct thrombin inhibitors (DTIs), lepirudin and argatroban, were introduced into the pharmacologic armamentarium through their approval for management of HIT (5).

HIT is a hypercoagulability state, with markedly elevated thrombin-antithrombin complexes (a marker of in vivo thrombin generation) (6). This state has certain treatment implications. For example, coumarin-associated skin necrosis is an otherwise rare complication of warfarin and other vitamin K antagonists (coumarins). However, HIT confers at least a 100-fold increase in the risk of coumarin necrosis, as the absolute risk of this complication may be as high as 5% to 10% in patients with acute HIT treated with warfarin and other agents versus a background rate of less than 0.02% (7). Similarly, the transition period from DTI therapy to coumarin anticoagulation also poses a relatively high-risk situation for thrombotic events (8), including coumarin-associated necrosis (9,10).

HIT PATHOGENESIS

HIT is an adverse drug effect characterized by thrombocytopenia that is caused by in vivo immunoglobulin G (IgG)-mediated platelet activation, with increased risk of thrombosis (Fig. 1) (11). HIT is autoimmune-like, since the target antigen is a multimolecular complex

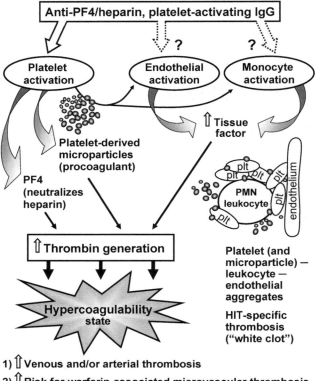

Figure 1 Pathogenesis of HIT. Illustrated are two potential explanations for thrombosis in HIT. Activation of platelets (plts) by anti-PF4/heparin IgG antibodies ("HIT antibodies"), leading to formation of procoagulant, platelet-derived microparticles, and neutralization of heparin by PF4 released from activated platelets, leads to marked increase in thrombin generation ("hyper-coagulability state"), characterized by an increased risk of venous and/or arterial thrombosis, as well as increased risk for coumarin-associated microthrombosis (venous limb gangrene, skin necrosis). However, it is also possible that unique mechanisms operative in HIT explain unusual thromboses, such as arterial "white clots." For example, HIT antibodies have been shown to activate endothelium and monocytes (leading to cell surface tissue factor expression, although this stimulation may be largely "indirect" through poorly-defined mechanisms involving platelet activation and, possibly, formation of platelet-derived microparticles). Further, aggregates of platelets and PMN leukocytes have been described in HIT. To what extent these cooperative interactions between platelets, platelet-derived microparticles, PMN leukocytes, monocytes, and endothelium lead to arterial (or venous) thrombotic events in HIT, either in large or small vessels, remains unclear. *Abbreviations:* HIT, heparin-induced thrombocytopenia; PMN, polymorphonuclear; PF4, platelet factor 4; plts, platelets. *Source*: From Ref. 11.

of the "self" protein, platelet factor 4 (PF4)—a (cationic) member of the C-X-C subfamily of chemokines—and (anionic) heparin, through charge interactions (12,13). Large PF4/heparin/IgG complexes are formed in situ on platelet surfaces and produce platelet activation because of cross-linking of platelet FcγIIa receptors (14). The degree of platelet activation is intense, resulting in thromboxane generation, granule release, and generation of procoagulant, platelet-derived microparticles (15). Anti-PF4/heparin antibodies of immunoglobulin M (IgM) and immunoglobulin A class are not pathogenic (16) because they cannot activate platelets via FcγIIa receptors. Besides platelet activation, there is evidence for "pancellular" activation (endothelium, monocytes), and neutralization of the anticoagulant effect of heparin by PF4 released from activated platelets (11).

DEFINITION AND TERMINOLOGY

HIT can be defined as any clinical event (or events) best explained by the presence of platelet-activating anti-PF4/heparin antibodies ("HIT antibodies") in a patient who is receiving, or who has recently received, heparin (17). Thrombocytopenia is the most common event in HIT, and is observed in at least 90% of patients, depending on how thrombocytopenia is defined. Most patients with HIT develop thrombosis (2–4,17).

HIT is a clinicopathologic syndrome (17). Thus, diagnosis requires one or more *clinical* events (e.g., thrombocytopenia, thrombosis) bearing a temporal association with *pathologic* HIT antibody formation. Hence, a patient suspected to have HIT but in whom antibodies cannot be detected does not have the diagnosis. Indeed, some disorders mimic HIT closely ("pseudo-HIT"), pointing to the role of laboratory testing for HIT antibodies (18). An increasingly recognized problem is the presence of non-platelet-activating anti-PF4/heparin antibodies that can lead to a false diagnosis of HIT (16,19).

FREQUENCY

Four factors influence the frequency of developing HIT (listed in decreasing order of importance): duration of heparin use (especially beyond seven days); type of heparin [unfractionated heparin (UFH) > low-molecular-weight heparin (LMWH) > fondaparinux)]; type of patient population (surgical > medical > obstetrical/pediatric); and patient sex (females > males) (2,20–25). Thus, the "typical" patient with HIT is a female receiving postsurgery thromboprophylaxis with UFH for more than one week (risk, 1–5%). Despite its higher risk in females, HIT is rare in pregnancy (25). HIT usually reflects "point immunization" resulting from heparin given perioperatively, and so a course of heparin that continues beyond two weeks is unlikely to cause HIT, if it has not already done so by day 14. Thus, HIT is rare in chronic hemodialysis, but more often complicates acute hemodialysis, particularly in postoperative or other proinflammatory settings. HIT occurs in about 0.1% to 0.5% of medical patients receiving UFH for treatment of venous thrombosis, and in a similar frequency in postoperative patients receiving LMWH prophylaxis (24). The 10- to 15-fold reduced risk of HIT with LMWH compared with UFH among postoperative patients (especially women) (22) is in part explained by a lower risk of forming "strong" platelet-activating HIT antibodies by LMWH (2,21). Although the antithrombin-binding pentasaccharide anticoagulant, fondaparinux, is approximately as immunogenic as LMWH, it does not form well the antigens on PF4, and may therefore have a lower risk of HIT compared with LMWH (23). Nevertheless, HIT has been reported with fondaparinux treatment (26).

CLINICAL PICTURE

HIT is a distinctive syndrome compared with immune-mediated thrombocytopenia due to other drugs, such as quinine, vancomycin, and glycoprotein IIb/IIIa antagonists (27) (Fig. 2). Although these other agents typically produce severe thrombocytopenia and mucocutaneous hemorrhage, death or long-term disability are rare. In contrast, HIT usually evinces a moderate degree of thrombocytopenia, and petechiae are not seen; nevertheless, long-term sequelae or even death from thrombosis are not uncommon.

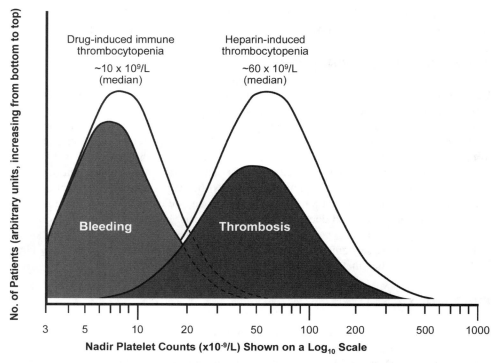

Figure 2 Clinical picture of HIT versus classic drug-induced immune-mediated thrombocytope-nia. "Classic" drug-induced immune-mediated thrombocytopenia (e.g., caused by quinine, vancomycin, or glycoprotein IIb/IIIa antagonists, among other drugs) typically produces severe thrombocytopenia (median platelet count nadir, about 10×10^9/L) and associated mucocutaneous bleeding. In contrast, HIT typically results in mild-to-moderate thrombocytopenia (median platelet count nadir, 60×10^9/L) and associated venous or arterial thrombosis. Note that the heights of the two peaks are not drawn to scale, as HIT is much more common than all other causes of drug-induced immune-mediated thrombocytopenia combined. *Abbreviation:* HIT, heparin-induced thrombocytopenia. *Source*: Modified from Ref. 27.

Thrombocytopenia

The median platelet count nadir in HIT is approximately 60×10^9/L (4,17,27,28). Most patients develop a 50% or greater fall in the platelet count (20). In postoperative patients, the appropriate "baseline" platelet count is *not* the preoperative platelet count, but rather the highest *post*operative platelet count immediately preceding the platelet count fall indicating HIT (20,28).

Timing

HIT represents a transient immune response triggered by heparin (29). The antibodies are first detectable beginning four or five days after the immunizing heparin exposure, which usually is UFH given during or soon after surgery or other inflammatory situations. The earliest onset of the platelet count fall is typically five days after beginning the immunizing heparin exposure (usual range, day 5–10). Since the median time for the platelet count to fall by 50% or more is about two days, this means that thrombocytopenia is usually apparent about 7 to 14 days after beginning the inciting course of heparin. This profile, called "typical-onset" HIT, occurs in about 70% of patients (29).

"Rapid-onset" HIT is the presenting feature in about one-quarter of patients, and is defined as a drop in platelet count rapidly (usually within 24 hours) of beginning a course of heparin, or increasing the dose during ongoing heparin therapy (29). This occurs because the patient already has circulating HIT antibodies, a result of *recent* exposure to heparin, generally within the past few weeks or months.

"Delayed-onset" HIT is used to describe a patient whose platelet count only begins to fall *after* all heparin has been stopped (30,31). This is caused by unusually high levels of antibodies that can activate platelets without the need for pharmacologic heparin, possibly because the antibodies recognize PF4 bound to platelet-associated chondroitin sulfate (32).

"Spontaneous" HIT is a rare disorder in which a patient develops a clinical profile strongly suggestive of HIT and in whom high levels of HIT antibodies can be detected, despite no plausible history of recent (or even remote) heparin exposure (33).

Thrombosis and Other Sequelae

Thrombosis is the most important complication of HIT (Lists A) (28). The occurrence of thrombosis during or soon after stopping heparin therapy should prompt consideration of the diagnosis of HIT, since in some studies of postsurgical thromboprophylaxis with heparin, the development of symptomatic thrombosis indicated an approximate 50% risk of HIT (34).

List A   Thrombotic Complications of HIT
Venous thrombosis: Deep-vein thrombosis (DVT)[a], pulmonary embolism (PE)[a], venous
    limb gangrene, adrenal vein thrombosis[b], cerebral venous (dural sinus) thrombosis
Arterial thrombosis: Limb artery thrombosis, cerebral artery thrombosis, myocardial
    infarction, mesenteric artery thrombosis, miscellaneous artery thromboses (e.g.,
    renal artery thrombosis, spinal artery thrombosis)
Coumarin necrosis:[c] Venous limb gangrene, "classic" skin necrosis (subdermal and
    dermal necrosis, usually in non-acral sites, e.g., breast, abdominal wall, thigh, calf,
    or forearm); characterized by microvascular thrombosis
Skin lesions at heparin injection sites: Necrotizing skin lesions, erythematous skin lesions
    (plaques)
Anaphylactoid reactions post-intravenous bolus heparin:[d] Inflammatory (fever, chills,
    rigors, flushing), cardiac (chest pain or tightness, hypertension, tachycardia, cardiac
    arrest), respiratory (dyspnea, tachypnea, respiratory arrest), neurologic (pounding
    headache, transient global amnesia), gastrointestinal (large-volume diarrhea)
Overt (decompensated) disseminated intravascular coagulation (DIC):
    Laboratory: elevated prothrombin time, decreased fibrinogen, positive protamine
    sulfate paracoagulation assay, greatly elevated D-dimer levels, red cell fragments,
    normoblasts (nucleated red cells), increased lactate dehydrogenase
    Clinical: digital ischemic necrosis, venous limb gangrene, livedo reticularis

---

[a] DVT and PE are the two most common thrombotic sequelae of HIT.

[b] Adrenal vein thrombosis is the key factor accounting for adrenal hemorrhagic infarction.

[c] HIT is a risk factor for coumarin necrosis, particularly, venous limb gangrene.

[d] Anaphylactoid reactions characteristically begin 5–30 minutes after intravenous bolus heparin injection (rarely, after subcutaneous injection of LMWH).

The probability of thrombosis in HIT increases with the magnitude of the platelet count fall: Approximately half of patients exhibiting a 50% fall in platelet count develop thrombosis, whereas the risk increases to about 90% if the platelet count falls by 90% (17,34,35).

Lower-limb DVT is the most common thrombotic event in HIT, with approximately half of these patients exhibiting symptomatic PE (4,28). Upper-limb thrombosis is also common, and typically occurs at a central venous catheter site (36). Adrenal vein thrombosis manifests as adrenal hemorrhagic necrosis; when bilateral, this can cause death due to adrenal crisis (26,28). Cerebral venous (dural sinus) thrombosis is a rare but well-documented complication of HIT (31).

Arterial thrombosis is the "classic" presentation of HIT, which presumably reflected a diagnostic referral bias (since HIT was first discovered by vascular surgeons) (5). Lower limb artery thrombosis is most common, followed by thrombotic stroke and myocardial infarction (4,28). The ratio of venous to arterial thromboses in HIT is about 4:1 (4,17).

Microvascular thrombosis, most often manifesting as acral (distal extremity) ischemic necrosis despite palpable or doppler-identifiable pulses, can complicate especially severe HIT with overt (decompensated) DIC (28) (In contrast, limb artery thrombosis with platelet-rich "white clots" presents with absent pulses). Laboratory features can include elevated prothrombin time [international normalized ratio (INR)], hypofibrinogenemia, red cell fragmentation, and leukoerythroblastosis. However, in most cases, microvascular thrombosis is *iatrogenic*, as a result of coumarin therapy. The explanation is severe protein C depletion due to vitamin K antagonism together with failure of the coumarin to inhibit intense thrombin generation (6,7,9,10). A laboratory hallmark of coumarin-induced venous limb gangrene is a *supra*therapeutic INR, usually > 4.0, with acral ischemic necrosis in the same limb affected by symptomatic DVT. The explanation for the marked elevation in INR is a parallel severe decrease in factor VII. Less often, the non-acral presentation of coumarin-induced "skin necrosis" occurs with HIT (37). As discussed later, avoiding coumarin during the acute (thrombocytopenic) phase of HIT is one of the key tenets of management (1).

Other less common—although characteristic—clinical features of HIT include necrotizing and non-necrotizing skin lesions at heparin injection sites (38), acute anaphylactoid reactions following intravenous heparin bolus administration (28,39), and overt DIC (28,31).

CLINICAL SCORING SYSTEM FOR HIT

In evaluating a patient for possible HIT, a clinical scoring system may be of help (40). One system, the *4 Ts*, evaluates (*i*) *t*hrombocytopenia, (*ii*) its *t*iming, (*iii*) presence of *t*hrombosis (or other sequelae of HIT), and (*iv*) whether o*t*her plausible explanations for thrombocytopenia or thrombosis are present. Each criterion can be scored as 0, 1, or 2, depending on how well it fits HIT. A low score (three or fewer points) makes HIT unlikely (<2%). In some settings, a high score predicts a high likelihood of HIT (40).

LABORATORY DETECTION OF HIT ANTIBODIES

Laboratory detectability of HIT antibodies is a sine qua non of HIT diagnosis. There are two complementary ways to detect antibodies: (*i*) platelet activation assays, and (*ii*) PF4-dependent immunoassays (41). In general, the more abnormal the test result, the more likely the patient is to have HIT, given a certain pretest probability of having this diagnosis (19,21,42). Also, *acute* serum or plasma must be tested, as HIT antibodies are transient (29).

Platelet Activation Assays

HIT antibodies can be detected on the basis of their highly characteristic heparin- and Fcγ receptor-dependent platelet-activating properties. The typical platelet activation profile is "strong" platelet activation at pharmacologic (0.1–0.3 U/mL) but not at high heparin levels (100 U/mL). Washed platelet activation assays, e.g., the platelet serotonin-release assay (SRA) and the heparin-induced platelet activation (HIPA) test, have excellent operating characteristics (i.e., high sensitivity-specificity tradeoff) (21). Certain technical aspects of these assays are key to performance, such as "washing" the donor platelets in apyrase-containing buffer (so as to maintain sensitivity to adenosine diphosphate), using platelets from donors selected because their platelets react well to HIT antibodies, and utilizing "weak" positive control sera (to ensure the platelets are sufficiently reactive in any given experiment) (41,43). In contrast, conventional platelet aggregometry (using citrate-anticoagulated platelet-rich plasma) has a relatively low sensitivity for HIT (50–80%) (41), and is not recommended.

Enzyme-Immunoassays

PF4-dependent enzyme-immunoassays (EIAs) utilize PF4/heparin or PF4/polyvinyl sulfonate as targets. PF4-dependent EIAs are very sensitive for clinical HIT (~99%); hence, a negative test essentially rules out the diagnosis (16,41). Although EIAs are more sensitive than platelet activation assays for detecting anti-PF4/heparin antibodies, this is not an advantage, as more clinically *in*significant antibodies are detected, including non-platelet-activating IgA and IgM class antibodies in certain assays (potential for overdiagnosis). Indeed, only about half of all patient sera referred for testing for HIT antibodies in those of whom a positive EIA is obtained will also yield a positive result in a washed platelet-activation assay (16,19,21). In all likelihood, these patients do not have HIT, as their thrombosis risk is low, and an alternate explanation for thrombocytopenia is apparent (19).

Rapid Immunoassays

Two "rapid assays" for HIT based on particle agglutination have been developed (41). A "particle gel immunoassay" utilizes PF4/heparin complexes bound to red polystyrene beads; if anti-PF4/heparin antibodies are present, these often (but not always) result in agglutination of the polystyrene beads, which is evident when centrifugation is unable to cause migration of the beads through sephacryl gel. Unlike the EIAs, a negative test does not necessarily rule out HIT. This assay is not currently available in the United States. Another rapid assay, the "Particle ImmunoFiltration Assay" (PIFA), is being marketed in the United States, but its operating characteristics for HIT are poor (44).

Iceberg Model

The "iceberg" model of HIT (Fig. 3) indicates that only a small subset of anti-PF4/heparin antibodies evince pathogenicity; analogously, only a small portion (10%) of an iceberg protrudes above the waterline. Indeed, in one serosurveillance study, only 1 in 10 heparin-treated patients who formed antibodies (identified by EIA) developed clinical HIT (21). Even among patients who are tested because of some clinical suspicion of HIT, about half

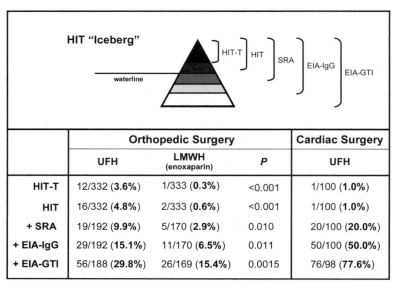

	Orthopedic Surgery			Cardiac Surgery
	UFH	LMWH (enoxaparin)	*P*	UFH
HIT-T	12/332 (**3.6%**)	1/333 (**0.3%**)	<0.001	1/100 (**1.0%**)
HIT	16/332 (**4.8%**)	2/333 (**0.6%**)	<0.001	1/100 (**1.0%**)
+ SRA	19/192 (**9.9%**)	5/170 (**2.9%**)	0.010	20/100 (**20.0%**)
+ EIA-IgG	29/192 (**15.1%**)	11/170 (**6.5%**)	0.011	50/100 (**50.0%**)
+ EIA-GTI	56/188 (**29.8%**)	26/169 (**15.4%**)	0.0015	76/98 (**77.6%**)

Figure 3 Iceberg model of HIT. The upper panel depicts a generic "iceberg," illustrating the interrelationship of clinical HIT with formation of anti-PF4/heparin antibodies detected by the platelet SRA, an enzyme-immunoassay that detects IgG class antibodies against PF4/heparin complexes (EIA-IgG), and a commercial EIA (from GTI, Inc., Waukesha, Wisconsin, U.S.) that detects antibodies of all three major immunoglobulin classes (IgG, IgA, IgM) against PF4/polyanion (EIA-GTI). The portion of the iceberg above the "waterline" depicts clinical HIT (HIT), including the subgroup with associated thrombosis (HIT-T). The lower panel illustrates the event rates for clinical HIT (HIT), HIT-associated thrombosis (HIT-T), in relation to the frequencies of antibody formation (for three different assays), observed in three clinical settings: UFH or LMWH thromboprophylaxis during orthopedic surgery (data shown are from a randomized controlled trial) (2,20,21) and UFH thromboprophylaxis postcardiac surgery (prospective cohort study) (45,46). + indicates positive test. *Abbreviations:* HIT, heparin-induced thrombocytopenia; SRA, serotonin release assay; EIA, enzyme-immunoassay; UFH, unfractionated heparin; LMWH, low-molecular-weight heparin; PF4, platelet factor 4. *Source*: From Ref. 24.

with a positive EIA do *not* have HIT on the basis of two considerations: (*i*) washed platelet activation assays yield negative results and (*ii*) the clinical profile suggests a more plausible explanation for the thrombocytopenia (16,19).

Interpretation of HIT Antibody Testing

Results of HIT antibody tests must be interpreted in the appropriate clinical context of pretest probability, the particular test performed, and the specific result obtained. Thus, a rigorous definition of HIT requires (*i*) the pretest probability to be intermediate or high, and (*ii*) a strong positive test for HIT antibodies, preferably using a washed platelet activation assay [e.g., >50% serotonin release (normal <20% release)]. However, despite its suboptimal specificity, in at least 80% to 90% of cases, an EIA result is nonetheless very informative as the diagnosis of HIT can be effectively ruled out (i.e., negative EIA), or effectively ruled in [EIA optical density (OD) >2.00 units (normal, <0.40 OD units) in an intermediate/high pretest probability situation]. However, when a positive EIA is obtained in a low probability setting, or a weak/moderate-positive EIA result (e.g., 0.4–2.0 OD units in some laboratories) occurs in a patient with a higher score, referral to a laboratory that performs a high-quality platelet activation assay can be helpful.

TREATMENT

The strong association between HIT and thrombosis, and the tendency for thrombotic events to occur early in the disease course, mean that many—perhaps most—patients have symptomatic thrombosis when HIT is diagnosed (2,4,17,20,24,27–29). Further, there is evidence that isolated HIT—defined as HIT recognized because of a platelet count decline (and without clinically-apparent thrombosis)—is subsequently complicated by thrombosis in one-third to one-half of cases (1,17,24,35). These concepts support the recommendation that a highly probable (or confirmed) diagnosis of HIT should be treated with an alternative non-heparin anticoagulant even in the absence of clinically apparent thrombosis (1). List B summarizes this and other principles of HIT management (47).

List B Principles of HIT Management—when HIT Is Strongly Suspected or Has Been Confirmed

Two *Do's*
  1. *Do* stop all heparin (including low-molecular-weight heparin and heparin administered as "flushes").
  2. *Do* start an alternative non-heparin anticoagulant, generally in therapeutic doses, e.g., danaparoid (not available in the United States), lepirudin, or argatroban (bivalirudin and fondaparinux are rational therapies, but supporting data are sparse and anecdotal, and these therapies are "off-label" for HIT).

Two *Don'ts*
  3. *Don't* give warfarin (or other coumarins) during the acute phase of HIT; if warfarin has already been started when HIT is diagnosed, vitamin K (e.g., 10 mg over 30 min by intravenous route) should be administered.
  4. *Don't* give prophylactic platelet transfusions.

Two *Diagnostics*
  1. *Diagnosis* laboratory support: Test for HIT antibodies (in 80–90% of cases, an EIA is sufficient to rule in or to rule out HIT in the appropriate clinical context; in the remaining cases, patient serum should be referred to a laboratory experienced in performed a washed platelet activation assay, e.g., serotonin release assay).
  2. *Diagnosis* of DVT: perform duplex ultrasonography to investigate for lower-limb DVT (the most common thrombotic sequela of HIT).

Source: Modified from Ref. 47

Alternative Non-Heparin Anticoagulants

Three alternative non-heparin anticoagulants—danaparoid, lepirudin, and argatroban (listed in order of market entry)—are approved for treatment of HIT (although approvals vary by jurisdiction) (1,48–50). A fourth agent, bivalirudin, is approved in the specific setting of anticoagulation during percutaneous transluminal coronary angioplasty, the most frequent type of percutaneous coronary intervention (PCI); it is also indicated for PCI with provisional use of glycoprotein IIb/IIIa antagonist therapy, and for patients with, or at risk of, HIT (with or without thrombosis) undergoing PCI (51). There are major differences in mechanism of action and pharmacologic properties between the antithrombin-dependent anticoagulant, danaparoid, and the (antithrombin-independent) DTIs, as well as among the DTIs themselves (Table 1) (1,48–53).

Only danaparoid was evaluated for HIT using a randomized controlled trial design, where it showed superior efficacy versus dextran-70, without major bleeding

Table 1 Comparison of Danaparoid with Direct Thrombin Inhibitor (DTI) Therapy for HIT

Feature	Danaparoid[a]	Direct thrombin inhibitors (DTIs)[b]	Comment
Mechanism of action	Indirect (AT-mediated) inhibition of factor Xa (minor thrombin inhibition)	Direct inhibition of thrombin (IIa); relative affinity for IIa: lepirudin > bivalirudin > argatroban	Theoretically, thrombin inhibition could compromise activated protein C generation in some circumstances
Influence on immune complexes	Both increase and decrease in HIT Ab-induced platelet activation reported in presence of danaparoid	No effect (theoretically, DTIs would not be expected to affect formation of PF4/glycosaminoglycan/IgG-immune complexes on platelet surface)	Theoretically, disruption of PF4-containing immune complexes by danaparoid could be therapeutically beneficial (52)
Half-life	Long (25h for anti-factor Xa inhibition)	Short: lepirudin, 80 min; argatroban, 45 min; bivalirudin, 25 min	Potential for abrupt rebound of hypercoagulability after stopping DTI (49)
Drug elimination	Predominantly renal	Variable: lepirudin, renal; argatroban, hepatobiliary; bivalirudin, proteolysis > renal	Minor (~30%) and major (>90%) dose reductions with danaparoid and lepirudin, respectively, for patients with severe renal failure (1)
Laboratory monitoring	Chromogenic anti-factor Xa level	Activated partial thromboplastin time (APTT); limited availability of direct drug assays	Use of APTT as a surrogate marker for estimating DTI levels can be problematic in some clinical circumstances (10, 49)
Influence on INR	No significant effect	DTIs prolong INR, as follows: argatroban > bivalirudin > lepirudin	Greater molar DTI levels required for anticoagulant effect (argatroban > bivalirudin > lepirudin) explain corresponding prolongation of the INR (53)

[a]Danaparoid is neither approved (nor currently available) for treatment of HIT in the United States
[b]DTIs = lepirudin, bivalirudin, argatroban.
Abbreviations: Ab, antibody; APTT, activated partial thromboplastin time; AT, antithrombin, DTI, direct thrombin inhibitor; INR, international normalized ratio; PF4, platelet factor 4.

complications (54). Danaparoid also exhibited superior efficacy, and reduced major bleeding, compared with controls (ancrod, warfarin, or both), in a historically-controlled retrospective study of patients with HIT confirmed by the SRA (55). An intriguing feature of danaparoid is that in therapeutic concentrations it often inhibits HIT antibody–induced platelet activation (52); the clinical relevance, if any, of this effect, or the contrary property of increasing antibody-induced platelet activation ("in vitro cross-reactivity") is uncertain.

Data supporting efficacy of the two DTIs, lepirudin and argatroban, evaluated in prospective cohort studies, and compared against historical controls, are presented in Table 2A (HIT-associated thrombosis) (1,56–60) and Table 2B (isolated HIT) (1,58–61). These agents appear to reduce the risk of thrombosis, compared with controls, although at the expense of increased bleeding.

Two other agents—bivalirudin and fondaparinux—are rational therapies for acute HIT (1,51,62,63), but little controlled data are available to support their use for acute HIT (64). On rare occasions, fondaparinux appears to cause HIT (26,65,66).

Warfarin Is Contraindicated During Acute HIT

Acute HIT is a risk factor for warfarin (coumarin) necrosis, manifesting either as venous limb gangrene or classic skin necrosis (6,7,10,28,37). The pathogenesis is microvascular thrombosis due to depletion of the vitamin K-dependent natural anticoagulant, protein C, together with increased thrombin generation from HIT (6,7).

Venous limb gangrene is characterized by (*i*) an underlying hypercoagulability disorder such as HIT or adenocarcinoma; (*ii*) acral (distal extremity) necrosis in a limb affected by DVT; and (*iii*) a supratherapeutic INR that is usually >4.0 (surrogate marker for severe protein C depletion) (6,7,67). In contrast, skin necrosis is characterized by the involvement of skin/subcutaneous tissues at central (non-acral) sites, e.g., breast, abdomen, thigh, calf (7).

Warfarin therapy is inimical to successful management of HIT for four reasons: (*i*) it does not inhibit HIT-associated hypercoagulability, (*ii*) it can lead to necrosis through protein C depletion, (*iii*) its prolongation of the activated partial thromboplastin time (APTT) can result in underdosing of DTI therapy (which is usually monitored by the APTT) (10), and (*iv*) the effect of warfarin on the INR is exacerbated by DTIs (especially argatroban), with the potential for a clinician to conclude incorrectly that a patient is adequately anticoagulated with warfarin too early during the DTI-warfarin overlap (1,6,7,53).

Treatment Overview

The treatment approach for acute HIT is to achieve sufficient anticoagulation with a rapidly acting non-heparin anticoagulant, usually given in therapeutic doses. Further, according to the 2008 ACCP guidelines (1), it is recommended that warfarin be avoided or postponed until substantial resolution of thrombocytopenia has occurred (usually, to a platelet count of 150×10^9/L or greater), that warfarin therapy only be started with low maintenance doses (maximum first dose, 5 mg), and that there be a minimum overlap of at least five days between non-heparin anticoagulation and warfarin. Further, for patients receiving warfarin at the time of diagnosis of HIT, vitamin K (10 mg p.o. or 5–10 mg IV) should be given.

Table 2A Summary of Studies of Efficacy and Safety of DTIs (Lepirudin, Argatroban) as Treatment of Thrombosis Complicating HIT

Study	Intervention/Dosing	New thrombosis	Amputation	Composite[a]	Major bleeds	Comment
Lubenow et al. 2005 (56)	Lep: Bolus 0.4 mg/kg; 0.15 mg/kg/h[b] Con: variable	Lep: 15/214 (7%) Con: 19/75 (25%) RR = 0.28 (0.15, 0.52) $P < 0.001$	Lep: 12/214 (6%) Con: 6/75 (8%) RR = 0.70 (0.27, 1.80) $P = 0.58$	Lep: 41/214 (19%) Con: 30/75 (40%) RR = 0.48 (0.32, 0.71) $P < 0.001$	Lep: 33/214 (15%)[c] Con: 5/75 (7%) RR = 2.31 (0.94, 5.71) $P = 0.072$	Pooled analysis of HAT-1, -2, -3 studies; analysis from start of treatment; all patients tested positive for HIT Abs
Lewis et al. (58–60)	Arg: 2 µg/kg/min (no bolus)[d] Con: variable	Arg: 58/373 (16%) Con: 16/46 (35%) RR = 0.45 (0.28, 0.71) $P = 0.0032$[e]	Arg: 53/373 (14%) Con: 5/46 (11%) RR = 1.26 (0.53, 2.99) $P = 0.81$	Arg: 158/373 (42%) Con: 26/46 (57%) RR = 0.75 (0.57, 0.99) $P = 0.083$[f]	Arg: 30/373 (8%)[c] Con: 1/46 (2%) RR = 3.70 (0.52, 26.5) $P = 0.23$	Pooled analysis of Arg-911, -915, and -915X studies[g]

Note: 95% CIs are provided for RRs (risk ratios); P values are Fishers exact test, 2-tailed, unless otherwise indicated.

[a]Composite end point: all-cause mortality, all-cause limb amputation, and/or new thrombosis (each patient counted only once).

[b]APTT adjusted to 1.5–2.5-times baseline APTT; mean lepirudin treatment duration was 15.8 days (for 214 lepirudin-treated patients).

[c]Major bleeding, expressed *per treatment day*, was 0.97% for lepirudin, and 1.25% for argatroban.

[d]APTT adjusted to 1.5–3.0-times baseline APTT; mean argatroban treatment duration was 6.6 days (for 373 argatroban-treated patients).

[e]$P < 0.001$ by log rank test (time-to-event analysis for proportion of patients event-free: note that 376, rather than 373, patients used for this analysis, as 3 patients initially deemed ineligible were subsequently determined to be eligible for analysis) (60).

[f]$P = 0.014$ and $P = 0.008$ for Arg-911 and Arg-915/915X studies, respectively, by log rank analysis (58, 59); P value for pooled data not available.

[g]Patients did not require positive test for HIT Abs: 65% of argatroban-treated patients tested positive for HIT Abs in Arg-911 study (58); data not available for the Arg-915/915X studies (59).

Abbreviations: Abs, antibodies; APTT, activated partial thromboplastin time; Arg, argatroban; Con, control; HAT, heparin-associated thrombocytopenia; Lep, lepirudin.

Source: Modified from Ref. 1.

Table 2B Summary of Studies of Efficacy and Safety of DTIs (Lepirudin, Argatroban) as Treatment of Isolated HIT

Study	Intervention/Dosing	New thrombosis	Amputation	Composite[a]	Major bleeds	Comment
Lubenow et al. 2004 (61)	Lep: No bolus; 0.10 mg/kg/h[b] Con: variable	Lep: 4/91 (4%) Con: 7/47 (15%) RR = 0.30 (0.09, 0.96) $P = 0.045$	Lep: 3/91 (3%) Con: 0/47 (0%) RR = 3.65 (0.19, 69.3) $P = 0.55$	Lep: 18/91 (20%) Con: 14/47 (30%) RR = 0.66 (0.36, 1.21) $P = 0.22$	Lep: 13/91 (14%)[c] Con: 4/47 (9%) RR = 1.68 (0.58, 4.86) $P = 0.42$	Pooled analysis of HAT-1, -2, -3 studies (all patients tested positive for HIT Abs)
Lewis et al. (58–60)	Arg: 2 μg/kg/min (no bolus)[d] Con: variable	Arg: 24/349 (7%) Con: 33/147 (22%) RR = 0.31 (0.19, 0.50) $P < 0.001$	Arg: 11/373 (3%) Con: 4/147 (3%) RR = 1.16 (0.37, 3.58) $P = 1.00$	Arg: 94/349 (27%) Con: 57/147 (39%) RR = 0.69 (0.53, 0.91) $P = 0.010$	Arg: 15/349 (4%) Con: 12/147 (8%) RR = 0.53 (0.25, 1.10) $P = 0.088$	Pooled analysis of Arg-911, -915, and -915X studies[e]

95% CIs are provided for RR's (risk ratios); P values are Fisher's exact test, 2-tailed, unless otherwise indicated.

[a]Composite end point: all-cause mortality, all-cause limb amputation, and/or new thrombosis (each patient counted only once).

[b]APTT adjusted to 1.5–2.5-times baseline APTT; also, mean lepirudin treatment duration was 13.9 days (pooled data).

[c]Major bleeding, expressed *per treatment day*, was 1.03% for lepirudin, and 0.84% for argatroban.

[d]APTT adjusted to 1.5–3.0-times baseline APTT; also, mean argatroban treatment duration was 5.2 days (pooled data).

[e]Patients did not require positive test for HIT Abs (50% of argatroban-treated patients tested positive for HIT Abs in the Arg-911 study; data not available for Arg-915 study).

Abbreviations: Abs, antibodies; APTT, activated partial thromboplastin time; Arg, argatroban; Con, control; HAT, heparin-associated thrombocytopenia; Lep, lepirudin

Source: Modified from Ref. 1.

Intravenous danaparoid is recommended to start with an initial bolus (2250 U for a patient weighing 60–75 kg), followed by a relatively high initial infusion rate (400 U/h for four hours, then 300 U/h for four hours), and then a somewhat lower constant infusion rate of 200 U/h (150 U/h for renal insufficiency), with subsequent intermittent boluses and/or dose rate increases (if subtherapeutic) or downward adjustments in infusion rate (if supratherapeutic) made on the basis of anti-factor Xa levels, if available (usual therapeutic range, 0.5–0.8 anti-factor Xa U/mL) (1). Subsequent warfarin overlap with danaparoid is straightforward, as the lack of effect of danaparoid on INR and its long half-life, make transition to warfarin relatively easy.

Recent studies (54,68) and expert opinion support using lepirudin dosing that is substantially *less* than that indicated in the manufacturers' package insert. For example, whereas the package insert recommends (for patients with normal renal function) an initial bolus (0.4 mg/kg) followed by an infusion starting at a rate of 0.15 mg/kg/h, the recent ACCP guidelines recommend avoiding the initial bolus and starting lepirudin at a dose of between 0.05 and 0.10 mg/kg/h (i.e., about one-third to two-third of the package insert dose). Similarly, the package insert dosing for argatroban (2 µg/kg/min without an initial bolus) should also be reduced (e.g., 0.5–1.2 µg/kg/min) in patients within intensive care unit settings or with congestive heart failure, besides the known situation of hepatobiliary disease (in which case a starting dose of 0.5 µg/kg/min is also recommended by the manufacturer). Besides reducing the risk of major bleeding, initial lower doses of DTI therapy may help to avoid thrombotic events by reducing the potential for interruption of therapy (because of supratherapeutic APTT values), with subsequent "rebound" in severe HIT-associated hypercoagulability (49).

In general, the initial parenteral anticoagulant (danaparoid or DTI) should be continued until the platelet count has reached a stable plateau within the normal range. This often takes *at least* one to two weeks. As already stated, warfarin (if given) should not be started until the platelet count has substantially recovered (usually, 150×10^9/L or greater). The ultimate duration of anticoagulant therapy depends mainly on the type of thrombotic event(s), if any. For patients with extensive DVT or PE, treatment for six months or more (usually with warfarin) may be appropriate. In contrast, for a patient with "isolated HIT" who demonstrates platelet count recovery to a stable plateau within two weeks, it is reasonable to simply discontinue the danaparoid or DTI, in the absence of lower-limb DVT (by ultrasonography) or any other indication for longer-term anticoagulation. Some physicians, however, prefer to administer warfarin or other anticoagulation for a few weeks after recovery of HIT, even in the absence of thrombosis. A theoretical approach (not yet described in the literature) would be to ensure transition from DTI therapy to fondaparinux and thus avoid warfarin completely. Since fondaparinux does not "cross-react" with HIT antibodies and is administered by subcutaneous injection, it could also facilitate discharge from hospital, besides avoiding the risks of vitamin K antagonism during management of acute HIT.

PREVENTION OF HIT AND ITS SEQUELAE

Platelet count monitoring for HIT is rational in certain higher risk situations, e.g., postoperative UFH thromboprophylaxis beyond four days. Here, *at least* every-other-day platelet count monitoring until day 14 or stopping heparin (whichever comes first) is suggested (1). Somewhat less frequent monitoring (e.g., twice or thrice weekly from day 4 to 14 while receiving UFH or LMWH) is suggested when the risk of HIT is lower, e.g., UFH prophylaxis or therapy in medical patients, or LMWH prophylaxis in postoperative patients. In settings where the risk is very low (e.g., LMWH treatment or prophylaxis in medical patients or during pregnancy; anticoagulation with fondaparinux), routine platelet count monitoring for HIT is not recommended (1). Regardless of the clinical situation, an urgent platelet count is usually appropriate when a patient who is receiving heparin—or who has recently received heparin—develops symptomatic thrombosis (1,17,34,35).

The reduced risk of HIT with LMWH (or fondaparinux) prophylaxis among postoperative patients—compared with UFH—suggests that HIT is a potentially preventable adverse drug reaction. It is uncertain whether there is also a reduced risk of HIT in medical patients given LMWH rather than UFH. This is either because the absolute risk of HIT is sufficiently low in medical patients that a true difference between the two heparin preparations is difficult to prove (the most likely situation) (69), or perhaps because no difference exists.

REPEAT HEPARIN EXPOSURE DESPITE PREVIOUS HIT

For patients with a previous history of HIT who have an important indication for heparin (e.g., cardiac or vascular surgery), it is recommended that they use heparin, provided that antibodies are no longer detectable, or (in emergencies) that sufficient time has elapsed from the episode of HIT (>2 or 3 months) so that clinically significant levels of antibodies are unlikely to be present (1,29). The basis for this recommendation is that it takes a minimum of five days to form clinically significant levels of HIT antibodies— even in patients with previous HIT—thus permitting safe intraoperative exposure. Further, there is no evidence that a patient with previous HIT is anymore likely to form high levels of HIT antibodies upon reexposure than anyone else. However, in situations where an alternative anticoagulant agent is available and safe (e.g., postoperative prophylaxis with danaparoid, fondaparinux, or warfarin), this may be preferred.

CONCLUSIONS AND FUTURE DIRECTIONS

The potential of heparin to induce a profound hypercoagulability state, and particularly of warfarin to exacerbate its clinical impact (e.g., coumarin-associated microvascular thrombosis), represents a striking paradox of anticoagulant therapy. Thus, new anticoagulants under development, such as oral factor Xa and/or thrombin inhibitors, have the potential both to reduce the risk of HIT (by leading to less use of heparin), as well as to simplify HIT therapy and even improve outcomes (by avoiding the risks of overlapping coumarin treatment).

ACKNOWLEDGMENTS

Some of the studies cited (2–7,10,11,15,17–24,26–31,33,34,36–47,49,51,53,55,63,65,67,69) were supported by the Heart and Stroke Foundation of Ontario (operating grants #A2449, #T2967, B3763, #T4502, #T5207, and #T6157).

REFERENCES

1. Warkentin TE, Greinacher A, Koster A, et al. Treatment and prevention of heparin-induced thrombocytopenia. American College of Chest Physicians evidence based clinical practice guidelines (8th edition). Chest 2008; 133(6 suppl):340s–380s.

2. Warkentin TE, Levine MN, Hirsh J, et al. Heparin-induced thrombocytopenia in patients treated with low-molecular-weight heparin or unfractionated heparin. N Engl J Med 1995; 332 (20):1330–1335.

3. Warkentin TE. Management of heparin-induced thrombocytopenia: a critical comparison of lepirudin and argatroban. Thromb Res 2003; 110(2–3):73–82.

4. Warkentin TE, Kelton JG. A 14-year study of heparin-induced thrombocytopenia. Am J Med 1996; 101(5):502–507.

5. Warkentin TE. History of heparin-induced thrombocytopenia. In: Warkentin TE, Greinacher A, eds. Heparin-Induced Thrombocytopenia. 4th ed. New York: Informa Healthcare USA, 2007:1–19.

6. Warkentin TE, Elavathil LJ, Hayward CPM, et al. The pathogenesis of venous limb gangrene associated with heparin-induced thrombocytopenia. Ann Intern Med 1997; 127(9):804–812.

7. Warkentin TE. Coumarin-induced skin necrosis and venous limb gangrene. In: Colman RW, Marder VJ, Clowes AW, et al., eds. Hemostasis and Thrombosis: Basic Principles and Clinical Practice. 5th ed. Philadelphia: Lippincott Williams & Wilkins, 2006:1663–1671.

8. Bartholomew JR, Hursting MJ. Transitioning from argatroban to warfarin in heparin-induced thrombocytopenia: an analysis of outcomes in patients with elevated international normalized ratio. J Thromb Thrombolysis 2005; 19(3):183–188.

9. Smythe MA, Warkentin TE, Stephens JL, et al. Venous limb gangrene during overlapping therapy with warfarin and a direct thrombin inhibitor for immune heparin-induced thrombocytopenia. Am J Hematol 2002; 71(1):50–52.

10. Warkentin TE. Should vitamin K be administered when HIT is diagnosed after administration of coumarin? J Thromb Haemost 2006; 4(4):894–896.

11. Warkentin TE. An overview of the heparin-induced thrombocytopenia syndrome. Semin Thromb Hemost 2004; 30(3):273–283.

12. Greinacher A, Pötzsch B, Amiral J, et al. Heparin-associated thrombocytopenia: isolation of the antibody and characterization of a multimolecular PF4-heparin complex as the major antigen. Thromb Haemost 1994; 71(2):247–251.

13. Greinacher A, Gopinadhan M, Guenther JU, et al. Close approximation of two platelet factor 4 tetramers by charge neutralization forms the antigens recognized by HIT antibodies. Arterioscler Thromb Vasc Biol 2006; 26(10):2386–2393.

14. Kelton JG, Sheridan D, Santos A, et al. Heparin-induced thrombocytopenia: laboratory studies. Blood 1988; 72(3):925–930.

15. Warkentin TE, Hayward CPM, Boshkov LK, et al. Sera from patients with heparin-induced thrombocytopenia generate platelet-derived microparticles with procoagulant activity: an explanation for the thrombotic complications of heparin-induced thrombocytopenia. Blood 1994; 84(11):3691–3699.

16. Greinacher A, Juhl D, Strobel U, et al. Heparin-induced thrombocytopenia: a prospective study on the incidence, platelet-activating capacity and clinical significance of anti-PF4/heparin antibodies of the IgG, IgM, and IgA classes. J Thromb Haemost 2007, 5(8):1666–1673.

17. Warkentin TE. Heparin-induced thrombocytopenia: pathogenesis and management. Br J Haematol 2003; 121(4):535–555.

18. Warkentin TE. Pseudo-heparin-induced thrombocytopenia. In: Warkentin TE, Greinacher A, eds. Heparin-Induced Thrombocytopenia. 4th ed. New York: Informa Healthcare USA, 2007, 261–282.

19. Lo GK, Sigouin CS, Warkentin TE. What is the potential for overdiagnosis of heparin-induced thrombocytopenia? Am J Hematol 2007; 82(12):1037–1043.

20. Warkentin TE, Roberts RS, Hirsh J, et al. An improved definition of immune heparin-induced thrombocytopenia in postoperative orthopedic patients. Arch Intern Med 2003; 163(20):2518–2524.

21. Warkentin TE, Sheppard JI, Moore JC, et al. Laboratory testing for the antibodies that cause heparin-induced thrombocytopenia: how much class do we need? J Lab Clin Med 2005; 146 (6):341–346. .

22. Warkentin TE, Sheppard JI, Siguoin CS, et al. Gender imbalance and risk factor interactions in heparin-induced thrombocytopenia. Blood 2006; 108(9):2937–2941.

23. Warkentin TE, Cook RJ, Marder VJ, et al. Anti-platelet factor 4/heparin antibodies in orthopedic surgery patients receiving antithrombotic prophylaxis with fondaparinux or enoxaparin. Blood 2005; 106(12):3791–3796.
24. Warkentin TE, Lee DH. Frequency of heparin-induced thrombocytopenia. In: Warkentin TE, Greinacher A, eds. Heparin-Induced Thrombocytopenia. 4th ed. New York: Informa Healthcare USA, 2007, 67–116.
25. Fausett MB, Vogtlander M, Lee RM, et al. Heparin-induced thrombocytopenia is rare in pregnancy. Am J Obstet Gynecol 2001; 185(1):148–152.
26. Warkentin TE, Maurer BT, Aster RH. Heparin-induced thrombocytopenia associated with fondaparinux. N Engl J Med 2007; 356(25):2653–2654.
27. Warkentin TE. Drug-induced immune-mediated thrombocytopenia: from purpura to thrombosis. N Engl J Med 2007; 356(9):891–893.
28. Warkentin TE. Clinical picture of heparin-induced thrombocytopenia. In: Warkentin TE, Greinacher A, eds. Heparin-Induced Thrombocytopenia. 4th ed. New York: Informa Healthcare USA, 2007, 21–66.
29. Warkentin TE, Kelton JG. Temporal aspects of heparin-induced thrombocytopenia. N Engl J Med 2001; 344(17):1286–1292.
30. Warkentin TE, Kelton JG. Delayed-onset heparin-induced thrombocytopenia and thrombosis. Ann Intern Med 2001; 135(7):502–506.
31. Warkentin TE, Bernstein RA. Delayed-onset heparin-induced thrombocytopenia and cerebral thrombosis after a single administration of unfractionated heparin. N Engl J Med 2003; 348 (11):1067–1069.
32. Rauova L, Zhai L, Kowalska MA, et al. Role of platelet surface PF4 antigenic complexes in heparin-induced thrombocytopenia pathogenesis: diagnostic and therapeutic implications. Blood 2006; 107(6):2346–2353.
33. Warkentin TE, Makris M, Jay RM, et al. A spontaneous prothrombotic disorder resembling heparin-induced thrombocytopenia. Am J Med 2008; 121(7):632–636.
34. Warkentin TE. Think of HIT when thrombosis follows heparin. Chest 2006; 130(3): 631–632.
35. Greinacher A, Farner B, Kroll H, et al. Clinical features of heparin-induced thrombocytopenia including risk factors for thrombosis. A retrospective analysis of 408 patients. Thromb Haemost 2005; 94(1):132–135.
36. Hong AP, Cook DJ, Sigouin CS, Warkentin TE. Central venous catheters and upper-extremity deep-vein thrombosis complicating immune heparin-induced thrombocytopenia. Blood 2003; 101(8):3049–3051.
37. Warkentin TE, Sikov WM, Lillicrap DP. Multicentric warfarin-induced skin necrosis complicating heparin-induced thrombocytopenia. Am J Hematol 1999; 62(1):44–48.
38. Warkentin TE. Heparin-induced skin lesions. Br J Haematol 1996; 92(2):494–497.
39. Warkentin TE, Hirte HW, Anderson DR, et al. Transient global amnesia following intravenous heparin bolus therapy is caused by heparin-induced thrombocytopenia. Thromb Haemost 1994; 97(5):489–491.
40. Lo GK, Juhl D, Warkentin TE, et al. Evaluation of pretest clinical score (4 T's) for the diagnosis of heparin-induced thrombocytopenia in two clinical settings. J Thromb Haemost 2006; 4(4): 759–765.
41. Warkentin TE, Sheppard JI. Testing for heparin-induced thrombocytopenia antibodies. Transfus Med Rev 2006; 20(4):259–272.
42. Warkentin TE, Sheppard JI, Moore JC, et al. Quantitative interpretation of optical density measurements using PF4-dependent enzyme-immunoassays. J Thromb Haemost 2008; 6(8): 1304–1312.
43. Warkentin TE, Hayward CPM, Smith CA, et al. Determinants of donor platelet variability when testing for heparin-induced thrombocytopenia. J Lab Clin Med 1992; 120(3):371–379.
44. Warkentin TE, Sheppard JI, Raschke R, et al. Performance characteristics of a rapid assay for anti-PF4/heparin antibodies: the particle immunofiltration assay. J Thromb Haemost 2007; 5(11): 2308–2310.

45. Warkentin TE. Sheppard JI, Horsewood P, Simpson PJ, Moore JC, Kelton JG et al. Impact of the patient population on the risk for heparin-induced thrombocytopenia. Blood 2000; 96 (5):1703–1708.

46. Warkentin TE, Sheppard JI. No significant improvement in diagnostic specificity of an anti-PF4/polyanion immunoassay with use of high heparin confirmatory procedure. J Thromb Haemost 2006; 4(1):281–282.

47. Warkentin TE, Greinacher A, eds. Six treatment principles of HIT (Appendix 12). In: Heparin-induced thrombocytopenia; 4th ed. New York, Informa Healthcare USA, 2007:p. 544.

48. Chong BH, Magnani HN. Danaparoid for the treatment of heparin-induced thrombocytopenia. In: Warkentin TE, Greinacher A, eds. Heparin-Induced Thrombocytopenia. 4th ed. New York: Informa Healthcare USA, 2007:319–343.

49. Greinacher A, Warkentin TE. The direct thrombin inhibitor hirudin. Thromb Haemost 2008; 99(5):819–829.

50. Lewis BE, Hursting MJ. Argatroban therapy in heparin-induced thrombocytopenia. In: Warkentin TE, Greinacher A, eds. Heparin-Induced Thrombocytopenia. 4th ed. New York: Informa Healthcare USA, 2007:379–408.

51. Warkentin TE, Greinacher A, Koster A. Bivalirudin. Thromb Haemost 2008; 99(5):830–839.

52. Chong BH, Ismail F, Cade J, et al. Heparin-induced thrombocytopenia: studies with a new low molecular weight heparinoid, Org 10172. Blood 1989; 73(6):1592–1596.

53. Warkentin TE, Greinacher A, Craven S, et al. Differences in the clinically effective molar concentrations of four direct thrombin inhibitors explain their variable prothrombin time prolongation. Thromb Haemost 2005; 94(5):958–964.

54. Chong BH, Gallus AS, Cade JF, et al. Prospective randomized open-label comparison of danaparoid with dextran 70 in the treatment of heparin-induced thrombocytopenia with thrombosis: a clinical outcome study. Thromb Haemost 2001; 86(5):1170–1175.

55. Lubenow N, Warkentin TE, Greinacher A, et al. Results of a systematic evaluation of treatment outcomes for heparin-induced thrombocytopenia in patients receiving danaparoid, ancrod, and/or coumarin explain the rapid shift in clinical practice in the 1990s. Thromb Res 2006; 117 (5):507–515.

56. Lubenow N, Eichler P, Lietz T, et al. Lepirudin in patients with heparin-induced thrombocytopenia—results of the third prospective study (HAT-3) and a combined analysis of HAT-1, HAT-2, and HAT-3. J Thromb Haemost 2005; 3(11):2428–2436.

57. Greinacher A, Eichler P, Lubenow N, et al. Heparin-induced thrombocytopenia with thromboembolic complications: meta-analysis of two prospective trials to assess the value of parenteral treatment with lepirudin and its therapeutic aPTT range. Blood 2000; 96(3):846–851.

58. Lewis BE, Wallis DE, Berkowitz SD, et al. Argatroban anticoagulant therapy in patients with heparin-induced thrombocytopenia. Circulation 2001; 103(14):1838–1843.

59. Lewis BE, Wallis DE, Leya F, et al. Argatroban anticoagulation in patients with heparin-induced thrombocytopenia. Arch Intern Med 2003; 163(15):1849–1856.

60. Lewis BE, Wallis DE, Hursting MJ, et al. Effects of argatroban therapy, demographic variables, and platelet count on thrombotic risks in heparin-induced thrombocytopenia. Chest 2006; 129 (6):1407–1416.

61. Lubenow N, Eichler P, Lietz T, et al. Lepirudin for prophylaxis of thrombosis in patients with acute isolated heparin-induced thrombocytopenia: an analysis of 3 prospective studies. Blood 2004; 104(10):3072–3077.

62. Bradner JE, Eikelboom JW. Emerging anticoagulants and heparin-induced thrombocytopenia: indirect and direct factor Xa inhibitors and oral thrombin inhibitors. In: Warkentin TE, Greinacher A, eds. Heparin-Induced Thrombocytopenia, 4th ed. New York: Informa Healthcare USA, 2007, 441–461.

63. Warkentin TE. Fondaparinux versus direct thrombin inhibitor therapy for the management of heparin-induced thrombocytopenia (HIT)—bridging the River Coumarin. Thromb Haemost 2008; 99(1):2–3.

64. Lobo B, Finch C, Howard A, et al. Fondaparinux for the treatment of patients with acute heparin-induced thrombocytopenia. Thromb Haemost 2008; 99(1):208–214.

65. Warkentin TE, Lim W. Can heparin-induced thrombocytopenia be associated with fondaparinux use? Reply to a rebuttal. J Thromb Haemost 2008; 6:1243–1246.
66. Rota E, Bazzan M, Fantino G. Fondaparinux-related thrombocytopenia in a previous low-molecular-weight heparin (LMWH)-induced heparin-induced thrombocytopenia (HIT). Thromb Haemost 2008; 99(4):779–781.
67. Warkentin TE. Venous limb gangrene during warfarin treatment of cancer-associated deep venous thrombosis. Ann Intern Med 2001; 135(8 pt 1):589–593.
68. Tardy B, Lecompte T, Boelhen F, et al. Predictive factors for thrombosis and major bleeding in an observational study in 181 patients with heparin-induced thrombocytopenia treated with lepirudin. Blood 2006; 108(5):1492–1496.
69. Warkentin TE, Greinacher A. So, does low-molecular-weight heparin cause less heparin-induced thrombocytopenia than unfractionated heparin or not? Chest 2007; 132(4):1108–1110.

17

Emerging Links Between Thrombosis, Inflammation, and Angiogenesis: Key Role of Heparin and Low-Molecular-Weight Heparins

Shaker A. Mousa
The Pharmaceutical Research Institute, Albany College of Pharmacy/Medicine, Albany, New York, U.S.A.

INTRODUCTION

Heparin was discovered in 1916 by Jay McLean and William Henry Howell, but was not used in humans until 1935 (1,2). It was originally isolated from canine liver cells, hence its name (*"hepar"* is Greek for liver). Howell isolated a water-soluble polysaccharide anticoagulant, which was also termed "heparin," although it was distinct from the previously isolated phosphatide preparations. The first human trials of heparin began in 1935 and, by 1937, it was clear that Connaught's heparin was a safe, readily available, and effective anticoagulant (3).

Current commercial heparin is extracted from porcine intestine. Heparin is produced by basophils and mast cells, which are abundant in the intestinal mucosa. Heparin acts as an anticoagulant, preventing the formation of new or extension of existing thrombi. Heparin also accelerates thrombolysis when used in conjunction with fibrinolytics (4,5). In recent years, the potential limitations of heparin for the prevention and treatment of thromboembolic disorders have been revealed. These limitations have prompted the development of heparin derivatives, such as low-molecular-weight heparin (LMWH), which have expanded the options for the management of thromboembolic disorders and enhanced the safety of therapy. In the United States, LMWHs are currently approved for the prophylaxis and treatment of deep-vein thrombosis (DVT). LMWHs are also indicated for the management of unstable angina and non-ST-elevation myocardial infarction (MI) (6–9). In addition to the approved uses, LMWHs are currently being tested for several other indications (Table 1).

Table 1 Potential Utility of Heparin Beyond Anticoagulation

Disease states sensitive to heparin	Heparin's effect in experimental models	Clinical status
Adult respiratory distress syndrome	Reduces cell activation and accumulation in airways, neutralizes mediators and cytotoxic cell products, and improves lung function in animal models.	Clinical trials
Allergic rhinitis	Effects as for adult respiratory distress syndrome, although no specific nasal model has been tested.	Clinical trial
Asthma	As for adult respiratory distress syndrome, however, it has also been shown to improve lung function in experimental models.	Clinical trials
Cancer	Inhibits tumor growth, metastasis, and angiogenesis and increases survival time in animal models.	Anecdotal report and clinical trials
Inflammatory bowel disease	Inhibits inflammatory cell transport in general. No specific model tested.	Clinical trials

HEPARIN VS. LMWH

LMWHs exhibit improved pharmacodynamic and pharmacokinetic profiles over unfractionated heparin (UFH), including subcutaneous (SC) bioavailability; lower protein binding; longer half-life; variable number of antithrombin III binding sites; variable glycosaminoglycan contents; variable anti-serine protease activities (anti-Xa, anti-IIa, anti-Xa/anti-IIa ratio, and anti-other coagulation factors); and variable potency in releasing TFPI from vascular endothelial cells (10–16). For these reasons, over the last decade LMWHs have increasingly replaced UFH in the prevention and treatment of venous thromboembolic (VTE) disorders. Randomized clinical trials have demonstrated that individual LMWHs used at optimized dosages are at least as effective as and probably safer than UFH. The convenient once- or twice-daily SC dosing regimen, without the need for monitoring, has encouraged the wide use of LMWHs. It is well established that different LMWHs vary in their physical and chemical properties because of the differences in their methods of manufacturing. These differences translate into differences in their pharmacodynamic and pharmacokinetic characteristics (17,18).

EMERGING LINKS BETWEEN THROMBOSIS AND INFLAMMATION: ROLE OF HEPARIN/LMWH

Several lines of evidence have demonstrated the interplay between activated platelets and the coagulation system. Platelet activation triggers a conformational change in the platelet GPIIb/IIIa receptor that endows it with the capacity to bind fibrinogen. By bridging platelets together, platelet-bound fibrinogen mediates platelet aggregation. Activated platelets also interact with leukocytes. Platelet-leukocyte cohesion causes leukocyte activation. Once activated, platelets also provide a surface onto which coagulation factors assemble and promote thrombin generation. Thrombin then serves as a potent platelet and leukocyte activator.

Interplay among the coagulation system, platelets, and the vessel wall promotes thrombosis. Depending upon shear, the proportion of platelets and fibrin in thrombi varies.

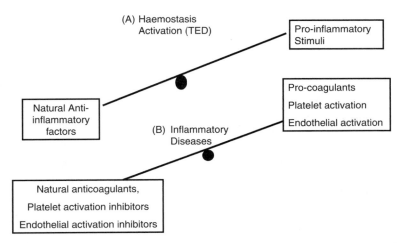

Figure 1 Illustration of hemostasis activation in inflammatory diseases and increased inflammation in TED. Imbalance between pro-inflammatory and natural anti-inflammatory mediators is shown in TED patients. In contrast, imbalance between procoagulant and natural anticoagulant mediators is shown in inflammatory disorders. *Abbreviation*: TED, thromboembolic disorders.

Venous thrombi, which form under low-shear conditions, are rich in fibrin, whereas arterial thrombi, which form under high shear, are composed predominantly of platelets.

Sepsis can trigger pro-inflammatory stimuli that lead to thrombosis. For example, endotoxin liberated from *Escherichia coli* or other bacteria can induce the release of tissue necrosis factor (TNF)-α and other cytokines (Fig. 1) that can activate leukocytes. Increased expression of L-selectin on the leukocyte surface and soluble L-selectin in the plasma can serve as surrogate markers of leukocyte activation. Activation of leukocytes results in tissue factor (TF) expression, which initiates coagulation and up-regulates TNF-α production (Fig. 1). This leads to a hypercoaguable state characterized by thrombin generation. Thrombin activates platelets and induces P-selectin expression on the platelet surface. Soluble P-selectin can serve as a surrogate marker of platelet activation (19).

Inflammatory cytokines can induce endothelial cell insult, leading to the expression of adhesion molecules, such as vascular adhesion molecule-1 (VCAM-1), intracellular adhesion molecule-1 (ICAM-1), and E-selectin. The emerging links between thrombosis, angiogenesis, and inflammation in vascular, cardiovascular, and inflammatory disorders are illustrated in Fig. 2. Both Figures 1 and 2 illustrate and support the interplay between inflammation-angiogenesis-thrombosis and the potential role of TF/VIIa in these processes. The impact of heparin-releasable TFPI is highlighted in Fig. 3.

Heparin and LMWH have anti-inflammatory activity in addition to their anticoagulant effects (20,21). In animal models, heparin disaccharides inhibit TNF-α production by macrophages and decrease immune inflammation (22). Heparin accelerates mucosal healing in colitis and has other anti-inflammatory effects (23–28).

Potential Anti-inflammatory Mechanisms of Heparin/LMWH

LMWH is used in the treatment and prevention of thrombotic and thromboembolic conditions like DVT, pulmonary embolism (PE), and crescendo angina (29–31). Additionally, heparin/LMWH possesses non-anticoagulant properties, including modulation of various proteases, anti-complement activity, and anti-inflammatory actions.

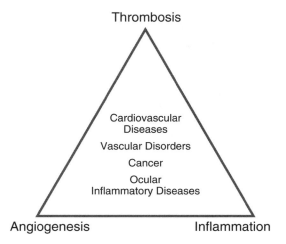

Figure 2 Emerging links between thrombosis, angiogenesis, and inflammation in vascular, cardiovascular, and inflammatory diseases. Interplay between thrombosis, inflammation, and angiogenesis is shown in various vascular-related disorders.

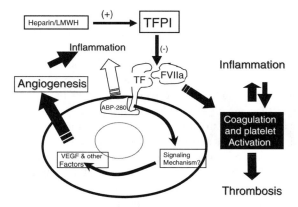

Figure 3 TF/VIIa in angiogenesis, inflammation, and thrombosis: impact of heparin-releasable endothelial cell TFPI in the modulation of these processes. *Abbreviation*: TF, tissue factor.

Inhaled heparin has been shown to reduce the early phase of the asthmatic reaction and to suppress allergen-induced bronchial hyperreactivity. Heparin also inhibits the acute cutaneous reaction due to allergens. The ubiquitous distribution of heparin in tissue spaces may serve to limit inflammatory responses in various tissues where leukocytes accumulate after an inflammatory challenge. It is interesting that heparin is found in high concentrations in the gastrointestinal tract and the lung (29,30), the two organs exposed to the external environment.

A few studies have reported an effect of heparin on reactive oxygen species' (ROS) generation (32) and cytokine secretion (33) by leukocytes, in vitro. It has been recently demonstrated that heparin, when injected intravenously into healthy subjects at a dose of 10,000 IU, inhibits ROS generation by mononuclear cells (MNCs) and polymorphonucleocytes (PMNs) (34). Heparin has been also shown, in a series of experiments using *N*-acetyl heparin, to protect the heart from ischemia-reperfusion injury both in vivo and in vitro, independently of its antithrombin mechanism (35,36). It was suggested that this protection may be due to a reduction in complement activation-mediated injury to the heart (36). Since ischemia-reperfusion injury may also be mediated by oxidative damage (37), it is possible that the protective effect of heparin may be due to an inhibition of ROS generation. A reduction in superoxide radical formation by heparin is likely to allow greater bioavailability of nitric oxide (NO) for vasodilatation. In fact, heparin has been shown to exert a vasodilatory effect in normal subjects (38). Increased bioavailability of NO may have an additional beneficial effect; inhibition of leukocyte adhesion to the endothelium, which would, in turn, inhibit or retard inflammation (39). In addition, NO inhibits the pro-inflammatory transcription factor-nuclear factor (NF-κB), which plays a central role in the triggering and coordinating of both innate and adaptive immune responses.

Heparin/LMWH and Asthma

Heparin exists in mast cells where it is thought to control the release of allergic mediators, such as histamine, in addition to its direct anti-inflammatory effects. Hence, the potential utility of heparin inhalation in asthma was evaluated by various groups. Heparin may attenuate mast cell degranulation by blocking internal calcium release. Heparin may also reduce eosinophil recruitment directly by preventing mast cell mediator release or indirectly by down-regulating adhesion molecule expression, thereby limiting eosinophil migration into the nasal mucosa (40–42). Furthermore, heavily anionic heparin may inactivate platelet-activating factor, a cationic protein with potent chemotactic activity for human eosinophils. Intranasal heparin has been shown to attenuate the nasal response to an allergic challenge in subjects with rhinitis (40–42). More studies are needed to better define the anti-inflammatory properties of heparin so as to optimize its use in allergic diseases, such as rhinitis and asthma.

Small, clinical trials have evaluated the utility of heparin in a range of inflammatory diseases, including rheumatoid arthritis, bronchial asthma (43,44), and inflammatory bowel disease (Table 1). Heparin was used at doses that are unlikely to produce hemorrhagic complications (45). Although more work is needed, it is likely that the anti-inflammatory actions of heparin are distinct from its anticoagulant activity (46,47).

Heparin/LMWH and Inflammatory Bowel Diseases

Under various experimental and clinical conditions, heparin was found to actively reduce the process of leukocyte recruitment to sites of injury or application of inflammatory stimuli. Carr (48) provide insight into the mechanism responsible for the anti-migratory action of heparin. In fact, intravital microscopy techniques have allowed direct observation of inflamed microvascular beds with definition of the paradigm of white blood cell extravasation. Leukocyte's interaction with the endothelium of an inflamed post-capillary venule is initially intermittent and dynamic (cell rolling); then becomes static (firm adhesion), and is finally followed by diapedesis (49). Using the potent cytokine, TNF-α, to promote this cascade of events in vivo, Salas and colleagues reported (47) that heparin down-regulated TNF-α-induced leukocyte rolling, adhesion, and migration into gut tissue without affecting changes in vascular permeability. These data extend and confirm previous studies in which heparin reduced leukocyte adhesion to vascular endothelial cells in vitro (50) and recruitment of inflammatory cells into other tissues during an experimental inflammatory reaction (47).

Several uncontrolled studies have suggested that heparin may be useful in the clinical management of both ulcerative colitis and Crohn's disease. Although these studies included only a limited number of patients, they demonstrated apparent beneficial effects of heparin with no associated hemorrhagic complications (45,51–57). In addition, heparin has been shown to prevent macroscopic inflammatory lesions in an animal model of experimental colitis. However, the molecular mechanisms by which heparin may help patients with inflammatory bowel disease are unknown.

A large body of evidence supports the concept that heparin has anti-inflammatory actions, which include modulation of some of the pathophysiological effects of endotoxin and TNF-α, such as neutrophil migration, edema formation, pulmonary hypertension, and hypoxemia (20–23,25). Moreover, heparin has been shown to suppress selected neutrophil functions, such as superoxide generation (26) and chemotaxis in vitro (27,28), to reduce eosinophil migration (26) and to diminish vascular permeability (58,59). Among the mechanisms that may account for the anti-inflammatory actions of heparin, binding of this glycosaminoglycan to adhesion molecules expressed on the surface of activated endothelial cells and/or leukocytes has been proposed. Recent in vitro studies have demonstrated the ability of heparin to effectively bind to endothelial P-selectin, but not E-selectin (20,60), as well as L-selectin and CD11b/CD18 expressed on neutrophils (60–62). Taken together, these reports suggest that the therapeutic actions of heparin observed in patients with inflammatory bowel disease may involve attenuation of inflammatory processes, as well as suppression of the hypercoaguable state associated with exacerbation of these disorders, effects that may promote mucosal repair.

EMERGING LINKS BETWEEN THROMBOSIS AND CANCER: KEY ROLE OF HEPARIN/LMWH

The association between coagulation system activation and systemic thrombosis in human cancers (Table 2) has been recognized for over a century since Trousseau's original description of migratory thrombophlebitis complicating gastrointestinal malignancy (64). In recent years, an improved appreciation of the interdependency of the coagulation system and malignant behavior has led to an understanding of how an activated coagulation system may enhance cancer cell growth (65). While this does not establish causality or even a biologic association, it is of interest that a recent Danish study showed that patients with cancer, who developed venous thrombosis during the course of their disease, had significantly shorter cancer-related survival than similar patients who remained thrombosis free (66). Resting on a greater strength of evidence, some, but not all studies, have documented improved cancer-related survival in patients treated with anticoagulants compared with those not receiving anticoagulants (67–72).

Table 2 Mechanisms of Tumor-Mediated Hypercoaguable States

Malignant tumor promotes the following

- Tumor cell surface TF
- Macrophage TF
- Expression of cell surface phospholipids that support coagulation activation
- Other tumor-mediated platelet activation and accumulation
- Tumor-induced endothelial cell activation
- Tumor-mediated monocyte activation
- Tumor-mediated fibrin generation

Abbreviation: TF, tissue factor.
Source: Modified from Ref. 63.

A recent study suggests that thromboembolic events are important predictors of cancer (71). Cancer screening in patients without identifiable risk factors for thrombosis might improve the prognosis of cancer patients (66,71). Thrombin generation and fibrin formation are often detectable in patients with malignancy who are at increased risk of thromboembolic complications (71–77). Most importantly, fibrin formation is also involved in the processes of tumor spread and metastasis. Activation of blood coagulation in cancer is a complex phenomenon, involving many different pathways of the hemostatic system and numerous interactions of the tumor cell with other blood cells, including platelets, monocytes, and endothelial cells. Tumor cells possess the capacity to interact with all parts of the hemostatic system. They can directly activate the coagulation cascade by producing their own procoagulant factors, or they can stimulate the prothrombotic properties of other blood cell components.

The etiology of thrombosis in malignancy is multifactorial; mechanisms include the release of procoagulants by tumor cells plus other predisposing factors, leading to a hypercoagulable state that is amplified by chemotherapeutic and radiotherapeutic agents (72–77). Unexplained thromboembolism may be an early indicator of the presence of a malignant tumor before signs and symptoms of the tumor itself become obvious (Table 2).

Hemostatic abnormalities are present in a majority of patients with metastatic cancer. These abnormalities can be categorized as increased platelet aggregation and activation, abnormal activation of the coagulation cascade, increased levels of plasminogen activator inhibitor type 1 (PAI-1), and decreased hepatic synthesis of anticoagulant proteins, such as protein C and antithrombin. Activation of the coagulation cascade is mediated through expression of TF and other procoagulants from the plasma membrane vesicles of tumor cells (72,74,77). Increasing evidence suggests that thrombotic episodes may also precede the diagnosis of cancer by months or years, thus representing a potential marker for occult malignancy (73). Recently, emphasis has been given to the potential risk of cancer therapy (both surgery and chemotherapy) in enhancing the risk for thromboembolic disease (74,76). Postoperative DVT is more frequent in patients who have undergone surgery for malignant diseases than for other disorders. On the other hand, both chemotherapy and hormone therapy are associated with an increased thrombotic risk, which can be prevented by low-dose oral anticoagulation (78,79). The procoagulant activities of tumor cells have been extensively studied; specific tumor procoagulants could represent a prognostic marker of malignancy.

Reports from animal studies have indicated that metastasis can be inhibited by UFH. There have also been clinical reports suggesting survival benefits from UFH and LMWH that go beyond their antithrombotic effects. Evidence from several experiments has suggested various possible antineoplastic mechanisms for heparin and heparin derivatives (Table 3). However, the primary antineoplastic mechanism for heparin still remains to be clinically defined. Several heparin-derived compounds demonstrate anti-inflammatory, anti-allergic, and anti-metastasis activities (Table 4).

Heparin/LMWH in Platelets–Cancer Cell Adhesion and Angiogenesis/Metastasis

Activated platelets not only release angiogenic growth factors, but also contain anti-angiogenic factors. Therefore, the balance between pro- and anti-angiogenic factors may be critical, and it has been proposed that activated platelets in cancer contribute to tumor angiogenesis in the tumor microenvironment (80–82). Growth factors in platelets include the following: vascular endothelial growth factor (VEGF), basic fibroblast growth factor (bFGF), and platelet-derived growth factor (PDGF) (80–82). A role for platelets in tumor

Table 3 Heparin Effect in Cancer

Inhibits	Stimulates
• Angiogenesis	• Immune system
• Proteases	• Differentiation and apoptosis
• Growth factors	• NO production
• Coagulation factors	• TFPI release
• Oncogene expression	
• Free radical generation	
• Inflammation via NF-κB	

Abbreviation: NO, nitric oxide.
Source: Modified from Ref. 63.

Table 4 Effect of Heparin-derived Compounds Compared to Heparin

Heparin-derived compounds	Heparin-derived compounds compared to heparin	Biological activities
Heparin tetrasaccharide	Non-anticoagulant, non-immunogenic, orally active	Anti-allergic
Pentosan polysulfate	Plant derived, little anticoagulant activity, anti-inflammatory, orally active	Anti-inflammatory, anti-adhesive, anti-metastatic
Phosphomannopentanose sulfate	Potent inhibitor of heparanase activity	Anti-metastatic, anti-angiogenic, anti-inflammatory
Selectively chemically O-desulfated heparin	Non-anticoagulant	Anti-inflammatory, anti-allergic, anti-adhesive

biology has been suggested (83). Serum levels of VEGF have been shown to correlate with platelet counts during chemotherapy (84). Platelet–tumor cell interactions are believed to be important in tumor metastasis. Tumor cell TF expression enhances metastasis and angiogenesis, and is primarily responsible for tumor-induced thrombin generation and the formation of tumor cell–platelet aggregates. Activated platelets express and release CD40 ligand (CD40L), which induces endothelial TF expression by ligation to CD40. Recent data suggested that, in malignancy, the increase in cellular TF activity via CD40 (tumor cell)-CD40L (platelet) interactions may enhance intravascular coagulation and hematogenous metastasis (85). Inhibition of experimental metastasis and tumor growth was demonstrated in animals by inducing thrombocytopenia or with antiplatelet therapies (86,87).

Cancer disturbs cellular activities that maintain multicellular organisms; namely, growth, differentiation, apoptosis, and tissue integrity. There are numerous clinical and experimental observations showing that invasion results from the cross talk between cancer cells and host cells (i.e., platelets, myofibroblasts, endothelial cells, and leukocytes, all of which are themselves invasive). In bone metastasis, host osteoclasts serve as targets for therapy. The molecular analysis of invasion-associated cellular activities (namely, homotypic and heterotypic cell-cell adhesion, cell-matrix interactions, and ectopic survival, migration, and proteolysis) reveals branching signal transduction pathways with extensive networks between individual pathways. The role of proteolysis in invasion is not limited to the breakdown of the extracellular matrix, but also includes cleavage of pro-invasive fragments from cell-surface glycoproteins (GPs).

In vivo, tumor cells interact with a variety of host cells, such as endothelial cells and platelets, and these interactions are mediated by integrins GPIIb/IIIa and $\alpha v\beta 3$. In a xenograft model, m7E3 Fab$_2$ binds to both human tumor and host platelet GPIIb/IIIa and endothelial $\alpha v\beta 3$ integrins, thus serving as an anti-angiogenic and antitumor agent. Data have suggested that combined blockade of GPIIb/IIIa and $\alpha v\beta 3$ affords significant anti-angiogenic and antitumor benefits (88).

Classic studies have indicated that the formation of tumor cell–platelet complexes in the bloodstream is important in facilitating the metastasis process. Metastasis in animal models can be inhibited by heparin, and retrospective analyses suggest that heparin use in human cancer may be beneficial (89).

Role of Coagulation in Angiogenesis and its Modulation by Heparin/LMWH

The coagulation system, which is activated in most cancer patients, plays an important role in tumor biology. It may make a substantial contribution to tumor angiogenesis, which represents an imbalance in the normal mechanisms that allow organized healing after injury (90). The recently recognized, but steadily growing, knowledge of the relationship between the coagulation and angiogenesis pathways has research and clinical implications. Manipulation of these systems may minimize both the neo-angiogenesis factors essential for tumor growth and associated thromboembolic complications.

Angiogenesis is a process that is dependent on coordinated production of stimulatory and inhibitory (angiostatic) molecules, and any imbalance in this regulatory circuit might lead to the development of a number of angiogenesis-mediated diseases. The steps in the angiogenesis process include activation, adhesion, migration, proliferation, and transmigration of endothelial cells across cell matrices to or from new capillaries and from existing vessels. A combined defect, representing overproduction of positive regulators of angiogenesis and a deficiency in endogenous angiostatic mediators, has been documented in tumor angiogenesis, psoriasis, rheumatoid arthritis, and other neo-vascularization-mediated disorders (91,92).

In various experimental models, LMWH has been shown to have potent anti-angiogenesis effects, inhibit tumor growth, and suppress metastasis (59,63,93). Additionally, the heparin-sensitive endothelial P-selectin has been shown to be involved in metastasis (94). Many cancer patients have hemostatic abnormalities that predispose them to develop platelet activation and fibrin formation, leading to clinical or subclinical thrombosis (95,96). Thus, cancer leads to thrombosis, which enhances the metastatic spread of tumor cells. Heparin is effective and safe for thromboprophylaxis, and LMWH works just as well or better than UFH.

TF has been implicated in the up-regulation of pro-angiogenic factors, such as VEGF, by tumor cells. This reflects a complex interaction between tumor cells, macrophages, and endothelial cells, leading to TF expression, fibrin formation, and tumor angiogenesis (97). A recent study has suggested that thrombin generation occurs via the extrinsic (TF dependent) coagulation pathway on cell surfaces and that some chemotherapeutic agents are able to up-regulate TF mRNA and protein expression in cancer cells (98).

The processes of blood coagulation and the generation of new blood vessels both play crucial roles in wound healing. Platelets, for example, are the first line of defense during vascular injury and contain at least a dozen promoters of angiogenesis, which can be secreted into the surrounding vasculature when platelets are activated by thrombin (87). It follows that these pathways are also intricately linked within human tumors. Targeting both the coagulation and angiogenesis pathways may provide more potent antitumor effect than targeting either pathway alone. Elucidation of the TF signaling pathway using tumor cells as a model system should provide new insights into the cellular biology of TF that might be applied to signaling in endothelial cells, smooth muscle cells, and fibroblasts. With new anticoagulants that selectively target TF and/or TF-VIIa complex (88,89,99), an understanding of this pathway might provide a rational basis for the use of these drugs to prevent and/or reduce angiogenesis-related disorders, tumor-associated thrombosis, and the positive feedback loop between thrombosis and cancer (100).

Activation of the blood coagulation system stimulates the growth and dissemination of cancer cells through multiple mechanisms, and anticoagulant drugs inhibit the progression of certain cancers. Laboratory data on the effects of anticoagulants in various tumors suggest that this treatment approach has considerable potential in some cancers but not others. For example, renal cell carcinoma (RCC) is one of a small number of human tumor types in which the tumor cell contains an intact coagulation pathway leading to thrombin generation and conversion of fibrinogen to fibrin immediately adjacent to viable tumor cells (101). Similar observations have been made in melanoma, ovarian cancer, and small-cell lung cancer but not in breast, colorectal, and non-small-cell lung cancers (102). On the basis of the relatively unique features of the interaction of RCC with the coagulation system, RCC might respond to anticoagulation therapy in a similar manner as small-cell lung cancer and melanoma. Hence, an anticoagulant that inhibits at the TF/VIIa level may improve efficacy and safety in inhibiting tumor-associated thrombosis, angiogenesis, and metastasis.

Several potent pro-angiogenesis factors, including TF, FGF2, VEGF, and interleukin (IL)-8, are recognized to promote pathological angiogenesis (97). Heparin counters these factors, although the inhibitory effect occurs through different mechanisms. In the presence of heparin, Zhang et al. (103) showed that TFPI activity is enhanced and the stimulatory effects of TF on angiogenesis are reduced. Chemokines have positively charged domains (104), and heparin might exhibit its inhibitory effect on IL-8 by binding these positive domains. In addition to angiogenesis, another key component of metastasis is the adhesion of cells to areas away from the primary tumor growth. Selectins and integrins are families of cellular components that mediate cell adhesion and are involved in a complex cascade of events following endothelial cell activation mediated by tumor cells. Studies have shown that heparin inhibited selectin and integrin-mediated interactions with tumor cells (105).

Tinzaparin, anti-VIIa, and TFPI have been shown to modulate angiogenesis-related processes, including in vitro endothelial tube formation and in vivo angiogenesis that is mediated either by angiogenic factors and/or by cancer cells (93). The agents have comparable inhibitory effects on endothelial cell tube formation, and they block FGF2 as well as other pro-angiogenesis factors-induced angiogenesis in the chick chorioallantoic membrane (CAM) model. Additionally, a significant inhibition of colon or lung carcinoma–induced angiogenesis, tumor growth, and regression was demonstrated with tinzaparin, anti-VIIa, and recombinant tissue factor pathway inhibitor (r-TFPI) (93). These studies suggest that tinzaparin, anti-VIIa, and tinzaparin-releasable TFPI play a role in the regulation of angiogenesis and tumor growth (93,15).

Tumor Factors Predicting Sensitivity to Anticoagulants

The various tumor types differ in the nature of their interactions with the coagulation system; in this regard, there are two types of tumors: those that activate the coagulation system directly and those that trigger coagulation activation indirectly via a paracrine mechanism. Tumors in the first group include RCC, melanoma, ovarian, and small-cell lung cancers. These tumors over-express procoagulant molecules such as TF and cancer procoagulant. Tumors in the second group, on the other hand, tend to activate systemic coagulation by releasing cytokines (e.g., TNF-α and IL-1-β) that, in turn, stimulate the production of procoagulant molecules on the surface of circulating monocytes. Examples of these tumor types include breast, colorectal, and non-small-cell lung cancers. On the basis of this difference in the biology of coagulation activation, one would predict that tumors in the first group might be more likely to respond to anticoagulants that interfere with TF/VIIa than would tumors in the second group. In support of this hypothesis, anticoagulants have had significant activity in melanoma and small-cell lung cancer, but not in breast, colorectal, and non-small-cell lung cancers in prospective trials (67–70,90).

Vascular Endothelial TFPI and Tumor Dissemination: Role of Heparin

Metastasis is the most deleterious event that leads to mortality of cancer patients (106). Using the B16 melanoma metastasis model in mice, SC injection of tinzaparin before intravenous injection of melanoma cells reduced lung tumor formation (94). Similarly, intravenous injection of TFPI prior to tumor cell injection also reduced B16 lung metastasis and abolished tumor cell–induced thrombocytopenia. These results support the potential role of LMWH and its releasable TFPI in tumor growth, angiogenesis, and metastasis (107). Heparin and LMWH are proposed to inhibit tumor metastasis via different mechanisms (108,109). Heparin and its improved version, LMWH, are effective in releasing endogenous TFPI, which in turn inhibits angiogenesis and tumor metastasis. Recent studies from our laboratory demonstrated that non-anticoagulant heparin derivatives that are devoid of any effect on factor Xa or IIa but sustain potent TFPI endothelial cell–releasing activity are effective inhibitors of angiogenesis and tumor metastasis (110).

POTENTIAL COMBINATION OF ANTICOAGULANT AND ANTIPLATELET IN CANCER

The key role of both fibrin and platelets in tumor survival, angiogenesis, and metastasis cannot be denied (98,111). It might be justified to inhibit both platelet and coagulation activation in the setting of cancer based on the details discussed earlier in this chapter about the key role of platelet and coagulation in the amplification of tumor progression via different complex processes. In that regard, synergistic benefits were demonstrated with a combination of anticoagulant and antiplatelet agents at adjusted doses (112). It is predicted that anticoagulants, with or without antiplatelet agents, such as aspirin, will be more commonly used as supplements for treatment of cancer patients and other patients at high risk for thrombosis. Additionally, heparin derivatives may prove to be more effective than anticoagulants that target only a single clotting enzyme in cancer prevention and treatment.

CONCLUSIONS

Heparin and its improved version, LMWH, have polypharmacological actions that extend beyond their recognized anticoagulant effects. Monitoring the true pharmacokinetic (113), in addition to the multiple pharmacodynamic profiles of heparin and LMWH, will facilitate the development of various forms of heparin, LMWH, and generic heparins.

Available uncontrolled data suggest that heparin may be effective in steroid-resistant ulcerative colitis, producing complete clinical remission in over 70% of patients after an average of four to six weeks of therapy. Although these results are promising, confirmatory studies are needed in larger numbers of patients. LMWH was used in a single trial in patients with steroid-refractory ulcerative colitis and yielded results similar to those observed with heparin. Since a prothrombotic state has been described in inflammatory bowel disease and microvascular intestinal occlusion appears to play a role in its pathogenesis, it is reasonable to assume that part of the beneficial effect of heparin may be a result of its anticoagulant properties. However, beyond its well-known anticoagulant activity, heparin also exhibits a broad spectrum of immune-modulating and anti-inflammatory properties, by inhibiting the recruitment of neutrophils and by reducing pro-inflammatory cytokines. In conclusion, heparin or heparin derivatives may represent a safe therapeutic option for severe, steroid-resistant ulcerative colitis and other inflammatory disorders. Randomized, controlled trials are needed to explore this possibility.

Clinical trials have suggested that LMWH improves survival of cancer patients with DVT. These findings need to be confirmed in a large multicenter trial in patients with defined tumor types and tumor stage. Recent studies from our laboratory have highlighted the role of LMWH, anti-factor VIIa, and r-TFPI in the modulation of angiogenesis, tumor growth, and tumor metastasis. Whether these agents alone, or in combination with antiplatelet agents, will be helpful in cancer patients remains to be established.

REFERENCES

1. Linhardt RJ. Heparin: an important drug enters its seventh decade. Chem Ind 1991; 50:45–47.
2. Marcum JA. The origin of the dispute over the discovery of heparin. J Hist Med Allied Sci 2000; 55:37–66.
3. Rutty CJ. Miracle Blood Lubricant: Connaught and the Story of Heparin, 1928–1937. Health Heritage Research Services. March 24, 2008. Available at: http://www.healthheritageresearch.com. Accessed May 21, 2007.
4. Bjork I, Lindahl U. Mechanism of the anticoagulant action of heparin. Mol Cell Biochem 1982; 48:161–182.
5. Hirsh J, Raschke R. Heparin and low-molecular-weight heparin: the Seventh ACCP Conference on Antithrombotic and Thrombolytic Therapy. Chest 2004; 126:188S–203S.
6. Weitz JI. Low-molecular-weight heparins. N Engl J Med 1997; 337:688–698.
7. Mousa SA, Fareed JW. IBC's 11th Annual International Symposium: advances in anticoagulant, antithrombotic and thrombolytic drugs. Exp Opin Invest Drugs 2001; 10:157–162.
8. Mousa SA. Comparative efficacy of different low-molecular-weight heparins (LMWHs) and drug interactions with LMWH: implications for management of vascular disorders. Semin Thromb Hemost 2000; 26(suppl 1):39–46.
9. Aguilar D, Goldhaber SZ. Clinical uses of low-molecular-weight heparins. Chest 1999; 115:1418–1423.
10. Hirsh J, Levine MN. Low molecular weight heparin. Blood 1992; 79:1–17.
11. Nielsen JI, Ostergaard P. Chemistry of heparin and low molecular weight heparin. Acta Chir Scand Suppl 1988; 543:52–56.
12. Linhardt RJ, Gunay NS. Production and chemical processing of low molecular weight heparins. Semin Thromb Hemost 1999; 25(suppl 3):5–16.
13. Emanuele RM, Fareed J. The effect of molecular weight on the bioavailability of heparin. Thromb Res 1987; 48:591–596.
14. Brieger D, Dawes J. Production method affects the pharmacokinetic and ex vivo biological properties of low molecular weight heparins. Thromb Haemost 1997; 77:317–322.

15. Mousa SA, Mohamed S. Inhibition of endothelial cell tube formation by the low molecular weight heparin, tinzaparin, is mediated by tissue factor pathway inhibitor. Thromb Haemost 2004; 92:627–633.

16. Mousa SA, Fareed J, Iqbal O, et al. Tissue factor pathway inhibitor in thrombosis and beyond. Methods Mol Med 2004; 93:133–155.

17. Boneu B, Caranobe C, Cadroy Y, et al. Pharmacokinetic studies of standard unfractionated heparin, and low molecular weight heparins in the rabbit. Semin Thromb Hemost 1988; 14:18–27.

18. Sutor AH, Massicotte P, Leaker M, et al. Heparin therapy in pediatric patients. Semin Thromb Hemost 1997; 23:303–319.

19. Taheri SA, Lazar L, Haddad G, et al. Diagnosis of deep venous thrombosis by use of soluble necrosis factor receptor. Angiology 1998; 49:537–541.

20. Nelson RM, Cecconi O, Roberts WG, et al. Heparin oligosaccharides bind L- and P-selectin and inhibit acute inflammation. Blood 1993; 82:3253–3258.

21. Lantz M, Thysell H, Nilsson E, et al. On the binding of tumor necrosis factor (TNF) to heparin and the release in vivo of the TNF-binding protein I by heparin. J Clin Invest 1991; 88: 2026–2031.

22. Tyrell DJ, Kilfeather S, Page CP. Therapeutic uses of heparin beyond its traditional role as an anticoagulant. Trends Pharmacol Sci 1995; 16:198–204.

23. Hocking D, Ferro TJ, Johnson A. Dextran sulfate and heparin sulfate inhibit platelet-activating factor-induced pulmonary edema. J Appl Physiol 1992; 72:179–185.

24. Darien BJ, Fareed J, Centgraf KS, et al. Low molecular weight heparin prevents the pulmonary hemodynamic and pathomorphologic effects of endotoxin in a porcine acute lung injury model. Shock 1998; 9:274–281.

25. Meyer J, Cox CS, Herndon DN, et al. Heparin in experimental hyperdynamic sepsis. Crit Care Med 1993; 21:84–89.

26. Hiebert LM, Liu JM. Heparin protects cultured arterial endothelial cells from damage by toxic oxygen metabolites. Atherosclerosis 1990; 83:47–51.

27. Matzner Y, Marx G, Drexler R, et al. The inhibitory effect of heparin and related glycosaminoglycans on neutrophil chemotaxis. Thromb Haemost 1984; 52:134–137.

28. Bazzoni G, Beltran Nunez A, Mascellani G, et al. Effect of heparin, dermatan sulfate, and related oligo-derivatives on human polymorphonuclear leukocyte functions. J Lab Clin Med 1993; 121:268–275.

29. Vancheri C, Mastruzzo C, Armato F, et al. Intranasal heparin reduces eosinophil recruitment after nasal allergen challenge in patients with allergic rhinitis. J Allergy Clin Immunol 2001; 108:703–708.

30. Diamant Z, Timmers MC, van der Veen H, et al. Effect of inhaled heparin on allergen-induced early and late asthmatic responses in patients with atopic asthma. Am J Respir Crit Care Med 1996; 153:1790–1795.

31. Garrigo J, Danta I, Ahmed T. Time course of the protective effect of inhaled heparin on exercise-induced asthma. Am J Respir Crit Care Med 1996; 153:1702–1707.

32. Gaffney A, Gaffney P. Rheumatoid arthritis and heparin. Br J Rheumatol 1996; 35:808–809.

33. Bowler SD, Smith SM, Lavercombe PS. Heparin inhibits the immediate response to antigen in the skin and lungs of allergic subjects. Am Rev Respir Dis 1993; 147:160–163.

34. Dwarakanath AD, Yu LG, Brookes C, et al. 'Sticky' neutrophils, pathergic arthritis, and response to heparin in pyoderma gangrenosum complicating ulcerative colitis. Gut 1995; 37: 585–588.

35. Petitou M, Herault JP, Bernat A, et al. Synthesis of thrombin-inhibiting heparin mimetics without side effects. Nature 1999; 398:417–422.

36. Tyrrell DJ, Horne AP, Holme KR, et al. Heparin in inflammation: potential therapeutic applications beyond anticoagulation. Adv Pharmacol 1999; 46:151–208.

37. Salas A, Sans M, Soriano A, et al. Heparin attenuates TNF-alpha induced inflammatory response through a CD11b dependent mechanism. Gut 2000; 47:88–96.

38. Panes J, Perry M, Granger DN. Leukocyte-endothelial cell adhesion: avenues for therapeutic intervention. Br J Pharmacol 1999; 126:537–550.

39. Lever R, Hoult JR, Page CP. The effects of heparin and related molecules upon the adhesion of human polymorphonuclear leucocytes to vascular endothelium in vitro. Br J Pharmacol 2000; 129:533–540.

40. Gaffney PR, Doyle CT, Gaffney A, et al. Paradoxical response to heparin in 10 patients with ulcerative colitis. Am J Gastroenterol 1995; 90:220–223.

41. Gaffney P, Gaffney A. Heparin therapy in refractory ulcerative colitis—an update. Gastroenterology 1996; 110:A913.

42. Evans RC, Rhodes JM. Treatment of corticosteroid-resistant ulcerative colitis with heparin: a report of nine cases. Gut 1995; 37:A49.

43. Brazier F, Yzet T, Duchmann J, et al. Effect of heparin treatment on extra-intestinal manifestations associated with inflammatory bowel diseases. Gastroenterology 1996; 110: A872.

44. Brazier F, Yzet T, Boruchowicz A, et al. Treatment of ulcerative colitis with heparin. Gastroenterology 1996; 110:A872.

45. Dupas J, Brazier F, Yzet T, et al. Treatment of active Crohn's disease with heparin. Gastroenterology 1996; 110:A900.

46. Folwaczny C, Spannagl M, Wiebecke W, et al. Heparin in the treatment of the highly active inflammatory bowel disease (IBD). Gastroenterology 1996; 110:A908.

47. Teixeira MM, Hellewell PG. Suppression by intradermal administration of heparin of eosinophil accumulation but not oedema formation in inflammatory reactions in guinea-pig skin. Br J Pharmacol 1993; 110:1496–1500.

48. Carr J. The anti-inflammatory action of heparin: heparin as an antagonist to histamine, bradykinin and prostaglandin E1. Thromb Res 1979; 16:507–516.

49. Koenig A, Norgard-Sumnicht K, Linhardt R, et al. Differential interactions of heparin and heparan sulfate glycosaminoglycans with the selectins. Implications for the use of unfractionated and low molecular weight heparins as therapeutic agents. J Clin Invest 1998; 101:877–889.

50. Diamond MS, Alon R, Parkos CA, et al. Heparin is an adhesive ligand for the leukocyte integrin Mac-1 (CD11b/CD1). J Cell Biol 1995; 130:1473–1482.

51. Benimetskaya L, Loike JD, Khaled Z, et al. Mac-1 (CD11b/CD18) is an oligodeoxynucleotide-binding protein. Nat Med 1997; 3:414–420.

52. Majerus P, Broze J, Miletich J. Anticoagulant, thrombolytic and antiplatelet drugs. In: Hardman J, Limbird L, Molinoff P, et al., eds. The Pharmacological Basis of Therapeutics. 9th ed. New York: McGraw-Hill, 1996:1341–1359.

53. Silverstein R. Drugs affecting homeostasis. In: Munson P, Mueller R, Breeze G, eds. Munson's Principles of Pharmacology. New York: Chapman & Hall, 1995:1123–1143.

54. Theroux P, Waters D, Qiu S, et al. Aspirin versus heparin to prevent myocardial infarction during the acute phase of unstable angina. Circulation 1993; 88:2045–2048.

55. Itoh K, Nakao A, Kishimoto W, et al. Heparin effects on superoxide production by neutrophils. Eur Surg Res 1995; 27:184–188.

56. Attanasio M, Gori AM, Giusti B, et al. Cytokine gene expression in human LPS- and IFNgamma-stimulated mononuclear cells is inhibited by heparin. Thromb Haemost 1998; 79: 959–962.

57. Dandona P, Qutob T, Hamouda W, et al. Heparin inhibits reactive oxygen species generation by polymorphonuclear and mononuclear leucocytes. Thromb Res 1999; 96:437–443.

58. Friedrichs GS, Kilgore KS, Manley PJ, et al. Effects of heparin and N-acetyl heparin on ischemia/reperfusion-induced alterations in myocardial function in the rabbit isolated heart. Circ Res 1994; 75:701–710.

59. Black SC, Gralinski MR, Friedrichs GS, et al. Cardioprotective effects of heparin or N-acetylheparin in an in vivo model of myocardial ischaemic and reperfusion injury. Cardiovasc Res 1995; 29:629–636.

60. Lucchesi BR, Kilgore KS. Complement inhibitors in myocardial ischemia/reperfusion injury. Immunopharmacology 1997; 38:27–42.

61. Hawari FI, Shykoff BE, Izzo JL, Jr. Heparin attenuates norepinephrine-induced venocon-striction. Vasc Med 1998; 3:95–100.
62. De Caterina R, Libby P, Peng HB, et al. Nitric oxide decreases cytokine-induced endothelial activation. Nitric oxide selectively reduces endothelial expression of adhesion molecules and proinflammatory cytokines. J Clin Invest 1995; 96:60–68.
63. Mousa SA, Mohamed S. Anti-angiogenic mechanisms and efficacy of the low molecular weight heparin, tinzaparin: anti-cancer efficacy. Oncol Rep 2004; 12:683–688.
64. Trousseau A. Phlegmasia alba dolens. In: Baillier JB, ed. Clinique Medicale de l'Hotel-Dieu de Paris. London: New Syndenham Society, 1865:94.
65. Schiller H, Bartscht T, Arlt A, et al. Thrombin as a survival factor for cancer cells: thrombin activation in malignant effusions in vivo and inhibition of idarubicin-induced cell death in vitro. Int J Clin Pharmacol Ther 2002; 40:329–335.
66. Sorensen HT, Mellemkjaer L, Olsen JH, et al. Prognosis of cancers associated with venous thromboembolism. N Engl J Med 2000; 343:1846–1850.
67. Caine GJ, Lip GY. Anticoagulants as anticancer agents? Lancet Oncol 2002; 3:591–592.
68. Lebeau B, Chastang C, Brechot JM, et al. Subcutaneous heparin treatment increases survival in small cell lung cancer. "Petites Cellules" Group. Cancer 1994; 74:38–45.
69. Chahinian AP, Propert KJ, Ware JH, et al. A randomized trial of anticoagulation with warfarin and of alternating chemotherapy in extensive small-cell lung cancer by the Cancer and Leukemia Group B.J Clin Oncol 1989; 7:993–1002.
70. Thornes R. Coumarins, melanoma and cellular immunity. In: McBrien DCH, Slater TF, eds. Protective Agents in Cancer. London: Academic Press, 1983:43–56.
71. Saba HI, Khalil FK, Morelli GA, et al. Thromboembolism preceding cancer: a correlation study. Am J Hematol 2003; 72:109–114.
72. Goldberg RJ, Seneff M, Gore JM, et al. Occult malignant neoplasm in patients with deep venous thrombosis. Arch Intern Med 1987; 147:251–253.
73. Baron JA, Gridley G, Weiderpass E, et al. Venous thromboembolism and cancer. The Lancet 1998; 351:1077–1080.
74. Rickles FR, Edwards RL. Activation of blood coagulation in cancer: Trousseau's syndrome revisited. Blood 1983; 62:14–31.
75. Levine MN. Prevention of thrombotic disorders in cancer patients undergoing chemotherapy. Thromb Haemost 1997; 78:133–136.
76. Falanga A. Mechanisms of hypercoagulation in malignancy and during chemotherapy. Haemostasis 1998; 28(suppl 3):50–60.
77. Kakkar AK, DeRuvo N, Chinswangwatanakul V, et al. Extrinsic-pathway activation in cancer with high factor VIIa and tissue factor. Lancet 1995; 346:1004–1005.
78. Simonneau G, Sors H, Charbonnier B, et al. A comparison of low-molecular-weight heparin with unfractionated heparin for acute pulmonary embolism. The THESEE Study Group. Tinzaparine ou Heparine Standard: Evaluations dans l'Embolie Pulmonaire. N Engl J Med 1997; 337:663–669.
79. Koopman MM, Prandoni P, Piovella F, et al. Treatment of venous thrombosis with intravenous unfractionated heparin administered in the hospital as compared with subcutaneous low-molecular-weight heparin administered at home. The Tasman Study Group. N Engl J Med 1996; 334:682–687.
80. Pintucci G, Froum S, Pinnell J, et al. Trophic effects of platelets on cultured endothelial cells are mediated by platelet-associated fibroblast growth factor-2 (FGF-2) and vascular endothelial growth factor (VEGF). Thromb Haemost 2002; 88:834–842.
81. Manegold PC, Hutter J, Pahernik SA, et al. Platelet-endothelial interaction in tumor angiogenesis and microcirculation. Blood 2003; 101:1970–1976.
82. Werther K, Christensen IJ, Nielsen HJ. Determination of vascular endothelial growth factor (VEGF) in circulating blood: significance of VEGF in various leucocytes and platelets. Scand J Clin Lab Invest 2002; 62:343–350.
83. Verheul HM, Pinedo HM. Tumor growth: a putative role for platelets? Oncologist 1998; 3:II.

84. Verheul HM, Hoekman K, Luykx-de Bakker S, Platelet: transporter of vascular endothelial growth factor. Clin Cancer Res 1997; 3:2187–2190.

85. Amirkhosravi A, Amaya M, Desai H, et al. Platelet-CD40 ligand interaction with melanoma cell and monocyte CD40 enhances cellular pro-coagulant activity. Blood Coagul Fibrinolysis 2002; 13:505–512.

86. Gasic GJ, Gasic TB, Stewart CC. Antimetastatic effects associated with platelet reduction. Proc Natl Acad Sci U S A 1968; 61:46–52.

87. Karpatkin S, Pearlstein E, Ambrogio C, et al. Role of adhesive proteins in platelet tumor interaction in vitro and metastasis formation in vivo. J Clin Invest 1988; 81:1012–1019.

88. Trikha M, Zhou Z, Timar J, et al. Multiple roles for platelet GPIIb/IIIa and alphavbeta3 integrins in tumor growth, angiogenesis, and metastasis. Cancer Res 2002; 62:2824–2833.

89. Varki NM, Varki A. Heparin inhibition of selectin-mediated interactions during the hematogenous phase of carcinoma metastasis: rationale for clinical studies in humans. Semin Thromb Hemost 2002; 28:53–66.

90. Dvorak HF, Senger DR, Dvorak AM. Fibrin as a component of the tumor stroma: origins and biological significance. Cancer Metastasis Rev 1983; 2:41–73.

91. Levine M, Hirsh J, Gent M, et al. Double-blind randomised trial of a very-low-dose warfarin for prevention of thromboembolism in stage IV breast cancer. Lancet 1994; 343:886–889.

92. Mousa SA, Mousa AS. Angiogenesis inhibitors: current & future directions. Curr Pharm Des 2004; 10:1–9.

93. Amirkhosravi A, Mousa SA, Amaya M, et al. Antimetastatic effect of tinzaparin, a low-molecular-weight heparin. J Thromb Haemost 2003; 1:1972–1976.

94. Ludwig RJ, Boehme B, Podda M, et al. Endothelial P-selectin as a target of heparin action in experimental melanoma lung metastasis. Cancer Res 2004; 64:2743–2750.

95. Falanga A, Rickles FR. Pathophysiology of the thrombophilic state in the cancer patient. Semin Thromb Hemost 1999; 25:173–182.

96. Markus G. The role of hemostasis and fibrinolysis in the metastatic spread of cancer. Semin Thromb Hemost 1984; 10:61–70.

97. Ruf W, Mueller BM. Tissue factor in cancer angiogenesis and metastasis. Curr Opin Hematol 1996; 3:379–384.

98. Paredes N, Xu L, Berry LR, et al. The effects of chemotherapeutic agents on the regulation of thrombin on cell surfaces. Br J Haematol 2003; 120:315–324.

99. Pinedo HM, Verheul HM, D'Amato RJ, et al. Involvement of platelets in tumour angiogenesis? Lancet 1998; 352:1775–1777.

100. Chambers AF, MacDonald IC, Schmidt EE, et al. Steps in tumor metastasis: new concepts from intravital videomicroscopy. Cancer Metastasis Rev 1995; 14:279–301.

101. Wojtukiewicz MZ, Zacharski LR, Memoli VA, et al. Fibrinogen-fibrin transformation in situ in renal cell carcinoma. Anticancer Res 1990; 10:579–582.

102. Zacharski LR, Wojtukiewicz MZ, Costantini V, et al. Pathways of coagulation/fibrinolysis activation in malignancy. Semin Thromb Hemost 1992; 18:104–116.

103. Zhang Y, Deng Y, Luther T, et al. Tissue factor controls the balance of angiogenic and antiangiogenic properties of tumor cells in mice. J Clin Invest 1994; 94:1320–1327.

104. Engelberg H. Actions of heparin in the atherosclerotic process. Pharmacol Rev 1996; 48: 327–352.

105. Borsig L, Wong R, Feramisco J, et al. Heparin and cancer revisited: mechanistic connections involving platelets, P-selectin, carcinoma mucins, and tumor metastasis. Proc Natl Acad Sci U S A 2001; 98:3352–3357.

106. Chambers AF. The metastatic process: basic research and clinical implications. Oncol Res 1999; 11:161–168.

107. Mousa SA. Anticoagulants in thrombosis and cancer: the missing link. Expert Rev Anticancer Ther 2002; 2:227–233.

108. Varki A, Varki NM. P-selectin, carcinoma metastasis and heparin: novel mechanistic connections with therapeutic implications. Braz J Med Biol Res 2001; 34:711–717.

109. Engelberg H. Actions of heparin that may affect the malignant process. Cancer 1999; 85: 257–272.
110. Mousa SA, Linhardt R, Francis JL, et al. Anti-metastatic effect of a non-anticoagulant low-molecular-weight heparin versus the standard low molecular weight heparin, enoxaparin. Thromb Haemost 2006; 96(6):816–821.
111. Rickles FR, Levine MN. Epidemiology of thrombosis in cancer. Acta Haematol 2001; 106:6–12.
112. El-Naggar MM, Mousa SA, inventors; PatentStorm, assignee. Prevention and treatment of tumor growth, metastasis, and thromboembolic complications in cancer patients. US patent 6 908 907. June 21, 2005.
113. Mousa SA, Zhang F, Aljada A, Pharmacokinetics and pharmacodynamics of oral heparin solid dosage form in healthy human subjects. J Clin Pharmacol 2007; 47:1508–1520.

18
Oral Direct Factor Xa Inhibitors

Alexander G. G. Turpie
Department of Medicine, Hamilton Health Sciences, Ontario, Canada

INTRODUCTION

Anticoagulants are recommended for the prevention and treatment of venous thromboembolism (VTE) and the prevention of thromboembolic events in patients with chronic conditions, including atrial fibrillation (AF) and acute coronary syndromes (ACS) (1–4). VTE can manifest as deep vein thrombosis (DVT) and pulmonary embolism (PE) and is a significant cause of morbidity and mortality among patients undergoing general or major orthopedic surgery (2,5). Without prophylaxis, these patients are at high risk of a thromboembolic event (2).

Available therapeutic options for anticoagulation currently encompass the long-established vitamin K antagonists (VKAs), low molecular weight heparins (LMWHs), and the more recently added fondaparinux (a synthetic pentasaccharide), among others. Despite the efficacy of these agents, they have a number of limitations. For example, the majority require parenteral administration, which is difficult once patients leave a hospital setting. Warfarin, which is administered orally, has a narrow therapeutic window, multiple food and drug interactions, inter-patient variability and is associated with an increased risk of bleeding, with frequencies of fatal and major or minor bleeding during administration approximately five times higher than expected without warfarin (6,7). These properties necessitate regular coagulation monitoring and dose adjustment. Thus, there is clearly an unmet need for safe, effective, and convenient oral anticoagulants that do not require monitoring and are therefore more suitable for long-term use.

This chapter provides an overview of a new class of oral anticoagulants—active-site-directed Factor Xa (FXa) inhibitors. Rivaroxaban and apixaban (Fig. 1) are direct FXa inhibitors in the advanced stages of clinical development, and others (DU-176b, LY517717, betrixaban, and YM150) are in earlier stages of development.

TARGET OF ACTION FOR NOVEL ANTICOAGULANTS

Established anticoagulation agents are characterized by actions on multiple enzymes within the coagulation pathway. More recently, efforts to find new approaches to anticoagulation have focused on a single target within the coagulation cascade and an

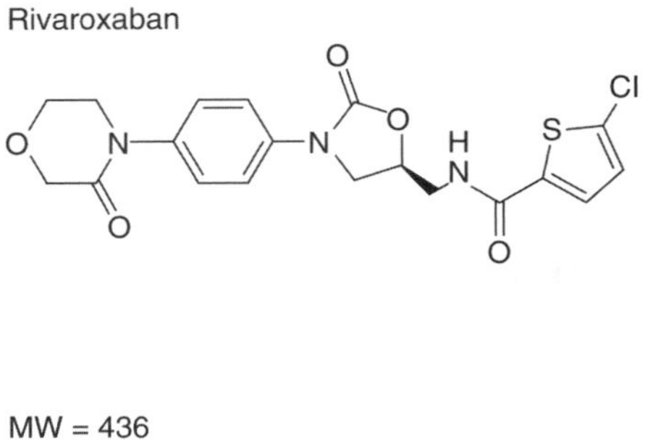

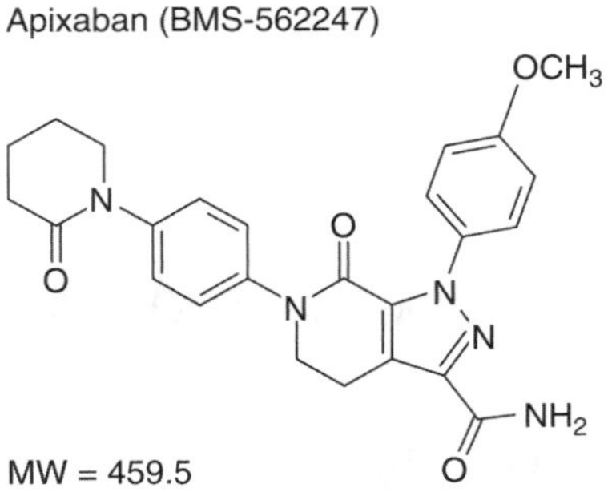

Figure 1 Structures of rivaroxaban and apixaban. *Source*: From Ref. 8.

appealing target is FXa, which plays an integral role in clot formation by virtue of its position at the convergence point of the intrinsic and extrinsic pathways. Fondaparinux is a selective, but indirect, FXa inhibitor that has provided proof-of-principle for selective FXa inhibition by demonstrating efficacy in the treatment and prevention of VTE in patients undergoing total hip replacement (THR), total knee replacement (TKR), or hip fracture surgery in the treatment of symptomatic VTE and in the management of ACS (9–11). However, like many conventional anticoagulants, fondaparinux relies on a parenteral mode of administration.

Thrombin is positioned downstream of FXa in the coagulation cascade and is also a rational site of action for novel anticoagulants. The parenterally administered direct thrombin inhibitors (DTIs) that have been approved for clinical use are effective but limited by a narrow therapeutic window (12). With the exception of desirudin, which is licensed for VTE prevention in patients undergoing THR, the use of these DTIs is restricted to patients undergoing percutaneous coronary interventions and for the treatment of heparin-induced thrombocytopenia (HIT) (12). The oral DTI ximelagatran, developed to address the limitations of the above agents, became available in Europe in 2004, but hepatotoxicity concerns led to its withdrawal in 2006 (13). Several other DTIs are currently under investigation [e.g., oral dabigatran etexilate (Boehringer Ingelheim)].

Theoretical and empirical evidence points toward FXa as a more attractive target for anticoagulation than downstream thrombin (14). For example, FXa is the key enzyme in the amplification of thrombin generation (one molecule of FXa results in the generation of >1000 thrombin molecules) and is therefore the rate-limiting step for this process (15). Consequently, blockade of FXa has the potential to limit thrombin-mediated coagulation. In addition, the effects of FXa are limited to promoting coagulation and inflammation, whereas thrombin has varied roles in addition to its procoagulant properties, including activation of the protein C anticoagulation pathway, promotion of cell proliferation, and both positive and negative effects on inflammation (16–18). Thus, thrombin inhibition may produce more effects on processes other than coagulation than FXa inhibition. Dose-finding evidence suggests a wider therapeutic window for FXa inhibitors than for DTIs (19–23). Moreover, a relationship between the cessation of DTI administration and rebound thrombin generation has been observed (24). The resulting increase in thrombin has been shown to exceed levels before or during DTI administration and may be associated with deleterious consequences, such as the initiation of ischemic events (24). Because of these issues, extensive research in the anticoagulant arena has been dedicated to the development of small-molecule, oral, direct FXa inhibitors.

ISSUES IN THE CLINICAL DEVELOPMENT
OF NOVEL ANTICOAGULANTS

The large body of literature charting the efficacy and safety of conventional anticoagulants has informed the development of novel anticoagulants, including the oral, direct FXa inhibitors. The balance between efficacy and safety (bleeding events in particular) is a primary concern in the clinical development of such agents. In order to assess this objectively and to allow comparisons between novel and established agents, several factors need to be taken into consideration when designing clinical trials in addition to the requirement for well-defined efficacy and safety endpoints (8). For example, variable criteria for the interpretation of venograms, the choice of dosage and administration schedules, and VTE rates used for sample size calculations will all influence study outcomes. It is general practice to establish proof-of-principle for novel anticoagulants in dose-finding studies undertaken within the short-term clinical setting of thromboprophylaxis after major orthopedic surgery (THR or TKR) (8,25). Patients undergoing THR or TKR represent a large study population in whom the high risk of VTE is well documented and fairly well characterized, thus allowing for better definitions of efficacy endpoints. Furthermore, because of the requirement for initial inpatient care, bleeding can be monitored and controlled. Finally, because such surgery is elective, patients are otherwise healthy. Once assessed in short-term studies, novel anticoagulants are often evaluated in a longer-term setting, such as VTE treatment, or stroke prevention in patients with AF. To establish the therapeutic range in these patient populations, dose-ranging studies are generally performed in phase II studies of symptomatic VTE patients, because the event rate for patients with AF in phase II studies is likely to be too low to allow selection of a safe and effective dose. However, in some cases such as the PETRO and PETRO-Ex studies for the prevention of stroke in patients with AF, phase II studies were performed to determine the safest and most efficacious dose to be used in phase III studies (26).

ORAL, DIRECT FACTOR Xa INHIBITORS IN THE ADVANCED
STAGES OF CLINICAL DEVELOPMENT

Rivaroxaban

Rivaroxaban (Xarelto®, Bayer HealthCare AG and Ortho-McNeil) is in development for the prevention and treatment of thromboembolic disorders, including VTE prevention following orthopedic surgery, VTE prevention in the medically ill, treatment of DVT and PE, treatment of ACS, and the prevention of stroke in patients with AF.

Preclinical Development

In vitro studies in human plasma established that rivaroxaban is a potent inhibitor of fluid-phase FXa [inhibitory constant (K_i) 0.4 nM] with a >10,000-fold greater selectivity for FXa than for other related serine proteases (27). Rivaroxaban also effectively inhibits FXa incorporated within the prothrombinase complex and clot-associated FXa activity (27,28).

As an FXa inhibitor, rivaroxaban does not inhibit thrombin-induced platelet aggregation, but it attenuates tissue factor–induced platelet aggregation indirectly, through inhibition of thrombin generation (29). Rivaroxaban and apixaban inhibit tissue factor–induced platelet aggregation in vitro more potently than enoxaparin (an indirect FXa/thrombin inhibitor) or fondaparinux (an indirect FXa inhibitor) (29).

The antithrombotic efficacy of rivaroxaban has been demonstrated in various animal models of arterial or venous thrombosis across doses that do not prolong bleeding times (27,30,31). In a venous stasis model, rivaroxaban reduced thrombus formation by 50% (ED_{50}) at a dose of 0.1 mg/kg (27). In a rabbit venous thrombosis model, thrombus growth was markedly inhibited by rivaroxaban, with no significant increase in bleeding times (31). Oral administration of rivaroxaban to rats or rabbits with arteriovenous (AV) shunts reduced thrombus formation (ED_{50} 5.0 mg/kg and 0.6 mg/kg, respectively). At the ED_{50}, FXa was inhibited by 74%, and the prothrombin time (PT) was prolonged 3.2-fold in rats; for rabbits the values were 92% and 1.2-fold, respectively. Bleeding times in both species were not significantly affected at antithrombotic doses (27). In a mouse model of ferric chloride ($FeCl_3$)-induced arterial thrombosis, rivaroxaban reduced thrombus formation by 86% at a dose of 3 mg/kg, an effect that was considerably greater than the reduction observed with 10 mg/kg fondaparinux (47%) (30). There was a similar difference between these two agents in the rabbit AV-shunt model; thrombus formation was inhibited by 83% with 3 mg/kg rivaroxaban, whereas the maximum reduction at the highest dose of fondaparinux (10 mg/kg) was 59%. Rivaroxaban prevented tissue factor–induced thromboembolic death in mice in a dose-dependent manner, with 97% survival at a rivaroxaban dose of 1 mg/kg, whereas the survival rate of mice given fondaparinux was very low (17% survival at a dose of 3 mg/kg and 20% survival at a dose of 10 mg/kg) (30).

When combined with acetylsalicylic acid (ASA) or clopidogrel, the antithrombotic potency of rivaroxaban is enhanced (32,33). For example, rivaroxaban (0.3 mg/kg) inhibited thrombus formation in the rats (AV-shunt model) by 60%, whereas inhibition with clopidogrel (1 mg/kg) was 29%. When the two drugs were given concomitantly, thrombus inhibition increased to 72% (33). A higher dose of clopidogrel (3 mg/kg) prolonged bleeding times that were enhanced in combination with rivaroxaban, suggesting a higher bleeding risk with higher clopidogrel doses. In the same model, ASA (3 mg/kg) alone inhibited thrombus formation by 20%; when administered with rivaroxaban, inhibition increased to 52%, without affecting bleeding times (32).

The favorable efficacy/bleeding ratio observed for rivaroxaban in animal models suggests a wide therapeutic window (27). Consistent with this, an in vivo comparison of anticoagulants with different mechanisms of action suggested that rivaroxaban had the most favorable risk/benefit ratio (34).

Pharmacokinetics and Pharmacodynamics

In healthy subjects and patients undergoing orthopedic surgery, rivaroxaban displays predictable pharmacokinetics and pharmacodynamics (Table 1). Two phase I studies in

Table 1 Summary of Rivaroxaban and Apixaban

	Rivaroxaban (8,32,33,35)	Apixaban (36–40)
Oral bioavailability (%)	~80% in humans	Chimps (51%); dogs (88%); rats (43%)
t_{max} (h)	2–4	1.5–3.5
K_i (nM)	0.4	0.08
Reversible	Yes	Yes
$t_{1/2}$ (h)	9–12	8–15
Mode of excretion	2/3 metabolized by the liver; 1/3 excreted unchanged by the kidneys	~70% in feces and 25% renal

Abbreviations: K_i, inhibitory constant; $t_{1/2}$, half-life; t_{max}, time to maximum plasma concentration.

healthy adult male subjects assessed rivaroxaban in single doses ranging from 1.25 to 80 mg ($n = 108$) or multiple total daily doses ranging from 5 to 60 mg ($n = 68$) (35,36). In the single-dose study, peak plasma concentrations were achieved rapidly (within 2 hours of administration) and dose-dependent increases in plasma concentrations were observed at rivaroxaban doses ≥ 10 mg (41). The half-life was between 7.6 and 9.1 hours for the 10 to 40 mg tablets. In the multiple-dose study, peak plasma concentrations were observed to increase dose-proportionally (42). For all doses, peak concentrations were achieved after 3 to 4 hours. The half-life ranged between 5.8 and 9.2 hours at steady state (day 7).

Plasma levels of rivaroxaban correlate well with both inhibition of FXa activity and prolongation of PT (Pearson's correlation coefficients of 0.950 and 0.958, respectively), as assessed in healthy subjects who received multiple doses of rivaroxaban across a wide dose range (42). The pharmacodynamic effects of rivaroxaban (as measured by endogenous thrombin potential) are sustained for 24 hours after single oral doses, thus supporting once-daily dosing (43).

Age, gender, and bodyweight have not been shown to exert clinically significant effects on the pharmacokinetic or pharmacodynamic profiles of rivaroxaban (44,45). A randomized, single-blind study of the effect of age (>75 years vs. 18–45 years) and gender on the pharmacology and tolerability of a 10-mg dose of rivaroxaban in healthy subjects ($n = 34$) suggests that fixed doses of rivaroxaban are appropriate irrespective of age or gender (44). In a study of 48 healthy subjects, divided into three groups on the basis of their weight (≤ 50 kg, 70–80 kg, and ≥ 120 kg), who received 10 mg of rivaroxaban, differences in pharmacokinetic and pharmacodynamic parameters between the lowest and the highest weight groups were either not detected or were very small (45). Consistent with these observations, rivaroxaban demonstrated predictable pharmacodynamic and pharmacokinetic profiles in patients undergoing major orthopedic surgery in the phase II trials described below. There were good correlations between peak rivaroxaban plasma concentrations and FXa inhibition and PT prolongation. In patients undergoing THR, these predictable and consistent profiles were observed irrespective of the dosing regimen [once daily (od) or twice daily (bid)] (35). As in healthy subjects, age, renal function, and weight had minimal effects on the pharmacokinetics of rivaroxaban (46). These analyses suggested that for the prevention of VTE, fixed dosing with rivaroxaban 10 mg od should be feasible in all patients without an increased risk of VTE or bleeding, irrespective of age, renal impairment, or body weight.

The effects of food and gastric pH-altering agents (frequently used by the elderly) on rivaroxaban (at doses of 5–20 mg) have been studied in healthy males (47). The half-life of rivaroxaban (ranging from 6 to 9 hours in healthy young subjects and from 9 to 13 hours in healthy elderly subjects) (44) was unaffected by food intake, and there was no effect of antacids or ranitidine on the absorption and exposure to rivaroxaban (47).

Rivaroxaban has a dual mode of elimination: one-third is excreted unchanged via the kidneys and the remaining two-thirds of the drug is metabolized by the liver; there are no major or active circulating metabolites (48). A study of 32 subjects revealed that mild hepatic impairment (Child-Pugh A) had no effect on the pharmacokinetics or pharmacodynamics of rivaroxaban (10 mg). In subjects with moderate hepatic impairment (Child-Pugh B), the decrease in total body clearance resulted in increases in the area under the plasma concentration–time curve and maximum plasma concentration (least-squares-mean ratios 2.27 and 1.27, respectively), compared with healthy controls. This led to moderately increased FXa inhibition and prolongation of PT (49). Thus, patients with severe renal or hepatic impairment have been excluded from clinical trials with rivaroxaban (50–58).

Cross-reactivity with HIT antibodies has not been demonstrated with rivaroxaban. Furthermore, the agent does not interact with or mobilize platelet factor 4 (PF4) on platelets, and, therefore, is unlikely to induce the conformational changes in PF4 necessary for cross-reaction with HIT antibodies (59). In addition, rivaroxaban has been shown to block the release of PF4 from activated platelets (59).

Characterizing drug–drug interactions is of paramount importance in a clinical environment such as VTE prevention, which often requires concomitant administration of different drugs. Evidence shows that rivaroxaban has a low propensity for clinically relevant drug–drug interactions with ASA, the nonsteroidal anti-inflammatory drug naproxen, the cardiac glycoside digoxin, and the antiplatelet agent clopidogrel (36,60–62). Coadministration of ASA (100 mg) had modest effects on the pharmacokinetics of rivaroxaban in healthy males, as demonstrated by the minimal difference in maximum plasma concentrations and half-life values achieved for rivaroxaban alone, compared with the combination (126.3 µg/L vs. 133.4 µg/L and 9.3 hours vs. 8.2 hours, respectively) (36). Similar effects on the pharmacokinetics of rivaroxaban were observed upon coadministration with naproxen (500 mg), digoxin (0.375 mg), and clopidogrel (300 mg followed by 75 mg) (60–62). Although there was a significant prolongation of bleeding time in a few subjects receiving the combination of clopidogrel and rivaroxaban, the overall results suggest that they may be administered together (62). A modest additive effect on anti-FXa activity and PT prolongation following coadministration of rivaroxaban 10 mg and enoxaparin 40 mg has been reported, but was not considered to be clinically important (37).

Thromboprophylaxis after Major Orthopedic Surgery

Four dose-finding clinical studies (one phase IIa and three phase IIb) have assessed the potential efficacy and safety of rivaroxaban for thromboprophylaxis in patients undergoing major orthopedic surgery. All four studies assessed rivaroxaban relative to conventional anticoagulants and measured the composite of the incidence of any DVT or objectively confirmed nonfatal PE or all-cause mortality as the primary endpoint and major bleeding as the primary safety endpoint.

The proof-of-principle for rivaroxaban in VTE prevention was established in the phase IIa study, which was a randomized, open-label, dose-escalation study of rivaroxaban doses between 2.5 and 30 mg bid, and 30 mg od in patients undergoing THR surgery (50). At the doses investigated, the primary efficacy endpoint occurred in 10.2% to 23.8% of patients receiving rivaroxaban and in 16.8% of patients receiving enoxaparin. The results in the od dosing arm of the study were consistent with those in the bid dosing arm, suggesting the feasibility of od dosing in this patient population.

The three phase IIb studies employed a randomized, double-blind, double-dummy, dose-ranging design to investigate the safety and efficacy of rivaroxaban at total daily doses of 5 to 60 mg (starting 6–8 hours after surgery) relative to enoxaparin in patients undergoing THR or TKR (52–54). In two of these studies, 722 patients undergoing elective THR and 621 patients undergoing elective TKR were randomized to a bid regimen of rivaroxaban (2.5–30 mg) or subcutaneous enoxaparin (30 mg bid initiated post-operatively in the knee study or 40 mg od initiated pre-operatively in the hip study) (52,53). Patients received rivaroxaban or enoxaparin for an additional five to nine days, and DVT was assessed by bilateral venography. The observed incidence of the primary efficacy endpoint in patients undergoing THR was similar to, or lower, for rivaroxaban

(7–15% of patients) than that for enoxaparin (17% of patients) (52). In the TKR study, the primary efficacy endpoint occurred in 23% to 40% of the rivaroxaban group and in 44% of the enoxaparin group (53). Significant dose–response relationships between rivaroxaban and the primary efficacy endpoint were not apparent in either study, which may reflect the high efficacy with the lower doses. For both studies, the incidence of major bleeding with rivaroxaban increased dose-dependently, and the observed incidence of major bleeding in each rivaroxaban dose group was similar to that for enoxaparin. These studies suggested that rivaroxaban (5–20 mg) had similar efficacy and safety to either enoxaparin regimen.

The third phase IIb trial compared the more convenient od regimen of rivaroxaban (5–40 mg, initiated 6–8 hours post-operatively) with the standard enoxaparin regimen (40 mg od, starting the evening before surgery) in 873 patients undergoing THR (54). As with the previous phase IIb trials, administration was continued for five to nine days. The observed incidence of the primary efficacy endpoint was lower in all rivaroxaban dose groups relative to enoxaparin (6.4–14.9% vs. 25.2%, respectively). The primary efficacy endpoint did not show a significant dose–response relationship with rivaroxaban, whereas a relationship was evident for the secondary endpoint of major VTE (composite of proximal DVT, PE, and VTE-related death; $p = 0.0072$); the incidence of major VTE was 8.5% for rivaroxaban 5 mg, but in other rivaroxaban dose groups it was similar to that in the enoxaparin group (0.9–2.7% vs. 2.8%). The primary safety endpoint (major post-operative bleeding) ranged from 0.7% to 5.1% in the rivaroxaban group [with a significant dose-response relationship ($p = 0.039$)] and was 1.9% for enoxaparin. The results from this study further supported the feasibility of the od dosing regimen. Thus, the 10 mg od dose (which was within the range identified in the bid studies) was considered to provide the optimal balance between efficacy and safety and was therefore selected as the most appropriate dose for further study in phase III trials. There has been no evidence of liver safety issues associated with rivaroxaban in completed phase II and phase III studies.

The fixed-dose 10 mg od regimen is currently under investigation in phase III studies of rivaroxaban for the prevention of VTE after major orthopedic surgery. The RECORD program (REgulation of Coagulation in major Orthopedic surgery reducing the Risk of DVT and PE) was initiated in December 2005 and enrolled more than 12,500 patients worldwide to participate in four multicenter, randomized, active-controlled, double blind studies of rivaroxaban prophylaxis in patients undergoing THR (RECORD1 and RECORD2) and TKR (RECORD3 and RECORD4) (NCT00329628; NCT00332020; NCT00361894; NCT00362232). The studies were designed with the same efficacy and safety endpoints. The primary efficacy endpoint is the composite of DVT, nonfatal PE, and all-cause mortality; the secondary efficacy endpoints include a composite of proximal DVT, nonfatal PE, and VTE-related death.

RECORD3 was the first randomized, double-blind, phase III trial to be completed in the RECORD program. This study compared rivaroxaban 10 mg od (initiated 6–8 hours post-operatively) with enoxaparin 40 mg od (initiated before surgery) for 10 to 14 days in 2531 patients undergoing TKR (58). Rivaroxaban was significantly more effective in the prevention of VTE after TKR. The primary endpoint occurred significantly less frequently in the rivaroxaban arm (9.6% vs. 18.9%, relative risk reduction 49%; $p < 0.001$), as did the secondary endpoints of major VTE (relative risk reduction 62%; $p = 0.016$) and symptomatic VTE (relative risk reduction 62%; $p = 0.005$). Rates of major bleeding were similarly low in both groups.

In the RECORD1 trial, 4541 patients undergoing THR were randomized to receive rivaroxaban 10 mg od (initiated 6–8 hours post-operatively) or enoxaparin 40 mg od (initiated before surgery) for 35±4 days (56). The incidence of the primary efficacy endpoint was 1.1% for rivaroxaban and 3.7% for enoxaparin (relative risk reduction 70%; $p < 0.001$). There was also a marked reduction in the occurrence of the secondary endpoint of major VTE for rivaroxaban compared with enoxaparin (0.2% and 2.0%, respectively; relative risk reduction 88%; $p < 0.001$). The observed incidence of symptomatic VTE was similar between rivaroxaban and enoxaparin (0.3% and 0.5%, respectively; $p = 0.22$). The incidence of major and nonmajor bleeding events was similar between treatment groups.

The RECORD2 trial, which randomized 2509 patients undergoing THR, compared an extended rivaroxaban regimen of 35±4 days (as for RECORD1) with an enoxaparin regimen limited to 10 to 14 days' duration (55). For patients in the extended rivaroxaban regimen group, the incidence of the primary efficacy endpoint was 2.0% compared with 9.3% in the short-term enoxaparin group (relative risk reduction 79%; $p < 0.001$). The occurrence of major VTE was also significantly lower with rivaroxaban than with enoxaparin (0.6% vs. 5.1%; $p < 0.001$). The incidence of symptomatic VTE was also lower in patients receiving extended thromboprophylaxis with rivaroxaban, compared with short-term therapy with enoxaparin (0.2% vs. 1.2%; $p = 0.009$). The safety profile in RECORD2 was consistent with that in RECORD1 and RECORD3, with similar incidences of bleeding events in the extended rivaroxaban regimen group versus the short-term enoxaparin group.

These three phase III studies demonstrate that a fixed, od, unmonitored dose of rivaroxaban provides a safe and effective option for short-term and extended thromboprophylaxis after major orthopedic surgery. In the RECORD4 study, patients undergoing TKR were randomized to receive rivaroxaban 10 mg od or enoxaparin 30 mg bid initiated after surgery (North American regimen). This study was completed recently and results were reported at the 9th EFORT congress in Nice (http://www.efort.org/cdrom2008/F85.pdf).

VTE Treatment

Rivaroxaban was also assessed for the treatment of VTE in two randomized, phase IIb, double-blind, dose-ranging studies of rivaroxaban administered for 12 weeks in patients with acute, symptomatic proximal DVT (without PE) (51,57). Patients were randomized to receive rivaroxaban od or bid [total daily doses of 20–60 mg (ODIXa-DVT) and 20–40 mg (EINSTEIN-DVT)] or open-label standard therapy of initial parenteral unfractionated heparin (UFH) or LMWH and a VKA. These two studies of more than 1150 patients suggested that the efficacy of rivaroxaban for the treatment of proximal DVT was similar to that achieved with standard anticoagulation therapy, with no significant dose–response relationship for the primary efficacy endpoints and low rates of VTE recurrence. At all doses in both studies, rivaroxaban was associated with a low rate of bleeding events (1.7–3.3% and 0.0–1.5% in ODIXa-DVT and EINSTEIN-DVT, respectively), similar to the rates with standard therapy (0.0% and 1.5%, respectively). Furthermore, there was no signal for compromised liver safety with rivaroxaban. Thus, the results of these two studies suggest that rivaroxaban has similar efficacy and safety to standard therapy for the treatment of proximal DVT, with a low incidence of recurrent VTE.

On the basis of the above results, phase III VTE treatment studies with rivaroxaban are underway. Because thrombus burden was reduced to a greater extent with bid than with od dosing of rivaroxaban in the acute setting (up to three weeks), an intensified bid regimen of rivaroxaban will be used for the initial three-week treatment period in these studies. The od and bid regimens of rivaroxaban had efficacy similar to that of standard therapy at three months; therefore, rivaroxaban will be given long term in a convenient od dose (20 mg). Two phase III, non-inferiority studies are investigating the efficacy and safety of rivaroxaban given for 3, 6, or 12 months compared with standard anticoagulant therapy in patients with confirmed acute, symptomatic, proximal DVT (EINSTEIN-DVT) or PE (EINSTEIN-PE), respectively (NCT00440193 and NCT00439777). A total of approximately 6200 patients are being enrolled and the primary outcome measure is symptomatic, recurrent VTE. The EINSTEIN-EXT study is a placebo-controlled, event-driven, superiority extension study that will investigate the efficacy and safety of rivaroxaban in approximately 1300 patients with symptomatic DVT or PE who have already completed 6 or 12 months of therapy with rivaroxaban or standard therapy (NCT00439725).

Clinical Development in Other Indications

Following on from the promising findings in the VTE treatment studies, phase III studies of long-term, od rivaroxaban for stroke prevention in patients with AF are underway. On the basis of the VTE studies, a fixed dose of rivaroxaban 20 mg od was considered suitable for investigation in the AF study (ROCKET-AF; NCT00403767). This randomized, double-blind study has been designed to assess the efficacy and safety of rivaroxaban 20 mg od relative to dose-adjusted warfarin for the prevention of stroke in approximately 14,000 patients with AF. Additionally, patients with moderate renal impairment (creatinine clearance between 30 and 49 mL/min) entering the study will receive a lower fixed dose of rivaroxaban of 15 mg od. Two pilot phase Ib studies were conducted in Japanese patients with AF to determine whether ethnic differences influence the safety and pharmacology of rivaroxaban and a phase III trial of rivaroxaban 15 mg od (10 mg od for patients with moderate renal impairment) relative to warfarin for the prevention of stroke in this patient population is in progress (NCT00494871).

A large dose-finding, randomized, double-blind, placebo-controlled phase II study is also underway to investigate the efficacy and safety of rivaroxaban alone or in combination with ASA or ASA and thienopyridine, for the secondary prevention of fatal and nonfatal cardiovascular events in patients with recent ACS (ATLAS ACS; NCT00402597).

Apixaban

Apixaban (BMS-562247, DPC-AG0023; Bristol-Myers Squibb) is in clinical development for the prevention of VTE in patients undergoing THR and TKR, in patients with advanced metastatic cancer and in medically ill patients, secondary prevention in patients with ACS, the prevention of stroke in non valvular AF, and the treatment of VTE. Apixaban is a follow-up to razaxaban (an aminobenzisoxazole with high affinity for the active site of FXa) (8). Clinical development of razaxaban was stopped following a phase II trial in patients undergoing TKR, in which the three higher dosages of razaxaban caused major bleeding (38). Apixaban has an improved pharmacological profile relative to razaxaban.

Preclinical Development

In purified systems and in plasma, apixaban has been shown to be a highly potent and selective direct inhibitor of FXa (K_i 0.08 nM) (63). Apixaban dose-dependently prolongs FXa-mediated clotting assays. The human plasma concentrations required to double the PT and activated partial thromboplastin time (aPTT) are 3.6 and 7.4 μM, respectively.

In animal studies, apixaban demonstrates high oral bioavailability (51%, 88%, and 34% in chimpanzees, dogs, and rats, respectively) (39). It has a small volume of distribution, low systemic clearance, and a low potential for the formation of reactive metabolites. The primary metabolite defined in vitro is the O-demethylated product. Apixaban is eliminated via multiple pathways; 70% of the compound is eliminated in the feces and 25% is eliminated via the renal pathway (40).

In a rabbit venous thrombosis model, apixaban revealed potent antithrombotic activity; apixaban inhibited venous thrombus formation in a dose-dependent manner, with a half maximal inhibitory concentration (IC_{50}) value of 0.16 μM (64). In this study, apixaban did not influence blood pressure or heart rate, suggesting that apixaban does not have relevant hemodynamic effects. Bleeding times at doses inhibiting 80% of thrombus formation (ID_{80}) were increased by 9%, with apixaban and 516% with warfarin.

Pharmacokinetics and Pharmacodynamics

In two double-blind, randomized, placebo-controlled, dose-escalation studies in healthy male subjects, oral apixaban demonstrated predictable pharmacokinetics with single doses ranging from 0.5 to 50 mg and with multiple doses ranging from 2.5 to 25 mg bid and 10 or 20 mg od for seven days (65,66). Maximum plasma concentrations were achieved 1.5 to 3.5 hours after oral administration of apixaban. Exposure and clotting times increased dose-proportionately and, for the latter, tracked the plasma concentration–time profile. After administration of a 50 mg oral dose of apixaban, the aPTT, international normalized ratio, and modified PT increased by 1.2-, 1.5-, and 2.6-fold, respectively. Similar increases in these parameters were observed after administration of apixaban 25 mg bid for seven days (1.2-, 1.5-, and 3.2-fold, respectively). The terminal half-life of apixaban ranged from 8 to 15 hours with multiple dosing and 3.6 to 27 hours with single dosing.

Thromboprophylaxis after Major Orthopedic Surgery

The efficacy and safety of apixaban for the prevention of VTE in patients undergoing TKR was evaluated in a phase IIb trial (APROPOS) (40,67). In this study, 1217 patients were randomized to receive one of six doses of apixaban (5 mg, 10 mg, or 20 mg, administered od or bid), open-label enoxaparin 30 mg bid, or warfarin for 10 to 14 days. Apixaban and enoxaparin were initiated 12 to 24 hours after surgery, whereas warfarin was started in the evening of the day of surgery. Rates of VTE and all-cause mortality, the primary efficacy endpoint, were significantly lower in the combined apixaban groups (8.6%) than in either the enoxaparin or warfarin groups [15.6% ($p < 0.02$) and 26.6% ($p < 0.001$), respectively]. For individual apixaban arms, the relative risk reduction in the primary endpoint ranged from 21% to 69% compared with enoxaparin and from 53% to 82% compared with warfarin. The primary safety endpoint of major bleeding was similar between treatment groups, with the rate of major bleeding in the apixaban group ranging from 0% (2.5 mg bid) to 3.3% (20 mg od) compared with 0% in both comparator groups.

Using data from the above study, exposure–clinical outcome modeling was conducted to identify the optimal dosing regimen of apixaban for phase III studies. Individual apixaban exposure from the six dose arms was estimated from a population pharmacokinetic model, and exposure–clinical relationships were analyzed by logistic regression. It was concluded that a 2.5 mg bid dosing regimen of apixaban provided the optimal benefit–risk profile relative to other assessed apixaban dosing regimens. Consequently, this regimen was selected for phase III studies (68).

The ADVANCE program includes three ongoing phase III studies of apixaban compared with enoxaparin for the prevention of VTE in patients undergoing major orthopedic surgery. Two of these studies will investigate short-term administration (12 days) of apixaban in patients undergoing TKR, with each study enrolling approximately 3000 patients (ADVANCE-1; NCT00371683, ADVANCE-2 NCT00452530). The third study is assessing extended administration (35 days) of apixaban in approximately 4000 patients undergoing THR (ADVANCE-3; NCT00423319). All three studies are designed with the same primary efficacy outcome (a combination of asymptomatic and symptomatic DVT, nonfatal PE, and all-cause mortality) and study completion is scheduled for 2008 (ADVANCE-1) and 2009 (ADVANCE-2 and ADVANCE-3).

VTE Treatment

A recent double-blind, randomized, dose-finding trial investigated the efficacy and safety of apixaban in patients with confirmed DVT (proximal DVT or extensive calf DVT) (69). In total, 520 patients were randomized to receive one of three dosing regimens of apixaban (5 or 10 mg bid or 20 mg od) or conventional therapy (LMWH or fondaparinux followed by dose-adjusted VKA) for 84 to 91 days. The frequency of the primary efficacy endpoint (composite of symptomatic recurrent VTE and deterioration of the thrombotic burden, as assessed by repeat bilateral compression ultrasound and perfusion lung scan) was similar in the apixaban 5 mg bid and 10 mg bid groups (6.0% and 5.6%, respectively) and lower in the apixaban 20 mg od group (2.6%). The primary efficacy outcome rate was 4.2% for standard therapy. Rates for the primary safety endpoint (the composite of major and clinically relevant nonmajor bleeding) were similar between apixaban (5 mg bid, 8.6%; 10 mg bid, 4.3%; 20 mg od, 7.3%) and standard therapy (7.9%). Findings from this study suggest that, like rivaroxaban, apixaban is a potential therapeutic option for the treatment of VTE, and two phase III trials are currently being planned for this indication (http://clinicaltrials.gov; NCT00633893, NCT00643201).

Clinical Development in Other Indications

A placebo-controlled, phase II pilot study is in progress to investigate apixaban (2.5 mg, 10 mg, or 20 mg od for 12 weeks) for the prevention of thromboembolic events in patients undergoing treatment for advanced cancer (ADVOCATE; NCT00320255). The efficacy and safety of a 30-day regimen of apixaban compared with enoxaparin for the prevention of VTE in acutely medically ill patients has been initiated in a phase III study (ADOPT; NCT00457002). The primary outcome measure in the 6500 patients to be enrolled is the composite of VTE and VTE-related death.

Results from the VTE treatment studies were instrumental in the initiation of an extensive phase II and phase III program in other clinical indications. Two phase III studies of apixaban for stroke prevention in AF are in progress. One is designed to evaluate the efficacy and safety of apixaban versus warfarin in preventing stroke and systemic embolism in 15,000 patients with non valvular AF and at least one additional risk factor for stroke (ARISTOTLE; NCT00412984). The second trial is assessing whether apixaban is superior to ASA in preventing stroke or systemic embolism in 5600 patients with AF and at least one additional risk factor for stroke who refuse or are unsuitable for treatment with a VKA (AVERROES; NCT00496769).

A large phase II, placebo-controlled study is examining the efficacy and safety of apixaban (2.5 mg bid or 10 mg od administered for 26 weeks) in patients with recent ACS (APPRAISE-I; NCT00313300).

Table 2 Summary of FXa Inhibitors in Early Clinical Development

	DU-176b (70–72)	LY517717 (71,73)	Betrixaban (74)	YM150 (75)
Oral bioavailability (%)	~50	~25–82	47	Not available
t_{max} (h)	1.0–1.5	Not available	Not available	Not available
K_i (nM)	0.56	5	0.1	31
Reversible	Yes	Not reported	Not reported	Not reported
$t_{1/2}$ (h)	8.6–10.7	Elimination $t_{1/2}$ ~27	19	Not reported
Mode of excretion	Mainly renal route	Mainly gastrointestinal route	Unchanged in bile	Not reported

Abbreviations: K_i, inhibitory constant; $t_{1/2}$, half-life; t_{max}, time to maximum plasma concentration.

ORAL, DIRECT FACTOR Xa INHIBITORS IN EARLY CLINICAL DEVELOPMENT

In addition to rivaroxaban and apixaban, there are several agents at various early stages of clinical development (Table 2). These novel agents vary in their pharmacokinetic and pharmacodynamic properties.

DU-176b

DU-176b (Daiichi Sankyo) is an oral, direct FXa inhibitor in early clinical development for the prophylaxis and treatment of thrombotic disorders. It is a potent inhibitor of FXa (K_i 0.56 nM), with a 10,000-fold higher selectivity for FXa than for thrombin (76). DU-176b dose-dependently prolongs clotting times, and decreases thrombin generation (77) and platelet aggregation (70,76).

The antithrombotic effects of DU-176b have been demonstrated in animal models of venous and arterial thrombosis (76,78). Unlike the indirect FXa inhibitor fondaparinux, which required more than a 100-fold higher dose to inhibit arterial thrombosis compared with venous thrombosis, DU-176b was able to inhibit arterial and venous thrombosis at the same dose range (0.05–1.25 mg/kg/h) (79). Furthermore, comparisons between DU-176b and conventional anticoagulants (UFH, LMWHs, and warfarin) in rat models of venous thrombosis and hemorrhage suggest a wider therapeutic window for DU-176b because it has a lower risk of bleeding (80). The dose required for 50% inhibition of thrombus formation by DU-176b was 10-fold lower than the dose required to double bleeding time, whereas the dose difference for the other agents was 2-fold or less (80). The potential for combination with antiplatelet or fibrinolytic drugs was demonstrated in rat models of arterial and venous thrombosis. In these models, DU-176b potentiated the antithrombotic effects of ticlopidine or tissue plasminogen activator (78).

A phase I study in 12 healthy adults demonstrated that DU-176b was able to reduce thrombus formation ex vivo in a Badimon chamber. The antithrombotic effects of DU-176b were sustained for up to 5 hours, with maximum inhibition of FXa activity occurring 1.5 hours after administration (77).

Two phase II studies investigating the efficacy and safety of DU-176b for the prevention of VTE after THR are underway (NCT003982162, NCT00107900). In a phase II study of the prevention of stroke in AF, patients will receive DU-176b or warfarin for three months (NCT00504556). Studies in patients with ACS and VTE are in the planning stages.

LY517717

LY517717 (Lilly) is an indol-6-yl-carbonyl derivative in development for the treatment and prophylaxis of thromboembolic disorders. It is an FXa inhibitor (K_i 5 nM) with 1000-fold higher selectivity for FXa than other serine proteases and high oral availability (71).

In human subjects, the anticoagulant activity of LY517717 peaked within 0.5 to 4 hours of administration, and a terminal half-life of approximately 27 hours was observed, with the gastrointestinal tract as the main elimination route (73).

A phase II, double-blind, parallel-group, dose-ranging study of LY517717 was undertaken in 511 patients undergoing THR or TKR. LY517717 was investigated at doses of 25, 50, 75, 100, 125, or 150 mg od (initiated after surgery) relative to enoxaparin (40 mg od initiated before surgery) (73). The primary efficacy endpoint was a composite of DVT detected by mandatory bilateral venography at the end of the study treatment (days 5–9) and objectively confirmed symptomatic DVT and/or PE occurring during the treatment period. LY517717 doses of 25 to 75 mg were ineffective and were therefore terminated prematurely. For the higher doses of LY517717, the incidences of VTE were 19% (100 mg), 19% (125 mg), and 16% (150 mg) compared with 21% for enoxaparin, indicating that LY517717 at these doses was non-inferior to enoxaparin according to prespecified criteria. Bleeding events were uncommon across all doses of LY517717 and the enoxaparin group.

Further development of LY517717 is planned: phase III trials in prevention of VTE are expected to begin in 2009, and two other indications are also being pursued.

Betrixaban

Betrixaban [PRT054021 (MLN-1021), Portola] is a potent inhibitor of FXa (K_i 0.117 nM), with a bioavailability of 47% and a half-life of 19 hours. The antithrombotic activity of betrixaban, demonstrated in different animal models of arterial and venous thrombosis, has been shown to occur at doses that inhibit thrombin generation in human blood (81). The ability of betrixaban to maintain vessel patency after $FeCl_3$-induced arterial injury in rats was compared with those of enoxaparin or clopidogrel, while its capacity to inhibit thrombus mass in rabbits was compared with that of enoxaparin and to inhibit platelet deposition in baboons also were assessed. The efficacy of betrixaban compared favorably to supratherapeutic levels of enoxaparin or clopidogrel.

A phase I dose-escalation study in 64 subjects revealed that betrixaban had minimal interactions with food and predictable pharmacokinetics and pharmacodynamics (74). Furthermore, betrixaban undergoes minimal renal excretion because it is predominantly eliminated unchanged in the bile (82).

In a phase IIa proof-of-concept study (EXPERT), betrixaban was investigated at doses of 15 or 40 mg od relative to enoxaparin 30 mg bid (post-operatively) administered for 10 to 14 days in a randomized, partly blinded study for the prevention of VTE in 215 patients undergoing TKR (82). The primary efficacy endpoint was the incidence of VTE (symptomatic DVT or PE or asymptomatic DVT on a mandatory venogram) on days 10 to 14. The rates of VTE were 20% and 15% in patients receiving betrixaban 15 and 40 mg, respectively, and 10% in patients receiving enoxaparin. There were no reports of major bleeding events in patients receiving betrixaban, whereas 2% of patients in the enoxaparin group had major bleeding events. Dose selection will be evaluated further in a large, dose-ranging study.

Further clinical studies for the prevention and treatment of VTE, stroke prevention in AF, and secondary prevention of stroke and myocardial infarction are planned.

YM150

YM150 (Astelas) is in development for the prevention of VTE. YM150 has a major active metabolite, YM-222741, and K_i values against FXa are 31 nM and 20 nM for YM150 and YM-222741, respectively (83). In animal models of venous and arterial thrombosis, YM150 demonstrated dose-dependent antithrombotic effects and prolongation of PT (83). In an AV-shunt thrombosis model in rabbits, plasma concentrations for YM150 were much lower than for YM-2221714 (less than 125 ng/mL vs. 3641 ng/mL after dosing at 10 mg/kg), suggesting that the active metabolite is mainly responsible for the antithrombotic effects in vivo.

A randomized, open-label, phase IIa dose-escalation trial in 178 patients undergoing THR assessed YM150 at doses of 3, 10, 30, or 60 mg od, given 6 to 10 hours after surgery for 7 to 10 days, relative to enoxaparin 40 mg od (initiated before surgery). The primary endpoint was major and/or clinically relevant nonmajor bleeding and the main efficacy endpoint was the composite of DVT detected by mandatory bilateral venography performed within 24 hours of the last dose of study medication, confirmed symptomatic DVT or nonfatal PE and/or all-cause mortality. There were no major bleeding events during the study and 3 clinically relevant nonmajor bleeding events [YM150 3 mg, 1 event (2.9%); YM150 10 mg, 2 events (5.7%)]. VTE incidence was dose-dependent, ranging from 52% with YM150 3 mg to 19% with YM150 60 mg ($p = 0.006$, logistic regression analysis); the incidence of VTE in the enoxaparin group was 39% (84).

A phase IIb study to determine the optimal dosing of YM150 (5–120 mg od) for the prevention of VTE after THR has been completed recently (75). The incidence of the primary efficacy endpoint (composite of DVT, symptomatic VTE, PE, and death up to day 7–10 of treatment) ranged from 31.7% to 13.3% and decreased significantly with increasing doses of YM150 ($p = 0.0002$). The primary safety endpoint (major bleeding up to day 7–10 of treatment) occurred in 0.1% of patients receiving YM150. The study included an open-label enoxaparin 40 mg arm for which the incidences of the primary efficacy and safety endpoints were 18.9% and 0.6%, respectively. A phase IIa study has been initiated to investigate the safety and tolerability of YM150 in patients undergoing TKR (NCT00408239). A further phase II study will assess the pharmacokinetics, pharmacodynamics, and safety and tolerability of YM150 in an AF patient population (NCT00448214).

CONCLUSIONS

The use of anticoagulants is a critical element in the optimal management of patients at high risk of thromboembolic events, such as those undergoing major orthopedic surgery. However, currently available anticoagulants are inconvenient, costly, and are associated with adverse effects on patient safety. In addition, and despite guideline recommendations, not all eligible patients receive appropriate therapy, which may explain why the clinical burden of VTE is still considerable (85–87). Barriers to the use of appropriate thromboprophylaxis include the belief by some surgeons that pharmacological prophylaxis increases the risk of bleeding (88) and the use of asymptomatic VTE as a primary outcome (assessment of efficacy) in the clinical trials (89). In addition, in patients at risk of VTE, thromboprophylaxis should be given beyond the standard duration recommended in international or national guidelines, and many surgeons have concerns about adherence and adverse events in the outpatient setting (90,91). Thus, there is a clear unmet need for orally administered agents for both short-term and extended use that are predictable, convenient, and effective without compromising patient safety. This is particularly important in view of the expanding number of patients at risk of thromboembolic disorders, resulting from an ageing population and an increasing pool of individuals requiring orthopedic surgery.

Oral, direct FXa inhibitors have been the focus of extensive research, and accumulating evidence supports the potential for these novel anticoagulants to meet the current unmet need for therapies that can effectively prevent and treat thromboembolic events in all patient groups. They do not have the drawbacks associated with VKA (including warfarin), such as risk of hemorrhage and difficulties in administration (i.e., the need for frequent monitoring). Therefore, they would be easier to use in the outpatient setting, which would help reduce the burden associated with thromboembolic disorders.

REFERENCES

1. Buller HR, Agnelli G, Hull RD, et al. Antithrombotic therapy for venous thromboembolic disease: the Seventh ACCP Conference on Antithrombotic and Thrombolytic Therapy. Chest 2004; 126:401S–428S.
2. Geerts WH, Bergqvist D, Pineo GF, et al. Prevention of venous thromboembolism: American College of Chest Physicians Evidence-Based Clniical Practice Guidelines (8th Edition). Chest 2008; 126:381S–453S.
3. Albers GW, Amarenco P, Easton JD, et al. Antithrombotic and thrombolytic therapy for ischemic stroke: the Seventh ACCP Conference on Antithrombotic and Thrombolytic Therapy. Chest 2004; 126:483S–512S.
4. Harrington RA, Becker RC, Ezekowitz M, et al. Antithrombotic therapy for coronary artery disease: the Seventh ACCP Conference on Antithrombotic and Thrombolytic Therapy. Chest 2004; 126:513S–548S.
5. Lindblad B, Eriksson A, Bergqvist D. Autopsy-verified pulmonary embolism in a surgical department: analysis of the period from 1951 to 1988. Br J Surg 1991; 78:849–852.
6. Ansell J, Hirsh J, Poller L, et al. The pharmacology and management of the vitamin K antagonists: the Seventh ACCP Conference on Antithrombotic and Thrombolytic Therapy. Chest 2004; 126:204S–233S.
7. Wells PS, Holbrook AM, Crowther NR, et al. Interactions of warfarin with drugs and food. Ann Intern Med 1994; 121:676–683.
8. Eriksson BI, Quinlan DJ. Oral anticoagulants in development: focus on thromboprophylaxis in patients undergoing orthopaedic surgery. Drugs 2006; 66:1411–1429.
9. Glaxo SmithKline. Arixtra (fondaparinux sodium) prescribing information. http://us.gsk.com/products/assets/us_arixtra.pdf 2005.
10. Yusuf S, Mehta SR, Chrolavicius S, et al. Comparison of fondaparinux and enoxaparin in acute coronary syndromes. N Engl J Med 2006; 354:1464–1476.
11. Yusuf S, Mehta SR, Chrolavicius S, et al. Effects of fondaparinux on mortality and reinfarction in patients with acute ST-segment elevation myocardial infarction: the OASIS-6 randomized trial. JAMA 2006; 295:1519–1530.
12. Weitz JI, Hirsh J, Samama MM. New anticoagulant drugs: the Seventh ACCP Conference on Antithrombotic and Thrombolytic Therapy. Chest 2004; 126:265S–286S.
13. AstraZeneca. AstraZeneca decides to withdraw Exanta. AstraZeneca Press Release, 14 February 2006. http://www.astrazeneca.com/pressrelease/5217.aspx 2006.
14. Ansell J. Factor Xa or thrombin: is factor Xa a better target? J Thromb Haemost 2007; 5:60–64.
15. Mann KG, Brummel K, Butenas S. What is all that thrombin for? J Thromb Haemost 2003; 1:1504–1514.
16. Esmon CT. The protein C pathway. Chest 2003; 124:26S–32S.
17. Vesey DA, Cheung CW, Kruger WA, et al. Thrombin stimulates proinflammatory and proliferative responses in primary cultures of human proximal tubule cells. Kidney Int 2005; 67:1315–1329.

18. Tarzami ST, Wang G, Li W, et al. Thrombin and PAR-1 stimulate differentiation of bone marrow-derived endothelial progenitor cells. J Thromb Haemost 2006; 4:656–663.

19. Bauer KA. New anticoagulants: anti IIa vs anti Xa – is one better? J Thromb Thrombolysis 2006; 21:67–72.

20. Ezekowitz MD, Reilly P, Nehmiz G, et al. Dabigatran with or without concomitant aspirin compared with warfarin alone in patients with nonvalvular atrial fibrillation (PETRO study). Am J Cardiol 2007; 100:1419–1426.

21. Eriksson BI, Dahl OE, Rosencher N, et al. Oral dabigatran etexilate vs. subcutaneous enoxaparin for the prevention of venous thromboembolism after total knee replacement: the RE-MODEL randomized trial. J Thromb Haemost 2007; 5:2175–2177.

22. Friedman RJ, Caprini JA, Comp PC, et al. Dabigatran etexilate versus enoxaparin in preventing venous thromboembolism following total knee arthroplasty (RE-MOBILIZE). J Thromb Haemost 2007; 5:Abstract O-W-051.

23. Eriksson BI, Dahl OE, Rosencher N, et al. Dabigatran etexilate versus enoxaparin for prevention of venous thromboembolism after total hip replacement: a randomised, double-blind, non-inferiority trial. Lancet 2007; 370:949–956.

24. Hermans C, Claeys D. Review of the rebound phenomenon in new anticoagulant treatments. Curr Med Res Opin 2006; 22:471–481.

25. CPMP. Guideline on clinical investigation of medicinal products for prophylaxis of high intra- and post-operative thromboembolic risk. http://www.emea.europa.eu/pdfs/human/ewp/70798en.pdf 2006.

26. The Petro-Ex Investigators. . Safety and efficacy of extended exposure to several doses of a new oral direct thrombin inhibitor dabigatran etexilate in atrial fibrillation. Cerebrovasc Dis 2006; 21:Abstract 5.

27. Perzborn E, Strassburger J, Wilmen A, et al. *In vitro* and *in vivo* studies of the novel antithrombotic agent BAY 59-7939 – an oral, direct Factor Xa inhibitor. J Thromb Haemost 2005; 3:514–521.

28. Depasse F, Busson J, Mnich J, et al. Effect of BAY 59-7939 – a novel, oral, direct Factor Xa inhibitor – on clot-bound Factor Xa activity *in vitro*. J Thromb Haemost 2005; 3:P1104.

29. Perzborn E, Lange U. Rivaroxaban – an oral, direct Factor Xa inhibitor – inhibits tissue factor-mediated platelet aggregation. J Thromb Haemost 2007; 5:P-W-642.

30. Perzborn E, Arndt B, Harwardt M, et al. Antithrombotic efficacy of BAY 59-7939 – an oral, direct Factor Xa inhibitor – compared with fondaparinux in animal arterial thrombosis and thromboembolic death models. Eur Heart J 2005; 26(abstract supplement):481.

31. Biemond BJ, Perzborn E, Friederich PW, et al. Prevention and treatment of experimental thrombosis in rabbits with rivaroxaban (BAY 59-7939) – an oral, direct factor Xa inhibitor. Thromb Haemost 2007; 97:471–477.

32. Perzborn E, Fischer E, Lange U. Combining rivaroxaban with acetylsalicylic acid increases antithrombotic potency without affecting bleeding times in animal models. J Thromb Haemost 2007; 5:P-W-639.

33. Perzborn E, Fischer E, Lange U. Rivaroxaban – a novel, oral, direct Factor Xa inhibitor – enhanced the antithrombotic effects of clopidogrel in rats. J Thromb Haemost 2007; 5:P-W-641.

34. Perzborn E, Arndt B, Fischer E, et al. An *in vivo* risk-benefit comparison of the effects of rivaroxaban – an oral, direct Factor Xa inhibitor – with thrombin inhibitors, warfarin and clopidogrel. J Thromb Haemost 2007; 5:P-W-638.

35. Mueck W, Eriksson B, Borris L, et al. Rivaroxaban for thromboprophylaxis in patients undergoing total hip replacement: comparison of pharmacokinetics and pharmacodynamics with once- and twice-daily dosing. Blood 2006; 108:Abstract 903.

36. Kubitza D, Becka M, Mueck W, et al. Safety, tolerability, pharmacodynamics, and pharmacokinetics of rivaroxaban – an oral, direct Factor Xa inhibitor – are not affected by aspirin. J Clin Pharmacol 2006; 46:981–990.

37. Kubitza D, Becka M, Voith B, et al. Effect of enoxaparin on the safety, tolerability, pharmacodynamics and pharmacokinetics of BAY 59-7939 – an oral, direct Factor Xa inhibitor. J Thromb Haemost 2005; 3:P1704.

38. Lassen MR, Davidson BL, Gallus AS, et al. A phase II randomized, double-blind, five-arm, parallel-group, dose-response study of a new oral directly-acting Factor Xa inhibitor, razaxaban, for the prevention or deep vein thrombosis in knee replacement surgery. Blood 2003; 102: Abstract 41.

39. He K, He B, Grace JE, et al. Preclinical pharmacokinetic and metabolism of apixaban, a potent and selective Factor Xa inhibitor. Blood 2006; 108:Abstract 910.

40. Lassen MR, Davidson BL, Gallus A, et al. On behalf of the apixaban investigators. A phase II randomized, double-blind, eight-arm, parallel-group, dose-response study of apixaban, a new oral Factor Xa inhibitor for the prevention of deep vein thrombosis in knee replacement surgery. Blood 2006; 108:Abstract 574.

41. Kubitza D, Becka M, Voith B, et al. Safety, pharmacodynamics, and pharmacokinetics of single doses of BAY 59-7939, an oral, direct factor Xa inhibitor. Clin Pharmacol Ther 2005; 78: 412–421.

42. Kubitza D, Becka M, Wensing G, et al. Safety, pharmacodynamics, and pharmacokinetics of BAY 59-7939 – an oral, direct Factor Xa inhibitor – after multiple dosing in healthy male subjects. Eur J Clin Pharmacol 2005; 61:873–880.

43. Graff J, von Hentig N, Misselwitz F, et al. Effects of the oral, direct Factor Xa inhibitor rivaroxaban on platelet-induced thrombin generation and prothrombinase activity. J Clin Pharmacol 2007; 47:1398–1407.

44. Kubitza D, Becka M, Mueck W, et al. The effect of extreme age, and gender, on the pharmacology and tolerability of rivaroxaban – an oral, direct Factor Xa inhibitor. Blood 2006; 108:Abstract 905.

45. Kubitza D, Becka M, Zuehlsdorf M, et al. Body weight has limited influence on the safety, tolerability, pharmacokinetics, or pharmacodynamics of rivaroxaban (BAY 59-7939) in healthy subjects. J Clin Pharmacol 2007; 47:218–226.

46. Mueck W, Eriksson BI, Bauer KA, et al. Population pharmacokinetics and pharmacodynamics of rivaroxaban – an oral, direct Factor Xa inhibitor – in patients undergoing major orthopaedic surgery. Clin Pharmacokinet 2008; in press.

47. Kubitza D, Becka M, Zuehlsdorf M, et al. Effect of food, an antacid, and the H2 antagonist ranitidine on the absorption of BAY 59-7939 (rivaroxaban), an oral, direct Factor Xa inhibitor, in healthy subjects. J Clin Pharmacol 2006; 46:549–558.

48. Weinz C, Schwartz T, Pleiss U, et al. Metabolism and distribution of [14C]BAY 59-7939 – an oral, direct Factor Xa inhibitor – in rat, dog and human. Drug Metab Rev 2004; 36:Abstract 196.

49. Halabi A, Kubitza D, Zuehlsdorf M, et al. Effect of hepatic impairment on the pharmacokinetics, pharmacodynamics and tolerability of rivaroxaban – an oral, direct Factor Xa inhibitor. J Thromb Haemost 2007; 5:P-M-635.

50. Eriksson BI, Borris LC, Dahl OE, et al. Dose-escalation study of rivaroxaban (BAY 59-7939) – an oral, direct Factor Xa inhibitor – for the prevention of venous thromboembolism in patients undergoing total hip replacement. Thromb Res 2007; 120:685–693.

51. Buller HR. Once-daily treatment with an oral, direct Factor Xa inhibitor – rivaroxaban (BAY 59-7939) – in patients with acute, symptomatic deep vein thrombosis. The EINSTEIN-DVT dose-finding study. Eur Heart J 2006; 27(Abstract supplement):761.

52. Eriksson BI, Borris L, Dahl OE, et al. Oral, direct Factor Xa inhibition with BAY 59-7939 for the prevention of venous thromboembolism after total hip replacement. J Thromb Haemost 2006; 4:121–128.

53. Turpie AGG, Fisher WD, Bauer K, et al. An oral, direct Factor Xa inhibitor – BAY 59-7939 – for prophylaxis against venous thromboembolism after total knee replacement: a dose-ranging study. J Thromb Haemost 2005; 3:2479–2486.

54. Eriksson BI, Borris LC, Dahl OE, et al. A once-daily, oral, direct Factor Xa inhibitor, rivaroxaban (BAY 59-7939), for thromboprophylaxis after total hip replacement. Circulation 2006; 114:2374–2381.

55. Kakkar AK, Brenner B, Dahl OE, Eriksson BI, et al. Extended duration rivaroxaban versus short-term enoxaparin for the prevention of venous thromboembolism after total hip arthroplasty: a double-blind, randomised controlled trial. Lancet 2008; 372:31–39.

56. Eriksson BI, Borris LC, Friedman RJ, et al. Rivaroxaban versus enoxaparin for thromboprophylaxis after hip arthroplasty. N Engl J Med 2008; 358:2765–2775.

57. Agnelli G, Gallus A, Goldhaber SZ, et al. Treatment of proximal deep-vein thrombosis with the oral direct Factor Xa inhibitor rivaroxaban (BAY 59-7939): the ODIXa-DVT (oral direct Factor Xa inhibitor BAY 59-7939 in patients with acute symptomatic deep-vein thrombosis) study. Circulation 2007; 116:180–187.

58. Lassen MR, Ageno W, Borris LC, et al. Rivaroxaban for thromboprophylaxis after total knee arthroplasty. N Engl J Med 2008; 358:2776–2785.

59. Walenga JM, Jeske WP, Prechel M. Potential of the Factor Xa inhibitor rivaroxaban for the anticoagulation management of patients with heparin-induced thrombocytopenia. J Thromb Haemost 2007; 5:P-M-648.

60. Kubitza D, Becka M, Zuehlsdorf M, et al. No interaction between the novel, oral direct Factor Xa inhibitor BAY 59-7939 and digoxin. J Clin Pharmacol 2006; 46:Abstract 11.

61. Kubitza D, Becka M, Mueck W, et al. Rivaroxaban (BAY 59-7939) – an oral, direct Factor Xa inhibitor – has no clinically relevant interaction with naproxen. Br J Clin Pharmacol 2007; 63: 469–476.

62. Kubitza D, Becka M, Mueck W, et al. Co-administration of rivaroxaban – a novel, oral, direct Factor Xa inhibitor – and clopidogrel in healthy subjects. Eur Heart J 2007; 28:Abstract 189.

63. Luettgen JM, Bozarth TA, Bozarth JM, et al. *In vitro* evaluation of apixaban, a novel, potent, selective and orally bioavailable Factor Xa inhibitor. Blood 2006; 108:Abstract 4130.

64. Wong PC, Watson CA, Crain EJ, et al. Effects of the Factor Xa inhibitor apixaban on venous thrombosis and hemostasis in rabbits. Blood 2006; 108:Abstract 917.

65. Frost C, Nepal S, Mosqueda-Garcia R, et al. Apixaban, an oral direct Factor Xa inhibitor:single-dose safety, pharmacokinetics and pharmacodynamics in healthy volunteers. J Thromb Haemost 2007; 5:P-M-665.

66. Frost C, Yu Z, Moore K. Apixaban, an oral direct Factor Xa inhibitor: multiple-dose safety, pharmokinetics and pharmaccodynamics in healthy subjects. J Thromb Haemost 2007; 5:P-M-664.

67. Lassen MR, Davidson BL, Gallus A, et al. The efficacy and safety of apixaban, an oral, direct factor Xa inhibitor, as thromboprophylaxis in patients following total knee replacement. J Thromb Haemost 2007; 5:2368–2375.

68. Feng Y, Li LY, Shenker A, et al. Exposure-clinical outcome modeling and simulation to facilitate dose selection of apixaban in subjects undergoing elective total knee replacement surgery. J Thromb Haemost 2007; 5:P-M-663.

69. Buller HR. A dose finding study of the oral direct Factor Xa inhibitor apixaban in the treatment of patients with acute symptomatic deep vein thrombosis – the Botticelli investigators. J Thromb Haemost 2007; 5:O-S-003.

70. Shibano T, Tsuji N, Kito F, et al. Effects of DU-176b, a novel direct factor Xa inhibitor on prothrombinase activity and platelet aggregation *in vitro*. J Thromb Haemost 2007; 5:P-T-642.

71. Spyropoulos AC. Investigational treatments of venous thromboembolism. Expert Opin Investig Drugs 2007; 16:431–440.

72. Morishima Y, Fukuda T, Honda Y. Activated prothrombin complex concentrate, recombinant factor VIIa and factor IX reverse the prolonged clotting time induced by DU-176b, a direct factor Xa inhibitor, in human plasma. J Thromb Haemost 2007; 5:P-T-639.

73. Agnelli G, Haas S, Ginsberg JS, et al. A phase II study of the oral factor Xa inhibitor LY517717 for the prevention of venous thromboembolism after hip or knee replacement. J Thromb Haemost 2007; 5:746–753.

74. Turpie AG. Oral, direct Factor Xa inhibitors in development for the prevention and treatment of thromboembolic diseases. Arterioscler Thromb Vasc Biol 2007; 27:1238–1247.

75. Eriksson BI, Turpie AGG, Lassen M, et al. Once daily YM150, an oral direct Factor Xa inhibitor, for prevention of venous thromboembolism in patients undergoing elective primary hip replacement. Blood 2007; 110:Abstract 309. Oral presentation at ASH 2007.

76. Morishima Y, Furugohri T, Isobe K, et al. *In vitro* characteristics, anticoagulant effects and *in vivo* antithrombotic efficacy of a novel, potent and orally active direct factor Xa inhibitor, DU-176b. Blood 2004; 104:Abstract 1862.

77. Zafar MU, Vorchheimer DA, Gaztanaga J, et al. Antithrombotic effects of factor Xa inhibition with DU-176b: Phase-I study of an oral, direct factor Xa inhibitor using an *ex-vivo* flow chamber. Thromb Haemost 2007; 98:883–888.

78. Morishima Y, Furugohri T, Honda Y, et al. Antithrombotic properties of DU-176b, a novel orally active Factor Xa inhibitor: inhibition of both arterial and venous thrombosis, and combination effects with other antithrombotic agents. J Thromb Haemost 2005; 3:PO511.

79. Fukuda T, Matsumoto C, Honda Y, et al. Antithrombotic properties of DU-176b, a novel, potent and orally active direct Factor Xa inhibitor in rat models of arterial and venous thrombosis: comparison with fondaparinux, an antithrombin dependent Factor Xa inhibitor. Blood 2004; 104:Abstract 1852.

80. Furugohri T, Honda Y, Matsumoto C, et al. Antithrombotic and hemorrhagic effects of DU-176b, a novel, potent and orally active direct Factor Xa inhibitor: a wider safety margin compared to heparins and warfarin. Blood 2004; 104:Abstract 1851.

81. Abe K, Siu G, Edwards S, et al. Animal models of thrombosis help predict the human therapeutic concentration of PRT54021, a potent oral Factor Xa inhibitor. Blood 2006; 108: Abstract 901.

82. Turpie AG, Gent M, Bauer K, et al. Evaluation of the Factor Xa (FXa) inhibitor, PRT054021 (PRT021), against enoxaparin in a randomized trial for the prevention of venous thromboembolic events after total knee replacement (EXPERT). J Thromb Haemost 2007; 5: P-T-652.

83. Iwatsuki Y, Shigenaga T, Moritani Y, et al. Biochemical and pharmacological profiles of YM150, an oral direct Factor Xa inhibitor. Blood 2006; 108:Abstract 911.

84. Eriksson BI, Turpie AG, Lassen MR, et al. A dose escalation study of YM150, an oral direct factor Xa inhibitor, in the prevention of venous thromboembolism in elective primary hip replacement surgery. J Thromb Haemost 2007; 5:1660–1665.

85. Brenkel IJ, Cook RE. Thromboprophylaxis in patients undergoing total hip replacement. Hosp Med 2003; 64:281–287.

86. Brenkel IJ, Hyers TM. Thromboprophylaxis in patients undergoing hip replacement: a survey of British orthopaedic surgeons. J Bone Joint Surg Br 2004; 87-B(suppl. III):301–302.

87. Walker N, Rodgers A, Gray H. Changing patterns of pharmacological thromboprophylaxis use by orthopaedic surgeons in New Zealand. ANZ J Surg 2002; 72:335–338.

88. Salvati EA, Pellegrini VD Jr., Sharrock NE, et al. Recent advances in venous thromboembolic prophylaxis during and after total hip replacement. J Bone Joint Surg Am 2000; 82:252–270.

89. Caprini JA, Hyers TM. Compliance with antithrombotic guidelines. Manag Care 2006; 15: 49–66.

90. Anderson FA, Jr., White K. Prolonged prophylaxis in orthopedic surgery: insights from the United States. Semin Thromb Hemost 2002; 28(suppl 3):43–46.

91. Lieberman JR, Hsu WK. Prevention of venous thromboembolic disease after total hip and knee arthroplasty. J Bone Joint Surg Am 2005; 87:2097–2112.

19
Direct Thrombin Inhibitors

Menaka Pai
Department of Adult Hematology, Princess Margaret Hospital, University of Toronto, Toronto, Ontario, Canada

Mark A. Crowther
Department of Medicine, St. Joseph's Hospital, McMaster University, Hamilton, Ontario, Canada

INTRODUCTION

Most of the currently available anticoagulants used for the prevention and treatment of venous and arterial thromboembolism require antithrombin for their anticoagulant effect and (with the exception of fondaparinux) produce their anticoagulant effect by inhibiting multiple coagulation factors. Heparin, LMWH, and warfarin all produce at least a component of their anticoagulant effect by inhibiting thrombin. The conversion of the zymogen precursor prothrombin to thrombin is the final common pathway of blood coagulation. Thrombin is a versatile enzyme. It not only converts fibrinogen to fibrin, but also activates FXIII, rendering fibrin resistant to fibrinolysis. With the assistance of thrombomodulin, thrombin cleaves protein C and thrombin-activatable fibrinolysis inhibitor (TAFI) as well. Thrombin upregulates its own production by activating FVIII and FV, cofactors for tenase and prothrombinase, as well as FXI and FVII. It also acts as a platelet agonist. In this way, thrombin is able to provide positive feedback and amplify hemostasis. Thrombin's ubiquitous role in maintaining hemostasis makes it a prime target for newer, more specific anticoagulant drugs.

DTIs bind thrombin with high affinity, preventing the interaction of thrombin with its substrates. Licensed DTIs include hirudin, bivalirudin, and argatroban; a number of novel products are in development. Theoretical advantages of DTIs include activity against fibrin-bound thrombin, less nonspecific-binding to proteins and platelets, lack of a requirement for a cofactor, an absence of natural inhibitors, and a wider therapeutic window. As a result of their predictable pharmacokinetic profile and reduced specific and nonspecific protein binding, the oral DTIs also have the potential to be used without laboratory monitoring—a major advantage over current oral anticoagulants (1,2).

PARENTERAL DIRECT THROMBIN INHIBITORS

Hirudins

Hirudin is the principal anticoagulant in the saliva of the medicinal leech (*Hirudo medicinalis*). Hirudin consists of a single polypeptide chain of 65 amino acids, with a sulfate group that increases affinity for thrombin. Natural hirudin was used as an anticoagulant during dialysis in the 1920s; however, extraction of the crude substance was costly. Various recombinant hirudins have since been developed. Lepirudin and desirudin are produced in yeast using recombinant technology. Their structure is similar to natural hirudin, though the absence of the sulfate group reduces their activity (3–5). Hirudins are bivalent DTIs—they bind thrombin with high affinity, forming noncovalent, essentially irreversible, 1:1 stoichiometric complexes. Binding occurs at exosite 1 (substrate-binding site) and the apolar-binding site located near the catalytic site of thrombin (5–7).

Hirudins are administered either intravenously or subcutaneously. Their plasma half-life is approximately one to two hours, and they distribute widely in the extravascular space. Peak concentrations are achieved approximately three to four hours after administering subcutaneous injection (3). Clearance is primarily through the kidneys, so dose adjustment is required in the setting of impaired renal function (3,8).

Monitoring hirudin is problematic because plasma levels must be determined using enzyme-linked immunosorbent assays (ELISA), which are costly and limited in availability. Because there is evidence that elevated levels of hirudin are associated with bleeding, monitoring is required to avoid excessive anticoagulation. Hirudin prolongs the activated partial thromboplastin time (APTT), and thus the APTT is widely used to monitor hirudin therapy; an APTT 1.5 to 2.5 times the patient's or laboratory's baseline APTT is frequently targeted. Many centers create an APTT-hirudin standard curve, allowing indirect measurement of hirudin plasma levels.

Lepirudin is the hirudin licensed for use in patients with heparin-induced thrombocytopenia (HIT), with thrombosis. In this setting, the recommended drug level is 0.6 to 1.4 mg/mL. This range, however, is not evidence based and, in practice, it is difficult to achieve this level because the correlation between the APTT-level and the plasma–lepirudin level is not linear. Thus, with high drug levels, the APTT reaches a plateau (9–11). The ecarin clotting time (ECT) has also been used to monitor lepirudin, particularly in the setting of cardiopulmonary bypass. The ECT versus lepirudin standard curve is linear, even with the high lepirudin levels required during this procedure (11–13). However, there is no clinical evidence that targeting particular ECTs reduces either bleeding or anticoagulant failure.

Bleeding is the most common side effect of the hirudins. Major bleeding occurs in 18% to 20% of patients receiving lepirudin for treatment of HIT. Clinical use of commercially available hirudins is complicated by the development of antibodies. Thus, over 40% of lepirudin-treated patients develop antibodies against lepirudin of the IgG class (14). These antibodies form one to four weeks after starting treatment and most are not associated with any adverse clinical outcomes. However, in approximately 10% of lepirudin-treated patients, the antibodies delay the clearance of lepirudin, thereby enhancing its anticoagulant effect (14). Anaphylaxis, which can be fatal, has also been reported in patients receiving intravenous bolus lepirudin for treatment of HIT (15).

Lepirudin is currently approved in the United States, Canada, and the European Union for the treatment of HIT, complicated by thrombosis. Approval is based on the findings of three prospective, historically-controlled cohort studies, HAT-1, HAT-2, and

HAT-3. These studies found that, compared with historical controls, lepirudin reduced the frequency of the composite endpoint of all-cause mortality, new thrombosis, or limb amputation in patients with HIT. Lepirudin was also associated with significantly reduced new thrombosis (16–18). For patients with HIT complicated by thrombosis, lepirudin is administered as a continuous infusion of 0.15 mg/kg/hr adjusted to a target APTT at 1.5 to 2.5 times the patient's baseline or the mean of the laboratory normal range. An intravenous bolus of 0.4 mg/kg may be administered as well (17,19,20). Lepirudin is also used off-label for thromboprophylaxis in patients with acute isolated HIT, on the basis of findings that it reduces the composite endpoint of all-cause mortality, new thrombosis, and limb amputation in this group as well (21). In this setting, the recommended dose is a continuous infusion of 0.1 mg/kg/hr with no bolus, adjusted to a target APTT of 1.5 to 2.5 times the patient's baseline or the mean of the laboratory normal range (20).

Lepirudin has also been studied in the setting of non-ST-segment acute coronary syndrome (ACS). When compared with heparin in 10,141 patients with ACS, lepirudin not only significantly reduced the incidence of cardiovascular death, refractory angina, or new myocardial infarction (MI) at seven days from 6.7% to 5.6%, but also significantly increased the rate of major bleeding from 0.7% to 1.2%. Lepirudin has not been approved for use in ACS, but these results support the hypothesis that hirudins are superior to heparin in preventing recurrent ischemia, but highlight their narrow therapeutic window (22). Because of the excess bleeding, lepirudin was not licensed for this indication.

Desirudin is a hirudin used for thromboprophylaxis in patients undergoing elective hip or knee surgery. In this setting the recommended adult dose is 15 mg subcutaneously twice daily. The first dose is recommended to be given after induction of anesthesia and 5 to 15 minutes prior to surgery. Desirudin is used for 9 to 12 days, or until the patient is fully ambulant. Unlike lepirudin, monitoring of desirudin is not necessary.

Like lepirudin, bleeding is the most common side effect of desirudin. When receiving desirudin for thromboprophylaxis, approximately 10% of patients also develop antibodies against hirudin of the IgG class. These antibodies have not been associated with altered plasma concentrations of desirudin, deep vein thrombosis (DVT), pulmonary embolism, allergic reactions, or hemorrhage (23).

Desirudin is currently approved in Europe for thromboprophylaxis in patients undergoing elective hip or knee surgery. Approval is based on the findings of two multicenter, randomized, double-blind trials. In the first study, desirudin 15 mg subcutaneously twice daily was compared with unfractionated heparin (UHF) 5000 international units three times daily, in patients undergoing primary elective total hip replacement. The duration of treatment was 8 to 11 days. The primary endpoint was a thromboembolic event, confirmed by venography, during the treatment period. The total population was 445 patients. Desirudin was associated with a significantly lower rate of DVT (7% vs. 41%, $p < 0.0001$) and proximal DVT (3% vs. 29%, $p < 0.0001$). During a six-week follow-up period, pulmonary embolism was confirmed in four patients, all of whom had received heparin. There was no significant difference in bleeding between the groups (24). In the second study, desirudin 15 mg subcutaneously twice daily was compared to enoxaparin 40 mg subcutaneously once daily in patients undergoing elective total hip replacement. The duration of treatment was 8 to 12 days, and DVT during the treatment period was verified by mandatory bilateral venography. Desirudin was associated with a significantly lower rate of proximal DVT (4.5% vs. 7.5%, $p = 0.01$) and overall DVT (18.4% vs. 25.5%, $p = 0.001$). There was no significant difference in bleeding, transfusion requirements, or thrombocytopenia between the groups (25).

Bivalirudin

A hirudin analogue, bivalirudin is a 20 amino-acid synthetic polypeptide. Bivalirudin has several key similarities to hirudin. Bivalirudin is also a bivalent DTI, with its N-terminus moiety binding to the active site of thrombin and its C-terminus moiety binding to exosite 1. Bivalirudin binds thrombin with high affinity to form a 1:1 stoichiometric complex. However, once bound, thrombin cleaves the Arg–Pro bond in the N-terminus of bivalirudin. This allows for recovery of thrombin activity, with fibrinogen competing with the bivalirudin remnant for thrombin (26–28).

Bivalirudin is administered intravenously and has a half-life of 25 minutes (29). Unlike hirudin, only 20% of bivalirudin is excreted via the kidneys. The primary route of elimination is by enzymatic degradation by proteases (30).

Both the APTT and the activated clotting time (ACT) have been used to monitor bivalirudin.

Bivalirudin has been licensed as an alternative to heparin in patients undergoing percutaneous coronary interventions (PCI), and for patients with HIT who require PCI. A prospective trial comparing bivalirudin with high-dose heparin in 1261 patients demonstrated a lower rate of death, MI, or repeat revascularization at seven days (6.2% vs. 7.9%, $p = 0.039$). The rate of major hemorrhage, retroperitoneal bleeding, and the need for blood transfusion was also lower with bivalirudin than with heparin (3.5% vs. 9.3%, $p < 0.001$) (31). The REPLACE-1 trial compared bivalirudin to heparin in 1056 patients undergoing coronary stenting with any one of the GP IIb/IIIa inhibitors. In this study, the protocol used an intravenous bolus of 1.0 mg/kg of bivalirudin and a subsequent four-hour infusion rate of 2.5 mg/kg/hr. There was a trend toward a reduction in the combined endpoint of death, MI, or revascularization with bivalirudin at 48 hours. There was no difference in major bleeding (32). REPLACE-2, a randomized, double-blind, active-controlled trial, randomized 6010 patients to either bivalirudin with provisional use of GP IIb/IIIa blockage or heparin with planned GP IIb/IIIa blockage. The intravenous bolus dose of bivalirudin was lowered to 0.75 mg/kg and the subsequent four-hour infusion rate was 1.75 mg/kg/hr. Bivalirudin was as effective as heparin plus GP IIb/IIIa inhibition in reducing death, MI, and revascularization. Bivalirudin was also associated with a significant reduction in the incidence of bleeding and thrombocytopenia (33).

The acute catheterization and urgent intervention triage strategy (ACUITY) trial studied patients with moderate to high risk unstable angina or non-ST-elevation MI undergoing early invasive management (angiography with 72 hours, followed by triage to PCI, coronary artery bypass surgery or medical management). As many as 13,819 patients were randomized to UFH or enoxaparin plus GPIIb/IIIa inhibitors, bivalirudin plus GPIIb/IIIa inhibitors, or bivalirudin alone. The primary endpoint was a composite of death, MI, unplanned revascularization for ischemia, and non-CABG major bleeding at 30 days. The secondary endpoint examined the same variables at one year. At 30 days, bivalirudin alone was noninferior to heparin (either UFH or enoxaparin), plus GPIIb/IIIa inhibitors in terms of mortality and the primary endpoint. It was also associated with significantly less bleeding. At one year, bivalirudin was still noninferior to heparin in terms of the primary endpoint and mortality rates. However, bivalirudin either alone or with GPIIb/IIIa inhibitors, continued to be associated with significantly less bleeding. The results were similar in patients triaged to medical management, PCI, or coronary artery bypass surgery. The ACUITY trial showed a strong association between major bleeding in the first 30 days and the risk of death over one year. (hazard ratio 3.77, $p < 0.0001$) (34). Given that early bleeding is significantly associated with long-term prognosis in patients with ACS, bivalirudin's association with decreased bleeding makes it a favorable agent in this population.

Argatroban

Argatroban is a potent agent that stands apart among the parenteral DTIs, as a univalent inhibitor that binds reversibly only to the active site of thrombin. It is a synthetic heterocyclic derivative of L-arginine, and inhibits both free and clot-bound thrombin (35).

Argatroban is administered intravenously, and reaches steady state levels within one to three hours. Its half-life is approximately 45 minutes. Argatroban is metabolized by the liver. Therefore, its clearance is reduced in patients with moderate hepatic impairment, as defined by a Child-Pugh score over 6. The half-life of argatroban in these individuals is increased threefold. For this reason, significant reductions in argatroban dose are required for individuals with moderate hepatic impairment, and the drug is contraindicated in patients with severe hepatic dysfunction. No dose adjustment is needed in the setting of renal impairment (36,37).

Argatroban increases the APTT, PT/INR, thrombin time, ECT, and ACT in a dose-dependent fashion. Its anticoagulant effect is monitored using the APTT, with a target of 1.5 to 3.0 times baseline. Many laboratories generate an argatroban-specific standard curve, allowing estimation of argatroban levels using the APTT. This approach has not been formally compared with the recommended method of APTT monitoring (38).

The major side effect of argatroban is bleeding. Because there is no specific antidote, excessive bleeding can only be managed by stopping the argatroban infusion and providing supportive therapy. In patients with normal hepatic function, the anticoagulant effect of argatroban disappears two to four hours after stopping the infusion. However, the anticoagulant effects of argatroban may persist for up to 24 hours in patients with hepatic impairment.

In patients with normal hepatic function, argatroban is given as an intravenous infusion at a dose of 2 µg/kg/min, with no initial bolus. Subsequent dose adjustments should be made to achieve an APTT of 1.5 to 2.0 times the baseline value. A major challenge of argatroban is its effect on the PT/INR. When overlapped with warfarin, the PT/INR is prolonged beyond what would be expected with warfarin alone, making dose adjustment of either drug difficult. When argatroban is infused at low doses (< 2 µg/kg/min) and the thromboplastin reagent used in the PT/INR assay has an ISI of 0.88 to 2.13, the INR prolongation attributable to warfarin alone can be teased out (39). Warkentin et al. have published guidelines for conversion from argatroban to warfarin. They suggest initiating warfarin using the expected daily dose, and monitoring the INR daily. If higher than 2 µg/kg/min, the argatroban infusion should be temporarily reduced to this level four to six hours before the INR is measured. If the INR is less than 4.0, the authors suggest continuing concomitant therapy. If the INR is greater than 4.0, the argatroban infusion should be stopped and the INR repeated four to six hours later. This second measurement reflects the true therapeutic range for warfarin alone. If the INR is too low, the argatroban infusion should be resumed. If the INR is within the therapeutic range, the argatroban infusion can be discontinued (40). Arpino et al. have also described the use of the chromogenic factor X level to monitor warfarin therapy in patients receiving concomitant argatroban. They suggest that a chromogenic factor X level of 45% or less is a reliable predictor that the INR would be therapeutic when argatroban therapy is discontinued. Using a cutoff of 45% or less to predict an INR of 2.0 or greater, absent of argatroban influence, has a sensitivity of 93%, a specificity of 78%, and an accuracy of 89% (41).

Two multicenter phase III prospective trials of argatroban in HIT have been completed. They found that when compared with historical controls, patients on argatroban had reduced rates of thrombosis and death due to thrombosis, without an increase in bleeding (42,43). On the basis of these findings, argatroban has been approved for treatment of thrombosis and for thromboprophylaxis in patients with HIT. Argatroban is also approved in the United States for PCI in patients with HIT (2,44).

Argatroban has been shown to provide adequate and safe anticoagulation in patients with HIT undergoing PCI (44). There is now emerging data supporting the use of argatroban in patients without HIT undergoing PCI. A 2007 multicenter, prospective pilot study evaluated the efficacy and safety of argatroban in combination with the GP IIb/IIIa inhibitors abciximab or eptifibatide in 152 patients. The primary efficacy endpoint (a composite of death, MI, or urgent revascularization at 30 days) occurred in 2.6% of patients, and major bleeding occurred in 1.3% of patients (45). This pilot study showed that argatroban in combination with GP IIb/IIIa inhibition was an adequate anticoagulant with an acceptable bleeding risk; however, additional studies must be done.

ORAL DIRECT THROMBIN INHIBITORS

Overview

Current anticoagulant practice dates to the 1940s, when oral vitamin K antagonists were first used for the prevention and treatment of thromboembolism. All currently available oral anticoagulants produce their anticoagulant effect by interfering with posttranslational processing of four vitamin K–dependent clotting proteins, factors VII, IX, X, and prothrombin (46). Oral anticoagulants also block the posttranslational modification of two naturally occurring anticoagulants, proteins C and S. Vitamin K antagonists act as competitive antagonists to two enzymes that catalyze the conversion of vitamin K from the epoxide to the reduced form. Reduced vitamin K is required for γ-carboxylation of glutamine residues found on the amino-termini of vitamin K-dependent clotting factors (46). γ-Carboxylation is necessary for interaction of these proteins with calcium, an essential step in the assembly of coagulation factor complexes on phospholipid surfaces.

Oral vitamin K antagonists are effective antithrombotic drugs. For example, warfarin reduces the risk of stroke in patients with atrial fibrillation by about 70%, and lowers the risk of recurrent DVT by about 90% (47,48). However, oral vitamin K antagonists have four major drawbacks: (*i*) delayed onset of anticoagulation, because it takes several days to lower the levels of the vitamin K-dependent into the therapeutic range (49); (*ii*) multiple drug and food interactions render the anticoagulant response unpredictable so that coagulation monitoring is essential (50); (*iii*) reversal of the anticoagulant effect of vitamin K antagonists is slow unless supplemental vitamin K and/or fresh frozen plasma is given because it takes time to regenerate normal or near normal levels of the vitamin K–dependent clotting factors; and (*iv*) decreases in the levels of proteins C or protein S, on initiation of oral anticoagulant therapy, can precipitate skin necrosis in individuals whose baseline levels of proteins C or S are reduced (51–53).

Currently, there are no safe and effective orally available alternatives to the vitamin K antagonists. Aspirin and other orally active antiplatelet agents reduce the risk of thrombosis in a variety of patient populations, including those with atherosclerotic vascular diseases. However, antiplatelet agents are less effective than warfarin or parenteral anticoagulants in many patients at high risk of thrombosis (54,55). Orally available heparin formulations are undergoing clinical trials, but their utility remains to be proven. Chemical manipulation of existing parenteral DTIs has led to the production of orally active DTIs (Table 1).

Table 1 Properties of Direct Thrombin Inhibitors

Drug	Approved indications	Route of administration	Plasma half-life	Clearance
Bivalirudin	PCI in patients with or without HIT	Intravenous	25 min	Kidney, liver
Lepirudin	HIT complicated by thrombosis	Intravenous	60 min	Kidney
Desirudin	Thromboprophylaxis in elective hip or knee replacement surgery (Europe only)	Subcutaneous	120 min	Kidney
Argatroban	Thromboprophylaxis in HIT, HIT complicated by thrombosis, PCI (United States.) only	Intravenous	45 min	Liver
Dabigatran	None in United States. Orthopedic prophylaxis in Canada and Europe	Oral	12 hr	Kidney

Abbreviations: PCI, percutaneous coronary intervention; HIT, heparin-induced thrombocytopenia.

Oral DTIs have the potential to overcome many of the limitations of the vitamin K antagonists. For example, DTIs have a rapid onset of action and their anticoagulant effect is dose-dependent. Because they target only a single enzyme, DTIs may have a wider therapeutic window than vitamin K antagonists (56). With short half-lives, the anticoagulant effect of oral DTIs is rapidly reversible, and because these agents have no effect on the levels of proteins C or S, there is no danger of skin necrosis.

Ximelagatran

Ximelagatran, the orally available prodrug of the univalent DTI melagatran, was the first drug in this class to generate widespread interest. Randomized controlled trials demonstrated that ximelagatran was at least as effective as warfarin or LMWH for thromboprophylaxis in the setting of hip or knee arthroplasty (57,58). Ximelagatran was also shown to be as effective as warfarin in preventing stroke or systemic embolism in the setting of atrial fibrillation (59). However, questions were raised about ximelagatran's safety profile. The open-label SPORTIF III trial compared ximelagatran with warfarin for prevention of stroke and systemic embolism in 3407 patients with nonvalvular atrial fibrillation. Though ximelagatran was shown to be noninferior to warfarin in preventing stroke and systemic embolism, serum alanine aminotransferase levels rose to greater than three times the upper limit of normal in 6% of individuals in the ximelagatran group and greater than five times the upper limit of normal in 3.4% of individuals in the ximelagatran group. This liver enzyme elevation generally occurred within six months and tended to decline whether or not treatment continued (60). The double-blind SPORTIF V trial compared ximelagatran with warfarin for prevention of stroke and systemic embolism in 3922 patients with nonvalvular atrial fibrillation. Serum alanine aminotransferase levels again rose to greater than three times the upper limit of normal in 6.0% of individuals in the ximelagatran group, and tended to decline whether or not treatment continued. However, there was one clearly documented case and one suggestive case of fatal liver disease (59). SPORTIF III and SPORTIF V concluded that fixed-dose ximelagatran without anticoagulation monitoring was noninferior to dose-adjusted warfarin in preventing stroke or systemic embolism (the primary endpoint), but even the conclusion of noninferiority was called into question when their data were reanalyzed using more conservative criteria. Reanalysis revealed that the SPORTIF trials had overestimated the warfarin event rate, and thus overcalculated the noninferiority margin (the clinically acceptable worst case loss in efficacy). This potentially biased the trials toward noninferiority. The data from SPORTIF V and SPORTIF III were pooled. However, the heterogeneity in the magnitude of efficacy observed in the two trials and the difference in their design—double-blind versus open label—argued against pooling their data. Significant safety concerns regarding increased liver toxicity without a significant offsetting advantage in major bleeding led the Food and Drug Administration to reject the sponsor's application for ximelagatran in 2004. In 2006, the sponsoring company decided to withdraw ximelagatran from the market and terminate its development. The ximelagatran experience illustrated the difficulties inherent in designing noninferiority trials and the importance of considering toxicity when developing new drugs.

Currently, there are a number of orally available DTIs still undergoing clinical development. The most advanced agent is dabigatran etexilate, which is the orally available prodrug of the synthetic DTI, dabigatran (Fig. 1).

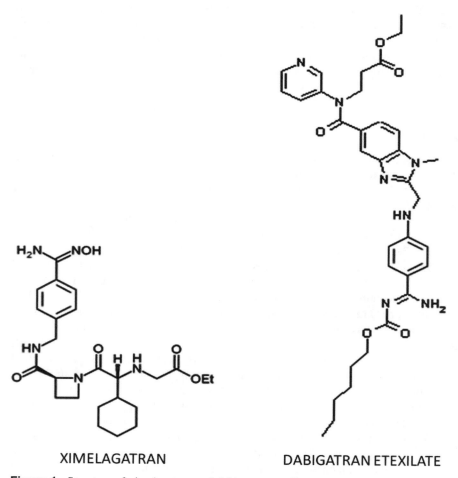

XIMELAGATRAN   DABIGATRAN ETEXILATE

Figure 1 Structure of ximelagatran and dabigatran etexilate.

Dabigatran Etexilate

Like ximelagatran, dabigatran etexilate is a double prodrug. It has a bioavailability of about 6% after oral administration. Once absorbed, the drug is rapidly converted by esterases to dabigatran, whose levels peak in approximately one to two hours. Dabigatran is a small molecule, reversible inhibitor that binds to the active site of thrombin. The half-life of dabigatran is approximately 12 hours, and it is primarily eliminated via the kidneys (61). The half-life is prolonged in the elderly, reflecting their impaired renal function (62). The pharmacokinetics and pharmacodynamics of dabigatran are not influenced by aspirin, and because the cytochrome P450 enzymes and other hepatic oxidoreductases are not involved in dabigatran's metabolism, it does not interfere with drugs that are metabolized by the P450 enzyme system (61).

Dabigatran produces a predictable anticoagulant response. Therefore, routine coagulation monitoring is unlikely to be necessary. Dabigatran prolongs the ECT, APTT, and PT/INR in a dose-dependent fashion (62,63). Because these widely available tests have not been used in the clinical setting for monitoring, the target levels are unknown.

The major side effect of dabigatran is hemorrhage. No specific antidote is available. Consequently, bleeding complications must be managed symptomatically. Although not well studied, dialysis or hemoperfusion likely removes this compound from the circulation, and the administration of activated coagulation factor complexes such as FEIBA™, Autoplex, or recombinant activated factor VII (factor VIIa), may overcome its anticoagulant effect (11,64).

Several clinical trials have demonstrated dabigatran's antithrombotic effect. The phase II Boehringer Ingelheim Study in Thrombosis II (BISTRO II) trial, compared oral dabigatran with enoxaparin as thromboprophylaxis after total hip or total knee replacement (65). Dabigatran was administered at doses of 50 mg, 150 mg, or 225 mg twice daily, or 300 mg once daily for 6 to 10 days. A significant dose-dependent decrease in VTE occurred with increasing doses of dabigatran etexilate. Overall VTE rates were 28.5% in patients receiving 50 mg of dabigatran twice daily, 17.4% in patients receiving 150 mg of dabigatran twice daily, 13.1% in patients receiving 225 mg of dabigatran twice daily, 16.6% in patients receiving 300 mg of dabigatran once daily, and 24% in patients receiving enoxaparin. The risk of serious bleeding with dabigatran increased in a dose-dependent manner as well, but did not reach statistical significance at any dose. Serious bleeding occurred in 0.3% of patients receiving 50 mg of dabigatran twice daily, 4.1% of patients receiving 150 mg of dabigatran twice daily, 4.8% of patients receiving 225 mg of dabigatran twice daily, and 4.7% of patients receiving 300 mg of dabigatran once daily. Serious bleeding occurred in 2.0% of patients receiving enoxaparin.

The RE-NOVATE study demonstrated that dabigatran etexilate was as effective as enoxaparin for the prevention of VTE after total hip replacement, with a similar safety profile (66). This double-blind, noninferiority trial randomized 3494 patients to treatment for 28 to 35 days with dabigatran etexilate 220 mg or 150 mg once daily, or subcutaneous enoxaparin 40 mg once daily. The primary efficacy outcome was the composite of total VTE, and all cause mortality. Both doses of dabigatran etexilate were noninferior to enoxaparin, with the primary efficacy outcome occurring in 6.7% of patients in the enoxaparin group versus 6.0% of patients in the dabigatran etexilate 220-mg group, and 8.6% of patients in the 150-mg group. There was no significant difference in major bleeding rates with either dose of dabigatran etexilate compared with enoxaparin. There was no difference in the frequency of liver enzyme elevation.

The subsequent RE-MODEL trial reproduced these results in 2076 patients undergoing total knee replacement (67). The primary efficacy outcome occurred in 37.7%

of the enoxaparin group versus 36.4% of the dabigatran etexilate 220-mg group and 40.5% of the 150-mg group. Both doses of dabigatran etexilate were thus noninferior to enoxaparin. The incidence of major bleeding did not differ significantly between the three groups (1.3% vs. 1.5% and 1.3%, respectively), and there were no significant differences in liver enzyme elevation.

The RE-MOBILIZE trial was similar in design to the RE-MODEL trial. However, RE-MOBILIZE was performed in North America, and because of labeling requirements, dabigatran was compared to a higher dose of enoxaparin (60 mg). In contrast to RE-MODEL, RE-MOBILIZE failed to show equivalence for a composite endpoint of proximal DVT, distal DVT, PE, and all-cause mortality. The primary efficacy outcome occurred in 25.3% of the enoxaparin group, 31.1% of the dabigatran 220 mg-group, and 33.7% of the dabigatran 150-mg group. The difference in the results of RE-MODEL and RE-MOBILIZE has been attributed to the incidence of asymptomatic DVT in the latter trial, detected by protocol, required venography at the end of therapy. Major VTE did occur at similar rates across all treatment groups in RE-MOBILIZE (3.0% and 3.4% for 150-mg and 220-mg dabigatran etexilate, respectively, vs. 2.2% enoxaparin). Although major bleeding events were more common in the enoxaparin group (1.4%) compared with the dabigatran 220-mg group (0.6%) and the dabigatran 150-mg group (0.6%), these differences were not statistically significant (68).

Warfarin is often used for thromboprophylaxis after knee arthroplasty in centers in North America, but it has not been directly compared with dabigatran in a clinical trial.

Oral DTIs have the potential to revolutionize the treatment of acute venous thrombosis. Single-agent, unmonitored therapy would substantially reduce the complexity and might reduce the cost of treating this common clinical problem. Dabigatran is currently undergoing phase III development for initial and long-term treatment of patients with established VTE. A phase III trial evaluating dabigatran for prevention of cardioembolic events in patients with atrial fibrillation is also underway. Dabigatran was licensed in Canada and Europe for orthopedic prophylaxis in the spring of 2008.

CONCLUSION

Thrombin plays a central role in the initiation and propagation of thrombus. Therefore, DTIs are a powerful alternative to traditional anticoagulants. Their ability to specifically bind circulating and fibrin-bound thrombin, lack of a requirement for a cofactor, absence of natural inhibitors, and wide therapeutic window are particular advantages. DTIs have already found roles in thromboprophylaxis, in anticoagulation during PCI, and in the management of heparin-induced thrombocytopenia. Yet there are unresolved challenges with the DTIs. Monitoring intravenous DTIs is challenging and nonstandardized, and there is no antidote for rapidly reversing the effect of DTIs. There were concerns that ximelagatran's hepatotoxicity was a class effect common to all oral DTIs. There has been no evidence to date that dabigatran etexilate causes hepatotoxicity, but experience with ximelagatran underscores the need to be vigilant for unexpected side effects. Thrombin is ubiquitous in the body, playing a part in coagulation, anticoagulation, inflammation, and cellular proliferation. It is not known if long-term thrombin blockade will impair these latter two processes. The anti-inflammatory and antiproliferative effects of anticoagulants are currently viewed to be beneficial, however, the long-term consequences are not yet known. It is also not known how DTIs compare with direct FXa inhibitors. FXa has a limited role in coagulation, solely controlling thrombin generation. However, the activation of one molecule of FX results in the generation of 1000 molecules of thrombin.

On a molar basis, activated FX is more thrombogenic than thrombin, and inhibiting coagulation prior to thrombin formation may be more effective than inhibiting coagulation afterwards (69). There have been no head-to-head clinical trials of DTIs versus direct FXa inhibitors. At this time, both classes of drugs appear promising. Continued study of oral DTIs is particularly vital, as they have the potential to overcome many of the limitations of vitamin K antagonists. Even if oral DTIs prove to be no more effective than vitamin K antagonists, treatment will be streamlined if the need for laboratory monitoring can be reduced or eliminated.

REFERENCES

1. Weitz JI. Factor Xa or thrombin: is thrombin a better target? J Thromb Haemost 2007; 5(suppl 1):65–67.
2. Warkentin TE. Bivalent direct thrombin inhibitors: hirudin and bivalirudin. Best Pract Res Clin Haematol 2004; 17(1):105–125.
3. Markwardt F, Nowak G, Sturzebecher J. Clinical pharmacology of recombinant hirudin. Haemostasis 1991; 21(suppl 1):133–136.
4. Markwardt F. Past, present, and future of hirudin. Haemostasis 1991; 21(suppl 1):11–26.
5. Markwardt F. Hirudin as alternative anticoagulant: a historical review. Semin Thromb Hemost 2002; 28(5):405–414.
6. Salzet M. Leech thrombin inhibitors. Curr Pharm Des 2002; 8(7):493–503.
7. Romisch J, Diehl KH, Hoffmann D, et al. Comparison of in vitro and in vivo properties of r-hirudin (HBW 023) and a synthetic analogous peptide. Haemostasis 1993; 23(5):249–258.
8. Nowak G, Bucha E, Goock T, et al. Pharmacology of r-hirudin in renal impairment. Thromb Res 1992; 66(6):707–715.
9. Nurmohamed MT, Berckmans RJ, Morrien-Salomons WM, et al. Monitoring anticoagulant therapy by activated partial thromboplastin time: hirudin assessment. An evaluation of native blood and plasma assays. Thromb Haemost 1994; 72(5):685–692.
10. Hafner G, Roser M, Nauck M. Methods for the monitoring of direct thrombin inhibitors. Semin Thromb Hemost 2002; 28(5):425–430.
11. Greinacher A. Lepirudin for the treatment of heparin-induced thrombocytopenia. In: Warkentin TE, Greinacher A, eds.. Heparin-Induced Thrombocytopenia. 2nd ed., New York: Marcel Dekker Inc, 2004:397–436.
12. Potzsch B, Madlener K, Seelig C, et al. Monitoring of r-hirudin anticoagulation during cardiopulmonary bypass: assessment of the whole blood ecarin clotting time. Thromb Haemost 1997; 77(5):920–925.
13. Iqbal O, Tobu M, Aziz S, et al. Successful use of recombinant hirudin and its monitoring by ecarin clotting time in patients with heparin-induced thrombocytopenia undergoing off-pump coronary artery revascularization. J Card Surg 2005; 20(1):42–51.
14. Eichler P, Friesen HJ, Lubenow N, et al. Antihirudin antibodies in patients with heparin-induced thrombocytopenia treated with lepirudin: incidence, effects on aPTT, and clinical relevance. Blood 2000; 96(7):2373–2378.
15. Greinacher A, Lubenow N, Eichler P. Anaphylactic and anaphylactoid reactions associated with lepirudin in patients with heparin-induced thrombocytopenia. Circulation 2003; 108(17): 2062–2065.
16. Lubenow N, Eichler P, Lietz T, et al. Lepirudin in patients with heparin-induced thrombocytopenia: results of the third prospective study (HAT-3) and a combined analysis of HAT-1, HAT-2, and HAT-3. J Thromb Haemost 2005; 3(11):2428–2436.
17. Greinacher A, Volpel H, Janssens U, et al. Recombinant hirudin (lepirudin) provides safe and effective anticoagulation in patients with heparin-induced thrombocytopenia: a prospective study. Circulation 1999; 99(1):73–80.

18. Greinacher A, Eichler P, Lubenow N, et al. Heparin-induced thrombocytopenia with thromboembolic complications: meta-analysis of 2 prospective trials to assess the value of parenteral treatment with lepirudin and its therapeutic aPTT range. Blood 2000; 96(3):846–851.

19. Weitz JI. A novel approach to thrombin inhibition. Thromb Res 2003, 109(suppl 1):S17–S22.

20. Warkentin TE, Greinacher A. Heparin-induced thrombocytopenia: recognition, treatment, and prevention: the Seventh ACCP Conference on Antithrombotic and Thrombolytic Therapy. Chest 2004; 126(suppl 3):311S–337S.

21. Lubenow N, Eichler P, Lietz T, et al. Lepirudin for prophylaxis of thrombosis in patients with acute isolated heparin-induced thrombocytopenia: an analysis of 3 prospective studies. Blood 2004; 104(10):3072–3077.

22. Effects of recombinant hirudin (lepirudin) compared with heparin on death, myocardial infarction, refractory angina, and revascularisation procedures in patients with acute myocardial ischaemia without ST elevation: a randomised trial. Organisation to Assess Strategies for Ischemic Syndromes (OASIS-2) Investigators. Lancet 1999; 353(9151):429–438.

23. Greinacher A, Eichler P, Albrecht D, et al. Antihirudin antibodies following low-dose subcutaneous treatment with desirudin for thrombosis prophylaxis after hip-replacement surgery: incidence and clinical relevance. Blood 2003; 101(7):2617–2619.

24. Eriksson BI, Ekman S, Lindbratt S, et al. Prevention of thromboembolism with use of recombinant hirudin: results of a double-blind, multicenter trial comparing the efficacy of desirudin (Revasc) with that of unfractionated heparin in patients having a total hip replacement. J Bone Joint Surg Am 1997; 79(3):326–333.

25. Eriksson BI, Wille-Jorgensen P, Kalebo P, et al. A comparison of recombinant hirudin with a low-molecular-weight heparin to prevent thromboembolic complications after total hip replacement. N Engl J Med 1997; 337(19):1329–1335.

26. Parry MA, Maraganore JM, Stone SR. Kinetic mechanism for the interaction of Hirulog with thrombin. Biochemistry 1994; 33(49):14807–14814.

27. Bartholomew JR. Bivalirudin for the treatment of heparin-induced thrombocytopenia. In: Warkentin TE, Greinacher A, eds. Heparin-Induced Thrombocytopenia. 2nd ed. New York: Marcel Dekker, 2004:475–508.

28. Bates SM, Weitz JI. Direct thrombin inhibitors for treatment of arterial thrombosis: potential differences between bivalirudin and hirudin. Am J Cardiol 1998; 82(8B):12P-18P.

29. Fox I, Dawson A, Loynds P, et al. Anticoagulant activity of Hirulog, a direct thrombin inhibitor, in humans. Thromb Haemost 1993; 69(2):157–163.

30. Robson R. The use of bivalirudin in patients with renal impairment. J Invasive Cardiol 2000; 12(suppl F):33F-36F.

31. Bittl JA, Chaitman BR, Feit F, et al. Bivalirudin versus heparin during coronary angioplasty for unstable or postinfarction angina: final report reanalysis of the Bivalirudin Angioplasty Study. Am Heart J 2001; 142(6):952–959.

32. Lincoff AM, Bittl JA, Kleiman NS, et al. Comparison of bivalirudin versus heparin during percutaneous coronary intervention (the Randomized Evaluation of PCI Linking Angiomax to Reduced Clinical Events [REPLACE]-1 trial). Am J Cardiol 2004; 93(9):1092–1096.

33. Lincoff AM, Kleiman NS, Kereiakes DJ, et al. Long-term efficacy of bivalirudin and provisional glycoprotein IIb/IIIa blockade vs. heparin and planned glycoprotein IIb/IIIa blockade during percutaneous coronary revascularization: REPLACE-2 randomized trial. JAMA 2004; 292(6):696–703.

34. Stone GW, Ware JH, Bertrand ME, et al. Antithrombotic strategies in patients with acute coronary syndromes undergoing early invasive management: one-year results from the ACUITY trial. JAMA 2007; 298(21):2497–2506.

35. Berry CN, Girardot C, Lecoffre C, et al. Effects of the synthetic thrombin inhibitor argatroban on fibrin- or clot-incorporated thrombin: comparison with heparin and recombinant hirudin. Thromb Haemost 1994; 72(3):381–386.

36. Swan SK, Hursting MJ. The pharmacokinetics and pharmacodynamics of argatroban: effects of age, gender, and hepatic or renal dysfunction. Pharmacotherapy 2000; 20(3):318–329.

37. Swan SK, St Peter JV, Lambrecht LJ, et al. Comparison of anticoagulant effects and safety of argatroban and heparin in healthy subjects. Pharmacotherapy 2000; 20(7):756–770.

38. Love JE, Ferrell C, Chandler WL. Monitoring direct thrombin inhibitors with a plasma diluted thrombin time. Thromb Haemost 2007; 98(1):234–242.

39. Sheth SB, DiCicco RA, Hursting MJ, et al. Interpreting the International Normalized Ratio (INR) in individuals receiving argatroban and warfarin. Thromb Haemost 2001; 85(3):435–440.

40. Greinacher A, Warkentin TE. Treatment of heparin-induced thrombocytopenia: an overview. In: Warkentin TE, Greinacher A, eds. Heparin-Induced Thrombocytopenia. 3rd ed. New York: Informa Healthcare, 2007:283–317.

41. Arpino PA, Demirjian Z, Van Cott EM. Use of the chromogenic factor X assay to predict the international normalized ratio in patients transitioning from argatroban to warfarin. Pharmacotherapy 2005; 25(2):157–164.

42. Lewis BE, Wallis DE, Leya F, et al. Argatroban anticoagulation in patients with heparin-induced thrombocytopenia. Arch Intern Med 2003; 163(15):1849–1856.

43. Lewis BE, Wallis DE, Berkowitz SD, et al. Argatroban anticoagulant therapy in patients with heparin-induced thrombocytopenia. Circulation 2001; 103(14):1838–1843.

44. Lewis BE, Matthai WH Jr, Cohen M, et al. Argatroban anticoagulation during percutaneous coronary intervention in patients with heparin-induced thrombocytopenia. Catheter Cardiovasc Interv 2002; 57(2):177–184.

45. Cruz-Gonzalez I, Sanchez-Ledesma M, Baron SJ, et al. Efficacy and safety of argatroban with or without glycoprotein IIb/IIIa inhibitor in patients with heparin induced thrombocytopenia undergoing percutaneous coronary intervention for acute coronary syndrome. J Thromb Thrombolysis 2007, July 15 Epub.

46. Furie B, Bouchard BA, Furie BC. Vitamin K-dependent biosynthesis of γ–carboxyglutamic acid. Blood 1999; 3(6):1798–1808.

47. Kearon C, Gent M, Hirsh J, et al. A comparison of three months of anticoagulation with extended anticoagulation for a first episode of idiopathic venous thromboembolism. N Engl J Med 1999; 340(12):901–907.

48. Hart RG, Sherman DG, Easton JD, et al. Prevention of stroke in patients with nonvalvular atrial fibrillation. Neurology 1998; 51(3):674–681.

49. Harrison L, Johnston M, Massicotte MP, et al. Comparison of 5–mg and 10–mg loading doses in initiation of warfarin therapy. Ann Intern Med 1997; 126(2):133–136.

50. Ansell J, Hirsh J, Dalen J, et al. Managing oral anticoagulant therapy. Chest 2001; 119(suppl 1): 22S-38S.

51. Shetty HG, Backhouse G, Bentley DP, et al. Effective reversal of warfarin-induced excessive anticoagulation with low dose vitamin K1. Thromb Haemost 1992; 67(1):13–15.

52. Hirsh J, Dalen JE, Anderson DR, et al. Oral anticoagulants: mechanism of action, clinical effectiveness, and optimal therapeutic range. Chest 1998; 114(suppl 5):445S-469S.

53. Conlan MG, Bridges A, Williams E, et al. Familial type II protein C deficiency associated with warfarin-induced skin necrosis and bilateral adrenal hemorrhage. Am J Hematol 1988; 29(4): 226–229.

54. Gent M, Hirsh J, Ginsberg JS, et al. Low-molecular-weight heparinoid orgaran is more effective than aspirin in the prevention of venous thromboembolism after surgery for hip fracture. Circulation 1996; 93(1):80–84.

55. Risk factors for stroke and efficacy of antithrombotic therapy in atrial fibrillation: analysis of pooled data from five randomized controlled trials. Arch Intern Med 1994; 154(13):1449–1457.

56. Elg M, Gustafsson D, Carlsson S. Antithrombotic effects and bleeding time of thrombin inhibitors and warfarin in the rat. Thromb Res 1999; 94(3):187–197.

57. Francis CW, Davidson BL, Berkowitz SD, et al. Ximelagatran versus warfarin for the prevention of venous thromboembolism after total knee arthroplasty: a randomized, double-blind trial. Ann Intern Med 2002; 137(8):648–655.

58. Eriksson BI, Bergqvist D, Kalebo P, et al. Ximelagatran and melagatran compared with dalteparin for prevention of venous thromboembolism after total hip or knee replacement: the METHRO II randomised trial. Lancet 2002; 360(9344):1441–1447.

59. Albers GW, Diener HC, Frison L, et al. Ximelagatran vs. warfarin for stroke prevention in patients with nonvalvular atrial fibrillation: a randomized trial. JAMA 2005; 293(6):690–698.
60. Olsson SB. Stroke prevention with the oral direct thrombin inhibitor ximelagatran compared with warfarin in patients with nonvalvular atrial fibrillation (SPORTIF III): randomised controlled trial. Lancet 2003; 362(9397):1691–1698.
61. Blech S, Ebner T, Ludwig-Schwellinger E. The metabolism and disposition of the oral direct thrombin inhibitor, dabigatran, in humans. Drug Metab Dispos 2007; 36(2):386–399.
62. Stangier J, Stahle H, Rathgen K, et al. Pharmacokinetics and pharmacodynamics of the direct oral thrombin inhibitor dabigatran in healthy elderly subjects. Clin Pharmacokinet 2008; 47(1): 47–59.
63. Wienen W, Stassen JM, Priepke H, et al. In-vitro profile and ex-vivo anticoagulant activity of the direct thrombin inhibitor dabigatran and its orally active prodrug, dabigatran etexilate. Thromb Haemost 2007; 98(1):155–162.
64. Wienen W, Stassen JM, Priepke H, et al. Effects of the direct thrombin inhibitor dabigatran and its orally active prodrug, dabigatran etexilate, on thrombus formation and bleeding time in rats. Thromb Haemost 2007; 98(2):333–338.
65. Eriksson BI, Dahl OE, Buller HR, et al. A new oral direct thrombin inhibitor, dabigatran etexilate, compared with enoxaparin for prevention of thromboembolic events following total hip or knee replacement: the BISTRO II randomized trial. J Thromb Haemost 2005; 3(1):103–111.
66. Eriksson BI, Dahl OE, Rosencher N, et al. Dabigatran etexilate versus enoxaparin for prevention of venous thromboembolism after total hip replacement: a randomised, double-blind, non-inferiority trial. Lancet 2007; 370(9591):949–956.
67. Eriksson BI, Dahl OE, Rosencher N, et al. Oral dabigatran etexilate vs. subcutaneous enoxaparin for the prevention of venous thromboembolism after total knee replacement: the RE-MODEL randomized trial. J Thromb Haemost 2007; 5(11):2178–2185.
68. Dabigatran etexilate versus enoxaparin in preventing venous thromboembolism following total knee arthroplasty. 07 Jul 13; Geneva, Switzerland: 2007 Congress of the International Society on Thrombosis and Hemostasis, 2007.
69. Ansell J. Factor Xa or thrombin: is factor Xa a better target? J Thromb Haemost 2007; 5(suppl 1):60–64.

20
Modulators of the Protein C Pathway

Charles T. Esmon
Howard Hughes Medical Institute, Oklahoma Medical Research Foundation, Oklahoma City, Oklahoma, U.S.A.

INTRODUCTION

The protein C anticoagulant pathway consists of several proteins whose mechanisms of action are distinct from other antithrombotic agents and hence offer potentially novel approaches to the treatment of thrombotic diseases. At present, there is limited human clinical data related to the treatment of thrombosis with components of the pathway. There are a number of congenital and acquired deficiency states, however, that provide potential insights into how the system might be utilized. To understand the application of this pathway to thrombotic disease, it is useful to consider our current view of its mechanism of action. There are a substantial number of reviews on this area for those wishing additional information from this author (1–3) or others (4–20). A recent review on the cytoprotective influences of activated protein C (APC) is particularly insightful (21).

MODULATORS OF THE PROTEIN C PATHWAY

The coagulation cascade is illustrated in Figure 1 with the regulatory events associated with the protein C pathway illustrated to the right of the schematic. In this highly simplified view, coagulation is triggered by the tissue factor (TF)-factor VIIa complex. This complex can then activate either factor X or factor IX. The factor VIIIa–factor IXa complex can then activate factor X. Factor Xa generated by either mechanism can then complex with factor Va to activate prothrombin. Factors Va and VIIIa are critical to the amplification of the coagulation response. The protein C pathway is designed to block this amplification by inactivating these two critical cofactors, factors Va and VIIIa. To accomplish this, thrombin binds to thrombomodulin (TM) on the surface of the endothelium and then generates the anticoagulant, APC. Protein C activation by the thrombin-TM complex is further enhanced by protein C binding to EPCR, a process that enhances protein C activation in vivo approximately 20-fold (24). APC complexes with protein S to inactivate factors Va and VIIIa, thus shutting down the propagation phase of the coagulation response. For simplicity the activation of factors VII, VIII and V are not shown in this figure. It is relevant to point out that the precursors of the activated cofactors of the factor V and factor VIII/von Willebrand factor complex are much more resistant to inactivation than factors Va or VIIIa (4–6,25,26). Reports have indicated that factor V, but not factor Va can serve as a cofactor to further accelerate the inactivation of the cofactors (22). By regulating the cofactors, the protein C pathway complements the

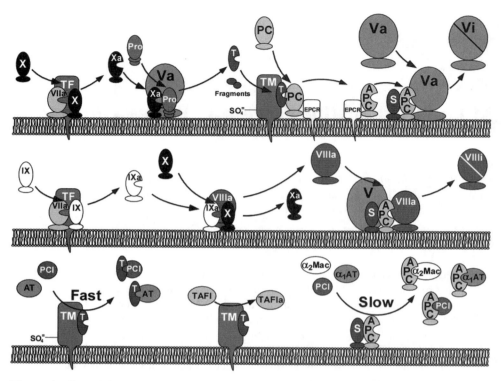

Figure 1 Coagulation is initiated when TF is exposed to blood. This can occur either as the result of monocyte activation or exposure of the blood to extravascular cells. For simplicity, factor designations are not used in the figure, i.e., factor VIIa becomes VIIa. The TF-VIIa complex can then activate either factor X (*top row*) or IX (*middle row*). These, in turn, form complexes with factors Va and VIIIa, respectively, probably on the surface of the activated platelet. The Xa-Va complex leads to explosive T formation. Unchecked, the thrombin would cause platelet activation, fibrin deposition and initiate an inflammatory cascade. All steps to this point occur much better on negatively charged phospholipids. These can be made available by complement activation of the cells and by other agents that mobilize intracellular calcium. Several potent natural anticoagulant factors exist including the heparin-antithrombin mechanism responsible for the inhibition of factor Xa and T and the TF pathway inhibitor mechanism responsible for the control of the TF-factor VIIa complex. Because the impact of inflammation on these pathways is less characterized than the protein C pathway, emphasis is placed on the latter pathway for purposes of this review. The protein C anticoagulant pathway is triggered when T binds to TM on the surface of the endothelium (*top row, center*). This complex does not appear to need negatively charged phospholipids, especially when the EPCRis present. Once APC is generated, it can either remain bound to EPCR or dissociated to S. The APC-S complex can then inactivate factors Va or VIIIa. In the case of factor VIIIa, the reaction is stimulated by V (22).

In addition to playing a role in the regulation of the coagulation cascade *per se*, TM serves other functions shown on the third level of the figure. TM accelerates thrombin inhibition by AT and PCI, thus providing a mechanism for clearance of thrombin from the circulation. Thus, when TM is downregulated by inflammatory mediators, proteolysis and oxidation, thrombin inhibition is compromised. In addition, TM can accelerate the activation of TAFI. In its active form, this procarboxypeptidase B has been shown to inhibit fibrinolysis. This loss of the fibrin stabilization resulting from TM downregulation may compensate in part for the loss of anticoagulant functions of TM. The APC is then cleared from the circulation by α_2-Mac α1-AT and PCI. Of importance to inflammation, α1-AT behaves as an acute phase reactant, and with respect to the hemostatic balance, functions primarily as an inhibitor of APC and therefore should shift the balance slightly in favor of clot formation. *Abbreviations*: TF, tissue factor; T, thrombin; EPCR, endothelial cell protein C receptor; APC, activated protein C; S, protein S; V, factor V; AT, antithrombin; PCI, protein C inhibitor; α_2-Mac, α_2-macroglobulin; α1-AT, α1-antitrypsin. *Source*: From Ref. 23.

vast array of proteinase inhibitors whose function it is to regulate the protease components of the coagulation cascade.

A potential complication in application of this system to the treatment of thrombotic disease is that there is a common factor V variant (Factor V Leiden) that is resistant to proteolytic inactivation by APC (4–10). This trait, commonly referred to as APC resistance, is caused by a substitution of Gln at residue 506 in factor V. This corresponds to the first cleavage site in factor Va (27–29). Even in the homozygous form, the risk of thrombosis is lower in patients with the Factor V Leiden mutation than it is in those with protein C deficiency. This likely reflects the fact that failure of APC to cleave factor Va at Arg506 slows, but does not prevent, the inactivation of factor Va, and this difference is largely eliminated in the presence of protein S (29).

A schematic diagram of the components of the protein C pathway is presented in Figure 2 and a more complete schematic representation of the protein C pathway is shown

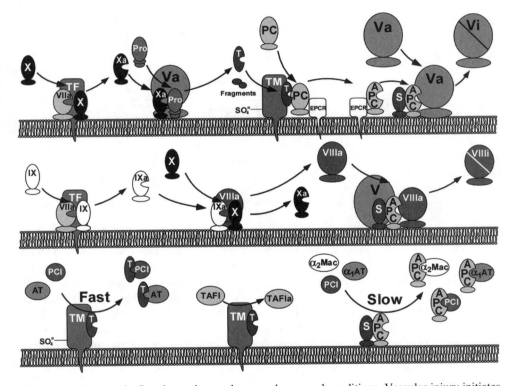

Figure 2 The protein C anticoagulant pathway under normal conditions. Vascular injury initiates Proactivation that results in T formation. Pro activation involves complex formation between Va and Xa. Thrombin then binds to TM on the lumen of the endothelium, illustrated by the heavy line, and the thrombin-TM complex converts PC to APC. Thrombin bound to TM can be rapidly inactivated by ATIII and the thrombin-antithrombin III complex then rapidly dissociates from TM. APC binds to S on cellular surfaces. The APC-S complex then converts factor Va to an Vi, illustrated by the slash through the larger part of the two-subunit factor Va molecule. Protein C and APC interact with an EPCR. This association may concentrate the zymogen and enzyme near the cell surface and facilitate the function of the pathway, but this has yet to be shown directly. S circulates in complex with C4bBP, which may in turn bind SAP. APC is inhibited by forming complexes with PCI, α_1AT, or α_2-macroglobulin (not shown). See text for a more complete discussion. *Abbreviations*: Pro, prothrombin; T, thrombin; Va, factor Va; Xa, factor Xa; TM, thrombomodulin; PC, protein C; APC, activated protein C; S, protein S; Vi, inactive complex; ATIII, antithrombin III; SAP, serum amyloid P; PCI, protein C inhibitor; α_1AT, α_1-antitrypsin. *Source*: Modified from Ref. 30.

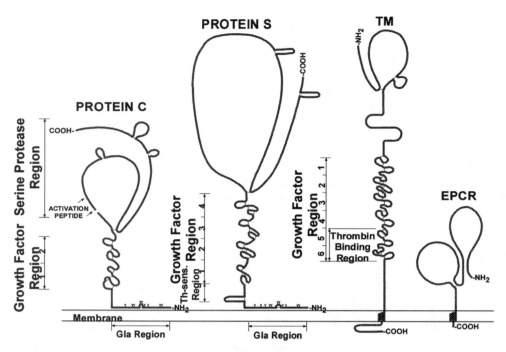

Figure 3 Schematic representation of protein C, protein S, the EPCR, and TM. The vitamin K–dependent Gla residues of protein C and protein S are indicated by small Y-shaped symbols. Formation of these Gla residues is essential for full activity of protein C and protein S. The EPCR domain structure is based on homology to the CD1 family, and the disulfide pairing remains to be documented experimentally. *Abbreviations*: EPCR, endothelial cell protein C receptor; Gla, γ-carboxyglutamic acid; Th.-sens., thrombin sensitive. *Source*: Modified from Ref. 31.

in Figure 3. The protein C pathway is triggered when thrombin binds to TM. This complex exhibits altered macromolecular specificity. Thus, the complex rapidly activates protein C, but fails to promote coagulation reactions, including platelet activation (32), fibrinogen clotting (33), and activation of factor V (33) and XIII activation (34). The basis for the specificity switch is illustrated in Figure 4. In addition, thrombin bound to TM is inhibited more rapidly by antithrombin (38) and the protein C inhibitor (39). The acceleration of the inhibition by antithrombin is dependent on the presence of a chondroitin sulfate moiety that can be covalently attached to TM (15,38,40), while the acceleration of the reaction with protein C inhibitor is not (39). Thus, TM not only triggers the anticoagulant pathway, but also directly blocks most of the procoagulant activities of thrombin and facilitates thrombin inactivation. Once thrombin is bound to antithrombin, the complex rapidly dissociates from TM. These features render the protein C pathway a potent, multifaceted, on demand anticoagulant system.

The image of TM as strictly anticoagulant in nature is clouded by some apparent contradictions. One exception to this general rule is factor XI. Thrombin can activate factor XI in a reaction that is accelerated about 20-fold by TM (41). Given that TM accelerates thrombin inactivation, the net effect of thrombin binding to TM on factor XI activation may be minimal. Another confusing paradox is that TM accelerates the thrombin-dependent activation of TAFI; a procarboxypeptidase B–like enzyme, that once activated, serves as a fibrinolytic inhibitor (42). TAFIa, however, has potent anti-inflammatory functions, which may offset its modest inhibitory effects on fibrinolysis.

Thrombin-TM Complex

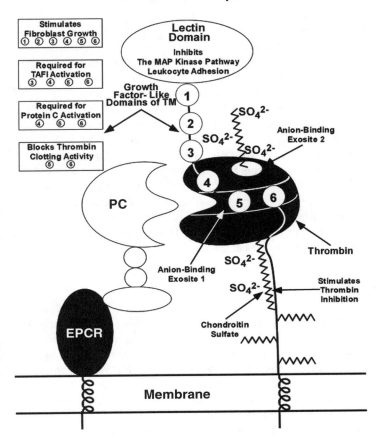

Figure 4 A model of the protein C activation complex. The small balls labeled 1–6 correspond to the EGF-like repeats in thrombomodulin, the extended structure rising from the membrane contains O-linked glycosylation sites (*shown as zigzag lines*) and is the site of attachment of the chondroitin sulfate moiety, depicted by the zigzag line with the terminal sulfate. This complex cleaves protein C to release a 12-residue peptide from the amino terminus of its heavy chain C (not shown), which leads to activation. Both protein C and activated protein C interact with the activation complex (36,37). Lectin refers to the lectin-like amino-terminal domain of thrombomodulin. *Source*: From Ref. 38.

Furthermore, TM also accelerates the inactivation of prourokinase (43,44). Despite data indicating that the thrombin-TM complex leads to the inhibition of fibrinolysis, there is evidence that APC facilitates fibrinolysis in vivo (33,45,46). Thus, the influence of TM on the fibrinolytic system remains uncertain.

Once the thrombin-TM complex activates protein C, the resultant APC can inactivate factor Va or VIIIa. This process requires protein S. The APC-protein S complex functions on membrane surfaces expressing negatively charged phospholipid. The membrane specificity of the factor Va inactivation complex differs somewhat from that reported for prothrombin in that the activity of the complex is potently augmented by phosphatidylethanolamine or cardiolipin in the membrane (47). In purified systems under standard conditions, protein S only enhances factor Va inactivation about twofold. Factor Xa can protect factor Va and factor IXa can protect factor VIIIa from inactivation by APC; protein S largely eliminates these protective effects (48,49).

One of the unusual properties of APC is that it circulates with a long half-life, ≈ 15 min (50), and is slowly inactivated in plasma (51) by protein C inhibitor, α_1-antitrypsin, and in a Ca^{2+}-dependent fashion by α_2-macroglobulin and α_2-antiplasmin (51). The slow clearance impacts on the mechanisms involved in APC function. Once generated, APC can circulate throughout the vasculature, presumably serving "sentry" duty by inactivating any cofactors on the membrane surfaces. This contrasts to the rapid clearance and inactivation by other coagulation factors, like thrombin, which are inactivated by a single pass through the microcirculation (52).

The ability of APC to elude the masses of plasma proteinase inhibitors endows the enzyme with therapeutic potential. There are distinct theoretical differences between protein C and APC as therapeutic agents. In the case of protein C, the generation of anticoagulant activity increases with increasing thrombin challenge. This has been clearly documented in baboons where the amount of APC generated is approximately equivalent to the thrombin dose (36). Thrombin is rapidly neutralized and thus additional protein C activation ceases once thrombin generation is effectively controlled. From all of the available data, the protein C concentration in vivo is far below saturation (below Km). Thus, the system could be augmented by infusing additional protein C.

POTENTIAL THERAPEUTIC USES OF TM

The combined capacity of TM to block coagulation, activate protein C, and promote thrombin inhibition suggests that it could be a useful antithrombotic agent. In inflammatory settings, TM decreases NFκB and MAP kinase signaling in endothelium (53) and inhibits complement activation (37). TM has also been shown to inhibit HMGB 1-mediated activation of RAGE (54), a process that likely contributes to organ dysfunction in a number of settings. In cell culture, TM is down regulated by inflammatory cytokines raising the possibility that TM downregulation contributes to the thrombotic tendencies associated with inflammation. Downregulation of TM has been more difficult to demonstrate in vivo than in cell culture (55–57), but has been observed in certain settings (58–60). This downregulation can be influenced by many factors, including interleukin 4 (61) and retinoic acid (62,63), making our understanding of this potentially important phenomenon very incomplete. Nonetheless, the suggestion that TM supplementation would be useful during thrombotic complications, especially those associated with an underlying inflammatory condition, is attractive.

In animal models, soluble TM has been shown to block TF-induced disseminated intravascular coagulation (DIC) in rats (64) or endotoxin-mediated DIC (65) and to attenuate the pulmonary vascular injury that ensues (66). As was the case in primates (67), active site blocked factor Xa, which is a potent antithrombotic, failed to protect the animals from lung injury, suggesting a protein C pathway specific response in addition to the anticoagulant effect (66). APC also blocked lung injury in this model (68), suggesting that the TM effect was mediated by increased APC formation.

TM with or without chondroitin sulfate was effective in blocking TF-mediated DIC (64). Although TM containing chondroitin sulfate was more effective on a mass basis, it was cleared more rapidly from the circulation than TM without chondroitin sulfate (20 minutes versus 1 hour). TM appeared to have less effect on the bleeding time than heparin. When expressed as the concentration required to double the bleeding time versus that required to block the decrease in platelet count by 50%, TM with chondroitin sulfate was about threefold better than heparin, while TM without chondroitin sulfate was twofold better than heparin.

TM was also shown to be effective in a rat arterio-venous shunt thrombosis model. In this model, approximately 0.1 mg/kg of TM gave inhibition of thrombus mass equivalent to 10 units/kg standard heparin (69). Thrombus formation in the injured, ligated inferior vena cava of the rat was also prevented with soluble TM, in this case lacking chondroitin sulfate (70,71). In this model, TM blocked thrombosis at concentrations that doubled the bleeding time, whereas effective antithrombotic doses of hirudin or heparin resulted in bleeding times more than six times the control.

Soluble TM has been evaluated in small numbers of patients. In one trial, soluble TM (ART 123) decreased DIC in septic patients and produced fewer bleeding complications than did heparin (72). There was also a trend towards improved survival. A second study evaluated ART 123 in patients undergoing elective hip replacement surgery (73). In this open label, sequention dose-finding study, patients were given subcutaneous ART 123 two to four hours after surgery. Because of the long half-life, only those receiving the lowest dose of ART 123 were given a second dose of drug on day 6. On the basis of venographic assessment of deep vein thrombosis, ART 123 appeared to reduce the risk of deep vein thrombosis. However, there was no control group in this study. These findings suggest that soluble TM is worthy of further investigation.

When immobilized on surfaces, TM renders them non-thrombogenic in vitro, a finding predicted based on its antithrombotic properties (74). The author is unaware of any in vivo testing of these surfaces.

PROTEIN C AS AN ANTITHROMBOTIC

Limited information is available about the use of protein C in the treatment of thrombotic disease in humans. Much of our knowledge has been gathered from the treatment of congenital deficiencies. Homozygous protein C deficiency results in life-threatening thrombotic complications in infancy, which usually manifests as purpura fulminas, or microvascular thrombosis of the skin capillaries. These skin lesions are not prevented with heparin (75). In contrast, replacement therapy with protein C has been shown to prevent further progression of the lesions, which then heal (76,77,123,124).

The skin lesions in patients with warfarin-induced skin necrosis resemble those in patients with homozygous protein C deficiency. The biochemical basis for this similarity is that protein C is a vitamin K–dependent protein the levels of which decline more rapidly than those of prothrombin and factor IX after starting warfarin. This creates a hypercoagulable window that favors procoagulant events. Consistent with this proposal, coagulation activation peptide levels rise transiently soon after the administration of warfarin (78). In addition to suggesting that protein C concentrate might be a logical treatment for patients with warfarin-induced skin necrosis, the data also suggest that protein C supplementation might be an effective method for safely enhancing the antithrombotic effectiveness of warfarin, with less bleeding risk than increased warfarin doses. This proposal remains to be tested. A universal observation, however, is that in experimental animals, even those subjected to open chest surgery (79), APC causes relatively little bleeding at doses that are antithrombotic (79–81). The basis for this observation is uncertain, but may be related to the fact that APC is only an effective anticoagulant at low levels of TF (as might be generated within the vasculature) and that high levels of TF (such as those in the extravascular space) may overcome its anticoagulant effects.

Both congenital protein C deficiency and warfarin-induced acquired deficiency manifest themselves in microvascular thrombosis. The other situation in which microvascular thrombosis is common is inflammation-mediated DIC responses. Several lines of evidence provide a strong rationale for the use of protein C in the treatment of gram-negative septic shock, especially when purpura-like lesions are evident, such as those in seriously ill patients with menigococcemia. The suggestions that protein C or APC might be of use in this system comes from the observation that thrombin infusion into dogs subsequently challenged with lethal doses of *Escheria coli* prevented DIC and improved survival (82). With the subsequent recognition that the thrombin infusion might be functioning by activating protein C, we tested the ability of APC to prevent the lethal response to *E. coli* in baboons. APC protected the animals from death, DIC, and organ dysfunction (83). In contrast, if the protein C pathway was blocked, sublethal doses of *E. coli* resulted in death (83,84), and the animals had much higher levels of circulating TNFα than control animals given the same numbers of *E. coli*. Restoration of the protein C system prevented the DIC, organ damage, and elaboration of elevated cytokine levels. Taken together, these results suggest that protein C is a major regulator of microvascular thrombosis and that the system modulates the inflammatory response by as-yet-unknown mechanisms. In humans with meningococcemia, protein C consumption correlates better with the formation of the purpura-like lesions and death than other markers (85).

Given the link between protein C deficiency and microvascular thrombosis, it was logical to examine the utility of protein C supplementation in the treatment of septic shock. Eleven children with severe manifestations of septic shock, mostly due to meningococcemia, have been treated with protein C. In general, protein C infusion resulted in normalization of circulating protein C levels and reversal of organ dysfunction, including rapid improvement in the level of consciousness and renal function (86). The benefits of this treatment do not appear to be restricted to patients with meningococcemia. One patient with septic shock, DIC, and protein C consumption secondary to a group A β-hemolytic streptococcal and varicella infection improved rapidly after protein C infusion (87). While these results are promising and consistent with the current basic and physiological understanding of the protein C system, a larger clinical trial is needed to verify the validity of this approach.

Potential mechanisms by which protein C might influence the septic shock process include the regulation of thrombin formation at the vessel surface or modulation of the inflammatory response. There are several observations that provide suggestions that this system can modulate inflammation. In vitro, APC has been reported to inhibit tumor necrosis factor elaboration by monocytes (88), to bind to these cells, probably via a specific receptor, and to prevent interferon γ-mediated Ca^{2+} transients and cellular proliferation (89) and to inhibit leukocyte adhesion to selectins (90). An endothelial cell protein C–binding protein, structurally related to major histocompatibility (MHC) class 1 molecules, has been identified and shown to be downregulated by TNF (91). The exact mechanisms by which the protein C pathway modulates inflammatory responses remain obscure, but each or all of these effects may contribute to the effectiveness of this system in limiting damage caused by the host response to infection.

In addition to being able to modulate sepsis, the system itself is sensitive to modulation by inflammatory mediators. These changes are depicted in Figure 5. In cell culture, TNF can downregulate the expression of TM (92) and the endothelial cell protein C receptor (EPCR) (93) and can lead to protein S consumption (93–95) and increased levels of C4bBP (11,96). Major basic protein from eosinophils can inhibit TM function (97). Proteolytic release of TM from the endothelium also occurs in shock and inflammatory disease (98–101). The downregulation of TM induced by inflammatory agents is less pronounced in vivo than in cell culture (55–57), although this process does seem to occur in villitis (60) and allograft organ rejection (59,102).

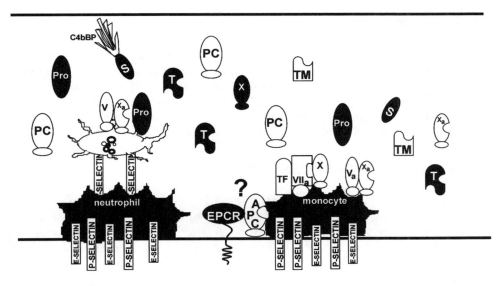

Figure 5 The protein C pathway after inflammation. In this model, inflammatory mediators lead to the disappearance of thrombomodulin from the endothelial cell surface. Endothelial cell leukocyte adhesion molecules, P-selectin or E-selectin, are synthesized or expressed on endothelial or platelet surfaces. TF is expressed on monocytes and binds VIIa, and this complex converts X to Xa, which forms complexes with Va to generate T from Pro. Elevated circulating levels of C4bBP results in little free protein S. Because little APC is generated, and the little that is formed has limited activity because S levels are low, Va is not inactivated and prothrombin complexes are stabilized. This results in ongoing thrombin generation and subsequent thrombosis. See text for discussion. *Abbreviations*: TF, tissue factor; VIIa, factor VIIa; X, factor X; Xa, factor Xa; T, thrombin; Pro, prothrombin; APC, activated protein C; S, protein S; SAP, serum amyloid P. *Source*: Modified from Ref. 31.

ACTIVATED PROTEIN C IN SEPSIS

APC (Xigris) is now FDA approved for the treatment of patients with severe sepsis and failure of two or more organs. On the basis of the original clinical trial (103), Xigris treatment reduced the relative risk of death by 19.4% with virtually all of the benefit occurring in the more severely ill patients (APACHE II scores of 25 or greater). One of the complications of Xigris in sepsis is the increased risk of severe bleeding. On the basis of earlier studies comparing APC with other highly specific anticoagulants (67), APC was more effective at preventing organ failure than the other anticoagulants. This suggests that the beneficial effects of APC may reflect functions other than anticoagulation, thereby raising the possibility of generating APC mutants that have reduced anticoagulant activity yet retain the "other properties." These beneficial properties include anti-inflammatory, vascular protective and cytoprotective functions. Such mutants have now been generated in Dr. John Griffin's laboratory and tested in Dr. Hartmut Weiler's laboratory. These mutants have been shown to prevent bacterially induced sepsis in mouse models (104). The results indicate that the cytoprotective activities of APC were of comparable or greater importance in these models of sepsis than its anticoagulant activity. The cytoprotective activity of APC required EPCR and protease-activated receptors (PAR)-1 (104).

ACTIVATED PROTEIN C IN STROKE

The cytoprotective activity of APC suggests that it might be beneficial in stroke. Consistent with this possibility, APC has been shown to protect neurons from the toxic effects of tissue plasminogen activator (105). APC was protective in murine models of stroke (106). In stroke, as in sepsis, the cytoprotective effects of the APC required the presence of EPCR and PAR-1. It appears that APC signaling through the EPCR-PAR-1 mechanism elicits a series of responses distinct from those initiated by thrombin activation of PAR-1, reviewed in (21).

PROTEIN S AS AN ANTITHROMBOTIC

Protein S serves as a cofactor for APC and also can block the assembly of the prothrombin activation complex by binding to factor Va and Xa (99–101,107–109). In addition, factor Xa and IXa protect factor Va and VIIIa, respectively, from inactivation by APC; protein S largely overcomes this protection. No data is presently available to determine which of these functions is most relevant physiologically. Depletion of protein S from plasma, however, has little influence on coagulation times in the absence of APC, whereas depletion of protein S decreases the anticoagulant response to APC about 10-fold, suggesting that the APC-dependent activities may be more important.

As a therapeutic, protein S has not been studied extensively. Warfarin-induced skin necrosis has been described in patients with protein S deficiency (110) and patients with homozygous protein S deficiency may develop purpura fulminans (111). Free and total protein S levels are often low in septic shock or in patients with extensive thrombosis (93,95,112). Therefore, it is reasonable to infer that protein S may have antithrombotic activity, especially in patients whose levels are low due to their underlying disease process.

Support for this concept has been obtained in a baboon model of *E. coli*-induced septic shock. Animals given 10% of the lethal dose of *E. coli* exhibit only an acute phase response. If free protein S is reduced by infusion of C4bBP or an antibody to protein S, infusion of the sublethal doses of bacteria lead to death, organ failure and either DIC or microvascular thrombosis (84). Supplementation with sufficient protein S to return the protein S levels to normal protects the animals from death and DIC. It should be pointed out, however, that the clinical experience to date with protein C infusion suggests that it is effective without simultaneous protein S supplementation. As these clinical trials continue, it will be important to determine whether patients who fail to respond to protein C infusion have unusually low protein S levels. Mutants of protein C have been generated that maintain full or increased anticoagulant activity without a dependence on protein S (113), but no in vivo results have been reported with these mutants.

PROTEIN C AND ARTERIAL THROMBOSIS

Studies done by Hanson and Harker in baboons have shown that APC is effective at preventing platelet and fibrin accretion on vascular grafts at arterial flow rates. The concentration required to inhibit platelet accretion had little effect on the bleeding time (81). This model is highly thrombin dependent because direct thrombin inhibitors block platelet accretion. Paradoxically, when thrombin is infused systemically, platelet accretion decreases (35). This response was due primarily, if not exclusively, to activation of protein C since the protective effect of thrombin in this study was eliminated by an antibody that blocks protein C activation. These studies raise the possibility that APC might be effective at preventing arterial thrombosis. It should be noted, however,

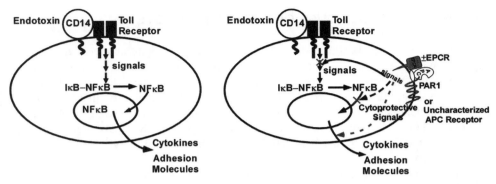

Figure 6 The role of APC in modulating the inflammatory response. APC interacts with the cell surface either through EPCR and then signals through PAR-1 to produce cytoprotective mediators. There may also be one or more distinct activated protein C receptors involved in downregulating the inflammatory response. This generates signals that block NFκB nuclear translocation and decrease NFκB through modulation of transcript levels of several of the components of this signaling pathway. See the text for further discussion.

that protein C deficiency is usually associated with venous or microvascular thrombosis, rather than arterial occlusion. This could be due to the requirement for development of arteriosclerosis before arterial thrombosis can occur and, therefore, protein C may not be observed as a risk factor in the heterozyogous state. In the homozygous situation, the microvascular and venous thrombotic complications dominate.

PROTEIN C IN REPERFUSION INJURY

Whenever thrombin is generated in the microvasculature, protein C activation occurs. This situation could arise in ischemia, a hypothesis supported by animal experiments. Thus, when the left anterior descending coronary artery was occluded in pigs (79) or dogs, protein C activation occurred within two minutes and activation was restricted to the region at risk. If protein C activation was blocked with a monoclonal antibody, left ventricular function did not recover as rapidly or completely from the ischemic injury and ventricular fibrillation often occurred. APC infusion appeared to improve recovery of left ventricular function, although under the conditions of these experiments, this difference did not reach statistical significance. These data raise the possibility that APC or protein C supplementation might diminish reperfusion injury. Theoretically, this would be an especially attractive approach in patients with downregulated thrombomodulin. Patients with coronary artery disease have been reported to have elevated TNF levels (114), which could induce local thrombomodulin downregulation. This has been suggested to occur in transplant rejection (58). It should be emphasized that protein C activation in response to ischemia has not been documented to be due to the thrombin-TM complex. Other activators are possible. For instance, it has been shown that protein C can be activated and subsequently inactivated by plasmin (115,116).

ACTIVATED PROTEIN C IN INFLAMMATORY BOWEL DISEASE

TM and EPCR are downregulated in mouse models of inflammatory bowel disease (117). Treatment of these mice with APC improved disease outcome with reduced weight loss and improvement in the disease activity index and histopathological changes. At least some of these improvements are likely a refection of attenuation of thrombosis.

AMPLIFYING THE RESPONSE OF THE PROTEIN C SYSTEM

The apparent safety and efficacy of this pathway in experimental animals suggests that supplementation with components of the system may provide safe and effective antithrombotic therapy. An alternative approach is to enhance the natural system. Recently, two approaches have been extensively exploited to accomplish this goal. First, a protein C mutant has been designed that activates rapidly with thrombin in the absence of TM (118). Thrombin-induced activation is sufficiently rapid that the mutant exerts an anticoagulant effect in plasma, an activity not seen with wild-type protein C in the absence of TM.

A second approach is to modify thrombin. Several functions of thrombin are potential aids in eliciting a selective response. In principle, one could eliminate the fibrinogen-clotting activity of thrombin or increase its capacity to activate protein C. Enhanced protein C activation could involve TM-dependent or -independent mechanisms and several thrombin mutants with one or more of these properties have been identified (119,120). A particularly promising mutant has been studied in vivo. Its capacity to clot fibrinogen or activate platelets are 40- and 50-fold lower than those of wild-type thrombin, respectively, yet the mutant still retains about 50% of its protein C activating capacity in the presence of TM (121). In addition, reactivity with antithrombin is reduced sevenfold. In vivo, this thrombin mutant generated the anticoagulant response observed previously with normal thrombin but induced less fibrinogen consumption.

CONCLUSIONS AND FUTURE DIRECTIONS

The protein C system offers promise as a target for novel antithrombotic agents. The system appears to be especially important in the control of microvascular thrombosis and hence might provide the agents of choice for treatment of these diseases. Although limited, clinical data suggest that protein C supplementation is safe and effective in congenital deficiencies, warfarin-induced skin necrosis and gram-negative sepsis. APC is approved for the treatment of severe sepsis. As more is learned about the specific functions of the system, (Fig. 6) our capacity to select patients who will benefit from treatment is likely to improve. In addition to its anticoagulant function, there is increasing evidence that the protein C pathway also has an important anti-inflammatory role. As the anti-inflammatory activity of this pathway is better defined, methods to exploit this activity may provide novel treatments for stroke, inflammatory bowel disease, and possibly diabetes (122).

REFERENCES

1. Esmon CT, Schwarz HP. An update on clinical and basic aspects of the protein C anticoagulant pathway. Trends Cardiovasc Med 1995; 5:141–148.
2. Esmon CT. Thrombomodulin as a model of molecular mechanisms that modulate protease specificity and function at the vessel surface. FASEB J 1995; 9:946–955.
3. Esmon CT, Fukudome K. Cellular regulation of the protein C pathway. Semin Cell Biol 1995; 6: 259–268.
4. Fulcher CA, Gardiner JE, Griffin JH, et al. Proteolytic inactivation of human factor VIII procoagulant protein by activated protein C and its analogy with factor V. Blood 1984; 63:486–489.
5. Koedam JA, Meijers JCM, Sixma JJ, et al. Inactivation of human factor VIII by activated protein C. Cofactor activity of protein S and protective effect of von Willebrand factor. J Clin Invest 1988; 82:1236–1243.

6. Eaton D, Rodriguez H, Vehar GA. Proteolytic processing of human factor VIII. Correlation of specific cleavages by thrombin, factor Xa, and activated protein C with activation and inactivation of factor VIII coagulant activity. Biochemistry 1986; 25:505–512.

7. Griffin JH, Evatt B, Wideman C, et al. Anticoagulant protein C pathway defective in majority of thrombophilic patients. Blood 1993;82:1989–1993.

8. Halbmayer W-M, Haushofer A, Schon R, et al. The prevalence of poor anticoagulant response to activated protein C (APC resistance) among patients suffering from stroke or venous thrombosis and among healthy subjects. Blood Coagul Fibrinol 1994;5:51–57.

9. Bertina RM, Koeleman BPC, Koster T, et al. Mutation in blood coagulation factor V associated with resistance to activated protein C. Nature 1994; 369:64–67.

10. Dahlbäck B. Physiological anticoagulation. Resistance to activated protein C and venous thromboembolism. J Clin Invest 1994; 94:923–927.

11. Dahlbäck B. Protein S and C4b-binding protein: Components involved in the regulation of the protein C anticoagulant system. Thromb Haemost 1991; 66:49–61.

12. Davie EW, Fujikawa K, Kisiel W. The coagulation cascade: Initiation, maintenance and regulation. Biochemistry 1991; 30:10363–10370.

13. Walker FJ, Fay PJ. Regulation of blood coagulation by the protein C system. FASEB J 1992; 6: 2561–2567.

14. Pabinger I, Brucker S, Kyrle PA, et al. Hereditary deficiency of antithrombin III, protein C and protein S: prevalence in patients with a history of venous thrombosis and criteria for rational patient screening. Blood Coagul Fibrinol 1992; 3:547–553.

15. Bourin MC, Lindahl U. Glycosaminoglycans and the regulation of blood coagulation. Biochem J 1993; 289:313–330.

16. Alving BM, Comp PC. Recent advances in understanding clotting and evaluating patients with recurrent thrombosis. Am J Obstet Gynecol 1992; 167:1184–1191.

17. Reitsma PH, Poort SR, Bernardi F, et al. Protein C deficiency: a database of mutations. For the Protein C & S subcommittee of the scientific and standardization committee of the international society on thrombosis and haemostasis. Thromb Haemost 1993; 69:77–84.

18. Castellino FJ. Human protein C and activated protein C. Trends Cardiovasc Med 1995; 5:55–62.

19. Reitsma PH, Bernardi F, Doig RG, et al. Protein C deficiency: A database of mutations, 1995 update. Thromb Haemost 1995; 73(5):876–879.

20. Van de Wouwer M, Collen D, Conway EM. Thrombomodulin-Protein C-EPCR system integrated to regulate coagulation and inflammation. Arterioscler Thromb Vasc Biol 2004; 24: 1374–1383.

21. Mosnier LO, Zlokovic BV, Griffin JH. The cytoprotective protein C pathway. Blood 2007; 109:3161–3172.

22. Shen L, Dahlbäck B. Factor V and protein S as synergistic cofactors to activated protein C in degradation of factor VIIIa. J Biol Chem 1994; 269:18735–18738.

23. Esmon CT, Cell mediated events that control blood coagulation and vascular injury. Ann Rev Cell Biology. 1993; 9:1–26.

24. Taylor FB Jr., Peer GT, Lockhart MS, et al. EPCR plays an important role in protein C activation in vivo. Blood 2001; 97:1685–1688.

25. Walker FJ, Sexton PW, Esmon CT. Inhibition of blood coagulation by activated protein C through selective inactivation of activated factor V. Biochim Biophys Acta 1979; 571:333–342.

26. Kalafatis M, Rand MD, Mann KG. The mechanism of inactivation of human factor V and human factor Va by activated protein C. J Biol Chem 1994; 269:31869–31880.

27. Kalafatis M, Bertina RM, Rand MD, et al. Characterization of the molecular defect in factor V^{R506Q}. J Biol Chem 1995; 270(8):4053–4057.

28. Billy D, Willems GM, Hemker HC, et al. Prothrombin contributes to the assembly of the factor Va-factor Xa complex at phosphatidylserine-containing phospholipid membranes. J Biol Chem 1995; 270:26883–26889.

29. Rosing J, Hoekema L, Nicolaes GAF, et al. Effects of protein S and factor Xa on peptide bond cleavages during inactivation of factor Va and factor Va^{R506Q} by activated protein C. J Biol Chem 1995; 270:27852–27858.

30. Esmon CT. The protein C anticoagulant pathway. Arterioscl Thromb 1992; 12(2):135.
31. Esmon CT. The roles of protein C and thrombomodulin in the regulation of blood coagulation. J Biol Chem 1989; 264:4743–4746.
32. Esmon NL, Carroll RC, Esmon CT. Thrombomodulin blocks the ability of thrombin to activate platelets. J Biol Chem 1983; 258:12238–12242.
33. Esmon CT, Esmon NL, Harris KW. Complex formation between thrombin and thrombomodulin inhibits both thrombin-catalyzed fibrin formation and factor V activation. J Biol Chem 1982; 257:7944–7947.
34. Polgar J, Lerant I, Muszbek L, et al. Thrombomodulin inhibits the activation of factor XIII by thrombin. Thromb Res 1986; 43:585–590.
35. Hanson SR, Griffin JH, Harker LA, et al. Antithrombotic effects of thrombin-induced activation of endogenous protein C in primates. J Clin Invest 1993; 92:2003–2012.
36. Van de Wouwer M, Plaisance S, De Vriese A, et al. The lectin-like domain of thrombomodulin interferes with complement activation and protects against arthritis. Thromb Haemost 2006; 8:1813–1824.
37. Esmon CT. Molecular events that control the protein C anticoagulant pathway. Thromb Haemost 1993; 70(1):29.
38. Parkinson JF, Koyama T, Bang NU, et al. Thrombomodulin: an anticoagulant cell surface proteoglycan with physiologically relevant glycosaminoglycan moiety. Adv Exp Med Biol 1992; 313:177–188.
39. Rezaie AR, Cooper ST, Church FC, et al. Protein C inhibitor is a potent inhibitor of the thrombin-thrombomodulin complex. J Biol Chem 1995; 270:25336–25339.
40. Lin J-H, McLean K, Morser J, et al. Modulation of glycosaminoglycan addition in naturally expressed and recombinant human thrombomodulin. J Biol Chem 1994; 269(40): 25021–25030.
41. Gailani D, Broze GJ Jr. Factor XI activation in a revised model of blood coagulation. Science 1991; 253:909–912.
42. Bajzar L, Manuel R, Nesheim ME. Purification and characterization of TAFI, a thrombin-activable fibrinolysis inhibitor. J Biol Chem 1995; 270:14477–14484.
43. Molinari A, Giogetti C, Lansen J, et al. Thrombomodulin is a cofactor for thrombin degradation of recombinant single-chain urokinase plasminogen activator in vitro and in a perfused rabbit heart model. Thromb Haemost 1992; 67:226–232.
44. de Munk GAW, Parkinson JF, Groeneveld E, et al. Role of the glycosaminoglycan component of thrombomodulin in its acceleration of the inactivation of single-chain urokinase-type plasminogen activator by thrombin. Biochem J 1993; 290:655–659.
45. Krishnamurti C, Young GD, Barr CF, et al. Enhancement of tissue plasminogen activator-induced fibrinolysis by activated protein C in endotoxin-treated rabbits. J Lab Clin Med 1991; 118:523–530.
46. Gruber A, Harker LA, Hanson SR, et al. Antithrombotic effects of combining activated protein C and urokinase in nonhuman primates. Circulation 1991; 84:2454–2462.
47. Smirnov MD, Esmon CT. Phosphatidylethanolamine incorporation into vesicles selectively enhances factor Va inactivation by activated protein C. J Biol Chem 1994; 269:816–819.
48. Regan LM, Lamphear BJ, Huggins CF, et al. Factor IXa protects factor VIIIa from activated protein C. J Biol Chem 1994; 269:9445–9452.
49. Solymoss S, Tucker MM, Tracy PB. Kinetics of inactivation of membrane-bound factor Va by activated protein C. J Biol Chem 1988; 263:14884–14890.
50. Comp PC, Esmon CT. Generation of fibrinolytic activity by infusion of activated protein C into dogs. J Clin Invest 1981; 68:1221–1228.
51. Heeb MJ, Gruber A, Griffin JH. Identification of divalent metal ion-dependent inhibition of activated protein C by alpha$_2$–macroglobulin and alpha$_2$–antiplasmin in blood and comparisons to inhibition of factor Xa, thrombin, and plasmin. J Biol Chem 1991; 266: 17606–17612.
52. Lollar P, Owen W. Clearance of thrombin from the circulation in rabbits by high-affinity binding sites on endothelium. J Clin Invest 1980; 66:1222–1230.

53. Conway EM, Van de Wouwer M, Pollefeyt S, et al. The lectin-like domain of thrombomodulin confers protection from neutrophil-mediated tissue damage by suppressing adhesion molecule expression via nuclear factor kB and mitogen-activated protein kinase pathways. J Exp Med 2002; 196:565–577.

54. Abeyama K, Stern DM, Ito Y, et al. The N-terminal domain of thrombomodulin sequesters High mobility group-B1 Protein, a novel anti-inflammatory mechanism. J Clin Invest 2005; 115:1267–1274.

55. Laszik Z, Carson CW, Nadasdy T, et al. Lack of suppressed renal thrombomodulin expression in a septic rat model with glomerular thrombotic microangiopathy. Lab Invest 1994; 70:862–867.

56. Semeraro N, Triggiani R, Montemurro P, et al. Enhanced endothelial tissue factor but normal thrombomodulin in endotoxin-treated rabbits. Thromb Res 1993; 71:479–486.

57. Drake TA, Cheng J, Chang A, et al. Expression of tissue factor, thrombomodulin, and E-selectin in baboons with lethal E. coli sepsis. Am J Pathol 1993; 142:1458–1470.

58. Hancock WW, Tanaka K, Salem HH, et al. TNF as a mediator of cardiac transplant rejection, including effects on the intragraft protein C/protein S/thrombomodulin pathway. Transplant Proc 1991; 23:235–237.

59. Faulk WP, Gargiulo P, Bang NU, et al. Immunopathology of hemostasis in allografted human kidneys. Blood 1987; 70(5)(suppl 1):371a (abstr).

60. Labarrere CA, Esmon CT, Carson SD, et al. Concordant expression of tissue factor and Class II MHC antigens in human placental endothelium. Placenta 1990; II:309–318.

61. Kapiotis S, Besemer J, Bevec D, et al. Interleukin-4 counteracts pyrogen-induced downregulation of thrombomodulin in cultured human vascular endothelial cells. Blood 1991; 78:410–415.

62. Dittman WA, Nelson SC, Greer PK, et al. Characterization of thrombomodulin expression in response to retinoic acid and identification of a retinoic acid response element in the human thrombomodulin gene. J Biol Chem 1994; 269:16925–16932.

63. Koyama T, Hirosawa S, Kawamata N, et al. All-trans retinoic acid upregulates thrombomodulin and down regulates tissue-factor expression in acute promyelocytic leukemia cells: Distinct expression of thrombomodulin and tissue factor in human leukemic cells. Blood 1994; 84(9):3001–3009.

64. Nawa K, Itani T, Ono M, et al. The glycosaminoglycan of recombinant human soluble thrombomodulin affects antithrombotic activity in a rat model of tissue factor-induced disseminated intravascular coagulation. Thromb Haemost 1992; 67:366–370.

65. Gonda Y, Hirata S, Saitoh K-I, et al. Antithrombotic effect of recombinant human soluble thrombomodulin on endotoxin-induced disseminated intravascular coagulation in rats. Thromb Res 1993; 71:325–335.

66. Uchiba M, Okajima K, Murakami K, et al. Recombinant human soluble thrombomodulin reduces endotoxin-induced pulmonary vascular injury via protein C activation in rats. Thromb Haemost 1995; 74:1265–1270.

67. Taylor FB Jr., Chang ACK, Peer GT, et al. DEGR-factor Xa blocks disseminated intravascular coagulation initiated by Escherichia coli without preventing shock or organ damage. Blood 1991; 78:364–368.

68. Murakami K, Okajima K, Uchiba M, et al. Activated protein C attenuates endotoxin-induced pulmonary vascular injury by inhibiting activated leukocytes in rats. Blood 1996; 87:642–647.

69. Aoki Y, Takei R, Mohri M, et al. Antithrombotic effects of recombinant human soluble thrombomodulin (rhs-TM) on arteriovenous shunt thrombosis in rats. Am J Hematol 1994; 47:162–166.

70. Solis MM, Cook C, Cook J, et al. Intravenous recombinant soluble human thrombomodulin prevents venous thrombosis in a rat model. J Vasc Surg 1991; 14:599–604.

71. Solis MM, Vitti M, Cook J, et al. Recombinant soluble human thrombomodulin: A randomized, blinded assessment of prevention of venous thrombosis and effects on hemostatic parameters in a rat model. Thromb Res 1994; 73:385–394.

72. Saito H, Maruyama I, Shimazaki S, et al. Efficacy and safety of recombinant human soluble thrombomodulin (ART-123) in disseminated intravascular coagulation: results of a phase III, randomized, double-bind clinical trial. J Thromb Haemost 2007; 5:31–41.

73. Kearon C, Comp P, Douketis J, et al. Dose–response study of recombinant human soluble thrombomodulin (ART-123) in the prevention of venous thromboembolism after total hip replacement. J Thromb Haemost 2005; 3:962–968.

74. Kishida A, Ueno Y, Maruyama I, et al. Immobilization of human thrombomodulin onto biomaterials. Comparison of immobilzation methods and evaluation of antithrombogenicity. ASAIO Journal 1994; 40:M840–M845.

75. Sills RH, Marlar RA, Montgomery RR, et al. Severe homozygous protein C deficiency. J Pediatrics 1984; 105:409–413.

76. Dreyfus M, Masterson M, David M, et al. Replacement therapy with a monoclonal antibody purified protein C concentrate in newborns with severe congenital protein C deficiency. Sem Thromb Hemost 1995; 21:371–381.

77. Muller F-M, Ehrenthal W, Hafner G, et al. Purpura fulminans in severe congenital protein C deficiency: monitoring of treatment with protein C concentrate. Eur J Pediatr 1996; 155: 20–25.

78. Conway EM, Bauer KA, Barzegar S, et al. Suppression of hemostatic system activation by oral anticoagulants in the blood of patients with thrombotic diatheses. J Clin Invest 1987; 80: 1535–1544.

79. Snow TR, Deal MT, Dickey DT, et al. Protein C activation following coronary artery occlusion in the in situ porcine heart. Circulation 1991; 84:293–299.

80. Emerick SC, Murayama H, Yan SB, et al. Preclinical pharmacology of activated protein C. In: Holcenber JS, Winkelhake JL, eds. The Pharmacology and Toxicology of Proteins, UCLA Symposia on Molecular and Cellular Biology. Alan R. Liss, Inc., 1987:351–367.

81. Gruber A, Griffin JH, Harker LA, et al. Inhibition of platelet-dependent thrombus formation by human activated protein C in a primate model. Blood 1989; 73:639–642.

82. Taylor FB Jr., Chang A, Hinshaw LB, et al. A model for thrombin protection against endotoxin. Thromb Res 1984; 36:177–185.

83. Taylor FB Jr., Stern DM, Nawroth PP, et al. Activated protein C prevents E. coli induced coagulopathy and shock in the primate. Circulation 1986; 74:65–256 (abstr).

84. Taylor F, Chang A, Ferrell G, et al. C4b-binding protein exacerbates the host response to Escherichia coli. Blood 1991; 78:357–363.

85. Powars D, Larsen R, Johnson J, et al. Epidemic meningococcemia and purpura fulminans with induced protein C deficiency. Clin Infect Dis 1993; 17:254–261.

86. Rivard GE, David M, Farrell C, et al. Treatment of purpura fulminans in meningococcemia with protein C concentrate. J Pediatr 1995; 126(4):646–652.

87. Gerson WT, Dickerman JD, Bovill EG, et al. Severe acquired protein C deficiency in purpura fulminans associated with disseminated intravascular coagulation: treatment with protein C concentrate. Pediatrics 1993; 91:418–422.

88. Grey ST, Tsuchida A, Hau H, et al. Selective inhibitory effects of the anticoagulant activated protein C on the responses of human mononuclear phagocytes to LPS, IFN-gamma, or phorbol ester. J Immunol 1994; 153:3664–3672.

89. Hancock WW, Grey ST, Hau L, et al. Binding of activated protein C to a specific receptor on human mononuclear phagocytes inhibits intracellular calcium signaling and monocyte-dependent proliferative responses. Transplantation 1995; 60:1525–1532.

90. Grinnell BW, Hermann RB, Yan SB. Human protein C inhibits selectin-mediated cell adhesion: Role of unique fucosylated oligosaccharide. Glycobiology 1994; 4:221–226.

91. Fukudome K, Esmon CT. Identification, cloning and regulation of a novel endothelial cell protein C/activated protein C receptor. J Biol Chem 1994; 269:26486–26491.

92. Dittman WA. Thrombomodulin: Biology and potential cardiovascular applications. Trends Cardiovasc Med 1991; 1:331–336.

93. Heeb MJ, Mosher D, Griffin JH. Activation and complexation of protein C and cleavage and decrease of protein S in plasma of patients with intravascular coagulation. Blood 1989; 73: 455–461.

94. Bourin MC, Lundgren-Åkerlund E, Lindahl U. Isolation and characterization of the glycosaminoglycan component of rabbit thrombomodulin proteoglycan. J Biol Chem 1990; 265:15424–15431.

95. Fourrier F, Chopin C, Goudemand J, et al. Septic shock, multiple organ failure, and disseminated intravascular coagulation. Compared patterns of antithrombin III, protein C, and protein S deficiencies. Chest 1992; 101:816–823.

96. D'Angelo A, Vigano-D'Angelo S, Esmon CT, et al. Acquired deficiencies of protein S: Protein S activity during oral anticoagulation, in liver disease and in disseminated intravascular coagulation. J Clin Invest 1988; 81:1445–1454.

97. Mukai HY, Ninomiya H, Ohtani K, et al. Major basic protein binding to thrombomodulin potentially contributes to the thrombosis in patients with eosinophilia. Br J Haematol 1995; 90:892–899.

98. Takano S, Kimura S, Ohdama S, et al. Plasma thrombomodulin in health and diseases. Blood 1990; 76:2024–2029.

99. Karmochkine M, Boffa MC, Piette JC, et al. Increase in plasma thrombomodulin in lupus erythematosus with antiphospholipid antibodies. Blood(Lett) 1992; 79:837–838.

100. Asakura H, Jokaji H, Saito M, et al. Plasma levels of soluble thrombomodulin increase in cases of disseminated intravascular coagulation with organ failure. Am J Hematol 1991; 38: 281–287.

101. Wada H, Ohiwa M, Kaneko T, et al. Plasma thrombomodulin as a marker of vascular disorders in thrombotic thrombocytopenic purpura and disseminated intravascular coagulation. Am J Hematol 1992; 39:20–24.

102. Tsuchida A, Salem H, Thomson N, et al. Tumor necrosis factor production during human renal allograft rejection is associated with depression of plasma protein C and free protein S levels and decreased intragraft thrombomodulin expression. J Exp Med 1992; 175:81–90.

103. Bernard GR, Vincent JL, Laterre PF, et al. Efficacy and safety of recombinant human activated protein C for severe sepsis. New Engl J Med 2001; 344:699–709.

104. Kerschen EJ, Fernandez JA, Cooley BC, et al. Endotoxemia and sepsis mortality reduction by non-anticoagulant-activated protein C. J Exp Med 2007; 204:2439–2448.

105. Cheng T, Liu D, Griffin JH, et al. Activated protein C blocks p53–mediated apoptosis in ischemic human brain endothelium and is neuroprotective. Nature Medicine 2003; 9:338–342.

106. Shibata M, Kumar SR, Amar A, et al. Anti-inflammatory, antithrombotic, and neuroprotective effects of activated protein C in a murine model of focal ischemic stroke. Circulation 2001; 103:1799–1805.

107. Heeb MJ, Rosing J, Bakker HM, et al. Protein S binds to and inhibits factor Xa. Proc Natl Acad Sci U S A 1994; 91:2728–2732.

108. Heeb MJ, Mesters RM, Tans G, et al. Binding of protein S to factor Va associated with inhibition of prothrombinase that is independent of activated protein C. J Biol Chem 1993; 268:2872–2877.

109. Hackeng TM, van't Veer C, Meijers JCM, et al. Human protein S inhibits prothrombinase complex activity on endothelial cells and platelets via direct interactions with factors Va and Xa. J Biol Chem 1994; 269(33):21051–21058.

110. Goldberg SL, Orthner CL, Yalisove BL, et al. Skin necrosis following prolonged administration of coumarin in a patient with inherited protein S deficiency. Am J Hematol 1991; 38:64–66.

111. Marlar RA, Neumann A. Neonatal purpura fulminans due to homozygous protein C or protein S deficiencies. Sem Thromb Hemost 1990; 16:299–309.

112. Nguyen P, Reynaud J, Pouzol P, et al. Varicella and thrombotic complications associated with transient protein C and protein S deficiencies in children. Eur J Pediatr 1994; 153:646–649.

113. Smirnov MD, Safa O, Regan L, et al. A chimeric protein C containing the prothrombin Gla domain exhibits increased anticoagulant activity and altered phospholipid specificity. J Biol Chem 1998; 273:9031–9040.

114. Maury CPJ, Teppo A-M. Circulating tumour necrosis factor alpha (Cachectin) in myocardial infarction. J Int Med Res 1989; 225:333–336.

115. Bajaj SP, Rapaport SI, Maki SL, et al. A procedure for isolation of human protein C and protein S as by-products of the purification of factors VII, IX, X and prothrombin. Prep Biochem 1983; 13:191–214.

116. Varadi K, Philapitsch A, Santa T, et al. Activation and inactivation of human protein C by plasmin. Thromb Haemost 1994; 71:615–621.

117. Scaldaferri FF, Sans M, Vetrano S, et al. Crucial role of the protein C pathway in governing microvascular inflammation in inflammatory bowel disease. J Clin Invest 2007; 117:1951–1960.

118. Richardson MA, Gerlitz B, Grinnell BW. Enhancing protein C interaction with thrombin results in a clot- activated anticoagulant. Nature 1992; 360:261–264.

119. Wu Q, Sheehan JP, Tsiang M, et al. Single amino acid substitutions dissociate fibrinogen-clotting and thrombomodulin-binding activities of human thrombin. Proc Natl Acad Sci U S A 1991; 88:6775–6779.

120. Le Bonniec BF, Esmon CT. Glu-192 [to] Gln substitution in thrombin mimics the catalytic switch induced by thrombomodulin. Proc Natl Acad Sci U S A 1991; 88:7371–7375.

121. Gibbs CS, Coutré SE, Tsiang M, et al. Conversion of thrombin into an anticoagulant by protein engineering. Nature 1995; 378:413–416.

122. Isermann B, Vinnikov IA, Madhusudhan T, et al. Activated protein C protects against diabetic nephropathy by inhibiting endothelial and podocyte apoptosis. Nature Medicine 2007; 13: 1349–1358.

123. Muntean W, Finding K, Gamillscheg A, et al. Multiple thromboses and coumarin-induced skin necrosis in a child with anticardiolipin antibodies: Effects of protein C concentrate administration. Thrombosis and Haemostasis 1991; 65:2017 (abstr).

124. Schramm W, Spannagl M, Bauer KA, et al. Treatment of coumarin-induced skin necrosis with a monoclonal antibody purified protein C concentrate. Arch Dermatol 1993; 129:753–756.

21

Factor IXa Inhibitors

Richard C. Becker and Mark Chan
Department of Medicine, Divisions of Cardiology and Hematology, Duke University Medical Center, Duke University School of Medicine, and Duke Clinical Research Institute, Durham, North Carolina, U.S.A.

Emily L. Howard
Department of Pathology, College of Medicine, University of Arkansas for Medical Sciences, Little Rock, Arkansas, U.S.A.

Kristian C. D. Becker
Department of Molecular Biology, Cell Biology and Biochemistry, Boston University, Boston, Massachusetts, U.S.A.

Christopher P. Rusconi
Regado Biosciences, Inc., Durham, North Carolina, U.S.A.

INTRODUCTION

Coagulation is a complex process in which circulating soluble proteins, cellular elements, and tissue-based proteins interface to form an insoluble clot at sites of vascular injury. While this dynamic process represents a teleologically distinct, adaptive response that is critical to survival following localized vessel trauma, clot formation may also be undesirable. For example, tissue perfusion compromising thrombosis within the coronary or cerebrovascular beds is the proximate cause of myocardial infarction (MI) and ischemic stroke, respectively. Moreover, common procedures such as percutaneous coronary intervention, hemodialysis, blood pheresis, cardiac valve replacement, and extracorporeal circulatory support systems may themselves incite coagulation. Accordingly, pharmacotherapies that attenuate clot formation safely, effectively, and selectively assume a priority for practicing clinicians.

Herein, we summarize the current landscape of factor IX_a (FIX_a) inhibitors as an emerging and novel class of anticoagulants.

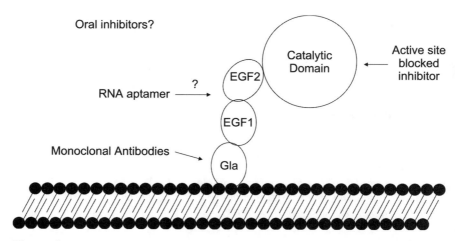

Figure 1 Factor IX is a vitamin K-dependent coagulation protease with six distinct structural-functional domains: AP (activation peptide), EGF 1 and 2 (epidermal growth factor), Gla (glutamic acid), catalytic domain, and hydrophobic domain. The hydrophobic domain (not shown) is exposed following calcium binding and anchors factor IX to the cell surface. *Source*: With permission from Ref. 96.

CELL-BASED MODELS OF COAGULATION

Coagulation in vivo is best characterized as a cell-based, coordinated, and integrated series of events (1) with three distinct phases: *initiation*, *priming*, and *propagation* (Fig. 1). Coagulation is initiated when tissue factor (TF) binds and activates factor VII, a coagulation protease circulating under normal (physiologic) conditions in plasma. Vascular injury exposes constitutively expressed, TF-bearing cells to blood. TF expression can also be upregulated on monocytes and vascular endothelial cells by bacterial antigens and byproducts (2), inflammatory cytokines (3), and tumor necrosis factor (4).

The TF/VIIa complex, also referred to as the "extrinsic tenase" complex, activates factors IX (5) and X. FIXa is relatively stable and diffuses toward activated platelets. In contrast, factor Xa is unstable in plasma and is rapidly inhibited by TF pathway inhibitor (TFPI) and antithrombin (AT) (6,7). On the surface of TF-bearing cells, factor V is complexed with factor Xa. The factor Xa/Va complex, in turn, generates a small but sufficient amount of thrombin to cause platelet activation (8).

In the *priming phase*, platelets and protein cofactors are activated by thrombin. Thrombin binds and cleaves platelet protease-activated receptors 1 and 4 (PAR1 and PAR4), triggering a signaling cascade that catalyzes further platelet activation (9–13) and release of factor V from platelet α granules. In addition, thrombin activates factors V, VIII (14), and XI (15).

Thrombin generation is maximized on the surface of platelets during the *propagation* phase. Primed, activated platelets bind the factor IXa/VIIIa "intrinsic tenase" complex. Additional IXa is generated by factor XIa on the platelet surface (15). The factor IXa/VIIIa complex, in physical proximity to factor Va, recruits factor X to the platelet surface for activation. The Xa/Va complex on the platelet surface is protected from inhibition by TFPI and AT (16–18). Activation of factor X by the factor IXa/VIIIa complex is nearly 50 times more efficient than its activation by the TF/VIIa complex (19). The platelet factor Xa/Va complex then generates a "burst" of thrombin, resulting in a stable fibrin-platelet clot.

FACTOR IX STRUCTURE AND BIOCHEMISTRY

FIX is synthesized in the liver where it undergoes vitamin K–dependent carboxylation of glutamate residues. It circulates in the plasma as a single-chain 57-kDa zymogen with a half-life of 18 to 24 hours. The zymogen has six domains: the amino terminal Gla domain containing 12 γ-carboxyglutamic acid residues (residues 1–40), a hydrophobic region (residues 41–46), two epidermal growth factors (EGF)-like domains (EGF-1 residues 47–84 and EGF-2 residues 85–127), an activation peptide (residues 146–180), and a serine protease domain in the carboxy terminus (residues 181–415) (20). The protease is activated by cleavage of peptide bonds following Arg145 and Arg180, releasing a 10-kDa activation peptide. The resulting protease consists of a 17-kDa light chain, linked via a cysteine bond to a 30-kDa heavy chain containing the active site (Fig. 1).

The Gla domain is essential for cellular membrane binding. With calcium binding, the Gla residues are turned "inward" to coordinate calcium ion flux (21), exposing a hydrophobic patch that inserts into the membrane lipid bilayer, anchoring FIX to the cell surface (21,22). The two EGF-like domains of FIX position the catalytic domain above the cell surface (20). Disruption of the EGF domains causes reduced binding of factors VIIa-TF (23) and VIIIa, with reduced activation of factor X (24–26).

The catalytic domain of FIX consists of a substrate-binding groove surrounded by six surface loops. The active site has surprisingly low activity toward substrates compared with other coagulation enzymes; however, binding of factor VIIIa provokes a conformational change of the active site, triggering high enzyme activity (27,28). The surface loops are important for structural integrity and interactions with factors X (29) and VIIIa (20,25,26).

Sodium plays an important role in modulating both the amidolytic and proteolytic activities of thrombin. Though the optimal amidolytic activity of factor Xa also requires Na^+, its proteolytic activity within the prothrombinase complex is minimally affected by the monovalent cation. In contrast to both thrombin and factor Xa, FIXa binds to its cofactor VIIIa and exhibits normal catalytic activity within the intrinsic Xase complex— entirely independent of Na^+ (29).

FIX is inactivated and regulated by multiple factors, including AT, nexin-2/amyloid β protein precursor, (30) neutrophil elastase, (31) and protein Z-dependent protease inhibitor (32). Clearance of FIX from the circulation is mediated by low-density lipoprotein receptor-related protein (LRP), an endocytic receptor on hepatocytes (33).

The importance of FIX in hemostatic regulation is highlighted by the clinically relevant manifestations of inherited and acquired deficiency states, such as Christmas disease or hemophilia B (34). A severe bleeding tendency is typically associated with <1% FIX activity. A moderate bleeding risk is incurred among individuals with 1% to 5% FIX activity, while 5% to 40% FIX activity causes a relatively modest hemostatic defect (35).

Factor IXa: Angiogenesis, Wound Healing, and Vascular Repair

FIXa plays a role in a range of biologic functions including angiogenesis, wound healing, and vascular repair. Hemophilia B mice subjected to punch biopsies have delayed macrophage infiltration and wound healing, develop subcutaneous hematomas, and exhibit increased angiogenesis compared with wild-type mice (36). Perivascular TF expression is downregulated during wound healing, reducing the likelihood of thrombosis within developing neovessels, but increasing the vulnerability to bleeding (37). Restoring a normal concentration of FIXa with replacement therapy improves thrombin generation and shortens the time to wound healing (38), but does not normalize vascular remodeling and angiogenesis.

Factor IX Enzyme Kinetics in Cell-Based Models of Coagulation

The relative contribution of individual coagulation proteins and protein complexes assembled on TF-bearing cells, platelets, and other phospholipid-containing or phospholipid-expressing surfaces to thrombin generation is an important consideration for both hemostasis and thrombosis. Allen and colleagues reported a fourfold increase of thrombin generation with FIX levels ranging from 0% to 200% (of normal plasma concentration) (39). This relationship is in sharp contrast to *ex vivo* experiments with factor X, wherein maximal rate, peak, and total thrombin generation is achieved with concentrations between 0% and 1% factor X.

Factor IX–Platelet Interactions

The contribution of platelets to hemostasis and thrombosis is incontrovertible; however, emerging evidence supports the presence of several distinct platelet populations within a developing thrombus—each with specific functional roles (40). Not all platelets express phosphatidyl serine at their outer surface following activation, and prolonged tyrosine phosphorylation downregulates αIIbβ3. Considered collectively, these observations suggest that platelets are programmed for either aggregation or procoagulant activity—characterized by the efficient binding of Gla domain containing coagulation factors, thrombin generation, and fibrin formation.

After decades of study, our understanding of coagulation continues to grow rapidly. FIXa, viewed originally as a protein responsible solely for clot formation, also plays a fundamental role in platelet-mediated hemostasis. Using FIX knockout mice, Gui and colleagues showed that platelet-rich hemostatic plug formation in response to vascular injury was markedly impaired in the absence of FIX activity (41). The platelet thrombus remained immature and easily dispersed, suggesting that the factor IXa/VIIIa complex may play a pivotal role in amplifying thrombin generation that is initiated by the TF-VIIa complexes after vascular injury.

The binding of factors IX and IXa to thrombin-activated human platelets is well described (42), with 300 to 400 FIX- and FIXa-binding sites per platelet. In the presence of factors VIII and X, the affinity of receptors for FIXa increases fivefold. Asn89, Ile90, and Val107 residues within loops 1 and 2 of the EGF-2 domain of FIXa may be particularly important for platelet interactions and for the assembly of a factor X-activating complex on the surface of activated platelets (43). The expression of PAR-1-stimulated, FIXa-binding sites on platelets is dependent on release of calcium from internal stores, producing sustained and pronounced calcium transients (44).

GENETICS OF FACTOR IX

The gene-encoding FIX is a 40-kb sequence that resides within the X chromosome at Xq27.1 between base pairs 138,440,561 and 138,473,283. The FIX gene includes eight exons and seven introns, and its complete nucleotide sequence was first reported in 1985 (45). The major transcription start site of FIX in human liver tissue is located at nucleotide −176 (46), a considerable distance 5′ upstream from the originally reported site (47). The human liver synthesizes only one mRNA species composed of 205 bases for the 5′ untranslated region (UTR), 1383 bases for the prepro FIX, a stop codon, and 1392 bases for the 3′ UTR. Exons I, II, and III encode the prepro leader sequence, Gla domain, and aromatic amino acid stack domain (44). Exons IV and V encode the two consecutive

EGF-like domains, whereas exons VI, VII, and VIII encode the activation peptide and the serine protease catalytic domain.

FIX gene regulation is mediated by elements within the 5′ flanking region, various intron sequences, and the 3′ UTR (48). The basic promoter sequence necessary for the maximal expression of FIX resides in the 5′ end sequence extending up to nucleotide −416. There are multiple negative regulatory elements (silencers) upstream to the basic promoter sequence within the 5′ flanking sequence, up to nucleotide −6900 (48). Sequential activation of these upstream silencers can suppress FIX production to below 3% (48).

An unusual form of hemophilia, hemophilia B Leyden, shows a dramatic improvement in FIX expression with the onset of puberty. This unique phenotype is caused by a series of 11 mutations clustered within the Leyden-specific (LS) region, a short sequence spanning nucleotides −40 to +20 within the 5′ region of the FIX gene (48). The Leyden phenotype appears to be androgen sensitive, and the increase in androgen levels during puberty has been implicated as a mechanism through which FIX expression is increased (46). The LS region of the normal FIX gene binds (*i*) three proteins at three specific footprint (FP) sequences, FP-I, FP-II, and FP-III, of which FP-III spans nucleotides −34 to −23; (*ii*) a protein known as CCAAT/enhancer-binding protein (C/EBP) in normal individuals; and (*iii*) an alternative protein FP-III′ when there are mutations of nucleotides −20 and −21 (49). FP-III′ interacts with androgen receptors via protein-protein interactions, resulting in sensitization of the FIX gene to androgens, which then stimulate expression of FIX mRNA (49).

The seven introns within the FIX gene, especially the first intron sequence, contain important enhancers of FIX gene expression. Vectors containing FIX cDNA and the first intron alone can produce up to seven- to ninefold higher mRNA levels compared with vectors lacking the first intron sequence (48). Within the 1.4 kb long 3′ UTR region, the most important regulatory elements lie within small regions containing the FIX polyadenylation signal sequences (45). The polyA tail stabilizes and prevents degradation of all mRNAs produced by the FIX gene. The importance and functional role of these regulatory elements are supported by the ability of FIX expression vectors lacking most of the 3′ UTR except for small polyadenylation signal sequences to induce high levels of FIX mRNA (46).

There is considerable variation in the levels of circulating FIX, with up to threefold differences seen among healthy individuals (50). FIX levels tend to be higher in older individuals and in women taking oral contraceptives. The contribution of non-environmental heritable factors in determining FIX levels has been estimated at 39% on the basis of a study of 398 Caucasian subjects from 21 extended Spanish pedigrees (51). Within the same population, Khachidze and colleagues identified a total of 27 candidate polymorphisms within the functional domains of the FIX gene, including three polymorphisms within cis elements responsible for the increase in FIX levels with ageing. However, the investigators did not identify significant difference in mean FIX levels associated with individual genotypes (52).

An estrogen-sensitive polymorphism within the FIX promoter region, the −698C/T polymorphism, contributes to variation in FIX levels among women, but not men. Adams and colleagues found higher mean FIX levels in CC homozygotes (123 IU/dl) compared with heterozygotes (116 IU/dl) and TT homozygotes (96 IU/dl) in women, but not among men (53). Subsequent transfection of gene vectors containing the −698C allele into liver-derived and erythroleukemic cell lines increased the expression of FIX in the presence of estrogenic factors, but not in their absence. Raised levels of estrogen in women using oral contraceptives and other estrogen formulations are consistent with these observations and raise the possibility that women carrying two copies of the FIX −698C allele may be more susceptible to estrogen-related thrombotic events.

Several investigators have also reported a direct and linear relationship between circulating FIX levels and age. In longitudinal analyses of transgenic mice, Kurachi and colleagues identified two regulatory elements, AE59 and AE39, which contributed to age-related changes in FIX gene expression (54). Because FIX clearance from the circulation is not significantly affected by age, regulation of plasma levels is achieved primarily by improved stabilization of gene transcription and a consequent age-dependent increase in FIX mRNA levels. AE59, present in the 5′ upstream region, is responsible for age-stable expression of the FIX gene, while AE39, present in the middle of the 3′ UTR, is responsible for age-associated elevation of FIX mRNA levels in the liver. Several biologic parameters, including triglycerides, factor VIII levels, and body mass index, and an important environmental factor (smoking) are also associated with elevated levels of FIX (52).

Factor IX Plasma Levels and Thrombosis Phenotypes

The pivotal role of FIXa in each successive stage of coagulation, coupled with its requirement for platelet thrombus formation and thrombin generation in animal models of arterial injury, supports a biologically plausible argument for FIXa as a risk factor for myocardial infarction (MI). In the study of MIs Leiden (SMILE), which included 560 men <70 years of age with a first MI and 646 control subjects, mean FIX activity was higher in patients than in controls, particularly in those younger than age 55 (55). Similarly, FIX activation peptide, which is released upon activation of FIX, was measured in relation to coronary heart disease–related events among 2997 men between 50 and 63 years of age (56). Increased FIX activation peptide levels were found to be an independent predictor of coronary heart disease events as an endpoint, with a one standard deviation increase in FIX activation peptide level corresponding to an adjusted hazard ratio of 1.20 (95% confidence interval 1.00–1.43) for the endpoint. Whether FIXa represents an inherited, acquired, or combined risk trait requires further investigation (52).

FACTOR IXa INHIBITORS

Active-Site Competitive Antagonists

Mechanism of Action

The earliest investigation of FIXa inhibitors was based on an active-site competitive antagonist—IXai. To generate IXai, the active site of IXa is blocked by incubation with glutamyl-glycyl-arginyl-chloromethylketone (57), yielding a protein without functional anticoagulant activity.

Preclinical Data

Intravenous infusion of IXai inhibited thrombosis in a canine model of coronary thrombosis in a dose-dependent fashion and produced less bleeding than unfractionated heparin (57). A rabbit model of synthetic patch angioplasty also showed effective anticoagulation with limited bleeding from puncture sites produced in synthetic vascular grafts (58). In a rabbit model of arterial thrombosis, IXai inhibited thrombus formation although it appeared to be less effective than active site-blocked Xa (Xai) (59).

In a canine model of cardiopulmonary bypass, IXai produced effective anti-coagulation, limited fibrin formation in the extracorporeal circuit, and diminished blood loss compared with unfractionated heparin (60). Similar results were observed in a primate model of cardiopulmonary bypass (61).

The IXai active-site competitive inhibitor exhibited anticoagulant effects in a rat model of stroke (62). Platelet and fibrin deposition following occlusion of the middle cerebral artery was markedly reduced after IXai administration. In addition, intracerebral hemorrhage occurred with decreased frequency when compared with either tissue plasminogen activator or unfractionated heparin. Of particular interest, IXai was protective even after the onset of stroke, suggesting that microvascular thrombosis occurs after occlusion of a major cerebral vessel and may be attenuable with FIXa-directed therapy.

Clinical Experience

To date, clinical trials of FIXai have not been conducted.

Monoclonal Antibodies

Mechanism of Action

Monoclonal antibodies are currently used for the treatment of cancer, autoimmune disease, and allergy. Murine antibodies are "humanized" by fusing the variable region or the complementarity-determining regions of the murine antibody with the heavy chain of human antibodies. Humanized monoclonal antibodies are generally well tolerated.

Preclinical Data

Several antibodies directed against the Gla domain of FIX have been developed. The 10C12 antibody contains a variable region joined to F(ab′)2 fragments. X-ray crystallography subsequently confirmed that the 10C12 antibody recognized the Ca^{2+}-stabilized Gla domain of FIX (23). The 10C12 clone was an effective anticoagulant, prolonging the activated partial thromboplastin time and also inhibiting platelet-mediated clotting in vitro (63). It effectively inhibited arterial thrombosis in a rabbit model of carotid artery injury without increasing blood loss from a standardized cutaneous incision (64).

A humanized monoclonal antibody directed against FIX was subsequently developed by SmithKline Beecham (presently Glaxo-Smith-Kline). SB 249417 is a chimeric molecule with human IgG1 fused to the complementarily determining region of a murine monoclonal antibody BC2, directed against the human FIX Gla domain (65,66). In a rat arterial thrombosis model, the antibody produced significant reductions in thrombus formation with modest prolongation of the activated partial thromboplastin time (aPTT). In a murine stroke model (67), SB 249417 reduced infarct volume and was associated with reduced neurologic deficits compared with tissue-type plasminogen activator. Pharmacokinetic studies in cynomolgus monkeys showed an elimination phase half-life of 3.8 days. Suppression of FIX activity and prolongation of the aPTT were rapid and dose dependent (68).

Clinical Experience

A phase I clinical trial with SB 249417 has been completed (69). Designed as a single-blind, randomized, placebo-controlled, single intravenous infusion, dose-escalating trial, the study was undertaken to establish pharmacokinetic and pharmacodynamic properties. The antibody displayed a dose-dependent effect on clotting times, with a maximal effect at completion of a 50-minute continuous infusion. There were no major safety concerns.

RNA Aptamers

Mechanism of Action

Aptamers (L. *aptus*, to fit) are short oligonucleotides (<100 bases) selected for their ability to bind a chosen target, typically, a protein or small molecule (70). The identification of an RNA aptamer possessing high affinity and specificity to a target protein begins with screening of a large combinatorial RNA library using systematic evolution of ligands by exponential enrichment (SELEX) (71). A complex between RNA and the selected target protein (or small molecule) involves a three-dimensional folding of the RNA such that it is complementary with the surface of the target protein. The molecular recognition of a target protein by an aptamer can involve several types of RNA-protein interactions, including hydrogen bonding, salt bridges, van der Waals forces, and stacking with aromatic amino acids (72).

Preclinical Data

Using SELEX, Rusconi and colleagues (74) isolated an aptamer (9.3t) specific for FIXa from a library of 10^{14} modified RNA species. For plasma stability, polyethylglycerol (PEG)-9.3t or cholesterol (Ch)-9.3t was attached to the 5' end. In vitro binding studies showed that the aptamer bound factors IX (75) and IXa with high affinity and (74,75) exhibited minimal affinity for the structurally related proteins, factors VII, X, or XI, or protein C. In vitro studies showed that PEG-9.3t inhibited activation of factor X by factor VIIIa/IXa complex. In human plasma, PEG-9.3t prolonged the aPTT. The aptamer blocked activation of FIX by factor VIIa, but not by factor XIa. Since factor VIIa binds FIX via the Gla and EGF domains, Gopinath and colleagues suggested that the aptamer may interact with the EGF domain (75).

Rusconi and colleagues subsequently synthesized an RNA antidote (5.2) to the FIXa aptamer. The antidote oligonucleotide was able to reverse 9.3t-induced anticoagulation in human plasma. Antidote 5.2 acted rapidly (<10 minutes) in a dose-dependent fashion and reversed the aptamer's effect for over five hours (76).

Animal studies have validated these in vitro findings. Ch-9.3t prolongs the aPTT in pigs, and this effect was reversed rapidly and durably after administration of antidote 5.2 (77). Aptamer Ch-9.3t prevented thrombosis in a murine model of arterial injury and induced bleeding after murine tail transection, which was rapidly terminated with antidote 5.2 (76).

In a porcine model of cardiopulmonary bypass, the fIXa aptamer/antidote pair was compared with unfractionated heparin and protamine (77). The aptamer produced an immediate elevation of both plasma and whole blood clotting times but a more modest anticoagulant effect [aPTT 177 seconds; activated clotting time (ACT) 294 seconds] compared with unfractionated heparin (aPTT >400 seconds; ACT >400 seconds). The clotting times returned toward pretreatment values within five minutes of antidote injection. The study also suggested several advantages of the aptamer/antidote pair, including reduced generation of thrombin and inflammatory mediators Interleukin (IL) (IL-1β, IL-6), reduced postoperative hemorrhage, and improved cardiac output (77).

The anti-IXa aptamer-antidote pair 9.3t and its antidote 5-2 were subsequently optimized at Regado Biosciences for in vivo stability and manufacturability to generate the REG-1 anticoagulation system, RB006 (drug) and RB007 (antidote).

Clinical Experience

Regado-1A was a subject-blinded, dose escalation, placebo-controlled study that randomized 85 healthy volunteers to receive a bolus of drug (FIX aptamer—RB006) or placebo, followed three hours later by a bolus of antidote (RB007) or placebo (78). Among subjects treated with RB006, the aPTT and ACT increased rapidly in a dose-dependent fashion, and the observed pharmacodynamic effect was stable over a three-hour time period. An escalation of RB006 dose prompted a stepwise inhibition of FIX activity, with a 99% loss correlating *ex vivo* with a 2.9-fold increase in the aPTT.

Administration of RB007 after RB006 caused a rapid (one to five minutes) and durable return of the aPTT to baseline values. There was no evidence of rebound thrombin generation following antidote administration. Overall, RB006 and RB007 were well tolerated.

Regado-1B evaluated the safety, tolerability, and pharmacodynamic profile of the REG-1 system (the aptamer and its antidote) in a multicenter, randomized, double-blind, placebo-controlled study, assigning 50 patients with stable coronary artery disease (CAD) taking aspirin and/or clopidogrel to four dose levels of RB006 (15, 30, 50, and 75 mg) and RB007 (30, 60, 100, and 150 mg). The median age was 61 years, and 80% of patients were male. RB006 produced a dose-dependent increase in the aPTT; the median aPTT values measured 10 minutes after a single intravenous bolus of 15, 30, 50, or 75 mg of RB006 were 29.2 seconds (95% CI 28.1–29.8), 34.6 seconds (30.9–40.0), 46.9 seconds (40.3–51.1), and 52.2 seconds (46.3–58.6), respectively ($p < 0.0001$; normal range 27–40 seconds). RB007 returned the aPTT to baseline levels within a median of one (1–2) minute, with no rebound increase through seven days. No major bleeding or other serious adverse events occurred (79).

The Regado-1C study randomized 39 healthy human subjects in a double-blind fashion to either three consecutive weight-adjusted, drug antidote treatment cycles or double placebo. Each treatment cycle consisted of an intravenous bolus—0.75 mg/kg RB006, followed an hour later by an ascending dose of RB007, ranging from a 0.125 to a 2:1 antidote:drug ratio (0.094 mg/kg to 1.5 mg/kg RB007). Serial clinical and coagulation assessments were performed through 14 days post randomization. A total of 30 subjects received three drug antidote cycles, while eight subjects received double placebo injections. Repeat doses of RB006 achieved highly reproducible aPTT prolongation and prompt reversal following RB007 administration (Fig. 2). There was a graded response to varying doses of antidote, showing an ability to titrate anticoagulant response and reversibility. There were no major bleeding or other serious adverse events (80).

Potential clinical applications for this injectable FIXa-specific drug antidote system include percutaneous and surgical coronary revascularization procedures, bridging therapy for elective noncardiac surgery in patients on coumadin therapy, the prophylaxis and treatment of venous and arterial thromboembolic disorders, and the maintenance of hemodialysis circuit patency. A subcutaneous formulation, which is currently being studied, may extend the pharmacodynamic half-life of the drug, therefore minimizing the number of daily injections and enabling home use. A key concern will be the potential for equipment-related thrombosis, a phenomenon that has hindered the clinical development of other specific coagulation protease inhibitors (81).

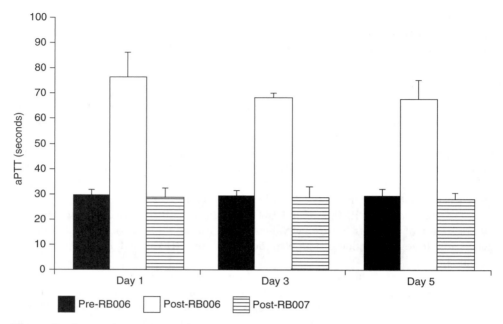

Figure 2 Consecutive doses of RB006 (aptamer) (0.75 mg/kg) given over 3 cycles (every other day) produced a consistent prolongation of the aPTT and a prompt return to baseline (normal) values following administration of RB007 (antidote). *Source*: From Ref. 80.

ORAL FACTOR IXA INHIBITORS

TTP889

Mechanism of Action

TTP889 is an orally available, small-molecule, selective partial antagonist of factor IX/IXa manufactured by Transtech Pharma (Winston-Salem, North Carolina, U.S.). The mechanism of action for the compound has not been published.

Preclinical Data

There are no preclinical data in the published literature.

Clinical Experience

Transtech Pharma has completed phase I and early phase II clinical trials at MDS Pharma Sciences in Nebraska (www.ttpharma.com). The drug was reported to be safe and demonstrated a predictable pharmacokinetic profile with a circulating half-life of approximately 20 hours in phase I studies of healthy volunteers (82).

The FIXIT study group conducted a phase II clinical trial to determine the safety and antithrombotic efficacy of TTP889 in patients at risk for venous thromboembolism. This multicenter, placebo-controlled trial enrolled 261 hip fracture surgery patients. After receiving routine anticoagulant prophylaxis for one week, patients were randomized to three weeks of extended venous thomboembolism (VTE) prophylaxis with daily oral doses of TTP889 or placebo (83). Because there was no significant difference between treatment groups in the composite primary outcome of venographic or symptomatic deep vein thrombosis or pulmonary embolism at the end of the study period, the investigators considered this a negative study. However, TTP889 had no effect on markers of thrombin generation (prothrombin fragment 1 + 2 and thrombin-antithrombin complex) and fibrin degradation (D-dimer) compared with placebo, despite the use of TTP889 dose levels considered sevenfold higher than that required to prevent venous thrombosis in animal models. This apparent lack of pharmacodynamic effect raises concerns about the appropriateness of the dose of TTP889 selected for this phase II human study.

Factor IX-Binding Proteins

Mechanism of Action

An intriguing discovery is the isolation of natural anticoagulants from snake venom. There is a family of homologous proteins that complex with FIX [IX-binding proteins (bp)], factor X (X-bp), or both (IX/X-bp). The family includes habu IX-bp and habu IX/X-bp of *Trimeresurus flavoviridis,* eichis IX/X-bp of *Echis carinatus leucogaster,* and acutus X-bp of *Deinagkistrodon acutus* (84). The venom of *Agkistrodon acutus* contains agkisacutacin, a homologous protein that binds both platelet glycoprotein Ib and coagulation factors IX and X (85). These proteins have similar structures with disulfide-linked heterodimers of C-type lectin-like subunits. X-ray crystallographic studies suggest that binding occurs with the Gla domains of factors IX and/or X. In vitro studies with IX-bp from *T. flavorviridis* showed anticoagulant activity with prolongation of the aPTT and interference of FIXa binding to phosphatidyl serine on the plasma membrane (86). These proteins represent a potential platform for future drug development.

Preclinical Data

To date, no preclinical studies with isolated FIX-bp have been published.

Clinical Experience

No clinical trials with isolated FIX-bp have been performed.

Heparin Compounds

The structural homology between factors IXa and Xa suggested that heparin compounds, particularly unfractionated heparin, may exert an inhibitory effect on intrinsic tenase activity. Indeed, the available data show that AT is the predominant inhibitor of FIXa in plasma. The rate of FIXa inhibition by AT is increased by pentasaccharide, with the maximal increase in the rate of inhibition reaching two orders of magnitude (87). In the presence of calcium, full-length heparin produces an additional 10-fold increase in the rate of FIXa inhibition. Considered collectively, heparin-mediated FIXa inhibition is achieved by two distinct and complimentary mechanisms—pentasaccharide-induced conformational change in AT and heparin-associated bridging of AT to FIXa (referred to as a template effect).

FIXa contains a heparin-binding site, and kinetic data suggest that five basic residues, Arg^{233}, Arg^{165}, Lys^{230}, Arg^{126}, and Arg^{170} are spatially aligned in a manner optimal for interactions (88). Residue Lys^{98}, specifically the 99-loop of FIXa, is particularly important in allosteric modulation of the heparin-binding exosite (89), providing a mechanistic rationale for heparin's ability to inhibit intrinsic tenase by disrupting the interaction between FIXa and the A_2 domain of factor VIIIa (90), as well as the resulting complexes' interaction with factor Xa (91). The preclinical data and clinical experience with heparin compounds have been published previously (92).

Table 1 Summary of Factor IXa Inhibitors

Class of drug	Mechanism of action	Pharmacodynamics	Pharmacokinetics	Phase of development
Active site–blocked inhibitors				
FIXai	Competitive inhibitor with active site blocked by chemical modification	Dose dependent	90-min half-life in primate model	Preclinical trials with animal models
Oral inhibitors				
TTP889	Partial inhibition of FIX/FIXa to a maximum of 90%	IC50 1.5 μM Dose dependent	20-hr half-life in humans	Phase II clinical trial completed
Monoclonal antibodies				
10C12	Ab against Gla domain	Kd 2 nM Dose dependent		Preclinical trials with animal models
SB 249417	Humanized murine Ab against Gla domain	Kd 20 nM Dose dependent	90-hr half-life in primates	Phase I clinical trial completed
RNA aptamers				
RB006	Oligonucleotide aptamer binds FIX/FIXa	Kd 3–5 nM Dose dependent	Pharmacodynamic half-life of 12–24 hr (dose dependent)	Phase I clinical trials completed; Phase II pilot completed
RB007 (RB006 antidote)	Complementary oligonucleotide binds aptamer	Not available	Reversal within 10 min	Phase I clinical trials completed
FIX-binding proteins				
Eichis IX/X-bp	Binds Gla domain	Kd 7 nM	Not available	In vitro assays
Habu IX-bp	Binds Gla domain	Not available	Not available	In vitro assays
Habu IX/X-bp	Binds Gla domain	Not available	Not available	In vitro assays
Agkisacutacin IX-bp	Binds Gla domain	Not available	Not available	In vitro assays

Source: Adapted from Ref. 96.

Thus, heparin compounds inhibit FIXa by AT-dependent and AT-independent mechanisms (93).

COAGULATION MEASUREMENT TOOLS

The administration of a FIX inhibitor as pharmacotherapy for thrombotic disorders or to facilitate extracorporeal circulation may require a coagulation measurement tool for dose selection, drug titration, and/or documentation of either drug clearance or gauged neutralization. FIX antigen levels can be determined using commercially available ELISA methods (94). Similarly, assays of FIX activity are widely available. Such tests use either a traditional mixing platform or a chromogenic assay that detects factor Xa, a correlate of FIXa activity (95).

A predictable dose-pharmacodynamic response, reflected in aPTT measurements, and correlation with FIX activity using an *ex vivo* calibration curve was observed in the Regado-1A study (78). The analysis indicated that a 1.1-fold increase in aPTT was equivalent to a 35% to 40% loss of FIX activity; a 1.3-fold increase represented a loss of 80% activity; a 2.1-fold increase represented a loss of 98% activity; and a 2.9-fold increase in aPTT correlated with a loss of >99% of FIX activity. ACT measurements followed a similar response; however, the dose activity—clotting time relationship was less robust than with the aPTT. Prothrombin time was not affected by FIX inhibition. Similar relationships were observed in Regado 1B—a study of patients with stable CAD (79). In Regado-1C, a whole blood aPTT assay was shown to correlate with plasma-based measurements; however, an ability to guide REG-1 dosing with whole blood aPTT measurement tools will require further investigation (80). Given that other FIXa inhibitors do not prolong or only modestly prolong the aPTT, the monitoring and interpretation of coagulation measures will likely be specific for each drug or mechanistically related drug class.

SUMMARY AND FUTURE DIRECTIONS

FIX plays a fundamental role in coagulation reactions triggered by either TF/factor VIIa or contact-initiated activation (Table 1). To date, RNA aptamers represent the newest, and perhaps, most promising generation of FIXa inhibitors. The RNA aptamer/antidote pair (REG-1) is an attractive system that produced effective anticoagulation and rapid reversal in animal models of thrombosis and bleeding, respectively. Phase I clinical trials have exhibited the requisite safety and pharmacokinetic and pharmacodynamic results to inform phase II investigations.

ACKNOWLEDGMENTS

The authors wish to acknowledge Bruce Sullenger, Ph.D. for his contributions to aptamer science, oligonucleotide antidotes, and FIXa-directed inhibitors.

REFERENCES

1. Monroe DM. Platelets and thrombin generation. Arterioscler Thromb Vasc Biol 2002; 22: 1381–1389.
2. Gregory SA, Morrissey JH, Edgington TS. Regulation of tissue factor gene expression in the monocyte procoagulant response to endotoxin. Mol Cell Biol 1989; 9:2752–2755.

3. Schecter AD, Rollins BJ, Zhang YJ, et al. Tissue factor is induced by monocyte chemoattractant protein-1 in human aortic smooth muscle and THP-1 cells. J Biol Chem 1997; 272:28568–28573.

4. Conway EM, Bach R, Rosenberg RD, et al. Tumor necrosis factor enhances expression of tissue factor mRNA in endothelial cells. Thromb Res 1989; 53:231–241.

5. Komiyama Y, Pedersen AH, Kisiel W. Proteolytic activation of human factors IX and X by recombinant human factor VIIa: effects of calcium, phospholipids, and tissue factor. Biochemistry 1990; 29:9418–9425.

6. Broze GJ Jr., Warren LA, Novotny WF, et al. The lipoprotein-associated coagulation inhibitor that inhibits the factor VII-tissue factor complex also inhibits factor Xa: insight into its possible mechanism of action. Blood 1988; 71:335–343.

7. Rapaport SI. The extrinsic pathway inhibitor: a regulator of tissue factor-dependent blood coagulation. Thromb Haemost 1991; 66:6–15.

8. Monroe DM, Hoffman M, Roberts HR. Transmission of a procoagulant signal from tissue factor-bearing cells to platelets. Blood Coagul Fibrinolysis 1996; 7:459–464.

9. Liu LW, Vu TK, Esmon CT, et al. The region of the thrombin receptor resembling hirudin binds to thrombin and alters enzyme specificity. J Biol Chem 1991; 266:16977–16980.

10. Vu TK, Hung DT, Wheaton VI, et al. Molecular cloning of a functional thrombin receptor reveals a novel proteolytic mechanism of receptor activation. Cell 1991; 64:1057–1068.

11. Vu TK, Wheaton VI, Hung DT, et al. Domains specifying thrombin-receptor interaction. Nature 1991; 353:674–677.

12. Brass LF, Hoxie JA, Manning DR. Signaling through G proteins and G protein-coupled receptors during platelet activation. Thromb Haemost 1993; 70:217–223.

13. Brass LF, Manning DR, Cichowski K, et al. Signaling through G proteins in platelets: to the integrins and beyond. Thromb Haemost 1997; 78:581–589.

14. Pieters J, Lindhout T, Hemker HC. In situ-generated thrombin is the only enzyme that effectively activates factor VIII and factor V in thromboplastin-activated plasma. Blood 1989; 74:1021–1024.

15. Oliver JA, Monroe DM, Roberts HR, et al. Thrombin activates factor XI on activated platelets in the absence of factor XII. Arterioscl Thromb Vasc Biol 1999; 19:170–177.

16. Scandura JM, Walsh PN. Factor X bound to the surface of activated human platelets is preferentially activated by platelet-bound factor IXa. Biochemistry 1996; 35:8903–8913.

17. Franssen J, Salemink I, Willems GM, et al. Prothrombinase is protected from inactivation by tissue factor pathway inhibitor: competition between prothrombin and inhibitor. Biochem J 1997; 323(pt 1):33–37.

18. Rezaie AR. Prothrombin protects factor Xa in the prothrombinase complex from inhibition by the heparin-antithrombin complex. Blood 2001; 97:2308–2313.

19. Lawson JH, Kalafatis M, Stram S, et al. A model for the tissue factor pathway to thrombin. I. An empirical study. J Biol Chem 1994; 269:23357–23366.

20. Mathur A, Zhong D, Sabharwal AK, et al. Interaction of Factor IXa with Factor VIIIa. Effects of protease domain ca2+ binding site, proteolysis in the autolysis loop, phospholipid, and factor X. J Biol Chem 1997; 272:23418–23426.

21. Freedman SJ, Blostein MD, Baleja JD, et al. Identification of the phospholipid binding site in the vitamin k-dependent blood coagulation protein factor IX. J Biol Chem 1996; 271:16227–16236.

22. Huang M, Furie BC, Furie B. Crystal structure of the calcium-stabilized human factor IX Gla domain bound to a conformation-specific anti-factor IX antibody. J Biol Chem 2004; 279:14338–14346.

23. Zhong D, Smith KJ, Birktoft JJ, et al. First epidermal growth factor-like domain of human blood coagulation factor IX is required for its activation by factor VIIa/tissue factor but not by factor XIa. Proc Natl Acad Sci U S A 1994; 91:3574–3578.

24. Christophe OD, Lenting PJ, Kolkman JA, et al. Blood coagulation factor IX residues Glu78 and Arg94 provide a link between both epidermal growth factor-like domains that is crucial in the interaction with factor VIII light chain. J Biol Chem 1998; 273:222–227.

25. Celie PH, Lenting PJ, Mertens K. Hydrophobic contact between the two epidermal growth factor-like domains of blood coagulation factor IX contributes to enzymatic activity. J Biol Chem 2000; 275:229–234.

26. Kolkman JA, Christophe OD, Lenting PJ, et al. Surface loop 199–204 in blood coagulation factor IX is a cofactor-dependent site involved in macromolecular substrate interaction. J Biol Chem 1999; 274:29087–29093.

27. Mutucumarana VP, Duffy EJ, Lollar P, et al. The active site of factor IXa is located far above the membrane surface and its conformation is altered upon association with factor VIIIa. A fluorescence study. J Biol Chem 1992; 267:17012–17021.

28. Kolkman JA, Lenting PJ, Mertens K. Regions 301–303 and 333–339 in the catalytic domain of blood coagulation factor IX are factor VIII-interactive sites involved in stimulation of enzyme activity. Biochem J 1999; 339(pt 2):217–221.

29. Gopalakrishna K, Rezaie AR. The influence of sodium ion binding on factor IXa activity. Thromb Haemost 2006; 95:936–941.

30. Schmaier AH, Dahl LD, Rozemuller AJ, et al. Protease nexin-2/amyloid beta protein precursor. A tight-binding inhibitor of coagulation factor IXa. J Clin Invest 1993; 92:2540–2555.

31. Samis JA, Kam E, Nesheim ME, et al. Neutrophil elastase cleavage of human factor IX generates an activated factor IX-like product devoid of coagulant function. Blood 1998; 92: 1287–1296.

32. Heeb MJ, Cabral KM, Ruan L. Down-regulation of factor IXa in the factor Xase complex by protein Z-dependent protease inhibitor. J Biol Chem 2005; 280:33819–33825.

33. Neels JG, van Den Berg BM, Mertens K, et al. Activation of factor IX zymogen results in exposure of a binding site for low-density lipoprotein receptor-related protein. Blood 2000; 96:3459–3465.

34. Bowen DJ. Haemophilia A and Haemophilia B: molecular insights. Mol Pathol 2002; 55:1–18.

35. Roberts HR, Escobar M, White G. Hemophilia a and hemophilia B. In: Lichtman MA, Beutler E, eds. Williams Hematology. 7th ed. New York: McGraw-Hill, 2006:1867–1886.

36. Hoffman M, Harger A, Lenkowski A, et al. Cutaneous wound healing is impaired in hemophilia B. Blood 2006; 108:3053–3060.

37. McDonald AG, Yang K, Roberts HR, et al. Perivascular tissue factor is down-regulated following cutaneous wounding: implications for bleeding in hemophilia. Blood 2008; 111: 2046–2048.

38. McDonald A, Hoffman M, Hedner U, et al. Restoring hemostatic thrombin generation at the time of cutaneous wounding does not normalize healing in hemophilia B. J Thromb Haemost 2007; 5:1577–1583.

39. Allen GA, Wolberg AS, Oliver JA, et al. Impact of procoagulant concentration on rate, peak and total thrombin generation in a model system. J Thromb Haemost 2004; 2:402–413.

40. Munnix IC, Kuijpers MJ, Auger J, et al. Segregation of platelet aggregatory and procoagulant microdomains in thrombus formation: regulation by transient integrin activation. Arterioscler Thromb Vasc Biol 2007; 27:2484–2490.

41. Gui T, Reheman A, Funkhouser WK, et al. In vivo response to vascular injury in the absence of factor IX: examination in factor IX knockout mice. Thromb Res 2007; 121:225–234.

42. Ahmad SS, Rawala-Sheikh R, Walsh PN. Comparative interactions of factor IX and factor IXa with human platelets. J Biol Chem 1989; 264:3244–3251.

43. Yang X, Chang YJ, Lin SW, et al. Identification of residues Asn89, Ile90, and Val107 of the factor IXa second epidermal growth factor domain that are essential for the assembly of the factor X-activating complex on activated platelets. J Biol Chem 2004; 279:46400–46405.

44. London FS, Marcinkiewicz M, Walsh PN. PAR-1-stimulated factor IXa binding to a small platelet subpopulation requires a pronounced and sustained increase of cytoplasmic calcium. Biochemistry 2006; 45:7289–7298.

45. Yoshitake S, Schach BG, Foster DC, et al. Nucleotide sequence of the gene for human factor IX (antihemophilic factor B). Biochemistry 1985; 24:3736–3750.

46. Kurachi S, Furukawa M, Salier JP, et al. Regulatory mechanism of human factor IX gene: protein binding at the Leyden-specific region. Biochemistry 1994; 33:1580–1591.
47. Anson DS, Choo KH, Rees DJ, et al. The gene structure of human anti-haemophilic factor IX. EMBO J 1984; 3:1053–1060.
48. Kurachi K, Kurachi S. Regulatory mechanism of the factor IX gene. Thromb Haemost 1995; 73: 333–339.
49. Crossley M, Ludwig M, Stowell KM, et al. Recovery from hemophilia B Leyden: an androgen-responsive element in the factor IX promoter. Science 1992; 257:377–379.
50. Lowe GD, Rumley A, Woodward M, et al. Epidemiology of coagulation factors, inhibitors and activation markers: the Third Glasgow MONICA Survey. I. Illustrative reference ranges by age, sex and hormone use. Br J Haematol 1997; 97:775–784.
51. Souto JC, Almasy L, Borrell M, et al. Genetic determinants of hemostasis phenotypes in Spanish families. Circulation 2000; 101:1546–1551.
52. Khachidze M, Buil A, Viel KR, et al. Genetic determinants of normal variation in coagulation factor (F) IX levels: genome-wide scan and examination of the FIX structural gene. J Thromb Haemost 2006; 4:1537–1545.
53. Adams B, Western AK, Winship PR. Identification and functional characterization of a polymorphic oestrogen response element in the human coagulation factor IX gene promoter. Br J Haematol 2008; 140:241–249.
54. Kurachi S, Deyashiki Y, Takeshita J, et al. Genetic mechanisms of age regulation of human blood coagulation factor IX. Science 1999; 285:739–743.
55. Doggen CJ, Rosendaal FR, Meijers JC. Levels of intrinsic coagulation factors and the risk of myocardial infarction among men: opposite and synergistic effects of factors XI and XII. Blood 2006; 108:4045–4051.
56. Miller GJ, Ireland HA, Cooper JA, et al. Relationship between markers of activated coagulation, their correlation with inflammation, and association with coronary heart disease (NPHSII). J Thromb Haemost 2008; 6:259–267.
57. Benedict CR, Ryan J, Wolitzky B, et al. Active site-blocked factor IXa prevents intravascular thrombus formation in the coronary vasculature without inhibiting extravascular coagulation in a canine thrombosis model. J Clin Invest 1991; 88:1760–1765.
58. Spanier TB, Oz MC, Madigan JD, et al. Selective anticoagulation with active site blocked factor IXa in synthetic patch vascular repair results in decreased blood loss and operative time. ASAIO J 1997; 43:M526–M530.
59. Wong AG, Gunn AC, Ku P, et al. Relative efficacy of active site-blocked factors IXa, Xa in models of rabbit venous and arterio-venous thrombosis. Thromb Haemost 1997; 77: 1143–1147.
60. Spanier TB, Oz MC, Minanov OP, et al. Heparinless cardiopulmonary bypass with active-site blocked factor IXa: a preliminary study on the dog. J Thorac Cardiovasc Surg 1998; 115: 1179–1188.
61. Spanier TB, Chen JM, Oz MC, et al. Selective anticoagulation with active site-blocked factor IXA suggests separate roles for intrinsic and extrinsic coagulation pathways in cardiopulmonary bypass. J Thorac Cardiovasc Surg 1998; 116:860–869.
62. Choudhri TF, Hoh BL, Prestigiacomo CJ, et al. Targeted inhibition of intrinsic coagulation limits cerebral injury in stroke without increasing intracerebral hemorrhage. J Exp Med 1999; 190:91–99.
63. Suggett S, Kirchhofer D, Hass P, et al. Use of phage display for the generation of human antibodies that neutralize factor IXa function. Blood Coagul Fibrinolysis 2000; 11:27–42.
64. Refino CJ, Jeet S, DeGuzman L, et al. A human antibody that inhibits factor IX/IXa function potently inhibits arterial thrombosis without increasing bleeding. Arterioscler Thromb Vasc Biol 2002; 22:517–522.
65. Feuerstein GZ, Patel A, Toomey JR, et al. Antithrombotic efficacy of a novel murine antihuman factor IX antibody in rats. Arterioscler Thromb Vasc Biol 1999; 19:2554–2562.

66. Toomey JR, Blackburn MN, Storer BL, et al. Comparing the antithrombotic efficacy of a humanized anti-factor IX(a) monoclonal antibody (SB 249417) to the low molecular weight heparin enoxaparin in a rat model of arterial thrombosis. Thromb Res 2000; 100:73–79.
67. Toomey JR, Valocik RE, Koster PF, et al. Inhibition of factor IX(a) is protective in a rat model of thromboembolic stroke. Stroke 2002; 33:578–585.
68. Benincosa LJ, Chow FS, Tobia LP, et al. Pharmacokinetics and pharmacodynamics of a humanized monoclonal antibody to factor IX in cynomolgus monkeys. J Pharmacol Exp Ther 2000; 292:810–816.
69. Chow FS, Benincosa LJ, Sheth SB, et al. Pharmacokinetic and pharmacodynamic modeling of humanized anti-factor IX antibody (SB 249417) in humans. Clin Pharmacol Ther 2002; 71: 235–245.
70. Ellington AD, Szostak JW. In vitro selection of RNA molecules that bind specific ligands. Nature 1990; 346:818–822.
71. Tuerk C, Gold L. Systematic evolution of ligands by exponential enrichment: RNA ligands to bacteriophage T4 DNA polymerase. Science 1990; 249:505–510.
72. Hermann T, Patel DJ. Adaptive recognition by nucleic acid aptamers. Science 2000; 287: 820–825.
73. Patel DJ, Suri AK, Jiang F, et al. Structure, recognition and adaptive binding in RNA aptamer complexes. J Mol Biol 1997; 72:55–64.
74. Rusconi CP, Scardino E, Layzer J, et al. RNA aptamers as reversible antagonists of coagulation factor IXa. Nature 2002; 419:90–94.
75. Gopinath SC, Shikamoto Y, Mizuno H, et al. A potent anti-coagulant RNA aptamer inhibits blood coagulation by specifically blocking the extrinsic clotting pathway. Thromb Haemost 2006; 95:767–771.
76. Rusconi CP, Roberts JD, Pitoc GA, et al. Antidote-mediated control of an anticoagulant aptamer in vivo. Nat Biotechnol 2004; 22:1423–1428.
77. Nimjee SM, Keys JR, Pitoc GA, et al. A novel antidote-controlled anticoagulant reduces thrombin generation and inflammation and improves cardiac function in cardiopulmonary bypass surgery. Mol Ther 2006; 14:408–415.
78. Dyke CK, Steinhubl SR, Kleiman NS, et al. First-in-human experience of an antidote-controlled anticoagulant using RNA aptamer technology: a phase 1a pharmacodynamic evaluation of a drug-antidote pair for the controlled regulation of factor IXa activity. Circulation 2006; 114: 2490–2497.
79. Chan MY, Cohen MG, Rusconi CP, et al. A phase ib randomized study of antidote-controlled modulation of factor ixa activity in patients with stable coronary artery disease. Circulation 2008; 117:2865–2874.
80. Chan MY, Rusconi CP, Alexander JH, et al. A randomized, repeat dose, pharmacodynamic, and safety study of an antidote-controlled factor IXa inhibitor. A randomized, repeat dose, pharmacodynamic, and safety study of an antidote-controlled factor IXa inhibitor. J Thromb Haemost 2008; 6:789–796.
81. Califf RM. Fondaparinux in ST-segment elevation myocardial infarction: the drug, the strategy, the environment, or all of the above? JAMA 2006; 295:579–580.
82. Rothlein R, Shen JM, Naser N, et al. TTP889, a novel orally active partial inhibitor of FIXa inhibits clotting in two A/V shunt models without prolonging bleeding times. Blood 2005; 106: 1886 (abstr).
83. Eriksson BI, Dahl OE, Lassen MR, et al. Partial factor IXa inhibition with TTP889 for prevention of venous thromboembolism: an exploratory study. J Thromb Haemost 2008; 6:457–463.
84. Atoda H, Kaneko H, Mizuno H, et al. Calcium-binding analysis and molecular modeling reveal echis coagulation factor IX/factor X-binding protein has the Ca-binding properties and Ca ion-independent folding of other C-type lectin-like proteins. FEBS Lett 2002; 531:229–234.
85. Li WF, Chen L, Li XM, et al. A C-type lectin-like protein from Agkistrodon acutus venom binds to both platelet glycoprotein Ib and coagulation factor IX/factor X. Biochem Biophys Res Commun 2005; 332:904–912.

86. Li YF, Spencer FA, Becker RC. Comparative efficacy of fibrinogen and platelet supplementation on the in vitro reversibility of competitive glycoprotein IIb/IIIa (alphaIIb/beta3) receptor-directed platelet inhibition. Am Heart J 2001; 142:204–210.

87. Wiebe EM, Stafford AR, Fredenburgh JC, et al. Mechanism of catalysis of inhibition of factor IXa by antithrombin in the presence of heparin or pentasaccharide. J Biol Chem 2003; 278: 35767–35774.

88. Yang L, Manithody C, Rezaie AR. Localization of the heparin binding exosite of factor IXa. J Biol Chem 2002; 277:50756–50760.

89. Neuenschwander PF, Williamson SR, Nalian A, et al. Heparin modulates the 99-loop of factor IXa: effects on reactivity with isolated Kunitz-type inhibitor domains. J Biol Chem 2006ssss; 281: 23066–23074.

90. Yuan QP, Walke EN, Sheehan JP. The factor IXa heparin-binding exosite is a cofactor interactive site: mechanism for antithrombin-independent inhibition of intrinsic tenase by heparin. Biochemistry 2005; 44:3615–3625.

91. Misenheimer TM, Buyue Y, Sheehan JP. The heparin-binding exosite is critical to allosteric activation of factor IXa in the intrinsic tenase complex: the role of arginine 165 and factor X. Biochemistry 2007; 46:7886–7895.

92. Ginsberg JS. Pharmacology of heparin-related compounds and coumarin derivatives. In: Loscalzo J, Schafer AL, eds. Thrombosis and Hemorrhage. 3rd ed. Philadelphia: Lippincott Williams & Wilkins, 2003:937–994.

93. Sheehan JP, Kobbervig CE, Kirkpatrick HM. Heparin inhibits the intrinsic tenase complex by interacting with an exosite on factor IXa. Biochemistry 2003; 42:11316–11325.

94. Janatpour KA, Gosselin RC, Owings JT, et al. Laboratory comparison of the VisuLize IX antigen assay with the Asserachrome IX antigen assay. Lab Hematol 2006; 2:152–155.

95. Cunningham MT, Brandt JT, Chandler WL, et al. Quality assurance in hemostasis: the perspective from the College of American Pathologists proficiency testing program. Semin Thromb Hemost 2007; 33:250–258.

96. Howard EL, Becker KC, Rusconi CP, et al. Factor IXa inhibitors as novel anticoagulants. Arterioscl Thromb Vasc Biol 2007; 27:722–727.

22

Contact-Activation Pathways as Targets for New Anticoagulants

David Gailani
Departments of Pathology and Medicine, Vanderbilt University, Nashville, Tennessee, U.S.A.

Thomas Renné
Institute of Clinical Biochemistry and Pathobiochemistry, Julius-Maximilians-University of Würzburg, Würzburg, Germany

Andras Gruber
Departments of Biomedical Engineering and Medicine, Oregon Health and Science University, Portland, Oregon, U.S.A.

INTRODUCTION

Exposure of mammalian blood to surfaces carrying a negative charge triggers a series of reactions involving activation of the plasma protease zymogens factor XII, factor XI, and plasma prekallikrein (PK), and cleavage of the plasma glycoprotein high-molecular-weight kininogen (HK) (Fig. 1) (1–3). These proteins are traditionally referred to as contact factors, and the processes involved in their activation are called contact-activation reactions because a charged surface is needed for them to proceed optimally. Contact activation triggers several host defense mechanisms in vitro, including blood coagulation (Fig. 2) and liberation of vasoactive/proinflammatory kinins from HK (Fig. 1) (1–3). In fact, factors XI (4) and XII (5) were initially identified as missing components of plasma in patients with inherited abnormalities of surface-initiated coagulation. Deficiency of PK (6) or HK (7), components of the kallikrein-kinin system, also causes a defect in surface-mediated coagulation. Despite the clear importance of the contact factors to surface-initiated clotting in vitro, a role for contact activation in normal blood coagulation (hemostasis) in vivo appears unlikely.

Plasma coagulation, as depicted in the classic cascade/waterfall model (Fig. 2), involves a series of sequential proteolytic reactions that can be initiated by two distinct mechanisms (8,9). When the vascular endothelium is breached, activated factor VII (factor VIIa) in plasma binds to tissue factor (TF), an integral membrane protein normally expressed on cells underlying the endothelium. The factor VIIa/TF complex (the extrinsic

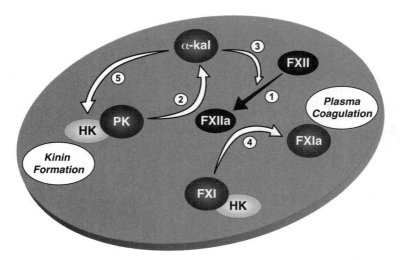

Figure 1 Contact-activation reactions. Contact activation is initiated by the slow activation of FXII to FXIIa, probably by autoactivation, when plasma is exposed to a negatively charged surface (*reaction 1*). Reciprocal activation of PK to α-kal by FXIIa (*reaction 2*), and FXII by α-kal (*reaction 3*) enhances FXII activation. FXIIa promotes coagulation through conversion of FXI to FXIa (*reaction 4*). α-kal also cleaves HK to liberate bradykinin (*reaction 5*). Note that HK is required for proper binding of PK and FXI to the contact surface. *Abbreviations*: FXII, factor XII; FXIIa, α-factor XIIa; PK, prekallikrein; α-kal, α-kallikrein; FXIa, factor XIa; FXI, factor XI; HK, high-molecular-weight kininogen.

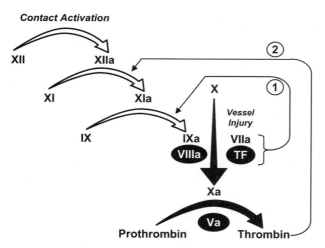

Figure 2 Plasma coagulation. The bold arrows indicate reactions involving proteolytic conversion of the zymogens of plasma serine proteases (*designated by Roman numerals*) to active proteases (*designated by Roman numerals followed by "a"*). Nonenzymatic cofactors are indicated by numerals in black ovals. White arrows indicate reactions of the classic intrinsic pathway and bold black arrows the activation of factor X and prothrombin. The thin black line designated "1" represents activation of factor IX by the factor VIIa/tissue factor (TF) complex, while the thin line labeled "2" indicates activation of factor XI by thrombin.

pathway of coagulation) activates factor X, which then converts prothrombin to the protease α-thrombin. α-thrombin mediates many reactions, including fibrin formation and activation of platelets, the major constituents of normal and pathologic thrombi. Alternatively, activation of factor X can be initiated through contact activation, by the sequential activation of factor XII, factor XI, and ultimately factor IX, which collectively comprise the intrinsic pathway of coagulation.

Although they provide an accurate description of the major protease-substrate interactions that occur during surface-initiated coagulation in vitro, the linear sequence of events in the classic intrinsic pathway does not adequately explain clinical syndromes associated with specific factor-deficiency states. Congenital deficiency of factor IX or its cofactor, factor VIII, causes the severe bleeding disorder hemophilia; which indicates an important role for the intrinsic pathway in hemostasis (10). However, complete deficiency of one of the three proteins involved in initiating contact activation (factor XII, PK, or HK) has not been linked to a hemostatic abnormality in any species, suggesting that these proteins do not contribute significantly to coagulation in vivo (11–12). To complicate matters, one-third to one-half of individuals with factor XI deficiency have a bleeding diathesis, but the pattern of abnormal bleeding is distinctly different from that observed in hemophilia (discussed below) (11–12). Indeed, because of the bleeding diathesis associated with factor XI deficiency, and the absence of bleeding with factor XII, PK, or HK deficiency, many experts no longer classify factor XI as a contact factor.

The discrepancies between the cascade/waterfall model and the clinical phenotypes can be explained by observations that the intrinsic pathway factors downstream from factor XII can be activated by more than one mechanism (Fig. 2) (13). Thus, the differences in the syndromes associated with factor IX and factor XI deficiency are attributable to the fact that factor IX is also a major substrate for the factor VIIa/TF complex (13–16). Similarly, factor XI may be activated by multiple proteases, including activated factor XII (factor XIIa), α-thrombin, and activated factor XI (factor XIa), reconciling the excessive bleeding that occurs in some factor XI-deficient patients and the absence of abnormal bleeding in those with factor XII deficiency (12,17,18). The kallikrein-kinin-generating mechanism of plasma is also being defined in terms distinct from classic contact activation (3). For example, mast-cell proteases such as elastase and tryptase, and the heat shock protein HSP90 facilitate kinin cleavage via factor XII-independent mechanisms (19,20). Similarly, the lysosomal protease prolylcarboxypeptidase activates PK with a K_m that is ~250-fold lower than that for factor XIIa-mediated PK activation (3,21). Understandably then, recent models have tended to assign more limited roles to contact activation in coagulation and kinin generation (13,22). The fact that members of the order *cetacea* (whales and dolphins) lack factor XII, yet possess other components of the plasma coagulation system shown in Figure 2, reinforces the impression that this protein, and thus contact activation, is not required for normal clot formation at a wound site (23,24).

Given that the contact factors do not appear to be required for hemostasis, it seems reasonable to postulate that these proteins also play a limited role in arterial and venous thrombosis. However, recent studies in animal models raise the possibility that the intrinsic pathway, perhaps triggered by contact activation, contributes substantively to pathologic coagulation. This chapter will review the evidence that the contact factors and the intrinsic pathway contribute to thrombotic disease in humans, discuss the role of these factors in animal models of thrombosis and consumptive coagulopathies, and cover recent information on development of therapeutic agents targeting components of the contact system.

CONTACT FACTORS AND THROMBOTIC DISEASE IN HUMANS

Studies examining the contributions of the contact factors and the intrinsic pathway of coagulation to thrombosis in humans generally fall into two categories: (1) large epidemiologic studies looking for variation in risk within the broad normal range for a plasma protein, and (2) comparisons of differences in disease risk between the general population and a relatively small group of patients with inherited deficiency of a plasma factor. Interestingly, data from the two types of studies support opposite conclusions in some instances. Congenital deficiencies of intrinsic pathway factors are relatively rare. Deficiency of factor VIII (hemophilia A—1 in 5000–10,000 male births) or factor IX (hemophilia B—1 in 30,000 male births) are the most common inherited abnormalities of thrombin generation, and over 50% of such patients have severe deficiency of factor VIII or IX (<1% of normal plasma levels) (25). Factor XI deficiency was originally thought to occur at a rate of ~1 per million individuals, although recent studies suggest that milder forms may be relatively common (26,27). Severe factor XI deficiency (<15% of normal plasma levels) is particularly common in Jewish people, with an incidence of 1 in 450 in Ashkenazi Jews (28). Accurate data for the incidences of factor XII, PK, or HK deficiencies are not available.

Contact Factors and the Intrinsic Pathway in Venous Thromboembolic Disease in Humans

In current models of coagulation, initiation of fibrin formation is triggered by factor VIIa/TF–mediated activation of factor X and prothrombin (Fig. 2), while sustained generation of thrombin requires factor IX (in conjunction with factor VIIIa) and, in some cases, factor XI (13,22,29). Bleeding in factor IX or factor XI deficiency, therefore, can be viewed as a failure of consolidation of coagulation, rather than as a defect in its initiation (22). Sustained thrombin generation through factors IX and XI may result in modifications of fibrin that render thrombi more resistant to fibrinolytic degradation (29). The antifibrinolytic effect of factor XI may be manifest through thrombin-mediated activation of a metalloproteinase called TAFI (thrombin-activatable fibrinolysis inhibitor), which proteolytically modifies fibrin by cleavage after lysine residues, resulting in downregulation of the fibrinolytic system (30–32). Given the procoagulant and antifibrinolytic roles proposed for the intrinsic pathway, dysregulation of one or more components of this system would be expected to contribute to thromboembolism. A relationship between plasma levels of intrinsic pathway proteins and thrombosis is most clearly observed in the venous circulation, where thrombi tend to be relatively fibrin rich.

In humans, correlations between plasma-factor levels and risk of venous thrombosis or thromboembolism have been demonstrated in case-controlled studies for factors VIII (33), IX (34), and XI (35). Factor VIII levels above the upper limit of normal (1.5 International Units/mL) were associated with an odds ratio of approximately five for venous thromboembolism (33), and most subsequent prospective studies support the concept that high factor VIII levels are a moderate risk factor for venous thrombosis (36). In the Leiden Thrombophilia Study, plasma factor IX (34) or factor XI (35) levels in the upper 10% of the normal distribution were associated with an ~twofold increased risk of venous thromboembolism compared with the remainder of the population, independent of other inherited risk factors. A recent analysis of single nucleotide polymorphisms (SNPs) in a subpopulation of the Leiden study revealed linkage between several SNPs, plasma factor XI level, and deep-vein thrombosis, consistent with a genetic influence on factor levels and predisposition to thrombosis (37). Cumulatively, these results are consistent with observations that venous thrombosis is rare in patients with factor VIII or IX deficiency (38). Venous thrombosis may also be infrequent in patients with factor XI deficiency (39), although the low incidence of this disorder in the general population makes it difficult to determine if it is protective against this condition.

Establishing a relationship between plasma levels of factor XII and venous thrombotic disease has been difficult, with multiple studies and case reports presenting conflicting results. Congenital factor XII deficiency has appeared in the differential diagnosis of inherited hypercoagulable disorders in reviews dating back to the death of John Hageman, the index case for severe factor XII deficiency, as a consequence of pulmonary embolism after lower extremity trauma (40). Contact activation enhances fibrinolysis in plasma in vitro, and activated PK (α-kallikrein) (41,42), factor XIIa (42,43), and factor XIa (44) are weak activators of plasminogen, converting it to plasmin, the major mediator of fibrinolysis. These observations have led to the speculation that a defect in contact activation may increase thrombotic risk. Indeed, it has been postulated that the absence of bleeding in factor XII–, PK–, or HK–deficient patients may reflect a defect in fibrinolysis that offsets any reduction in thrombin generation associated with the deficiency (45,46). While thrombotic events do occur in patients with moderate or severe factor XII deficiency, recent surveys suggest that other congenital or acquired risk factors account for most cases (47), and case-controlled studies done in Switzerland (48) and The Netherlands (49) failed to find a correlation between factor XII deficiency and adverse outcomes. As with severe factor XI deficiency, the number of patients with severe factor XII deficiency is relatively small in the general population, making it difficult to establish strong statistical correlations with disease.

There is a paucity of information regarding the effects of PK and HK levels on venous thrombotic risk in humans. In a study performed in East Kent in the United Kingdom, plasma levels of contact factor measured in 300 patients on stable warfarin therapy at least three months after a venous thromboembolic event, were compared with those in an equal number of age- and gender-matched controls (50). The patient population had significantly lower levels of factor XII, but higher levels of HK than controls, while the PK levels were similar in the two groups.

In summary, available data suggest that components of the intrinsic pathway that are required for hemostasis in humans (i.e., factors VIII, IX, and XI) influence the risk of venous thromboembolism. This is in keeping with the importance of these proteins in fibrin formation and stabilization. A correlation between plasma levels of the contact proteins (factor XII, HK, and PK) and venous thrombotic disease has not been clearly established.

Contact Factors and the Intrinsic Pathway in Arterial Thrombotic Disease in Humans

Pathologic thrombi in the arterial circulation tend to be relatively rich in platelets compared with venous thrombi. Contact factors and the intrinsic pathway could hypothetically affect the risk of atherothrombotic disease by influencing atherogenesis and/or by promoting the formation of a thrombus at the site of plaque rupture. While there are studies that indicate that hemophilia retards the development of atherosclerosis to some degree in humans (51) and mice (52), in general severe congenital coagulopathies, including hemophilia (53), type III von Willebrand disease (54), and Glanzmann thrombasthenia (absence or dysfunction of the platelet α_{IIb}/β_3 integrin) (55) do not appear to protect humans from atherosclerotic disease.

The contributions of elevated plasma factor VIII levels to coronary artery and cerebrovascular diseases have been addressed in several large studies (reviewed in reference 36) with conflicting results. Interpretation of such studies is complicated by the fact that plasma factor VIII levels fluctuate over short time periods in response to a variety of stresses, and because plasma levels are influenced by the physical association of factor VIII with von Willebrand factor, a contributor to arterial thrombosis (36). Longitudinal studies in patients with hemophilia in the Netherlands demonstrated a lower incidence of myocardial infarction (MI) in such patients compared with controls, with an 80% reduction in mortality from coronary artery disease (56,57). This suggests that factor VIII or IX deficiency may inhibit acute formation of thrombi at sites of plaque rupture. Two recent reviews emphasized that that there are case reports describing MI in hemophiliacs, raising the possibility that MI may be more frequent than previously suspected (58,59). Many of the cases of MI were associated with factor replacement or with the use of prothrombotic prothrombin complex concentrates. Thus, while the data do not allow firm conclusions to be drawn regarding an association between factor VIII or IX levels and risk for arterial thrombosis in general, a significant deficiency of one these proteins may provide some degree of protection from acute arterial thrombotic events.

The relationship between factor XI and arterial disease in humans has been addressed in several studies. In the Study of Myocardial Infarction—Leiden (SMILE), men with plasma factor XI levels in the highest quintile had an ~twofold increased risk of MI compared with those whose factor XI levels were in the lowest quintile (60). Factor XI activity above the normal range was also a risk factor for stroke and transient ischemic attacks in a retrospective analysis of patients under the age of 55 (61). Santamaria et al. reported on a possible synergistic effect between elevated factor XI levels and dyslipidemia in 218 patients with ischemic stroke, with an odds ratio of 6.4 compared with dyslipidemic controls who had normal factor XI levels (62). Recently, Butenas et al. demonstrated that both TF and factor XIa are increased in plasma in three-quarters of patients with stable angina and a history of MI, and in essentially all patients with acute coronary syndromes, suggesting that factor XIa may be a marker for atherosclerotic disease (63).

While the epidemiologic data from the general population suggest that factor XI contributes to acute arterial thrombosis, studies involving Jewish patients with severe factor XI deficiency suggest a more complex phenomenon. In a retrospective study of 96 Israeli patients over the age of 35 years with severe factor XI deficiency, the incidence of MI did not differ statistically from what was expected in the general population (64). The control population in this analysis appears to include age-matched survivors and nonsurvivors of MI, while the factor XI–deficient patients obviously were all alive. Considering that one-third of MI patients die from their acute event, and no patient in the factor XI–deficient group had died from an MI at the time of the study, this study may not exclude the possibilities that: (*i*) the incidence of MI is actually higher in factor XI deficiency but patients who died of MI were not included in the study, or (*ii*) factor XI deficiency does not change the incidence of MI but may lower the likelihood of a fatal event. In a study of 115 patients with severe factor XI deficiency (a population similar to the one in the MI study) a significantly lower risk for ischemic stroke was observed compared with age- and sex-matched controls (65). As with the earlier study, no protective effect of factor XI deficiency was observed with regard to MI. These studies involving severely deficient patients raise the interesting possibilities that factor XI may be more important for thrombus formation in the carotid arteries or the heart (the origins of most emboli that occlude cerebral vessels), or in driving fibrin formation during ischemia/reperfusion injury after a cerebral vascular occlusive event, than for thrombus formation superimposed on a disrupted atherosclerotic coronary artery plaque.

As in the case of venous thrombosis, the contribution of factor XII to arterial thrombotic disease in humans is controversial. In the SMILE project, an inverse relationship was noted between plasma factor XII and the risk of MI, with an odds ratio for the highest quintile of factor XII levels of 0.4 compared with the lowest quintile (60). Furthermore, a high factor XI level combined with a low factor XII level was associated with the highest risk of MI (odds ratio 6.4) (60). A study from Austria, which included more than 8500 individuals, observed a similar inverse association between factor XII levels and heart disease (66). In addition to death from cardiovascular disease, overall mortality increased as factor XII levels decreased. While this suggests a detrimental effect for lower factor XII levels within the normal range, curiously, mortality for patients with severe factor XII deficiency (1–10% of normal level) was similar to that for the population median. This suggests a fundamental difference between severe and moderate factor XII deficiency, a possibility that has implications for therapeutic targeting of this protein. It is possible that a low factor XII level is a risk marker, as opposed to a risk factor, for cardiovascular disease (67).

While there appears to be an inverse association between total plasma factor XII levels and arterial disease, elevated levels of factor XIIa have been associated with an increased risk of coronary heart disease in one study (68), and were a prognostic risk factor for recurrent coronary events in a second (69). It is not clear if factor XIIa formation contributed directly to thrombotic events in these patients, or was a consequence of thrombosis and the resultant tissue ischemia. In contrast, a case-control analysis from the Second Northwick Park Heart Study indicated that low factor XIIa levels determined by measuring factor XIIa in complex with C1-inhibitor, were associated with an increased risk of coronary artery disease and stroke in middle-aged men (70). Antibodies to factor XII and reduced factor XII levels have been associated with antiphospholipid antibodies (APA) and thrombosis and pregnancy loss in the APA syndrome (71,72). APAs are common in the general population, and may be prevalent in patients with apparently low factor XII levels. If verified in future studies, this association will need to be taken into account when planning studies examining the relationship between factor XII levels and thrombotic disease.

Arterial thrombotic events have been reported in patients with PK or HK deficiency, but the rarity of these conditions does not allow us to draw conclusions beyond the observation that deficiency was not absolutely protective in the individual cases. In one study, plasma factor XI, PK, and HK levels were elevated in 200 survivors of MIs compared with healthy controls, with the strongest association being for PK (73). PK is an acute phase protein and, thus, it is not clear if elevated levels represent a baseline prothrombotic risk factor or increase in response to tissue ischemia and injury.

At this point, it does not appear that levels of intrinsic pathway factors, or deficiencies of these proteins, have a major impact on the development of atherosclerosis. Hemophilia appears to provide protection from acute arterial events, although correlations between plasma levels of factor VIII or IX and arterial disease in the general population are not as evident. An association between factor XI levels and arterial disease has been identified in several studies. However, severe deficiency does not appear to be protective against acute thrombosis in all cases.

CONTACT FACTORS IN ANIMAL MODELS OF VASCULAR DISEASE

The intriguing and often contradictory data from studies in humans have been a driving force for the development of models to test the contributions of the contact factors and the intrinsic pathway to thrombosis under more controlled conditions. Studies in several animal species have been performed. Mice homozygous for gene deletions of factors XI (74), XII (75), and HK (76) have been established, and comparisons with factor IX–deficient mice

(77) have been instrumental in changing our perspective on the roles of the contact factors in thrombosis. The bleeding disorders associated with the gene deletions in mice are relatively similar to the corresponding clinical conditions in humans, with a few important differences that need to be kept in mind. As with their human counterparts, murine plasma lacking factor IX, XI, XII, or HK will demonstrates a prolonged time to clot formation in a partial thromboplastin time (PTT) assay where coagulation is triggered by contact activation. Factor IX–null mice will exsanguinate when the tip of the tail is amputated with a scalpel (tail bleeding time—TBT) (77,78), consistent with the severe bleeding seen in hemophiliacs. However, the spontaneous bleeding typical of severe hemophilia in humans is relatively infrequent in mice with factor VIII deficiency (a disorder similar to factor IX deficiency) (79). Instead, spontaneous bleeding in mice tends to involve subcutaneous tissue or the thoracic cavity (80), rather than joints and soft tissues as seen in humans. Factor XI–deficient mice have normal TBTs (74,78), and no obvious bleeding diathesis. About one-third to one-half of humans with severe factor XI deficiency have excessive bleeding after trauma or surgery, particularly if the oropharynx or urinary tract is involved (81). As discussed, predilection for bleeding in these areas may be related to premature fibrinolytic degradation of thrombus due to the loss of sustained thrombin generation through factor XI (29,30,81). Factor XI–deficient mice have not been systematically challenged by injury to the oropharynx or urinary tract, so it is not known if this protein serves a similar function in these animals. Hemostasis in factor XII– or HK–deficient mice, as in their human counterparts, appears to be normal (75,76). A PK-deficient mouse line has not been described. There is no evidence of a bleeding diathesis in brown Norway Katholiek rats, which have a plasma PK level that is about 30% of the normal value because of severe HK deficiency (PK is bound to HK in plasma) (82). The following sections review recent literature on the role of contact factors and factor IX in models of thrombosis, cerebral ischemia-reperfusion injury, and sepsis.

Models of Arterial Thrombosis

In 2003, Gruber and Hanson demonstrated that inhibition of factor XI with a polyclonal antibody affected thrombus formation in TF-coated Gortex^{TM} (polytetrafluoroethylene) grafts introduced into arteriovenous shunts in baboons (*Papio anubis*) (83). While initiation of thrombus formation on the surface of the graft was not affected by factor XI inhibition, three-dimensional growth of the thrombus was markedly inhibited. The inhibitory effect was comparable to that produced by a large dose of heparin which significantly prolonged the bleeding time. We subsequently observed a similar phenomenon in factor XI deficient mice. Application of ferric chloride (FeCl$_3$) to the exterior of a blood vessel causes significant damage to the endothelial lining resulting in rapid occlusion of the vessel (84). Several variations of this technique have been used to study thrombus formation in rodents. Using relatively low FeCl$_3$ concentrations, we demonstrated that factor XI deficiency protects mice from carotid artery occlusion to a similar extent as does complete factor IX deficiency or a supratherapeutic dose of heparin (78). The important implication of the studies in baboons and mice is that the contribution of a coagulation protease to hemostasis may not be an accurate indicator of its importance in thrombosis. A subsequent study using intravital microscopy demonstrated a pronounced reduction in platelet accumulation into thrombi formed in arterioles after laser-induced injury in factor XI–null mice, with only a modest effect on fibrin deposition (85,86). These results are consistent both with the earlier baboon studies (83), and with recent work demonstrating that inhibition of factor XI with an antibody retards growth of platelet aggregates after arterial endothelial injury in rabbits (87).

While the studies described above implicate factor XI in arterial thrombus formation, they do not address how factor XI is activated during this process. A comparison of results in factor XI– and factor XII–null mice supports the unexpected conclusion that contact activation or another factor XII–dependent process is involved. Factor XII–deficient mice have a marked defect in occlusive thrombus formation in response to FeCl$_3$-induced injury of mesenteric vessels, and after ligature injury or mechanical endothelial denudation of the carotid artery (88). Intravital microscopy studies in which the mesenteric arteries and veins were treated with FeCl$_3$ clearly demonstrate instability of large platelet aggregates that prevent vessel occlusion (88). Factor XI–deficient mice had an identical phenotype to the factor XII–null animals in this study. A subsequent comparison of factor XII–deficient mice and factor IX– or factor XI–deficient animals in the FeCl$_3$-carotid artery injury model (unpublished observations) confirmed the potent antithrombotic effect of factor XII deficiency. Thus, factor XII and factor XI are essential for thrombus propagation in arteries in mice, suggesting that the classic intrinsic pathway of coagulation (factors XII, XI, and IX) may be operating during pathologic thrombus growth. The trigger for activation of factor XII after FeCl$_3$-induced injury has not been established, but could be collagen in subendothelial layers of the vessel that are exposed upon injury (89), or an activity associated with platelets (90). Kannemeier and colleagues recently demonstrated that extracellular RNA augments activation of the contact proteases (91). Using the FeCl$_3$-injury model in mice, they demonstrated that RNA, probably released from damaged cells, associates with fibrin-rich thrombi in the carotid artery, and showed that pretreatment of animals with intravenous RNAse delayed formation of occlusive thrombi.

The importance of HK to thrombus formation in mice has recently been described. Mice have two kininogen genes (*mKng1* and *mKng2*), in contrast to the single gene in humans. Merkulov et al. reported that mice homozygous for null deletions of the *mKng1* gene have complete absence of HK in plasma (76). *mKng1*$^{-/-}$ animals show delayed time to carotid artery occlusion in a Rose Bengal/laser injury model (76,84). The injury in this model is probably less severe than that produced by FeCl$_3$, resulting in less collagen exposure (89), and it is not clear if HK deficiency provides the degree of protection observed in the FeCl$_3$ injury model with factor XII or factor XI–null mice. Indeed, factor XII–deficient mice were not protected from cerebral ischemia induced by Rose Bengal/laser injury, suggesting that this model may not be optimal for assessing intrinsic pathway–mediated thrombosis (92). Mice of the B6:129S7 genetic background (but not other backgrounds) lacking the bradykinin B2 receptor have prolonged bleeding times and a delay in time to thrombosis (93), suggesting that loss of bradykinin may contribute in some manner to the delayed time to thrombus formation observed in *mKng1*$^{-/-}$ animals. In stark contrast, studies in brown Norway Katholiek rats with very low plasma HK levels suggest that HK has antithrombotic properties (94). Thrombus formation after mechanical denudation of the endothelial lining of the abdominal aorta was greater in the HK-deficient rats than in controls, and the effect could be reversed by infusing cleaved human HK or components of HK. It must be recognized that HK-deficient rats have a significant deficiency of PK as a consequence of HK deficiency, and the contribution of PK deficiency to this model is not clear. Furthermore, rats express a rodent-specific kininogen (T-kininogen) that has no equivalent in humans, making it difficult to extrapolate results in rats to humans.

The findings in the baboon and mouse arterial models indicate that there is a fundamental difference in formation of a normal "hemostatic" clot and a pathologic thrombus that occludes the vessel. During hemostasis, clot formation is triggered by exposure of blood to TF and basement membranes, which induces fibrin formation and

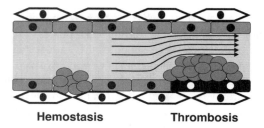

Hemostasis   **Thrombosis**

Figure 3   The role of factors XII and XI in pathologic (occlusive) thrombus formation. Pictured is a schematic diagram of a blood vessel, with healthy vascular endothelial cells represented by gray rectangles, cells in the vessel wall expressing TF by hexagons, and damaged/activated vascular endothelial cells by black rectangles. During normal hemostasis at the site of a wound where the vascular endothelium is disrupted (*left*), a clot consisting primarily of platelets (*gray ovals*) and fibrin forms in response to exposure to extravascular TF and components of the basement membrane. This process does not require factor XII and in many cases does not require factor XI. The vascular injury in the murine thrombosis models discussed in this chapter appears to initiate a different process (*right*). Here, a platelet-rich aggregate accumulates within the lumen of the blood vessel, and the three-dimensional growth of the aggregate to form an occlusive thrombus is dependent on factor XII and factor XI. It is possible that as the vessel narrows and shear forces increase (*arrows*), factor XII and factor XI are required for local thrombin generation or platelet activation to sustain thrombus growth.

platelet activation (Fig. 3). Thrombus formation is at least in part an extravascular event under these conditions. In contrast, occlusive thrombi form intraluminally. Studies in mice expressing low levels of TF clearly demonstrate that this protein is required for both normal hemostasis and thrombus propagation in arterial occlusion models (95,96). In contrast to the situation during normal hemostasis, factor XII and factor XI are required for occlusive thrombus propagation. It is possible that that these proteases contribute to thrombin generation on the surface of the enlarging thrombus (see Factor XIa Inhibitors— below). A thrombus growing within the lumen of an artery will be subjected to increasing shear as the lumen narrows (Fig. 3), and factors XII and XI may promote fibrin formation/ stabilization and/or platelet activation in this environment. It is not clear at this point, however, whether a process similar to classic contact activation is involved, or if novel pathways are operating.

Models of Venous Thromboembolism

There are relatively fewer animal model studies addressing the role of factor XI in venous thrombosis. Minnema et al. demonstrated that experimentally induced clots in the jugular veins of rabbits treated with a polyclonal factor XI antibody were nearly twice as susceptible to endogenous fibrinolytic degradation as were clots in untreated animals (97). Feuerstein et al. demonstrated that inhibiting factor IX affected injury-induced venous thrombus formation in rats (98). Administration of the antibody immediately after injury resulted in a fourfold reduction in the mass of venous thrombi associated with a relatively modest prolongation of the PTT clotting time compared with a bolus of heparin. In another study, factor XI–deficient mice developed significantly smaller venous thrombi after FeCl$_3$ injury to the inferior vena cava than did wild-type mice (99). The thrombi that form after FeCl$_3$-induced injury are rich in platelets, resembling the thrombi that form in the arterial injury model described above. This is different from deep-vein thrombi that form in humans, which tend to be relatively platelet poor, so the implications for human pathophysiology remain to be determined. In a model of lethal pulmonary thrombembolism induced by intravenous infusion of collagen and epinephrine, factor XII–deficient mice exhibited reduced mortality and had significantly fewer pulmonary thrombi than wild-type controls (88). A substantial amount of work remains to be done before we can draw firm conclusions on the role of the contact factors in the rodent venous thrombembolism models.

Models of Cerebral Ischemia-Reperfusion Injury

The use of anticoagulants and antifibrinolytic agents for treatment of acute cerebrovascular events is limited by the catastrophic consequences of therapy-associated hemorrhage. Because inhibition of intrinsic pathway reactions, and particularly inhibition of contact factors, should be associated with significantly less bleeding than with currently available therapies, there is considerable interest in studying the role of the intrinsic pathway in ischemia-reperfusion injury. After transient occlusion of the middle cerebral artery (MCA), Choudri et al. examined the consequences of factor IX inhibition on infarct size, fibrin and platelet deposition, and cerebral hemorrhage in mice (100). Factor IX inhibition was achieved by infusion of active site–inhibited factor IXa, a competitive inhibitor of factor IXa. Treated animals had significantly reduced infarct size and less fibrin and platelet deposition compared with controls. As important, the treated animals did not develop reperfusion-associated intracranial bleeding, in contrast to mice treated either with tissue plasminogen activator (tPA) or with heparin.

Kleinschnitz and colleagues subsequently examined the importance of factors XII and XI to cerebral ischemia/reperfusion injury in mice in a transient MCA occlusion model (101). Deficiency of either protease markedly reduced ischemic injury compared with wild-type animals, with significantly lower mortality and residual neurologic deficit. Fibrin deposition in the microvasculature of vessels within the ischemic zone was markedly reduced in the factor XII– or XI–deficient animals. When human factor XII was infused into factor XII–deficient mice, cerebral injury was comparable to what was observed in wild-type controls. Postreperfusion intracerebral hemorrhage, determined by T2-weighted nuclear magnetic resonance images, was observed in wild-type mice but not in factor XII– or factor XI–deficient mice.

Taken as a whole, the data suggest that the contribution of factor XII to cerebral injury during ischemia-reperfusion may be mediated through the intrinsic pathway, thereby raising the possibility that contact activation could be involved in this process. We do not have any direct evidence from HK-deficient mice that this protein is involved in ischemia-reperfusion injury, although the importance of bradykinin, a product of HK cleavage, has been addressed. Three studies examining bradykinin B2 receptor-null mice in ischemia-reperfusion generated discrepant conclusions (102–104). Studies with HK-deficient mice will be important in clarifying the role of HK and bradykinin in this model. It is possible that factor XII contributes to ischemia-reperfusion injury through mechanisms unrelated to factor XI activation. In addition to effects on kallikrein/kinin formation (105), factor XIIa and factor XIIa fragments may prime the extrinsic pathway of coagulation through activation of factor VII (106), and initiate other proteolytic cascades involving complement (107) and fibrinolysis (108), which could contribute to thrombosis and inflammation, thereby aggravating ischemia-reperfusion-related damage.

Models of Sepsis and Endotoxemia

Using enzyme-linked immunosorbant assays that measure complexes between contact proteases and plasma inhibitors, it was demonstrated that factor XII, factor XI, and PK are activated in humans with sepsis (109,110). What is not clear is whether contact proteases contribute to the disseminated intravascular coagulation (DIC) that accompanies this syndrome. Pixley et al. examined the effects of sepsis on contact factors in baboons treated with a lethal dose of *Escherichia coli* (111). There was a significant decrease in HK levels, but no changes in the levels of factor XII, factor XI, or PK. Subsequent work demonstrated that blocking factor XII with an antibody had a significant effect on hypotension, fibrinolysis, and markers of inflammation, but not on DIC (112,113). One animal treated with anti-factor XII antibody survived. While these studies suggest an important role for factor XII, and perhaps contact activation, in the pathophysiology of sepsis, they do not provide strong support for a substantive contribution to DIC in this syndrome. It should be noted, however, that the antibody used in this study did not completely inhibit factor XII, and it is possible that more effective inhibition may have an impact on DIC and possibly survival.

Tucker et al. recently presented data indicating that factor XI has a significant role in the pathogenesis of DIC and the pathophysiology of sepsis in mice (114). In this study, the cecum was ligated and punctured, resulting in polymicrobial peritonitis and sepsis. Two to four days after injury, 87% of wild-type mice died and had clear evidence of DIC, with decreases in platelet counts and fibrinogen and increases in plasma thrombin-antithrombin (TAT) complexes 24 hours post injury compared with levels in animals subjected to sham surgery. Mortality was significantly reduced in factor XI–deficient mice (54%, $p = 0.0001$ compared with wild type), and length of survival among animals that ultimately died was greater, with most deaths occurring between days 3 and 6 ($p < 0.001$). Factor XI–deficient mice had smaller decreases in platelet count and smaller increases in TAT complexes, with an increase in fibrinogen compared to baseline, probably as a response to inflammation. An assessment of factor XII– and HK-null mice in this model will be critical for determining if the contribution of factor XI to sepsis is due to contact activation.

THERAPUETIC TARGETING OF CONTACT FACTORS

The data from primate and rodent studies have stimulated interest in developing inhibitors that target contact activation for treatment or prevention of thromboembolic disease, with an emphasis on inhibitors of factors XIa and XIIa. Nearly all of the published nonproprietary information on this topic concerns factor XIa inhibitors, and this will be discussed in the following section. The favored strategy is to design compounds that target the active sites of the proteases. Factor XIa, factor XIIa, and α-kallikrein are all trypsin-like enzymes that are members of the chymotrypsin family of serine proteases, and their catalytic domains have structural similarities. Factor XI and PK, which share 58% identity in amino acid sequence, are products of a gene duplication event involving a common ancestral gene. Inhibitors designed against the active sites of factor XIa or α-kallikrein, therefore, often have substantial activity against the other protease. While generation of compounds with long half-lives that can be taken orally is a long-term goal, the literature currently describes compounds administered by intravenous infusion.

Factor XIa Inhibitors

Structures are now available for the factor XIa catalytic domain in complex with the inhibitors benzamidine (115), ecotin (a pan-serine protease inhibitor from *E. coli*) (116), and the Kunitz protease domain of protease nexin-2 (117), facilitating design of small molecule inhibitors. Phenyl boronic acids and functionalized aryl boronic acids weakly inhibit serine proteases through formation of a tetrahedral boronate ester with the hyrodxyl group of the protease active site serine residue. Lazarova and colleagues reported on the synthesis and characterization of several factor XIa inhibitors based on aryl boronic acid (118). The most potent compounds had IC50s in the 1 to 10 μM range, with varying degrees of activity (10 to >100 μM) against other proteases such as factor Xa, thrombin, and trypsin.

Using peptidomimetic strategies, small tripeptide factor XIa inhibitors have been developed with IC50s for the target protease in the low nanomolar range. Lin et al. presented data on a promising compound (designated compound 32) with an IC50 of 6 nM for factor XIa, and comparable activity against α-kallikrein (10 nM) and trypsin (12 nM), but with considerably higher values for factor Xa (1.6 μM), thrombin (2.0 μM), and factor VIIa (38 μM) (119). This compound had a selective effect on the PTT assay in human plasma, with little effect on TF-triggered clotting through the extrinsic pathway. Compound 32 limited venous thrombus formation in rats with an efficacy comparable to a 50 unit/kg bolus of heparin. A related molecule, compound 37, demonstrated efficacy similar to that of heparin, without prolonging bleeding in a rat mesenteric artery bleeding time model. The same group prepared factor XIa inhibitors that are analogs of α-ketothiazole arginine (120) in an effort to develop agents that are smaller than the peptidic inhibitors described above (119). Some of these compounds have IC50s in the hundreds of nanomolar range, and may serve as scaffolds for further refinement. The specificity and in vivo activity of the α-ketothiazole arginine compounds have not been reported.

Schumacher and coworkers reported on the properties of a small molecule protease inhibitor (BMS-262084) with a β-lactam structure that covalently binds to the active site of serine proteases (121). The compound was originally identified as a tryptase inhibitor (122), and was subsequently found to interfere with plasma clotting in the PTT assay. In purified enzyme systems, BMS-262084 inhibits human factor XIa and human tryptase with IC50s of 2.8 and 5 nM, respectively, and also has activity against trypsin (IC50 50 nM). The IC50 for α-kallikrein is 200-fold greater than for factor XIa, and values for other coagulation (thrombin, factors IXa, Xa, XIIa, and factor VIIa/TF) and fibrinolytic (tPA, urokinase, plasmin) proteases are at least 170-fold greater. BMS-262084 is relatively less potent in plasma assays, but doubled the PTT in human plasma at a concentration of ~140 nM. TF-induced coagulation was unaffected at concentrations up to 100 μM. BMS-262084 is 15-times more potent in human plasma than in rat plasma, but still exhibited a selective effect on the PTT in rats. With a loading dose of 12 mg/kg, followed by a continuous infusion of 12 mg/kg/hr, the compound reduced thrombus weight by ~75% in a rat carotid artery thrombosis model, and showed even greater efficacy in a vena cava thrombosis model. Compared with vehicle, the drug did not increase bleeding in the cuticle, mesenteric artery, or renal bleeding models. In contrast, a dose of heparin with similar antithrombotic efficacy significantly increased bleeding.

Results with compounds such as BMS-262084 show the promise of small molecule active site inhibitors of factor XIa as therapeutic agents. However, enhanced specificity for factor XIa may also be achieved by targeting portions of the molecule remote from the active site that are required for activation of the protease or binding of natural macromolecular substrates. Antibodies to factor XI have been successfully used to create transient states of factor XI deficiency in primates (83) and rabbits (87,97), and have provided compelling evidence that therapeutic targeting of factor XI may be beneficial as an antithrombotic strategy. Recently, Tucker et al. presented data on the effects of a murine monoclonal antihuman factor XI antibody on thrombus formation in the baboon femoral arteriovenous shunt model described in the section on Models of Arterial

Thrombosis (123). Preliminary work with this antibody showed that it does not block cleavage of a small chromogenic substrate by factor XIa, indicating that the active site of the protease is not occupied in the presence of the antibody. A single intravenous infusion of the antibody (2 mg/kg) in baboons reduced the plasma factor XI activity level (as measured in a PTT assay) to <5% of normal for approximately one week. Compared with untreated animals, factor XI inhibition significantly reduced platelet and fibrin deposition (39–59% and 83–89%, respectively) in Gortex grafts coated with collagen (wall shear rate 265/sec) introduced into an AV shunt. Peak levels of TAT complex and β-thromboglobulin (a marker of platelet activation) in blood sampled immediately downstream from the growing thrombus were significantly lower in antibody-treated animals than in controls (38-fold and 7-fold, respectively). Consistent with intravital microscopy work in factor XI–deficient mice, thrombi that formed in antibody-treated baboons were unstable and fragmented. Narrower grafts (wall shear rate 2120/sec) consistently occluded in 30 minutes when introduced into the AV shunts of untreated animals, but did not occlude in antibody-treated animals.

This work demonstrates that targeting the factor XIa molecule at sites other than the active site is a viable strategy for developing a specific antithrombotic compound. Taken as a whole, the data in baboons also strongly indicate that factor XI contributes to thrombus stability under high shear through enhancement of thrombin generation, leading to fibrin formation and platelet activation. Interestingly, levels of the fibrin degradation product D-dimer in blood sampled immediately downstream from thrombi did not change appreciably in treated or untreated animals, indicating that the proposed role for factor XI as an inhibitor of fibrinolysis during hemostasis (12,29,30) may not be as important during arterial thrombus formation.

Factor XIIa and Prekallikrein Inhibitors

There is currently limited information in the public domain regarding inhibitors of factor XIIa and α-kallikrein. D-Pro-Phe-Arg-chormethyl ketone is a tripeptide-based inhibitor of trypsin-like serine proteases with particularly high activity against factor XIIa and α-kallikrein (101,124,125). The chloromethyl ketone group forms covalent bonds with the active site serine and histidine residues of the protease catalytic triad, resulting in irreversible inhibition. Kleinschnitz et al. tested D-Pro-Phe-Arg-chormethyl ketone in the transient MCA occlusion model described under Models of Cerebral Ischemia-reperfusion Injury, and found that this compound limited ischemia/reperfusion to a similar extent as congenital factor XII deficiency, without causing excessive bleeding (101). Patients with hereditary angioedema (HAE) experience acute life-threatening episodes of soft tissue swelling associated with an increase in bradykinin production (126). Three forms of HAE, designated types I, II, and III, have been described. The type III form is associated with factor XII mutations. D-Pro-Phe-Arg-chormethyl ketone completely blocked the enhanced factor XIIa activity in the plasma of patients with type III HAE caused by a factor XII Thr328Arg amino acid substitution (127). While the pathophysiologic mechanism of type III HAE is not completely understood, this observation suggests that factor XII inhibitors may be useful in preventing the consequences of vascular leak associated with HAE.

α-Kallikrein is thought to play an important role in formation of angioedema in patients with types I and II HAE associated with deficiency or dysfunction of the serpin C1-inhibitor, a regulator of contact-activation proteases (126). DX-88 is a Kunitz type inhibitor isolated from a phage display library that was developed as a specific inhibitor of α-kallikrein to treat patients with HAE (128). When administered prior to, or during transient MCA occlusion in mice, this compound markedly reduced cerebral ischemic volume, with less cerebral swelling and neurologic deficit (129). Delay in administration of DX-88 until 30 minutes after reperfusion or in animals with permanent occlusions of the MCA did not improve outcome. This study suggests that inhibition of α-kallikrein during the early phases of cerebral ischemia may reduce reperfusion injury and, given the results with factor XII and factor XI deficient mice in this model, raises the possibility of a role for α-kallikrein in a contact activation–like process in this setting. It should be recognized that while DX-88 is a potent and relatively specific inhibitor of α-kallikrein (apparent $K_i < 50$ pM), the apparent K_i for inhibition of factor XIa is ~100 nM (128), and the plasma drug levels attained in this study may have had a significant effect on factor XIa activity. It is possible, therefore, that the beneficial effects of the inhibitor in the ischemia-reperfusion model may have been due, at least in part, to inhibition of factor XIa.

CONCLUSIONS

The modest bleeding disorder associated with factor XI deficiency, and the absence of a bleeding diathesis in patients with factor XII, PK, or HK deficiency, have understandably contributed to a relative lack of enthusiasm in the past for the potential of these proteins as therapeutic targets for treating or preventing thrombotic disease. However, recent work in animal models has strengthened the concept that a protein's contribution to pathologic coagulation is not necessarily reflected in its contribution to hemostasis. This work, in combination with epidemiologic data from patient populations, has kindled an interest in developing therapeutic agents to target the proteases of the intrinsic pathway and contact activation. At this point it is not possible to definitively state which protease or proteases may be the best therapeutic targets, nor is it clear in which clinical situations such treatments will be most useful. An argument could be made that inhibition of a secondary pathway for sustaining thrombin generation may have limited application in the treatment of acute thrombotic events, such as deep venous thromboses, in which thrombin generation may be mediated primarily through factor VIIa/TF. However, the impressive effects of factor XII and factor XI deficiency/inhibition on the stability of platelet-rich thrombi suggest that targeting these proteases may be beneficial as prophylaxis in patients with a history of coronary artery disease, stroke, or atrial fibrillation, with the substantial added benefit of a relatively low risk of treatment-related bleeding complications. Furthermore, given the lack of severe bleeding associated with deficiencies of the contact factors, agents inhibiting these proteins may find a role in clinical situations where the bleeding risk of anticoagulation is particularly high, such as in DIC or acute stroke. Many outstanding questions will undoubtedly be addressed over the coming years as new compounds targeting the contact factors advance through preclinical and clinical trials.

ACKNOWLEDGMENTS

The authors are grateful to the National Heart, Lung, and Blood Institute; the American Heart Association; and the Deutsche Forschungsgmeinschaft for their generous support of this research.

REFERENCES

1. Cochrane CG, Griffin JH. The biochemistry and pathophysiology of the contact system of plasma. Adv Immunol 1982; 33:241–306.
2. Colman RW, Schmaier AH. Contact system: a vascular biology modulator with anticoagulant, profibrinolytic, antiadhesive, and proinflammatory attributes. Blood 1997; 90:3819–3843.

3. Schmaier AH, McCrae KR. The plasma kallikrein-kinin system: its evolution from contact activation. J Thromb Haemost 2007; 5:2323–2329.

4. Rosenthal R, Dreskin O, Rosenthal N. New hemophilia-like disease caused by deficiency of a third plasma thromboplastin factor. Proc Soc Exp Biol Med 1953; 82:171–174.

5. Ratnoff O, Colopy J. A familial hemorrhagic trait associated with a deficiency of a clot promoting fraction of plasma. J Clin Invest 1955; 34:602–613.

6. Wuepper K. Prekallikrein deficiency in man. J Exp Med 1973; 138:1345–1355.

7. Colman R, Bagdasarian A, Talamo R, et al. Williams trait: Human kininogen deficiency with diminished levels of plasminogen proactivator and prekallikrein associated with abnormalities of the Hageman factor-dependent pathways. J Clin Invest 1975; 56:1650–1662.

8. Macfarlane R. An enzyme cascade in the blood clotting mechanism, and its function as a biochemical amplifier. Nature 1964; 202:498–499.

9. Davie E, Ratnoff O. Waterfall sequence for intrinsic clotting. Science 1964; 145:1310–1313.

10. Lozier JN, Kessler CM. Clinical aspects and therapy of hemophilia. In: Hoffman R, Benz E, Shattil S, Furie B, Cohen H, Silberstein L, McGlave P eds. Hematology: Basic Principles and Practice, 4th ed. New York: Churchill Livingstone, 2005:2047.

11. Saito H. Contact factors in health and disease. Semin Thromb Hemost 1987; 13:36–49.

12. Gailani D, Broze GJ. Factor XI and the contact system. In Scriver CR, Beaudet AL, Sly WS, Valle D, Childs B, Kinzler KW, Vogelstein B eds. The Metabolic and Molecular Bases of Inherited Disease. 8th ed. New York: McGraw-Hill, 2001:4433.

13. Davie E, Fujikawa K, Kisiel W. The coagulation cascade: initiation, maintenance and regulation. Biochemistry 1991; 30:10363–70.

14. Osterud B, Rapaport SI. Activation of factor IX by the reaction product of tissue factor and factor VII: additional pathway for initiating blood coagulation. Proc Natl Acad Sci USA 1977; 74: 5260–5264.

15. Mackman N. Role of tissue factor in hemostasis, thrombosis, and vascular development. Arterioscler Thromb Vasc Biol 2004; 24:1015–1022.

16. Morrissey JH. Tissue factor: a key molecule in hemostatic and nonhemostatic systems. Int J Hematol 2004; 79:103–108.

17. Naito K, Fujikawa K. Activation of human blood coagulation factor XI independent of factor XII. Factor XI is activated by thrombin and factor XIa in the presence of negatively charged surfaces. J Biol Chem 1991; 266:7353–7358.

18. Gailani D, Broze GJ, Jr. Factor XI activation in a revised model of blood coagulation. Science 1991; 253:909–912.

19. Kozik A, Moore RB, Potempa J, et al. A novel mechanism for bradykinin production at inflammatory sites. Diverse effects of a mixture of neutrophil elastase and mast cell tryptase versus tissue and plasma kallikreins on native and oxidized kininogens. J Biol Chem 1998; 273: 33224–33229.

20. Joseph K, Tholanikunnel BG, Kaplan AP. Heat shock protein 90 catalyzes activation of the prekallikrein-kininogen complex in the absence of factor XII. Proc Natl Acad Sci USA 2002; 99: 896–900.

21. Shariat-Madar Z, Mahdi F, Schmaier AH. Recombinant prolylcarboxypeptidase activates plasma prekallikrein. Blood 2004; 103:4554–4561.

22. Broze G, Girard T, Novotny W. Regulation of coagulation by a multivalent Kunitz-type inhibitor. Biochemistry 1990; 29:7539–7546.

23. Robinson A, Kropatkin M, Aggeler P. Hageman factor (factor XII) deficiency in marine mammals. Science 1969: 166: 1420–1422.

24. Semba U, Shibuya Y, Okabe H, et al. Whale Hageman factor (factor XII): prevented production due to pseudogene conversion. Thromb Res 1998; 90:31–37.

25. Kessler CM, Mariani G. Clinical manifestations and therapy of the hemophilias. In Colman RW, Marder VJ, Clowes AW, George JN, Goldhaber SZ, eds. Hemostasis and Thrombosis: Basic Principles and Clinical Practice. 5th ed. Philadelphia: Lippincott, Williams & Wilkins, 2006:887.

26. Bolton-Maggs PH, Peretz H, Butler R, et al. A common ancestral mutation (C128X) occurring in 11 non-Jewish families from the UK with factor XI deficiency. J Thromb Haemost 2004; 2: 918–924.

27. Zivelin A, Bauduer F, Ducout L, et al. Factor XI deficiency in French Basques is caused predominantly by an ancestral Cys38Arg mutation in the factor XI gene. Blood 2002; 99: 2448–2454.

28. Peretz H, Mulai A, Usher S, et al. The two common mutations causing factor XI deficiency in Jews stem from distinct founders: one of ancient Middle Eastern origin and another of more recent European origin. Blood 1997; 90:2654–2659.

29. von dem Borne P, Meijers J, Bouma, BN. Feedback activation of factor XI by thrombin in plasma results in additional formation of thrombin that protects fibrin clots from fibrinolysis. Blood 1995; 86:3035–3042.

30. von dem Borne PA, Bajzar L, Meijers JC, et al. Thrombin-mediated activation of factor XI results in a thrombin-activatable fibrinolysis inhibitor-dependent inhibition of fibrinolysis. J Clin Invest 1997; 99:2323–2327.

31. Bajzar L, Moser J, Nesheim M. TAFI, or plasma carboxypeptidase B, couples the coagulation and fibrinolytic cascades through the thrombin-thrombomodulin complex. J Biol Chem 1996; 271: 16603–16608.

32. Bouma BN, Meijers JC. Role of blood coagulation factor XI in down regulation of fibrinolysis. Curr Opin Hematol 2000; 7:266–272.

33. Koster T, Blann AD, Breit E, et al. Role of clotting factor VIII in effect of von Willebrand factor on occurrence of deep-vein thrombosis. Lancet 1995; 345:152–155.

34. Van Hylckama Vlieg A, van der Linden IK, Bertina RM, et al. High levels of factor IX increase risk of venous thrombosis. Blood 2000; 95:3678–3682.

35. Meijers J, Tekelenburg W, Bouma B, et al. High levels of coagulation factor XI as a risk factor for venous thrombosis. N Engl J Med 2000; 342:696–701.

36. Martinelli I. von Willebrand factor and factor VIII as risk factors for arterial and venous thrombosis. Semin Hematol. 2005; 42:49–55.

37. Bezemer ID, Bare LA, Doggen CJ, et al. Gene variants associated with deep vein thrombosis. JAMA 2008; 299:1306–1314.

38. Girolami A, Scandellari R, Zanon E, et al. Non-catheter associated venous thrombosis in hemophilia A and B. A critical review of all reported cases. J Thromb Thrombolysis 2006; 21: 279–284.

39. Girolami A, Ruzzon E, Tezza F, et al. Arterial and venous thrombosis in rare congenital bleeding disorders: a critical review. Haemophilia 2006; 12:345–351.

40. Ratnoff OD. The George M. Kober lecture. The legacy of John Hageman: new dividends. Trans Assoc Am Phys 1985; 98:151–161.

41. Colman RW. Activation of plasminogen by human plasma kallikrein. Biochem Biophys Res Commun 1969; 35:273–279.

42. Mandle R, Kaplan AP. Hageman factor substrates. Human plasma prekallikrein: mechanisms of activation of Hageman factor and participation in Hageman factor-dependent fibrinolysis. J Biol Chem 1977; 252:6097–6104.

43. Goldsmith G, Saito H, Ratnoff OD. The activation of plasminogen by Hageman FXII (factor XII) and Hageman factor fragments. J Clin Invest 1978; 62:54–60.

44. Mandle RJ, Kaplan AP. Hageman factor-dependent fibrinolysis: generation of fbrininolytic activity by the interaction of human activated factor XI and plaminogen. Blood 1979; 54:850–862.

45. Kaplan AP. Intrinsic coagulation, thrombosis, and bleeding. Blood 1996; 87:2090.

46. Pedicord DL, Seiffert D, Blat Y. Feedback activation of factor XI by thrombin does not occur in plasma. Proc Natl Acad Sci USA 2007; 104:12855–12860.

47. Girolami A, Randi ML, Gavasso S, et al. The occasional venous thromboses seen in patients with severe (homozygous) FXII deficiency are probably due to associated risk factors: a study of prevalence in 21 patients and review of the literature. J Thromb Thrombolysis 2004; 17: 139–143.

48. Zeerleder S, Schloesser M, Redondo M, et al. Reevaluation of the incidence of thromboembolic complications in congenital factor XII deficiency—a study on 73 subjects from 14 Swiss families. Thromb Haemost 1999; 82:1240–1246.

49. Koster T, Rosendaal FR, Briet E, et al. John Hageman's factor and deep-vein thrombosis: Leiden thrombophilia Study. Br J Haematol 1994; 87:422–424.

50. Gallimore MJ, Harris SL, Jones DW, et al. Plasma levels of factor XII, prekallikrein and high molecular weight kininogen in normal blood donors and patients having suffered venous thrombosis. Thromb Res 2004; 114:91–96.

51. Bilora F, Zanon E, Petrobelli F, et al. Does hemophilia protect against atherosclerosis? A case-control study. Clin Appl Thromb Hemost 2006; 12:193–198.

52. Khallou-Laschet J, Caligiuri G, Tupin E, et al. Role of the intrinsic coagulation pathway in atherogenesis assessed in hemophilic apolipoprotein E knockout mice. Arterioscler Thromb Vasc Biol. 2005; 25:123–126.

53. Sramek A, Reiber JH, Gerrits WB, et al. Decreased coagulability has no clinically relevant effect on atherogenesis: observations in individuals with a hereditary bleeding tendency. Circulation 2001; 104:762–767.

54. Sramek A, Bucciarelli P, Federici AB, et al. Patients with type 3 severe von Willebrand disease are not protected against atherosclerosis: results from a multicenter study in 47 patients. Circulation 2004; 109:740–744.

55. Shpilberg O, Rabi I, Schiller K, et al. Patients with Glanzmann thrombasthenia lacking platelet glycoprotein alpha(IIb)beta(3) (GPIIb/IIIa) and alpha(v)beta(3) receptors are not protected from atherosclerosis. Circulation 2002; 105:1044–1048.

56. Rosendaal FR, Briet E, Stibbe J, et al. Haemophilia protects against ischaemic heart disease: a study of risk factors. Br J Haematol 1990; 75:525–530.

57. Triemstra M, Rosendaal FR, Smit C, et al. Mortality in patients with hemophilia. Changes in a Dutch population from 1986 to 1992 and 1973 to 1986. Ann Intern Med 1995; 123:823–827.

58. Girolami A, Randi ML, Ruzzon E, et al. Myocardial infraction, other arterial thrombosis and invasive coronary procedures in Haemophilia B: a critical evaluation of case reports. J Thromb Thrombolysis 2005; 20:43–46.

59. Girolami A, Ruzzon E, Fabris C, et al. Myocardial infarction and other arterial occlusions in hemophilia A patients. A cardiological evaluation of all 42 cases reported in the literature. Acta Haematol 2006; 116:120–125.

60. Doggen CJ, Rosendaal FR, Meijers JC. Levels of intrinsic coagulation factors and the risk of myocardial infarction among men: opposite and synergistic effects of factors XI and XII. Blood 2006; 108:4045–4051.

61. Yang DT, Flanders MM, Kim H, et al. Elevated factor XI activity levels are associated with an increased odds ratio for cerebrovascular events. Am J Clin Pathol 2006; 126:411–415.

62. Santamaría A, Oliver A, Borrell M, et al. Higher risk of ischaemic stroke associated with factor XI levels in dyslipidaemic patients. Int J Clin Pract 2007; 61:1819–1823.

63. Butenas S, Undas A, Gissel MT, et al. Factor XIa and tissue factor activity in patients with coronary artery disease. Thromb Haemost 2008; 99:142–149.

64. Salomon O, Steinberg D, Dardik R, et al. Inherited factor XI deficiency confers no protection against acute myocardial infarction. J Thromb Haemost 2003; 1:658–661.

65. Salomon O, Steinberg DM, Koren-Morag N, et al. Reduced incidence of ischemic stroke in patients with severe factor XI deficiency. Blood 2008; 111:4113–4117.

66. Endler G, Marsik C, Jilma B, et al. Evidence of a U-shaped association between FXII activity and overall survival. J Thromb Haemost 2007; 5:1143–1148.

67. Kanaji T. Lower factor XII activity is a risk marker rather than a risk factor for cardiovascular disease: a rebuttal. J Thromb Haemost; 2008; 6:1053–1054.

68. Zito F, Drummond F, Bujac SR, et al. Epidemiological and genetic associations of activated factor XII concentration with factor VII activity, fibrinopeptide A concentration, and risk of coronary heart disease in men. Circulation 2000; 102:2058–2062.

69. Grundt H, Nilsen DW, Hetland O, et al. Activated factor 12 (FXIIa) predicts recurrent coronary events after an acute myocardial infarction. Am Heart J 2004; 147:260–266.

70. Govers-Riemslag JW, Smid M, Cooper JA, The plasma kallikrein-kinin system and risk of cardiovascular disease in men. J Thromb Haemost 2007; 5:1896–1903.
71. Jones DW, Gallimore MJ, MacKie IJ, et al. Reduced factor XII levels in patients with the antiphospholipid syndrome are associated with antibodies to factor XII. Br J Haematol 2000; 110: 721–726.
72. Jones DW, Nichols PJ, Donohoe S, et al. Antibodies to factor XII are distinct from antibodies to prothrombin in patients with the anti-phospholipid syndrome. Thromb Haemost 2002; 87: 426–430.
73. Merlo C, Wuillemin WA, Redondo M, et al. Elevated levels of plasma prekallikrein, high molecular weight kininogen and factor XI in coronary heart disease. Atherosclerosis 2002; 161:261–267.
74. Gailani D, Lasky NM, Broze GJ, Jr. murine model of factor XI deficiency. Blood Coagul Fibrinolysis 1997; 8:134–144.
75. Pauer HU, Renne T, Hemmerlein B, et al. Targeted deletion of murine coagulation factor XII gene-a model for contact phase activation in vivo. Thromb Haemost 2004; 92:503–508.
76. Merkulov S, Zhang WM, Komar AA, et al. Deletion of murine kininogen gene 1 (mKng1) causes loss of plasma kininogen and delays thrombosis. Blood 2008; 111:1274–1281.
77. Lin HF, Maeda N, Smithies O, et al. A coagulation factor IX-deficient mouse model for human hemophilia B. Blood. 1997; 90:3962–3966.
78. Wang X, Cheng Q, Xu L, et al. Effects of factor IX or factor XI deficiency on ferric chloride-induced carotid artery occlusion in mice. J Thromb Haemost 2005; 3:695–702.
79. Bi L, Sarkar R, Naas T, et al. Further characterization of factor VIII-deficient mice created by gene targeting: RNA and protein studies. Blood 1996; 88:3446–3450.
80. Muchitsch EM, Turecek PL, Zimmermann K, et al. Phenotypic expression of murine hemophilia. Thromb Haemost 1999; 82:1371–1373.
81. Asakai R, Chung DW, Davie EW, et al. Factor XI deficiency in Ashkenazi Jews in Israel. N Engl J Med 1991; 325:153–158.
82. Oh-ishi S, Hayashi I, Satoh K, et al. Prolonged activated partial thromboplastin time and deficiency of high molecular weight kininogen in brown Norway rat mutant (Katholiek strain). Thromb Res 1984; 33:371–377.
83. Gruber A, Hanson SR. Factor XI-dependence of surface- and tissue factor-initiated thrombus propagation in primates. Blood 2003; 102:953–955.
84. Westrick RJ, Winn ME, Eitzman DT. Murine models of vascular thrombosis (Eitzman series). Arterioscler Thromb Vasc Biol 2007; 27:2079–2093.
85. Furie B, Furie BC. Thrombus formation in vivo. J Clin Invest 2005; 115:3355–3362.
86. Baird TR, Gailani D, Furie B, et al. Factor XI deficient mice have reduced platelet accumulation and fibrin deposition after laser injury. Blood 2004; 104:66a.
87. Yamashita A, Nishihira K, Kitazawa T, et al. Factor XI contributes to thrombus propagation on injured neointima of the rabbit iliac artery. J Thromb Haemost 2006; 4:1496–1501.
88. Renne T, Pozgajova M, Gruner S, et al. Defective thrombus formation in mice lacking coagulation factor XII. J Exp Med 2005; 202:271–281.
89. Falati S, Patil S, Gross PL, et al. Platelet PECAM-1 inhibits thrombus formation in vivo. Blood 2006; 107:535–441.
90. Johne J, Blume C, Benz PM, et al. Platelets promote coagulation factor XII-mediated proteolytic cascade systems in plasma. Biol Chem 2006; 387:173–178.
91. Kannemeier C, Shibamiya A, Nakazawa F, et al. Extracellular RNA constitutes a natural procoagulant cofactor in blood coagulation. Proc Natl Acad Sci USA 2007; 104:6388–6393.
92. Kleinschnitz C, Braeuninger S, Pham M, et al. Blocking of platelets or intrinsic coagulation pathway-driven thrombosis does not prevent cerebral infarctions induced by photothrombosis. Stroke 2008; 39:1262–1268.
93. Shariat-Madar Z, Mahdi F, Warnock M, et al. Bradykinin B2 receptor knockout mice are protected from thrombosis by increased nitric oxide and prostacyclin. Blood 2006; 108:192–199.
94. Hassan S, Sainz IM, Khan MM, et al. Antithrombotic activity of kininogen is mediated by inhibitory effects of domain 3 during arterial injury in vivo. Am J Physiol Heart Circ Physiol 2007; 292:2959–2965.

95. Pawlinski R, Pedersen B, Erlich J, et al. Role of tissue factor in haemostasis, thrombosis, angiogenesis and inflammation: lessons from low tissue factor mice. Thromb Haemost 2004; 92: 444–450.

96. Day SM, Reeve JL, Pedersen B, et al. Macrovascular thrombosis is driven by tissue factor derived primarily from the blood vessel wall. Blood 2005; 105:192–198.

97. Minnema MC, Friederich PW, Levi M, et al. Enhancement of rabbit jugular vein thrombolysis by neutralization of factor XI. In vivo evidence for a role of factor XI as an anti-fibrinolytic factor. J Clin Invest 1998; 101:10–14.

98. Feuerstein GZ, Toomey JR, Valocik R, et al. An inhibitory anti-factor IX antibody effectively reduces thrombus formation in a rat model of venous thrombosis. Thromb Haemost 1999; 82: 1443–1445.

99. Wang X, Smith PL, Hsu MY, et al. Effects of factor XI deficiency on ferric chloride-induced vena cava thrombosis in mice. J Thromb Haemost 2006; 4:1982–1988.

100. Choudhri TF, Hoh BL, Prestigiacomo CJ, et al. Targeted inhibition of intrinsic coagulation limits cerebral injury in stroke without increasing intracerebral hemorrhage. J Exp Med 1999; 190: 91–99.

101. Kleinschnitz C, Stoll G, Bendszus M, et al. Targeting coagulation factor XII provides protection from pathological thrombosis in cerebral ischemia without interfering with hemostasis. J Exp Med 2006; 203:513–518.

102. Groger M, Lebesgue D, Pruneau D, et al. Release of bradykinin and expression of kinin B2 receptors in the brain: role for cell death and brain edema formation after focal cerebral ischemia in mice. J Cereb Blood Flow Metab 2005; 25:978–989.

103. Xia CF, Smith RS Jr., Shen B, et al. Postischemic brain injury is exacerbated in mice lacking the kinin B2 receptor. Hypertension 2006; 47:752–761.

104. Kleinschnitz C, Austinat M, Bader M, et al. Deficiency of bradykinin receptor B2 is not detrimental in experimental stroke. Hypertension 2008; 51:e41.

105. Renné T, Schuh K, Muller-Esterl W. Local bradykinin formation is controlled by glycosaminoglycans. J Immunol 2005; 175:3377–3385.

106. Radcliffe R, Bagdasarian A, Colman R, et al. Activation of bovine factor VII by hageman factor fragments. Blood 1977; 50:611–617.

107. Ghebrehiwet B, Randazzo BP, Dunn JT, et al. Mechanisms of activation of the classical pathway of complement by Hageman factor fragment. J Clin Invest 1983; 71:1450–1456.

108. Ichinose A, Fujikawa K, Suyama T. The activation of pro-urokinase by plasma kallikrein and its inactivation by thrombin. J Biol Chem 1986; 261:3486–3489.

109. Nuijens JH, Huijbregts CC, Eerenberg-Belmer AJ, et al. Quantification of plasma factor XIIa-Cl-inhibitor and kallikrein-Cl-inhibitor complexes in sepsis. Blood 1988; 72:1841–1848.

110. Wuillemin WA, Fijnvandraat K, Derkx BH, et al. Activation of the intrinsic pathway of coagulation in children with meningococcal septic shock. Thromb Haemost 1995; 74:1436–1441.

111. Pixley RA, DeLa Cadena RA, Page JD, et al. Activation of the contact system in lethal hypotensive bacteremia in a baboon model. Am J Pathol 1992; 140:897–906.

112. Pixley RA, De La Cadena R, Page JD, et al. The contact system contributes to hypotension but not disseminated intravascular coagulation in lethal bacteremia. In vivo use of a monoclonal anti-factor XII antibody to block contact activation in baboons. J Clin Invest 1993; 91:61–68.

113. Jansen PM, Pixley RA, Brouwer M, et al. Inhibition of factor XII in septic baboons attenuates the activation of complement and fibrinolytic systems and reduces the release of interleukin-6 and neutrophil elastase. Blood 1996; 87:2337–2344.

114. Tucker EI, Gailani D, Hurst S, et al. Survival advantage of coagulation factor XI deficient mice in peritoneal sepsis. J Infect Dis 2008; 198:271–274.

115. Jin L, Pandey P, Babine RE, et al. Mutation of surface residues to promote crystallization of activated factor XI as a complex with benzamidine: an essential step for the iterative structure-based design of factor XI inhibitors. Acta Crystallogr D Biol Crystallogr 2005; 61: 1418–1425

116. Jin L, Pandey P, Babine RE, et al. Crystal structures of the FXIa catalytic domain in complex with ecotin mutants reveal substrate-like interactions. J Biol Chem 2005; 280:4704–4712.

117. Navaneetham D, Jin L, Pandey P, et al. Structural and mutational analyses of the molecular interactions between the catalytic domain of factor XIa and the Kunitz protease inhibitor domain of protease nexin 2. J Biol Chem 2005; 280:36165–36175.
118. Lazarova TI, Jin L, Rynkiewicz M, et al. Synthesis and in vitro biological evaluation of aryl boronic acids as potential inhibitors of factor XIa. Bioorg Med Chem Lett 2006; 16:5022–5027.
119. Lin J, Deng H, Jin L, et al. Design, synthesis, and biological evaluation of peptidomimetic inhibitors of factor XIa as novel anticoagulants. J Med Chem 2006; 49:7781–7791.
120. Deng H, Bannister TD, Jin L, et al. Synthesis, SAR exploration, and X-ray crystal structures of factor XIa inhibitors containing an alpha-ketothiazole arginine. Bioorg Med Chem Lett. 2006; 16: 3049–3054.
121. Schumacher WA, Seiler SE, Steinbacher TE, et al. Antithrombotic and hemostatic effects of a small molecule factor XIa inhibitor in rats. Eur J Pharmacol 2007; 570:167–174.
122. Sutton JC, Bolton SA, Hartl KS, et al. Synthesis and SAR of 4-carboxy-2-azetidinone mechanism-based tryptase inhibitors. Bioorg Med Chem Lett 2002; 12:3229–3233.
123. Tucker EI, Marzec UM, White TC, et al. Prevention of vascular graft occlusion and thrombus-associated thrombin generation by inhibition of factor XI. Blood (in press). PMID: 18945968.
124. Kettner C, Shaw E. Inactivation of trypsin-like enzymes with peptides of arginine chloromethyl ketone. Methods Enzymol 1981; 80:826–842.
125. Tans G, Janssen-Claessen T, Rosing J, et al. Studies on the effect of serine protease inhibitors on activated contact factors. Application in amidolytic assays for factor XIIa, plasma kallikrein and factor XIa. Eur J Biochem 1987; 164:637–642.
126. David AE. Hereditary angioedema: A current state-of-the-art revivew, III: mechanisms of hereditary angioedema. Ann Allergy Asthma Immunol 2008; 100(1 suppl 2):S7–S12.
127. Cichon S, Martin L, Hennies HC, et al. Increased activity of coagulation factor XII (Hageman factor) causes hereditary angioedema type III. Am J Hum Genet 2006; 79:1098–1104.
128. Williams A, Baird LG. DX-88 and HAE: A developmental perspective. Transfus Apher Sci 2003; 29:255–258.
129. Storini C, Bergamaschini L, Gesuete R, et al. Selective inhibition of plasma kallikrein protects brain from reperfusion injury. J Pharmacol Exp Ther 2006; 318:849–854.

23
Overview of Antiplatelet Therapy

Shaker A. Mousa
*The Pharmaceutical Research Institute, Albany College of Pharmacy/Medicine,
Albany, New York, U.S.A.*

James T. Willerson
*Health Science Center at Houston, The University at Texas, Cullen Cardiovascular
Research Laboratories at Texas Heart Institute, Baylor College of Medicine, and
The University of Texas M.D. Anderson Cancer Center, Houston, Texas, U.S.A.*

Robert P. Giugliano
*Cardiovascular Division, Brigham and Women's Hospital, Harvard Medical
School, Boston, Massachusetts, U.S.A.*

BACKGROUND

Platelets play a key role in arterial thrombosis (Fig. 1), where platelet activation and aggregation are the proximate events associated with acute coronary syndromes (ACS), stroke, and peripheral artery disease (PAD) (1–7). Platelet adhesion to injured vascular endothelium leads to platelet activation, which is further amplified by various platelet agonists, including arachidonic acid, thromboxane A_2, adenosine disphosphate (ADP), thrombin, serotonin, and collagen (6–8). Aspirin was the first antiplatelet drug to provide insight into the role of platelets in health and disease (7,9). Since its development in 1899 and subsequent elucidation of mechanism of action, thromboxane A_2 blockade has been one of the most well-known antiplatelet paradigms (9). Aspirin inhibits the formation of thromboxane by irreversibly inhibiting COX-1 via acetylation of the serine-529 peptide, the requisite site for the formation of thromboxane from arachidonic acid. It was not until the late 1970s that aspirin was widely recognized for its therapeutic benefit in cardiovascular disease (3,10). Aspirin is known to reduce the risk of myocardial infarction (MI), lower the risk of developing ischemic stroke, and decrease mortality in patients with vascular disease (11). Aspirin is presently recommended for the management of acute MI and unstable angina and is an effective therapeutic agent for secondary prevention of ischemic events (Fig. 2) (12,13).

Following the discovery of the clinical utility of aspirin in the treatment of cardiovascular disease, a number of other antiplatelet agents were developed and tested (Table 1). The first ADP-receptor antagonist, ticlopidine (14), demonstrated antithrombotic

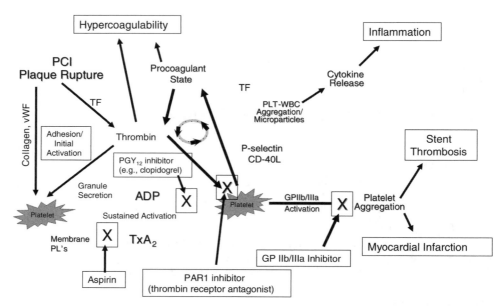

Figure 1 Central role of platelets in the genesis of thrombus formation. During either de novo plaque rupture or with intracoronary balloon inflation during percutaneous coronary intervention (PCI), platelets may be activated via release of tissue factor and formation of thrombin (which can be blocked by thrombin receptor antagonists) or, more directly, via collagen and von-willebrand factor. Platelets then secrete a variety of substances that potentiate thrombus formation, including thromboxane A_2 (TxA2) inhibited by aspirin and granules that act via ADP (inhibited by thienopyridienes) to activate other platelets. Activated platelets then promote: (*i*) a procoagulant state in their interaction with leukocytes and the clotting cascade, (*ii*) a proinflammatory state via release of P-selectin, CD-40 ligand, and other inflammatory mediators, and (*iii*) platelet-rich thrombosis via fibrinogen binding of platelet GP IIb/IIIa receptors resulting in platelet aggregation. *Source*: From Ref. 1.

benefits but was occasionally associated with the development of neutropenia, aplastic anemia, and thrombotic thrombocytopenic purpura (15). With the discovery of the second thienopyridine ADP-receptor antagonist, clopidogrel, antiplatelet therapy via alteration of this platelet functional pathway held promise with efficacy comparable to ticlopidine, but with a better safety profile (16,17). Clopidogrel was shown to be associated with a lower incidence of neutropenia and thrombotic thrombocytopenic purpura (18). With the development of various antiplatelet therapies, consideration was given to the therapeutic strategy of combining different antiplatelet agents (19,20). One of the earliest examples of the clinical success of such dual antiplatelet therapy was Aggrenox®, a combination of a low-dose aspirin with dipyridamole for stroke prevention (21). Combination of aspirin and clopidogrel have also been shown to be useful in treating and preventing vascular events (see below).

A more recent target of antiplatelet therapy relates to fibrinogen displacement in existing thrombi to prevent further platelet cross-linking and thrombosis via the platelet glycoprotein (GP) IIb/IIIa complex (22–25). Abciximab, tirofiban, and eptifibatide are examples of GPIIb/IIIa receptor inhibitors that have demonstrated clinical benefits in various trials (26–31) and have been incorporated into current American College of Cardiology/American Heart Association (ACC/AHA) treatment guidelines for unstable angina/non-ST elevation MI (32). Unfortunately, phase III clinical trial evaluation of oral

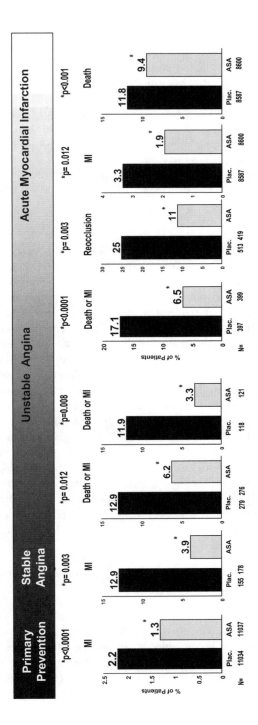

Figure 2 Aspirin across the spectrum of CAD. Aspirin has been demonstrated to substantially reduce the risk of death or myocardial infarction in a wide variety of patients with CAD, ranging from patients with stable angina through acute ST-segment elevation myocardial infarction. *Abbreviation*: CAD, coronary artery disease. *Source*: From Ref. 12.

Table 1 Classification of Selected Antiplatelet Agents and Common Indications

Class/drug	Most common clinical indications
Cyclooxygenase (COX) inhibitors	
Aspirin	Chronic and acute coronary, cerebral, and peripheral vascular disease
Triflusal	Secondary prevention of vascular events
Phosphodiesterase inhibitors	
Dipyridamole	Stroke prevention, prosthetic cardiac valves
Pentoxifylline	Peripheral vascular disease
Cilostazol	Peripheral vascular disease, intracoronary stenting
Thienopyridienes	
Ticlopidine	Stroke prevention, intracoronary stenting
Clopidogrel	Acute and chronic coronary artery disease, intracoronary stenting, chronic atherosclerosis
Intravenous glycoprotein IIb/IIIa antagonists	
Abciximab	Percutaneous coronary intervention
Eptifibatide	Acute coronary syndromes, percutaneous coronary intervention
Tirofiban	Acute coronary syndromes

GP IIb/IIIa inhibitors was halted after several studies showed no benefit or increased mortality coupled with higher rates of bleeding (33).

In several different clinical populations, the combination of dual antiplatelet therapy has been tested to achieve optimal efficacy with minimal adverse affects. Aspirin has been combined with the thienopyridine, clopidogrel, in different doses and at different durations to assess its effectiveness compared with aspirin alone (34). Improved efficacy has not always been the case and, in some cases, dual antiplatelet therapy carries a significant hemorrhagic risk (35). When combining clopidogrel with aspirin, there are several factors that must be carefully weighed against the benefits. Each agent should individually demonstrate a significant benefit, and the combination should have greater benefit/risk ratio as compared to each one alone. When combining the agents at different doses, one should be able to demonstrate improved efficacy without a compromise of safety. During a hospitalization, use of triple antiplatelet therapy (aspiring, clopidogrel, and intravenous GP IIb/IIIa inhibitor) may be indicated in patients at highest risk, who undergo an early invasive approach, although current treatment guidelines note that the body of evidence supporting such "triple" therapy is not as extensive and, hence, consider this a class IIa recommendation with level of evidence B (32). Furthermore, any incremental benefit must be counterbalanced by an increase risk in bleeding complications, as antiplatelet agents are combined.

MEDICAL NEED

Antiplatelet agents represent a key class of drugs that are of proven value in arterial thromboembolic disorders (36,37). There is a need for effective and safe antiplatelet agents, or their combinations, to provide predictable therapeutic benefit, dosage flexibility, and unique pharmacologic profiles, such as rapid onset in acute thrombotic states as well as sustained antiplatelet effect in chronic platelet-activating states (e.g., poststent placement). Aspirin, clopidogrel, or their combination has demonstrated improved clinical outcomes in certain unique settings, and the search for additional antiplatelet agents is ongoing. Current studies suggest that, combination antiplatelet therapy with existing agents is best considered a use-adapted strategy, with the greatest clinical benefit of combination therapy realized in acute, platelet-activating, and prothrombotic states (38,39).

The agents discussed in this chapter are not without shortcomings, and their limitations are a backdrop to the studies discussed. Aspirin resistance, a phenomenon described clinically as a lack of desired response while the patient is receiving aspirin, may affect $\geq 20\%$ of the population. On the basis of genetic polymorphism, noncompliance, or concomitant administration of a competing medication (NSAID), aspirin resistance remains an uncontrolled variable without a laboratory definition (40,41).

Clopidogrel, a prodrug, suffers from a delayed onset, a limitation that can be partially overcome by dose loading, a strategy used in some of the discussed studies. Other thienopyridines, such as prasugrel, which do not exhibit this limitation, are just now completing phase III clinical studies (42). There is also evidence that the dose benefit of clopidogrel co-therapy may also be disease related; as in the case of type 2 diabetes, in which 60% of the patients demonstrated platelet reactivity after receiving twice the standard maintenance dose of typical clopidogrel therapy (43). In the case of aspirin, clopidogrel noncompliance is also a serious clinical-confounding element, and in the presence of drug-eluting stents, is strongly associated with subsequent mortality. Regardless of the development of antiplatelet agents, full clinical benefit can only be realized by parallel strategies in patient education to ensure medication compliance (44).

CURRENT RESEARCH GOALS

The bar has already been raised for therapeutic regimens employing aspirin, clopidogrel, and their combination. Antiplatelet therapies with enhanced efficacy and parallel safety profiles are desired, but such goals may be mutually exclusive and difficult to attain (Table 2). Such was the case in the recent TRITON-TIMI-38 (Trial to Assess Improvement in Therapeutic Outcomes by Optimizing platelet Inhibition with Prasugrel Thrombolysis in Myocardial Infarction 38) study (42), in which enhanced antiplatelet therapy with a rapidly acting, potent thienopyridine, prasugrel, while associated with a significant reduction in ischemic events compared to clopidogrel, was accompanied by a

Table 2 Promising New Antiplatelet Therapies in Development

Class/drug	Current agents	Potential advantages over current agent
PGY$_{12}$ inhibitors	Clopidogrel, ticlopidine	
Prasugrel		Faster onset, greater antiplatelet effect, less variable response
AZD6140		Reversible, faster onset and offset, greater antiplatelet effect
Cangrelor (IV)		Reversible, shorter half-life, faster onset, greater antiplatelet effect, less variable response
PAR-1 (thrombin receptor antagonist)		
SCH 530348	None	Greater antiplatelet effect, less variable response, lower risk of bleeding

significant risk of fatal and life-threatening bleeding. Newer antiplatelet agents that target a different mechanism are also being developed and studied in addition to aspirin and clopidogrel (45). The major challenges faced by these newer agents include not only the difficulty in proving incremental meaningful clinical benefit but also doing so at a minimum of increase bleeding risk and on a background of contemporary therapies, which themselves continue to evolve.

SCIENTIFIC RATIONALE

The search for ADP-receptor antagonists, with rapid-onset and short half-lives or those that are reversible, would allow for urgent surgical procedures to overcome the limitations of clopidogrel. Furthermore, antiplatelet agents that work via collagen receptors, serotonin receptors, or thrombin receptors may have additional value and the ability to complement current antiplatelet therapy. However, the prohibitive cost of clinical trials demonstrating significant differences to current antiplatelet therapies might limit the development of new antiplatelet targets.

COMPETITIVE ENVIRONMENT AND POTENTIAL DEVELOPMENT ISSUES

A significant impediment to the development and clinical application of antiplatelet therapies is the prohibitive cost of the clinical trials and the potential risk involved in attaining clinical superiority and safety over existing regimens. The recruitment and study of a large number of patients for a prolonged period of time may be necessary to demonstrate a modest clinical benefit, as was the case in the CAPRIE (Clopidogrel vs. Aspirin in Patients at Risk of Ischemic Events) study, which employed 19,185 patients and demonstrated an 8.7% relative-risk reduction ($p = 0.043$) in comparison with the control group over three years (39).

SUMMARY AND CONCLUSIONS

Platelets are the principal effectors of cellular hemostasis and key mediators in the pathogenesis of thrombosis. A variety of membrane receptors determine platelet reactivity with numerous agonists and adhesive proteins, and, therefore, represent key targets for the development of antiplatelet drug therapies. In this regard, several rapid-onset and rapid-offset reversible ADP antagonists are in clinical development, including reversible oral (46) and rapid-acting intravenous (47), $P2Y_{12}$ receptor antagonists. Novel inhibitors of platelet adhesion in early development are targeting von-willebrand factor (VWF)-GPIb/IX and collagen-GPVI interaction. Since platelet aggregation also plays such a critical role in the pathogenesis of arterial thrombosis, more potent agents that interfere with platelet aggregation via other pathways (e.g., mediated via the thrombin receptor) are also under clinical investigations (45).

However, the major limitation to treatment with multiple antiplatelet agents is the increased bleeding risk associated with the enhanced antiplatelet effect, as is exemplified by the clinical conundrum in patients with ACS who may need to undergo CABG surgery. Aspirin and clopidogrel irreversibly inhibit platelet function, with the maximal antiplatelet effect occurring after three to five days. The increased risk of procedural bleeding arising from dual aspirin and clopidogrel administration immediately prior to

CABG surgery raises the question of whether clopidogrel should be routinely given to patients presenting with ACS. In light of the current recommendation to discontinue clopidogrel at least five days prior to elective CABG surgery, the emergency physician is likely to avoid clopidogrel in case the patient may require urgent cardiac surgery. Delaying clopidogrel therapy until coronary revascularization has been performed would, however, deprive patients of the early clinical benefits of the drug. These limitations might be solved with the availability of a rapid-onset and rapid-offset ADP antagonists.

One issue that deserves further discussion is the duration of therapy. There is conflicting evidence between the MATCH (48) and CARESS (49) trials as to the optimal duration of antiplatelet therapy in cerebrovascular disease. For coronary artery disease, the CHARISMA (50) trial failed to show benefit of long-term clopidogrel in the overall trial population, although the 80% of patients with clinical evident atherothrombosis experienced a modest reduction (12% RRR, $p = 0.046$) of the primary endpoint, and emerging data with drug-eluting stents suggest that dual antiplatelet therapy may be required even beyond one year (51). Clearly, additional studies are necessary to evaluate optimal antiplatelet therapy combinations and duration of therapies to permit maximal benefit with the minimum of harm in our patients with cardiovascular disease. The following chapters provide detailed information on the clinically most useful antiplatelet agents as well as several classes of novel antiplatelet drugs in development.

ABBREVIATIONS

ACS, acute coronary syndrome; CABG, coronary artery bypass grafting; CARESS, Clopidogrel and Aspirin for Reduction of Emboli in Symptomatic carotid Stenosis; CHARISMA, Clopidogrel for High Artherothrombotic Risk and Ischemic Stabilization, Management, and Avoidance; CLARITY-TIMI, Clopidogrel as Adjunctive Reperfusion Therapy-Thrombolysis in Myocardial Infarction; COMMIT, Clopidogrel and Metoprolol in Myocardial Infarction Trial; CURE, Clopidogrel in Unstable angina to prevent Recurrent Events; MATCH, Management of Atherothrombosis with Clopidogrel in High-Risk Patients with Recent Transient Ischemic Attack or stroke; MI, myocardial infarction; PCI, percutaneous coronary intervention; TIA, transient ischemic attack.

REFERENCES

1. Gubrel PA, Tantry US. The relationship of platelet reactivity to the occurance of post-stenting ischemic events: emergence of a new cardiovascular risk factor. Rev Cardiovasc Med 2006; 7 (suppl 4):520–528.
2. Jamieson DG, Parekh A, Exekowitz MD. Review of antiplatelet therapy in secondary prevention of cerebrovascular events: a need for direct comparison between antiplatelet agents. J Cardiovasc Pharmacol Ther 2005; 10:153–161.
3. Antiplatelet Trialist' Collaboration. Collaborative overview of randomized trials of antiplatelet therapy-I: prevention of death, myocardial infarction, and stroke by prolonged antiplatelet therapy in various categories of patients. Br Med J 1994; 308:81–106.
4. Fitzgerald DJ, Roy L, Catella F, et al. Platelet activation in unstable coronary disease. N Engl J Med 1986; 315:983–989.
5. Fuster V, Steele PM, Chesebro JH. Role of platelets and thrombosis in coronary atherosclerotic disease and sudden death. J Am Coll Cardiol 1985; 5:175B–184B.
6. Hamm CW, Bliefield W, Kupper W, et al. Biochemical evidence of platelet activation in patients with persistent unstable angina. J Am Coll Cardiol 1987; 10:998–1004.

7. Mousa SA, Bennett JS. Platelets in health and disease: platelet GPIIb/IIIa structure and function: recent advances in antiplatelet therapy. Drugs Future 1996; 21:1141–1154.

8. Mousa SA, Giugliano R. Antiplatelet therapies: platelet GPIIb/IIIa antagonists and beyond. In: Sasahara AA, ed. New Therapeutic Agents in Thrombosis. New York: Marcel Dekker, 2003: 341–347.

9. Born GV, Gorog P, Begent NA. The biologic background to some therapeutic uses of aspirin. Am J Med 1983; 74:2–9.

10. Mousa SA. Antiplatelet therapies: platelet GPIIb/IIIa antagonists and beyond. Curr Pharm Design 2003; 9:2317–2322.

11. Hart RH. Aspirin wars: the optimal dose of aspirin to prevent stroke. Stroke 1996; 27:585–587.

12. Cannon CP, Fuster V. Thrombogenesis, antithrombotic, and thrombolytic therapy. In: Fuster V, Alexander RW, O'Rourke R, eds. The Heart. 10th ed. New York: McGraw Hill, 2001.

13. Hennekens CH, Sechenova O. Dose of aspirin in the treatment and prevention of cardiovascular disease: current and future directions. J Cardiovasc Pharmacol Ther 2006; 11:170–176.

14. Haynes RB, Sandler RS, Larson EB, et al. A critical appraisal of ticlopidine, a new antiplatelet agent: effectiveness and clinical indications for prophylaxis of atherosclerotic events. Arch Intern Med 1992; 152:1376–1380.

15. Love BB, Biller J, Gent M. Adverse hematological effects of ticlopidine: prevention, recognition, and management. Drug Saf Int J Med Toxicol Drug Exp 1998; 9:89–98.

16. Creager MA. Results of the CAPRIE trial: efficacy and safety of clopidogrel. Clopidogrel versus aspirin in patients at risk of ischemic events. Vasc Med 1998; 3:257–260.

17. Moussa I, Oetgen M, Roubin G, et al. Effectiveness of clopidogrel and aspirin versus ticlopidine and aspirin in preventing stent thrombosis after coronary-stent implantation. Circulation 1999; 99:2364–2366.

18. Hankey GJ, Sudlow CL, Dunbabin DW. Thienopyridine derivatives (ticlopidine, clopidogrel) versus aspirin for preventing stroke and other serious vascular events in high vascular risk patients. Cochrane Database Syst Rev 2000; 2:CD001246.

19. Bednar MM, Quilley J, Russell SR, et al. The effect of oral antiplatelet agents on tissue plasminogen activator-mediated thrombolysis in a rabbit model of thromboembolic stroke. Neurosurgery 1996; 39:352–359.

20. Nicolau DP, Tessier PR, Nightingale CH. Beneficial effect of combination antiplatelet therapy on the development of experimental *Staphylococcus aureus* endocarditis. Int J Antimicrob Agents 1999; 11:159–161.

21. Lenz TL, Hilleman DE. Aggrenox: a fixed-dose combination of aspirin and dipyridamole. Ann Pharmacother 2000; 34:1283–1290.

22. Mousa SA. Antiplatelet therapies: recent advances in the development of platelet glycoprotein IIb/IIIa antagonists. Curr Interv Cardiol Rep 1999; 1:243–252.

23. Mousa SA. Antiplatelet therapies: from aspirin to GPIIb/IIIa-receptor antagonists and beyond. Drug Discov Today 1999; 4:552–561.

24. Pytela R, Pierschbacher MS, Ginsberg MH, et al. Platelet membrane glycoprotein IIb/IIIa: member of a family of RGD specific adhesion receptors. Science 1986; 231:1559–1562.

25. Philips DR, Charo IF, Scarborough RM. GPIIb/IIIa: the responsive integrin. Cell 1991; 65:359–362.

26. The EPIC investigators. Use of a monoclonal antibody directed against the platelet glycoprotein IIb/IIIa receptor in high-risk coronary angioplasty. N Engl J Med 1994; 330:956–961.

27. Hayes R, Chesebro JH, Fuster V, et al. Antithrombotic effects of abciximab. Am J Cardiol 2000; 85:1167–1172.

28. Neumann FJ, Kastrati A, Schmitt C, et al. Effect of glycoprotein IIb/IIIa receptor blockade with abciximab on clinical and angiographic restenosis rate after the placement of coronary stents following acute myocardial infarction. J Am Coll Cardiol 2000; 35:915–921.

29. Lincoff AM, Califf RM, Van De Werf F, et al. Global use of strategies to open coronary arteries investigators (GUSTO): mortality at 1 year with combination platelet glycoprotein IIb/IIIa inhibition and reduced-dose fibrinolytic therapy versus conventional fibrinolytic therapy for acute myocardial infarction: GUSTO V randomized trial. JAMA 2002; 288:2130–2135.

30. Januzzi JL Jr. Benefits and safety of tirofiban among acute coronary syndrome patients with mild to moderate renal insufficiency: results from the Platelet Receptor Inhibition in Ischemic Syndrome Management in Patients Limited by Unstable Signs and Symptoms (PRISM-PLUS) trial. Circulation 2002; 105:2361–2366.

31. Fitchett DH, Langer A, Armstrong PW, et al. Interact trial long-term follow-up investigators: randomized evaluation of the efficacy of enoxaparin versus unfractionated heparin in high-risk patients with non-ST-segment elevation acute coronary syndromes receiving the glycoprotein IIb/IIIa inhibitor eptifibatide. Long-term results of the Integrilin and Enoxaparin Randomized Assessment of Acute Coronary Syndrome Treatment (INTERACT) trial. Am Heart J 2006; 151:373–379.

32. Anderson JL, Adams CD, Antman EM, et al. ACC/AHA 2007 Guidelines for the Management of Patients With Unstable Angina/Non-ST-Elevation Myocardial Infarction: a report of the American College of Cardiology/American Heart Association Task Force on Practice Guidelines (Writing Committee to Revise the 2002 Guidelines for the Management of Patients with Unstable Angina/Non-ST-Elevation Myocardial Infarction) developed in collaboration with the American College of Emergency Physicians, the Society for Cardiovascular Angiography and Interventions, and the Society of Thoracic Surgeons endorsed by the American Association of Cardiovascular and Pulmonary Rehabilitation and the Society for Academic Emergency Medicine. J Am Coll Cardiol 2007; 50(7):e1–e157.

33. Chew DP, Bhatt DL, Sapp S, et al. Increased mortality with oral platelet glycoprotein IIb/IIIa antagonists: a meta-analysis of phase III multicenter randomized trials. Circulation 2001; 103: 201–206.

34. Steinhubl SR, Berger PB, Mann JT III, et al. Credo investigators: clopidogrel for the reduction of events during observation. Early and sustained dual oral antiplatelet therapy following percutaneous coronary intervention: a randomized controlled trial. JAMA 2002; 288:2411–2420.

35. Classics investigators. Double-blind study of the safety of clopidogrel with and without a loading dose in combination with aspirin compared with ticlopidine in combination with aspirin after coronary stenting. The clopidogrel aspirin stent international cooperative study (CLASSICS). Circulation 2000; 102:624–629.

36. Rothwell PM. Lessons from MATCH for future randomized trials in the secondary prevention of stroke. Lancet 2004; 364:305–307.

37. Payne DA, Jones CI, Hayes PD, et al. Beneficial effects of clopidogrel combined with aspirin in reducing cerebral emboli in patients undergoing carotid endarterectomy. Circulation 2004; 109:1476–1481.

38. Hirsh J, Bhatt DL. Comparative benefits of clopidogrel and aspirin in high-risk patient populations: lessons from the CAPRIE and CURE studies. Arch Intern Med 2004; 164:2106–2110.

39. Caprie investigators. A randomized, blinded, trial of clopidogrel versus aspirin in patients at risk of ischemic events. Lancet 1996; 348:1329–1339.

40. Cadroy Y, Bossavy JP, Thalamas C, et al. Early potent antithrombotic effect with combined aspirin and a loading dose of clopidogrel on experimental arterial thrombogenesis in humans. Circulation 2000; 101:2823–2828.

41. Coma-Canella I, Velasco A, Castano S. Prevalence of aspirin resistance measured by PFA-100. Int J Cardiol 2005; 101(1):71–76.

42. Wiviott SD, Braunwald E, McCabe CH, et al. The TRITON-TIMI-38 investigators prasugrel versus clopidogrel in patients with acute coronary syndromes. N Engl J Med 2007; 357:2001–2015.

43. Angliolillo DJ, Shoemaker SB, Desai B, et al. Randomized comparison of a high clopidogrel maintenance dose in patients with diabetes mellitus and coronary artery disease: results of the Optimizing Antiplatelet Therapy in Diabetes Mellitus (OPTIMUS) study. Circulation 2007; 115(6): 708–716.

44. Spertus JA, Kettelkamp R, Vance C, et al. Prevalence, predictors, and outcomes of premature discontinuation of thienopyridine therapy after drug-eluting stent placement: results from the PREMIER registry. Circulation 2006; 113(24):2803–2809.

45. Anderluh M. Dolenc MS. Thrombin receptor antagonists: recent advances in PAR-1 antagonist development. Curr Med Chem 2002; 9:1229–1250.

46. Cannon CP, Husted S, Harrington RA, et al. Safety, tolerability, and initial efficacy of AZD6140, the first reversible oral adenosine diphosphate receptor antagonist, compared with clopidogrel, in patients with non-ST-segment elevation acute coronary syndrome: primary results of the DISPERSE-2 trial. J Am Coll Cardiol 2007; 50:1844–1851.

47. Greenbaum AB, Grines CL, Bittl JA, et al. Initial experience with an intravenous P2Y$_{12}$ platelet receptor antagonist in patients undergoing percutaneous coronary intervention: results from a 2-part, phase II, multicenter, randomized, placebo- and active-controlled trial. Am Heart J 2006; 151:689, e1–e10.

48. Diener HC, Bogousslavsky J, Brass LM, et al. Match investigators. Aspirin and clopidogrel compared with clopidogrel alone after recent ischemic stroke or transient ischemic attack in high-risk patients. Randomized, double-blind, placebo-controlled trial. Lancet 2004; 364:331–337.

49. Markus HS, Droste DW, Kaps M, et al. Dual antiplatelet therapy with clopidogrel and aspirin in symptomatic carotid stenosis evaluated using Doppler embolic signal detection: the Clopidogrel and Aspirin for Reduction of Emboli in Symptomatic Carotid Stenosis (CARESS) trial. Circulation 2005; 111:2233–2240.

50. Bhatt DL, Fox KA, Hacke W, et al. The Charisma investigators: clopidogrel and aspirin versus aspirin alone for the prevention of atherothrombotic events. N Engl J Med 2006; 354: 1706–1711.

51. Garg P, Mauri L. The conundrum of late and very late stent thrombosis following drug-eluting stent implantation. Curr Opin Cardiol 2007; 22:565–571.

24

Markers of Platelet Function

Udaya S. Tantry
Sinai Center for Thrombosis Research, Sinai Hospital of Baltimore, Baltimore, Maryland, U.S.A.

Paul A. Gurbel
Sinai Center for Thrombosis Research, Sinai Hospital of Baltimore and Johns Hopkins University School of Medicine, Baltimore, Maryland, U.S.A.

INTRODUCTION

Our understanding of the central role of platelet function in the genesis of thrombotic events has stimulated the development of novel antiplatelet agents targeting specific pathways involved in adhesion, activation, and aggregation (1). The results of recent clinical trials evaluating $\alpha_{IIb}\beta_3$ (GPIIb/IIIa) blockers and $P2Y_{12}$ receptor inhibitors have supported the concept that improved platelet inhibition significantly attenuates ischemic event occurrence. However, the prevalence of recurrent thrombotic events still remains high (2,3) Moreover, the "one size fits all" approach employed in these clinical trials has also demonstrated that agents associated with superior platelet inhibition are also linked to increased bleeding. Recent translational research studies have strongly supported the relation of high on-treatment platelet reactivity to the occurrence of ischemic events including stent thrombosis, and a potential threshold level associated with event occurrence has been reported (4,5). The present strategy of treating all patients with the same dose of antiplatelet agents may be flawed. At one end of the spectrum, selected patients with excessively low platelet reactivity may bleed, while other patients with high platelet reactivity may have ischemic events. These concerns will be addressed by future strategies based on the measurement of platelet function and thrombotic potential in the individual patient. Platelet reactivity is a quantifiable and modifiable risk factor (5). The determination of a therapeutic target of platelet reactivity associated with reduced thrombotic risk and bleeding events remains an elusive and overall understudied goal at this time. Thus, the measurement of platelet function that optimally correlates with patient outcomes has assumed increased importance in cardiovascular medicine.

Previously, platelet function measurements were largely confined to the assessment of patients with inherited platelet dysfunction associated with bleeding and the assessment of patients with bleeding complications after cardiovascular surgery to determine optimal therapy. However, recent advancements in understanding the critical role of platelets in cardiovascular thrombotic events and the significance of platelet function attenuation in reducing ischemic risks have led to the development of various methods, including point-of-care assays, to measure platelet reactivity (4). Establishing a relation between measurable factors in blood indicating platelet reactivity and activation (the presence of vulnerable blood) to the patient's vulnerability of developing an acute thrombotic event is one of the major goals of cardiovascular research. The characterization of mechanisms responsible for the transition from an asymptomatic stable disease state to a more severe disease state would be an important step in the prevention and treatment of cardiovascular disease. Nevertheless, platelet function measurement is complicated by various factors such as (*i*) the numerous redundant pathways by which platelets are activated, (*ii*) the intimate interaction of the platelet with coagulation processes and other blood cells, (*iii*) the fact that platelets' function must be immediately determined following blood drawing, and (*iv*) artifactual activation by selected anticoagulants, blood-drawing techniques, and preparation methods. Moreover, there is no available standardized platelet function test that uniformly emulates in vivo thrombus generation. In other words, a bench to bedside approach using a simple and standardized method of platelet function that accurately assesses the individual patient's thrombogenic potential for personalized antiplatelet therapy remains elusive. The present discussion will highlight the current markers of platelet function that may prove useful in the identification of patients with cardiovascular disease who are at greatest risk for disease progression and acute thrombosis.

ROLE OF PLATELETS IN THROMBOSIS

Under normal conditions, anucleate circulating platelets are in a quiescent state. Healthy vascular endothelium prevents thrombosis by producing antithrombotic factors such as CD39 (ADPase), prostaglandin I_2, nitric oxide, heparin, matrix metalloproteinase-9 (MMP-9), protein S, thrombomodulin, and tissue-type plasminogen activator (t-PA) (6). Under normal physiological conditions, circulating platelets adhere to the injured vessel wall and facilitate subsequent healing processes that maintain vessel wall integrity and limit bleeding. In addition to a well-defined role in hemostasis and thrombosis, platelets are involved in wound healing, atherosclerosis progression, inflammation, tumor metastasis, and immune-mediated host defenses (7,8).

Under the pathological condition of atherosclerosis associated with dysfunctional endothelium, uncontrolled platelet activation leads to occlusive thrombus generation and subsequent ischemic complications. Atherosclerotic plaque rupture and endothelial denudation that occurs in acute coronary syndromes and during percutaneous interventions result in the exposure of the subendothelial matrix and the release of factors facilitating platelet adhesion and activation. Under high-shear conditions present in arterial blood vessels, initial platelet adhesion requires binding of the GPIb/IX/V receptor to von Willebrand Factor (vWF) immobilized on collagen; the GPVI receptor directly binds to collagen. The subsequent intracellular signaling events, particularly downstream from GPVI, lead to activation of $\alpha_2\beta_1$ (GPIa/IIa) and $\alpha_{IIb}\beta_3$ receptors and the release of important secondary agonists, TxA_2 and ADP. The activated $\alpha_2\beta_1$ receptor by directly binding to collagen and the activated $\alpha_{IIb}\beta_3$ receptor by binding to immobilized vWF ensures stable platelet adhesion to the injured vessel wall (9,10). Additionally,

Table 1 Platelet Granule Secretion

α-granule contents	
Adhesion molecules	P-selection (CD62P), von Willebrand factor, fibrinogen, fibronectin, $\alpha_{IIb}\beta_3$, vitronectin receptor ($\alpha_V\beta_3$), thrombospondin-1, PECAM-1
Chemokines	MIP-1α(CCL-3), RANTES (CCL-5), MCP-3 (CCL-7), CXCL-1 (growth-regulated oncogene-α), CXCL4, ENA-78 (CXCL5)
Cytokine-like proteins	IL-8 (CXCL8), β-thromboglobulin, CD40L.
Fibrinolytic pathway	PAI-1, TFPI, α2-macroglobulin
Coagulation factors	Fibrinogen, protein S, factors V, VII, VIII, XI, XIII
Growth factors	PDGF, TGF-β, EGF
Dense-granule contents	
Nucleotides	ATP, ADP, GTP, GDP
Amines	Serotonin, histamine
Ions	Calcium, magnesium, phosphate
Membrane proteins	Granulophysin (CD63), (LAMPs)

Abbreviations: ADP, adenosine diphosphate; PECAM, platelet endothelial cell adhesion molecule; CXCL4, platelet factor-4; ENA, epithelial neutrophil-activating; IL, interleukin; PAI-1, plasminogen activator inhibitor-1; TFPI, tissue factor pathway inhibitor; PDGF, platelet-derived growth factor; TGF, transforming growth factor; EGF, epidermal growth factor; RANTES, released upon activation T cell expressed and secreted; MCP, monocyte chemoattractant protein; LAMPs, lysosomal membrane proteins.

activated platelets bind to exposed vWF through the vitronectin receptor ($\alpha_V\beta_3$), to fibronectin through $\alpha_5\beta_1$ and activated $\alpha_{IIb}\beta_3$, to thrombospondin via GPIb/IX/V, to laminin through $\alpha_6\beta_1$ and GPVI receptors, and to fibrinogen and fibrin through activated $\alpha_{IIb}\beta_3$. All of the latter processes promote stable adhesion and aggregation (9,10).

Following adhesion, platelets form a single monolayer at the site of vessel wall injury and undergo activation. The activation process involves morphological changes coupled with intracellular calcium ion mobilization. Reorganization of the cytoskeleton occurs that changes the discoid shape to a spherical shape with peudopods. Finally, there is secretion of granule contents. Shape change results in an increased platelet surface area available for coagulation processes and the exposure of various receptors such as $\alpha_{IIb}\beta_3$ and $\alpha_2\beta_1$, platelet endothelial cell adhesion molecule (PECAM)-1, intercellular cell adhesion molecule (ICAM)-2, CD40L, and P-selectin. Specific receptors play important roles in homotypic (platelet-platelet) and heterotypic (platelet-leukocyte) aggregation and the modulation of leukocyte function. The secretion and exposure of contents from lysosomes, α-granules, and dense granules mediate thrombosis, coagulation, and inflammation (Tables 1 and 2) (9–12). Furthermore, platelet activation also results in the release of procoagulant and pro-inflammatory microparticles and certain chemokines that play important roles in inflammation (9–12).

Thromboxane (Tx)-A_2 is produced from membrane phospholipids, and ADP is released from dense granules following initial platelet adhesion and activation. Through autocrine and paracrine mechanisms, these two locally generated secondary agonists play a critical role in sustaining platelet activation that results in stable aggregation and robust thrombus generation at the site of vessel wall injury. It has been proposed that sustaining platelet activation of the $\alpha_{IIb}\beta_3$ receptor and platelet procoagulant activity are critically dependent on signaling downstream from the $P2Y_{12}$ receptor, an important receptor of ADP (10). The latter concept is supported by (*i*) the demonstration of superior clinical

Table 2 Platelet Adhesion and Activation-Related Molecules, Functions, and Measurements

Molecule	Molecule recognized: location	Function	Measurement
P-selectin	PSGL-1: platelets, leukocytes, endothelium	Platelet-platelet aggregation, platelet-leukocyte aggregation and inflammation, tissue factor exposure	Flow cytometry
	Mac-1: leukocytes		ELISA and MAP— soluble P-selection
CD40L	CD40, $\alpha_{IIb}\beta_3$: platelets CD 40: endothelium, leukocytes Mac-1: leukocytes	As above	Flow cytometry ELISA and MAP— soluble CD40L
ICAM-2	Lymphocyte function-associated antigen-1, LFA-1 and Mac-1: leukocytes	Leukocyte recruitment	Flow cytometry
GPVI	Collagen: endothelium	Adhesion and activation does not require divalent cations	Adhesion experiments (see text)
$\alpha_2\beta_1$	Collagen: endothelium	Adhesion requires divalent cations	Adhesion experiments (see text)
$\alpha_{IIb}\beta_3$	Fibrin, fibrinogen	Platelet-platelet aggregation, platelet-endothelial/leukocyte binding	Flow cytometry, radioligand binding
	Mac-1 and $\alpha_v\beta_3$ through fibrinogen: leukocytes and endothelium		
GPIbα	vWF, P-selectin, thrombin: platelets, endothelium Mac-1: leukocytes	Platelet adhesion and leukocyte binding	Adhesion experiments (see text) Flow cytometry
PSGL-1	P-selection; platelets, endothelial cells	Platelet adhesion, platelet-endothelial/leukocyte binding	Adhesion experiments, platelet-leukocyte aggregates

Abbreviations: ICAM, intercellular cell adhesion molecule; PSGL, P-selectin glycoprotein ligand; LFA-1, lymphocyte function-associated antigen-1; ELISA, enzyme-linked immunoabsorbent assays.

efficacy associated with dual antiplatelet therapy of clopidogrel and aspirin compared with aspirin therapy alone, (*ii*) demonstration of adverse ischemic events associated with high on-treatment ADP-induced platelet reactivity, and (*iii*) superior clinical outcomes with respect to ischemia observed in patients treated with the more potent $P2Y_{12}$ receptor blockers (Fig. 1) (4,5).

Plaque rupture also results in tissue factor release and the generation of small amounts of thrombin, a coagulation factor, and the most potent primary platelet agonist. Thrombin production further promotes the formation of a procoagulant platelet surface where subsequently large amounts of thrombin are produced through coagulation processes. Finally, thrombin converts fibrinogen to fibrin that ultimately leads to the formation of a fibrin network and a stable occlusive platelet-fibrin clot (9,10).

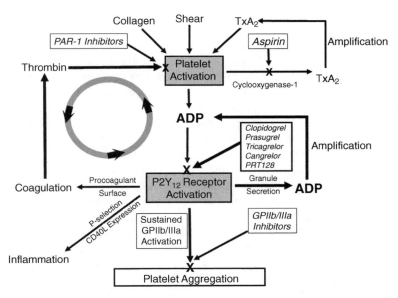

Figure 1 Central role of ADP in modulating multiple pathways leading to the occurrence of thrombosis. ADP is involved in the amplification of the platelet response to other agonists leading to GPIIb/IIIa activation. Platelet activation also affects leukocyte function through P-selectin and CD40L expression and the generation of thrombin, leading to a cycle of platelet activation-coagulation and thrombin generation.

MARKERS OF PLATELET FUNCTION

Platelet Count

Determination of a direct platelet count should accompany the quantitative analysis of platelet function to eliminate the influence of low platelet counts (<100,000 platelets/uL). This measurement may be more meaningful when accompanied by a measurement of mean platelet volume, since abnormal platelet volume has been associated with adverse clinical events (13). In addition, elevated platelet counts and increased numbers of young platelets observed immediately following cardiac surgery may, in part, explain aspirin resistance through uninhibited COX-2 expression (14). Platelet number can be measured easily using automated analyzers (e.g., Beckman Coulter, Fullerton, California, U.S., Ichor PlateletWorks, Helena Laboratories, Beaumont, Texas, U.S., and Thrombelastography, Haemonetics Corp., Braintree, Massachusetts, U.S.). Single-platelet counting after specific agonist stimulation of whole blood has been used to evaluate the effects of antiplatelet drugs (15).

Bleeding Time

Measurement of bleeding time was the first laboratory method to assess platelet function. The bleeding time is not recommended as a screening test or as a tool to quantify antiplatelet effects, since it is associated with poor reproducibility, specificity, and sensitivity (16). The bleeding time has largely been replaced by turbidimetric aggregation assays and point-of-care tests.

Platelet Adhesion

In vitro models of platelet adhesion are available as research tools to study the role of adhesion receptors and intracellular signaling in thrombosis and also to assess the effects of antiplatelet agents. Early adhesion studies were performed with platelets isolated from patients lacking specific adhesion receptor expression or from knockout mice (17). In current models, adhesion proteins such as collagen, fibrinogen, or other adhesion-related molecules are first immobilized on glass or plastic surfaces, and platelet binding is monitored in either static or under flow conditions. In addition, cultured human umbilical vein endothelial cells have also been used in platelet adhesion studies (18).

In static adhesion assays, $\alpha_2\beta_1$ has been studied using monomeric collagen, whereas GPVI has been studied using collagen-related peptides or convulxin. In static experiments using fibrillar collagen, cation-chelating agents have been used to inhibit $\alpha_2\beta_1$ activity since cations are essential for $\alpha_2\beta_1$ but not GPVI binding. Static assays and aggregation methods have used ristocetin and orbotrocetin to study the shear-dependent adhesion processes of GPIb binding to vWF (19). These assays are conducted by either using specific fluorescent or radiolabeled ligands or the measurement of light transmission in microtiter plates or platelet-rich plasma.

Various techniques are available to study platelet adhesion under flow conditions. Important methods include the use of laminar flow devices (tubular, annular, or parallel-plate flow chambers) with high-resolution microscopy (20). In these experiments, platelets are labeled with fluorescent dyes such as fluorescein isothiocyanate, Fluo3, DM505, or rhodamine (21,22). Quantitative assessment of thrombus generation on collagen or other adhesion-related molecule-coated surfaces in real time can then be performed. These experiments have greatly enhanced our knowledge regarding the role of various collagen receptors and have also aided in the development of novel antiplatelet agents.

In vivo murine models using intravital fluorescence microscopy are available to study the role of platelets in intravascular thrombus generation (23). Using a piezoelectric thickness shear model biosensor coated with collagen fibers, a novel assay has been developed to study platelet function at different phases of adhesion, activation, and aggregation in real time (24). In addition, platelets shed surface receptors that mediate adhesion. Plasma levels of collagen receptors are measured by enzyme-linked immuno-assays. High levels of soluble GPVI receptors and also GPVI polymorphisms have been correlated with recurrent thrombotic events (25,26).

Shape Change

Platelet shape change is the first measurable physiological change following stimulation by agonists and has been quantified by aggregometry using the Michal and Born method (27). Intracellular calcium mobilization is measured using specific fluorescent calcium ion sensing indicators such as fura-2 detected by flow cytometry assays or fluorescence spectrophotometry (28).

Platelet Activation

Various terms such as "platelet activation," "increased platelet reactivity," and "greater platelet aggregation" have been used to indicate increased platelet function in cardiovascular disease states. Platelet activation is an in vivo phenomenon and is clinically measured by ex vivo methods. The detection in plasma or whole blood of (*i*) platelets expressing activation-dependent receptors, (*ii*) platelet microparticles,

Platelet activation and reactivity to agonists
are interrelated processes.

Platelet activation is an in vivo process
measured primarily by ex vivo methods

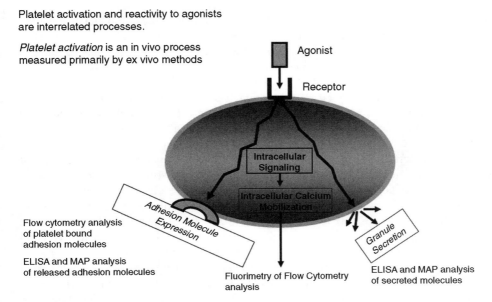

Figure 2 Platelet activation occurs after exposure to agonists that stimulate a cascade of intracellular signaling events. Platelet activation can be assessed by measuring (*i*) the expression of surface molecules, (*ii*) soluble surface markers, (*iii*) intracellular calcium mobilization, and (*iv*) secreted granule contents.

(*iii*) released soluble activation-dependent molecules, and (*iv*) other granule contents are all evidence of in vivo platelet activation. Platelet activation is measured by flow cytometry using labeled monoclonal antibodies that specifically bind to receptors present on activated platelets and microparticles. Soluble markers released from the activated platelet surface or from granules are measured by enzyme-linked immunosorbent assays (ELISA) and multianalyte profiling (MAP) methods (Fig. 2).

Platelet Reactivity

In patients on antiplatelet therapy, platelet reactivity—the response of platelets to various stimuli—is most often measured by ex vivo aggregation in the presence of an anticoagulant. Platelet aggregation in these experiments is primarily mediated by the activated $\alpha_{IIb}\beta_3$ receptor binding to fibrinogen. The stimuli for activation in these experiments include (*i*) primary agonists (e.g., collagen, thrombin), (*ii*) secondary agonists (e.g., ADP, TxA_2, serotonin, epinephrine) that are released following platelet activation, or (*iii*) shear in the presence of agonists.

The degree of platelet reactivity following antiplatelet therapy has been quantified by (*i*) conventional light transmittance aggregometry (LTA) in platelet-rich plasma, (*ii*) impedence aggregometry in whole blood (29), (*iii*) light transmittance where platelet binding to fibrinogen-coated beads occurs in whole blood (VerifyNow®, Accumetrics, San Diego, California, U.S.) (30), (*iv*) time to aperture occlusion in assays that employ shear-induced blood flow through the aperture [Platelet Function Analyzer-100® (PFA), Dade-Behring, Miami, Florida, U.S.; Placor, PlaCor Inc., Plymouth, Minnesota, U.S.] (31,32), (*v*) platelet-fibrin clot tensile strength measured by thrombelastography (Haemonetics Corp., Braintree, Massachusetts, U.S.) (33), (*vi*) real-time quantification of platelet aggregate size (Perfusion Chamber Analysis, Portola Pharmaceuticals Inc., South San Francisco,

California, U.S.) (21), (*vii*) quantitative measurement of platelet adhesion and aggregation on polysterene plates under shear (34) (Cone and Platelet Analyzer®, Diamed, Cressier sur Morat, Switzerland), and (*viii*) quantitative measurement of agonist-induced platelet aggregates based on a light-scattering principle (35) (Thrombovision, Houston, Texas, U.S.). Platelet aggregation is most often measured by light transmittance aggregation in platelet-rich plasma. Turbidimetric aggregation has also been widely used to provide important information about inherited and acquired platelet function defects. Whole-blood impedence aggregometry has been reported to be associated with wider assay variability than turbidometric aggregation (4).

Since increased expression of activation-dependent molecules on the platelet surfaces accompanies heightened platelet reactivity to ex vivo stimuli, both measurements have been used synonymously in clinical trials to indicate elevated platelet function. Thus, these terms imply the same pathophysiologic concept—increased platelet responsiveness to stimuli that leads to activation and the formation of homotypic and heterotypic aggregates. Both of these measurements have been associated with an increased risk for thrombosis and subsequent ischemic complications.

The release of ADP from platelets during aggregation can be monitored by assaying ATP using the firefly luminescence assay. The latter method is performed with either whole blood or platelet-rich plasma. In this assay, ADP released from dense granules is converted to ATP, which then reacts with luciferin generating adenyl-luciferon. Light emitted by adenyl-luciferon is measured by a lumiaggregometer following oxidation, and its extent is proportional to the amount of ADP released from the dense granules (36).

IMPORTANT MARKERS OF PLATELET ACTIVATION

Activated $\alpha_{IIb}\beta_3$ Receptor (GPIIb/IIIa or CD41/CD61)

The binding of primary (collagen, vWF, and thrombin) and secondary agonists (ADP and TxA_2) to respective receptors leads to the inside-out signaling and finally to the activation of $\alpha_{IIb}\beta_3$. Fibrinogen and vWF are the main ligands for the activated $\alpha_{IIb}\beta_3$ receptor. However, fibronectin, vitronectin, thrombospondin, and CD40 ligand (CD40L) also bind to $\alpha_{IIb}\beta_3$ and facilitate firm platelet adhesion and stable platelet aggregation. Activated $\alpha_{IIb}\beta_3$ levels are determined by flow cytometry assays using specific PAC-1 antibodies that bind to the fibrinogen-binding site on activated platelets. Binding assays utilizing radiolabeled fibrinogen are also used to quantitate the extent of activated $\alpha_{IIb}\beta_3$ receptor expression (37,38).

P-selectin (CD-62P)

On activation, P-selectin molecules stored in α-granules are expressed on the platelet surface and are subsequently released into the circulation. Therefore, both platelet-bound and free (in plasma) P-selectin indicate platelet activation. Platelet-bound P-selectin is measured by flow cytometry using monoclonal antibodies, whereas soluble P-selectin is measured by ELISA or MAP assays. In addition to its role in thrombosis, P-selectin mediates leukocyte adhesion to endothelium that is critical for leukocyte infiltration into the subendothelium and progression of atherosclerosis and inflammation (39,40).

CD40 Ligand

CD40L is a transmembrane protein expressed on the surface of activated platelets and binds to $\alpha_{IIb}\beta_3$ via the KGR (Lys-Gly-Arg) sequence to trigger outside-in signaling and thrombus stabilization. In addition, released CD40L activates platelets by binding to platelet CD40 and induces an inflammatory response in endothelial cells by binding to endothelial CD40. The latter response subsequently leads to expression of adhesion molecules E-selectin, vascular cell adhesion molecule (VCAM)-1 and intercellular adhesion molecule (ICAM)-1, chemokines (IL-6) and monocyte chemoattractant protein (MCP)-1, and tissue factor. The primary source of soluble CD40L measured in plasma is activated platelets. Soluble CD40L is measured in plasma using ELISA or MAP methods whereas platelet-bound CD40L levels are low, thus limiting detection by flow cytometry analysis. Soluble CD40L levels have been correlated with cardiovascular risk studied during antiplatelet treatment and coronary interventions (41).

Platelet-Leukocyte Aggregates

Activated platelets adhere to leukocytes via P-selectin—P-selectin glycoprotein ligand (PSGL)-1, CD40-CD40L, and Mac-1 ($\alpha_M\beta_2$)-fibrinogen-$\alpha_{IIb}\beta_3$, and Mac-1-ICAM-2 interactions. Firm adhesion occurs through binding of Mac-1 to GPIb. Platelet-leukocyte (platelet-monocyte and platelet-neutrophil) aggregates are measured in whole blood by flow cytometry-based assays using a combination of platelet-specific and leukocyte-specific antibodies. It has been suggested that platelet-monocyte aggregates may be a more sensitive indicator of in vivo platelet activation than platelet-neutrophil or platelet-bound P-selectin measurements (42). Platelet-leukocyte aggregates are increased in various manifestations of cardiovascular diseases such as myocardial infarction, unstable angina and stable coronary artery disease, and following post-percutaneous interventions (43).

Thromboxane Metabolites

On activation, phospholipase A2 activity in platelets leads to the release of arachidonic acid from membrane phospholipids. Arachidonic acid is subsequently converted to prostaglandin H_2 by cyclooxygenase-1 and then to TxA_2 by thromboxane synthase. Released TxA_2 is converted to a stable metabolite, TxB_2, and is excreted in urine as 11-dehydro TxB_2. Both serum and urine thromboxane metabolites are measured by ELISA and radioimmunoassays or by chromatographic methods. Elevated thromboxane metabolites in serum and urine have been correlated with ischemic cardiovascular events and diabetes and have been used as an indication of aspirin resistance (44).

Platelet Procoagulant Activity

Following platelet activation, the procoagulant phosphotidyl serine surface is exposed and provides a suitable surface for attachment of coagulation factors and the generation of thrombin. Procoagulant platelets can be identified by flow cytometry analysis using fluorescent dye-labeled annexin-V (45). Platelet procoagulant activity is measured by a prothrombinase assay using a chromogenic substrate (46).

Platelet-Derived Microparticles

Platelet activation by agonists results in the production of microparticles or platelet fragments. These microparticles are identified by flow cytometry analysis as CD42-positive particles that are smaller than platelets (low forward angle light scatter) (47). These microparticles may be procoagulant, since they bind to coagulation-related protein molecules such as annexin V, or antibodies to coagulation factors (V or VII) (48).

Platelet Chemokines

After activation, platelets release various stored chemokines and cytokine-like factors into the circulation that promote inflammatory responses at the site of platelet adhesion. These factors include RANTES (released upon activation normal T cell expressed and secreted), platelet factor 4, IL-1β, and β-thromboglobulin (7–9). These molecules are measured by ELISA or MAP analysis in plasma samples. Recently, the critical role of platelet-derived stromal cell-derived factor (SDF)-1 in adhesion and differentiation of human CD34+ cells into endothelial progenitor cells has been demonstrated (49).

MEASUREMENT OF PLATELET FUNCTION TO ASSESS RESPONSIVENESS TO ANTIPLATELET THERAPY

Multiple signaling pathways mediate platelet activation and the occurrence of thrombotic events. Thus a treatment strategy designed to block a single pathway cannot be expected to prevent the occurrence of all events, and treatment failure following a single antiplatelet strategy alone is not sufficient evidence of drug resistance. "Resistance" or nonresponsiveness to an antiplatelet agent is provided by persistent activity of the specific target of the antiplatelet agent. Since the active metabolite of clopidogrel irreversibly inhibits the P2Y$_{12}$ receptor, evidence for nonresponsiveness to clopidogrel is provided by high posttreatment P2Y$_{12}$ reactivity. For aspirin, the identification of resistance utilizes laboratory technique that detects residual activity of the primary target COX-1 (50) (Fig. 3).

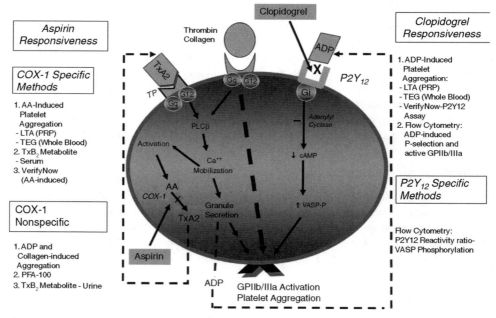

Figure 3 Mechanism of action and laboratory evaluation of clopidogrel and aspirin responsiveness. *Abbreviations*: AA, arachidonic acid; ADP, adenosine diphosphate; COX-1, cyclooxygenase-1; LTA, light transmittance aggregometry; PRP, platelet-rich plasma; PAC-1, activated GP IIb/IIIa receptor; PFA-100, platelet function analyzer-100; TP, thromboxane receptor; TxB2, thromboxane B2; TEG, thrombelastography; VASP-P, vasodilator-stimulated phosphoprotein phosphorylated.

Measurement of Clopidogrel Responsiveness

The most widely used laboratory evaluation of clopidogrel responsiveness is the ex vivo measurement of maximum ADP-induced platelet aggregation by LTA. In this method, maximum platelet aggregation in response to 5 and 20 μM ADP is determined in platelet-rich plasma before and after treatment with clopidogrel. Patients with an absolute difference in aggregation of <10% have been considered nonresponders, those with 10% to 30% considered semi-responders, and those with >30% considered responders (51,52). LTA is a cumbersome, time-consuming method that requires trained technicians. Although, ex vivo "final" platelet aggregation measured at six minutes following stimulation by ADP rather than maximum aggregation has been proposed as a more physiologically relevant measure of clopidogrel response, a recent study indicated that there was no difference in the estimation of clopidogrel responsiveness using both measurements (53,54).

Flow cytometric determination of P-selectin and activated GPIIb/IIIa receptor expression following ADP stimulation have been used to assess platelet inhibition by clopidogrel (51). Flow cytometry is also cumbersome and requires sophisticated methods and well-trained technicians. The PFA-100, thrombelastography (Platelet Mapping™ Assay, Haemoscope Corp., Skokie, Illinois, with ADP as the agonist), and the VerifyNow P2Y$_{12}$ Assay™ have been proposed as reproducible point-of-care methods to assess platelet inhibition by clopidogrel (4). These methods are undergoing investigation in clinical studies. The phosphorylation state of vasodilator-stimulated phosphoprotein (VASP) is a specific intracellular marker of clopidogrel-induced P2Y$_{12}$ receptor inhibition and is measured by flow cytometry. Permeation of the membrane and the use of monoclonal antibodies specific for phosphorylated VASP are required in this method (54). Recent translational research studies correlated clopidogrel nonrepsonsiveness or high on-treatment platelet reactivity to ADP with the occurrence of myocardial necrosis, stent thrombosis, and long-term ischemic events (4) (55–66) (Table 3).

Table 3 Studies Linking High On-Treatment Platelet Reactivity to ADP and Clopidogrel Nonresponsiveness to Adverse Clinical Event Occurrence

Study	Results	Clinical relevance
1. Matetzky et al. (55)	↓ Platelet inhibition	Recurrent ischemic events
2. Gurbel et al. (56)	↑ Platelet aggregation	Recurrent ischemic events
3. Gurbel et al. (57)	↑ Periprocedural platelet aggregation	Post-PCI myonecrosis
4. Bliden et al. (58)	↑ Pre-PCI platelet aggregation in patients on chronic clopidogrel therapy	1-yr recurrent ischemic events
5. Lev et al. (59)	Clopidogrel/aspirin-resistant patients	Post-PCI myonecrosis
6. Cuisset et al. (60)	↑ Platelet aggregation	30-day post-PCI events
7. Geisler et al. (61)	Clopidogrel low responders	3-mo MACE and death
8. Hocholzer et al. (62)	↑ Platelet aggregation (upper quartile)	30-day MACE
9. Price et al. (63)	↑ Posttreatment platelet reactivity (VerifyNow assay)	6-mo post-PCI events including stent thrombosis
10. Barragan et al. (64)	↑ P2Y$_{12}$ reactivity ratio (VASP-P assay)	Stent thrombosis
11. Gurbel et al. (65)	↑ P2Y$_{12}$ reactivity ratio (VASP-P assay) ↑ Platelet aggregation ↑ Stimulated GPIIb/IIIa expression	Stent thrombosis
12. Buonamici et al. (66)	↑ Platelet aggregation	Stent thrombosis

Abbreviations: PCI, percutaneous coronary intervention; MACE, major adverse cardiovascular events; VASP-P, phosphorylated vasodilator-stimulated phosphoprotein.

Measurement of Aspirin Responsiveness

Aspirin irreversibly inhibits platelet COX-1 activity that leads to thromboxane A_2-induced platelet aggregation. Laboratory methods for assessing platelet responsiveness to aspirin can be categorized as COX-1 specific and COX-1 nonspecific (4). COX-1-specific methods include arachidonic acid-induced platelet aggregation measured by LTA, thrombelastography using the Platelet Mapping™ assay (Haemonetics Corp., Braintree, Massachusetts, U.S.), VerifyNow, and enzyme-linked immunoassay determination of the stable metabolites of TxB_2 in serum. COX-1-nonspecific methods include ADP- and collagen-induced platelet aggregation as determined by LTA, the PFA-100 and enzyme-linked immunoassay determination of the stable metabolites of TxB_2 in urine. Recently, it was suggested that aspirin inhibits targets other than COX-1 in platelets, and aspirin responsiveness indicated by these pathways may be important in certain conditions and may correlate with clinical outcomes (67).

The assessment of aspirin resistance is highly assay dependent. Aspirin resistance is infrequent in compliant patients when measured by COX-1-specific assays (<5%). A higher prevalence of aspirin resistance has been associated with noncompliance and assessment by COX-1-nonspecific assays. The latter findings should be taken into account when interpreting the level of aspirin responsiveness and its relation to various clinical outcomes. In a recent randomized, double-blind, double-crossover investigation of relation of resistance to aspirin dosing in patients with stable coronary artery disease, 1% to 5% were aspirin resistant when COX-1-specific methods were used and up to 30% were resistant according to COX-1-nonspecific methods (67). Moreover, there was little consistency in the measurement of aspirin responsiveness between point-of-service assays in these patients receiving different doses of aspirin (67).

Aspirin resistance may also be associated with concomitant clopidogrel resistance (59). Patients identified as aspirin resistant have exhibited high platelet reactivity to collagen and ADP. These data suggest that the presence of a generalized high-platelet-reactivity phenotype indicated by VerifyNow assay may be associated with an increased risk for ischemic events (68). Similar to clopidogrel-resistant patients, patients with aspirin resistance have also been associated with an increased risk of ischemic event occurrence following coronary intervention (44,59,69–76) (Table 4).

Measurement of GPIIb/IIIa Inhibitor Responsiveness

The three approved GPIIb/IIIa inhibitors (abciximab, eptifibatide, and tirofiban) inhibit fibrinogen binding to activated GPIIb/IIIa receptors and subsequent agonist-induced platelet aggregation. These three GPIIb/IIIa inhibitors have distinct physical properties and have mechanisms of action other than inhibiting GPIIb/IIIa receptors. The pharmacodynamic and pharmacokinetic properties also differ between the agents (77). Platelet responsiveness to GPIIb/IIIa inhibitors has been assessed by multiple methods. The latter methods include (i) LTA to assess agonist-induced platelet aggregation (57,78), (ii) the Ultegra Rapid Platelet Function Analyzer point-of-care assay employing TRAP (thrombin receptor activator peptide) to stimulate platelet binding to fibrinogen-coated beads(79), and (iii) flow cytometry utilizing a phycoerythrin-conjugated D3 monoclonal antibody for fibrinogen to measure activated GPIIb/IIIa receptor occupancy (80). Since GPIIb/IIIa activation is critically dependent on calcium ions, ex vivo assays are often performed with Phe-Pro-Arg chloromethyl ketone (PPACK) as the anticoagulant.

Ex vivo studies indicated that GPIIb/IIIa inhibitors are associated with superior inhibition of agonist-induced platelet aggregation unlike aspirin and clopidogrel (57,78). In

Table 4 Studies Linking Aspirin Nonresponsiveness to Adverse Clinical Events

Investigators	n	Method	Clinical outcome
1. Lev et al. (59)	150 PCI	LTA (AA) RPFA-(cationic propyl gallate)	Elevated CK-MB
2. Mueller et al. (69)	100 PVD	Impedence aggregometry	An increase of 87% in incidence of reocclusion
3. Eikelboom et al. (44)	976 HOPE study	Urinary 11-dehydro-TxB_2	Increase in MI/stroke/death with increase in TxB_2
4. Gum et al. (70)	325 stable CAD	LTA (AA and ADP)	$3.12\times$ MI/stroke/death
5. Tantry et al. (71)	223 Elective PCI	LTA and TEG (AA)	Aspirin resistance = 0.4%, 1 patient with stent thrombosis
6. Chen et al. (72)	151 elective PCI	LTA (AA)	$2.9\times$ myonecrosis
7. Marcucci et al. (73)	146 MI/PCI	PFA-100 (coll/epi)	Increase in 1-yr MACE
8. Gianetti et al. (74)	175 SA/AMI	PFA-100 (coll/epi and ADP)	6-mo outcome, HR = 8.5
9. Foussas et al. (75)	612 SA/UA	PFA-100 (coll/epi)	1-yr CV death and rehospitalization, HR = 2.7
10. Borna et al. (76)	135 ACS	PFA-100 (coll/epi and ADP)	Aspirin resistance associated with STEMI

Abbreviations: LTA, light transmittance aggregometry; PVD, peripheral vascular disease; MI, myocardial infarction; Tx, thromboxane; AA, arachidonic acid; ADP, adenosine diphosphate; Coll, collagen; Epi, epinephrine; PFA, platelet function analyzer; RPFA, rapid platelet function analyzer; SA, stable angina, AMI, acute myocardial infarction; ACS, acute coronary syndrome; STEMI, ST-elevation myocardial infarction; HR, hazard ratio; MACE, major adverse cardiovascular events; HOPE, Heart Outcomes Prevention Evaluation; TEG, thrombelastography.

the COMPARE (comparision of platelet inhibition with abciximab, tirofiban and eptifibatide during percutaneous coronary intervention in acute coronary syndromes) study, distinct pharmacodynamic responses measured by ADP-induced platelet aggregation were observed with different GPIIb/IIIa inhibitors that were proposed to affect their relative efficacy in the treatment of acute coronary syndromes (78). Substantial interpatient variability and also variability in antiplatelet response to different GPIIb/IIIa inhibitors were observed in percutaneous coronary intervention (PCI) patients enrolled in the GOLD (AU-Assessing Ultegra) study. Platelet function inhibition $\geq 95\%$ at 10 minutes after the onset of therapy correlated with a significant reduction in the incidence of major adverse cardiovascular events (79). Distinct variability in receptor occupancy correlated with clinical outcomes in patients with ST-segment elevation myocardial infarction treated with eptifibatide and tenectplase in the INTEGRITI (integrilin and tenecteplase in acute myocardial infarction) substudy. Percent receptor occupancy was higher among patients with a patent coronary artery, those with TIMI (thrombolysis in myocardial infarction) myocardial perfusion grade 2/3, and those with complete ST-segment resolution at 60 minutes after onset of reperfusion therapy (80).

MEASUREMENT OF ADP-INDUCED PLATELET AGGREGATION TO ASSESS THROMBOTIC RISK

A Quantifiable and Modifiable Risk Factor

The ex vivo measurement of ADP-induced platelet aggregation as a risk factor with a potential threshold level has been explored in recent studies, since ADP is an important secondary agonist that plays a critical role in the amplification of platelet aggregation and finally occlusive thrombus formation. Preliminary evidence for a threshold of platelet reactivity, as measured by LTA after ADP stimulation that is associated with an increased risk of post-discharge ischemic events after PCI comes from three bodies of data: (*i*) A threshold of $\geq$50% periprocedural platelet aggregation in response to 20 μmol/L ADP has been associated with a greater likelihood of ischemic events during a six-month follow-up (56). (*ii*) A threshold level of $\geq$40% platelet aggregation in response to 20 μmol/L ADP has been associated with the occurrence of stent thrombosis (65). (*iii*) A threshold of $\geq$40% preprocedural platelet aggregation in response to 5 μmol/L ADP among patients receiving long-term clopidogrel and aspirin therapy before undergoing stenting was associated with the occurrence of ischemic events over the ensuing 12 months (58). These data suggest that the majority of ischemic events including stent thrombosis are associated in a stepwise fashion with a cutpoint of platelet function assessed by an ex vivo measurement (>40%) rather than in a continuous fashion.

These translational studies may provide a "testable" level of on-treatment platelet function to be studied in future investigations, similar to the international normalized ratio (INR) ranges established for warfarin therapy. Moreover, superior platelet inhibition associated with higher clopidogrel loading and maintenance doses and with new $P2Y_{12}$ receptor blockers strongly suggest that the aforementioned measurable or quantifiable risk factor (high on-treatment ADP-induced aggregation) is also a modifiable risk factor (5).

Limitations of Measuring Platelet Function in Isolation

The progressive development of multiple pathophysiological processes such as dysfunctional endothelium, inflammation, and hypercoagulability ultimately leads to the unstable plaque rupture, thrombus generation, and vessel occlusion. Thus, the evaluation of thrombotic risk by a single marker provides only partial indication of the complex underlying pathophysiology. Establishing a relation between measurable blood-borne factors to the patient's vulnerability for acute thrombosis is a major hurdle of ongoing investigations. The reliable characterization of mechanisms responsible for the transition from an asymptomatic disease state to the symptomatic disease state is an important step in the prevention of thrombotic cardiovascular disease (81). A multibiomarker profile may facilitate future studies of cardiovascular disease risk stratification. The proper assessment of antiplatelet responsiveness in this framework may enhance strategies directed at personalized antithrombotic treatment for the patient at greatest risk.

The majority of published studies to evaluate adverse ischemic event risk and the efficacy of antiplatelet therapy have measured platelet function in isolation. This approach may not provide the optimal assessment of risk. Therefore, in addition to measuring platelet function, the measurement of platelet-fibrin interactions together with assessment of thrombin generation kinetics may be more informative. In this regard, it was demonstrated that high maximum platelet-fibrin clot strength measured by thrombelastography was more strongly associated with the occurrence of six-month ischemic events following PCI than ADP-induced platelet aggregation (56).

In a recent study, patients with coronary artery disease who required stenting had markedly elevated levels of specific metalloproteinases (MMP-2 and MMP-9), metalloproteinase inhibitors (α2-macroglobulin and TIMP-1), inflammation markers [CRP (C-reactive protein), IL-6, IL-8, IL-10, RANTES, and TNF-β], endothelin, and PAI-1 compared with asymptomatic coronary artery disease patients. This study suggested that a specific biomarker profile may distinguish patients with progressive coronary atherosclerosis culminating in either elective or emergent PCI from the patients with quiescent disease (81). In another study, an important link between inflammation (as measured by CRP and IL-8), increased growth factor production (epidermal growth factor and vascular endothelial growth factor), and heightened thrombogenicity (platelet fibrin-clot strength and platelet aggregation) measured pre-procedurally in patients undergoing stenting was demonstrated (82).

Thrombin-induced platelet-fibrin clot strength, time to initial platelet-fibrin clot formation, CRP, prothrombotic factors (vWF and fibrinogen), and unstimulated and ADP-stimulated GPIIb/IIIa receptor expression were studied simultaneously in patients with asymptomatic stable CAD and in patients undergoing PCI for stable and unstable angina. There was an incremental increase in all parameters in unstable angina patients. A distinct pathophysiological state of heightened platelet function, hypercoagulability, and inflammation that marked the presence of unstable cardiovascular disease requiring intervention was demonstrated. Moreover, each stage was characterized by a distinct relationship between these parameters (83).

In summary, platelet function can be reliably quantified by a variety of established methods. Importantly, different assays of platelet function have been associated with thrombotic risk. The future challenge will be to establish the measurements that most closely predict adverse outcomes. A combination of assays that indicate the activity of multiple pathophysiological processes may enhance risk assessment. Diagnostic strategies may include measurements of the physical characteristics of the platelet-fibrin clot and biomarker profiling. Responsiveness to antiplatelet therapy will likely be quantified by measurements of platelet function with the potential establishment of a therapeutic window to guide antiplatelet dosing in the individual patient.

REFERENCES

1. Tantry US, Etherington E, Bliden KP, et al. Antiplatelet therapies; current strategies and future trends. Future Cardiol 2006; 2:343–366.
2. Mehta SR, Yusuf S, Peters RJ, et al. Clopidogrel in Unstable angina to prevent Recurrent Events trial (CURE) Investigators. Effects of pretreatment with clopidogrel and aspirin followed by long-term therapy in patients undergoing percutaneous coronary intervention: the PCI-CURE study. Lancet 2001; 358:527–533.
3. Wiviott SD, Braunwald E, McCabe CH, and the TRITON-TIMI 38 Investigators. Prasugrel versus clopidogrel in patients with acute coronary syndromes. N Engl J Med 2007; 357: 2001–2015.
4. Gurbel PA, Becker RC, Mann KG, et al. Platelet function monitoring in patients with coronary artery disease. J Am Coll Cardiol 2007; 50:1822–1834.
5. Gurbel PA. The relationship of platelet reactivity to the occurrence of post-stenting ischemic events: emergence of a new cardiovascular risk factor. Rev Cardiovasc Med 2006; 7(suppl 4):S20–S28.
6. Egbrink MG, Van Gestel MA, Broeders MA, et al. Regulation of microvascular thromboembolism in vivo. Microcirculation 2005; 12:287–300.
7. von Hundelshausen P, Weber C. Platelets as immune cells: bridging inflammation and cardiovascular disease. Circ Res 2007; 100:27–40.
8. Lindemann S, Krämer B, Seizer P, et al. Platelets, inflammation and atherosclerosis. J Thromb Haemost 2007; 1:(suppl 5): 203–211.
9. Ruggeri ZM, Mendolicchio GL. Adhesion mechanisms in platelet function. Circ Res 2007; 100:1673–1685.
10. Jackson SP. The growing complexity of platelet aggregation. Blood 2007; 109:5087–5095.
11. Reed GL. Platelet secretory mechanisms. Semin Thromb Hemost 2004; 30:441–450.
12. Zarbock A, Polanowska-Grabowska RK, Ley K. Platelet-neutrophil-interactions: linking hemostasis and inflammation. Blood Rev 2007; 21:99–111.

13. Huczek Z, Kochman J, Filipiak KJ, et al. Mean platelet volume on admission predicts impaired reperfusion and long-term mortality in acute myocardial infarction treated with primary percutaneous coronary intervention. J Am Coll Cardiol 2005; 46:284–290.

14. Zimmermann N, Kurt M, Wenk A, et al. Is cardiopulmonary bypass a reason for aspirin resistance after coronary artery bypass grafting?Eur J Cardiothorac Surg 2005; 27:606–610.

15. White MM, Krishnan R, Kueter TJ, et al. The use of the point of care Helena ICHOR/ Plateletworks and the Accumetrics Ultegra RPFA for assessment of platelet function with GPIIB-IIIa antagonists. J Thromb Thrombolysis 2004; 18:163–169.

16. Peterson P, Hayes TE, Arkin CF, et al. The preoperative bleeding time test lacks clinical benefit: College of American Pathologists' and American Society of Clinical Pathologists' position article. Arch Surg 1998; 133:134–139.

17. Schulz C, Schäfer A, Stolla M, et al. Chemokine fractalkine mediates leukocyte recruitment to inflammatory endothelial cells in flowing whole blood: a critical role for P-selectin expressed on activated platelets. Circulation 2007; 116:764–773.

18. Stevens JM. Platelet adhesion assays performed under static conditions. Methods Mol Biol 2004; 272:145–151.

19. Bockenstedt PL. Laboratory methods in hemostasis. In: Loscalzo J, Schafer AI, eds. Thrombosis and Hemorrhage. 2nd ed. Baltimore: Williams and Wilkins, 1998:517–580.

20. Polanowska-Grabowska R, Gear AR. Platelet adhesion assays under flow using matrix protein-coupled adhesion columns. Methods Mol Biol 2004; 272:153–163.

21. Stephens G, Gao D, Phillips DR, et al. Differential effects of anti-platelet drugs on thrombus formation and thrombus stability. J Thromb Haemost 2007; 5(suppl 2):O-W-034 (abstr).

22. Kulkarni S, Nesbitt WS, Dopheide SM, et al. Techniques to examine platelet adhesive interactions under flow. Methods Mol Biol 2004; 272:165–186.

23. Furie B, Furie BC. Thrombus formation in vivo. J Clin Invest 2005; 115:3355–3362.

24. Ergezen E, Appel M, Shah P, et al. Real-time monitoring of adhesion and aggregation of platelets using thickness shear mode (TSM) sensor. Biosens Bioelectron 2007; 23:575–582.

25. Arthur JF, Dunkley S, Andrews RK. Platelet glycoprotein VI-related clinical defects. Br J Haematol 2007; 139:363–372.

26. Ollikainen E, Mikkelsson J, Perola M, et al. Platelet membrane collagen receptor glycoprotein VI polymorphism is associated with coronary thrombosis and fatal myocardial infarction in middle-aged men. Atherosclerosis 2004; 176:95–99.

27. Michal F, Born GV. Effect of the rapid shape change of platelets on the transmission and scattering of light through plasma. Nat New Biol 1971; 231:220–222.

28. Ohlmann P, Hechler B, Cazenave JP, et al. Measurement and manipulation of [Ca2+]i in suspensions of platelets and cell cultures. Methods Mol Biol 2004; 273:229–250.

29. Ivandic BT, Giannitsis E, Schlick P, et al. Determination of aspirin responsiveness by use of whole blood platelet aggregometry. Clin Chem 2007; 53:614–619.

30. Smith JW, Steinhubl SR, Lincoff AM, et al. Rapid platelet-function assay: an automated and quantitative cartridge-based method. Circulation 1999; 99:620–625.

31. Harrison P. In vitro measurement of high-shear platelet adhesion and aggregation by the PFA-100. Methods Mol Biol 2004; 272:215–223.

32. Rao G, Placor PRT. Presented at XXIst Congress of International Society of Thrombosis and Haemostasis, Geneva, 2007.

33. Hobson AR, Agarwala RA, Swallow RA, et al. Thrombelastography: current clinical applications and its potential role in interventional cardiology. Platelets 2006; 17:509–518.

34. Savion N, Varon D. Impact—the cone and plate(let) analyzer: testing platelet function and anti-platelet drug response. Pathophysiol Haemost Thromb 2006; 35(1–2):83–88.

35. Kleiman N. Thrombovision approach to point-of-care platelet monitoring. Presented at XXIst Congress of International Society of Thropmbosis and Haemostasis, Geneva, 2007.

36. Higashi T, Isomoto A, Tyuma I, et al. Quantitative and continuous analysis of ATP release from blood platelets with firefly luciferase luminescence. Thromb Haemost 1985; 53:65–69.

37. Cox D, Seki J. Characterization of the binding of FK633 to the platelet fibrinogen receptor. Thromb Res 1998; 91:129–136.

38. Ginsberg MH, Frelinger AL, Lam SC, et al. Analysis of platelet aggregation disorders based on flow cytometric analysis of membrane glycoprotein IIb-IIIa with conformation-specific monoclonal antibodies. Blood 1990; 76:2017–2023.

39. Burger PC, Wagner DD. Platelet P-selectin facilitates atherosclerotic lesion development. Blood 2003; 101:2661–2666.

40. André P. P-selectin in haemostasis. Br J Haematol 2004; 126:298–306.

41. Ferroni P, Santilli F, Guadagni F, et al. Contribution of platelet-derived CD40 ligand to inflammation, thrombosis and neoangiogenesis. Curr Med Chem 2007; 14:2170–2180.

42. Michelson AD, Barnard MR, Krueger LA, et al. Circulating monocyte-platelet aggregates are a more sensitive marker of in vivo platelet activation than platelet surface P-selectin: studies in baboons, human coronary intervention, and human acute myocardial infarction. Circulation 2001; 104:1533–1537.

43. May AE, Langer H, Seizer P, et al. Platelet-leukocyte interactions in inflammation and atherothrombosis. Semin Thromb Hemost 2007; 33:123–127.

44. Eikelboom JW, Hirsh J, Weitz JI, et al. Aspirin-resistant thromboxane biosynthesis and the risk of myocardial infarction, stroke, or cardiovascular death in patients at high risk for cardiovascular events. Circulation 2002; 105:1650–1655.

45. Stuart MC, Reutelingsperger CP, Frederik PM. Binding of annexin V to bilayers with various phospholipid compositions using glass beads in a flow cytometer. Cytometry 1998; 33:414–419.

46. Hemker HC, Al Dieri R, Béguin S. Thrombin generation assays: accruing clinical relevance. Curr Opin Hematol 2004; 11:170–175.

47. Nomura S. Function and clinical significance of platelet-derived microparticles. Int J Hematol 2001; 74:397–404.

48. Morel O, Toti F, Hugel B, et al. Procoagulant microparticles: disrupting the vascular homeostasis equation? Arterioscler Thromb Vasc Biol 2006; 26:2594–2604.

49. Stellos K, Langer H, Daub K, et al. Platelet-derived stromal cell-derived factor-1 regulates adhesion and promotes differentiation of human CD34+ cells to endothelial progenitor cells. Circulation 2008; 117:206–215.

50. Gurbel PA, Tantry US. Aspirin and clopidogrel resistance: consideration and management. J Interv Cardiol 2006; 19(5):439–448.

51. Gurbel PA, Bliden KP, Hiatt BL, et al. Clopidogrel for coronary stenting: response variability, drug resistance, and the effect of pretreatment platelet reactivity. Circulation 2003; 107: 2908–2913.

52. Gurbel PA, Bliden KP, Hayes KM, et al. The relation of dosing to clopidogrel responsiveness and the incidence of high post-treatment platelet aggregation in patients undergoing coronary stenting. J Am Coll Cardiol 2005; 45:1392–1396.

53. Labarthe B, Théroux P, Angioï M, et al. Matching the evaluation of the clinical efficacy of clopidogrel to platelet function tests relevant to the biological properties of the drug. J Am Coll Cardiol 2005; 46:638–645.

54. Gurbel PA, Bliden KP, Etherington A, et al. Assessment of clopidogrel responsiveness: measurements of maximum platelet aggregation, final platelet aggregation and their correlation with vasodilator-stimulated phosphoprotein in resistant patients. Thromb Res 2007; 121:107–115.

55. Matetzky S, Shenkman B, Guetta V, et al. Clopidogrel resistance is associated with increased risk of recurrent atherothrombotic events in patients with acute myocardial infarction. Circulation 2004; 109:3171–3175.

56. Gurbel PA, Bliden KP, Guyer K, et al. Platelet reactivity in patients and recurrent events post-stenting: results of the PREPARE POST-STENTING Study. J Am Coll Cardiol 2005; 46: 1820–1826.

57. Gurbel PA, Bliden KP, Zaman KA, et al. Clopidogrel loading with eptifibatide to arrest the reactivity of platelets: results of the Clopidogrel Loading With Eptifibatide to Arrest the Reactivity of Platelets (CLEAR PLATELETS) study. Circulation 2005; 111:1153–1159.

58. Bliden KP, DiChiara J, Tantry US, et al. Increased risk in patients with high platelet aggregation receiving chronic clopidogrel therapy undergoing percutaneous coronary intervention: is the current antiplatelet therapy adequate? J Am Coll Cardiol 2007; 49:657–666.

59. Lev EI, Patel RT, Maresh KJ, et al. Aspirin and clopidogrel drug response in patients undergoing percutaneous coronary intervention: the role of dual drug resistance. J Am Coll Cardiol 2006; 47:27–33.

60. Cuisset T, Frere C, Quilici J, et al. High post-treatment platelet reactivity identified low-responders to dual antiplatelet therapy at increased risk of recurrent cardiovascular events after stenting for acute coronary syndrome. J Thromb Haemost 2006; 4:542–549.

61. Geisler T, Langer H, Wydymus M, et al. Low response to clopidogrel is associated with cardiovascular outcome after coronary stent implantation. Eur Heart J 2006; 27:2420–2425.

62. Hochholzer W, Trenk D, Bestehorn HP, et al. Impact of the degree of peri-interventional platelet inhibition after loading with clopidogrel on early clinical outcome of elective coronary stent placement. J Am Coll Cardiol 2006; 48:1742–1750.

63. Price JM, Wong GB, Valenica R, et al. Measurement of clopidogrel inhibition with a point-of-care assay identifies patients at risk for stent thrombosis after percutaneous coronary intervention. Am J Cardiol 2006; 98: 204M (abstr).

64. Barragan P, Bouvier JL, Roquebert PO, et al. Resistance to thienopyridines: clinical detection of coronary stent thrombosis by monitoring of vasodilator-stimulated phosphoprotein phosphorylation. Catheter Cardiovasc Interv 2003; 59:295–302.

65. Gurbel PA, Bliden KP, Samara W, et al. Clopidogrel effect on platelet reactivity in patients with stent thrombosis: results of the CREST Study. J Am Coll Cardiol 2005; 46:1827–1832.

66. Buonamici P, Marcucci R, Miglironi A, et al. Impact of platelet reactivity after clopidogrel administration on drug-eluting stent thrombosis. J Am Coll Cardiol 2007; 49:2312–2317.

67. Gurbel PA, Bliden KP, DiChiara J, et al. Evaluation of dose-related effects of aspirin on platelet function: results from the Aspirin-Induced Platelet Effect (ASPECT) study. Circulation 2007; 115:3156–3164.

68. Dichiara J, Bliden KP, Tantry US, et al. Platelet function measured by VerifyNow identifies generalized high platelet reactivity in aspirin treated patients. Platelets 2007; 18:414–423.

69. Mueller MR, Salat A, Stangl P, et al. Variable platelet response to low-dose ASA and the risk of limb deterioration in patients submitted to peripheral arterial angioplasty. Thromb Haemost 1997; 78:1003–1007.

70. Gum PA, Kottke-Marchant K, Welsh PA, et al. A prospective, blinded determination of the natural history of aspirin resistance among stable patients with cardiovascular disease. J Am Coll Cardiol 2003; 41:961–965.

71. Tantry US, Bliden KP, Gurbel PA. Overestimation of platelet aspirin resistance detection by thrombelastograph platelet mapping and validation by conventional aggregometry using arachidonic acid stimulation. J Am Coll Cardiol 2005; 46:1705–1709.

72. Chen W-H, Lee P-Y, Ng W, et al. Aspirin resistance is associated with a high incidence of myonecrosis after non-urgent percutaneous coronary intervention despite clopidogrel pretreatment. J Am Coll Cardiol 2004; 43:1122–1126.

73. Marcucci R, Paniccia R, Antonucci E, et al. Usefulness of aspirin resistance after percutaneous coronary intervention for acute myocardial infarction in predicting one-year major adverse coronary events. Am J Cardiol 2006; 98:1156–1159.

74. Gianetti J, Parri MS, Sbrana S, et al. Platelet activation predicts recurrent ischemic events after percutaneous coronary angioplasty: a 6 months prospective study. Thromb Res 2006; 118:487–493.

75. Foussas SG, Zairis MN, Patsourakos NG, et al. The impact of oral antiplatelet responsiveness on the long-term prognosis after coronary stenting. Am Heart J 2007; 154:676–681.

76. Borna C, Lazarowski E, van Heusden C, et al. Resistance to aspirin is increased by ST-elevation myocardial infarction and correlates with adenosine diphosphate levels. Thromb J 2005; 3:10.

77. Topol EJ, Byzova TV, Plow EF. Platelet GPIIb-IIIa blockers. Lancet 1999; 353:227–231.

78. Batchelor WB, Tolleson TR, Huang Y, et al. Randomized COMparison of platelet inhibition with abciximab, tiRofiban and eptifibatide during percutaneous coronary intervention in acute coronary syndromes: the COMPARE trial. Comparison Of Measurements of Platelet aggregation with Aggrastat, Reopro, and Eptifibatide. Circulation 2002; 106:1470–1476.

79. Steinhubl SR, Talley JD, Braden GA, et al. Point-of-care measured platelet inhibition correlates with a reduced risk of an adverse cardiac event after percutaneous coronary intervention: results of the GOLD (AU-Assessing Ultegra) multicenter study. Circulation 2001; 103:2572–2578.

80. Gibson CM, Jennings LK, Murphy SA, et al. INTEGRITI Study Group. Association between platelet receptor occupancy after eptifibatide (integrilin) therapy and patency, myocardial perfusion, and ST-segment resolution among patients with ST-segment-elevation myocardial infarction: an INTEGRITI (Integrilin and Tenecteplase in Acute Myocardial Infarction) substudy. Circulation 2004; 110:679–684.

81. Gurbel PA, Kreutz RP, Bliden KP, et al. Biomarker analysis by fluorokine multianalyte profiling distinguishes patients requiring intervention from patients with long-term quiescent coronary artery disease: a potential approach to identify atherosclerotic disease progression. Am Heart J 2007; 155:56–61.

82. Gurbel PA, Bliden KP, Kreutz KP, et al. Relation of platelet-fibrin clot strength, platelet reactivity, inflammation and growth factor release to thrombotic risk in patients undergoing stenting: a biomarker profile correlating vulnerable blood to vulnerable patient. J Thromb Haemost 2007; 5(suppl 2):P-W-683 (abstr).

83. Tantry US, Bliden KP, Kreutz RP, et al. Transition to an unstable coronary syndrome is marked by hypercoaguability, platelet activation, heightened platelet reactivity, and inflammation: results of the thrombotic risk progression (TRIP) study. J Am Coll Cardiol 2007; 49: 196A (abstr).

25

Intravenous Glycoprotein IIb/IIIa Antagonists

Jason N. Katz and Robert A. Harrington
Division of Cardiovascular Medicine, Duke University Medical Center and Duke Clinical Research Institute, Durham, North Carolina, U.S.A.

INTRODUCTION

One of the greatest advances in the care of patients with myocardial infarction (MI) has been recognition of the pivotal role of platelets in the pathophysiology of coronary thrombosis. Not only are platelets influential in thrombus propagation during acute coronary syndromes (ACS), but they are also key contributors to the enhanced thrombogenicity associated with the implantation of intracoronary stents. Consequently, platelets have become the primary targets for pharmacologic therapy in patients with cardiac ischemic syndromes.

One of the key mediators of platelet-specific adhesion is the glycoprotein (GP) IIb/IIIa receptor, which enhances platelet aggregation by facilitating binding between dimeric adhesion molecules such as fibrinogen and von Willebrands factor (vWF) when activated (1). Preclinical study suggests that occupation of approximately 80% of the activable receptors could result in clinically relevant inhibition of platelet-dependent thrombus formation (2). This notion led to the development of a variety of novel GP IIb/IIIa receptor antagonist compounds, which have now become an accepted and integral part of the cardiovascular clinician's antithrombotic armamentarium. In this chapter, we review the currently available intravenous GP IIb/IIIa inhibitors, discuss the evidence supporting their use, describe safety issues and potential complications of therapy, and suggest future directions of clinical investigation.

THE GLYCOPROTEIN IIb/IIIa INHIBITORS

Abciximab

Abciximab is a chimeric Fab fragment of a monoclonal antibody with high affinity for the GP IIb/IIIa receptor (3). Compared with the other inhibitors, abciximab is the largest agent with a molecular weight of approximately 50,000 daltons. The binding sites of abciximab are located at the β-chain of the GP IIb/IIIa receptor, but this inhibitor is too large to directly block the ligand-binding pocket. Instead, it blankets the receptor, causing a steric hindrance to ligand access.

Abciximab has the strongest affinity for the GP IIb/IIIa receptor and dissociates at a significantly slower rate than the other GP IIb/IIIa antagonists. Unbound drug is rapidly cleared from the plasma by proteolytic degradation, resulting in a very short plasma half-life (i.e., several minutes). The biologic half-life of abciximab ranges from 8 to 24 hours, depending on the patient. As a result, some number of GP IIb/IIIa receptors may still be occupied by drug up to two weeks after discontinuation of drug infusion. In the event of bleeding, the antithrombotic effects of abciximab cannot be rapidly reversed by discontinuing therapy; instead, the effects can be significantly diminished by exogenous platelet transfusion.

Eptifibatide

Eptifibatide is a typical competitive antagonist of the GP IIb/IIIa receptor, with its antiplatelet effects being concentration dependent. Unlike abciximab, it is a synthetic small-molecule inhibitor with an approximate molecular weight of 800 daltons. As a small molecule, it fits directly into the Arg-Gly-Asp binding pocket of the GP IIb/IIIa receptor, directly competing with the binding of ligands such as fibrinogen and vWF (4). The stoichiometry of the drug is >100:1 (100 molecules of drug to each receptor to achieve full GP IIb/IIIa blockade) compared with a ratio of 1.5:1 seen with the large-molecule antagonist abciximab (5). Eptifibatide rapidly dissociates from its receptor, is cleared by the kidneys largely as active drug, and has a plasma half-life of approximately 1.5 to 2.5 hours. The return of hemostatic-capable platelet function is largely dependent on clearance of the drug from the plasma compartment by the kidneys. Reversing the antithrombotic effects requires cessation of drug infusion. In the setting of normal renal function, normal hemostasis returns within 15 to 30 minutes after drug discontinuation (4); however, unlike abciximab, the platelet inhibitory effect of eptifibatide is not significantly influenced by platelet transfusion. This is due to the inability of exogenous platelets to overcome the robust stoichiometry of drug to receptor.

Tirofiban

Tirofiban is a small-molecule (molecular weight approximately 500 daltons) non-peptide mimetic that, like eptifibatide, is a competitive inhibitor of the GP IIb/IIIa receptor that has high specificity but relatively low affinity (4). It is also excreted by the kidneys, predominantly as unchanged drug. It rapidly dissociates from the receptor and has a biologic half-life of 1.5 to 2.5 hours. Restoration of hemostasis is best achieved by discontinuing the drug infusion.

Table 1 compares clinical characteristics of the commonly used intravenous GP IIb/IIIa receptor antagonists.

GLYCOPROTEIN IIb/IIIa INHIBITORS IN PERCUTANEOUS CORONARY INTERVENTIONS

The GP IIb/IIIa inhibitors have been studied extensively as adjunctive pharmacotherapy during percutaneous coronary intervention (PCI). Table 2 highlights the study design, methods, and outcomes for the major clinical trials in this therapeutic area.

Table 1 Clinical Characteristics of the Intravenous Glycoprotein IIb/IIIa Inhibitors

Inhibitor	Molecular weight	Mechanism of action	Stoichiometry[a]	Biologic half-life	Clearance	Proposed reversal of antithrombotic effects
Abciximab	~50,000 Da	Fab fragment of monoclonal antibody blankets receptor causing steric hindrance to ligands	1.5:1	8–24 hr	Unbound drug cleared by proteolytic degradation; slow dissociation from receptor	Platelet transfusion, FFP/ cryoprecipitate, FEIBA, vWF, rFVIIa, hemodialysis
Eptifibatide	~800 Da	Fits directly into Arg-Gly-Asp binding pocket to compete with ligand binding	100:1	1.5–2.5 hr	Rapid dissociation from receptor; predominant renal clearance	Discontinue infusion, FFP/ cryoprecipitate, vWF
Tirofiban	~500 Da	Nonpeptide mimetic; competitive inhibitor	100:1	1.5–2.5 hr	Rapid dissociation from receptor; predominant renal clearance	Discontinue infusion, FFP/ cryoprecipitate, vWF

[a]Molecules of drug: receptor to achieve complete GP IIb/IIIa blockade.
Abbreviations: FFP, fresh frozen plasma; FEIBA, factor 8 inhibitor bypassing activity; vWF, von Willebrand factor; rFVIIa, recombinant factor 7a.

Table 2 Major Trials of Intravenous GP IIb/IIIa Inhibitors for PCI

Trial	Year	N	Clinical setting	Trial design	Outcomes	Notes
EPIC (6)	1994	2099	PTCA or atherectomy	Abciximab vs. placebo	Abciximab reduced occurrence of death, MI, or need for urgent intervention by 35%	Benefit in major ischemic event reduction or elective revascularization maintained at 6-mo and 1 yr
EPILOG (7)	1997	2792	Elective or urgent PTCA	Abciximab + standard-dose UFH vs. abciximab + low-dose UFH vs. placebo + standard-dose UFH	Significant improvement in 30-day composite EP of death or MI in abciximab-treated patients	Benefit maintained at 6-mo and 1-yr follow-up
IMPACT-II (8)	1997	4010	Elective, urgent, or emergent PCI	Eptifibatide 135 µg/kg bolus, then 0.5 µg/kg/min infusion vs. eptifibatide 135 µg/kg bolus, then 0.75 µg/kg/min infusion vs. placebo	25–30% relative risk reduction in low-dose eptifibatide group for primary EP of death, MI, unplanned revascularization, or stent placement for abrupt closure	EP benefit not maintained at 6 mo
EPISTENT (9)	1998	2399	Elective or urgent stenting and PTCA	Stenting + abciximab vs. stenting + placebo vs. PTCA + abciximab	52% reduction in risk of primary ischemic EP in patients treated with stent + abciximab compared with placebo	
ESPRIT (10)	2000	2064	Elective PCI	Eptifibatide vs. placebo	Eptifibatide reduced primary EP (48-hour death, MI, urgent revascularization, or bailout GP IIb/IIIa therapy) by 37% and secondary EP (death, MI, or urgent TVR) at 30 days	Benefits maintained at 1 yr, and similar for all subgroups
TARGET (11)	2001	4809	Non-emergent PCI	Tirofiban vs. abciximab	At 30 days, abciximab found to be significantly superior to tirofiban in composite endpoint (death, MI, or need for urgent revascularization)	Observed benefit largely due to reductions in MI with abciximab; tirofiban dosing questioned

Trial	Year	N	Population	Comparison	Results	Notes
ISAR-REACT (12)	2004	2159	Stable, native-vessel CAD undergoing elective PCI	Abciximab + UFH vs. placebo + UFH	No difference in incidence of death, MI, or urgent TVR at 30 days	Clopidogrel pretreatment
ISAR-SWEET (13)	2004	701	Diabetic patients with stable CAD undergoing elective PCI	Abciximab + UFH vs. placebo + UFH	Reduction in angiographic restenosis with abciximab treatment at 7-mo median follow-up; no significant difference in death or MI at 1 yr	Clopidogrel pretreatment
ADVANCE (14)	2004	202	PCI (56% with ACS)	High-dose tirofiban vs. placebo	6-mo primary EP of death, MI, TVR, or bailout GP IIb/IIIa use significantly less frequent with tirofiban (20% vs. 35% for placebo)	Subgroup analysis showed no benefit for stable angina or in nondiabetics
ISAR-REACT 2 (15)	2006	2022	NSTE-ACS undergoing PCI	Abciximab + UFH vs. placebo + UFH	25% relative risk reduction in primary composite EP (death, MI, or urgent TVR) at 30 days in abciximab-treated patients	Clopidogrel pretreatment

Abbreviations: ACS, acute coronary syndromes; NSTE, non–ST segment elevation; CAD, coronary artery disease; EP, endpoint; GP, glycoprotein; MI, myocardial infarction; PCI, percutaneous coronary intervention; PTCA, percutaneous transluminal coronary angioplasty; TVR, target vessel revascularization; UFH, unfractionated heparin.

In the EPIC (evaluation of 7E3 for the prevention of ischemic complications) (6) trial, 2099 high-risk ACS patients undergoing either percutaneous transluminal coronary angioplasty (PTCA) or atherectomy were randomly assigned to receive placebo or abciximab therapy. Abciximab was given as a bolus of 0.25 mg/kg, followed by a 12-hour continuous infusion at 10 μg/min, and was found to reduce the occurrence of death, MI, or need for urgent intervention (repeat PTCA, stenting, intra-aortic balloon counterpulsation, or surgical revascularization) by 35%. At six months, there was a 23% reduction in the incidence of major ischemic events or elective revascularization in the abciximab group compared with placebo (27% vs. 35%, $p = 0.001$) (16), and this benefit was maintained at three years (17).

In EPILOG (evaluation in PTCA to improve long-term outcome with abciximab GP IIb/IIIa blockade) (7), nearly 3000 patients who underwent elective or urgent PTCA were randomly assigned to receive either abciximab with standard-dose, weight-adjusted heparin (100 units/kg initial bolus), abciximab with low-dose, weight-adjusted heparin (70 units/kg), or placebo with standard-dose, weight-adjusted heparin. The trial was terminated prematurely after showing a significant improvement in the composite endpoint of death or MI at 30 days in abciximab-treated patients. The benefit of abciximab was observed in both high- and low-risk individuals and was maintained at six-month and one-year follow-up (18). At one year, the incidence of the primary composite endpoint was 9.5% in the abciximab with standard-dose, weight-adjusted heparin group ($p < 0.001$) and 9.6% in the abciximab with low-dose, weight-adjusted heparin group ($p < 0.001$) versus 16.1% in the placebo with standard-dose, weight-adjusted heparin group. Each of the components of the composite endpoint was reduced to a similar extent.

An important finding among EPILOG patients was the lack of major bleeding differences between treatment groups. In fact, the lowest rates of hemorrhagic complications and red cell transfusions occurred in patients receiving abciximab with low-dose heparin (7). These findings suggested that, with lower doses of unfractionated heparin (UFH), the benefits of GP IIb/IIIa inhibition could be maintained while attenuating the bleeding risks seen in previous studies.

The influence of abciximab on outcomes in patients undergoing PCI was further assessed as part of the EPISTENT (evaluation of platelet inhibition in stenting) trial (9). In the cohort of patients who received an intracoronary stent during PCI, there was a 52% reduction in the risk of the primary ischemic endpoint (death, MI, or need for urgent revascularization) in the abciximab group compared with placebo. Furthermore, patients receiving balloon angioplasty plus abciximab had a 36% lower primary endpoint compared with the stent plus placebo group, highlighting the significant independent influence of GP IIb/IIIa antagonism. As the field of interventional cardiology advanced to incorporating more stenting in practice, EPISTENT was the first study to demonstrate the importance of maintaining an aggressive antiplatelet strategy (through GP IIb/IIIa receptor inhibition) regardless of the interventional method employed in revascularization.

There is also a robust body of evidence that supports the use of the small-molecule GP IIb/IIIa inhibitors during PCI. In the IMPACT-II (integrilin to minimize platelet aggregation and coronary thrombosis-II) trial (8), 4010 patients scheduled for elective, urgent, or emergent PCI were randomly assigned to receive placebo or adjunctive eptifibatide therapy in addition to aspirin and heparin. Patients received eptifibatide as a bolus of 135 μg/kg, followed by a continuous infusion of either 0.5 or 0.75 μg/kg/min. The primary endpoint, a composite of death, MI, or urgent target vessel revascularization (TVR) at 30 days, occurred in 11.4% of placebo-treated patients compared with 9.2% in the 135/0.5 eptifibatide group ($p = 0.06$) and 9.9% in the 135/0.75 eptifibatide group ($p = 0.22$). Using a treatment-received analysis, the 135/0.5 eptifibatide regimen resulted in a significant reduction in the composite endpoint (9.1% vs. 11.6%, $p = 0.035$), without a significant increase in bleeding events.

In ESPRIT (enhanced suppression of the platelet IIb/IIIa receptor with integrilin therapy) (10), 2064 patients were randomly assigned to receive placebo or eptifibatide immediately before elective PCI. The study was prematurely terminated because eptifibatide was found to reduce the primary composite endpoint (48-hour rate of death, MI, urgent revascularization, or need for bailout GP IIb/IIIa antagonist therapy) by 37% (6.6% vs. 10.5% for placebo, $p = 0.0015$), and significantly reduced the secondary composite endpoint (death, MI, or urgent TVR at 30 days) (6.8% vs. 10.5% for placebo, $p = 0.0034$) as well. Each of the individual components of the primary endpoint was reduced by eptifibatide therapy, and the benefit of GP IIb/IIIa antagonism was seen in all prespecified subgroups. Further analysis of the ESPRIT trial suggested that eptifibatide did not reduce the incidence of angiographic complications such as coronary dissection, distal embolization, or abrupt closure (19). However, the benefits of eptifibatide on reducing the risk of the major clinical outcomes were maintained at one-year follow-up, with a significantly reduced incidence of death or MI [8% vs. 12.4%, hazard ratio (HR) 0.83, $p = 0.001$] and a reduction in the combined endpoint of death, MI, or TVR (17.5% vs. 22%, HR 0.63, $p = 0.007$) (20).

The role of tirofiban among patients undergoing percutaneous revascularization was first studied in the randomized, double-blind, placebo-controlled RESTORE (randomized efficacy study of tirofiban for outcomes and restenosis) trial (21). RESTORE included 2139 patients with ACS who underwent coronary intervention within 72 hours of hospital presentation. Tirofiban was given as a 10 µg/kg intravenous bolus over three minutes, followed by a continuous infusion of 0.15 µg/kg/min for 36 hours. At 30 days, the primary composite endpoint of death, MI, angioplasty failure requiring surgical revascularization or unplanned stenting, or recurrent ischemia requiring repeat PTCA tended to be less frequent in the tirofiban arm compared with placebo (10.3% vs. 12.2%), resulting in a nonsignificant 16% relative risk (RR) reduction ($p = 0.160$). When only urgent or emergent repeat revascularization procedures were included in the endpoint analysis, tirofiban administration was associated with a nearly significant 24% RR reduction over placebo ($p = 0.052$).

The influence of tirofiban on outcomes with PCI was also studied in the ADVANCE (additive value of tirofiban administered with the high-dose bolus in prevention of ischemic complications during high-risk coronary angioplasty) trial (14). Of the 202 patients enrolled, over half underwent PCI in the setting of an ACS. At six months, the primary composite endpoint of death, MI, TVR, or bailout GP IIb/IIIa use was significantly less frequent with tirofiban (20% vs. 35% with placebo, $p = 0.01$). Subgroup analysis showed the greatest benefit in those with ACS and in those with diabetes mellitus.

Glycoprotein IIb/IIIa Antagonists and Clopidogrel Therapy for Percutaneous Coronary Intervention

In the more contemporary era of aggressive dual oral antiplatelet therapy, GP IIb/IIIa antagonism has also been studied in patients undergoing PCI. ISAR-REACT (intra-coronary stenting and antithrombotic regimen: rapid early action for coronary treatment) (12), ISAR-REACT 2 (15), and ISAR-SWEET (intracoronary stenting and antithrombotic regimen: abciximab a superior way to eliminate elevated thrombotic risk in diabetics) (13) all evaluated abciximab therapy in patients undergoing PCI following clopidogrel pretreatment. In ISAR-REACT, 2159 patients with stable, native-vessel CAD were randomly assigned to receive either abciximab plus heparin (70 units/kg initial bolus) or placebo plus heparin (100–140 units/kg initial bolus). At 30 days, there was no difference in the incidence of death, MI, or urgent TVR (4% in each group) (12). However, among patients with non–ST segment elevation (NSTE) undergoing PCI, ISAR-REACT 2 demonstrated a 25% RR reduction in the primary composite endpoint of death, MI, or urgent TVR at 30 days in those receiving abciximab ($p = 0.03$) (15). In an exclusively diabetic population (29% considered insulin dependent), angiographic follow-up at a median of seven months demonstrated reduced rates of restenosis among abciximab-treated patients (29% vs. 38% with placebo, $p = 0.01$). However, at one year, there was no significant difference in the incidence of death or MI (8.3% vs. 8.6% with placebo, $p = 0.91$) in this population (13).

To better define the influence of GP IIb/IIIa antagonism during revascularization, Anderson and others conducted a meta-analysis of eight contemporary PCI trials (22). Over 5000 patients were randomly assigned to a regimen of abciximab bolus and infusion therapy in addition to standard of care. A control cohort of 4136 patients randomly assigned to receive conventional therapy alone comprised the comparison group for analysis. Investigators found a significant mortality benefit with abciximab [HR 0.71, 95% confidence interval (CI) 0.57–0.89, $p = 0.003$]. An absolute reduction in mortality was estimated to be 0.5% at 30 days, 0.7% through six months, 0.9% at one year, and 1.8% at three years. Multivariable regression suggested that patients with advanced cardiovascular disease may derive the greatest mortality benefit from GP IIb/IIIa inhibition.

In aggregate, most clinical trials of GP IIb/IIIa antagonism in PCI support the use of adjunctive abciximab or eptifibatide therapy. While studies comparing the use of tirofiban with these other agents will be described in more detail later in this chapter, there is considerably less evidence to support the administration of tirofiban in PCI-treated patients.

Glycoprotein IIb/IIIa Inhibitors in Non–ST Segment Elevation Acute Coronary Syndromes

There has been substantial investigation into the use of GP IIb/IIIa inhibitors among patients with ACS. While there are compelling data to advocate the use of GP IIb/IIIa antagonism to improve ischemic outcomes in these individuals, clinical trial results have led to many questions regarding the optimal use of these agents. Table 3 shows design features and outcomes for the major clinical trials assessing GP IIb/IIIa inhibitors in ACS.

The previously described EPIC trial assessed abciximab therapy in high-risk ACS patients undergoing percutaneous coronary revascularization. While there were significant reductions in death, ischemic events, and the need for revascularization among abciximab-treated patients up to three years after randomization, post hoc analysis suggested that the greatest benefit of GP IIb/IIIa inhibition was seen in those with either refractory angina or evolving MI (17).

The benefits of abciximab in NSTE-ACS were further validated in the CAPTURE (chimeric 7E3 antiplatelet therapy in unstable angina refractory to standard treatment) study (23). Designed to assess whether abciximab, given 18 to 24 hours prior to PTCA, could improve outcomes in NSTE-ACS patients refractory to standard medical therapy, this trial found that the primary endpoint of death, MI, or urgent revascularization was significantly reduced in abciximab-treated individuals at 30 days (11.3% vs. 15.9%, $p = 0.012$). The benefit of abciximab was primarily due to a lower rate of both preprocedural and periprocedural MI associated with PTCA, and was seen predominantly in patients

Table 3 Major Trials of Intravenous Glycoprotein IIb/IIIa Inhibitors for NSTE-ACS

Trial	Year	N	Clinical setting	Trial design	Outcomes	Notes
CAPTURE (23)	1997	1265	NSTE-ACS patients with ischemia refractory to UFH, nitrates, and aspirin	Abciximab vs. placebo	Primary EP (death, MI, or urgent revascularization) lower in abciximab group at 30 days	Subgroup analysis found no benefit in troponin-negative patients
RESTORE (21)	1997	2139	ACS undergoing PCI within 72 hr	Tirofiban vs. placebo	Primary composite EP (death, MI, angioplasty failure requiring CABG or stenting, or recurrent ischemia requiring PTCA) significantly reduced by tirofiban at 30 days	No persistent difference at 6 mo
PRISM (24)	1998	3232	Unstable angina or NSTEMI	Tirofiban vs. UFH	Primary composite EP (death, MI, or refractory ischemia) reduced with tirofiban at 48 hr; no difference at 30 days	Subgroup analysis suggested greatest benefit in troponin-positive patients
PRISM-PLUS (25)	1998	1915	Unstable angina or non-Q-wave MI	Tirofiban vs. UFH vs. tirofiban + UFH	At 7 days, composite EP (death, MI, or refractory ischemia) significantly lower in tirofiban + UFH group; benefit remained significant at 30 days and 6 mo	Excess mortality seen in tirofiban-alone group
PURSUIT (26)	1998	11,000	Unstable angina or NSTEMI	Eptifibatide bolus + 1.3 µg/kg/min infusion vs. eptifibatide bolus + 2.0 µg/kg/min infusion vs. placebo	Eptifibatide associated with significantly lower 30-day event rate of death or nonfatal MI; benefit seen at 96 hr and persisted through 30 days	Subgroup analysis suggested no benefit in women
GUSTO IV-ACS (27)	2001	7800	Medically managed unstable angina patients	Abciximab bolus + 24-hr infusion vs. abciximab bolus + 48-hr infusion vs. placebo	Primary EP (death or MI) same in all 3 groups at 30 days	Lack of benefit persisted at 1 yr

Abbreviations: ACS, acute coronary syndromes; CABG, coronary artery bypass graft; EP, endpoint; MI, myocardial infarction; NSTE, non-ST segment elevation; ACS, acute coronary syndromes; NSTEMI, non-ST segment elevation MI; PCI, percutaneous coronary intervention; PTCA, percutaneous transluminal coronary angioplasty; UFH, unfractionated heparin.

with complex angiographic lesions. Abciximab was also found to decrease the likelihood of recurrent ischemia, as well as the total ischemic burden (24).

The role of tirofiban in the management of ACS was evaluated in both the PRISM (platelet receptor inhibition in ischemic syndrome management) (25) and PRISM-PLUS (platelet receptor inhibition in ischemic syndrome management in patients limited by unstable signs and symptoms) (28) trials. PRISM enrolled 3232 patients with unstable angina or NSTEMI treated with a predominantly conservative strategy. In this study, patients were randomly assigned to receive either heparin or tirofiban (0.6 µg/kg/min for 30 minutes, followed by 0.15 µg/kg/min for 48 hours). The primary composite endpoint (death, MI, or refractory ischemia) at 48 hours was significantly reduced with tirofiban (3.8% vs. 5.6% with heparin alone, $p = 0.01$), but was not statistically different at 30 days. There was, however, a significant reduction in overall mortality in the tirofiban cohort (2.3% vs. 3.6% with heparin alone, $p = 0.02$). To further define the optimal dosing strategy for tirofiban in ACS and to examine the influence of combined GP IIb/IIIa antagonism with anticoagulation, the PRISM-PLUS trial was subsequently conducted. A total of 1915 patients with either unstable angina or non-Q-wave MI were randomly assigned to receive either tirofiban, heparin, or both the agents. Tirofiban was given at a dose of 0.4 µg/kg/min for 30 minutes, then 0.1 µg/kg/min for at least 48 hours (maximum 108 hours, median duration 71 hours). The tirofiban-alone arm was prematurely discontinued because of an excess in mortality (4.6% vs. 1.1% for heparin alone, $p = 0.012$)—an unexpected finding that has since been quite influential in formulating current consensus advocating combined antiplatelet and anticoagulant therapies for patients with ACS. At seven days, the frequency of the composite endpoint in PRISM-PLUS (death, MI, or refractory ischemia) was significantly lower in the tirofiban plus heparin group compared with heparin alone (12.9% vs. 17.9%, $p = 0.004$), primarily because of a reduction in MI. The benefit of tirofiban plus heparin with respect to the primary endpoint remained significant at 30 days and six months, regardless of whether or not the patients were managed with a conservative or an early invasive approach. Subsequent analysis of the PRISM-PLUS data suggested that five independent risk factors—age >65 years, prior coronary artery bypass graft (CABG) surgery, antecedent aspirin use, antecedent β-blocker use, and ST segment depression at admission—could identify patients who would receive the greatest potential benefit from GP IIb/IIIa inhibition with tirofiban. Validating these results in a cohort of patients from the PRISM trial, investigators found no benefit in individuals with zero to one risk factor, but did find a 16% absolute risk reduction in death or ischemic events in those with at least four risk factors, suggesting that perhaps GP IIb/IIIa antagonism might best be reserved for the highest risk group of patients (29).

The role of eptifibatide in patients with ACS was examined in the PURSUIT (platelet GP IIb/IIIa in unstable angina: receptor suppression using integrilin therapy) trial (26). In this study, approximately 11,000 patients with unstable angina or NSTEMI were randomly assigned to receive eptifibatide or placebo in addition to standard of care with aspirin and heparin therapy. Eptifibatide was associated with a significantly lower 30-day event rate of death or nonfatal MI (14.2% vs. 15.7% for placebo, $p = 0.04$), and its effect was similar and consistent in all prespecified subgroups, with the exception of women. The benefit of GP IIb/IIIa antagonism was similar between those who underwent early PCI and those who were medically managed (30). Post hoc subgroup analysis suggested that the greatest benefit of eptifibatide was seen in those with unstable angina, particularly those who underwent early intervention (31).

More recently, GUSTO [global utilization of streptokinase and tissue plasminogen activator (tPA) for occluded coronary arteries] IV–ACS evaluated the role of abciximab in 7800 medically managed patients with unstable angina or NSTEMI (27). Patients were included if they had ischemic symptoms and either a positive cardiac troponin test or electrocardiographic ST segment depression. Patients were excluded if early angiography was planned as part of their initial management strategy or if they were to undergo planned revascularization within 30 days. Those enrolled in the trial were randomly assigned to receive abciximab bolus plus 24-hour infusion, abciximab bolus plus 48-hour infusion, or placebo. The primary endpoint of death or MI at 30 days was no different among the three groups (8.2% vs. 9.1% vs. 8.0%, respectively) (27), and this lack of benefit persisted at one year (32). Overall mortality was also similar for the three groups, implying no benefit with abciximab as initial therapy for medically managed patients without ST segment elevation.

Risk Stratification for Glycoprotein IIb/IIIa Antagonism in Acute Coronary Syndromes

While the majority of trials seem to support the use of GP IIb/IIIa inhibitors in ACS patients, conflicting data such as those seen in the GUSTO IV–ACS trial and the overall modest effect in broad patient populations have led many to question their routine use in the care of these patients. As a consequence, investigators have begun to search for patient-specific subgroups as a way to identify those who might consistently reap the greatest benefit from GP IIb/IIIa antagonism.

A review of the CAPTURE data suggested that patients with elevated cardiac troponins preferentially benefited from abciximab therapy compared with placebo (33). Similarly, in the PRISM trial, among the 28% of patients with elevated troponin I at admission, tirofiban significantly reduced the 30-day risk of death (1.6% vs. 6.2% for heparin, $p = 0.004$) and MI (2.7% vs. 6.8% for heparin, $p = 0.01$) regardless of whether or not an invasive approach was used. On the other hand, among trial participants with normal cardiac troponins, no benefit of tirofiban was seen with regard to death or MI at 30 days (34).

Newby et al. also showed that the treatment benefit of the GP IIb/IIIa inhibitor lamifiban in patients with NSTE-ACS was limited almost exclusively to individuals with an elevated troponin T, reducing the primary composite endpoint (death, MI, or severe recurrent ischemia at 30 days) from 19.4% to 11.0% ($p = 0.01$) in a prespecified subgroup analysis of the PARAGON-B (platelet IIb/IIIa antagonism for the reduction of acute coronary syndrome events in a global organization network) (35) clinical trial (36). Boersma et al. subsequently conducted a meta-analysis of all major randomized clinical trials assessing the impact of GP IIb/IIIa inhibitors in ACS (37). Investigators evaluated six trials (PRISM, PURSUIT, PRISM-PLUS, PARAGON-A (38), PARAGON-B, and GUSTO IV–ACS), which had enrolled over 31,000 patients. At 30 days, there was a 9% reduction in the odds of death or MI seen with antagonism of the GP IIb/IIIa receptor compared with placebo or control [odds ratio (OR) 0.91, 95% CI 0.84–0.98, $p = 0.015$]. Additionally, the absolute treatment benefits of these agents were greatest in high-risk patient cohorts, including those with elevated cardiac troponins (37). Among the 45% of patients with a positive cardiac troponin, GP IIb/IIIa inhibitors were associated with a 15% reduction in the odds of 30-day death or MI compared with placebo or control (OR 0.85, 95% CI 0.71–1.03).

Diabetic patients also appear to uniquely benefit from GP IIb/IIIa inhibition. Roffi et al. conducted a recent meta-analysis of the same six trials as Boersma et al., focusing specifically on the diabetic population (39). Among 6458 diabetic patients, platelet GP IIb/IIIa antagonism was associated with a significant mortality reduction at 30 days (4.6% vs. 6.2% with placebo, $p = 0.007$). Conversely, among 23,072 nondiabetic patients, there was no apparent survival benefit. However, it should be noted that, unlike Boersma's study, this was a subgroup analysis of pooled trial-level data; therefore, these observations should be considered exploratory only and warrant future prospective validation.

Questions still remain regarding the optimal use of GP IIb/IIIa inhibitors in ACS patients. Some of these will be addressed in more detail later in this chapter. The totality of the evidence suggests that the use of these agents, especially in high-risk patients and those with elevated cardiac troponins, is reasonable as adjunctive therapy for the treatment of patients presenting to the hospital with ACS. The current American College of Cardiology/American Heart Association (ACC/AHA) guidelines for the management of patients with unstable angina or NSTEMI reflect this consensus, giving the use of upstream intravenous GP IIb/IIIa inhibitors a class I recommendation when an initial invasive management approach is utilized (class Ia for abciximab, class Ib for eptifibatide or tirofiban), and a class Ib recommendation for upstream administration of eptifibatide or tirofiban when a conservative strategy is employed (class III for abciximab) (40).

Glycoprotein IIb/IIIa Inhibitors in ST Segment Elevation Myocardial Infarction

Another area of active investigation concerns the use of GP IIb/IIIa inhibitors for patients with ST segment elevation MI (STEMI). The majority of randomized clinical trials comparing intravenous GP IIb/IIIa inhibitors with placebo have evaluated abciximab therapy in STEMI, and are shown in Table 4.

Glycoprotein IIb/IIIa Inhibitors and Fibrinolysis for ST Segment Elevation Myocardial Infarction

The IMPACT-AMI (integrilin to minimize platelet aggregation and coronary thrombosis in acute MI) trial was conducted to determine the effect of eptifibatide on coronary arterial patency when used in conjunction with the fibrinolytic agent alteplase (tPA) (45). A total of 132 patients with acute MI receiving accelerated alteplase, heparin, and aspirin were randomly assigned to receive a bolus and continuous infusion of one of six doses of eptifibatide or placebo. GP IIb/IIIa inhibition was initiated within 30 minutes of fibrinolytic administration and continued for a total of 24 hours. Compared with placebo, the high-dose eptifibatide group (180 µg/kg bolus followed by 0.75 µg/kg/min infusion) had more complete 90-minute reperfusion than placebo [66% vs. 39% thrombolysis in MI (TIMI) 3 flow], and shorter mean time to electrocardiographic ST segment recovery (65 vs. 116 minutes for placebo). The composite in-hospital event rate, which included death, reinfarction, revascularization, heart failure, hypertension, and stroke, was equivalent in all groups.

The added benefit of abciximab with fibrinolytic therapy was also studied as part of the TIMI 14 trial (46). In this study, 888 patients with STEMI were randomly assigned to receive front-loaded alteplase (100 mg bolus), streptokinase plus abciximab, low-dose alteplase (15 mg bolus, followed by 35–50 mg over 30–60 minutes) plus abciximab, or abciximab alone. The primary endpoint of the incidence of TIMI 3 flow at 90 minutes was seen in 32% of those treated with abciximab alone, 34% to 46% of those receiving streptokinase plus abciximab, 61% to 76% of those treated with reduced-dose alteplase plus abciximab, and 57% of those receiving alteplase alone. Subsequent analysis of the TIMI 14 data suggested that the reduced-dose alteplase plus abciximab regimen resulted in improved microvascular reperfusion, as indicated by a higher rate of complete ($\geq 70\%$) ST segment resolution at 90 minutes (59% vs. 37% for alteplase alone, $p < 0.0001$) (50). Despite reducing the rate of angiographically evident thrombus and residual stenosis, the combination of abciximab and alteplase did not increase the incidence of major hemorrhage compared with alteplase alone (7% vs. 6%) (51).

Table 4 Major Trials of Intravenous Glycoprotein IIb/IIIa Inhibitors for STEMI

Trial	Year	N	Clinical setting	Trial design	Outcomes	Notes
RAPPORT (41)	1998	483	Primary PCI	Abciximab vs. placebo	At 7 and 30 days, abciximab had significant reduction in primary EP (death, MI, or any TVR)	No difference in primary EP at 6 mo
ISAR-2 (42)	2000	401	Primary PCI	Abciximab + low-dose UFH vs. standard-dose UFH	At 30 days, primary composite EP (death, reinfarction, or TLR) was lower with abciximab; not significant at 1 yr	No difference in angiographic restenosis at 6 mo or composite EP at 1 yr
CADILLAC (43)	2002	2082	Primary PCI	PTCA alone vs. PTCA + abciximab vs. stent alone vs. stent + abciximab	At 6 mo, composite EP (death, reinfarction, disabling stroke, or ischemia-driven TVR) significantly lower with stenting +/− abciximab	Difference in EP primarily due to lower ischemia-driven TVR
ADMIRAL (44)	2001	300	Primary PCI	Abciximab vs. placebo	Primary EP of death, recurrent MI, or urgent TVR lower in abciximab group at 30 days and 6 mo	Subgroup analysis indicated more marked benefit with "early" abciximab
IMPACT-AMI (45)	1997	132	Thrombolytic therapy	6 dosing regimens of eptifibatide + accelerated alteplase	Highest-dose eptifibatide group (180 µg/kg bolus + 0.75 µg/kg/min infusion) with greater TIMI 3 flow at 90 min	Composite in-hospital event rate equivalent in all groups
TIMI 14 (46)	1999	888	Thrombolytic therapy	Front-loaded alteplase vs. streptokinase + abciximab vs. low-dose alteplase + abciximab vs. abciximab alone	Incidence of TIMI 3 flow at 90 min greatest with alteplase + abciximab therapy	Similar findings in 2nd phase of study with reteplase + abciximab

(Continued)

Table 4 Major Trials of Intravenous Glycoprotein IIb/IIIa Inhibitors for STEMI (*Continued*)

Trial	Year	N	Clinical setting	Trial design	Outcomes	Notes
ASSENT-3 (47)	2001	6095	Thrombolytic therapy	Full-dose tenecteplase + enoxaparin vs. half-dose tenecteplase + low-dose UFH + abciximab vs. full-dose tenecteplase + standard-dose UFH	Primary EP (30-day mortality, in-hospital reinfarction, or in-hospital refractory ischemia) less common in the full-dose lytic + enoxaparin and half-dose lytic + UFH + abciximab groups	Lytic + abciximab had no survival advantage compared with full-dose lytic regimen at 30 days
GUSTO V (48)	2002	16,588	Thrombolytic therapy	Half-dose reteplase + abciximab vs. standard-dose reteplase	No difference in mortality at 30 days	No benefit at 1 yr and increased intracranial hemorrhage with combination therapy in those >75 yr old
INTEGRITI (49)	2003	180	Thrombolytic therapy	Full-dose tenecteplase vs. half-dose tenecteplase + eptifibatide	Combination therapy associated with nonsignificant trend toward improved arterial patency	Greater major hemorrhage with combination therapy

Abbreviations: EP, endpoint; MI, myocardial infarction; PCI, percutaneous coronary intervention; PTCA, percutaneous transluminal coronary angioplasty; STEMI, ST segment elevation MI; RAPPORT (ReoPro and primary PTCA organization and randomized trial) TLR, target lesion revascularization; TVR, target vessel revascularization; UFH, unfractionated heparin.

However, in large-scale trials evaluating the clinical benefits of abciximab with thrombolytic therapy, both GUSTO V (48) and ASSENT (assessment of the safety and efficacy of a new thrombolytic regimen)-3 (47) trials yielded mixed results. In GUSTO V, nearly 17,000 patients were randomly assigned to receive half-dose reteplase plus abciximab or standard-dose reteplase alone. There was no difference in 30-day mortality (5.6% vs. 5.9% for standard-dose reteplase, $p = 0.43$) (48) and no mortality benefit at one year (8.4% for both groups) (52). While rates of intracranial hemorrhage and nonfatal stroke were similar among the two groups, combination therapy was associated with a significant increase in intracranial bleeding in those over the age of 75 (53).

In ASSENT-3, 6095 patients with STEMI were randomly assigned to receive one of three regimens: full-dose tenecteplase and enoxaparin for up to seven days, half-dose tenecteplase with weight-adjusted, low-dose UFH and abciximab for 12 hours, or full-dose tenecteplase with weight-adjusted UFH for 48 hours. The primary endpoint of 30-day mortality, in-hospital reinfarction, or in-hospital refractory ischemia was less common in the first two groups (11.4% and 11.1% vs. 15.4% in the full-dose tenecteplase plus UFH group, $p = 0.002$), but combination therapy with a GP IIb/IIIa inhibitor and tenecteplase had no survival advantage at 30 days. Furthermore, rates of bleeding and transfusion were significantly increased (47). There were significantly more major bleeding events ($p = 0.002$) and more transfusions ($p = 0.001$) in the abciximab group, especially among diabetic patients and those >75 years of age, whose rates of major bleeding complications were increased threefold compared with the UFH group.

The ability of eptifibatide, in conjunction with alteplase, to improve TIMI flow in STEMI was studied in the INTRO-AMI (integrilin and reduced dose of thrombolytic in acute MI) trial (54). In the dose-finding phase of the trial enrolling 344 patients, the greatest incidence of TIMI 3 flow at angiography was seen in patients treated with a double-bolus eptifibatide (180 µg/kg followed by 90 µg/kg) regimen, followed by a 1.33 µg/kg/min infusion along with 50 mg of alteplase. The second phase of the trial, a dose confirmation evaluation, found that a double-bolus eptifibatide regimen followed by 48-hour infusion of 2 µg/kg/min along with 50 mg of alteplase was associated with improved quality and speed of reperfusion compared with standard alteplase alone. It should be noted that 30-day mortality was no different between the combined eptifibatide plus alteplase groups and the alteplase-only group (54).

Eptifibatide was also studied in association with reduced-dose tenecteplase during the INTEGRITI (integrilin and tenecteplase in acute MI) trial (49). In this study, 249 patients were randomly assigned to receive either full-dose tenecteplase or half-dose tenecteplase plus eptifibatide (180 µg/kg bolus, followed by 2 µg/kg/min infusion plus a repeat 180 µg/kg bolus 10 minutes later). When compared with tenecteplase alone, combination therapy was associated with a nonsignificant trend toward improved TIMI 3 flow (59% vs. 49%, $p = 0.15$), coronary arterial patency (85% vs. 77%, $p = 0.17$), and electrocardiographic ST segment resolution (71% vs. 61%, $p = 0.08$), with a trend toward increased major hemorrhage (7.6% vs. 2.5% with tenecteplase alone, $p = 0.14$) (49).

Glycoprotein IIb/IIIa Inhibitors and Primary Percutaneous Coronary Intervention for ST Segment Elevation Myocardial Infarction

One of the earliest studies of abciximab in STEMI was the RAPPORT (ReoPro and primary PTCA organization and randomized trial) trial, in which 483 patients were randomly assigned to receive either abciximab or placebo prior to coronary intervention (41). The primary composite endpoint of death, MI, and any TVR was significantly reduced at 7 and 30 days in the abciximab group compared with placebo (5.8% vs. 11.2%, $p = 0.03$), as was the incidence of unplanned bailout stenting (11.9% vs. 20.4% for placebo, $p = 0.008$). The beneficial effects of GP IIb/IIIa antagonism were entirely due to a reduction in the need for urgent revascularization. At six months, there was no difference in the two groups with respect to the primary endpoint and no difference in the incidence of TIMI 3 flow or elective repeat revascularization rates (41). Similarly, in ADMIRAL (abciximab before direct angioplasty and stenting in MI regarding acute and long-term follow-up), 300 patients with STEMI were randomly assigned to receive abciximab or placebo prior to primary PTCA or stenting (44). Immediately following the procedure and at six-month follow-up, TIMI 3 flow rates were more frequently seen in the abciximab group (95% vs. 86.7% for placebo, $p = 0.04$). The primary endpoint of death, recurrent MI, or urgent TVR was also lower in the abciximab group at both the 30-day (6% vs. 14.6% for placebo, $p = 0.01$) and six-month (7.4% vs. 16% for placebo, $p = 0.02$) time points. At the three-year follow-up, abciximab therapy was associated with a nonsignificant trend toward improvements in all-cause mortality (9.1% vs. 12.2% for placebo, $p = 0.36$) and death or reinfarction (11.8% vs. 16.9% for placebo, $p = 0.20$) (55).

Corroborating the findings of ADMIRAL, the ISAR-2 (intracoronary stenting and antithrombotic regimen-2) trial enrolled 401 patients undergoing primary stenting for STEMI who were randomly assigned to receive either standard-dose heparin or reduced-dose heparin plus abciximab (42). At 30 days, the incidence of the composite endpoint of death, reinfarction, or target lesion revascularization was significantly lower with abciximab (5% vs. 10.5% for heparin, $p = 0.038$). However, despite an absolute reduction in the composite endpoint with abciximab of 5.7% at one year, the results did not reach statistical significance. There was also no demonstrable difference in late lumen loss or angiographic restenosis at one year (43).

The CADILLAC (controlled abciximab and device investigation to lower late angioplasty complications) trial examined the impact of platelet GP IIb/IIIa inhibition on outcomes in acute MI patients treated with either PTCA or coronary stenting (56). The primary endpoint—a composite of death, reinfarction, disabling stroke, and ischemia-driven TVR—occurred in 20% of patients after PTCA, 16.5% after PTCA plus abciximab, 11.5% after stenting, and 10.2% after stenting plus abciximab ($p < 0.001$). This endpoint reduction was driven almost entirely by differences in rates of TVR, and there were no significant differences among the groups in the rates of death, stroke, or reinfarction.

Finally, in a meta-analysis of randomized trials comparing GP IIb/IIIa inhibition with placebo or control therapy in primary PCI for acute MI, Kandzari et al. demonstrated significant reductions in early adverse ischemic events with abciximab—a clinical benefit that was maintained up to six months after revascularization (56). In aggregate, these findings underscore the current guidelines, which support the use of adjunctive GP IIb/IIIa antagonism (class IIa for abciximab, class IIb for eptifibatide or tirofiban) prior to primary PCI (57).

Glycoprotein IIb/IIIa Inhibitors and Facilitated Percutaneous Coronary Intervention for ST Segment Elevation Myocardial Infarction

The results of ADMIRAL led to questions regarding the optimal timing of GP IIb/IIIa antagonism in primary PCI. Among ADMIRAL enrollees, a small subset of patients (26%) received early (ambulance or emergency department) GP IIb/IIIa antagonism. The benefit of abciximab in these patients was significantly greater at 30 days (RR 0.12 vs. 0.67) and at six months (RR 0.11 vs. 0.69) compared with those receiving drug just prior to intervention, suggesting a possible role for facilitated PCI in the management of STEMI patients (55).

Several other studies have contributed to our understanding of GP IIb/IIIa inhibitor use in facilitated PCI. TIGER-PA (tirofiban given in the emergency room before primary angioplasty) was a pilot study of 100 patients undergoing primary PCI randomly assigned to receive tirofiban in the emergency department or later in the catheterization laboratory (58). Early therapy was associated with significant improvements in several angiographic variables prior to PCI, including greater TIMI 3 flow rates (32% vs. 10%, $p = 0.007$) and lower corrected TIMI frame counts, but was underpowered to detect differences in bleeding or other concrete clinical outcomes. The On-TIME (ongoing tirofiban in MI evaluation) trial compared early versus late administration of tirofiban in a cohort of 507 patients with STEMI (59). The primary endpoint of TIMI 3 flow at angiography was not statistically significant between the two groups, although there was a significant difference in combined TIMI 2 and TIMI 3 flow (43% vs. 34%, $p = 0.04$), as well as the incidence of visualized thrombus at angiography (60% vs. 73%, $p = 0.002$). More robust data from larger clinical trials are needed before making any definitive statements about the efficacy of this pharmacologic approach, although a recent meta-analysis of randomized trials comparing facilitated with primary PCI for STEMI suggested that facilitated PCI was associated with greater rates of death (OR 1.38, 95% CI 1.01–1.87), nonfatal reinfarction (OR 1.71, 95% CI 1.16–2.51), urgent TVR (OR 2.39, 95% CI 1.23–4.66), and a particularly dramatic increase in hemorrhagic complications when employed in conjunction with fibrinolytic therapy (60).

In a meta-analysis of over 27,000 patients from 11 trials of adjunctive abciximab in STEMI, De Luca et al. found that abciximab was associated with a significant reduction in both short-term (2.4% vs. 3.4%, $p = 0.047$) and long-term (4.4% vs. 6.2%, $p = 0.01$) mortality compared with control (usually placebo) in patients in whom PCI was performed (61). However, no mortality benefit was seen in those treated with fibrinolysis. Abciximab was also associated with a significant reduction in 30-day reinfarction in all trials (2.1% vs. 3.3%, $p < 0.001$). Furthermore, abciximab therapy did not result in an increased risk of intracranial bleeding overall, but was associated with an increased risk of major bleeding complications when combined with fibrinolytic therapy (5.2% vs. 3.1%, $p < 0.001$) (61).

As a result of these studies and the De Luca meta-analysis, current recommendations advocate the use of periprocedural GP IIb/IIIa inhibitors for primary PCI. The most rigorous study has been with abciximab, although recent observational data suggest that the smaller-molecule agents may be more commonly used in practice (62). There are very limited data to support GP IIb/IIIa antagonism as an adjunct to fibrinolytic therapy, and safety issues related to severe bleeding still predominate. Consequently, GP IIb/IIIa inhibitors are not currently recommended when employing a fibrinolysis-based regimen for the treatment of STEMI (57). This strategy is given a class IIb indication for the prevention of reinfarction or complications of STEMI in select patients (anterior MI, age <75 years, and no risk factors for bleeding), though special mention is given to the lack of a demonstrable survival benefit attributed to this therapeutic approach (57).

HEAD-TO-HEAD COMPARISONS OF GLYCOPROTEIN IIb/IIIa INHIBITORS

Despite a considerable body of literature investigating the pharmacologic effects of GP IIb/IIIa inhibitors, there are very few studies prospectively comparing these agents. TARGET (do tirofiban and ReoPro give similar efficacy trial), enrolling 4809 patients who underwent non-emergent PCI, was designed to test for noninferiority of tirofiban compared with abciximab (11). At 30 days, abciximab was found to be significantly superior to tirofiban in the composite endpoint of death, MI, or need for urgent revascularization (6% vs. 7.6%, $p = 0.038$). The observed benefit was largely due to a significant reduction in MI (5.4% vs. 6.9%, $p = 0.04$) with abciximab, but improvements were also consistent across all of the endpoint components. Furthermore, the benefit of abciximab over tirofiban was preserved, without further accentuation or attenuation, up to six months of follow-up (63). In COMPARE (comparison of measurements of platelet aggregation with Aggrastat, ReoPro, and eptifibatide) (64), tirofiban produced significantly less platelet inhibition at 30 minutes than either abciximab or eptifibatide—a finding that some consider a plausible mechanistic explanation for the TARGET observations. However, critics argue that the tirofiban dosing used in these comparative studies was suboptimal, thus biasing the results.

TIMING OF GLYCOPROTEIN IIb/IIIa ANTAGONISM IN NON–ST SEGMENT ELEVATION ACUTE CORONARY SYNDROMES

The appropriate timing and implementation of GP IIb/IIIa inhibition in patients with NSTE-ACS remains another area of significant controversy. In over 65,000 U.S. patients, in whom data was collected as part of the CRUSADE (can rapid risk stratification of unstable angina patients suppress adverse outcomes with early implementation of the ACC/AHA guidelines) registry, only 35.5% of eligible individuals received early GP IIb/IIIa inhibitor therapy (65). Among those receiving a GP IIb/IIIa inhibitor, 32% of patients received early upstream therapy in the emergency department, 33% received therapy in the coronary care unit, 32% received drug in the cardiac catheterization laboratory, and 3% received therapy elsewhere. In this large, observational study, early GP IIb/IIIa antagonism resulted in a 2% absolute risk reduction in overall mortality (65).

Similarly, in the National Registry of Myocardial Infarction (NRMI) 4, only a quarter of eligible patients with NSTE-ACS received early GP IIb/IIIa inhibition within 24 hours of presentation. GP IIb/IIIa inhibitor therapy was associated with a 6.3% absolute reduction of in-hospital mortality, with a calculated number needed to treat (NNT) of 16 patients (66).

The ACUITY (acute catheterization and urgent intervention triage strategy) timing trial was the first prospective study to address the timing of GP IIb/IIIa antagonism (67). Among a cohort of patients with moderate- to high-risk ACS, individuals were randomly assigned to receive either routine upstream initiation of tirofiban or eptifibatide or deferred, selective use of GP IIb/IIIa inhibitor therapy. The composite ischemic endpoint at 30 days occurred in 7.9% of patients assigned to a deferred strategy compared with 7.1% of patients in the upstream therapy group (RR 1.12, 95% CI 0.97–1.29). The results did not meet criteria for noninferiority, though there was a numerical trend in regard to ischemia reduction favoring the upstream administration of GP IIb/IIIa antagonists. The deferred strategy, however, resulted in a significant decrease in 30-day rates of major bleeding (4.9% vs. 6.1%, $p < 0.001$).

While the ACC/AHA currently recommends the use of either early, upstream GP IIb/IIIa inhibition or clopidogrel therapy in lower-risk, troponin-negative patients, and both agents as upstream treatments for higher-risk, troponin-positive patients (class I recommendation) (40), timing of GP IIb/IIIa antagonism remains a controversial issue. To help bring clarity to this management dilemma, the EARLY-ACS (early GP IIb/IIIa inhibition in NSTE-ACS) trial was designed (68). With a target enrollment of over 10,000 patients, this prospective, randomized, double-blind study will be the largest to evaluate the utility of early GP IIb/IIIa antagonism in patients with high-risk NSTE-ACS in whom an invasive approach is planned. Patients will be randomly assigned to receive either early eptifibatide therapy or placebo (with provisional eptifibatide in the cardiac catheterization laboratory), beginning at least one calendar day prior to planned PCI. The primary efficacy endpoint is a 96-hour composite of all-cause mortality, nonfatal MI, recurrent ischemia requiring urgent revascularization, or need for thrombotic bailout with GP IIb/IIIa inhibition during PCI.

COMPLICATIONS OF GLYCOPROTEIN IIb/IIIa INHIBITION

Bleeding

Part of the challenge in maximizing the antithrombotic actions of any potential pharmacotherapeutic agent is balancing the anti-ischemic benefits with the risk of hemorrhage. Because of marked platelet inhibition, increased bleeding can be seen with any antagonists of the GP IIb/IIIa receptor, although rigorous investigation suggests that these agents do not significantly increase the risk of life-threatening bleeding relative to UFH alone. Karvouni et al. performed a meta-analysis of 19 randomized, placebo-controlled trials ($n = 20,137$) that included patients who received intravenous GP IIb/IIIa inhibitors in the setting of PCI (69). With regard to safety endpoints, major bleeding was significantly increased only in trials where heparin infusion was continued following intervention (RR 1.70, 95% CI 1.36–2.14). There was no excess bleeding, however, when heparin was discontinued (RR 1.02, 95% CI 0.85–1.24). In patients with ACS, Boersma's meta-analysis found that major bleeding complications were indeed increased by GP IIb/IIIa inhibition (2.4% vs. 1.4%, $p < 0.0001$), but intracranial bleeding was not (0.09% vs. 0.06%, $p = 0.40$) (37). In the STEMI population, a pooled analysis of results from 11 trials ($n = 27,115$) showed that abciximab therapy did not result in an increased risk of intracranial hemorrhage (0.61% vs. 0.62%, $p = 0.62$). Furthermore, major bleeding complications were not increased in patients treated with primary angioplasty, but were more common in individuals treated with a regimen that included fibrinolysis (5.2% vs. 3.1%, $p < 0.001$) (61).

Impact of Dosing on Risk of Bleeding

Recently, the impact of dosing errors on bleeding events with GP IIb/IIIa inhibitors has received increasing attention. PROTECT-TIMI (randomized trial to evaluate the relative protection against post-PCI microvascular dysfunction and post-PCI ischemia among antiplatelet and antithrombotic agents: thrombolysis in MI) 30 showed that, within the more controlled environment of clinical trials, GP IIb/IIIa dosing errors were quite common (70). Among patients who would have required a dose adjustment of eptifibatide based on a reduction in creatinine clearance, nearly half received an excessive dose. Furthermore, those who were given an increased dose had a 20% rate of major or minor bleeding and a 26.7% rate of transfusion compared with a 2.9% rate of bleeding and a 4% transfusion rate in patients who did not require dose adjustment.

Alexander et al. performed a prospective, observational analysis of 30,136 patients from the CRUSADE registry who had high-risk NSTE-ACS (71). Nearly 27% of patients received at least one dose of the GP IIb/IIIa inhibitor outside of the recommended dosing range. In this analysis, investigators found that factors associated with excessive dosing included advanced age, female sex, renal dysfunction, and low body weight.

In aggregate, these observations should emphasize the need to properly dose intravenous GP IIb/IIIa agents. In particular, careful attention should be paid to the renal function of treated patients, since several of these agents are cleared predominantly by the kidneys. It is also important to remember that dose adjustment differs even among the GP IIb/IIIa inhibitors. For the small-molecule agents, the dosage of tirofiban should be reduced when creatinine clearance falls below 30 mL/min, whereas eptifibatide is reduced for creatinine clearance values <50 mL/min.

Thrombocytopenia

The results of therapeutic trials using GP IIb/IIIa inhibitors have shown that all three commonly used agents are associated with the occurrence of thrombocytopenia (72). The incidence of clinically recognized thrombocytopenia ranges from 0.5% to 5%. In most instances, the decrease in platelet count occurs without harm to the patient. However, there are some data to suggest that the development of thrombocytopenia may be a marker for unfavorable outcomes (73,74). Most authorities suspect that thrombocytopenia is an immune-mediated process that typically occurs shortly after GP IIb/IIIa administration (75). With abciximab, however, this process can occur up to a week after therapy because abciximab remains bound to circulating platelets for several days and can have prolonged antibody stimulation (76). Furthermore, results of a registry assessing outcomes of abciximab readministration suggested an increased risk of thrombocytopenia with subsequent use (77).

The diagnostic and therapeutic management of GP IIb/IIIa inhibitor-treated patients with thrombocytopenia is very challenging because several other agents commonly used to combat ischemia can result in decreases in platelet counts. Both aspirin and clopidogrel can reduce platelet numbers, and heparin-induced thrombocytopenia (HIT) can complicate therapy as well. In addition, while GP IIb/IIa inhibitor-induced thrombocytopenia rarely results in significant hemorrhage, decreases in platelet count may prompt modification of a patient's antithrombotic regimen, facilitating worse ischemic outcomes.

In a pooled analysis of eight placebo-controlled, randomized trials, Dasgupta et al. reviewed the clinical course of patients with thrombocytopenia in the setting of ACS or PCI who were treated with GP IIb/IIIa antagonism (78). Abciximab increased mild thrombocytopenia (platelet count 90,000 to 100,000/µL) compared with placebo (4.2% vs. 2.0%, $p < 0.001$), and significantly increased the incidence of severe thrombocytopenia (platelet count <50,000/µL) (1.0% vs. 0.4% for placebo, OR 2.48, $p = 0.01$). On the other hand, the small-molecule GP IIb/IIIa inhibitors did not increase either mild or severe thrombocytopenia compared with placebo. It should be noted that no major bleeding events were reported in any of the patients with severe or even profound thrombocytopenia (platelet count <20,000/µL) (78).

Nonetheless, it is important for practicing clinicians to be vigilant in monitoring platelet counts, especially during the first 24 hours of therapy. Alternative causes of thrombocytopenia, including disseminated intravascular coagulopathy (DIC), HIT, and pseudothrombocytopenia, should be carefully considered when platelet counts suddenly decrease. Pseudothrombocytopenia, for instance, may account for over one-third of cases of low platelet counts in patients treated with abciximab in the setting of PCI (79). Despite being a benign clinical finding that has not been associated with bleeding, stroke, transfusion, or ischemia, failure to recognize this condition may result in unnecessary discontinuation of potentially life-saving therapies.

While no formal protocol exists to guide physicians in the management of drug-related thrombocytopenia, the presence of bleeding and/or hemodynamic instability should first be ascertained. If severe or life-threatening bleeding occurs, all antithrombotic therapy should be immediately discontinued, platelets should be transfused if <20,000/μL, and consideration should be given to packed red blood cell transfusion and/or replacement therapy (e.g., fresh frozen plasma, cryoprecipitate, or vWF). If no bleeding results from thrombocytopenia, one should consider discontinuing GP IIb/IIIa inhibitor therapy for platelet counts that drop below 50,000/μL. For situations of low to moderate, hemodynamically stable bleeding, one should consider discontinuing GP IIb/IIIa receptor antagonists for platelet counts <100,000/μL, red blood cell transfusion if clinically indicated, and platelet transfusion for counts <10 to 20,000/μL. Careful monitoring of blood counts is also imperative in the management of these patients.

Monitoring Platelet Inhibition with Glycoprotein IIb/IIIa Antagonists

In an effort to maximize the antiplatelet effects of the GP IIb/IIIa inhibitors while minimizing bleeding complications, recent attention has focused on the possibility of dosage targeting for individual patients. Unfortunately, there are currently no standard methods for patient-specific dose selection and titration, largely because of the lack of a universal point-of-care assay with established efficacy. Platelet function testing has been studied in coronary interventions supported by adjunctive GP IIb/IIIa antagonism (2), and has been shown to predict the incidence of major adverse cardiac events in abciximab-treated patients (80). While platelet function testing may have a future in tailoring pharmacotherapy, especially for individuals at increased risk for bleeding events, the requisite clinical trials correlating the degree of platelet inhibition with hard clinical endpoints have yet to be performed.

FUTURE DIRECTIONS AND CONCLUSIONS

While it is clear that the GP IIb/IIIa inhibitors have become a useful pharmacologic tool for the management of patients with acute cardiac ischemia and those undergoing PCI, many questions remain regarding the optimal use of these agents and the optimal candidates for treatment.

As previously mentioned, controversy remains regarding the appropriate timing of GP IIb/IIIa antagonism in the setting of NSTE-ACS. Clinicians are still divided between those who utilize upstream therapy and those who prefer to wait until the time of PCI before initiating a GP IIb/IIIa inhibitor. The results of EARLY-ACS should help to clarify the most appropriate timing for GP IIb/IIIa antagonism, as well as clopidogrel therapy, in patients with NSTE-ACS (68).

A meta-analysis by Montalescot et al. suggested that early administration of GP IIb/IIIa inhibitors in STEMI appeared to improve coronary arterial patency with favorable trends in clinical outcomes (81). However, these findings did not translate into clear clinical benefit in the one large, randomized trial that addressed this question. Initial reports from the FINESSE (facilitated intervention with enhanced reperfusion speed to stop events) trial, examining the influence of GP IIb/IIIa inhibitor therapy for facilitated PCI in acute STEMI, showed that early abciximab administration did not reduce ischemic endpoints compared with treatment immediately prior to angioplasty (82). Further investigation regarding the use of GP IIb/IIIa antagonists for facilitated PCI is needed.

There has also been considerable interest in bolus-only GP IIb/IIIa regimens. Early clinical series have suggested that single-bolus administration of these agents for patients undergoing PCI may result in lower in-hospital death, MI, repeat revascularization, and bleeding events (83,84). Deibele et al. have even investigated the use of single-dose intracoronary eptifibatide in a NSTE-ACS population undergoing PCI (85). While preliminary data appear promising, more robust prospective study is certainly warranted.

Finally, more recent data on the use of bivalirudin in both ACS and STEMI patients has called into question both the efficacy and safety of GP IIb/IIIa antagonism in conjunction with direct thrombin inhibition. The ACUITY trial, in patients with moderate- or high-risk NSTE-ACS, showed that bivalirudin alone was noninferior to the combination of heparin and a GP IIb/IIIa inhibitor in the composite ischemic endpoint of death, MI, or unplanned revascularization for ischemia (7.8% vs. 7.3% for heparin plus a GP IIb/IIIa inhibitor, $p = 0.32$). Furthermore, compared with the heparin and GP IIb/IIIa combination, bivalirudin resulted in significantly reduced rates of major bleeding (3.0% vs. 5.7%, $p < 0.001$) (86). In addition, the recently published HORIZONS-AMI (harmonizing outcomes with revascularization and stents in acute MI) study demonstrated that bivalirudin alone was associated with a significant reduction in 30-day major bleeding (4.9% vs. 8.3%, $p < 0.0001$) compared with heparin and GP IIb/IIIa inhibition, as well as a significant reduction in net adverse clinical events (87). There was, however, an early hazard of stent thrombosis when GP IIb/IIIa inhibitor therapy was omitted in favor of bivalirudin monotherapy. Thus far the ACC/AHA advocates either a thienopyridine or a GP IIb/IIIa antagonist as concomitant therapy when bivalirudin is employed for NSTE-ACS patients (40), and it remains to be seen how the results of HORIZONS-AMI will be applied to future iterations of the STEMI guidelines.

Though there is much left to learn about these potent antiplatelet agents, the GP IIb/IIIa inhibitors are now commonly used to supplement the care of ischemic patients. The most recent ACC/AHA guidelines give the use of this therapy a class I indication for NSTE-ACS patients undergoing PCI (in the absence of concomitant clopidogrel treatment) (40,57,88). With concomitant clopidogrel administration, the early (pre-angiography) use of GP IIb/IIIa inhibitors has a class IIa indication, and a class I indication for post-angiography use. On the other hand, eptifibatide and tirofiban are considered class IIb if a conservative management strategy is employed for patients with NSTE-ACS.

The ACC/AHA also considers abciximab a class IIa adjunctive agent for use during primary PCI, while tirofiban and eptifibatide are considered class IIb for STEMI patients treated invasively. Combination pharmacologic reperfusion therapy with abciximab and half-dose reteplase or tenecteplase can be considered for prevention of reinfarction or other complications of STEMI in selected patients (i.e., those with anterior MI, age <75 years, and no risk factors for hemorrhage; class IIb).

REFERENCES

1. Sabatine MS, Jang IK. The use of glycoprotein IIb/IIIa inhibitors in patients with coronary artery disease. Am J Med 2000; 109:224–237.
2. Steinhubl SR, Talley JD, Braden GA, et al. Point-of-care measured platelet inhibition correlates with a reduced risk of an adverse cardiac event after percutaneous coronary intervention: results of the GOLD (AU-Assessing Ultegra) multicenter study. Circulation 2001; 103:2572–2578.
3. Schrör K, Weber AA. Comparative pharmacology of GP IIb/IIIa antagonists. J Thromb Thrombolysis 2003; 15:71–80.

4. Tcheng JE. Differences among the parenteral platelet glycoprotein IIb/IIIa inhibitors and implications for treatment. Am J Cardiol 1999; 83:7E–11E.

5. Barrett JS, Murphy G, Peerlinck K, et al. Pharmacokinetics and pharmacodynamics of MK-383, a selective non-peptide platelet glycoprotein-IIb/IIIa receptor antagonist, in healthy men. Clin Pharmacol Ther 1994; 56:377–388.

6. The EPIC Investigators. Use of a monoclonal antibody directed against the platelet glycoprotein IIb/IIIa receptor in high-risk coronary angioplasty. N Engl J Med 1994; 330:956–961.

7. The EPILOG Investigators. Platelet glycoprotein IIb/IIIa receptor blockade and low-dose heparin during percutaneous coronary revascularization. N Engl J Med 1997; 336:1689–1696.

8. The IMPACT-II Investigators. Randomised placebo-controlled trial of effect of eptifibatide on complications of percutaneous coronary intervention: IMPACT-II. Lancet 1997; 349:1422–1428.

9. The EPISTENT Investigators. Randomised placebo-controlled and balloon-angioplasty-controlled trial to assess safety of coronary stenting with use of platelet glycoprotein-IIb/IIIa blockade. Lancet 1998; 352:87–92.

10. The ESPRIT Investigators. Novel dosing regimen of eptifibatide in planned coronary stent implantation (ESPRIT): a randomised, placebo-controlled trial. Lancet 2000; 356:2037–2044.

11. Topol EJ, Moliterno DJ, Herrmann HC, et al. Comparison of two platelet glycoprotein IIb/IIIa inhibitors, tirofiban and abciximab, for the prevention of ischemic events with percutaneous coronary revascularization. N Engl J Med 2001; 344:1888–1894.

12. Kastrati A, Mehilli J, Schühlen H, et al. A clinical trial of abciximab in elective percutaneous coronary intervention after pretreatment with clopidogrel. N Engl J Med 2004; 350:232–238.

13. Mehilli J, Kastrati A, Schuhlen H, et al. Randomized clinical trial of abciximab in diabetic patients undergoing elective percutaneous coronary interventions after treatment with a high loading dose of clopidogrel. Circulation 2004; 110:3627–3635.

14. Valgimigli M, Percoco G, Barbieri D, et al. The additive value of tirofiban administered with the high-dose bolus in the prevention of ischemic complications during high-risk coronary angioplasty: the ADVANCE trial. J Am Coll Cardiol 2004; 44:14–19.

15. Kastrati A, Mehilli J, Neumann FJ, et al. Abciximab in patients with acute coronary syndromes undergoing percutaneous coronary intervention after clopidogrel pretreatment: the ISAR-REACT 2 randomized trial. JAMA 2006; 295:1531–1538.

16. Topol EJ, Califf RM, Weisman HF, et al. Randomised trial of coronary intervention with antibody against platelet IIb/IIIa integrin for reduction of clinical restenosis: results at six months. Lancet 1994; 343:881–886.

17. Topol EJ, Ferguson JJ, Weisman HF, et al. Long-term protection from myocardial ischemic events in a randomized trial of brief integrin beta3 blockade with percutaneous coronary intervention. EPIC investigator group. Evaluation of platelet IIb/IIIa inhibition for prevention of ischemic complications. JAMA 1997; 278:479–484.

18. Lincoff AM, Tcheng JE, Califf RM, et al. Sustained suppression of ischemic complications of coronary intervention by platelet GP IIb/IIIa blockade with abciximab: one-year outcome in the EPILOG trial. Circulation 1999; 99:1951–1958.

19. Blankenship JC, Tasissa G, O'Shea JC, et al. Effect of glycoprotein IIb/IIIa receptor inhibition on angiographic complications during percutaneous coronary intervention in the ESPRIT trial. J Am Coll Cardiol 2001; 38:653–658.

20. O'Shea JC, Buller CE, Cantor WJ, et al. Long-term efficacy of platelet glycoprotein IIb/IIIa integrin blockade with eptifibatide in coronary stent intervention. JAMA 2002; 287:618–621.

21. The RESTORE Investigators. Effects of platelet glycoprotein IIb/IIIa blockade with tirofiban on adverse cardiac events in patients with unstable angina or acute myocardial infarction undergoing coronary angioplasty. Circulation 1997; 96:1445–1453.

22. Anderson KM, Califf RM, Stone GW, et al. Long-term mortality benefit with abciximab in patients undergoing percutaneous coronary intervention. J Am Coll Cardiol 2001; 37:2059–2065.

23. The CAPTURE Investigators. Randomised placebo-controlled trial of abciximab before and during coronary intervention in refractory unstable angina: the CAPTURE study. Lancet 1997; 349: 1429–1435.

24. Klootwijk P, Meij S, Melkert R, et al. Reduction of recurrent ischemia with abciximab during continuous ECG-ischemia monitoring in patients with unstable angina refractory to standard treatment (CAPTURE). Circulation 1998; 98:1358–1364.
25. The PRISM Study Investigators. A comparison of aspirin plus tirofiban with aspirin plus heparin for unstable angina. N Engl J Med 1998; 338:1498–1505.
26. The PURSUIT Trial Investigators. Inhibition of platelet glycoprotein IIb/IIIa with eptifibatide in patients with acute coronary syndromes. N Engl J Med 1998; 339:436–443.
27. The GUSTO IV-ACS Investigators. Effect of glycoprotein IIb/IIIa receptor blocker abciximab on outcome in patients with acute coronary syndromes without early coronary revascularisation: the GUSTO IV-ACS randomised trial. Lancet 2001; 357:1915–1924.
28. The PRISM-PLUS Study Investigators. Inhibition of the platelet glycoprotein IIb/IIIa receptor with tirofiban in unstable angina and non-Q-wave myocardial infarction. N Engl J Med 1998; 338:1488–1497.
29. Sabatine MS, Januzzi JL, Snapinn S, et al. A risk score system for predicting adverse outcomes and magnitude of benefit with glycoprotein IIb/IIIa inhibitor therapy in patients with unstable angina pectoris. Am J Cardiol 2001; 88:488–492.
30. Kleiman NS, Lincoff AM, Flaker GC, et al. Early percutaneous coronary intervention, platelet inhibition with eptifibatide, and clinical outcomes in patients with acute coronary syndromes. Circulation 2000; 101:751–757.
31. Chang WC, Harrington RA, Simoons ML, et al. Does eptifibatide confer a greater benefit to patients with unstable angina than those with non-ST segment elevation myocardial infarction? Insights from the PURSUIT trial. Eur Heart J 2002; 23:1102–1111.
32. Heeschen C, Dimmeler S, Hamm CW, et al. Soluble CD40 ligand in acute coronary syndromes. N Engl J Med 2003; 348:1104–1111.
33. Hamm CW, Heeschen C, Goldmann B, et al. Benefit of abciximab in patients with refractory unstable angina in relation to serum troponin T levels. N Engl J Med 1999; 340:1623–1629.
34. Heeschen C, Hamm CW, Goldmann B, et al. Troponin concentrations for stratification of patients with acute coronary syndromes in relation to therapeutic efficacy of tirofiban. Lancet 1999; 354:1757–1762.
35. Moliterno DJ. Patient-specific dosing of IIb/IIIa antagonists during acute coronary syndromes: rationale and design of the PARAGON B study. The PARAGON B International Steering Committee. Am Heart J 2000; 139:563–566.
36. Newby LK, Ohman EM, Christenson RH, et al. Benefit of glycoprotein IIb/IIIa inhibition in patients with acute coronary syndromes and troponin t-positive status: the paragon-B troponin T substudy. Circulation 2001; 103:2891–2896.
37. Boersma E, Harrington RA, Moliterno DJ, et al. Platelet glycoprotein IIb/IIIa inhibitors in acute coronary syndromes: a meta-analysis of all major randomised clinical trials. Lancet 2002; 359:189–198.
38. The PARAGON Investigators. International, randomized, controlled trial of lamifiban (a platelet glycoprotein IIb/IIIa inhibitor), heparin, or both in unstable angina. Platelet IIb/IIIa antagonism for the reduction of acute coronary syndrome events in a global organization network (PARAGON). Circulation 1998; 97:2386–2395.
39. Roffi M, Chew DP, Mukherjee D, et al. Platelet glycoprotein IIb/IIIa inhibitors reduce mortality in diabetic patients with non-ST-segment-elevation acute coronary syndromes. Circulation 2001; 104:2767–2771.
40. Anderson JL, Adams CD, Antman EM, et al. ACC/AHA 2007 Guidelines for the management of patients with unstable angina/non-ST-elevation myocardial infarction: a report of the American College of Cardiology/American Heart Association Task Force on Practice Guidelines (writing committee to revise the 2002 guidelines for the management of patients with unstable angina/non-st-elevation myocardial infarction) developed in collaboration with the American College of Emergency Physicians, the Society for Cardiovascular Angiography and Interventions, and the Society of Thoracic Surgeons endorsed by the American Association of Cardiovascular and Pulmonary Rehabilitation and the Society for Academic Emergency Medicine. J Am Coll Cardiol 2007; 50:e1–e157.

41. Brener SJ, Barr LA, Burchenal JE, et al. Randomized, placebo-controlled trial of platelet glycoprotein IIb/IIIa blockade with primary angioplasty for acute myocardial infarction. Circulation 1998; 98:734–741.

42. Neumann FJ, Kastrati A, Schmitt C, et al. Effect of glycoprotein IIb/IIIa receptor blockade with abciximab on clinical and angiographic restenosis rate after the placement of coronary stents following acute myocardial infarction. J Am Coll Cardiol 2000; 35:915–921.

43. Stone GW, Grines CL, Cox DA, et al. Comparison of angioplasty with stenting, with or without abciximab, in acute myocardial infarction. N Engl J Med 2002; 346:957–966.

44. Montalescot G, Barragan P, Wittenberg O, et al. Platelet glycoprotein IIb/IIIa inhibition with coronary stenting for acute myocardial infarction. N Engl J Med 2001; 344:1895–1903.

45. Ohman EM, Kleiman NS, Gacioch G, et al. Combined accelerated tissue-plasminogen activator and platelet glycoprotein IIb/IIIa integrin receptor blockade with Integrilin in acute myocardial infarction. Results of a randomized, placebo-controlled, dose-ranging trial. Circulation 1997; 95:846–854.

46. Antman EM, Giugliano RP, Gibson CM, et al. Abciximab facilitates the rate and extent of thrombolysis: results of the Thrombolysis in Myocardial Infarction (TIMI) 14 trial. Circulation 1999; 99:2720–2732.

47. The Assessment of the Safety and Efficacy of a New Thrombolytic Regimen (ASSENT)-3 Investigators. Efficacy and safety of tenecteplase in combination with enoxaparin, abciximab, or unfractionated heparin: the ASSENT-3 randomised trial in acute myocardial infarction. Lancet 2001; 358:605–613.

48. The GUSTO V Investigators. Reperfusion therapy for acute myocardial infarction with fibrinolytic therapy or combination reduced fibrinolytic therapy and platelet glycoprotein IIb/IIIa inhibition: the GUSTO V randomised trial. Lancet 2001; 357:1905–1914.

49. Giugliano RP, Roe MT, Harrington RA, et al. Combination reperfusion therapy with eptifibatide and reduced-dose tenecteplase for ST-elevation myocardial infarction: results of the integrilin and tenecteplase in acute myocardial infarction (INTEGRITI) phase II angiographic trial. J Am Coll Cardiol 2003; 41:1251–1260.

50. de Lemos JA, Antman AM, Gibson CM, et al. Abciximab improves both epicardial flow and myocardial reperfusion in ST-elevation myocardial infarction. Observations from the TIMI 14 trial. Circulation 2000; 101:239–243.

51. Gibson CM, de Lemos JA, Murphy SA, et al. Combination therapy with abciximab reduces angiographically evident thrombus in acute myocardial infarction: a TIMI 14 substudy. Circulation 2001; 103:2550–2554.

52. Lincoff AM, Califf RM, Van de Werf F, et al. Mortality at 1 year with combination platelet glycoprotein IIb/IIIa inhibition and reduced-dose fibrinolytic therapy vs conventional fibrinolytic therapy for acute myocardial infarction: GUSTO V randomized trial. JAMA 2002; 288:2130–2135.

53. Savonitto S, Armstrong PW, Lincoff AM, et al. Risk of intracranial haemorrhage with combined fibrinolytic and glycoprotein IIb/IIIa inhibitor therapy in acute myocardial infarction. Dichotomous response as a function of age in the GUSTO V trial. Eur Heart J 2003; 24:1807–1814.

54. Brener SJ, Zeymer U, Adgey AA, et al. Eptifibatide and low-dose tissue plasminogen activator in acute myocardial infarction: the integrilin and low-dose thrombolysis in acute myocardial infarction (INTRO AMI) trial. J Am Coll Cardiol 2002; 39:377–386.

55. The ADMIRAL Investigators. Three-year duration of benefit from abciximab in patients receiving stents for acute myocardial infarction in the randomized double-blind ADMIRAL study. Eur Heart J 2005; 26:2520–2523.

56. Kandzari DE, Hasselblad V, Tcheng JE, et al. Improved clinical outcomes with abciximab therapy in acute myocardial infarction: a systematic overview of randomized clinical trials. Am Heart J 2004; 147:457–462.

57. Antman EM, Anbe DT, Armstrong PW, et al. ACC/AHA guidelines for the management of patients with ST-elevation myocardial infarction: a report of the American College of Cardiology/American Heart Association Task Force on Practice Guidelines (committee to revise

the 1999 guidelines for the management of patients with acute myocardial infarction). J Am Coll Cardiol 2004; 44:E1–E211.

58. Lee DP, Herity NA, Hiatt BL, et al. Adjunctive platelet glycoprotein IIb/IIIa receptor inhibition with tirofiban before primary angioplasty improves angiographic outcomes: results of the tirofiban given in the emergency room before primary angioplasty (TIGER-PA) pilot trial. Circulation 2003; 107:1497–1501.

59. van't Hof AW, Ernst N, de Boer MJ, et al. Facilitation of primary coronary angioplasty by early start of a glycoprotein 2b/3a inhibitor: results of the ongoing tirofiban in myocardial infarction evaluation (On-TIME) trial. Eur Heart J 2004; 25:837–846.

60. Keeley EC, Boura JA, Grines CL. Comparison of primary and facilitated percutaneous coronary interventions for ST-elevation myocardial infarction: quantitative review of randomised trials. Lancet 2006; 367:579–588.

61. De Luca G, Suryapranata H, Stone GW, et al. Abciximab as adjunctive therapy to reperfusion in acute ST-segment elevation myocardial infarction: a meta-analysis of randomized trials. JAMA 2005; 293:1759–1765.

62. Gurm HS, Smith DE, Collins JS, et al. The relative safety and efficacy of abciximab and eptifibatide in patients undergoing primary percutaneous coronary intervention: insights from a large regional registry of contemporary percutaneous coronary intervention. J Am Coll Cardiol 2008; 51:529–535.

63. Moliterno DJ, Yakubov SJ, DiBattiste PM, et al. Outcomes at 6 months for the direct comparison of tirofiban and abciximab during percutaneous coronary revascularisation with stent placement: the TARGET follow-up study. Lancet 2002; 360:355–360.

64. Batchelor WB, Tolleson TR, Huang Y, et al. Randomized comparison of platelet inhibition with abciximab, tirofiban and eptifibatide during percutaneous coronary intervention in acute coronary syndromes: the COMPARE trial. Circulation 2002; 106:1470–1476.

65. Hoekstra JW, Roe MT, Peterson ED, et al. Early glycoprotein IIb/IIIa inhibitor use for non-ST-segment elevation acute coronary syndrome: patient selection and associated treatment patterns. Acad Emerg Med 2005; 12:431–438.

66. Peterson ED, Pollack CV Jr., Roe MT, et al. Early use of glycoprotein IIb/IIIa inhibitors in non-ST-elevation acute myocardial infarction: observations from the National Registry of Myocardial Infarction 4. J Am Coll Cardiol 2003; 42:45–53.

67. Stone GW, Bertrand ME, Moses JW, et al. Routine upstream initiation vs deferred selective use of glycoprotein IIb/IIIa inhibitors in acute coronary syndromes: the ACUITY Timing trial. J Am Med Assoc 2007; 297:591–602.

68. Giugliano RP, Newby LK, Harrington RA, et al. The early glycoprotein IIb/IIIa inhibition in non-ST-segment elevation acute coronary syndrome (EARLY ACS) trial: a randomized placebo-controlled trial evaluating the clinical benefits of early front-loaded eptifibatide in the treatment of patients with non-ST-segment elevation acute coronary syndrome—study design and rationale. Am Heart J 2005; 149:994–1002.

69. Karvouni E, Katritsis DG, Ioannidis JP. Intravenous glycoprotein IIb/IIIa receptor antagonists reduce mortality after percutaneous coronary interventions. J Am Coll Cardiol 2003; 41:26–32.

70. Kirtane AJ, Piazza G, Murphy SA, et al. Correlates of bleeding events among moderate- to high-risk patients undergoing percutaneous coronary intervention and treated with eptifibatide: observations from the PROTECT-TIMI-30 trial. J Am Coll Cardiol 2006; 47:2374–2379.

71. Alexander KP, Chen AY, Roe MT, et al. Excess dosing of antiplatelet and antithrombin agents in the treatment of non-ST-segment elevation acute coronary syndromes. JAMA 2005; 294:3108–3116.

72. Abrams CS, Cines DB. Thrombocytopenia after treatment with platelet glycoprotein IIb/IIIa inhibitors. Curr Hematol Rep 2004; 3:143–147.

73. McClure MW, Berkowitz SD, Sparapani R, et al. Clinical significance of thrombocytopenia during non-ST-elevation acute coronary syndrome. The platelet glycoprotein IIb/IIIa inhibitors in unstable angina: receptor suppression using integrilin therapy (PURSUIT) trial experience. Circulation 1999; 99:2892–2900.

74. Patel S, Patel M, Din I, et al. Profound thrombocytopenia associated with tirofiban: case report and review of the literature. Angiology 2005; 56:351–355.
75. Coons JC, Barcelona RA, Freedy T, et al. Eptifibatide-associated acute, profound thrombocytopenia. Ann Pharmacother 2005; 39:368–372.
76. Curtis BR, Swyers J, Divgi A, et al. Thrombocytopenia after second exposure to abciximab is caused by antibodies that recognize abciximab-coated platelets. Blood 2002; 99:2054–2059.
77. Tcheng JE, Kereiakes DJ, Lincoff AM, et al. Abciximab readministration: results of the ReoPro Readmission Registry. Circulation 2001; 104:870–875.
78. Dasgupta H, Blankenship JC, Wood GC, et al. Thrombocytopenia complicating treatment with intravenous glycoprotein IIb/IIIa receptor inhibitors: a pooled analysis. Am Heart J 2000; 140: 206–211.
79. Sane DC, Damaraju LV, Topol EJ, et al. Occurrence and clinical significance of pseudothrombocytopenia during abciximab therapy. J Am Coll Cardiol 2000; 36:75–83.
80. Mukherjee D, Chew DP, Robbins M, et al. Clinical application of procedural platelet monitoring during percutaneous coronary intervention among patients at increased bleeding risk. J Thromb Thrombolysis 2001; 11:151–154.
81. Montalescot G, Borentain M, Payot L, et al. Early vs late administration of glycoprotein IIb/IIIa inhibitors in primary percutaneous coronary intervention of acute ST-segment elevation myocardial infarction: a meta-analysis. JAMA 2004; 292:362–366.
82. Ellis SG. Report of the FINESSE trial findings. Paper presented at: European Society of Cardiology Congress, September 1–5, 2007, Vienna, Austria.
83. Marmur JD, Poludasu S, Agarwal A, et al. Bolus-only platelet glycoprotein IIb/IIIa inhibition during percutaneous coronary intervention. J Invasive Cardiol 2006; 18:521–526.
84. Fischell TA, Attia T, Rane S, et al. High-dose, single-bolus eptifibatide: a safe and cost-effective alternative to conventional glycoprotein IIb/IIIa inhibitor use for elective coronary interventions. J Invasive Cardiol 2006; 18:487–491.
85. Deibele AJ, Kirtane AJ, Pinto DS, et al. Intracoronary bolus administration of eptifibatide during percutaneous coronary stenting for non ST elevation myocardial infarction and unstable angina. J Thromb Thrombolysis 2006; 22:47–50.
86. Stone GW, McLaurin BT, Cox DA, et al. Bivalirudin for patients with acute coronary syndromes. N Engl J Med 2006; 355:2203–2216.
87. Stone GW, Witzenbichler B, Guagliumi G, et al. Bivalirudin during primary PCI in acute myocardial infarction. N Engl J Med 2008; 358:2280–2282.
88. Smith SC Jr., Feldman TE, Hirshfeld JW Jr., et al. ACC/AHA/SCAI 2005 guideline update for percutaneous coronary intervention—summary article: a report of the American College of Cardiology/American Heart Association Task Force on Practice Guidelines (ACC/AHA/SCAI writing committee to update the 2001 guidelines for percutaneous coronary intervention). Circulation 2006; 113:e166–e286.

26

Inhibitors of Platelet Adhesion: VWF-GP1b/IX and Collagen-GPVI Inhibitors

Robert G. Schaub

Preclinical Research and Development, Archemix Corporation, Cambridge, Massachusetts, U.S.A.

INTRODUCTION

Coagulation is a complex series of biochemical and cellular reactions that results in the polymerization of fibrin and formation of platelet/fibrin hemostatic plugs. In normal blood vessels, these interactions serve as the primary mechanism to control hemorrhage. However, when combined with vascular pathology of major arteries, such activation can result in thrombosis and life-threatening vascular occlusion (1,2). Platelets play a major role in mediating some of the earliest events of both hemostasis and thrombosis. Antiplatelet therapies have been anti-thrombotic targets and the source of effective therapies (3). Most of the antiplatelet drugs target platelet biochemical pathways. To date, only the glycoprotein IIb/IIIa (GPIIb/IIIa) antagonists have targeted platelet adhesion mechanisms and been approved for the treatment of acute coronary events (4–6). Although the GPIIb/IIIa antagonists have been shown to provide improved outcomes, their efficacy is complicated by bleeding at platelet-inhibitory doses. Over the past few years, increased interest has been directed toward other platelet adhesion mechanisms that might permit separation of platelet inhibition from bleeding. Two of these adhesion pathways, von Willebrand factor/GPIbα (VWF/GPIbα) and GPVI, will be discussed in this chapter (7).

von WILLEBRAND FACTOR AND GLYCOPROTEIN IB/V/IX

Structure and Function

von Willebrand Factor (VWF) is a heterogenous, multimeric, soluble plasma glycoprotein (GP) of high moleculer weight (~400,000 –>12,000,000 Da), composed of repeating 270-kDa subunits containing 2050 amino acid residues (8–10). VWF is synthesized and stored by megakaryocytes and endothelial cells and is present in plasma, platelets, the vascular endothelium and subendothelium (basement membrane). VWF stored in endothelial cells can be released into the circulation constitutively or upon exposure to vasopressin or thrombin (8–10). VWF has two major functions. It serves as the plasma carrier for factor VIII, the antihemophilic coagulation factor. It also facilitates platelet adhesion to vascular subendothelium and platelet aggregation stabilization via interaction of the VWF A1 domain with platelet GPIbα in the GPIb/IX/V complex. Plasma factor VIII-VWF is a complex consisting of factor VIII and VWF linked by noncovalent bonds, with the majority (99%) of the complex consisting of VWF. This factor VIII-VWF complex circulates as a unit, with VWF believed to act as a carrier for factor VIII that protects it from degradation (11).

The VWF A1 domain interacts with platelet GPIbα, a component of the GPIb/IX/V complex, to facilitate adhesion and subsequent aggregation of platelets (12–16). The GPIb-IX-V complex has been extensively studied with respect to oligomeric structure and physiological function and is comprised of four transmembrane polypeptides, GPIbα, GPIX, and GPV (17). The adhesion function of the GPIb-IX-V complex that interacts with VWF factor resides in each GPIbα chain. The GPIbα polypeptide is a type I transmembrane protein of 610 amino acids, of which the amino terminal ~290 amino acids have been shown to contain the VWF-binding region (18,19). While the crystal structures of the GPIbα-binding domain for VWF (VWF A1) and GPIbα have been determined separately (20,21), the co-complex crystal structure reveals two distinct regions of protein interactions. First, a small contact site on GPIbα located near the N-terminus consisting of a β-hairpin turn (β-finger), and second, a much larger and extensive region of GPIbα that undergoes a conformational change to a β-hairpin structure after complex formation (β-switch) (14). The conformational status of the β-switch of GPIbα appears to be a critical factor in determining the affinity of GPIbα for VWF. Several single amino acid substitutions of the GPIbα protein have been reported to alter the binding affinity of the protein for VWF. Close examination of these amino acids in the context of GPIbα/VWF interactions indicates that these "gain-of-function" mutations are likely to induce β-hairpin formation in the β-switch of GPIbα, thereby promoting protein-protein binding. In platelet-type (or pseudo) von Willebrand disease for instance, GPIbα mutations of Met 239 to Val (22–24) or Gly 233 to Val (25) result in increased affinity for circulating VWF (25,26). In fact, several additional amino acids of the β-switch region have been shown to promote stabilization and increased binding affinity to VWF (27). A highly anionic region spanning residues Glu 269-Glu 287 of GPIbα has also been implicated in facilitating binding to VWF. Biochemical and mutagenesis data of three posttranslationally sulfated tyrosine residues (Tyr 276, Tyr 278, Tyr279) suggest that these modified, negatively charged amino acids enhance binding to VWF and thrombin (28–30). Several recent reports, including co-crystal studies of GPIbα and thrombin, indicate that these residues are most important for facilitating thrombin binding (13,15,16).

After vascular injury, an essential first step in primary hemostasis is platelet adhesion, which leads to platelet activation and subsequent platelet aggregation via platelet GPIIb/IIIa interactions with fibrinogen, causing thrombus formation. VWF promotes platelet adhesion by binding to collagen in exposed vascular subendothelium via the A3 domain and to platelet GPIbα via the A1 domain. In addition, the GPIbα/VWF A1 domain interaction can serve to further enhance platelet/platelet interactions in areas of high shear stress. Under conditions of high shear stress, such as arterial blood flow, the interactions of VWF with the GPIbα/IX/V complex is considerably enhanced (31,32) (Fig. 1).

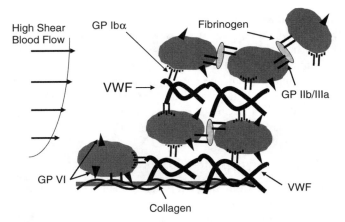

Figure 1 VWF promotes platelet adhesion by binding to collagen in exposed vascular subendothelium via the A3 domain and to platelet GPIbα via the A1 domain of multimeric VWF in areas of high shear stress where the interactions are considerably enhanced. GP VI may also interact at these sites, further promoting platelet adhesion to collagen and, in conjunction with GPIb, the activation of GPIIb/IIIa and thrombus growth. *Abbreviations*: VWF, von Willebrand factor; GP, glycoprotein.

Role of VWF and GPIbα in Thrombosis and Vascular Disorders

VWF has roles other than those involved in primary hemostasis, particularly in the pathogenesis of atherosclerosis and arterial thrombosis. A disruption in the continuity of the endothelial cells lining the artery wall, such as a plaque rupture, exposes subendothelial matrix components like collagen to arterial blood flow. Exposed collagen captures circulating VWF, causing the accumulation of immobilized VWF at subendothelial sites. In turn, this immobilized VWF, which is now subject to high fluid shear forces, becomes a receptor for platelet GPIbα. The VWF/GPIbα interaction causes platelets to roll along the damaged artery and eventually promotes secondary adhesion events that enable firm platelet adhesion. This process of platelet accumulation, the local conversion of circulating fibrinogen to its insoluble form, fibrin, and the upregulation of GPIIb/IIIa receptor on platelets promotes the local formation of a thrombus. It is important to note that the VWF/GPIbα interaction has evolved to be an adhesion event operative under high shear conditions and that some of the highest shear forces occur at sites of atherosclerotic lesions, where shear rate can be 40 times that of a normal artery. Conversely, under low shear conditions, such as in venous blood flow, the VWF/GPIbα adhesion mechanism is less essential, and other adhesion receptors such as GPIIb/IIIa and platelet collagen receptors can independently mediate platelet adhesion. It follows, therefore, that an agent that inhibits the VWF/GPIbα interaction will primarily have selectivity for blocking high shear arterial platelet adhesion and should have minimal impact on hemostasis in low shear blood flow.

VWF as a potential therapeutic target in thrombosis and vascular disorders has been gaining acceptance recently. An association between VWF release from endothelium and endothelial injury has been appreciated for many years from both animal model and human studies. Animal studies evaluating both large artery and arteriole thrombosis have demonstrated the important role of VWF/platelet interactions in thrombus formation and thrombus stabilization. Inhibition of these GPIbα/platelet interactions has profound anti-thrombotic effects, with low to moderate effects on bleeding time (31,33,34). More importantly, in the last few years, accumulating evidence has demonstrated that VWF has a similar impact on thrombosis in human coronary artery disease. Elevation of plasma VWF concentrations and reductions in PFA-100 closure times are associated with increased risk of recurrent acute coronary syndrome (ACS) in patients presenting with ACS and increased myocardial damage in acute myocardial infarction (AMI) patients (35–37). These data suggest that inhibition of the platelet activation by GPIbα/VWF interaction can have positive therapeutic benefit for patients with ACS.

Inhibition of von Willebrand Factor/Glycoprotein Ibα

Aurintricarboxylic acid, peptide fragments from the VWF A1 domain, and a soluble GPIb-IgG chimera have been agents used to demonstrate the anti-thrombotic potential of blocking VWF mediated platelet interactions in animal model studies (31,38–40). This summary will focus on studies that have been reported in the last seven years (Table 1).

GPG-290 is a recombinant protein consisting of the N-terminal 290 amino acids of human GPIbα with two gain-of-function mutations (G233V/M239V) that increase affinity for the A1 domain by 10-fold fused to human IgG1Fc. The Fc portion contains amino acid substitutions that reduce Fc effector function (31,40). GPG-290 is expressed as a homodimer linked by the two-disulfide bonds in the Fc hinge region. In vitro characterization studies have shown that GPG-290 has an enhanced affinity for the VWF A1 domain (Kd~12 nM) as compared with an identical molecule lacking the gain-of-function valine substitutions (Kd~270 nM). The in vivo anti-thrombotic and anti-hemostatic (bleeding time prolongation) and ex vivo platelet inhibitory effects of GPG-290 were evaluated in the canine Folts model of coronary thrombosis at doses of 10-, 25-, 50-, and 100-μg/kg IV bolus. In addition, the ability of Desmopressin (1-desamino-8-D-arginine vasopressin, DDAVP) to reverse the increased bleeding associated with a 500-μg/kg (10-fold the effective dose) GPG-290 dose by inducing the release of endothelial stores of VWF was also investigated. A single IV bolus of GPG-290 at doses of 25, 50, 100, and 500 μg/kg, which corresponds to plasma concentrations of 0.6 to 12.6 μg/mL, immediately abolished cyclic flow responses (CFRs) and restored the coronary blood flow for the entire 90-minute observation period in 67% to 100% of treated dogs. At the lowest dose of 10 μg/kg, GPG-290 abolished CFRs in 25% (2 out of 8) of the treated dogs. There was no significant bleeding time prolongation after GPG-290 administration at doses of 10, 25, 50, and 100 μg/kg. A moderate prolongation (~3-4-fold increase vs. baseline) was observed after 500-μg/kg GPG-290. GPG-290 at a dose of 25 μg/kg and above resulted in a dose-dependent inhibition on ex vivo platelet adhesion/aggregation mirrored by the significant adenosine diphosphate-collagen cartridge time (ADP-CT) prolongation in the Platelet Function Analyzer-100 (PFA-100), (Dade Behring, Miami, FL) at 10 and 90 minutes post administration. The ADP-CT prolongation caused by 500 μg/kg GPG-290 exceeded the PFA-100 maximal limit of 300 seconds at both the 10 and 90-minute time points. There was no significant change in either plasma VWF antigen (VWF:Ag) or VWF collagen binding (VWF:CB) after GPG-290 treatment. A single IV bolus of 500 μg/kg GPG-290 resulted in a three to fourfold increase in bleeding time, which peaked at 10 minutes and lasted for more than two hours. The prolonged bleeding time was normalized by infusion of 0.3-μg/kg DDAVP, which correlated with a 167% increase in plasma VWF:Ag level and a 198% increase in VWF:CB, as compared with their baseline levels. VWF multimer analysis confirmed that plasma high-molecular-weight VWF multimers were significantly increased 30 minutes post-DDAVP, and the increase persisted for two hours. DDAVP administration did not affect the coronary blood flow, and there was no recurrence of CFRs during the

Table 1 Summary: In Vivo Studies of GlycoproteinIbα/VWF Antagonists

Study title	Species, dose, and route of administration	Results
Abolition of cyclic flow variations in stenosed, endothelium-injured coronary arteries in nonhuman primates with a peptide fragment (VCL) derived from human plasma VWF/GPIb binding domain (39).	Baboon, IV 4-mg/kg bolus and 6 mg/kg/hr infusion for 90 min or 2-mg/kg bolus and 3 mg/kg/hr infusion for 90 min	High-dose animals had cyclic flow variations abolished in 7/8 during and for >3 hr following end of infusion. In low-dose group, 3/6 had cyclic flow abolished and reduced in the remaining animals. There was a slight increase in bleeding time and a reduction in botrocetin-induced aggregation.
Anti-thrombotic effects and bleeding risk of AJvW-2, a monoclonal antibody against human VWF (41).	Guinea pigs, 100 µg/kg IV vs. lamifiban (GPIIb/IIIa antagonist) at 1 mg/kg IV	AJvW-2 inhibited thrombus formation without increase in bleeding time. Lamifiban-inhibited thrombus formation with increased bleeding time.
Effect of a humanized monoclonal antibody to VWF in a canine model of coronary arterial thrombosis (33).	Dog, 0.1–1 mg/kg IV monoclonal VWF antibody AJW200 compared to abciximab at 0.8 mg/kg IV	AJW200 significantly inhibited cyclic flow reductions and botrocetin-induced platelet aggregation at 0.1 mg/kg. Prolongation of bleeding was observed at 0.3 to 1 mg/kg. Abciximab was effective inhibiting cyclic flow but produced significant prolongation of bleeding.
Pharmacokinetics and pharmacodynamics of AJW200, a humanized monoclonal antibody to VWF, in monkeys (34).	Cynomolgus monkeys, 0.3, 1, and 3 mg/kg IV vs. abciximab at 0.4 mg/kg IV	Sustained inhibition of ristocetin-induced platelet aggregation was observed over 24 hr, 6 days, and 2 wk after a single bolus injection of AJW200. Moderate prolongation of bleeding time was observed at 1 and 3 mg/kg. Abciximab produced markedly prolonged bleeding times combined with complete inhibition of ADP-induced platelet aggregation.
A humanized monoclonal antibody against VWF A1 domain inhibits VWF:RiCof activity and platelet adhesion in human volunteers (42).	Human volunteers, 0.01, 0.03, or 0.05 mg/kg IV	RiC of activity was reduced at 0.03 and 0.05 mg/kg 1 to 12 hr after infusion. Template bleeding time was unchanged. The PFA-100 showed inhibition up to 12 hr at the 0.05 mg/kg dose. This was the first study showing the effect of a monoclonal antibody that blocks GPIb/VWF in humans.
An anti-VWF A1 domain aptamer inhibits arterial thrombosis induced by electrical injury in cynomolgus macaques (43).	Cynomolgus monkeys 100–600 µg/kg IV bolus and 1–3.7 µg/kg/min IV infusion of ARC1779 anti-VWF A1 domain aptamer vs. 250 µg/kg and 0.3 µg/kg/min infusion of abciximab	ARC1779 demonstrated a dose-dependent inhibition of occlusive thrombus formation induced by electrical injury with efficacy comparable to abciximab at the higher doses with less bleeding.

(Continued)

Table 1 Summary: In Vivo Studies of GlycoproteinIbα/VWF Antagonists (*Continued*)

Study title	Species, dose, and route of administration	Results
First-in-human evaluation of anti-VWF therapeutic aptamer ARC1779 in healthy volunteers (44).	Human volunteers 0.05–1 mg/kg by IV bolus or slow infusion	Inhibition of VWF A1 binding activity was achieved with an EC90 value of 2.0 μg/mL and platelet function by PFA-100 was inhibited at an EC90 of 2.6 μg/mL. No bleeding complications were observed, and the drug was well tolerated. This is the first human evaluation of a novel aptamer antagonist of VWF.

Abbreviations: VWF, von Willebrand factor; RiCof, ristocetin cofactor; GP, glycoprotein; IV, intravenous.

entire two-hour post-DDAVP period. GPG-290 was also evaluated in combination with clopidogrel in a canine electrolytic injury thrombosis model (31). GPG-290 at doses of 100 and 500 μg/kg prolonged time to thrombotic occlusion by three to fivefold, respectively, compared with saline control combined with an increased patency over the four-hour observation period. In this study, clopidogrel was administered either as a standard daily therapeutic regimen started two days prior to experimental thrombosis or a pre-procedural loading dose regimen given three hours prior to experimental thrombosis. Animals on the daily therapeutic regimen had a threefold increase in time to occlusion, and those on the loading dose regimen, a fourfold increase in time to occlusion. The combination of 100-μg/kg GPG-290 with the daily therapeutic regimen increased time to occlusion to that comparable to the loading dose regimen and increased patency without increased bleeding, while a 100-μg/kg GPG-290 dose with the higher clopidogrel loading dose regimen caused increased bleeding combined with increased time to occlusion. The results of these studies suggest that the effect of GPIbα/VWF inhibition could be reversed with a currently approved (DDAVP) treatment regimen and that a lower clopidogrel dose combined with GPIbα/VWF inhibition could have improved efficacy with less bleeding risk.

Three VWF inhibitors have been in clinical trials this decade and two are currently in active clinical development. AJvW-2 is a murine monoclonal antibody to human VWF A1 domain that blocks the GPIbα/VWF interaction and has demonstrated anti-thrombotic activity in animal models (36,41). In order to reduce immunological responsen AJvW-2 was humanized and converted from an IgG1 to an IgG4. This humanized antibody (AJW200) exhibited similar inhibition of in vitro VWF-mediated platelet activation to AJvW-2 (34). In monkeys, AJW200 demonstrated dose proportional pharmacokinetics over a dose range of 0.03 to 3 mg/kg with half-life of 23 to 63 hours from lowest to highest dose. AJW200 inhibited ristocetin-induced platelet aggregation. Complete inhibition was observed from 0.3 mg and above, lasting from 24 hours at 0.3 mg/kg to 2 weeks at 3 mg/kg. There was a wide window in bleeding times with AJW200 treatment with little to minimal effect on bleeding time at doses of 0.1 and 0.3 mg/kg. However, a dose of 0.40-mg/kg abciximab was associated with a bleeding time that exceeded 30 minutes. Also, unlike AJW200, the platelet inhibition effect of abciximab was reversed after 24 hours (34). In a canine Folts cyclic flow model, AJW200 was found to inhibit cyclic flow at doses of 0.1 mg/kg, while abciximab was active at a dose of 0.8 mg/kg. Bleeding time increases were dose dependent, but only the 1-mg/kg AJW200 dose was comparable to abciximab. Inhibition of cyclic flow and platelet aggregation were observed at approximately 50% occupancy of VWF. Bleeding time was significantly prolonged when 80% to 100% of VWF was occupied (34). In human volunteer studies, AJW200 was infused into 24 healthy, normal male subjects aged 20 to 45 years at doses of 0.01, 0.03, and 0.05 mg/kg without clinically significant adverse events or immunogenicity. Blood samples were collected before and up to 28 days after infusion. Ristocetin cofactor (Ri:CoF) assays showed a significant reduction at one-hour post infusion compared with baseline that lasted for up to 12 hours. The template bleeding time was not significantly prolonged at all times and doses of AJW200. Platelet function as measured by the PFA-100 was reduced by up to three to six hours at the lower dose and 12 hours at the highest dose administered (42).

Another approach to blocking the GPIbα/VWF A1 domain interaction has been through the development of a nucleic acid aptamer (ARC1779), isolated using in vitro selection (SELEX) (45–49). The aptamer binds to the A1 domain of VWF with high affinity and potently inhibits VWF-dependent platelet aggregation. Aptamers are nucleic acid molecules with high affinity and specificity for a selected target molecule discovered through in vitro selection on the basis of their ability to fold into unique three-dimensional structures that promote binding to a target. The core aptamer portion of ARC1779 (MW ~13 kDa) is a 40-mer modified DNA/RNA oligonucleotide composed of 13 unmodified 2′-deoxy nucleotides, 26 modified 2′-O-methyl-nucleotides (to minimize endonuclease digestion), 1 inverted deoxythymidine (iT) nucleotide as a 3′-terminal "cap" (to minimize 3′-exonuclease digestion), and a single phosphorothioate (P = S) linkage between nucleotide positions mG20 and dT21 (to enhance affinity for VWF). The core 40-mer is synthesized with a hexylamine at the 5′-terminus as a reactive site for subsequent conjugation of a 20-kDa PEG moiety to form the active pharmaceutical ingredient ARC1779 (MW ~33 kDa). All concentrations and doses of ARC1779 are expressed on the basis of oligonucleotide mass, exclusive of PEG mass. Nonclinical studies evaluated platelet adhesion and thrombus inhibition. ARC1779 showed clear dose-dependent efficacy in a cynomolgus macaque model of electrical injury (EI). Using an intravenous bolus plus continuous infusion dosing regimen (0.3 mg/kg bolus + 0.0025 mg/kg/min infusion) that achieved mean plasma concentrations of 700 and 1300 nM, ARC1779 demonstrated efficacy comparable or superior to that of a previously published therapeutic dose of abciximab with respect to protection from thrombus formation and average time to occlusion. These data suggest that 700 nM is a pharmacologically effective target plasma concentration for ARC1779 (50,51).

Consistent with the dose-dependent efficacy of ARC1779 in the EI model, there was also a dose-dependent increase in template bleeding time. However, analysis of average template bleeding times during the course of these experiments revealed that while treatment with a plasma concentration of 1300-nM ARC1779 or abciximab significantly prolonged template bleeding times relative to saline control animals ($p < 0.001$), a plasma concentration of 700-nM ARC1779 did not increase bleeding times (43,50,51).

ARC1779 was evaluated in a randomized, double-blind, placebo-controlled study that evaluated doses of 0.05 to 1 mg/kg. A1 binding site blockade, platelet function, and concentration-time profiles were evaluated in addition to safety. Pharmacokinetic parameters were dose proportional with a mean apparent elimination half-life of two hours. Inhibition of VWF A1 binding activity was achieved with an EC90 value of 2.0 µg/mL and of platelet function using the PFA-100 with an EC90 value of 2.6 µg/mL. ARC1779 was generally well tolerated, and no bleeding was observed (44).

In unpublished observations, it has also been reported that targeting the VWF A1 domain with the recombinant nanobody ALX-0081, a novel class of antibody therapeutics, resulted in inhibition of VWF-mediated platelet activation at doses between 2 and 12 mg.

GLYCOPROTEIN VI

Glycoprotein VI Structure and Function

GPVI is a member of the immunoglobulin super family expressed on the surface of megakaryocytes and platelets. It is composed of 339 amino acids with an apparent molecular weight of 62 kDa because of glycosylation within the two extracellular IgG domains containing O-linked carbohydrate-rich regions. The tertiary structure of the protein is maintained by a Cys bond in each domain (52,53). GPVI covalently associates with the Fc receptor γ chain (FcRγ), which is required for its surface expression. Signaling by GPVI is via the FcR g immunoreceptor tyrosine activation motif (ITAM). The GPVI cytoplasmic tail contains a proline-rich motif that binds the Src homology 3 domain of the Src family tyrosine kinases Fyn and Lyn, thus promoting phosphorylation of the FcRγ ITAM and initiation of the signaling cascade through the binding of Syk. Syk activation results in the activation of a number of downstream pathways that culminate in activation of the integrin $\alpha_2\beta_1$ and subsequent $\alpha_{II}\beta_1$-induced platelet aggregation, release of ADP and thromboxane, expression of phosphytidylserine, and subsequent procoagulant activity (54). GPVI has been shown to associate with GPIbα in both resting and activated platelets (55). It has been suggested that these two molecules act together to promote platelet attachment to the extracellular matrix and the subsequent downstream platelet activation events (54,56–58) (Fig. 1).

GPVI Inhibition

No clinical trails have been reported to date with inhibitors of GPVI. However, a number of nonclinical animal studies have been performed with several types of specific GPVI inhibitor molecules. These data provide a useful understanding for the therapeutic potential of GPVI inhibition as well as to the role of GPVI in platelet activation and thrombosis (Table 2).

Nieswandt et al. have reported on the in vivo effect of a rat monoclonal (IgG2a) antibody (JAQ1) to mouse GPVI that results in GPVI depletion. The intact antibody resulted in limited inhibition of collagen-induced aggregation (59). Injection of JAQ1 or Fab fragments caused mild thrombocytopenia and resulted in a decrease in platelet counts of approximately 34% within 24 hours of treatment and a return to normal levels within 3 days of treatment. Platelets did not show any indication of activation as assessed by surface P-selectin expression or fibrinogen binding after JAQ1 injection, nor did they exhibit any indication of change in other GP surface proteins. A single 100-μg IP dose of JAQ1 resulted in 14 days inhibition of ex vivo collagen-induced aggregation using collagen concentrations as high as 50 μg/mL, while response to ADP and PMA was unaffected. Interestingly, in vitro inhibition of collagen-induced platelet aggregation was limited. Further evaluation of in vivo response determined that the binding of antibody for Fab to the platelet GPVI resulted in depletion of platelet GPVI. Collagen-induced adhesion was significantly reduced in these GPVI-depleted platelets. In addition, stimulation with platelets from JAQ1-treated mice with a combination of collagen and thrombin did not result in platelet expression of phosphatidylserine. Bleeding times of JAQ1-treated mice were significantly elevated over control mice (330 seconds vs. 158 seconds) but less than that seen following inhibition of GPIIb/IIIa (330 seconds vs. >600 seconds). Finally, the JAQ1-treated mice were protected against lethal pulmonary thromboembolism following injection of a combination collagen/epinephrine mixture. Control mice had 19 of 20 mice die within five minutes of injection. All mice treated with JAQ1 survived irrespective of

Table 2 Summary: In Vivo Studies of Glycoprotein VI Antagonists

Study title	Species, dose, route of administration	Results
Long-term anti-thrombotic protection by in vivo depletion of platelet GPVI in mice (59).	Mice, single 100-µg IP dose of a monoclonal GPVI antibody JAQ1	Produced a depletion of GPVI from platelets and abolished responses of platelets to collagen and collagen-related peptides. Mice were protected from lethal thromboembolism produced by injection of collagen and epinephrine.
Two-phase antithrombotic protection after anti-GPVI treatment in mice (60).	Mice, 20-µg IP dose followed by 100-µg IP after 3 hr of a monoclonal GPVI antibody JAQ1	Integrin $\alpha_{IIb}\beta_3$, P-selectin, and procoagulant activity were decreased on days 1 and 2 after injection, returning to normal by day 5. Mice were transiently protected from lethal tissue factor-induced pulmonary thromboembolism with 100% survival for treated vs. 40% for controls.
Soluble GPVI dimer inhibits platelet adhesion and aggregation to the injured vessel wall in vivo (61).	Mice, single 1- or 2-mg/kg IV dose of a GPVI-Fc fusion protein	Administration of 1 or 2 mg/kg of GPVI-Fc resulted in a modest increase in bleeding time or 11% and 21%, respectively. The carotid endothelium was denuded and platelet adhesion was followed. GPVI-Fc reduced platelet adhesion by 49% and 65%, respectively. Aggregation of adherent platelets was absent in animals treated with 2 mg/kg.
Ex vivo evaluation of anti-GPVI antibody in cynomolgus monkeys: Dissociation between antiplatelet aggregatory effect and bleeding time (62).	Cynomolgus monkeys, dose-escalating study (0.2–18.8 mg/kg) of OM2 monoclonal antibody to GPVI	A dose of 0.2-mg/kg inhibited collagen-induced aggregation by >80% with only a 1.3 × baseline increase in bleeding time, while a cumulative dose of 18.8 mg/kg increased bleeding time by 1.9 ×. Abciximab (0.35 mg/kg) increased bleeding time by 5 ×. A 0.4-mg/kg IV dose of OM2 inhibited platelet aggregation for 6 hr.
The Fab fragment of a novel anti-GPVI monoclonal antibody, OM4, reduces in vivo thrombosis without bleeding risk in rats (63).	Rat, 20-mg/kg IV dose of OM4 Fab antibody to GPVI	In a modified Folts model of cyclic flow, OM4 reduced the number of complete occlusions without prolongation of the tail- and nail-bleeding times compared with 7E3 Fab GPIIb/IIIa inhibitor (5 mg/kg) that doubled both bleeding times with a similar effect on number of complete occlusions.

Abbreviations: GP, glycoprotein; IV, intravenous.

treatment times of 3, 7, or 14 days before challenge. Histological evaluation confirmed that control mice had platelet-rich thrombi occluding a majority of large and small pulmonary arteries, while only a few thrombi were observed in the vessels of JAQ1-treated mice (59). Similar results were observed in mice with regard to tissue factor–induced pulmonary thromboembolism with 100% survival in treated mice versus 40% survival in the control group (60).

Studies of human monoclonal antibody-derived Fab fragments have also been reported (64). The antibody (9012.2) was obtained by immunizing mice with the cDNA, encoding soluble GPVI as a fusion protein. The antibody bound to human platelets, and GPVI transduced U937 cells. Its specificity was limited to primates with no binding to rodent platelets. The antibody did not bind GPVI after reduction, suggesting that the epitope is structural. Fab fragments and 9012.2 IgG induced platelet aggregation at concentrations of 150 and 2.5 μg/mL, respectively. This activation was inhibited when either anti-FcγRIIa or polyclonal anti-FPVI Fabs antibodies were included. Monovalent Fab fragments did not induce platelet aggregation or secretion and dose dependently inhibited collagen-induced platelet aggregation with full inhibition at 5- to 20-μg/mL Fab fragments. However, there was no inhibition of thrombin or thromboxane (U46619)-induced aggregation. Finally, 9012.2 Fab fragments were evaluated for their ability to inhibit platelet adhesion under flow conditions. Treatment with 50 μg/mL decreased the number of platelets and the translocation velocity at early times and the number and size of platelet aggregates at the later time points. The covered surface was reduced by 68% at one minute of perfusion.

An additional family of monoclonal antibodies (OM1–OM4) has also been reported (63,65). The effect of Fab fragment of the OM2 antibody was evaluated on ex vivo collagen-induced platelet aggregation and skin-bleeding time after intravenous injection in cynomolgus monkeys in a dose-escalation study. OM2 inhibited collagen-induced platelet aggregation (>80%) at the cumulative dose of 0.2 mg/kg with a slight prolongation of bleeding time (1.3 times baseline value). The highest dose tested (18.8 mg/kg) only prolonged bleeding time 1.9 times, while the GPIIb/IIIa antagonist abciximab prolonged bleeding time by 5.0 times at the lowest effective platelet inhibitory dose (0.35 mg/kg). A bolus injection of OM2 at 0.4 mg/kg produced potent inhibition of collagen-induced aggregation up to six hours after injection. The injection of OM2 Fab did not induce thrombocytopenia and GPVI depletion in monkeys (62). The OM4 antibody was found to cross-react with rat GPVI, allowing more detailed studies in this species. OM4 IgG caused acute thrombocytopenia, but OM4 Fab did not deplete platelet GPVI nor cause thrombocytopenia (63). Collagen-induced aggregation inhibition IC50 was 20 to 30 μg/mL. Of greater interest was the fact that OM4 Fab at a dose of 20 mg/kg reduced cyclic flow in a modified Folts model when given either before or after carotid injury without an increase in bleeding time (63). Massberg et al. (61) reported on the efficacy of a GPVI-Fc fusion molecule. A concentration of 800-μg/mL GPVI-Fc reduced human platelet adhesion to collagen by 37% to 44% at shear rates of 500 and 2000 sec^{-1}, respectively. Platelet adhesion to VWF was unaffected. Administration of 1 or 2 mg/kg of GPVI-Fc resulted in a modest increase in bleeding time, or 11% and 21%, respectively. These results were similar to that described with GPVI depletion described above. The effect of GPVI-Fc treatment on platelet recruitment was evaluated. Mice were pretreated with 1 or 2 mg/kg of GPVI-Fc or equimolar control Fc. The carotid endothelium was denuded, and platelet adhesion was followed by fluorescence microscopy. GPVI-Fc reduced platelet adhesion by 49% and 65%, respectively. Aggregation of adherent platelets was absent in animals treated with 2 mg/kg. This was confirmed by scanning electron microscopy and immunohistochemistry that showed significantly lower platelet accumulation and the presence of GPVI-Fc accumulated on the injured carotid surface.

SUMMARY

The past decade has seen a growing interest in targeting platelet adhesion and activation mediated through interactions of VWF with platelet GPIbα and collagen with platelet GPVI. The majority of the specific antagonists directed to these pathways have been biologics that include soluble ligands, soluble receptors, and antibodies. Animal model studies support the potential therapeutic value of inhibiting these pathways and suggest that effective doses are less likely to be associated with bleeding complications compared with current antiplatelet therapies. These findings have been supported by the limited clinical studies that have been reported in human volunteer studies. Two of these agents have entered clinical trials, and the results of these studies will be important to determinine the true therapeutic potential of inhibiting these platelet adhesion and activation pathways.

REFERENCES

1. Libby P. Current concepts of the pathogenesis of the acute coronary syndromes. Circulation 2001; 104:365–372.
2. Shah PK. Mechanisms of plaque vulnerability and rupture. J Am Coll Cardiol 2003; 41(4 suppl S): 15S–22S.
3. Mehta SR, Yusuf S. Short-and long-term oral antiplatelet therapy in acute coronary syndromes and percutaneous coronary intervention. J Am Coll Cardiol 2003; 41(4 suppl S):79S–88S.
4. Chew DP, Moliterno DJ. A critical appraisal of platelet glycoprotein IIb/IIIa inhibition. J Am Coll Cardiol 2000; 36:2028–2035.
5. Gurm HS, Smith DE, Collins JS, et al. The relative safety and efficacy of abciximab and eptifibatide in patients undergoing primary percutaneous coronary intervention. Insights from a large regional intervention. J Am Coll Cardiol 2008; 51:529–535.
6. Montalescot G, Borentain M, Payot L, et al. Early vs. late administration of glycoprotein IIb/IIIa inhibitors in primary percutaneous coronary interventions of acute ST-segment elevation of myocardial infarction: a meta-analysis. JAMA 2004; 292:362–366.
7. Jackson S. The growing complexity of platelet aggregation. Blood 2007; 109:5087–5095.
8. Wagner D. Cell biology of von Willebrand factor. Annu Rev Cell Biol 1990; 6:217–246.
9. Ruggeri ZM, and Ware J. von Willebrand factor. FASEB J 1993; 7:308–316.
10. Ruggeri Z. Perspectives series: cell adhesion in vascular biology - von Willebrand factor. J Clin Invest 1997; 99:559–564.
11. Weiss HJ, Sussman I, Hoyer LW. Stabilization of factor VIII in plasma by the von Willebrand factor. Studies on posttransfusion and dissociated factor VIII and in patients with von Willebrand's disease. J Clin Invest 1977; 60:390–404.
12. Sadler JE. Biomedicine. Contact: how platelets touch von Willebrand factor. Science 2002; 297:1128–1129.
13. Huizinga EG, Tsuji S, Romljn RAP, et al. Structures of glycoprotein Ibα and its complex with von Willebrand Factor A1 domain. Science 2002; 297:1176–1179.
14. Sadler JE. Structural biology: a ménage a trois in two configurations. Science 2003; 301:177–179.
15. Cilikel R, McClintock RA, Roberts JR, et al. Modulation of the α-thrombin function by distinct interactions with platelet glycoprotein Ibα. Science 2003; 301:218–221.
16. Dumas JJ, Kumar R, Seehra J, et al. Crystal structure of the GpIbα-thrombin complex essential for platelet aggregation. Science 2003; 301:222–226.

17. Andrews RK, Shen Y, Gardiner EE, et al. The glycoprotein Ib-IX-V complex in platelet adhesion and signaling. Thromb Haemost 1999; 82:357–364.
18. Handa M, Titani K, Holland LZ, et al. The von Willebrand factor-binding domain of platelet membrane glycoprotein Ib. Characterization by monoclonal antibodies and partial amino acid sequence analysis of proteolytic fragments. J Biol Chem 1986; 261:12579–12585.
19. Vicente V, Houghten RA, Ruggeri ZM. Identification of a site in the alpha chain of platelet glycoprotein Ib that participates in the von Willebrand factor binding. J Biol Chem 1990; 265:274–280.
20. Uff S, Clemetson JM, Harrison T, et al. Crystal structure of the platelet glycoprotein Ib (alpha) N-terminal domain reveals an unmasking mechanism for receptor activation. J Biol Chem 2002; 277:35657–35663.
21. Emsley J, Cruz H, Handin R, et al. Crystal structure of the von Willebrand Factor A1 domain and implications for the binding of platelet glycoprotein Ib. J Biol Chem 1998; 273: 10396–10401.
22. Murata M, Furihata K, Ishida F, et al. Genetic and structural characterization of an amino acid dimorphism in glycoprotein Ib alpha involved in platelet transfusion refractoriness. Blood 1992; 79:2086–3090.
23. Takahashi H, Murata M, Moriki T, et al. Substitution of Val for Met at residue 239 of platelet glycoprotein Ib alpha in Japanese patients with platelet-type von Willebrand disease. Blood 1995; 85:727–733.
24. Kunishima S, Heaton DC, Naoe T, et al. De novo mutation of the platelet glycoprotein Ib alpha gene in a patient with pseudo-von Willebrand disease. Blood Coagul Fibrinolysis 1997; 8:305–311.
25. Miller JL, Lyle VA, Cunningham D. Mutation of leucine-57 to phenylalanine in a platelet glycoprotein Ib alpha leucine tandem repeat occurring in patients with an autosomal dominant variant of Bernard-Soulier disease. Blood 1992; 79:439–446.
26. Weiss HJ, Meyer D, Rabinowitz R, et al. Pseudo-von Willebrand's disease. An intrinsic platelet defect with aggregation by unmodified human factor VIII/von Willebrand factor and enhanced adsorption of its high-molecular-weight multimers. N Engl J Med 1982; 306:326–333.
27. Dong J, Schade AJ, Romo GM, et al. Novel gain-of-function mutations of platelet glycoprotein Ib alpha by valine mutagenesis in the Cys209-Cys248 disulfide loop. Functional analysis under stasis and dynamic conditions. J Biol Chem 2000; 275:27663–27670.
28. Dong JF, Hyun W, Lopez JA. Aggregation of mammalian cells expressing the platelet glycoprotein (GP) Ib-IX complex and the requirement for tyrosine sulfation of GP Ib alpha. Blood 1995; 86:4175–4183.
29. Dong J, Ye P, Schade AJ, et al. Tyrosine sulfation of glycoprotein I(b)alpha. Role of electrostatic interactions in von Willebrand factor binding. J Biol Chem 2001; 276: 16690–16694.
30. Fredrickson BJ, Dong JF, McIntire LV, et al. Shear-dependent rolling on von Willebrand factor of mammalian cells expressing the platelet glycoprotein Ib-IX-V complex. Blood 1998; 92:3684–3693.
31. Hennan JK, Swillo RE, Morgan GW, et al. Pharmacologic inhibition of platelet vWF-GPIbα interaction prevents coronary artery thrombosis. Thromb Haemost 2006; 95:469–475.
32. Shida Y, Nishio K, Sugimoto M, et al. Functional imaging of shear-dependent activity of ADAMTS13 in regulating mural thrombus growth under whole blood flow conditions. Blood 2008; 111:1295–1298.
33. Kageyama S, Matsushita J, Yamamoto H. Effect of a humanized monoclonal antibody to von Willebrand factor in a canine model of coronary artery thrombosis. Eur J Pharmacol 2002; 443: 143–149.
34. Kageyama S, Yamamoto H, Nakazawa H, et al. Pharmacokinetics and pharmacodynamics of AJW200, a humanized monoclonal antibody to von Willebrand factor, in monkeys. Arterioscler Thromb Vasc Biol 2002; 22:187–192.
35. Goto S, Sakai H, Goto M, et al. Enhanced shear-induced platelet aggregation in acute myocardial infarction. Circulation 1999; 99:608–613.

36. Montalescot G, Philippe F, Ankri A, et al. Early increase of von Willebrand factor predicts adverse outcome in unstable coronary artery disease: beneficial effects of enoxaparin. Circulation 1998; 90:988–996.

37. Frossard M, Fuchs I, Leitner JM, et al. Platelet function predicts myocardial damage in patients with acute myocardial infarction. Circulation 2004; 110:1392–1397.

38. Strony J, Song A, Rusterholtz L, et al. Aurintricarboxylic acid prevents acute rethrombosis in a canine model of arterial thrombosis. Arterioscler Thromb Vasc Biol 1995; 15:359–366.

39. McGhie AI, McNatt J, Ezov N, et al. Abolition of cyclic flow variations in stenosed, endothelium-injured coronary arteries in nonhuman primates with a peptide fragment (VCL) derived from human plasma von Willebrand factor-glycoprotein Ib binding domain. Circulation 1994; 90:2976–2981.

40. Wadanoli M, Sako D, Shaw GD, et al. The von Willebrand factor antagonist (GPG-290) prevents coronary thrombosis without prolongation of bleeding time. Thromb Haemost 2007; 98:397–405.

41. Kageyama S, Yamamoto H, Nagano M, et al. Anti-thrombotic effects and bleeding risk of AJvW-2, a monoclonal antibody against human von Willebrand factor. Br J Pharmacol 1997; 122:165–171.

42. Machin SJ. A humanized monoclonal antibody against the vWF A1 domain inhibits vWF: RiCoF activity and platelet adhesion in human volunteers. J Thromb Haemost 2006; (suppl 1): 328.

43. Rottman JB, Gilbert M, Marsh HN, et al. An anti-von Willebrand Factor A1 domain aptamer inhibits arterial thrombosis induced by electrical injury in cynomolgus macaques. J Thromb Haemostas 2007; 5:P-S-664.

44. Gilbert JC, DeFeo-Fraulini T, Hutabarat RM, et al. Pharmacokinetics, pharmacodynamics, and safety of an anti-von Willebrand factor therapeutic aptamer, ARC1779, in healthy volunteers. Circulation 2007; 116:2678–2686.

45. Schneider D, Turek C, Gold L. Selection of high affinity RNA ligands to the bacteriophage R17 coat protein. J Mol Biol 1992; 228:862–869.

46. Joyce GF. In vitro evolution of nucleic acids. Curr Opin Struct Biol 1994; 4:331–336.

47. Klug SJ, Famulok M. All you wanted to know about SELEX. Mol Biol Rep 1994; 20:97–107.

48. Gold L. The SELEX process: a surprising source of therapeutic and diagnostic compounds. Harvey Lect 2003; 91:47–57.

49. Brody EN, Gold L. Aptamers as therapeutic and diagnostic agents. J Biotechnol 2000; 74:5–13.

50. Lagasse HAD, Merlino PG, Marsh HN, et al. Discovery and characterization of a potent neutralizing anti-VWF A1 domain specific aptamer. J Thromb Haemostas 2007; 5:P-S-665.

51. Merlino PG, Gilbert M, Lagasse H, et al. Inhibition of platelet function by the anti-von Willebrand factor aptamer, ARC1779. J Thromb Haemostas 2007; 5:P-M-346.

52. Clemetson JM, Polgar J, Magnenat E, et al. The platelet collagen receptor glycoprotein VI is a member of the immunoglobulin superfamily closely related to FcαR and the natural killer receptors. J Biol Chem 1999; 274:29019–29024.

53. Clemetson KJ, Clemetson JM. Platelet collagen receptors. Thromb Haemostast 2001; 86:189–197.

54. Samaha FF, Kahn ML. Novel platelet and vascular roles for immunoreceptor signaling. Arterioscler Thromb Vasc Biol 2006; 26:2588–2593.

55. Miura Y, Takahashi T, Jung SM, et al. Analysis of the interaction of platelet collagen receptor glycoprotein VI (GPVI) with collagen. J Biol Chem 2002; 277:46197–46204.

56. Arthur JF, Gardiner EE, Matzaris M, et al. Glycoprotein VI is associated with GPIb-IX-V on the membrane of resting and activated platelets. Thromb Haemost 2005; 93:716–723.

57. Nieswandt B, Watson SP. Platelet-collagen interaction: is GPVI the central receptor? Blood 2003; 102:449–461.

58. Varga-Szabo D, Pleines I, Nieswandt B. Cell adhesion mechanisms in platelets. Arterioscler Thromb Vasc Biol 2008; 28:403–412. [Epub 2008, Jan 3].

59. Nieswandt B, Schulte V, Bergmeier W, et al. Long-term anti-thrombotic protection by in vivo depletion of platelet glycoprotein VI in mice. J Exp Med 2001; 193:459–470.

60. Schulte V, Reusch HP, Pozgajova M, et al. Two-phase antithrombotic protection after anti-glycoprotein VI treatment in mice. Arterioscler Thromb Vasc Biol 2006; 26:1640–1647.
61. Massberg S, Konrad I, Bultmann A, et al. Soluble glycoprotein VI dimer inhibits platelet adhesion and aggregation to the injured vessel wall in vivo. FASEB J 2004; 18:397–399.
62. Matsumoto Y, Takizawa H, Nakama K, et al. Ex vivo evaluation of anti-GPVI antibody in cynomolgus monkeys: dissociation between anti-platelet aggregatory effect and bleeding time. Thromb Haemost 2006; 96:167–175.
63. Li H, Lockyer S, Concepcion A, et al. The Fab fragment of a novel anti-GPVI monoclonal antibody, OM4, reduces in vivo thrombosis without bleeding risk in rats. Arterioscler Thromb Vasc Biol 2007; 27:1199–1205.
64. Lecut C, Feeney LA, Kingsbury G, et al. Human platelet glycoprotein VI function is antagonized by monoclonal antibody-derived Fab fragments. J Thromb Haemost 2003; 1:2653–2662.
65. Matsumoto Y, Taizawa H, Gong X, et al. Highly potent anti-human GPVI monoclonal antibodies derived from GPVI knockout mouse immunization. Thromb Res 2007; 119:319–329.

27

Three Generations of Thienopyridines: Ticlopidine, Clopidogrel, and Prasugrel

Stephen D. Wiviott and Elliott M. Antman
Cardiovascular Division, Department of Medicine, Brigham and Women's Hospital, Harvard Medical School, Boston, Massachusetts, U.S.A.

BACKGROUND: ROLE OF THE PLATELET IN THROMBOSIS AND PLATELET RECEPTORS

Platelets play a key role in thrombosis and in the pathophysiology of ischemic syndromes related to coronary artery disease (CAD) and atherosclerotic vascular disease including peripheral vascular disease and cerebrovascular disease (1). Inactivated platelets circulate in a resting state until encountering activating substances such as thrombin and collagen. With the binding of these messenger molecules, platelets become activated, resulting in two major processes: shape change, which exposes more surface area for binding messengers and interaction with other circulating cells including platelets and leukocytes, and degranulation, which results in the release of secondary messengers, which further activates circulating platelet in a paracrine fashion. In addition to further platelet activation, release of signaling molecules including serotonin results in local vaso-constriction. Activation of platelets also results in the exposure of activated glycoprotein (GP) IIb/IIIa receptors allowing for fibrin-mediated cross-links of multiple platelets and formation of aggregates leading to an early platelet monolayer, which seals an injured vessel. In the setting of bleeding, this physiologic process serves a protective role; however, in the setting of atherosclerotic plaque rupture—either spontaneously or following percutaneous coronary intervention (PCI)—this process is central to the transition from stable CAD to unstable coronary syndromes including unstable angina (UA), non-ST-elevation myocardial infarction (NSTEMI), and ST-elevation MI (STEMI).

Among the multiple signaling molecules in this cascade of platelet activation and aggregation, adenosine diphosphate (ADP) is a central component. It is released from platelet-dense granules, and in its paracrine action this molecule results in amplification of the process regardless of how it is initiated. ADP binds to several receptors on the platelet surface including $P2Y_1$, and $P2Y_{12}$ (2). Each of these receptors plays a role in platelet activation and aggregation in addition to $P2X_1$ [an adenosine triphosphate (ATP) receptor], which supports shape change. The coactivation of both $P2Y_1$ and $P2Y_{12}$ is necessary for sustained platelet activation and aggregation in response to ADP (3). $P2Y_1$ activation initiates the process, and $P2Y_{12}$ amplifies and sustains activation. $P2Y_{12}$ is a G-protein-coupled seven transmembrane domain receptor that acts as a co-stimulator of platelets. Activation of the $P2Y_{12}$ receptor results in amplification of platelet activation regardless of the activating stimulus. As an amplifying receptor of an amplifying messenger (ADP), it is logical that this receptor could be an important target for management of thrombotic complications of platelet activation and aggregation (2). The inhibition of the $P2Y_{12}$ receptor results in both reduced platelet activation (resulting in less amplification of the effects of a given procoagulant stimulus) and inhibition of the expression of activated GP IIb/IIIa receptors, resulting in a reduction in platelet aggregation.

The thienopyridine antiplatelet agents (ticlopidine, clopidogrel, and prasugrel) (2) are irreversible inhibitors of the $P2Y_{12}$ receptor and are the subject of the current chapter. Each of these drugs is an inactive prodrug, which requires metabolic activation to expose the thiol moiety that directly and irreversibly binds to the $P2Y_{12}$ receptor and inactivates it. The metabolism of these drugs to their active metabolites plays a major role in the differences between agents in this class.

FIRST-GENERATION THIENOPYRIDINE: TICLOPIDINE

Ticlopidine was the first thienopyridine antiplatelet agent with widespread use in clinical practice. Initial development of this agent in comparison with aspirin was performed in patients with cerebrovascular and peripheral vascular disease. Ticlopidine was demonstrated to be superior to aspirin in the reduction of ischemic events in patients with previous transient ischemic attack or stroke in the Ticlopidine Aspirin Stroke Study (TASS) (4) and the Canadian American Ticlopidine Study (CATS) (5).

In a small study of patients with UA, the addition of ticlopidine to "standard therapy" resulted in a significant reduction in MI, foreshadowing a major use of thienopyridines (6). The major utility of ticlopidine, however, was demonstrated in combination with aspirin as dual antiplatelet therapy in the setting of PCI with intracoronary stenting (7–10) (Fig. 1). A series of trials of dual antiplatelet therapy in comparison with oral anticoagulant therapy (OAC), showing uniform and substantial benefits for the former, established a new standard of care for patients with PCI and coronary stenting. Further, these data helped to clarify the pathologic role of platelet activation and aggregation in the pathophysiology of ischemic complications following PCI. On the basis of these data, ticlopidine currently has two approved indications, the prevention of stroke in patients with prior stroke or risk for stroke and the prevention of subacute stent thrombosis in patients with coronary stents.

However, tolerability issues with ticlopidine including the potential for severe hematopoietic side effects such as bone marrow aplasia (12) limited its use, but led the way for the development and widespread use of the second-generation thienopyridine, clopidogrel, in PCI. Because of the side effect profile, ticlopidine has a limited role in the current clinical practice.

SECOND-GENERATION THIENOPYRIDINE: CLOPIDOGREL

Clopidogrel in PCI and Stenting

Building upon the knowledge based on the study of ticlopidine in PCI and the improved tolerability of clopidogrel (13), the second-generation thienopyridine has become the standard of care for dual antiplatelet therapy to support PCI. The Clopidogrel Aspirin Stent International Cooperative Study (CLASSICS) (11) trial compared ticlopidine plus aspirin

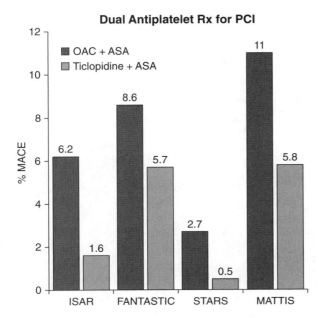

Figure 1 Major trials of the comparison of aspirin plus OAC on major adverse cardiac events in patients following PCI with stenting (*left panel*) , comparison of ticlopidine and clopidogrel in addition to aspirin in patients with coronary stenting (*right panel*) (11). Dual antiplatelet therapy showed significant benefit compared with oral anticoagulation. Ticlopidine and clopidogrel had similar benefits. *Abbreviation*: OAC, anticoagulant therapy. *Source*: From Refs. 7–10.

with clopidogrel (with or without a loading dose) plus aspirin in patients with successful stenting. The primary endpoint was safety and tolerability of the drug regimens. Clopidogrel was found to have a significantly better safety/tolerability profile, but no difference in recurrent ischemic events. Dual antiplatelet therapy with aspirin and clopidogrel has become the standard of care for all patients undergoing PCI with stenting regardless of indication, as supported by PCI guidelines (14). However, controversy remains regarding the timing and dose of clopidogrel as is discussed below.

Clopidogrel as Monotherapy

Similar to the earlier studies of ticlopidine, clopidogrel has been studied as monotherapy in comparison with aspirin in patients at risk for ischemic vascular events. More than 19,000 patients with atherosclerotic vascular disease manifested as either recent ischemic stroke, recent MI, or symptomatic peripheral arterial disease were randomized to either asprin (325 mg) or clopidogrel 75 mg for one to three years in the Clopidogrel versus Aspirin in Patients at Risk for Ischemic Events (CAPRIE) (15) trial. Patients treated with clopidogrel had a significant 0.5% absolute and 8.7% relative reduction in the composite endpoint of MI, ischemic stroke, or vascular death. Of significant importance, the CAPRIE trial demonstrated that clopidogrel was well tolerated without significant increases in hematopoetic side effects. This trial paved the way for approval of clopidogrel as the second thienopyridine available for clinical use.

Dual Antiplatelet Therapy with Aspirin and Clopidogrel

Like ticlopidine, the major utility of clopidogrel is in combination with aspirin as a component of a dual antiplatelet therapy strategy. The Clopidogrel in Unstable Angina to

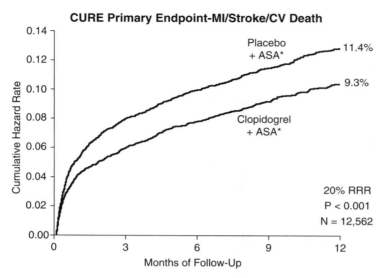

Figure 2 The primary efficacy results of the CURE trial. A significant 20% risk reduction was observed with clopidogrel plus aspirin compared with aspirin alone. *Source*: From Ref. 16.

Prevent Recurrent Events (CURE) trial tested clopidogrel plus aspirin compared with aspirin alone in more than 12,500 patients with UA or NSTEMI (16). The patients randomly assigned to clopidogrel had a 20% reduction in the primary endpoint of cardiovascular death, MI, or stroke (11.4% vs. 9.3%, Fig. 2). This was accompanied by an increase in major bleeding events (3.7% vs. 2.7%; RR = 1.38; $p = 0.001$); however, there was no difference in life-threatening bleeding (2.2% vs. 1.8%; $p = 0.13$) (16). A key substudy of CURE was the evaluation of more than 2500 patients enrolled in the main trial that underwent PCI, subsequently termed PCI-CURE (17). Clopidogrel plus aspirin appeared particularly effective in this population with a 30% relative reduction in the key composite endpoint of cardiovascular death, MI, and urgent revascularization, a finding that was persistent to one-year follow-up (17). On the basis of these studies, and others, the American College of Cardiology/American Heart Association (ACC/AHA) guidelines recommend dual antiplatelet therapy with aspirin and clopidogrel in patients with acute coronary syndromes for up to one year regardless of treatment strategy (medical, PCI, or surgery) (18).

Patients with STEMI were not included in the CURE trial, but they have a strong clinical trial evidence for the use of dual antiplatelet therapy including aspirin and clopidogrel. In the Clopidogrel as Adjunctive Reperfusion Therapy Clopidogrel as Adjunctive Reperfusion Therapy–Thrombolysis in Myocardial Infarction (CLARITY-TIMI 28) (19) trial, nearly 3500 subjects less than 75 years with STEMI and receiving fibrinolytic therapy were randomized to dual antiplatelet therapy with clopidogrel (a 300-mg loading dose followed by 75 mg daily in all subjects) and aspirin compared with aspirin alone. All subjects were to undergo planned coronary angiography following stabilization. The composite endpoint of death, MI, or an occluded infarct-related artery was highly statistically significantly reduced by 36% from 21.7% to 15.0%. This difference was not accompanied either by an increase in major bleeding nor a difference in intracranial hemorrhage (19). A key mechanistic observation from the CLARITY study was made by an analysis of ST-segment resolution, a noninvasive marker of reperfusion (20). This study demonstrated no increase in the rate of complete ST-segment resolution with clopidogrel therapy (38.4% vs. 36.6%), but there was a substantial benefit among those patients who achieved complete ST-segment resolution (OR 2.0, $p < 0.001$). This suggests that the mechanism of benefit of clopidogrel in this population was not the facilitation of fibrinolyisis for reperfusion, rather the prevention of reocclusion in patients who were successfully reperfused (20). Another key observation from CLARITY-TIMI 28 was that in subjects who underwent PCI, allocation to clopidogrel at the time of enrollment (pretreatment) was superior to clopidogrel given at the time of PCI. Pretreatment with clopidogrel resulted in a 46% relative reduction in the composite of death, recurrent MI, or stroke in the 30 days following PCI (21). These data, though not formally a randomized study, are perhaps the best rationale for pretreatment with clopidogrel prior to PCI.

The results of CLARITY-TIMI 28 were complemented by the report of the Clopidogrel and Metoprolol in Myocardial Infarction Trial/Second Chinese Cardiac Study (COMMIT/CCS-2) trial (22), a large simple trial of nearly 46,000 Chinese subjects with acute MI. Subjects were enrolled within 24 hours of MI and allocated to clopidogrel 75 mg daily plus aspirin or aspirin alone until hospital discharge. This short duration of clopidogrel administered without a loading dose resulted in a highly significant reduction in overall mortality from 10.1% to 9.2%. Severe bleeding as assessed by fatal bleeding, transfusion, or intracranial hemorrhage was not different between clopidogrel and placebo groups (22). These studies together, have resulted in the recommendation by national guidelines committees for the use of clopidogrel in patients with STEMI treated medically with or without fibrinolytic therapy (23).

While the data for dual antiplatelet therapy is consistent across the spectrum of acute coronary syndromes as noted above, more controversy surrounds the use of clopidogrel in patients with atherosclerosis in other vascular beds. Patients with peripheral arterial disease (PAD) and stroke (CVA) are at high risk not only for events related to the specific diseased vascular bed, but also to other vascular beds, including MI. In patients with noncardioembolic stroke (oral anticoagulation is indicated for secondary prevention of cardioembolic events), guidelines committees recommend either aspirin alone, clopidogrel alone, or the combination of aspirin and extended-release dipyridimole (24). The Management of Atherosclerosis with Clopidogrel in High-risk patients (MATCH) study (25) compared clopidogrel alone with clopidogrel plus aspirin in patients with a recent stroke or transient ischemic attack (TIA) with another high-risk feature (diabetes mellitus, MI, angina, PAD) and found that there was no significant difference in the primary outcome measure of stroke, MI, vascular death, or rehospitalization for ischemic events. However, there was an increased rate of life-threatening bleeding [2.6% vs. 1.3%; absolute risk increase 1.3% (95% CI 0.6 to 1.9)] in the dual antiplatelet therapy group (25). In patients with PAD, aspirin or clopidogrel are considered reasonable alternatives for the management of patients with PAD on the basis of the CAPRIE trial (26).

The Clopidogrel for High Atherosclerotic Risk and Ischemic Stabilization, Management, and Avoidance (CHARISMA) (27) study included more than 15,600 subjects, including more than 12,100 with "symptomatic" cardiovascular disease (CAD, PAD, or cerebrovascular disease) and approximately 3200 with no "symptomatic" disease, but multiple risk factors. These subjects were randomized to aspirin alone or dual antiplatelet therapy with aspirin and clopidogrel during long-term follow-up. Overall, the trial was neutral, showing a nonsignificant 7% lower relative rate of the primary endpoint of cardiovascular death, MI, or stroke (27), accompanied by a nonsignificant trend toward a higher rate of severe bleeding (1.7% vs. 1.2%, $p = 0.09$) (27). The results of the trial were disparate among those with "symptomatic" vascular disease in whom clopidogrel was demonstrated to have a marginally significant reduction in the primary endpoint (6.9%, vs. 7.9% with placebo; RR = 0.88; $p = 0.046$), whereas no benefit and a trend toward harm was seen in the patients with multiple risk factors alone (6.6%, vs. 5.5% with placebo; RR = 1.20, p = 0.20). Therefore, these data do not allow for the extension of dual antiplatelet therapy to the primary prevention of vascular events in a high-risk population; however, these data also do not discourage the long-term use in patients with established vascular disease who have another indication for longer-term therapy (including drug-eluting stents).

Pharmacologic Limitations of Clopidogrel

Despite the profound successes of clopidogrel alone and in combination with aspirin, for patients with atherosclerotic vascular disease, there are limitations of this agent that can impact clinical care (28). As noted above, clopidogrel is a prodrug that requires metabolism for its antiplatelet activity. As a result, the antiplatelet effects of clopidogrel have a delayed onset and substantial variability among patients. The peak antiplatelet effect of a standard 300-mg loading dose of clopidogrel can be expected within 6 to 24 hours after ingestion (29). As a result, a significant period of pretreatment with clopidogrel to achieve adequate antiplatelet therapy to support PCI is necessary. An analysis of the Clopidogrel for the Reduction of Events During Observation (CREDO) study showed that more than 12 hours of pretreatment was necessary before a significant benefit was seen (30,31). However, because clopidogrel irreversibly inactivates platelets, patients who at coronary angiograpy are found to have coronary anatomy appropriate for coronary artery bypass graft (CABG) remain at risk for bleeding for up to five to seven days (32). This creates a clinical conundrum for the treating physician who wishes to have adequate antiplatelet therapy at the time of PCI, but does not wish to expose a patient to delay or risk if a patient needs surgery. In addition to this issue, there is a biological variability in the antiplatelet response to clopidogrel, where some patients have a very limited (or no) antiplatelet response, sometimes termed "resistance" to clopidogrel (28,33–36). These data appear to be more than a laboratory curiosity as a growing number of studies have linked poor antiplatelet response to clopidogrel using a variety of measures to adverse clinical outcomes, particularly coronary ischemia and stent thrombosis (37–40).

Dose Modifications

In part, as a result of these limitations, several investigators have experimented with higher loading- (41–43) dose clopidogrel. These data suggest that 600 to 900 mg of clopidogrel achieve somewhat greater levels of platelet inhibition, more rapidly, and with slightly less variability; however, even with higher doses, some patients continue to have a limited response to clopidogrel (41–43). Clinical data to support the use of higher dose of clopidogrel is limited. One small 255 patient study of 600- versus 300-mg loading doses of clopidogrel prior to PCI demonstrated lower rates of peri-procedural MI in the patients receiving the higher dose (44). A large-scale study of high- versus standard-dose clopidogrel in acute coronary syndrome (ACS) patients with planned PCI, the Clopidogrel optimal loading dose Usage to Reduce Recurrent Events–Organization to Assess Strategies in Ischemic Syndromes (CURRENT-OASIS 7) trial tests the hypothesis that higher-dose clopidogrel will reduce ischemic events (45). Without the OASIS-7 data available, many clinicians have adopted and guidelines committees (14) have commented on the potential benefit for the use of higher loading–dose clopidogrel, usually 600 mg in patients undergoing PCI.

THIRD-GENERATION THIENOPYRIDINE: PRASUGREL

Prasugrel is a novel thienopyridine that is structurally somewhat similar to clopidogrel. However, modifications in some of the molecule's side chains (Fig. 3) result in substantially different metabolic, pharmacokinetic, and pharmacodynamic properties

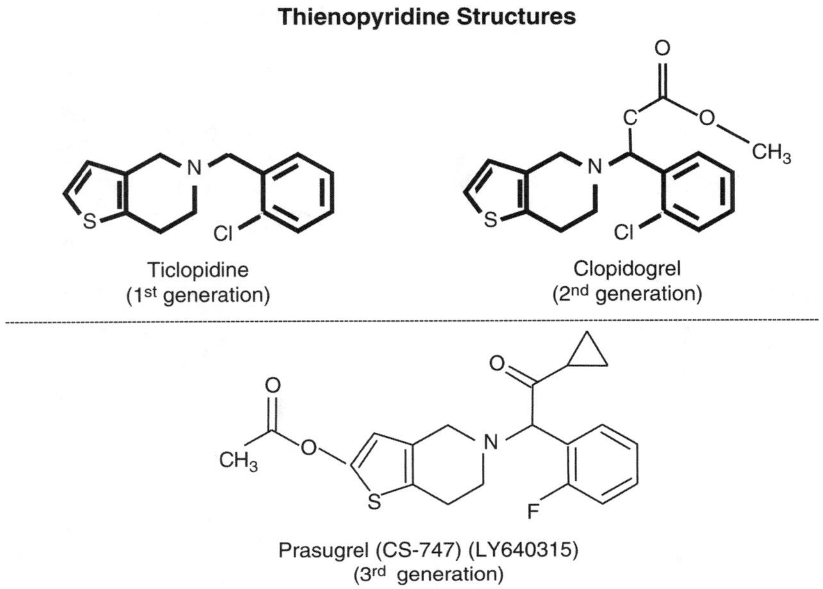

Thienopyridine Structures

Ticlopidine
(1st generation)

Clopidogrel
(2nd generation)

Prasugrel (CS-747) (LY640315)
(3rd generation)

Figure 3 Chemical structures of three generations of the inopyridines.

(46). After clopidogrel is absorbed, approximately 85% of the parent drug is inactivated by plasma esterases. Following this degradation, the remaining drug is metabolized in a two-step, cytochrome-dependent process (Fig. 4). In contrast, prasugrel is not degraded by esterases, the activation process is initiated by these enzymes and followed by a single-step cytochrome-dependent activation. These metabolic differences result in greater potency of prasugrel, more rapid and more consistent generation of the active metabolite, and less susceptibility to drugs or other substances that may interfere with hepatic cytochromes (46). This biology, results in the potential advantages of prasugrel as a more efficient, consistent, and potent thienopyridine than clopidogrel (29,48–50).

Clinical Data in Humans: Platelet Function Testing

In healthy aspirin-naive volunteers, prasugrel has been observed to be approximately ten times more potent than clopidogrel for both loading and maintenance dose regimens (46). The greater consistency of the effect of prasugrel was demonstrated in a crossover study of healthy volunteers (51). This study demonstrated higher levels of platelet inhibition with prasugrel 60 mg compared with clopidogrel 300 mg at each timepoint tested from 30 minutes to 24 hours, with a maximum inhibition of platelet aggregation (IPA) of approximately 78% with prasugrel compared with 35% with clopidogrel. As expected, a wide variability of response to clopidogrel was observed. All subjects who demonstrated a poor response to clopidogrel, responded robustly when treated with prasugrel after a washout period. The mechanistic underpinnings for this observation were more than a 10-fold greater concentration of the active metabolite of prasugrel than clopidogrel (46).

A phase 1b dose-ranging study compared prasugrel and clopidogrel dose regimens for four weeks in approximately 100 subjects with stable CAD receiving aspirin (52). Prasugrel-loading doses of 40 and 60 mg produced greater inhibition of platelet aggregation than 300 mg of clopidogrel by two hours. Maintenance doses of 10 and 15 mg achieved higher levels of platelet inhibition than 75 mg of clopidogrel daily.

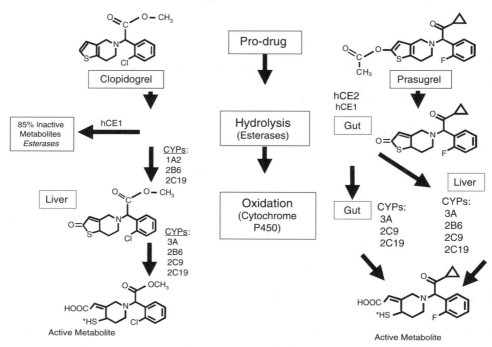

Figure 4 Differential metabolism of prasugrel and clopidogrel. Both drugs are prodrugs, which must be metabolically activated. Eighty-five percent of clopidogrel is inactivated prior to conversion, whereas no such inactivation occurs with prasugrel. *Source*: From Ref. 44,45.

Substantially, fewer subjects treated with prasugrel had IPA less than 20%, the study definition of "nonresponse." At four hours, 52% of clopidogrel-treated subjects had IPA less than 20% compared with 3% of prasugrel-treated subjects.

Prasugrel has also been shown to have a more rapid onset of action and greater platelet inhibition than high-dose clopidogrel. The Prasugrel in Comparision to Clopidogrel for Inhibition of Platelet Activation and Aggregation (PRINCIPLE)-TIMI 44 (53) study randomized approximately patients to prasugrel 60 mg or clopidogrel 600 mg prior to coronary angiography. If patients underwent PCI, they entered a four-week two-phase crossover study comparing 10 mg of prasugrel with 150 mg of clopidogrel. The primary endpoint of IPA to 20 μM ADP was significantly higher for prasugrel, both following loading and maintenance doses (Fig. 5), suggesting that prasugrel is even more potent than high-dose clopidogrel (53).

Clinical Trials Data

These pharmacologic characteristics of prasugrel, more rapid onset, more consistent and greater levels of platelet inhibition led to the hypothesis that prasugrel would reduce ischemic events in patients undergoing PCI. The initial test of this hypothesis was the Joint Utilization of Medications to Block platelets Optimally (JUMBO)-TIMI 26 trial (54). This phase II, dose-ranging safety study enrolled more than 900 patients into three loading/maintenance dose regimens of prasugrel, a low- (40 mg/7.5 mg), intermediate- (60 mg/10 mg), and high- (60 g/15 mg) dose regimens in comparison with clopidogrel

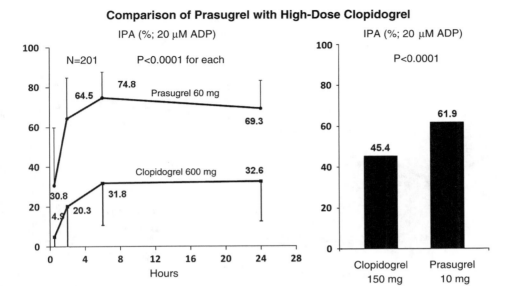

Figure 5 Primary results of the PRINCIPLE-TIMI 44 study (51). Prasugrel (60 mg) resulted in greater and more rapid onset of antiplatelet effect than clopidogrel (600 mg) in the acute phase (*left panel*). Prasugrel (10 mg resulted in higher levels of platelet inhibition than clopidogrel (150 mg) in the chronic phase (*right panel*).

(300 mg/75 mg). No significant difference between prasugrel and clopidogrel was observed for the key safety endpoint of TIMI major or minor bleeding (53). Minimal bleeding was increased with the highest dose regimen. Though, not significant, there was a trend toward fewer ischemic events with prasugrel.

The phase I and phase II data set the stage for the definitive test of prasugrel compared with clopidogrel in The Trial to Assess Improvement in Therapeutic Outcomes by optimizing Platelet Inhibition with Prasugrel (TRITON)-TIMI 38 (55). This trial enrolled more than 13,500 patients with ACS (including UA/NSTEMI and STEMI) and planned PCI, and randomized to prasugrel (60 mg/10 mg) compared with clopidogrel (300 mg/75 mg). Patients were followed for a median of 14.5 months. Treatment with prasugrel resulted in a highly significant 19% reduction in the primary composite endpoint of cardiovascular death, nonfatal MI, and nonfatal stroke from 12.1% to 9.9% ($p < 0.001$) (56) (Fig. 6). The reduction in the primary endpoint was largely driven by a 26% reduction in MI ($p < 0.001$). Cardiovascular death numerically favored prasugrel, and no effect was seen on CVA (Fig. 7). The secondary endpoint of urgent target vessel revascularization was reduced by 34%. These benefits were accompanied by an increase in the key safety endpoint of TIMI major bleeding not associated with CABG in subjects treated with prasugrel (2.4% vs. 1.8%, $p = 0.03$). This included increases in life-threatening and fatal bleeding. In the setting of the disparate results between improved ischemic endpoints and worse bleeding, a net benefit endpoint of all causes of death, nonfatal MI, nonfatal CVA, and nonfatal TIMI major bleeding was examined and favored prasugrel with a significant 13% lower rate. Three subgroups were identified as having a neutral (age > 75 years, weight < 60 kg) or adverse (prior CVA/TIA) net benefit profile. The net benefit endpoint in the approximately 80% of subjects without these features strongly favored prasugrel. In the groups with neutral net benefit, it may be possible to mitigate some of the risk with a lower maintenance dose of prasugrel. In TRITON-TIMI

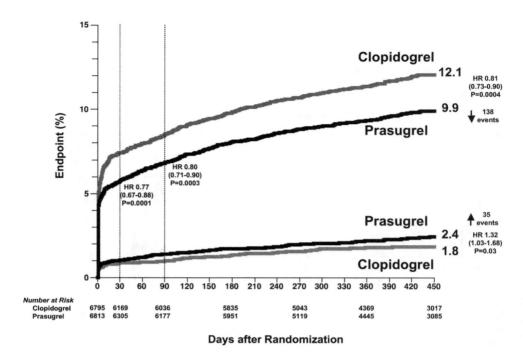

Figure 6 Primary efficacy and safety endpoints of the TRITON-TIMI 38 trial. A significant reduction in the primary endpoint was observed with prasugrel (*black line*) compared with clopidogrel (*gray line*), upper curves. A significant increase in TIMI major non-CABG bleeding was observed with prasugrel (black line) compared with clopidogrel (*gray line*), lower curves. *Abbreviation*: CABG, coronary artery bypass graft. *Source*: From Ref. 54.

Components of Endpoints

		Clopidogrel	Prasugrel	HR
CV Death, MI, Stroke		12.1	9.9	0.81
CV Death		2.4	2.1	0.89
Nonfatal MI		9.5	7.3	0.76
Nonfatal Stroke		1.0	1.0	1.02
All Cause Mortality		3.2	3.0	0.95
uTVR		3.7	2.5	0.66
Stent Thrombosis		2.4	1.1	0.48

0.5 ← Prasugrel Better   1   Clopidogrel Better → 2
HR

Figure 7 Selected endpoints of the TRITON-TIMI 38 trial (54). Kaplan-Meier event rates, hazard ratios, and confidence intervals are displayed. *Abbreviations*: CV, cardiovascular; MI, myocardial infarction; uTVR, urgent target vessel revascularization.

38, prasugrel decreased the rate of stent thrombosis, a rare but devastating consequence of PCI, by 52% (57). These findings were robust regardless of stent type, timing after the initial index procedures, and across many different clinical and procedural characteristics.

In addition to establishing the safety and efficacy of prasugrel, the TRITON-TIMI 38 study also is a proof of concept study. This trial demonstrated, for the first time in an adequately powered study, that a treatment regimen that achieved a faster, higher, and more consistent level of platelet inhibition than standard clopidogrel improved clinical ischemic outcomes. These data also further serve to highlight the importance of platelet activation and aggregation, the $P2Y_{12}$ receptor as a key target for therapy, and the thienopyridine class of drugs as important agents in the treatment of ACS.

SUMMARY AND FUTURE DIRECTIONS

Platelet activation and aggregation play key roles in ischemic complications of atherosclerotic vascular disease. ADP and the $P2Y_{12}$ ADP receptor play key roles in the amplification of these processes, and therefore serve as a key target of therapeutics. Ticlopidine, the first-generation thienopyridine, demonstrated the importance of this class of agents in a clinical setting, both compared with aspirin in secondary prevention and in combination with aspirin in coronary stenting. Tolerabilty and toxicity issues limited the utility of ticlopidine. Clopidogrel, the second-generation thienopyridine, was much better tolerated, and has been demonstrated to have similar effects to ticlopidine in PCI, and is an important part of the pharmacotherapy across the spectrum of ACS. Clopidogrel, despite profound successes, has been shown to have limited speed of onset and potency. These issues have been largely overcome by the third-generation thienopyridine, prasugrel. Prasugrel was shown to be superior to clopidogrel in patients with ACS undergoing PCI, including significant reductions in important ischemic events, but at the cost of more bleeding. Potential strategies to reduce this excess bleeding include dose modification in susceptible subgroups. In the future, it may be possible to identify patients more clearly than by baseline characteristics or disease state that have the greatest chance for benefit from these agents with the least potential for harm.

REFERENCES

1. Lange RA, Hillis LD. Antiplatelet therapy for ischemic heart disease. N Engl J Med 2004; 350:277–280.
2. Cattaneo M. Platelet P2 receptors: old and new targets for antithrombotic drugs. Expert Rev Cardiovasc Ther 2007; 5:45–55.
3. Storey F. The P2Y12 receptor as a therapeutic target in cardiovascular disease. Platelets 2001; 12:197–209.
4. Hass WK, Easton JD, Adams HP Jr., et al. A randomized trial comparing ticlopidine hydrochloride with aspirin for the prevention of stroke in high-risk patients. Ticlopidine Aspirin Stroke Study Group. N Engl J Med 1989; 321:501–507.
5. Gent M, Blakely JA, Easton JD, et al. The Canadian American Ticlopidine Study (CATS) in thromboembolic stroke. Lancet 1989; 1:1215–1220.
6. Balsano F, Rizzon P, Violi F, et al. Antiplatelet treatment with ticlopidine in unstable angina. A controlled multicenter clinical trial. The Studio della Ticlopidina nell'Angina Instabile Group. Circulation 1990; 82:17–26.
7. Bertrand ME, Legrand V, Boland J, et al. Randomized multicenter comparison of conventional anticoagulation versus antiplatelet therapy in unplanned and elective coronary stenting. The full anticoagulation versus aspirin and ticlopidine (fantastic) study. Circulation 1998; 98:1597–1603.

8. Leon MB, Baim DS, Popma JJ, et al. A clinical trial comparing three antithrombotic-drug regimens after coronary-artery stenting. Stent Anticoagulation Restenosis Study Investigators. N Engl J Med 1998; 339:1665–1671.

9. Schomig A, Neumann FJ, Kastrati A, et al. A randomized comparison of antiplatelet and anticoagulant therapy after the placement of coronary-artery stents. N Engl J Med 1996; 334:1084–1089.

10. Urban P, Macaya C, Rupprecht HJ, et al. Randomized evaluation of anticoagulation versus antiplatelet therapy after coronary stent implantation in high-risk patients: the multicenter aspirin and ticlopidine trial after intracoronary stenting (MATTIS). Circulation 1998; 98:2126–2132.

11. Elias M, Reichman N, Flatau E. Bone marrow aplasia associated with ticlopidine therapy. Am J Hematol 1993; 44:289–290.

12. Bhatt DL, Bertrand ME, Berger PB, et al. Meta-analysis of randomized and registry comparisons of ticlopidine with clopidogrel after stenting. J Am Coll Cardiol 2002; 39:9–14.

13. Bertrand ME, Rupprecht HJ, Urban P, et al. Double-blind study of the safety of clopidogrel with and without a loading dose in combination with aspirin compared with ticlopidine in combination with aspirin after coronary stenting: the clopidogrel aspirin stent international cooperative study (CLASSICS). Circulation 2000; 102:624–629.

14. Smith SC Jr., Feldman TE, Hirshfeld JW Jr., et al. ACC/AHA/SCAI 2005 guideline update for percutaneous coronary intervention-summary article: a report of the American College of Cardiology/American Heart Association Task Force on Practice Guidelines (ACC/AHA/SCAI Writing Committee to update the 2001 Guidelines for Percutaneous Coronary Intervention). Catheter Cardiovasc Interv 2006; 67:87–112.

15. CAPRIE Steering Committee. A randomised, blinded, trial of clopidogrel versus aspirin in patients at risk of ischaemic events (CAPRIE). Lancet 1996; 348:1329–1339.

16. Yusuf S, Zhao F, Mehta SR, et al. Effects of clopidogrel in addition to aspirin in patients with acute coronary syndromes without ST-segment elevation. N Engl J Med 2001; 345:494–502.

17. Mehta SR, Yusuf S, Peters RJ, et al. Effects of pretreatment with clopidogrel and aspirin followed by long-term therapy in patients undergoing percutaneous coronary intervention: the PCI-CURE study. Lancet 2001; 358:527–533.

18. Braunwald E, Antman EM, Beasley JW, et al. ACC/AHA guideline update for the management of patients with unstable angina and non-ST-segment elevation myocardial infarction-2002: summary article: a report of the American College of Cardiology/American Heart Association Task Force on Practice Guidelines (Committee on the Management of Patients With Unstable Angina). Circulation 2002; 106:1893–1900.

19. Sabatine MS, Cannon CP, Gibson CM, et al. Addition of clopidogrel to aspirin and fibrinolytic therapy for myocardial infarction with ST-segment elevation. N Engl J Med 2005; 352:1179–1189.

20. Scirica BM, Sabatine MS, Morrow DA, et al. The role of clopidogrel in early and sustained arterial patency after fibrinolysis for ST-segment elevation myocardial infarction: the ECG CLARITY-TIMI 28 Study. J Am Coll Cardiol 2006; 48:37–42.

21. Sabatine MS, Cannon CP, Gibson CM, et al. Effect of clopidogrel pretreatment before percutaneous coronary intervention in patients with ST-elevation myocardial infarction treated with fibrinolytics: the PCI-CLARITY study. JAMA 2005; 294:1224–1232.

22. Chen ZM, Jiang LX, Chen YP, et al. Addition of clopidogrel to aspirin in 45,852 patients with acute myocardial infarction: randomised placebo-controlled trial. Lancet 2005; 366:1607–1621.

23. Antman EM, Hand M, Armstrong PW, et al 2007. Focused Update of the ACC/AHA 2004 Guidelines for the Management of Patients With ST-Elevation Myocardial Infarction: a report of the American College of Cardiology/American Heart Association Task Force on Practice Guidelines: developed in collaboration With the Canadian Cardiovascular Society endorsed by the American Academy of Family Physicians: 2007 Writing Group to Review New Evidence and Update the ACC/AHA 2004 Guidelines for the Management of Patients With ST-Elevation Myocardial Infarction, Writing on Behalf of the 2004 Writing Committee. Circulation 2008; 117:(2)296–329.

24. Adams HP Jr, del Zoppo G, Alberts MJ, et al. Guidelines for the early management of adults with ischemic stroke: a guideline from the American Heart Association/American Stroke Association

Stroke Council, Clinical Cardiology Council, Cardiovascular Radiology and Intervention Council, and the Atherosclerotic Peripheral Vascular Disease and Quality of Care Outcomes in Research Interdisciplinary Working Groups: The American Academy of Neurology affirms the value of this guideline as an educational tool for neurologists. Circulation 2007; 115:e478–e534.

25. Diener HC, Bogousslavsky J, Brass LM, et al. Aspirin and clopidogrel compared with clopidogrel alone after recent ischaemic stroke or transient ischaemic attack in high-risk patients (MATCH): randomised, double-blind, placebo-controlled trial. Lancet 2004; 364:331–337.

26. Hirsch AT, Haskal ZJ, Hertzer NR, et al. ACC/AHA 2005 practice guidelines for the management of patients with peripheral arterial disease (lower extremity, renal, mesenteric, and abdominal aortic): a collaborative report from the American Association for Vascular Surgery/ Society for Vascular Surgery, Society for Cardiovascular Angiography and Interventions, Society for Vascular Medicine and Biology, Society of Interventional Radiology, and the ACC/ AHA Task Force on Practice Guidelines (Writing Committee to Develop Guidelines for the Management of Patients With Peripheral Arterial Disease): endorsed by the American Association of Cardiovascular and Pulmonary Rehabilitation; National Heart, Lung, and Blood Institute; Society for Vascular Nursing; TransAtlantic Inter-Society Consensus; and Vascular Disease Foundation. Circulation 2006; 113:e463–e654.

27. Bhatt DL, Fox KA, Hacke W, et al. Clopidogrel and aspirin versus aspirin alone for the prevention of atherothrombotic events. N Engl J Med 2006; 354:1706–1717.

28. O'Donoghue M, Wiviott SD. Clopidogrel response variability and future therapies: clopidogrel: does one size fit all? Circulation 2006; 114:e600–e606.

29. Weerakkody GJ, Jakubowski JA, Brandt JT, et al. Comparison of speed of onset of platelet inhibition after loading doses of clopidogrel versus prasugrel in healthy volunteers and correlation with responder status. Am J Cardiol 2007; 100:331–336.

30. Steinhubl SR, Berger PB, Mann JT 3rd, et al. Early and sustained dual oral antiplatelet therapy following percutaneous coronary intervention: a randomized controlled trial. JAMA 2002; 288:2411–2420.

31. Steinhubl SR, Darrah S, Brennan D, et al. Optimal duration of pretreatment with clopidogrel prior to PCI: data from the credo trial. Circulation 2003; 08-IV:374 (abstr).

32. Fox KA, Mehta SR, Peters R, et al. Benefits and risks of the combination of clopidogrel and aspirin in patients undergoing surgical revascularization for non-ST-elevation acute coronary syndrome: the Clopidogrel in Unstable angina to prevent Recurrent ischemic Events (CURE) Trial. Circulation 2004; 110:1202–1208.

33. Gurbel PA, Bliden KP. Durability of platelet inhibition by clopidogrel. Am J Cardiol 2003; 91:1123–1125.

34. Gurbel PA, Bliden KP, Hiatt BL, et al. Clopidogrel for coronary stenting: response variability, drug resistance, and the effect of pretreatment platelet reactivity. Circulation 2003; 7:908–913.

35. Jaremo P, Lindahl TL, Fransson SG, et al. Individual variations of platelet inhibition after loading doses of clopidogrel. J Intern Med 2002; 252:233–238.

36. Serebruany VL, Steinhubl SR, Berger PB, et al. Variability in platelet responsiveness to clopidogrel among 544 individuals. J Am Coll Cardiol 2005; 45:246–251.

37. Buonamici P, Marcucci R, Migliorini A, et al. Impact of platelet reactivity after clopidogrel administration on drug-eluting stent thrombosis. J Am Coll Cardiol 2007; 49:2312–2317.

38. Gurbel PA, Bliden KP, Samara W, et al. Clopidogrel effect on platelet reactivity in patients with stent thrombosis: results of the CREST Study. J Am Coll Cardiol 2005; 46:1827–1832.

39. Hochholzer W, Trenk D, Bestehorn HP, et al. Impact of the degree of peri-interventional platelet inhibition after loading with clopidogrel on early clinical outcome of elective coronary stent placement. J Am Coll Cardiol 2006; 48:1742–1750.

40. Wenaweser P, Dorffler-Melly J, Imboden K, et al. Stent thrombosis is associated with an impaired response to antiplatelet therapy. J Am Coll Cardiol 2005; 45:1748–1752.

41. Montalescot G, Sideris G, Meuleman C, et al. A randomized comparison of high clopidogrel loading doses in patients with non-ST-segment elevation acute coronary syndromes: the ALBION (Assessment of the Best Loading Dose of Clopidogrel to Blunt Platelet Activation, Inflammation and Ongoing Necrosis) trial. J Am Coll Cardiol 2006; 48:931–938.

42. Gurbel PA, Bliden KP, Hayes KM, et al. The relation of dosing to clopidogrel responsiveness and the incidence of high post-treatment platelet aggregation in patients undergoing coronary stenting. J Am Coll Cardiol 2005; 45:1392–1396.

43. von Beckerath N, Taubert D, Pogatsa-Murray G, et al. Absorption, metabolization, and antiplatelet effects of 300-, 600-, and 900-mg loading doses of clopidogrel: results of the ISAR-CHOICE (Intracoronary Stenting and Antithrombotic Regimen: Choose Between 3 High Oral Doses for Immediate Clopidogrel Effect) Trial. Circulation 2005; 112:2946–2950.

44. Patti G, Colonna G, Pasceri V, et al. Randomized trial of high loading dose of clopidogrel for reduction of periprocedural myocardial infarction in patients undergoing coronary intervention: results from the ARMYDA-2 (Antiplatelet therapy for Reduction of Myocardial Damage during Angioplasty) study. Circulation 2005; 111:2099–2106.

45. Mehta SR, Bassand JP, Chrolavicius S, et al. Design and rationale of CURRENT-OASIS 7: a randomized, 2 x 2 factorial trial evaluating optimal dosing strategies for clopidogrel and aspirin in patients with ST and non-ST-elevation acute coronary syndromes managed with an early invasive strategy. Am Heart J 2008; 156:(6):1080–1088.

46. Jakubowski JA, Winters KJ, Naganuma H, et al. Prasugrel: a novel thienopyridine antiplatelet agent. A review of preclinical and clinical studies and the mechanistic basis for its distinct antiplatelet profile. Cardiovasc Drug Rev 2007; 25:357–374.

47. Sugidachi A, Asai F, Ogawa T, et al. The in vivo pharmacological profile of CS-747, a novel antiplatelet agent with platelet ADP receptor antagonist properties. Br J Pharmacol 2000; 129:1439–1446.

48. Jakubowski JA, Matsushima N, Asai F, et al. A multiple dose study of prasugrel (CS-747), a novel thienopyridine P2Y(12) inhibitor, compared with clopidogrel in healthy humans. Br J Clin Pharmacol 2007; 63:421–430.

49. Sugidachi A, Ogawa T, Kurihara A, et al. The greater in vivo antiplatelet effects of prasugrel as compared to clopidogrel reflect more efficient generation of its active metabolite with similar antiplatelet activity to that of clopidogrel's active metabolite. J Thromb Haemost 2007; 5:1545–1551.

50. Brandt JT, Payne CD, Wiviott SD, et al. A comparison of prasugrel and clopidogrel loading doses on platelet function: magnitude of platelet inhibition is related to active metabolite formation. Am Heart J 2007; 153:66 e9–e16.

51. Jernberg T, Payne CD, Winters KJ, et al. Prasugrel achieves greater inhibition of platelet aggregation and a lower rate of non-responders compared with clopidogrel in aspirin-treated patients with stable coronary artery disease. Eur Heart J 2006; 27:1166–1173.

52. Wiviott SD, Trenk D, Frelinger AL, et al. Prasugrel compared with high loading- and maintenance-dose clopidogrel in patients with planned percutaneous coronary intervention: the prasugrel in comparison to clopidogrel for inhibition of platelet activation and aggregation-thrombolysis in myocardial infarction 44 trial. Circulation 2007; 116:2923–2932.

53. Wiviott SD, Antman EM, Winters KJ, et al. Randomized comparison of prasugrel (CS-747, LY640315), a novel thienopyridine P2Y12 antagonist, with clopidogrel in percutaneous coronary intervention: results of the Joint Utilization of Medications to Block Platelets Optimally (JUMBO)-TIMI 26 trial. Circulation 2005; 111:3366–3373.

54. Wiviott SD, Antman EM, Gibson CM, et al. Evaluation of prasugrel compared with clopidogrel in patients with acute coronary syndromes: design and rationale for the Trial to assess Improvement in Therapeutic Outcomes by optimizing platelet InhibitioN with prasugrel Thrombolysis In Myocardial Infarction 38 (TRITON-TIMI 38). Am Heart J 2006; 152:627–635.

55. Wiviott SD, Braunwald E, McCabe CH, et al. Prasugrel versus clopidogrel in patients with acute coronary syndromes. N Engl J Med 2007; 357:2001–2015.

56. Wiviott SD, Braunwald E, McCabe CH, et al. Intensive oral antiplatelet therapy for reduction of ischaemic events including stent thrombosis in patients with acute coronary syndromes treated with percutaneous coronary intervention and stenting in the TRITON-TIMI 38 trial: a subanalysis of a randomised trial. Lancet 2008; 371:1315–1316.

57. Herbert JM, Savi P. P2Y12, a new platelet ADP receptor, target of clopidogrel. Semin Vasc Med 2003; 3:113–122.

28

Direct P2Y$_{12}$ Antagonists

Marco Cattaneo
Unità di Ematologia e Trombosi, Ospedale San Paolo, Dipartimento di Medicina, Chirurgia e Odontoiatria, Università degli Studi di Milano, Milan, Italy

INTRODUCTION

Platelets play an important role in thrombus formation. They adhere to exposed subendothelial structures in response to vascular injury and become rapidly activated by interaction with thrombogenic substrates and agonists released or generated locally, such as adenosine-5′-diphosphate (ADP), thromboxane A$_2$, and thrombin. In this manner, they acquire the ability to bind soluble adhesive molecules that become the reactive surface for continuing platelet deposition (platelet aggregation).

ADP plays a key role in the process of platelet aggregate formation. Although it is a weak platelet agonist, when ADP is secreted from the platelet dense granules where it is stored, it amplifies the platelet responses induced by other platelet agonists. The amplifying effect of ADP on platelet aggregation accounts for the critical role played by ADP in hemostasis, as documented by the observation that patients lacking releasable ADP in granule stores or with congenital abnormalities of platelet, ADP receptors have a bleeding diathesis (1,2). In addition, ADP plays a key role in the pathogenesis of arterial thrombosis, because pharmacologic inhibition of ADP-induced platelet aggregation decreases the risk of arterial thrombosis (3). The transduction of the ADP signal involves its interaction with two platelet receptors, which belong to the family of purinergic P2 receptors (1,2,4).

Purinergic Receptors

Purinergic receptors are classified into P1, which are receptors for adenosine, and P2 receptors, which interact with purine and pyrimidine nucleotides (5). The P2 receptors are subdivided into two main groups: G protein-linked or "metabotropic," designated P2Y, and ligand-gated ion channels or "ionotropic," termed "P2X." P2Y receptors are seven-membrane-spanning proteins with a molecular mass of 41 to 53 kDa after glycosylation; their carboxyl terminal domain is on the cytoplasmic side, while the amino terminal domain is exposed to the extracellular environment. Common mechanisms of signal transduction are shared by most seven-membrane-spanning receptors, including activation of phospholipase C and/or regulation of adenylyl cyclase activity (3,5). P2X receptors are ligand-gated ion channels that mediate rapid changes in the membrane permeability of monovalent and divalent cations, including Na^+, K^+, and Ca^{2+}. P2X receptors range from 379 to 595 amino acids and have two transmembrane domains separated by a large extracellular region (3–5). Unlike the P2Y receptors, the amino and carboxyl terminal domains are both on the cytoplasmic side of the plasma membrane. Human platelets express at least three distinct purinergic P2 receptors stimulated by adenosine nucleotides: $P2Y_1$ and $P2Y_{12}$, which interact with ADP, and $P2X_1$, which interacts with ATP (3,4).

The Platelet P2Y Receptors for ADP

The transduction of the ADP signal involves pathways that are mediated by the G_q-coupled $P2Y_1$ receptor and by the G_i-coupled $P2Y_{12}$ receptor. Concomitant activation of both the G_q and G_i pathways by ADP is necessary to elicit normal platelet aggregation. Activation of the G_q pathway through $P2Y_1$ leads to platelet shape change and rapidly reversible aggregation, while activation of the G_i pathway through $P2Y_{12}$ elicits a slowly progressive and sustained platelet aggregation, not preceded by shape change. In vitro studies suggest that $P2Y_1$ and $P2Y_{12}$ appear to contribute to platelet function to a similar extent. Inhibition of $P2Y_1$ or $P2Y_{12}$ accomplishes similar degree of inhibition of thrombus formation on collagen-coated surfaces under different shear forces and of platelet aggregation induced by secretion-causing agonists in the light transmission aggregometer, or by high-shear stress in a viscometer or other instruments that mimic primary hemostasis in vitro (6,7). In addition to its role in ADP-induced platelet aggregation, $P2Y_{12}$ also mediates (i) the potentiation of platelet secretion induced by strong agonists, which is independent of the formation of large aggregates and thromboxane A_2 synthesis (8), (ii) the stabilization of thrombin-induced platelet aggregates (9,10), and (iii) the potentiation of the antiplatelet effects of the natural regulator of platelet function prostacyclin, which reduces platelet reactivity to agonists by increasing the platelet content of cyclic adenosine monophosphate (cAMP), mediated by the stimulation of adenylyl cyclase (Fig. 1) (11). This latter function of $P2Y_{12}$ may significantly contribute to the hemostatic impairment associated with $P2Y_{12}$ deficiency; in fact, it is plausible that higher platelet sensitivity to inhibition by prostacyclin in vivo may account for the more prolonged bleeding time in $P2Y_{12}$ knockout mice compared with $P2Y_1$ knockout (12–14). Inhibition of adenylyl cyclase by $P2Y_{12}$ may also be relevant to the formation of pathologic thrombi at sites of diseased arteries in vivo and on the effect of its pharmacologic inhibition. Therefore, the potentiation of the antiplatelet effect of PGI_2 in vivo may substantially contribute to the potent antithrombotic effect of thienopyridines and other $P2Y_{12}$ antagonists.

In contrast to $P2Y_1$, $P2Y_{12}$ has a very selective tissue distribution (15), making it an attractive molecular target for therapeutic intervention. Indeed, $P2Y_{12}$ is the target of efficacious antithrombotic agents such as the thienopyridines ticlopidine and clopidogrel, which are already used in clinical practice either alone or in combination with other antithrombotic drugs (2).

Thienopyridines

Ticlopidine and clopidogrel are structurally related compounds (Fig. 2), belonging to the thienopyridine family of $P2Y_{12}$ receptor antagonists; they are pro-drugs that are inactive in vitro and need to be metabolized in vivo by the hepatic cytochrome P-450 1A enzymatic pathway to active metabolites, which have very short half-lives. They irreversibly and specifically inhibit the function of the platelet $P2Y_{12}$ receptor (1,3,4,14). The ability of thienopyridines to inhibit platelet aggregation induced by several platelet agonists that induce platelet secretion is accounted for by suppression of the amplifying effect on platelet aggregation of ADP secreted from platelet dense granules (3). Treatment

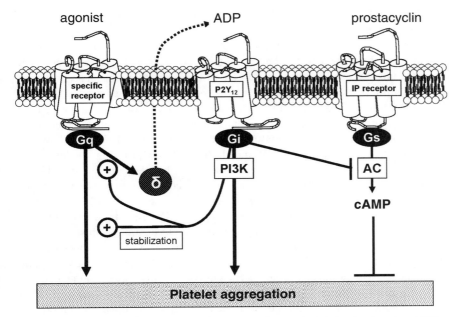

Figure 1 Roles of the platelet receptor for ADP, P2Y$_{12}$, in platelet function. P2Y$_{12}$, a seven-transmembrane receptor that is coupled to the inhibitory G protein G$_i$, induces platelet aggregation and amplifies the aggregation response that is induced by other agonists and/or receptors. In addition, P2Y$_{12}$ stabilizes the platelet aggregates and amplifies the secretion of platelet dense granules stimulated by secretion-inducing agonists (which are coupled to G$_q$). All the above functions are mediated by the activation of PI3K. Although P2Y$_{12}$ is coupled to inhibition of AC through G$_i$, this function is not causally related to P2Y$_{12}$-mediated platelet activation. However, it could have important implications in vivo, when platelets are exposed to the inhibitory prostaglandin PGI$_2$ (prostacyclin), which inhibits platelet aggregation by increasing platelet cyclic adenosine monophosphate (cAMP) through activation of AC mediated by the stimulatory G protein Gs; inhibition of AC by P2Y$_{12}$ counteracts the inhibitory effect of prostacyclin, thereby favoring the formation of platelet aggregates in vivo. Legend of symbols: green arrow, activation; truncated red line, inhibition; blue line ending with a (+), amplification; dotted black line, secretion. *Abbreviations*: cAMP, cyclic adenosine monophosphate; P13K, phosphoinositide 3-phosphate kinase; AC, adenylyl cyclase.

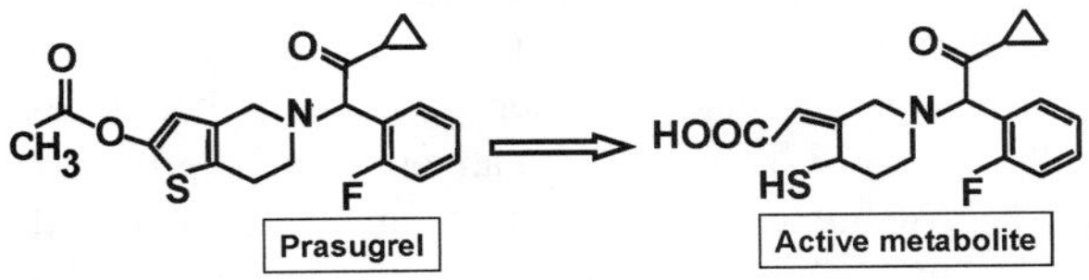

Figure 2 Chemical structures of prasugrel and its active metabolites.

with these thienopyridines renders thrombin-induced platelet aggregates more susceptible to de-aggregation and inhibits shear-induced platelet aggregation (16,17).

The use of ticlopidine and clopidogrel in the clinical setting, despite their proven antithrombotic activity, has some drawbacks. (*i*) The need for their metabolism to active metabolites accounts for their delayed antiplatelet effects: In fact, a maximum plateau of inhibition of ADP-induced platelet aggregation is observed four to five days after daily oral administration of 500 mg ticlopidine or 75 mg clopidogrel (2). It should be noted, however, that the delayed onset of action of clopidogrel can be reduced to about two to five hours by a loading dose of 300 mg to 600 mg (2). (*ii*) As a consequence of the irreversible inhibition of $P2Y_{12}$ function, the inhibitory effect of thienopyridines on circulating platelets lasts for approximately 8 to 10 days, which corresponds to the life span of a circulating platelet. Although the ability of thienopyridines to inhibit irreversibly $P2Y_{12}$ with their short-lived metabolites has theoretical advantages (18), it may represent a problem for patients who need to undergo coronary bypass surgery, because treatment with clopidogrel within five days of the procedure is associated with increased blood loss, reoperation for bleeding, increased transfusion requirements, and prolonged intensive care unit and hospital length of stay (19–21). (*iii*) Finally, there is a substantial interindividual variability in platelet inhibition by ticlopidine and clopidogrel, which is mostly due to interindividual differences in the extent of metabolism of the pro-drug to the active metabolite (2,22). Some studies demonstrated an association between insufficient platelet function inhibition by clopidogrel and heightened incidence of vascular events (23,24). Increasing the dose of clopidogrel in poor responders has been suggested (25). However, even at the high maintenance dose of 150 mg daily, there is still a high variability in response to the drug (26–28). In addition, safety issues should caution against the use of 150 mg clopidogrel daily, pending further data, not only because of the concern for an increase in the incidence of bleeding complications but also because the severe toxic effects such as bone marrow aplasia and microangiopathic thrombocytopenia that are associated with the chronic use of 75 mg q.d. clopidogrel [albeit much less frequently than 250 mg b.i.d. ticlopidine (2)] might be dose dependent. The above limitations of ticlopidine and clopidogrel have fostered the search for new $P2Y_{12}$ antagonists.

Prasugrel is a new thienopyridine compound (Fig. 2) with much faster onset of action and higher potency than clopidogrel, both reflecting more efficient conversion of the pro-drug to the active metabolite (2,29–32) (Fig. 2). Prasugrel has proven safe in a phase II trial (33). In addition, the phase III trial TRITON-TIMI 38 recently demonstrated that in patients with acute coronary syndromes (ACS) who need to undergo PCI, treatment with prasugrel (60 mg loading dose, followed by a 10 mg maintenance dose), compared with clopidogrel (300 mg loading dose followed by 75 mg maintenance dose), was associated with less ischemic events and more major and fatal bleeding complications (34). In addition, the PRINCIPLE-TIMI 44, which was not powered for clinical events, demonstrated that the same therapeutic regimen with prasugrel (60 mg loading dose plus 10 mg maintenance dose) was superior to higher clopidogrel doses (600 mg loading dose plus 150 mg maintenance dose) in terms of inhibition of $P2Y_{12}$-mediated platelet function (28).

Therefore, it appears that treatment with the new thienopyridine drug prasugrel is associated with faster and greater inhibition of platelet function and less interindividual variability of response as compared with clopidogrel even when given at higher doses than those commonly used and officially approved. However, the advent of prasugrel may not be sufficient to solve the problems associated with pharmacological inhibition of $P2Y_{12}$ with thienopyridines. In fact, in some clinical situations, inhibition of platelet aggregation by fast-acting and reversible antagonists with a short half-life might be preferable to irreversible inhibitors. Some direct $P2Y_{12}$ antagonists with such characteristics are currently under development.

DIRECT $P2Y_{12}$ ANTAGONISTS

Cangrelor

Pharmacokinetics and Pharmacodynamics

Cangrelor [N6-(2-methylthioethyl)-2-(3,3,3-trifluoropropylthio)-5′-adenylic acid, mono-anhydride with dichloromethylenebis (phosphonic acid)] (The Medicines Company, New

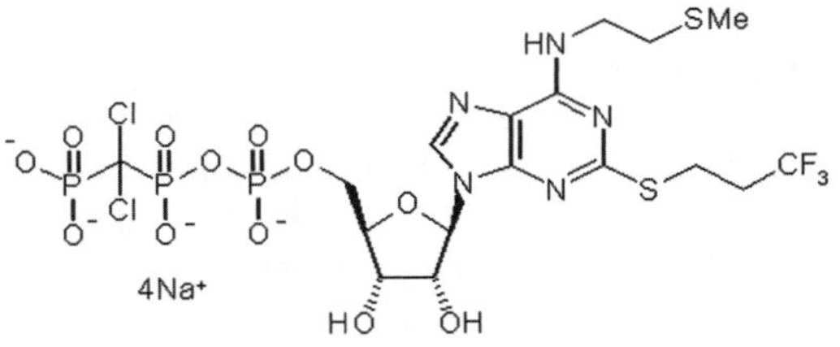

Figure 3 Chemical structures of ATP, AR-C69931MX (cangrelor), and AZD6140.

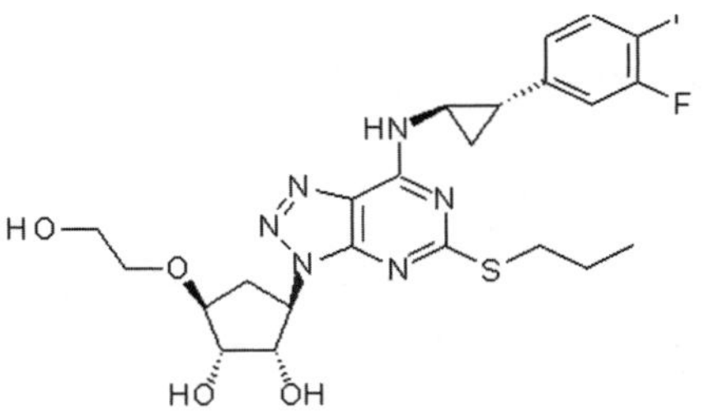

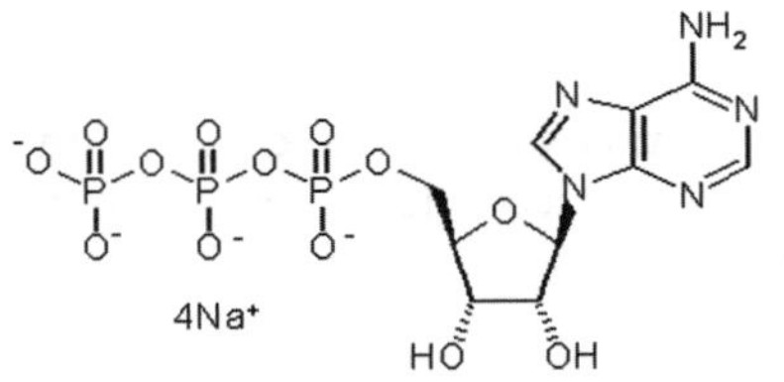

Jersey, U.S.), previously known as ARC69931[MX], belongs to a family of analogues of ATP that are relatively resistant to breakdown by ectonucleotidases and display high affinity for the P2Y$_{12}$ receptor (Fig. 3) (35). They are characterized by the presence of substitutions in the 2-position of the adenine ring, which increase the affinity properties of the molecule and of β,γ-methylene substitutions in the triphosphate part of the molecule, which increase the metabolic stability (35). Cangrelor is a potent inhibitor of ADP-induced aggregation of human-washed platelets (pIC$_{50}$ of 9.4 with 30 μM ADP). Initial studies showed that cangrelor displays no significant affinity for other P2 receptors at concentrations > 30 μM. However, more recent studies showed that it is a potent (IC$_{50}$ 4 nM), noncompetitive antagonist of P2Y$_{13}$, which is not expressed on the platelet membrane (36,37).

Experimental Thrombosis

In a model of cyclic flow reductions (CFRs) in the femoral artery of anesthetized male beagle dogs, cangrelor showed a better separation between antithrombotic effect and prolongation of the tongue bleeding time compared with clopidogrel and orbofiban (35). Cangrelor also displayed good antithrombotic effects in other models of experimental thrombosis, including a carotid artery thrombosis model in beagles (38), thrombosis of the rabbit mesenteric arteries induced by vessel wall puncture (39), and a Folts model in monkeys (40). In this last study, its antithrombotic efficacy was similar to that of SCH 602539, a selective PAR-1 receptor antagonist; interestingly, the simultaneous administration of the two antagonists, at doses that did not inhibit CFRs in any animal when administered alone, completely abolished CFRs in four of five animals.

Wang et al. provided evidence that the administration of cangrelor during fibrinolytic therapy can be of benefit in sustaining blood flow after myocardial infarction (MI) in a canine coronary electrolytic injury thrombosis model (41). After complete occlusion, fibrinolytic therapy was initiated by administering tissue plasminogen activator (t-PA) in the presence or absence of cangrelor given intravenously for two hours. All animals also received aspirin and heparin. Although cangrelor did not accelerate thrombolysis with t-PA, it prolonged reperfusion time and prevented both reocclusion and cyclic flow variations. Treatment with cangrelor was also associated with marked improvements in myocardial tissue blood flow and in microvascular perfusion, and with a 50% reduction in infarct size. Similar results were obtained at half-dosage t-PA, suggesting an additional role for cangrelor as a thrombolytic-sparing adjunct to reduce the risk of hemorrhagic complications. These observations are compatible with the demonstrations that $P2Y_{12}$ deficiency or its pharmacologic inhibition is associated with the formation of platelet aggregates that are loosely packed with few contact points (42) and would therefore be more easily affected by plasmin (43).

Clinical Pharmacology

Intravenous infusion of cangrelor was well tolerated in healthy volunteers, resulting in dose-dependent inhibition of ADP-induced platelet aggregation at doses up to 4 μg/kg/min (35) and, at the highest dose, in a 3.2- or 2.9-fold increase in the bleeding time in men and women. The short half-life (mean 2.6 minutes) resulted in a rapid reversal of both the platelet inhibitory effect and the effect on the bleeding time within 20 minutes after cessation of the infusion.

An open multicenter ascending-dose study in 39 ACS patients (44) showed dose-dependent and predictable plasma levels of cangrelor, resulting in complete or near-complete inhibition of 3 μmol/L ADP-induced platelet aggregation in all patients at doses of 2 μg/kg/min or higher. Bleeding times were increased three to fivefold at the 2 μg/kg/min, and approximately sevenfold at the 4 μg/kg/min dose. Although trivial bleeding was common in these patients (22,39), no major or minor bleeding was recorded as defined by the TIMI criteria.

A double-blind, placebo-controlled study of cangrelor as adjunctive therapy to aspirin and either heparin or low-molecular-weight heparin in patients with non-Q-wave MI showed that minor bleeding was slightly increased from 26% in the placebo-treated group to 38% in the cangrelor-treated group (45).

Greenbaum et al. more recently published a larger, two-part, phase II study, which assessed the safety and pharmacodynamics of cangrelor in patients undergoing PCI (46). The first part of the study enrolled 200 patients undergoing PCI, who were randomized to an 18 to 24-hour infusion of placebo, 1, 2, or 4 μg/kg/min cangrelor in addition to aspirin and heparin, beginning before the procedure. In the second part of the study, 199 additional patients were randomized to receive either cangrelor (4 μg/kg/min) or the anti-GPIIb/IIIa inhibitor abciximab, before the procedure. Combined major and minor bleeding through seven days follow-up occurred in 13% of patients who had been randomized to cangrelor and in 8% of patients randomized to placebo ($p = >0.05$) in the first part of the study, and in 7% receiving cangrelor compared with 10% receiving abciximab ($p = >0.05$) in the second part. Mean inhibition of platelet aggregation in response to 3 μmol/L ADP was complete both in the group of patients treated with cangrelor 4 μg/kg/min and in the group treated with abciximab (46). However, after termination of drug infusion, platelet aggregation returned to baseline values much faster in the cangrelor-treated group than in the abciximab-treated group, who still displayed significant inhibition of platelet aggregation 24 hours after termination of drug infusion (46).

The data of the study by Greenbaum et al. suggest that cangrelor may be very useful during the peri-procedural period in patients undergoing PCI. However, for long-term prevention, these patients should be treated with orally available agents. A recent paper demonstrated that the simultaneous administration of intravenous cangrelor with an oral

600 mg loading dose of clopidogrel prevents the expected inhibition of platelet aggregation by clopidogrel, presumably due to a competitive interaction between cangrelor and the active metabolite of clopidogrel at the P2Y$_{12}$ receptor level (47). Therefore, it was suggested that clopidogrel-loading dose should be administered after termination of cangrelor infusion (47). On the basis of the results of an in vitro study, which need to be confirmed in an ex vivo study (48), a similar problem can be predicted with the use of prasugrel during cangrelor infusion.

The STEP-AMI (safety, tolerability, and effect on patency in acute myocardial infarction) angiographic trial, assessed the safety and efficacy of cangrelor as an adjunct to t-PA in 92 patients with acute MI (49). All patients were treated with aspirin and heparin and were randomized to cangrelor alone (280 µg/min), full-dose t-PA alone (15 mg bolus followed by 0.75 mg/kg continuous infusion, up to 50 mg over 30 minutes, followed by 0.5 mg/kg up to 35 mg over 60 minutes, not to exceed 100 mg total), or cangrelor 35, 140, or 280 µg/min in conjunction with half-dose t-PA. The combination of cangrelor and half-dose t-PA resulted in similar 60-minute coronary patency as full-dose t-PA alone (55% vs. 50%, $p = >0.05$) and greater patency than with cangrelor alone (55% vs. 18%, $p < 0.05$) (49). Bleeding and adverse clinical events were comparable across the groups.

Comparison of Cangrelor with Clopidogrel

In a study that directly compared the effects of clopidogrel and cangrelor administration in patients with ischemic heart disease, Storey et al. showed that cangrelor infusion at 2 and 4 µg/mL/min resulted in near-complete inhibition of platelet aggregation measured at four minutes after the addition of 10 µM ADP, whereas four to seven days of clopidogrel treatment resulted in only approximately 60% inhibition (50). Addition of cangrelor in vitro to blood from the clopidogrel-treated patients resulted in near-complete inhibition of P2Y$_{12}$-dependent platelet function (51).

Cangrelor is currently being compared to clopidogrel in a phase III randomized, controlled, clinical study [clinical trial comparing cangrelor to clopidogrel in subjects who require (PCI CHAMPION-PCI)], which is enrolling patients requiring PCI. In a second randomized, controlled, phase III clinical trial [clinical trial comparing treatment with cangrelor (in combination with usual care) to usual care in subjects who require PCI (CHAMPION PLATFORM)], the effects of adding cangrelor to usual care in patients requiring PCI is evaluated.

AZD6140

Pharmacokinetics and Pharmacodynamics

AZD6140, (1S,2S,3R,5S)-3-{[(1R,2S)-2-(3,4-Difluorophenyl)cyclopropyl]amino}-5-(propylthio)-3H-[1,2,3,]-triazolo[4,5-d]pyrimidin-3-yl]-5-(2-hydroxyethoxy)cyclopentane-1,2-diol, has high affinity for P2Y$_{12}$ (Fig. 3). Efforts to find compounds for oral administration led first to the discovery of AR-C109318XX, the first oral, selective and stable, nonphosphate, competitive P2Y$_{12}$ antagonist. Further refinement to increase the oral bioavailability resulted in the discovery of the selective P2Y$_{12}$ competitive antagonist AZD6140, which is currently being developed as an oral antiplatelet agent. AR-C109318XX and AZD6140 both belong to the new chemical class cyclopentyl-triazolo-pyrimidines (Fig. 3) (35).

AZD6140 is a less potent P2Y$_{12}$ antagonist than cangrelor, with a pIC$_{50}$ value of 7.9 for inhibition of 30 µmol/L ADP-induced aggregation of human-washed platelets. AZD6140 displays no significant affinity for other P2 receptors at concentrations

>3 µmol/L (35). Preliminary studies suggest that AZD6140 and ADP bind independently to recombinant human $P2Y_{12}$, while the binding of the potent ADP analogue 2-methylthio ADP (2-MeSADP) overlaps with both (52).

Experimental Thrombosis

In in vitro experiments with human or mouse, blood perfused over collagen or collagen-containing atherosclerotic plaque material, AZD6140 dose-dependently reduced and destabilized thrombus formation and inhibited ADP- and collagen-induced thrombin generation (53).

In a model of CFRs in the femoral artery of anesthetized male beagles, AZD6140 displayed a good separation between the antithrombotic effect and the prolongation of the tongue bleeding time, which was intermediate between that of cangrelor and clopidogrel (35). The potency and specificity of AZD6140 inhibition of $P2Y_{12}$ was apparent in studies of laser-induced arterial thrombosis in mice, which showed that AZD6140 suppressed thrombus formation in $P2Y_{12}^{+/+}$ mice to similar levels seen in $P2Y_{12}^{-/-}$ mice (54). In addition, no further suppression of these responses was seen when AZD6140 was administered to $P2Y_{12}^{-/-}$ mice, consistent with selective inhibition of $P2Y_{12}$ (54).

In addition to its antiplatelet effects, AZD6140 potently inhibits adenosine uptake by erythrocytes. In an experimental in vivo model, AZD6140 caused the potentiation of both reactive hyperemia and adenosine-induced increase in coronary flow (55). These data suggest that treatment of ACS patients with AZD6140 may have additional benefits beyond inhibition of platelet aggregation by enhancing coronary blood flow.

Clinical Pharmacology

In a randomized, double blind, parallel-group dose-finding study [Dose-finding Investigative Study to assess the Pharmacodynamic Effects of AZD6140 in atherosclerotic disease (DISPERSE)], 200 stable atherosclerotic outpatients, on treatment with aspirin 75 to 100 mg once daily, received AZD6140 (50 mg b.i.d., 100 mg b.i.d., 200 mg b.i.d., or 400 mg q.d.) or clopidogrel 75 mg once daily for 28 days (56). The study showed that AZD6140 (100 mg b.i.d., 200 mg b.i.d., or 400 mg q.d.) rapidly and almost completely inhibited ADP-induced platelet aggregation both after the initial dose and at day 28. At these doses, AZD6140 more effectively inhibited platelet aggregation and with less variability than clopidogrel, both after the first dose and after 28 days of therapy. In addition, the inhibition of platelet aggregation by AZD6140 was very rapid (2 hours post-dose: final extent of aggregation, about 95%; maximal extent of aggregation, about 70%) compared with that of clopidogrel (2 hours post-dose: final extent of aggregation, about 15%; maximal extent of aggregation, about 10%). Only one major, nonfatal hemorrhage occurred in a patient treated with AZD6140 400 mg q.d.; the incidence of moderate and minor bleeding events was dose-related (29–51%) in AZD-treated patients and 32% in clopidogrel-treated patients. Other adverse events included dyspnea, dizziness, headache, and red blood cells in the urine. The incidence of dyspnea was dose related (reported in 10% of patients treated with AZD6140 50 mg b.i.d., 16% in patients treated with 200 mg b.i.d., and 20% in patients treated with 400 mg q.d.). None of the incidents of dyspnea was considered to be serious, and none was associated with congestive heart failure or bronchospasm (56).

The DISPERSE-2 study compared the safety of AZD6140 with that of clopidogrel in 990 patients with non ST elevation ACS NSTE-ACS, treated with aspirin and standard therapy for ACS, who were randomly assigned to AZD6140 90 mg b.i.d., AZD6140

180 mg b.i.d., and clopidogrel at the approved doses (300 mg loading dose plus 75 mg q. d. maintenance dose) for up to 12 weeks (57). The incidence of major bleedings was 6.9% in the clopidogrel group, 7.1% in the AZD6140 90 mg b.i.d. group ($p = 0.91$), and 5.1% in the AZD6140 180 mg b.i.d. group ($p = 0.35$, vs. clopidogrel). In a post hoc analysis of continuous electrocardiograms, mostly asymptomatic ventricular pauses longer than 2.5 seconds were more common in the group treated with AZD6140 180 mg b.i.d. (4.3%, 5.5%, and 9.9%; $p = 0.58$ and $p = 0.01$, vs. clopidogrel) (57). This study confirmed that dyspnea occurs more frequently with AZD6140 than with clopidogrel [clopidogrel = 6.5%; AZD6140 90 mg =10.5% ($p = 0.07$ vs. clopidogrel); AZD6140 = 15.8% ($p < 0.0002$ vs. clopidogrel)]. Again, the clinical impact appeared low, with few cases being considered serious or leading to discontinuation of treatment. The pathogenesis of dyspnea during AZD6140 treatment is unclear, although it has been hypothesized that it may be mediated by adenosine, which is the end product of the metabolism of ATP and its analogues (58).

Although the DISPERSE-2 study was not powered to detect differences in the incidence of MACE, it showed that AZD6140 180 mg b.i.d. may be more effective than clopiodgrel 75 mg daily in preventing them [incidence of cardiovascular (CV) death/MI/ stroke = 3.8% in the clopidogrel group, 4.3% in the AZD6140 90 mg group ($p = 0.71$ vs. clopidogrel), 1.9% in the AZD6140 180 mg group ($p = 0.17$)] (57). However, these data require confirmation from adequately powered, phase III trials.

A substudy of DISPERSE-2 showed that AZD6140 inhibited platelet aggregation in a dose-dependent fashion and both doses achieved greater levels of inhibition than clopidogrel (59). In addition, AZD6140 produced further suppression of platelet aggregation in patients who were currently receiving clopidogrel, confirming previous observations that clopidogrel treatment at the conventional doses does not inhibit a significant proportion of P2Y$_{12}$ receptors on the platelet membrane.

AZD6140 is currently under investigation in the phase III study PLATO (Platelet inhibition and patient Outcomes), a randomized, double-blind, parallel group, efficacy and safety study in which AZD6140 is being compared with clopidogrel for prevention of vascular events in patients with non-ST or ST-elevation ACS.

PRT060128

PRT060128 (or PRT128) is a direct-acting, reversible P2Y$_{12}$ inhibitor available for both intravenous and oral administration.

In a study in human volunteers, single oral doses of PRT060128 (10–800 mg) were administered to six groups of eight healthy subjects (6 active, 2 placebo) in a randomized, double-blind, dose-escalation study for the determination of tolerability, pharmacokinetic, and pharmacodynamic parameters (60). All doses were well tolerated with no serious or clinically important adverse events. The drug was well absorbed and had a terminal half-life of 12 hours. Drug concentrations increased dose proportionally up to 100 mg. Full inhibition of P2Y$_{12}$-dependent, ADP-induced platelet aggregation was obtained in a concentration-dependent manner with IC$_{50}$s of 980 ng/mL (maximum aggregation) and 450 ng/mL (at 6 minute endpoint). In a perfusion chamber assay, PRT060128 promoted thrombus destabilization and inhibited thrombus growth starting at 30 mg. The addition of aspirin to 30 mg PRT060128 accomplished complete thrombus destabilization and prevented the formation of large platelet aggregates, an effect, which was equivalent to that observed when PRT060128 was used alone at 100 mg (60).

Similar results were obtained in another randomized, double-blind study in which single intravenous doses of PRT060128 between 1 and 40 mg were administered over

20 minutes to five groups of eight healthy subjects (6 active, 2 placebo) (61). Complete inhibition of P2Y$_{12}$-dependent ADP-induced platelet aggregation was observed at 20 mg dose. Ex vivo thrombus formation on collagen-coated surfaces in a perfusion chamber was maximally inhibited by 40 mg PRT128 (61).

The in vitro addition of PRT060128 to blood samples from clopidogrel-treated healthy controls or diabetic patients undergoing coronary stent placement accomplished higher inhibition of ADP-induced platelet aggregation and of thrombus formation on collagen-coated surfaces (62).

CONCLUSION

In conclusion, the pharmacopeia of drugs inhibiting the platelet P2Y$_{12}$ receptor for ADP is rapidly expanding. In addition to ticlopidine and clopidogrel, well-known compounds of proven antithrombotic efficacy, a new thienopyridine, prasugrel, which is characterized by higher potency and faster onset of action, is currently under clinical evaluation. Two direct and reversible P2Y$_{12}$ antagonists, cangrelor, which can only be given intravenously, and AZD6140, which can be given orally, have rapid onset and reversal of platelet inhibition, which make them attractive alternatives to thienopyridines, especially when rapid inhibition of platelet aggregation or its quick reversal are required. A third compound, PRT060128, which can be given both orally and intravenously, is currently under development. Therefore, in the near future, physicians will have a panel of different P2Y$_{12}$ inhibitors to choose from, which will enable them to tailor the most appropriate antithrombotic therapy to the individual patient and risk situation.

REFERENCES

1. Cattaneo M. Inherited platelet-based bleeding disorders. J Thromb Haemost 2003; 1:1628–1636.
2. Cattaneo M, Gachet C. ADP receptors and clinical bleeding disorders. Arterioscler Thromb Vasc Biol 1999; 19:2281–2285.
3. Cattaneo M. ADP receptors antagonists. In: Michelson AD, ed. Platelets. San Diego: Academic Press, 2006:1127–1144.
4. Cattaneo M. The platelet P2 receptors. In: Michelson AD, ed. Platelets. San Diego: Academic Press, 2006:201–220.
5. Ralevic V, Burnstock G. Receptors for purines and pyrimidines. Pharmacol Rev 1998; 50:413–492.
6. Turner NA, Moake JL, McIntire LV. Blockade of adenosine diphosphate receptors P2Y(12) and P2Y(1) is required to inhibit platelet aggregation in whole blood under flow. Blood 2001; 98:3340–3345.
7. Cattaneo M, Savage B, Ruggeri ZM. Effects of pharmacological inhibition of the P2Y1 and P2Y12 ADP receptors on shear-induced platelet aggregation and platelet thrombus formation on a collagen-coated surface under flow conditions. Blood 2001; 98:239a (abstr).
8. Cattaneo M, Lecchi A, Lombardi R, et al. Platelets from a patient heterozygous for the defect of P2CYC receptors for ADP have a secretion defect despite normal thromboxane A2 production and normal granule stores: further evidence that some cases of platelet 'primary secretion defect' are heterozygous for a defect of P2CYC receptors. Arterioscler Thromb Vasc Biol 2000; 20:E101–E106.
9. Cattaneo M, Canciani MT, Lecchi A, et al. Released adenosine diphosphate stabilizes thrombin-induced human platelet aggregates. Blood 1990; 75:1081–1086.
10. Trumel C, Payrastre B, Plantavid M, et al. A key role of adenosine diphosphate in the irreversible platelet aggregation induced by the PAR1-activating peptide through the late activation of phosphoinositide 3-kinase. Blood 1999; 94:4156–4165.

11. Cattaneo M, Lecchi A. Inhibition of the platelet P2Y12 receptor for adenosine diphosphate potentiates the antiplatelet effect of prostacyclin. J Thromb Haemost 2007; 5:577–582.
12. Léon C, Hechler B, Freund M, et al. Defective platelet aggregation and increased resistance to thrombosis in purinergic P2Y(1) receptor-null mice. J Clin Invest 1999; 104:1731–1737.
13. Fabre JE, Nguyen M, Latour A, et al. Decreased platelet aggregation, increased bleeding time and resistance to thromboembolism in P2Y1-deficient mice. Nat Med 1999; 5:1199–202.
14. Andre P, Delaney SM, LaRocca T, et al. P2Y12 regulates platelet adhesion/activation, thrombus growth, and thrombus stability in injured arteries. J Clin Invest 2003; 112:398–406.
15. Hollopeter G, Jantzen HM, Vincent D, et al. Identification of the platelet ADP receptor targeted by antithrombotic drugs. Nature 2001; 409:202–207.
16. Cattaneo M, Akkawat B, Kinlough-Rathbone RL, et al. Ticlopidine facilitates the deaggregation of human platelets aggregated by thrombin. Thromb Haemost 1994; 71(1):91–94.
17. Cattaneo M, Lombardi R, Bettega D, et al. Shear-induced platelet aggregation is potentiated by desmopressin and inhibited by ticlopidine. Arterioscler Thromb 1993; 13(3):393–397.
18. Patrono C, Bachmann F, Baigent C, et al. European Society of Cardiology. Expert consensus document on the use of antiplatelet agents. The task force on the use of antiplatelet agents in patients with atherosclerotic cardiovascular disease of the European society of cardiology. Eur Heart J 2004; 25:166–181.
19. Yende S, Wunderink RG. Effect of clopidogrel on bleeding after coronary artery bypass surgery. Crit Care Med 2001; 29:2271–2275.
20. Hongo RH, Ley J, Dick SE, et al. The effect of clopidogrel in combination with aspirin when given before coronary artery bypass grafting. J Am Coll Cardiol 2002; 40:231–237.
21. Chen L, Bracey AW, Radovancevic R, et al. Clopidogrel and bleeding in patients undergoing elective coronary artery bypass grafting. J Thorac Cardiovasc Surg 2004; 128:425–431.
22. Cattaneo M. Aspirin and clopidogrel. Efficacy, safety and the issue of drug resistance. Arterioscler Thromb Vasc Biol 2004; 24:1980–1987.
23. Hochholzer W, Trenk D, Bestehorn HP, et al. Impact of the degree of peri-interventional platelet inhibition after loading with clopidogrel on early clinical outcome of elective coronary stent placement. J Am Coll Cardiol 2006; 48(9):1742–1750.
24. Buonamici P, Marcucci R, Migliorini A, et al. Impact of platelet reactivity after clopidogrel administration on drug-eluting stent thrombosis. J Am Coll Cardiol 2007; 49(24):2312–2317.
25. Smith SC Jr., Feldman TE, Hirshfeld JW Jr., et al. American College of Cardiology/American Heart Association Task Force on Practice Guidelines; ACC/AHA/SCAI Writing Committee to Update 2001 Guidelines for Percutaneous Coronary Intervention. ACC/AHA/SCAI 2005 guideline update for percutaneous coronary intervention: a report of the American College of Cardiology/American Heart Association Task Force on Practice Guidelines (ACC/AHA/SCAI Writing Committee to Update 2001 Guidelines for Percutaneous Coronary Intervention). Circulation 2006; 113:e166–e286.
26. von Beckerath N, Kastrati A, Wieczorek A, et al. A double-blind, randomized study on platelet aggregation in patients treated with a daily dose of 150 or 75 mg of clopidogrel for 30 days. Eur Heart J 2007; 28:1814–1819.
27. Angiolillo DJ, Shoemaker SB, Desai B, et al. Randomized comparison of a high clopidogrel maintenance dose in patients with diabetes mellitus and coronary artery disease: results of the Optimizing Antiplatelet Therapy in Diabetes Mellitus (OPTIMUS) study. Circulation 2007; 115(6):708–716.
28. Wiviott SD, Trenk D, Frelinger AL, et al. PRINCIPLE-TIMI 44 Investigators. Prasugrel compared with high loading- and maintenance-dose clopidogrel in patients with planned percutaneous coronary intervention: the Prasugrel in Comparison to Clopidogrel for Inhibition of Platelet Activation and Aggregation-Thrombolysis in Myocardial Infarction 44 trial. Circulation 2007; 116:2923–2932.
29. Niitsu Y, Jakubowski JA, Sugidachi A, et al. Pharmacology of CS-747 (Prasugrel, LY640315), a novel, potent antiplatelet agent with in vivo P2Y12 receptor antagonist activity. Semin Thromb Hemost 2005; 31:184–194.

30. Brandt JT, Payne CD, Wiviott SD, et al. A comparison of prasugrel and clopidogrel loading doses on platelet function: magnitude of platelet inhibition is related to active metabolite formation. Am Heart J 2007; 153(1):66.e9–e16.

31. Payne CD, Li YG, Small DS, et al. Increased active metabolite formation explains the greater platelet inhibition with prasugrel compared to high-dose clopidogrel. J Cardiovasc Pharmacol 2007; 50(5):555–562.

32. Sugidachi A, Ogawa T, Kurihara A, et al. The greater in vivo antiplatelet effects of prasugrel as compared to clopidogrel reflect more efficient generation of its active metabolite with similar antiplatelet activity to that of clopidogrel's active metabolite. J Thromb Haemost 2007; 5(7):1545–1551.

33. Wiviott SD, Antman EM, Winters KJ, et al. JUMBO-TIMI 26 Investigators. Randomized comparison of prasugrel (CS-747, LY640315), a novel thienopyridine P2Y12 antagonist, with clopidogrel in percutaneous coronary intervention: results of the Joint Utilization of Medications to Block Platelets Optimally (JUMBO)-TIMI 26 trial. Circulation 2005; 111(25):3366–3373.

34. Wiviott SD, Braunwald E, McCabe CH, et al. TRITON-TIMI 38 Investigators. Prasugrel versus clopidogrel in patients with acute coronary syndromes. N Engl J Med 2007; 357:2001–2015.

35. van Giezen JJJ, Humphries RG. Preclinical and clinical studies with selective reversible direct P2Y12 antagonists. Semin Thromb Hemost 2005; 31:195–204.

36. Marteau F, Le Poul E, Communi D, et al. Pharmacological characterization of the human P2Y13 receptor. Mol Pharmacol 2003; 64:104–112.

37. Fumagalli M, Trincavelli L, Lecca D, et al. Cloning, pharmacological characterization and distribution of the rat G-protein-coupled P2Y(13) receptor. Biochem Pharmacol 2004; 68:113–124.

38. Huang J, Driscoll EM, Gonzales ML, et al. Prevention of arterial thrombosis by intravenously administered platelet P2T receptor antagonist AR-C69931MX in a canine model. J Pharmacol Exp Ther 2000; 295:492–499.

39. van Gestel MA, Heemskerk JW, Slaaf DW, et al. In vivo blockade of platelet ADP receptor P2Y12 reduces embolus and thrombus formation but not thrombus stability. Arterioscler Thromb Vasc Biol 2003; 23:518–523.

40. Chintala M, Kurowski S, Vemulapalli S, et al. Efficacy of SCH 602539, a selective thrombin receptor antagonist, alone and in combination with cangrelor in a folts model of thrombosis in anesthetized monkeys. Eur Heart J 2007; 28:188 (abstr).

41. Wang K, Zhou X, Zhiou Z, et al. Blockade of the platelet P2Y12 receptor by AR-C69931MX sustains coronary artery recanalization and improves the myocardial tissue perfusion in a canine thrombosis model. Arterioscler Thromb Vasc Biol 2003; 23:357–362.

42. Humbert M, Nurden P, Bihour C, et al. Ultrastructural studies of platelet aggregates from human subjects receiving clopidogrel and from a patient with an inherited defect of an ADP-dependent pathway of platelet activation. Arterioscler Thromb Vasc Biol 1996; 16:1532–1543.

43. Nurden AT, Nurden P. Advantages of fast-acting ADP receptor blockade in ischemic heart disease. Arterioscler Thromb Vasc Biol 2003; 23(2):158–159.

44. Storey RF, Oldroyd KG, Wilcox RG. Open multicentre study of the P2T receptor antagonist AR-C69931MX assessing safety, tolerability and activity in patients with acute coronary syndromes. Thromb Haemost 2001; 85:401–407.

45. Jacobsson F, Swahn E, Wallentin L, et al. Safety profile and tolerability of intravenous ARC69931MX, a new antiplatelet drug, in unstable angina pectoris and non-Q-wave myocardial infarction. Clin Ther 2002; 24(5):752–765.

46. Greenbaum AB, Grines CL, Bittl JA, et al. Initial experience with an intravenous P2Y12 platelet receptor antagonist in patients undergoing percutaneous coronary intervention: results from a 2-part, phase II, multicenter, randomized, placebo- and active-controlled trial. Am Heart J 2006; 151(3):689.e1–689.e10.

47. Steinhubl SR, Oh JJ, Oestreich JH, et al. Transitioning patients from cangrelor to clopidogrel: pharmacodynamic evidence of a competitive effect. Thromb Res 2008; 121(4):527–534.

48. Dovlatova NL, Jakubowski JA, Sugidachi A, et al. Competition between reversible and irreversible p2y12 antagonists and its influence on adp-mediated platelet activation. J Thromb Hemost 2007; 5: (abstr P-S-340).

49. Greenbaum AB, Ohman EM, Gibson CM, et al. Preliminary experience with intravenous P2Y12 platelet receptor inhibition as an adjunct to reduced-dose alteplase during acute myocardial infarction: results of the Safety, Tolerability and Effect on Patency in Acute Myocardial Infarction (STEP-AMI) angiographic trial. Am Heart J 2007; 154(4):702–709.

50. Storey RF, Wilcox RG, Heptinstall S. Comparison of the pharmacodynamic effects of the platelet ADP receptor antagonists clopidogrel and AR-C69931MX in patients with ischaemic heart disease. Platelets 2002; 13(7):407–413.

51. Beham M, Fox S, Sanderson H, et al. Effect of clopidogrel on procoagulant activity in acute coronary syndromes: evidence for incomplete P2Y12 receptor blockade. Circulation 2002; 106: II-149–II-150.

52. Nilsson L, van Giezen JJJ, Greasley PJ. Evidence for distinct ligand-binding sites on recombinant human P2Y$_{12}$ receptors. Circulation 2006; 114 II–248 II (abstr 249).

53. Kuijpers MJE, Cosemans MEM, van der Meijden PEJ, et al. Inhibition of P2Y$_{12}$ by AZD6140 reduces thrombus formation and procoagulant activity on collagen and atherosclerotic plaques. J Thromb Haemost 2007; 5(suppl 2):P-W-275.

54. Patil SBG, Norman KE, Robins SJ, et al. Inhibition of thrombosis by AZD6140 via selective blockade of the P2Y$_{12}$ receptor in a murine laser-injury model. J Thromb Haemost 2007; 5(suppl 2):P-W-632.

55. Björkman J-A, Kirk I, van Giezen JJ. AZD6140 inhibits adenosine uptake into erythrocytes and enhances coronary blood flow after local ischemia or intracoronary adenosine infusion. Circulation, Oct 2007; 116: II (abstr 28).

56. Husted S, Emanuelsson H, Heptinstall S, Sandset PM, Wickens M, Peters G. Pharmacodynamics, pharmacokinetics, and safety of the oral reversible P2Y12 antagonist AZD6140 with aspirin in patients with atherosclerosis: a double-blind comparison to clopidogrel with aspirin. Eur Heart J 2006; 27:1038–1047.

57. Cannon CP, Husted S, Harrington RA, et al. Safety, tolerability, and initial efficacy of AZD6140, the first reversible oral adenosine diphosphate receptor antagonist, compared with clopidogrel, in patients with non-ST-segment elevation acute coronary syndrome: primary results of the DISPERSE-2 trial. J Am Coll Cardiol 2007; 50:1844–1851.

58. Serebruany VL, Stebbing J, Atar D. Dyspnoea after antiplatelet agents: the AZD6140 controversy. Int J Clin Pract 2007; 61(3):529–533.

59. Storey RF, Husted S, Harrington RA, et al. Inhibition of platelet aggregation by AZD6140, a reversible oral P2Y12 receptor antagonist, compared with clopidogrel in patients with acute coronary syndromes. J Am Coll Cardiol 2007; 50(19):1852–1856.

60. Gretler D, Conley P, Andre M, et al. "First In Human" experience with PRT060128, a new direct-acting, reversible, P2Y$_{12}$ inhibitor for intravenous and oral use. J Am Coll Cardiol 2007; 49:326A.

61. Lieu HD, Conley PB, Andre P, et al. Initial intravenous experience with PRT060128 (PRT128), an orally-available, direct-acting, and reversible P2Y$_{12}$ Inhibitor. J Thromb Haemost 2007; 5 (suppl 2):P-T-292.

62. Conley P, Jurek M, Stephens G, et al. A novel pharmacodynamic perfusion chamber assay reveals superior and unique antithrombotic activities of a direct-acting P2Y12 antagonist, PRT128, relative to clopidogrel. Blood 2006; 108:900 (abstr ASH Annual Meeting).

29

Nitric Oxide Donors as Platelet Inhibitors

Lina Badimon and Gemma Vilahur
Cardiovascular Research Center of Barcelona, CSIC-ICCC, Hospital de la Santa Creu i Sant Pau (UAB) and CIBEROBN (06/03), Instituto Salud Carlos III, Barcelona, Spain

INTRODUCTION

Under physiological conditions, the endothelium is inert for platelet activation and for the activation of the enzymatic components of the coagulation cascade. Endothelial thromboresistance is mainly derived from the coexistence of the following endothelium-related properties: (*i*) both platelets and endothelial cells are negatively charged, a characteristic that induces platelet cell repulsion; (*ii*) endothelial cells synthesize nitric oxide (NO), endothelial hyperpolarization factor (EHPF), and prostacyclin (PGI2), all of which are platelet inhibitors; (*iii*) endothelial cells constitutively express on their surface CD39 (an ecto-ADPase), thrombomodulin (disables thrombin action), and heparin sulfate (a glycosaminoglycan that activates antithrombin III); and (*iv*) healthy endothelium releases plasminogen activator, which in the presence of fibrin promotes fibrinolysis and resultant clot dissolution. Nevertheless, the presence and/or clustering of cardiovascular risk factors results in a breakdown of the endothelium's cardioprotective properties, resulting in endothelial activation/dysfunction (1). The hallmark of endothelial dysfunction is a decrease in NO bioavailability. Indeed, the NO pathway has multiple synergistic interactions with respect to cyclic nucleotide generation/degradation and protein phosphorylation in platelets and smooth muscle cells, which regulates several cardiovascular functions, including vascular tone, leukocyte adhesion and migration, prevention of smooth muscle cell proliferation, and inhibition of platelet activation and thrombus formation. In fact, it has been described that acute inhibition of endogenous NO production in humans causes rapid platelet activation in vivo, which can be reversed by the administration of an NO donor, thereby demonstrating that platelet function in vivo is rapidly regulated by NO bioavailability (2). In consideration of the physiological regulation of NO and the well-established pathological implications of decreased NO bioavailability, delivery of supplemental NO is an attractive therapeutic option to help prevent disease progression. Indeed, NO donor drugs represent a useful pathway for systemic NO delivery (3), and organic nitrates have been used for more than a century as

Table 1 Nitric Oxide Donors

NO donors		
Diazeniumdiolates (NONOates)		DEA/NO DETA/NONOate MAHMA NONOate Spermine-NONOate Proli-NONOate
Sodium nitroprusside		SNP
Molsidomine		SIN-1 (morpholinosidonimine)

S-nitrosothiols (RSNOs)		SNAP (S-nitroso-N-
		    acetylpenicillamine)
		SNVP (S-nitroso-N-valeryl-
		    D-penicillamine)
		GSNO (S-nitrosoglutathione)
		SNO-Cys
		SNO-Hcys
		RIG200
		SNO-albumin

Organic nitrates nitrite esters		GTN (nitroglycerin) ISMN (isosorbide mononitrate) ISDN (isosorbide dinitrate) PETN (pentaerythrityl tetranitrate) Nicorandil Amyl nitrite
Mesoionic oxatriazol derivatives		GEA-3162 GEA-3175
NO hybrid drugs	NO-NSAIDS	NCX 4016 NCX 4215
	NO-statins	NCX 6550 (pravastatin) NCX 6553 (fluvastatin)
	Other	SNO-captopril SNO-tissue plasminogen activator SNO-von Willebrand factor fragment SNO-diclofenac Nipradilol
Other NO donors		Zeolites OXINO B-NOD

Abbreviation: NO, nitric oxide.

effective therapies for symptomatic relief of cardiac ischemia. However, nitrates have limitations (4), and a number of alternative NO donor classes have emerged since the discovery that NO is an essential biological mediator (Table 1).

This chapter focuses on the current knowledge of NO's role in platelet function as well as the factors involved in NO modulation and provides an overview of the essential aspects of several NO donor compounds as platelet inhibitors.

BIOSYNTHESIS OF NO

The discovery of NO as endothelium-derived relaxing factor (EDRF) and its role in the cardiovascular system led to the Nobel Prize in Physiology and Medicine to F. Murat, R. Furchgott, and L. Ignarro in 1998 (5,6). NO is formed via the oxidative L-arginine pathway catalyzed by a family of enzymes termed "NO synthase" (NOS) isoenzymes. There are three isoforms of NOS, namely, NOS-1 [nNOS (neuronal NOS)]; NOS-2 [iNOS (inducible NO), or immunological NOS]; and NOS-3 [eNOS (endothelial NOS)]. Common features of the isoenzymes include binding domains for the substrates arginine and NADPH and also for five cofactors, FAD, FMN, heme, tetrahydrobiopterin (BH4), and Ca^{2+}/calmodulin (CaM).

Although endothelial cells are known to be the most important reservoir for eNOS, this enzyme is now known to be present in a variety of tissues, including brain hippocampus, lung, cardiac myocytes, the gastrointestinal tract, reproductive organs, the liver, megakaryocytes, and platelets. Indeed, NO is able to modulate a variety of physiological responses, including gene regulation, apoptosis, vascular smooth muscle cell (VSMC) relaxation and proliferation, neurotransmission, immune stimulation, and platelet function (7,8)

Platelets and endothelial cells constitutively express eNOS, yet extensive research has demonstrated that a wide variety of factors may dynamically influence both endothelial and platelet eNOS activity (9) and subsequent NO production (Fig. 1) (9,10). Within the three NOS isoforms, eNOS is most sensitive to activation in response to calcium (Ca^{2+})-elevating agonists. In fact, Ca^{2+}/(CaM) binding to eNOS controls via BH4 the electron flow from NADPH to flavins (FAD, FMN) and then to the iron/heme group of the enzyme. This so-called coupled eNOS, results in NO and L-citrulline release. Conversely, under pathological circumstances (e.g., absence of BH4), the intermediate electron reacts with molecular oxygen (instead of with L-citrulline), resulting in superoxide formation (the so-called uncoupled eNOS). eNOS activity, however, is not simply determined by the formation of a Ca^{2+}/CaM complex but rather by simultaneous changes in eNOS phosphorylation and the resulting changes in the accessibility Ca^{2+}/CaM to the binding domain. While eNOS endothelial activity in response to any stimuli is mainly dependent on Ser1177 and Thr495 residues phosphorylation, eNOS platelet activation is dependent merely on Ser1177 phosphorylation. Recently, several proteins such as heat shock protein (Hsp)-90, NOS3-interacting protein (NOSIP), NOS3 traffic inducer (NOSTRIN), β-actin, dynamin-2, and porin have been suggested to intervene also in eNOS activation (9,11,12).

NO's short half-life (~10 seconds) (13) limits its effects within a few microns of the site of its generation. Moreover, NO may be rapidly scavenged by the heme group of deoxyHb, forming a relatively stable complex nitrosylhemoglobin (Hb-NO), or by superoxide radicals. Hence, the transformation of NO to nitrites (NO^{2-})/nitrates (NO^{3-}) or to protein and non-protein S-nitrosothiols (RSNOs) complexes is crucial to protect NO from inactivation and allow NO to be stored and carried in the blood (Fig. 2) (14). Direct oxidation of NO forms nitrite, a process that is catalyzed in plasma by ceruloplasmin (15), whereas NO conversion to nitrate takes place via reaction with oxyhemoglobin's bound oxygen with meta-hemoglobin release (14). Conversely, interaction of NO with plasma albumin, glutathione (GSH), cysteine (Cys), or homocysteine (Hcy) derive in a variety of S-NO adducts [NO-albumin, S-nitrosoglutathione (GSNO), NO-Cys, NO-Hcy, respectively]. Release of NO from these endogenous NO reservoirs is strongly influenced by the availability of the parent compounds and by the redox status of plasma. For instance, under ischemic or hypoxic

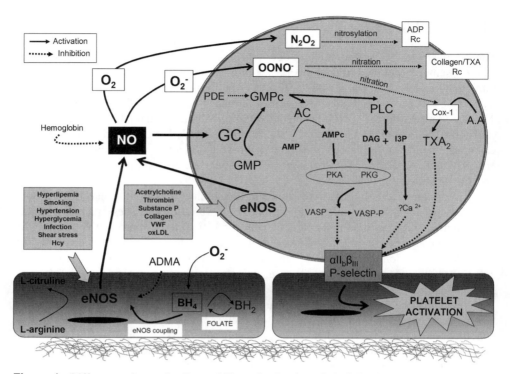

Figure 1 Different pathways leading to NO production in endothelial cells and platelets and NO effects on platelet signaling and function. Endothelial and platelet eNOS activation in response to several stimuli leads to NO production. NO may decrease platelet activation through cGMP-dependent and cGMP-independent mechanisms. NO activation of soluble guanylyl cyclase leads to GMPc formation, which in turn modulates the activity of several protein kinases that eventually decrease P-selectin and fibrinogen receptor activation. NO may also regulate platelet activation through mechanisms independent of the GC/GMPc axis via protein nitration and nitrosylation. *Abbreviations*: NO, nitric oxide; Aa, arachidonic acid; ADMA, asymmetric dimethylarginine; ADP, adenosine diphosphate; AC, adenylyl cyclase; camp, cyclic adenosine monohphosphate; Akt, protein kinase B; BH4, biopterin; cGMP, cyclic guanosine monophosphate; COX-1, cyclo-oxygenase-1; PKA and PKG, protein kinases; DAG, diacylglycerol; eNOS, endothelial nitric oxide synthase; GC, guanylyl cyclase; Hcy, hyperhomocysteinemia; I3P, inosytol triphosphate; PDE, phosphodiesterases; PLC, phospholipase C; TXA, thromboxane; VASP, vasodilator-stimulated phosphoprotein; NO, nitric oxide; VWF, von Willebrand factor.

conditions, nitrites and nitrates have the potential to be converted back to NO, thereby balancing NO availabiltiy (16). On the other hand, *S*-nitrosohomocysteine formation modulates homocystein-derived adverse effects in addition to reducing platelet activation and promoting vasorelaxation (17). However, in disease states where endothelial dysfunction and reduced eNOS activity are present, plasma levels of nitrates, nitrites, and S-NO adducts are often low (18).

It is generally thought that NO freely diffuses through cell membranes without need for a specific transporter. However, Herrera et al. (19) have recently reported that NO transport across cell membranes is facilitated by aquaporin-1 channels. Once in the endothelial cells, NO modulates the expression of several molecules rendering protection in the early steps of the atherosclerotic disease. For instance, NO reduces leukocyte vascular adhesion and further migration into the vessel by decreasing chemoattractant protein

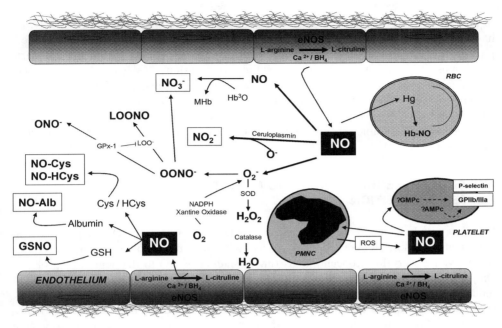

Figure 2 Metabolism of NO in the circulation. Release of NO to the bloodstream may be rapidly scavenged by the hemoglobin group of erythrocytes or by superoxide radicals present in the bloodstream forming H_2O_2 or $OONO^-$. In order to preserve NO inactivation and allow NO to be stored and carried in the blood, the transformation of NO to NO^{2-}, NO^{3-}, or to S-nitrosothiol complexes via Alb, GSH, Cys, or Hcy interaction is required. *Abbreviations*: NO, nitric oxide; $OONO^-$, perosynitrite; LOONO, lipid peroxynitrites; ROS, reactive oxygen species; GPx, glutathione peroxidases; LOO^-, peroxyl radicals; NO^{2-}, nitrites; nitrates, NO^{3-}, Alb, albumin; GSH, glutathione; Cys, cysteine; Hcy, homocysteine.

MCP-1 expression, surface adhesion molecules CD11/CD18, P-selectin, vascular cell adhesion molecule-1, and intercellular adhesion molecule-1 (20–22). Moreover, NO also prevents progression of atherosclerotic disease by diminishing endothelial permeability, thereby reducing the influx of lipoproteins into the vascular wall and therefore hampering low-density lipoprotein oxidation. On the other hand, paracrine release of NO toward adjacent VSMC is mainly involved in vascular dilation via the GC-cGMP pathway and, as opposed to endothelial cells, inhibition of VSMC migration. Conversely, NO release toward the vascular lumen is a potent inhibitor of platelet aggregation and adhesion, protecting the vessel from thrombotic complications. Platelet inhibition also prevents the release of platelet-derived growth factors that may further stimulate VSMC proliferation (23)

As already mentioned, in addition to being regulated by NO, platelets have the capacity to synthesize and release NO upon stimulation, although they do so in smaller amounts than endothelial cells (10). The presence of an L-arginine/NO-signaling pathway in human platelets was confirmed in seminal studies by Radomski et al. (24), and within the last few years, the role of platelet-derived NO has been receiving increasing attention (25). Evidence from in vitro systems and animal models suggest that platelet-derived NO modestly regulates primary platelet aggregation while markedly inhibiting secondary platelet recruitment, thus limiting the extent of thrombus formation (14,26–28). Within this context, relevant clinical data have ascertained the important role of platelet-derived NO in vascular diseases (14,26,27). Moreover, platelet NOS activity has an inverse correlation to total cholesterol, LDL cholesterol, and arterial blood pressure (29). Likewise, compared with healthy subjects, patients with acute coronary syndromes (15), diabetes (30), and essential hypertension (31) have shown reduced bioavailability of platelet-derived NO (32). Decrease of eNOS activity in diabetes accounts for enhanced eNOS glycosylation, which hides the enzyme phosphorylation sites, whereas hypertension has been associated with reduced L-arginine availability and enhanced eNOS-asymmetric dimethylarginine (i.e., endogenous L-arginine analogues) interaction (33).

MOLECULAR MECHANISMS OF NO-MEDIATED PLATELET INHIBITION

Reaction with heme-containing proteins is a fundamental aspect of NO biology. Many of the direct effects of NO are secondary to its ability to activate soluble guanylyl cyclase (GC), even at very low concentrations (nM). Binding of NO to the heme group of the enzyme catalyzes the conversion of GTP to the second messenger cGMP. The NO-induced cGMP signal modulates the intracellular activity of several protein kinases (PKG and PKA) that lead to calcium storage and vasodilator-stimulated phosphoprotein (VASP) phosphorylation. This in turn will drive the decrease of P-selectin surface expression and fibrinogen receptor (integrin αIIbβ3 or glycoprotein IIb/IIIa) activation (Fig. 1) (34). Indeed, NO-dependent VASP phosphorylation is an essential regulatory component of platelet function and correlates with inhibition of fibrinogen binding to glycoprotein IIb/IIIa (35), P-selectin expression, and platelet adhesion (36). Figure 1 shows the main NO/GC/cGMP targets involved in the inhibition of the platelet activation cascades (37–43).

With the increasing number of NO donors and components that inhibit the NO-cGMP-regulated signaling molecules, such as GC inhibitors, it has become evident that besides the cGMP-dependent activation cascade, effects of NO can be mediated by cGMP-independent mechanisms (44,45). The cGMP-independent mechanisms have not been clearly characterized, but protein nitrosylation and nitration have emerged as alternative mechanisms of NO-mediated platelet regulation (46). In this regard, it has recently been shown that NO inhibits platelet ADP receptor activation and exocytosis of platelet granules (dense, lysosomal, and α-granules) by nitrosylation. In the latter case, nitrosylation is brought about by a key component of the exocytic machinery, the N-ethylmaleimide-sensitive factor (NSF) (26). Conversely, peroxynitrite (ONOO$^-$), a reactive oxidant produced by the reaction of NO with superoxide anions (O^{2-}), is capable of nitrating amino acids, leading to cyclooxygenase-1 (COX-1) inhibition or a decrease in platelet receptors, including collagen and thromboxane receptors (Fig. 1) (47). Recently, NO has also been demonstrated to exert an cGMP-independent effect on integrin αIIbβ3 activation (48). NO has been concretely shown to induce S-nitrosylation of the cysteine residues of the β3 subunit, rendering the integrin unable either to interact with fibrinogen effectively or to affect its ability to transduce signals (49,50).

FACTORS THAT AFFECT THE BIOAVAILABILITY OF NO IN THE CARDIOVASCULAR SYSTEM

Strong evidence supports the association of cardiovascular risk factors (hypertension, diabetes, dyslipidemia, hyperhomocysteinemia, and smoking) (51–54) with a reduced NO bioavailability and an increase in platelet activation. This NO decrease may either result from a reduced eNOS activity or NO scavenging caused by the oxidative state commonly associated with cardiovascular disease (25). Besides eNOS and NO, the GC-cGMP axis may also be affected in several ways: the sGC or cGMP targets can be downregulated; the sGC's heme moiety can be oxidized or removed, rendering the enzyme insensitive to NO; and cGMP degradation can be accelerated by increased phosphodiesterase (PDE) activity.

The most important oxidant generators include NADPH oxidase, xantine oxidase, and uncoupled eNOS (Fig. 2). Reactive oxygen species (ROS; e.g., O^{2-}) may also be derived from the auto-oxidation of homocysteine to homocystine. In fact, hyper-homocysteinemia has been shown to promote oxidative stress by reducing the endogenous antioxidant glutathione peroxidases (GPx-1) and activating NADPH oxidase and uncoupled eNOS (55).

Under physiological conditions, ROS are chiefly counteracted by a group of nonenzymatic antioxidants (α-tocopherol, ascorbic acid, and glutathione) and antioxidant enzymes [superoxide dismutases (SODs), GPxs, and catalases]. However, the persistent generation of oxidants in disease states surmounts the endogenous antioxidant defense capacity, allowing O^{2-} to interact with NO and the consequent peroxynitrite ($ONNO^-$) formation (Fig. 2).

Paradoxically, low concentrations of peroxynitrite have been shown to exert antiplatelet effects under physiological conditions. Such effects are derived from peroxynitrite reaction with thiols (in cell membranes) or glucose (in the extracellular fluid), which results in synthesis of NO donors. Blood-borne NO donors may then counteract the vasoconstrictor and platelet-aggregatory activities of the parent oxidant (56,57). On the contrary, at high concentrations, peroxynitrite leads to oxidative inactivation of eNOS.

Increasing the bioavailability of NO and decreasing its inactivation are the goals in the prevention and reversal of cardiovascular disease. Successful strategies are shown in Figure 3 and include PPAR-α and PPAR-γ agonists, antioxidants, supplementation with L-arginine, tetrahydrobiopterin-BH4 or sepiapterin (precursor of BH4), statins, selective β1-adrenoreceptor antagonists, calcium channel blockers, angiotensin-converting enzyme (ACE) inhibitors, PDE inhibitors, NO donors, and regular physical exercise (58).

NO DONOR DRUGS

There are numerous different NO donor molecules that are classified according to their chemical structures and the manner in which they generate NO (Table 1). In general, NO donors may release NO spontaneously through thermal or photochemical self-decomposition (e.g., RSNOs, NONOates) or after metabolism or redox activation (e.g., organic nitrates, nitrites, sodium nitroprusside).

All classes of NO donor drugs have vasodilator properties, and Mellion et al. (59) were the first to demonstrate the ability of NO donor drugs to inhibit platelet function.

Organic Nitrates and Sodium Nitroprusside

As mentioned above, the nitrate–nitrite–NO pathway may be viewed as complementary to the classical L-arginine–NOS pathway (16). These pathways work partly in parallel, but when oxygen availability is reduced and NOS activity is decreased, nitrite reduction to NO becomes more pronounced. So, in pathological conditions, when regional and systemic ischemia prevails, it may be beneficial to support the nitrate and nitrite stores pharmacologically.

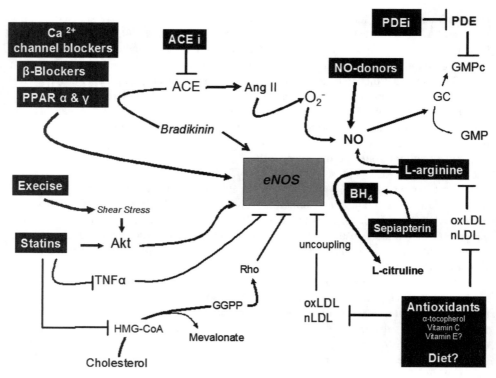

Figure 3 Schematic representation of factors modulating NO pathway. The figure emphasizes the fact that diverse, seemingly unrelated, cardioprotective interventions all operate by increasing the availability of NO, secondary either to increased NO generation or to decreased NO catabolism. *Abbreviations*: NO, nitric oxide; ACE, angiotensin-converting enzyme; Akt, protein kinase B; Ang II, angiotensin II; eNOS, endothelial nitric oxide synthase; GC, guanylyl cyclase; cGMP, cyclic guanosine monophosphate; eNOS, endothelial nitric oxide synthase; GGPP, geranyl-geraniol pyrophosphate; ox LDL, oxidized low-density lipoproteins; PDE, phosphodiesterase; statins, HMG CoA reductase inhibitors; TNF-α, tumor necrosis factor-α.

Nitrates (i.e., nitroglycerin, isosorbide 5-mononitrate, isosorbide dinitrate, amyl nitrite, nicorandil) have been used for many years acutely and orally in the symptomatic relief related to ischemic coronary heart disease, although their impact on cardiovascular mortality remains controversial (60). A meta-analysis found significant reduction in mortality when intravenous nitroglycerin or nitroprusside was used during acute course of myocardial infarction (61). In contrast, GISSI-III (62) and ISIS-4 (63) studies failed to show clinically beneficial effect of organic nitrates on mortality after myocardial infarction. Sodium nitroprusside can only be administered parenterally and thus has been primarily used for treatment of hypertensive crises and to relieve symptoms of heart failure.

Both compounds are viewed as pharmacological agents that release NO indirectly, requiring metabolic activity, biotransformation, and redox activation. Although the enzyme involved in NO delivery has yet to be definitively characterized, the cytochrome P450 system has been suggested to be implicated in NO delivery. In addition, the presence of intracellular thiols has shown to support the action of organic nitrates (58,64).

NO or related compounds generated by these nitrovasodilators not only activate sGC but can also affect the function of other proteins via nitrosation or interactions with metals (65). Nicorandil, in addition, combines NO release with potassium channel activation (66). Nitrate regimens currently in use may have antiplatelet effects. Indeed, short- and long-lasting administration of nitroglycerin and isosorbide dinitrate to patients suffering from coronary artery disease and acute myocardial infarction have resulted in a significant inhibition of platelet adhesion and aggregation (67,68). However, these effects are though to be generally weak relative to their vasodilatory activity probably because of a low platelet selectivity. In addition to nitrovasodilators' lack of cell-selectivity, the utility of organic nitrates has been limited by the onset of drug tolerance with prolonged administration, and chronic sodium nitroprusside treatment has been shown to develop thiocyanate toxicity (69). Although drug tolerance has yet to be solved, it has been associated with both a nitrate-mediated intracellular thiol depletion or an increase in ROS production (i.e., NO inactivation) (70). In the latter, organic nitrates promote oxidative stress partly through their potent vasodilatory and hypotensive actions, which activate the renin-angiotensin system that, in turn, promotes oxidative processes (Fig. 3) (22,71), or by induction of a dysfunctional eNOS gene expression that generates increased formation of superoxide rather than NO (23). Low-molecular-weight thiols, ascorbate, L-arginine, BH4, ACE inhibitors, and folate have thus been successfully used to reverse or prevent nitrate tolerance (72).

The platelet-inhibitory actions of organic nitrates cannot be separated from their effects on the vascular wall. Unwelcome hypotensive effects associated with the doses required to achieve platelet inhibition, however, have been a significant obstacle to surmount. Indeed, antiplatelet effects of organic nitrates remain controversial because of the supra-pharmacological doses required to inhibit platelet aggregation and the subsequent hypotensive side effects of the available formulations (73). We have previously reported that a new oral NO donor (LA419), a neutral sugar organic nitrate with protected thiol group, inhibits thrombosis without modifying hemodynamic parameters (74). Using an ex vivo porcine model of thrombosis, we have performed a direct comparison of the antiplatelet effectiveness of LA419 to isosorbide-5-mononitrate and the currently used ADP-receptor blocker, clopidogrel. We observed that LA419 exceeded the anti-thrombotic properties of isosorbide-5-mononitrate and provided additional anti-thrombotic properties to that of clopidogrel. Most importantly, these effects were observed without changes in blood pressure. On the basis of recent studies in our *laboratory* on the platelet proteome, it is likely that the presence of a thiol group within LA419's molecular structure conferred higher platelet selectivity and enabled LA419 to intracellularly deliver NO through platelet membrane protein disulfide isomerase (PDI) activation (see below) (75). Thereafter, we sought to evaluate LA419's antiplatelet effects ex vivo in healthy human subjects (76). LA419 rendered a high antithrombotic profile similar to that exerted by the GPIIb/IIIa antagonist abciximab (76). Indeed, when compared with placebo control, treatment with LA419 and abciximab was associated with a 62% and 73% reduction on thrombus size, respectively (76).

Diazeniumdiolates (NONOates)

Diazeniumdiolates, compounds of structure R1R2NN(O)=NOR3, which have also been called NONOates, have proved useful for treating an increasing diversity of medical disorders in relevant animal models. NONOates, are complexes of NO with nucleophiles that spontaneously generate NO in solution without previous metabolism. NONOates have different half-lives ranging from 2 seconds to 20 hours depending on the structure (77). Importantly, these solution half-lives tend to correlate very well with their pharmacological durations of action. Thus, while DEA/NO and MAHMA-NONOate are short acting and thus potent, NO donor–releasing drugs, DETA NONOate and SPERMINE NONOate, are more stable compounds (>1hour) with "weaker" but sustained effects (78,79). The vasodilator and antiplatelet activity displayed by most of the NONOates is mediated by the free NO (released on dissolution), which activates the GC-cGMP pathway in both endothelial cells and platelets. These NO donor drugs are used primarily for their vasodilator properties; however, an ability to inhibit platelet function in several animal models has also been demonstrated in most of the NONOates (80–82). Moreover, NO-releasing diazeniumdiolate-coated polymers, which have been used as vascular grafts in sheep, have proven to be thromboresistent prosthetic vascular implantation material (83). However, NONOates antiplatelet potential is limited by their short biological half-life.

S-Nitrosothiols

As highlighted in sections "Biosynthesis of NO" and "Factors That Affect the Bioavailability of NO in the Cardiovascular System" (Fig. 2), NO can be stored and carried in the blood as protein and non-protein RSNO (e.g., S-nitroso-N-acetylpenicillamine, S-nitrosohomocysteine, S-nitrosocysteine, and S-nitroso-albumin) (84), which protect NO from inactivation (85), and release NO depending on the "substrate" availability and oxidative plasma status. However, several enzymes and transporters have also been implicated in the intracellular delivery of NO from RSNOs (18). Among them, the platelet membrane-bound protein disulfide isomerase, PDI, deserves special attention (86). PDI is an enzyme that can catalyze three different reactions: isomerization of disulfide bonds, including thiol–disulfide exchange, reduction, and oxidation. By these means, PDI rapidly delivers NO-related signals into platelets from the donors (87).

To date, RSNOs have only been used intravenously in experimental models and small clinical trials (88). Because of the ability of RSNO to interact with membrane-bound platelet enzymes for further intraplatelet NO release, this platelet-specificity profile confers RSNO a high antiplatelet potential. Indeed, all RSNOs have shown to influence platelet function, mainly through a GC-cGMP pathway (89), with GSNO being the most potent platelet inhibitor. GSNO has been shown to reduce asymptomatic embolizations after carotid angioplasty without hypotensive episodes (88) and also to reduce markers of platelet activation such as P-selectin and fibrinogen GPIIb/IIIa receptor density without altering blood pressure in patients following percutaneous transluminal coronary angioplasty (90). In addition, GSNO has been shown to reduce neutrophil activation showing blood cell selectivity. Such cell selectivity makes GSNO inhibit platelet adhesion and aggregation to a greater extent than its effects on vascular tone (91,92). However, in some clinical conditions, no significant platelet inhibition by GSNO is likely observed, because the triggering stimulus surmounts GSNO antiplatelet properties at doses that do not affect blood pressure (93). In this regard, we have demonstrated in vitro and ex vivo the antithrombotic potential of two novel RSNO derivatives (LA810 and LA816) (74,94). Acute administration of LA810 exerted higher antiplatelet effects than equimolar doses of GSNO both in vitro and ex vivo, whereas intravenous LA816 administration provided additional platelet inhibitory effects to that achieved by combined oral administration of aspirin and clopidogrel. Most interestingly, all these effects were achieved with no concomitant adverse hemodynamic effects.

NO Hybrid Drugs

NO-NSAIDS NO-Releasing Aspirins

Nitro-aspirins (NCX-4016 and NCX-4215) are relatively new molecules in which an NO-releasing moiety is covalently linked to aspirin. The pharmacological rationale for the development of nitro-aspirins was based on the protective role of NO in the cardiovascular system and its cytoprotective effects on the gastrointestinal mucosa. Nitro-aspirins release both components after enzymatic metabolism, and it has been suggested that both aspirin acid and NO moieties are simultaneously released and exert their beneficial effects at the same time (95). Even more remarkably, it has been hypothesized that endothelial cells internalize NCX-4016 and that the release of NO occurs in the same intracellular compartments, an effect that may likely occur in platelets (96). However, properly conducted human pharmacokinetic studies are yet to be performed. Nitro-aspirins were also designed to prevent atherothrombotic disorders through complementary inhibition of different platelet activation pathways (i.e., aspirin-related COX suppression and NO-derived cGMP formation). In this regard, NCX-4215 and NCX-4016 were compared in vitro to aspirin with comparable results for maximal inhibition of arachidonic acid-stimulated platelet aggregation (97). However, NCX-4016 was the most efficient in inhibiting platelet activation induced by thrombin (97) and showed greater anti-inflammatory and analgesic activity, inhibition of cytokine release, and reduced monocyte-TF activity (98). Further phase I studies in healthy volunteers showed that NCX-4016 inhibited platelet COX-1 similarly to or slightly less than aspirin; however, in contrast to aspirin alone, NCX-4016 also decreased platelet aggregation induced by agonists not sensitive to aspirin such as U46619 (a stable analogue of TXA_2) or thrombin. Furthermore, NCX-4016 was able to suppress thrombin-induced platelet P-selectin expression, shear stress-induced platelet activation, glycoprotein IIb/IIIa activation (99), and the lipooxygenase pathway—events not affected by aspirin (100). NCX-4016 phase II studies have shown favorable effects on platelet activation parameters elicited by hyperglycemia in type 2 diabetes. None of the clinical studies reported thus far have suggested that NCX-4016 produced any relevant hypotensive side effects (101,102).

NCX-4016 has also shown to exert a number of anti-inflammatory activities beyond that of aspirin, reduce ischemia/reperfusion damage, correct endothelial dysfunction, and prevent oxygen radicals-induced vascular remodeling in animal models (101,103).

NO-Releasing Statins

Inhibitors of 3-hydroxy-3-methylglutaryl coenzyme A (HMG-CoA) reductase, statins, are widely used for the treatment of hypercholesterolemia. However, statins have been demonstrated to exert protective effects beyond lipid lowering, the so-called pleiotropic effects. Among these, eNOS restoration and anti-inflammatory and antiproliferative actions appear of relevance. Statins increase endothelial NO synthesis by stabilizing eNOS-mRNA with an increase in eNOS protein and by promoting eNOS activation via Ser1177/Thr495–Akt phosphorylation (104,105). Thus, with the aim of enhancing the non-lipid-lowering properties of selected statins, a NO-releasing moiety was introduced into the structure of pravastatin (NCX-6550) and fluvastatin (NCX-6553). This combination was expected to provide added therapeutic value, especially in those pathologies such as diabetes and atherosclerosis, where an impairment of endothelial function plays a crucial role in disease progression. In addition, Rosiello et al. (106) demonstrated the ability of nitrostatins to inhibit tissue factor expression and platelet aggregation in vitro and reduce thrombotic risk in a thromboembolism mouse model.

CONCLUDING REMARKS

The large body of evidence available to show that NO plays a critical role under a variety of physiological and pathological conditions has opened up the possibility of designing new drugs that are capable of delivering NO in the bloodstream. Moreover, the development of NO drug donors to favor site-specific delivery of NO and/or improve thromboresistivity is evolving and highly interesting (107–109). However, preclinical and clinical data are sparse. Additionally, the platelet NO/cGMP-dependent/independent signaling pathways still remain elusive, and more research is required to respond to unanswered questions. The use of specific transgenic mouse models and new insights at cellular-proteomic-genomic level will definitely help to better understand the role of NO on platelet pathophysiology. This new knowledge will enlighten new possibilities to develop new NO delivery systems that may largely contribute not only to improve clinical outcomes but also to reduce the severity of the disease.

ACKNOWLEDGMENTS

The writing of this chapter has been possible thanks to grants from PNS 2006-01091, CIBEROBN-Instituto de Salud Carlos III, y Cátedra de Investigación Catalana-Occidente, UAB (LB). GV is a Juan de la Cierva Investigator of the Ministerio de Educación y Ciencia (MEyC) of Spain.

REFERENCES

1. Badimon L, Martinez-Gonzalez J, Llorente-Cortes V, et al. Cell biology and lipoproteins in atherosclerosis. Curr Mol Med 2006; 6(5):439–456.
2. Schafer A, Wiesmann F, Neubauer S, et al. Rapid regulation of platelet activation in vivo by nitric oxide. Circulation 2004; 109(15):1819–1822.
3. Ignarro LJ, Napoli C, Loscalzo J. Nitric oxide donors and cardiovascular agents modulating the bioactivity of nitric oxide: an overview. Circ Res 2002; 90(1):21–28.
4. Warnholtz A, Tsilimingas N, Wendt M, et al. Mechanisms underlying nitrate-induced endothelial dysfunction: insight from experimental and clinical studies. Heart Fail Rev 2002; 7(4): 335–345.
5. Furchgott RF. Endothelium-derived relaxing factor: discovery, early studies, and identification as nitric oxide. Biosci Rep 1999; 19(4):235–251.
6. Ignarro LJ. Nitric oxide: a unique endogenous signaling molecule in vascular biology. Biosci Rep 1999; 19(2):51–71.
7. Loscalzo J, Vita J, eds. Nitric Oxide and the Cardiovascular System. Totowa, NJ: Humana Press, 2000.
8. Ignarro LJ, Cirino G, Casini A, et al. Nitric oxide as a signaling molecule in the vascular system: an overview. J Cardiovasc Pharmacol 1999; 34(6):879–886.
9. Gkaliagkousi E, Ritter J, Ferro A. Platelet-derived nitric oxide signaling and regulation. Circ Res 2007; 101(7):654–662.
10. Radomski MW, Palmer RM, Moncada S. Characterization of the L-arginine:nitric oxide pathway in human platelets. Br J Pharmacol 1990; 101(2):325–328.
11. Ji Y, Ferracci G, Warley A, et al. Beta-actin regulates platelet nitric oxide synthase 3 activity through interaction with heat shock protein 90. Proc Natl Acad Sci U S A 2007; 104(21): 8839–8844.
12. Sud N, Sharma S, Wiseman DA, et al. Nitric oxide and superoxide generation from endothelial NOS: modulation by HSP90. Am J Physiol Lung Cell Mol Physiol 2007; 293(6): L1444–L1453.
13. Gally JA, Montague PR, Reeke GN Jr., et al. The NO hypothesis: possible effects of a short-lived, rapidly diffusible signal in the development and function of the nervous system. Proc Natl Acad Sci U S A 1990; 87(9):3547–3551.
14. Freedman JE, Loscalzo J, Barnard MR, et al. Nitric oxide released from activated platelets inhibits platelet recruitment. J Clin Invest 1997; 100(2):350–356.

15. Freedman JE, Ting B, Hankin B, et al. Impaired platelet production of nitric oxide predicts presence of acute coronary syndromes. Circulation 1998; 98(15):1481–1486.

16. Lundberg JO, Weitzberg E, Gladwin MT. The nitrate-nitrite-nitric oxide pathway in physiology and therapeutics. Nat Rev Drug Discov 2008; 7(2):156–167.

17. Kang SS, Wong PW, Cook HY, et al. Protein-bound homocyst(e)ine. A possible risk factor for coronary artery disease. J Clin Invest 1986; 77(5):1482–1486.

18. Kleinbongard P, Dejam A, Lauer T, et al. Plasma nitrite concentrations reflect the degree of endothelial dysfunction in humans. Free Radic Biol Med 2006; 40(2):295–302.

19. Herrera M, Hong NJ, Garvin JL. Aquaporin-1 transports NO across cell membranes. Hypertension 2006; 48(1):157–164.

20. Zeiher AM, Fisslthaler B, Schray-Utz B, et al. Nitric oxide modulates the expression of monocyte chemoattractant protein 1 in cultured human endothelial cells. Circ Res 1995; 76(6): 980–986.

21. Kubes P, Suzuki M, Granger DN. Nitric oxide: an endogenous modulator of leukocyte adhesion. Proc Natl Acad Sci U S A 1991; 88(11):4651–4655.

22. Gauthier TW, Scalia R, Murohara T, et al. Nitric oxide protects against leukocyte-endothelium interactions in the early stages of hypercholesterolemia. Arterioscler Thromb Vasc Biol 1995; 15(10):1652–1659.

23. Draijer R, Atsma DE, van der Laarse A, et al. cGMP and nitric oxide modulate thrombin-induced endothelial permeability. Regulation via different pathways in human aortic and umbilical vein endothelial cells. Circ Res 1995; 76(2):199–208.

24. Radomski MW, Palmer RM, Moncada S. An L-arginine/nitric oxide pathway present in human platelets regulates aggregation. Proc Natl Acad Sci U S A 1990; 87(13):5193–5197.

25. Naseem KM, Riba R. Unresolved roles of platelet nitric oxide synthase. J Thromb Haemost 2008; 6(1):10–19.

26. Morrell CN, Matsushita K, Chiles K, et al. Regulation of platelet granule exocytosis by S-nitrosylation. Proc Natl Acad Sci U S A 2005; 102(10):3782–3787.

27. Williams RH, Nollert MU. Platelet-derived NO slows thrombus growth on a collagen type III surface. Thromb J 2004; (1): 2–11.

28. Storey RF, Heptinstall S. Laboratory investigation of platelet function. Clin Lab Haematol 1999; 21(5):317–329.

29. Ikeda H, Takajo Y, Murohara T, et al. Platelet-derived nitric oxide and coronary risk factors. Hypertension 2000; 35(4):904–907.

30. Rabini RA, Staffolani R, Fumelli P, et al. Decreased nitric oxide synthase activity in platelets from IDDM and NIDDM patients. Diabetologia 1998; 41(1):101–104.

31. Camilletti A, Moretti N, Giacchetti G, et al. Decreased nitric oxide levels and increased calcium content in platelets of hypertensive patients. Am J Hypertens 2001; 14(4 pt 1): 382–386.

32. Loscalzo J. Nitric oxide insufficiency, platelet activation, and arterial thrombosis. Circ Res 2001; 88(8):756–762.

33. Randriamboavonjy V, Fleming I. Endothelial nitric oxide synthase (eNOS) in platelets: how is it regulated and what is it doing there? Pharmacol Rep 2005; 57(suppl): 59–65.

34. Zhang J, Zhang J, Shattil SJ, et al. Phosphoinositide 3-kinase gamma and p85/ phosphoinositide 3-kinase in platelets. Relative activation by thrombin receptor or beta-phorbol myristate acetate and roles in promoting the ligand-binding function of alphaIIbbeta3 integrin. J Biol Chem 1996; 271(11):6265–6272.

35. Aszodi A, Pfeifer A, Ahmad M, et al. The vasodilator-stimulated phosphoprotein (VASP) is involved in cGMP- and cAMP-mediated inhibition of agonist-induced platelet aggregation, but is dispensable for smooth muscle function. Embo J 1999; 18(1):37–48.

36. Hauser W, Knobeloch KP, Eigenthaler M, et al. Megakaryocyte hyperplasia and enhanced agonist-induced platelet activation in vasodilator-stimulated phosphoprotein knockout mice. Proc Natl Acad Sci U S A 1999; 96(14):8120–8125.

37. Yuan SY. New insights into eNOS signaling in microvascular permeability. Am J Physiol Heart Circ Physiol 2006; 291(3):H1029–H1031.

38. Lucas KA, Pitari GM, Kazerounian S, et al. Guanylyl cyclases and signaling by cyclic GMP. Pharmacol Rev 2000; 52(3):375–414.
39. Pilz RB, Casteel DE. Regulation of gene expression by cyclic GMP. Circ Res 2003; 93(11): 1034–1046.
40. Ignarro LJ. Biological actions and properties of endothelium-derived nitric oxide formed and released from artery and vein. Circ Res 1989; 65(1):1–21.
41. Trepakova ES, Cohen RA, Bolotina VM. Nitric oxide inhibits capacitative cation influx in human platelets by promoting sarcoplasmic/endoplasmic reticulum Ca2+-ATPase-dependent refilling of Ca2+ stores. Circ Res 1999; 84(2):201–209.
42. Wang GR, Zhu Y, Halushka PV, et al. Mechanism of platelet inhibition by nitric oxide: in vivo phosphorylation of thromboxane receptor by cyclic GMP-dependent protein kinase. Proc Natl Acad Sci U S A 1998; 95(9):4888–4893.
43. Maurice DH, Haslam RJ. Molecular basis of the synergistic inhibition of platelet function by nitrovasodilators and activators of adenylate cyclase: inhibition of cyclic AMP breakdown by cyclic GMP. Mol Pharmacol 1990; 37(5):671–681.
44. Sogo N, Magid KS, Shaw CA, et al. Inhibition of human platelet aggregation by nitric oxide donor drugs: relative contribution of cGMP-independent mechanisms. Biochem Biophys Res Commun 2000; 279(2):412–419.
45. Boerrigter G, Burnett JC Jr. Nitric oxide-independent stimulation of soluble guanylate cyclase with BAY 41-2272 in cardiovascular disease. Cardiovasc Drug Rev 2007; 25(1):30–45.
46. Greenacre SA, Ischiropoulos H. Tyrosine nitration: localisation, quantification, consequences for protein function and signal transduction. Free Radic Res 2001; 34(6):541–581.
47. Blanchard-Fillion B, Souza JM, Friel T, et al. Nitration and inactivation of tyrosine hydroxylase by peroxynitrite. J Biol Chem 2001; 276(49):46017–46023.
48. Oberprieler NG, Roberts W, Riba R, et al. cGMP-independent inhibition of integrin alphaIIbbeta3-mediated platelet adhesion and outside-in signalling by nitric oxide. FEBS Lett 2007; 581(7):1529–1534.
49. Lahav J, Wijnen EM, Hess O, et al. Enzymatically catalyzed disulfide exchange is required for platelet adhesion to collagen via integrin alpha2beta1. Blood 2003; 102(6):2085–2092.
50. Essex DW. The role of thiols and disulfides in platelet function. Antioxid Redox Signal 2004; 6(4):736–746.
51. Heeschen C, Dimmeler S, Hamm CW, et al. Soluble CD40 ligand in acute coronary syndromes. N Engl J Med 2003; 348(12):1104–1111.
52. Schafer A, Fraccarollo D, Hildemann S, et al. Inhibition of platelet activation in congestive heart failure by aldosterone receptor antagonism and ACE inhibition. Thromb Haemost 2003; 89(6):1024–1030.
53. Winocour PD. Platelet abnormalities in diabetes mellitus. Diabetes 1992; 41(suppl 2):26–31.
54. Nimpf J, Wurm H, Kostner GM, et al. Platelet activation in normo- and hyperlipoproteine-mias. Basic Res Cardiol 1986; 81(5):437–453.
55. Lubos E, Loscalzo J, Handy DE. Homocysteine and glutathione peroxidase-1. Antioxid Redox Signal 2007; 9(11):1923–1940.
56. Brown AS, Moro MA, Masse JM, et al. Nitric oxide-dependent and independent effects on human platelets treated with peroxynitrite. Cardiovasc Res 1998; 40(2):380–388.
57. Naseem KM, Low SY, Sabetkar M, et al. The nitration of platelet cytosolic proteins during agonist-induced activation of platelets. FEBS Lett 2000; 473(1):119–122.
58. Napoli C, Ignarro LJ. Nitric oxide-releasing drugs. Annu Rev Pharmacol Toxicol 2003; 43: 97–123.
59. Mellion BT, Ignarro LJ, Ohlstein EH, et al. Evidence for the inhibitory role of guanosine 3′, 5′-monophosphate in ADP-induced human platelet aggregation in the presence of nitric oxide and related vasodilators. Blood 1981; 57(5):946–955.
60. Flaherty JT. Role of nitrates in acute myocardial infarction. Am J Cardiol 1992; 70(8):73B–81B.
61. Yusuf S, Collins R, MacMahon S, et al. Effect of intravenous nitrates on mortality in acute myocardial infarction: an overview of the randomised trials. Lancet 1988; 1(8594):1088–1092.

62. GISSI-3: effects of lisinopril and transdermal glyceryl trinitrate singly and together on 6-week mortality and ventricular function after acute myocardial infarction. Gruppo Italiano per lo Studio della Sopravvivenza nell'infarto Miocardico. Lancet 1994; 343(8906):1115–1122.

63. ISIS-4: a randomised factorial trial assessing early oral captopril, oral mononitrate, and intravenous magnesium sulphate in 58,050 patients with suspected acute myocardial infarction. ISIS-4 (Fourth International Study of Infarct Survival) Collaborative Group. Lancet 1995; 345(8951):669–685.

64. Gruetter CA, Gruetter DY, Lyon JE, et al. Relationship between cyclic guanosine 3': 5'-monophosphate formation and relaxation of coronary arterial smooth muscle by glyceryl trinitrate, nitroprusside, nitrite and nitric oxide: effects of methylene blue and methemoglobin. J Pharmacol Exp Ther 1981; 219(1):181–186.

65. Hess DT, Matsumoto A, Kim SO, et al. Protein S-nitrosylation: purview and parameters. Nat Rev Mol Cell Biol 2005; 6(2):150–166.

66. Patel DJ, Purcell HJ, Fox KM. Cardioprotection by opening of the K(ATP) channel in unstable angina. Is this a clinical manifestation of myocardial preconditioning? Results of a randomized study with nicorandil. CESAR 2 investigation. Clinical European studies in angina and revascularization. Eur Heart J 1999; 20(1):51–57.

67. Diodati J, Theroux P, Latour JG, et al. Effects of nitroglycerin at therapeutic doses on platelet aggregation in unstable angina pectoris and acute myocardial infarction. Am J Cardiol 1990; 66(7):683–688.

68. Sinzinger H, Virgolini I, O'Grady J, et al. Modification of platelet function by isosorbide dinitrate in patients with coronary artery disease. Thromb Res 1992; 65(3):323–335.

69. Friederich JA, Butterworth JFt. Sodium nitroprusside: twenty years and counting. Anesth Analg 1995; 81(1):152–162.

70. Parker JD. Nitrate tolerance, oxidative stress, and mitochondrial function: another worrisome chapter on the effects of organic nitrates. J Clin Invest 2004; 113(3):352–354.

71. Wada A, Ueda S, Masumori-Maemoto S, et al. Angiotensin II attenuates the vasodilating effect of a nitric oxide donor, glyceryl trinitrate: roles of superoxide and angiotensin II type 1 receptors. Clin Pharmacol Ther 2002; 71(6):440–447.

72. Kertland H. Nitrate tolerance–mechanisms and prevention. Conn Med 1993; 57(4):232–234.

73. Fitzgerald DJ, Roy L, Robertson RM, et al. The effects of organic nitrates on prostacyclin biosynthesis and platelet function in humans. Circulation 1984; 70(2):297–302.

74. Vilahur G, Segales E, Salas E, et al. Effects of a novel platelet nitric oxide donor (LA816), aspirin, clopidogrel, and combined therapy in inhibiting flow- and lesion-dependent thrombosis in the porcine ex vivo model. Circulation 2004; 110(12):1686–1693.

75. Vilahur G, Casani L, Badimon L. A thromboxane A2/prostaglandin H2 receptor antagonist (S18886) shows high antithrombotic efficacy in an experimental model of stent-induced thrombosis. Thromb Haemost 2007; 98(3):662–669.

76. Zafar MU, Vilahur G, Choi BG, et al. A novel anti-ischemic nitric oxide donor (LA419) reduces thrombogenesis in healthy human subjects. J Thromb Haemost 2007; 5(6):1195–1200.

77. Keefer LK. Progress toward clinical application of the nitric oxide-releasing diazeniumdiolates. Annu Rev Pharmacol Toxicol 2003; 43:585–607.

78. Wang GP, Cai TB, Taniguchi N. Nitric Oxide Donors: For Pharmaceutical And Biological Applications. Weinheim, Germany: Wiley-VCH Verlag GmbH & Co.KGaA, 2006.

79. Homer K, Wanstall J. In vitro comparison of two NONOates (novel nitric oxide donors) on rat pulmonary arteries. Eur J Pharmacol 1998; 356(1):49–57.

80. Diodati JG, Quyyumi AA, Hussain N, et al. Complexes of nitric oxide with nucleophiles as agents for the controlled biological release of nitric oxide: antiplatelet effect. Thromb Haemost 1993; 70(4):654–658.

81. Homer KL, Wanstall JC. Platelet inhibitory effects of the nitric oxide donor drug MAHMA NONOate in vivo in rats. Eur J Pharmacol 2003; 482(1–3):265–270.

82. Via LD, Francesconi M, Mazzucato M, et al. On the mechanism of the spermine-exerted inhibition on alpha-thrombin-induced platelet activation. Thromb Res 2000; 98(1):59–71.

83. Batchelor MM, Reoma SL, Fleser PS, et al. More lipophilic dialkyldiamine-based diazeniumdiolates: synthesis, characterization, and application in preparing thromboresistant nitric oxide release polymeric coatings. J Med Chem 2003; 46(24):5153–5161.

84. Rassaf T, Kleinbongard P, Preik M, et al. Plasma nitrosothiols contribute to the systemic vasodilator effects of intravenously applied NO: experimental and clinical Study on the fate of NO in human blood. Circ Res 2002; 91(6):470–477.

85. Stamler JS, Jaraki O, Osborne J, et al. Nitric oxide circulates in mammalian plasma primarily as an S-nitroso adduct of serum albumin. Proc Natl Acad Sci U S A 1992; 89(16):7674–7677.

86. Essex DW, Chen K, Swiatkowska M. Localization of protein disulfide isomerase to the external surface of the platelet plasma membrane. Blood 1995; 86(6):2168–2173.

87. Bell SE, Shah CM, Gordge MP. Protein disulfide-isomerase mediates delivery of nitric oxide redox derivatives into platelets. Biochem J 2007; 403(2):283–288.

88. Kaposzta Z, Baskerville PA, Madge D, et al. L-arginine and S-nitrosoglutathione reduce embolization in humans. Circulation 2001; 103(19):2371–2375.

89. Scatena R, Bottoni P, Martorana GE, et al. Nitric oxide donor drugs: an update on pathophysiology and therapeutic potential. Expert Opin Investig Drugs 2005; 14(7):835–846.

90. Langford EJ, Brown AS, Wainwright RJ, et al. Inhibition of platelet activity by S-nitrosoglutathione during coronary angioplasty. Lancet 1994; 344(8935):1458–1460.

91. Ramsay B, Radomski M, De Belder A, et al. Systemic effects of S-nitroso-glutathione in the human following intravenous infusion. Br J Clin Pharmacol 1995; 40(1):101–102.

92. Salas E, Langford EJ, Marrinan MT, et al. S-nitrosoglutathione inhibits platelet activation and deposition in coronary artery saphenous vein grafts in vitro and in vivo. Heart 1998; 80(2): 146–150.

93. Langford EJ, Parfitt A, de Belder AJ, et al. A study of platelet activation during human cardiopulmonary bypass and the effect of S-nitrosoglutathione. Thromb Haemost 1997; 78(6): 1516–1519.

94. Vilahur G, Baldellou MI, Segales E, et al. Inhibition of thrombosis by a novel platelet selective S-nitrosothiol compound without hemodynamic side effects. Cardiovasc Res 2004; 61(4):806–816.

95. Bolla M, Momi S, Gresele P, et al. Nitric oxide-donating aspirin (NCX 4016): an overview of its pharmacological properties and clinical perspectives. Eur J Clin Pharmacol 2006; 62(suppl 13): 145–154.

96. Fiorucci S, Mencarelli A, Mannucci R, et al. NCX-4016, a nitric oxide-releasing aspirin, protects endothelial cells against apoptosis by modulating mitochondrial function. Faseb J 2002; 16(12):1645–1647.

97. Lechi C, Gaino S, Tommasoli R, et al. In vitro study of the anti-aggregating activity of two nitroderivatives of acetylsalicylic acid. Blood Coagul Fibrinolysis 1996; 7(2):206–209.

98. Minuz P, Degan M, Gaino S, et al. NCX4016 (NO-aspirin) inhibits thromboxane biosynthesis and tissue factor expression and activity in human monocytes. Med Sci Monit 2001; 7(4):573–577.

99. Lechi C, Andrioli G, Gaino S, et al. The antiplatelet effects of a new nitroderivative of acetylsalicylic acid–an in vitro study of inhibition on the early phase of platelet activation and on TXA2 production. Thromb Haemost 1996; 76(5):791–798.

100. Gray PA, Warner TD, Vojnovic I, et al. Effects of non-steroidal anti-inflammatory drugs on cyclo-oxygenase and lipoxygenase activity in whole blood from aspirin-sensitive asthmatics vs healthy donors. Br J Pharmacol 2002; 137(7):1031–1038.

101. Gresele P, Momi S. Pharmacologic profile and therapeutic potential of NCX 4016, a nitric oxide-releasing aspirin, for cardiovascular disorders. Cardiovasc Drug Rev 2006; 24(2):148–168.

102. Wallace JL, Ignarro LJ, Fiorucci S. Potential cardioprotective actions of no-releasing aspirin. Nat Rev Drug Discov 2002; 1(5):375–382.

103. Gresele P, Momi S, Mezzasoma AM. NCX4016: a novel antithrombotic agent. Dig Liver Dis 2003; 35(suppl 2):S20–S26.

104. Martinez-Gonzalez J, Raposo B, Rodriguez C, et al. 3-hydroxy-3-methylglutaryl coenzyme a reductase inhibition prevents endothelial NO synthase downregulation by atherogenic levels of native LDLs: balance between transcriptional and posttranscriptional regulation. Arterioscler Thromb Vasc Biol 2001; 21(5):804–809.

105. Wu KK. Regulation of endothelial nitric oxide synthase activity and gene expression. Ann N Y Acad Sci 2002; 962:122–130.
106. Rossiello MR, Momi S, Caracchini R, et al. A novel nitric oxide-releasing statin derivative exerts an antiplatelet/antithrombotic activity and inhibits tissue factor expression. J Thromb Haemost 2005; 3(11):2554–2562.
107. Leopold JA, Loscalzo J. New developments in nitrosovasodilator therapy. Vasc Med 1997; 2(3): 190–202.
108. Ettenson DS, Edelman ER. Local drug delivery: an emerging approach in the treatment of restenosis. Vasc Med 2000; 5(2):97–102.
109. Bertrand OF, Sipehia R, Mongrain R, et al. Biocompatibility aspects of new stent technology. J Am Coll Cardiol 1998; 32(3):562–571.

30

The Interrelationship of Thrombin and Platelets—The Protease-Activated Receptor-1

Rohit Bhatheja and David J. Moliterno
Gill Heart Institute and Division of Cardiovascular Medicine, University of Kentucky, Lexington, Kentucky, U.S.A.

INTRODUCTION

Thrombin (factor IIa) is a serine protease that cleaves fibrinogen to fibrin and is the most potent stimulator of platelet aggregation. Thrombin has non-coagulation effects and interacts with multiple cell lines, including inflammatory, smooth muscle, and endothelial cells. Protease-activated receptors (PARs) represent a family of seven-transmembrane G-protein-coupled receptors (GPCRs), of which PAR-1 and PAR-4 have been identified on the platelets of primates. Platelet activation by thrombin's interaction with PAR-1 and PAR-4 has gained recent attention (1). The thrombin-platelet interaction is critical during endothelial injury, subsequent platelet reactivity, and release of various platelet products in the setting of acute coronary syndromes (ACS). Likewise, in the setting of balloon angioplasty and stenting, this interrelationship between serologic and cellular mediators of thrombosis is crucial to understand and control.

The purpose of this chapter is to review the present knowledge regarding the thrombin-PAR interaction, focusing primarily on the effect of PAR-1 in platelet biology and related clinical implications. Most of the work that has been done to understand the physiology of this receptor is based on small-animal experiments and may not translate into a similar beneficial profile in primates. This chapter will attempt to interpret these basic science data in a clinically applicable way.

THROMBIN

Thrombin plays a pivotal role in several different biological events, such as hemostasis, vasoreactivity, and cell proliferation. As part of the body's coagulation mechanism, it catalyzes the conversion of fibrinogen into fibrin and activates coagulation factors V, VIII, XI, and XIII. Thrombin, also known as factor IIa of the coagulation cascade, activates platelets to release pro-aggregatory mediators and express platelet adhesion molecules.

Thrombin has a host of other diverse physiological and regulatory functions. It is related to the digestive enzymes trypsin and chymotrypsin, and these proteases can activate PAR receptors in the gut. Thrombin also causes smooth muscle contraction and can activate other cell types such as endothelial cells, fibroblasts, neuronal, and mononuclear white blood cells (2), and is an important mediator in atherosclerosis (3) and restenosis (3–5). These pro-aggregatory, proliferative, and pro-inflammatory actions of thrombin are mediated by activation of specific cell surface receptors known as protease-activated receptors.

PLATELET PHYSIOLOGY

Normally, platelets are quiescent and form stable contacts only when there is a stimulus for platelet aggregation. Contact with the damaged endothelium and the underlying collagen activates them to release various chemokines that initiate the generation of platelet-rich thrombus. This primary physiological function during mechanical trauma, however, can lead to thrombotic vascular occlusion and major tissue ischemic damage in pathological conditions like atherosclerosis and ACS. Platelets also release many inflammatory mediators like P-selectin, CD40 ligand, platelet factor 4, transforming growth factor-β, thrombosponsin, and RANTES (regulated on activation, normal T-cell expressed and secreted), which are implicated in atherothrombosis (6), suggesting that inflammation and thrombosis are closely intertwined.

PLATELET RECEPTORS

Despite the high-shear blood flow, platelets attach to the injury site via its surface membrane receptors (Table 1) (7). These receptors respond to different types of stimuli, resulting in the release of paracrine factors, which in turn initiate the local cascade of

Table 1 Platelet Surface Receptors and Their Agonists in Platelet Adhesion, Activation, Aggregation, and Inhibition

Receptor	Agonist, Substrate, or Ligand	Response Phase
GPIb-IX-V	vWF	
$\alpha_2\beta_1$, GP VI	Collagen	
$\alpha_{IIb}\beta_3$	Fibrinogen, fibrin	Platelet adhesion
$\alpha_5\beta_1$	Fibronectin	
$\alpha_6\beta_1$	Laminin	
PAR-1, PAR4, GPIb-IX-V	Thrombin	Platelet activation
P2Y1, P2Y12	ADP	
TP	Thromboxane A2	
α_{2A}	Epinephrine	
$\alpha_{IIb}\beta_3$ (activated)	Fibrinogen, vWF, fibronectin	Platelet aggregation
SELPG, GPIb-IX-V	P-selectin	Platelet stabilization
$\alpha_{IIb}\beta_3$ (activated)	CD40 ligand	
PECAM-1	PECAM	Platelet inhibition

Abbreviations: ADP, adenosine diphosphate; GP, glycoprotein; PAR, protease-activated receptor; PECAM, platelet-endothelial cell adhesion molecule; PGI$_2$, prostaglandin I$_2$; vWF, von Willebrand Factor. *Source*: From Ref. 7.

platelet stimulation, secretion of inflammatory mediators, and finally aggregation to form the culprit platelet plug. Development of multiple antiplatelet agents was possible because of the presence of various receptors on the platelet surface. Aspirin has platelet anti-aggregatory effects due to its ability to inhibit the cyclooxygenase-dependent thromboxane-A2 synthesis in the platelets. Clopidogrel, a thienopyridine, has an anti-aggregatory effect on platelets via adenosine diphosphate (ADP) receptor antagonism. Even with the use of intravenous antiplatelet agents along with aspirin and clopidogrel, physiologic platelet inhibition may be incomplete (8). This has focused attention on newer platelet receptors to target therapies for optimal antiplatelet effect.

PROTEASE-ACTIVATED RECEPTORS

PARs are part of the superfamily of GPCRs (Fig. 1) (9). These are membrane proteins with an extracellular N-terminus, an intracellular C-terminus, and seven-transmembrane domains. GPCRs regulate the pathways for cell morphology, secretion, proliferation, migration, and adhesion in platelets, cardiomyocytes, and smooth muscle cells. Typically GPCRs undergo a conformational change on interaction of their N-termini with their ligands and relay the molecular signal to the cytoplasmic milieu. The G-protein is a heterotrimer made of single α-, β-, and γ-subunits. The α-subunit on human platelets has four members (Gs, Gi, G12, Gq), which have different actions. It is the Gq receptor that affects the intracellular signaling in platelets.

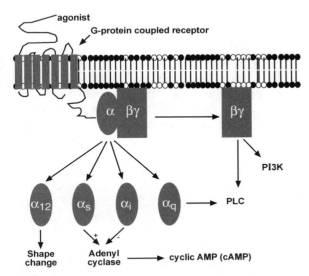

Figure 1 Illustration of the function of G-protein-coupled platelet receptors. Upon stimulation of the receptor by the appropriate agonist, there is a dissociation of heterotrimeric G-protein into a GTP-binding α-subunit and a β-γ heterodimeric subunit, each of which is then free to stimulate enzymes, which produce second messengers within the platelet. As examples, the G α-subclass 12/13 subunit induces platelet shape change, and the G α-subclass s and i subunits stimulate or inhibit adenyl cyclase activity, respectively. The G α-subclass q subunit responds to thrombin PAR interaction and activates phospholipase C–β. The separated G β-γ subunit also activates PLC-β as well as phosphatidylinositol 3-kinase. *Abbreviations*: PLC, phospholipase C; PI3K, phosphatidylinositol 3-kinase. *Source*: From Ref. 9.

PARs are somewhat unconventional; however, as they are enzymatically cleaved and expose an extracellular amino-terminus that serves as a tethered ligand, activating the PAR receptors themselves. Hence, the ligand is a part of the receptor itself rather than a separate molecule (10). The intracellular carboxy-terminus and the G-protein-coupling sites undergo phosphorylation, which leads to internalization and deactivation of the receptor. It is then degraded by lysosomes. Once lysed, PAR-1 is usually not recycled and requires resynthesis for further cellular effects.

The first PAR receptor on human platelets and the vascular endothelial cells were discovered and cloned in 1990 (10). Since then a total of four human PAR receptors have been sequentially identified. Of these, PAR-1 (10,11), PAR-3 (12), and PAR-4 (13,14) are activated by thrombin. PAR-2 is not a substrate for thrombin and is activated primarily by trypsin (15), tryptase (16), and coagulation factors Xa and VIIa (17). Of these receptors only PAR-1 and PAR-4 are found on human platelets. The PAR-1, 2, and 3 genes are encoded on chromosome 5q13, and PAR-4 genes are encoded on chromosome 19p12. Thrombin initiates a strong response in platelets, causing platelet aggregation and rapid stimulation of platelet procoagulant binding through PAR-1. With the same thrombin concentration, the responses mediated by PAR-4, however, are weaker and limited to platelet aggregation (18). This dual platelet receptor system may represent both the early and intense (PAR-1) platelet aggregation and the slow and late-phase (PAR-4) platelet aggregation. PAR-1 is a high-affinity receptor that can be activated at low levels of thrombin, unlike PAR-4, which is a low-affinity receptor requiring higher thrombin concentration for activation. The presence of PAR-1 on various other cell types including endothelial and vascular smooth muscle cells is responsible for its non-platelet actions (Table 2) (19).

STRUCTURE AND ACTIVATION OF PAR-1

PAR-1, historically known as the thrombin receptor, was cloned by expressing RNA from cells highly responsive to thrombin in *Xenopus* oocytes, thus creating the cDNA encoding the thrombin receptor (10). Sequencing identified the functional clone encoding a 425 amino acid protein typical of GPCR (PAR-1) that contained an N-terminal hydrophobic signal sequence, an extracellular 75 amino-acid domain, and a potential thrombin cleavage site: $LDPR^{41}$- $S^{42}FLLRN$ (i.e., arginine^{41}-serine^{42}).

PAR-1 has proved to be vital in thrombin-induced platelet activation and other thrombin-induced cellular events, and is the principal thrombin receptor on platelets. The number of PAR-1 receptors on resting platelets is variable, ranging from 547 to 2063 (mean 1276) copies per platelet in both males and females. Polymorphism of PAR-1 receptors has been described; however, this does not fully explain the inter-individual variability in receptor density (20).

Thrombin rapidly associates to the hirudin-like exodomain on the PAR-1 via its cationic hydrophobic groove (21). Once thrombin docks on the amino-terminus of PAR, it induces a conformational change (Fig. 2) (22). This facilitates binding of the anionic binding domain of thrombin to the specific PAR-1 cleavage sequence (23). Consequently, this binding cleaves the amino-terminal exodomain of PAR-1, exposing a new amino-terminus (beginning with SFLLRN) exodomain. The new amino-terminus hexapeptide recognition sequence acts as a tethered peptide ligand, which then binds intra-molecularly to the truncated receptor (i.e., itself) to effect transmembrane signaling via the cytoplasmic G-proteins. Depending on the rate and affinity of PAR-1 cleavage by

Table 2 PAR Subtypes and Their Associated Specific Sequences

	PAR-1	PAR-2	PAR-3	PAR-4
Activating protease	• Thrombin (50 pM) • Trypsin	• Trypsin (1 nM) • Tryptase (mast cell protease, 1 nM)	• Thrombin (0.2 nM)	• Thrombin (5 nM) • Trypsin (1 nM) • Plasmin • Cathepsin G
Inactivating proteases	• Leucocyte proteases: cathepsin G, Plasmin, and Proteinase 3 • Elastase • TACE-like MMP	• Cathepsin G • Plasmin • Proteinase 3 • Elastase		
Agonists	• SFLLRN • TFLLRN • RWJ-56110	• SLIGKV • SLIGRL • SFLLRN • Tc-LIGRLO		• GYPGKF • AYPGKF • Tc-YGPKF • Tc-LIGRL
Cell type	• Platelet • Smooth muscle • Endothelium • Epithelial • Fibroblasts • Myocytes • Neurons • Astrocytes	• Endothelial • Epithelial • Fibroblasts • Myocytes • Neurons • Astrocytes	• Endothelium • Myocytes • Astrocytes	• Platelet • Endothelium • Myocytes • Astrocytes
Tethered ligand sequence (human)	• SFLLRN	• SLIGKV	• TFRGAP	• GYPGQV
Vascular response	• Contractility • Inflammation • Proliferation • Repair • Embryonic development • Tissue remodeling	• Inflammation • Vasoregulation		• Platelet activation and thrombosis • Inflammation

Source: Modified from Ref. 19.

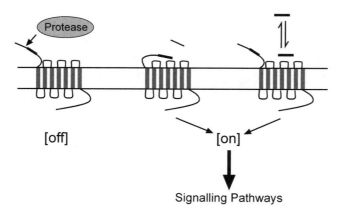

Figure 2 Thrombin (protease) attaches to the amino-terminus of PAR-1, causing a conformational change in the receptor. Binding of thrombin to the specific PAR-1 cleavage site cleaves this amino exodomain of PAR-1, exposing a new amino terminus. This terminus now acts as a tethered ligand, binding intramolecularly to the receptor, thus turning on transmembrane signaling. *Source*: From Ref. 22.

thrombin, there is calcium influx, which is pivotal in setting the momentum for platelet activation (Fig. 3) (24).

As thrombin is a protease (enzyme), it can link and activate more than one PAR molecule. Nonetheless, PAR-1 is not selective for thrombin and can be activated by other serine proteases, such as protein C, factor VIIa, and factor Xa. Also, proteolytic cleavage can be "nonproductive" despite receptor activation, as seen with cathepsin G (25) (released by activated neutrophils).

In contrast to reversible ligand binding, thrombin cleavage of PAR cannot be directly undone; once the previously hidden ligand is unmasked, the mechanisms for platelet desensitization are set into motion. This irreversible cleavage of the PAR with the creation of a new agonist that tethers to the receptor is a unique property of this receptor. Intracellular interaction of PAR with the α-subunit of the G-protein then activates phospholipase-C. This generates inositol triphosphate, mobilizing intracellular diacyl glycerol, which then activates the protein-kinase C that ultimately transcribes the cellular actions of the cell. The receptor function is then terminated by desensitization of the GPCR. Ligand activation of the receptor induces membrane translocation of G-protein receptor kinases (GRK) from the cytosol to the membrane (GRK3 and 5), which phosphorylates the receptor within the carboxy-terminus. This promotes membrane translocation of β-arrestins, that mediates uncoupling and desensitization of the PAR-1. As human platelets cannot resynthesize PAR, they are unable to repopulate their surfaces with more PAR-1 and do not respond to thrombin again. The presence of the PAR-4, however, may prolong the effect of thrombin (19). Some cells internalize and recycle their previously activated PAR receptors.

The synthetic peptide SFLLRN is a thrombin receptor–activating peptide (TRAP) that mimics the first six amino acids of the new amino-terminus unmasked by the cleavage of PAR-1 by thrombin. SFLLRN functions as a PAR-1 agonist independent of thrombin and proteolysis (26). It is 1000 times less effective than thrombin on platelets, and its action requires a high concentration of the agonist peptide in contrast to the picomolar concentrations required with thrombin (27). This property of SFLLRN and other similar peptides helped in uncovering the detailed mechanism of the agonist-platelet interaction. SFLLRN also has been used as a pharmacological probe of PAR function in various cell types.

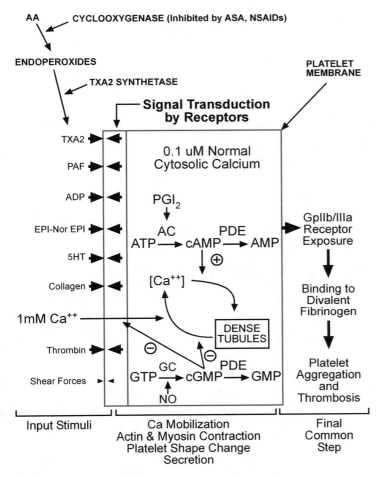

Figure 3 Various stimuli activate platelets by increasing the free cytosolic Ca^{2+} level. The enzyme AC converts ATP to cAMP. Subsequently, cAMP is broken by the enzyme phosphodiesterase down to AMP. Increased levels of cAMP are caused by PGI_2 binding to a specific receptor and stimulating AC; some Ca^{2+} is stored in the dense tubules. This reduces cytosolic-free Ca^{2+} and decreases the level of platelet activation. Similarly, GC coverts GTP to cyclic guanosine monophosphate that is converted to GMP via phosphodiesterase. Elevation of cGMP levels reduces free cytosolic Ca^2 by two mechanisms: Ca^{2+} is inhibited from entering the platelet from the plasma, and also Ca^{2+} is inhibited from leaving the dense tubules. Thus modulating free-cytosolic Ca^{2+} can increase or decrease platelet activity. The ultimate step in platelet-mediated thrombosis is the activation of the platelet glycoprotein IIb/IIIa fibrinogen receptor, which binds to fibrinogen and creates a platelet aggregate. *Abbreviations*: AC, adenylate cyclase; ATP, adenosine triphosphate; cAMP, cyclic adenosine monophosphate; PGI, prostacyclin; GC, guanylate cyclase; GTP, guansine triphosphate. *Source*: From Ref. 24.

THE ROLE OF PAR-1 INHIBITORS IN ATHEROTHROMBOSIS

PARs are the only signaling receptors that have been unequivocally identified for thrombin. They are present in many cell types and are implicated in the regulation of a number of vital functions (28), including hemostasis and thrombosis, tissue healing, inflammation, and endothelium-dependent vasomotor tone. Thrombin plays an important

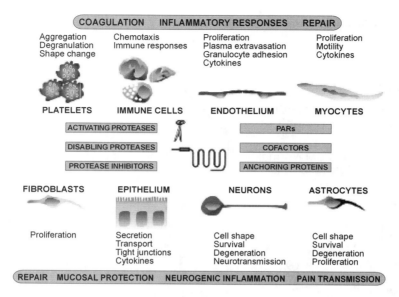

Figure 4 The role of PARs in different cell types. Signaling depends on the availability of proteases, which can activate or disable PARs, protease inhibitors, protease cofactors, and anchoring proteins. Proteases signal a wide variety of cells to regulate critically important biological processes, with implications for physiological regulation and disease. *Source*: From Ref. 19.

role as a cell-signaling effector molecule, most notably in atherosclerotic coronary disease where thrombosis, inflammation, and fibrinolysis are interconnected. Interruption of the thrombotic activities without hampering the hemostatic features is the key to the optimal therapeutic balance of any antithrombotic drug.

Although the interaction of thrombin and PAR-1 has many pleotropic effects and cardiovascular implications, platelet activation, recruitment, and thrombosis have clear relevance. Many of the non-platelet and non-thrombotic cardiovascular actions and its mechanisms have been described (Table 2; Fig. 4). Specific PAR inhibitors have helped elucidate actions of the receptor and of thrombin.

The PAR-1 inhibitor peptide RWJ-82259 (Johnson and Johnson, Spring House, Pennsylvania, U.S.) has been effective in inhibiting the thrombin-mediated smooth muscle cell response associated with vascular injury induced by balloon angioplasty of the common carotid artery of rat. Perivascular adventitial treatment with this compound causes a dose-dependent reduction in intimal area and thickness and a trend toward reduced luminal stenosis (Fig. 5) (29). PAR deficient mice also show a similar attenuated response to vascular injury (30). This anti-restenotic effect is independent of its effect on platelets, as mice platelets lack PAR-1 and exhibit normal platelet reactivity in the presence of PAR-1 antagonism. Similarly, antagonist RWJ-58259 has a beneficial effect on the injured carotid arteries of cynomolgus monkeys by diminishing thrombosis while maintaining neutrality on the hematological and coagulation parameters (31). This effect is independent of thrombin's proteolytic activity or platelet aggregation induced by other agonists like collagen. As human and non-human primates have a similar PAR expression profile on their platelets, these studies have clinical implications (32). Earlier animal studies have demonstrated that PAR antagonism inhibits thrombin, but not ADP or collagen-induced platelet aggregation and stimulation. There is also reduction in the cyclic flow in the carotid artery, which is primarily a platelet-dependent phenomenon,

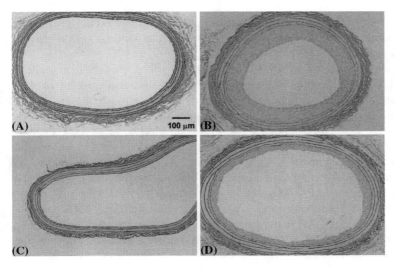

Figure 5 Rat carotid artery changes 14 days after vascular injury (restenosis model). RWJ-58259 (1, 5, or 10 mg) was suspended in 150 μL of a polymer gel and applied to the adventitia of the left common carotid, as it is not orally active. (**A**) Uninjured, vehicle-treated; (**B**) injured, vehicle-treated; (**C**) uninjured, RWJ-58259-treated; and (**D**) injured, RWJ-58259-treated. This suggests direct effect of PAR-1 inhibition on the vasculature by inhibiting the smooth muscle cell proliferation secondary to vascular injury. It is independent of the antiplatelet effect, as rat platelets lack PAR-1. *Source*: From Ref. 29.

thus reducing intravascular thrombus formation with minimal effect on bleeding time and no effect on coagulation time (33).

SCH 79797 (Schering-Plough, Kenilworth, New Jersey, U.S.) is an intravenous selective PAR-1 antagonist that was shown in a pilot study to limit myocardial reperfusion injury in rats (34). Clinical data regarding SCH 79797 are not available at this time.

SCH 530348 is a competitive PAR-1 antagonist that has been studied as oral antiplatelet therapy in patients with established vascular disease. This drug is derived from the bark of an Australian Magnolia plant *Galbulimima baccata*, which is mainly found in the tropical zones of Eastern Malaysia, New Guinea, northern Australia, and the Solomon Islands. It undergoes oxidative metabolism in the liver by the CYP3A4 enzymes and is 90% excreted in bile as the inactive metabolite. Hence, steady-state exposure to SCH 530348 is increased upon coadministration with potent CYP3A4 inhibitors (e.g., ketoconazole) and is decreased upon coadministration with potent CYP3A4 inducers (e.g., rifampin).

Clinical phase I studies have shown SCH 530348 to have rapid onset of action, with a potent (>90%) and prolonged (up to 72 hours) dose-related inhibition of TRAP-induced platelet aggregation with a good safety profile. Once-daily dosing of this drug appears adequate for the required antiplatelet effect (35). SCH 530348 is rapidly absorbed and distributed in the body but is excreted slowly (half-life of >100 hours). It takes 0.75 to 1.5 hours to achieve maximum plasma concentration after administration and an increased dose is associated with a faster onset of action and an increased inhibition of platelet aggregation. It has a sustained effect despite a decrease in plasma concentration; however, at concentrations below 5 to 10 ng/mL, the platelet function beings to recover. Thus, unlike aspirin, this drug is a reversible inhibitor of platelet aggregation. Phase II clinical studies have been completed with SCH 530348 and fast track evaluation designation by the FDA for secondary prevention of cardiovascular morbidity and mortality outcomes in at-risk patients has been granted (36).

TRA-PCI (Thrombin Receptor Antagonist in Percutaneous Coronary Intervention) was a clinical phase II, multicenter study of SCH 530348 on a background of dual antiplatelet and antithrombotic therapy among patients undergoing nonurgent PCI or cardiac catheterization. A total of 1030 patients were randomized in a 3:1 fashion to TRA drug ($n = 773$, loading with either 10, 20, or 40 mg) or to placebo ($n = 257$). Patients undergoing PCI and randomized to SCH 530348, received maintenance drug during the subsequent 60 days in a 1:1:1 randomization (0.1, 1, and 2.5 mg maintenance doses). PCI patients randomized to placebo received placebo over the 60-day treatment period. The safety of this orally administered PAR-1 antagonist as assessed by the TIMI classification of bleeding (primary safety endpoint) was confirmed in this study, as TRA was not associated with an increase in TIMI major or minor bleeding as compared with placebo ($n = 422$, 2.8%, vs. $n = 131$, 3.3%, $p = 0.77$). While not statistically significant, the 60-day death or major adverse cardiovascular event (MACE) rate (secondary efficacy endpoint) was reduced by 32% overall ($n = 25$, 5.9% versus $n = 13$, 8.6%), and myocardial infarction (MI) was reduced by 41% overall, with SCH 530348 as compared with placebo. Higher dose (40 mg) seemed to have more pronounced effect in reducing MACE and MI (46% and 52%, respectively) (37,38).

Having demonstrated the preliminary safety and tolerability of this molecule in phase II, SCH 530348/TRA is now being studied in the ACS population. TRACER (thrombin receptor antagonist for clinical event reduction in acute coronary syndrome) is a randomized, multicenter, 10,000-patient study. In this phase III trial, TRA will be administered (single loading dose of 40 mg followed by 2.5 mg/day vs. placebo) on a platform of standard medical therapy in a high-risk non-ST-elevation myocardial infarction (NSTEMI) ACS population. Patients will be followed for more than one year to assess the primary endpoint of cardiovascular death, MI, stroke, recurrent ischemia with re-hospitalization, and urgent coronary revascularization (39).

The efficacy of SCH 530348 in addition to standard of care in patients with established stable atherosclerotic disease is currently being studied in the thrombin receptor antagonist in secondary prevention of atherothrombotic ischemic events (TRA2P-TIMI50). In this multicenter, double blind, randomized, placebo-controlled trial, the composite outcome of cardiovascular death, MI, stroke, and urgent coronary revascularization will be studied among ~20,000 patients with coronary artery disease, ischemic cerebrovascular disease, and symptomatic peripheral vascular disease (40). Patients will be randomized to SCH 530348 2.5 mg daily or placebo and followed for at least one year.

E5555

E5555 (Eisai, Tokyo, Japan) is another orally active PAR-1 antagonist that is in phase II of development. It has been studied in animal models and shown to affect restenosis and limit hypercontractile vascular states associated with subarachnoid hemorrhage (41). E5555 has been shown to inhibit thrombin-induced platelet aggregation in a dose-dependent manner with maximum effects achieved at six hours after single administration (42). In a pilot study, the drug was taken by 40 healthy male volunteers for 10 days. At single doses of 50 mg or greater there was more than 80% platelet aggregation inhibition and the duration of inhibition was dose-dependently prolonged with E5555 administration. At drug-steady state, after 100 and 200 mg repeated administration, platelet aggregation induced by 2 units/mL of thrombin was near completely eliminated, even 24 hours after administration. It did not affect ADP-induced platelet aggregation, coagulation time, or bleeding time, and had no significant adverse effects, abnormalities, or changes in vital signs, ECG findings, or clinical laboratory tests. Two additional phase II trials enrolling together ~800 patients are currently underway to assess the safety and tolerability of E5555 and its effect on intravascular inflammation and thrombosis in subjects with coronary artery disease (43) and those with an ACS (44).

As these molecules specifically interfere with the intramolecular binding of the tethered ligand sparing the proteolytic effects of thrombin, they may be considered "super selective thrombin receptor antagonists." This represents a promising lead for further investigation in this field.

APROTININ AND PAR-1

Aprotinin was developed as a drug that would prevent excessive bleeding complications and at the same time is antithrombotic. It is a 56-amino acid, non-specific serine protease inhibitor that has been used during cardiopulmonary bypass to prevent post-operative bleeding by preserving platelet function. It also inhibits plasmin and can act as an antifibrinolytic. Counterintuitive as it may seem, this thrombin inhibitor has been observed to reduce bleeding complications during cardiopulmonary bypass operations. Thrombin receptor–agonist protein-6 is a synthetic peptide chain that mimics the SFLLRN domain of the PAR-1 and can activate PAR-1 without the cleavage of exodomain. During cardiopulmonary bypass, thrombin generated in the bypass circuit can activate and cleave PAR-1, rendering it unresponsive to TRAP. Post-operatively, however, in patients with increased bleeding there is a significant reduction in the TRAP-induced platelet activation, suggesting that decreased PAR-1 responsiveness or desensitization by thrombin may be the cause of excessive bleeding (45). Thus, a strategy focused on limiting or inhibiting the effects of thrombin may help decrease the risk of postoperative bleeding in patients undergoing cardiac surgery.

One way to inhibit the action of thrombin on platelets would be to inhibit its receptor, PAR-1. Aprotinin is unique in theoretically balancing hemostatic and antithrombotic properties by selectively preventing thrombin-induced proteolysis of PAR-1 and not affecting platelet activation by other non-proteolytic agonists (e.g., collagen, epinephrine) (46). Aprotinin reduces postoperative bleeding while maintaining platelet aggregation (47), even in patients on clopidogrel undergoing coronary artery bypass graft surgery (48). In addition to reduction in blood transfusion, aprotinin is also associated with reduced incidence of perioperative stroke (49) and cognitive function that may be related to its anti-inflammatory and neuroprotective effects (50). The phase III trial of aprotinin (51) demonstrated platelet transfusions to be associated with higher mortality, stroke, use of vasopressors, and postoperative infection. Longer operating time and redo-surgery may have stimulated more thrombin generation leading to the PAR-1 deficiency and, thus, significantly increased stroke risk. However, patients who did not require platelet transfusion were more likely to have been administered full-dose aprotinin.

On the other hand, in a select group of patients, high-dose aprotinin was associated with increased thrombosis, renal failure, and higher bleeding rates (52). Recent data have questioned the safety of aprotinin in patients undergoing coronary artery bypass graft surgery. In a retrospective analysis of 33,517 patients receiving aprotinin versus 44,682 who received aminocaproic acid, there was 64% higher risk of inpatient mortality in the aprotinin treated group (relative risk, 1.64; 95% CI, 1.50 to 1.78). Postoperative revascularization and dialysis were more frequent among recipients of aprotinin than among recipients of aminocaproic acid (53). A large Canadian study comparing use of aprotinin versus aminocaproic acid or tranexamic acid during cardiac surgery was halted because of similar safety concerns and an increased 30-day mortality in the aprotinin group (54).

Although the Cochrane meta-analysis of 211 randomized controlled trials involving a total of 20,781 patients found no significantly increased risk of MI or death from any cause for aprotinin use (55), and the need for blood transfusions is reduced by aprotinin (56), the above safety concerns in the absence of convincing new data makes it difficult to prescribe this drug.

MATRIX METALLOPROTEINASES AND PAR

Recent evidence suggests that each phase of the atherosclerotic process may be mediated by a series of enzymes called matrix metalloproteinases (MMP), which are the main physiological regulators of the extracellular matrix (57). Acute inflammatory response (58) at the site of plaque rupture is associated with the release of proteolytic enzymes causing plaque instability and is a prelude to the onset of clinical events.

MMP are a group of 25 structurally related zinc-dependent non-serine proteases. They are anchored to the cell surface to be excreted into the extracellular milieu to cleave extracellular matrix structures like collagen, elastins, proteoglycans, and glycoproteins. Of these, collagenases including MMP-1 (collagenase-1), MMP-8 (neutrophil collagenase, collagenase-2), and MMP-13 (collagenase-3) are present in human atheromas especially in the vulnerable atherosclerotic plaque. MMP-1 is implicated in human atherosclerotic carotid atherosclerosis causing intraplaque hemorrhage (59) and also in coronary lesions, leading to increased circumferential stress in the fibrous plaque. This action may play a role in the pathogenesis of plaque rupture and acute ischemic syndromes (60).

Studies have shown that MMP-1 cleaves PAR-1 at the proper site for receptor activation, generating robust PAR-1-dependent calcium signaling in tumor cells (61). This mechanism suggests that the increased oxidative stress and pro-inflammatory signaling of MMP-1 in the atherosclerotic plaque may be due to PAR-1. Inhibition of MMP-1 holds promise for therapeutic intervention in treating atherosclerotic cardiovascular disease. This inhibition may translate into plaque stabilization, as seen with statin therapy, arresting the smoldering inflammatory activity within the atheroma. However, at this time, no preclinical or early clinical data are available.

PAR-1 IN VASOMOTOR TONE, SMOOTH MUSCLE CELLS, AND CARDIOMYOCYTES

Platelets secrete pro-and anti-angiogenic factors that aid wound healing and also tumor growth. PAR-1 activation is associated with release of pro-angiogenic vascular endothelial growth factor and also inhibition of endostatin, which inhibits angiogenesis (62). This appears to be due to counter-regulatory modulation of the release of angiogenic factors by PAR-1 and PAR-4, independent of the action of thrombin.

PAR-1 stimulation in human coronary arteries shows endothelium-dependent vasorelaxation, which is inversely affected by atherosclerosis burden. There is a graded decrease in the vasodilatory and a reciprocal increase in the vasoconstrictive response with increasing intimal thickening and atherosclerosis (63). Although there may be an

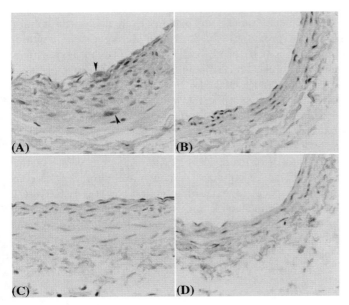

Figure 6 Immunohistochemical labeling of PAR-1 in WT and PAR-1$^{-/-}$ mice 14 days after vascular injury. (**A**) Injured carotid artery from a WT mouse (note *brown label* through the neointima at *arrowheads*); (**B**) corresponding uninjured carotid artery from the same WT mouse, showing little or no label in the media; (**C**) injured carotid artery from a PAR-1$^{-/-}$ mouse (note the absence of label for PAR-1); (**D**) corresponding uninjured carotid artery from the same PAR-1$^{-/-}$ mouse, which also did not label for PAR-1. *Abbreviation*: WT, wild type. *Source*: From Ref. 67.

initial increase in coronary blood flow, it is followed by a sustained decrease. This contractile effect can also lead to depressed ventricular function (64). Denuded endothelium generates a strong contractile response, suggestive of PAR-1-mediated calcium influx in the smooth muscle (65). These smooth muscle effects, which can affect vascular tone, are independent of PAR-related platelet effects.

The pro-angiogenic effects of thrombin are also seen with other PAR-1 activators, and involve amplification of the response of vascular endothelial growth factor by upregulation of its receptors (KDR and flt-1) (66). Smaller vessel caliber and attenuated neointimal response is seen with PAR-1-deficient mice, suggesting a role of PAR-1 in regulation of vascular matrix after vascular injury (Fig. 6) (67). It has recently become clear that PAR-1 is implicated in reperfusion arrhythmias (68), increased myocyte contraction (69), myocyte cell elongation typical of volume-overloaded dilated cardiomyopathy (70), and cardiac fibroblast proliferation (71).

CONCLUSION

Vascular injury is associated with an exuberant prothrombotic state, which can compromise the vessel patency. This response, in the physiological state, is opposed by antithrombotic molecules like PGI2, nitric oxide, thrombomodulin, heparin sulfate, and tissue plasminogen activator normally present on the endothelium (71). The presence of multiple receptors on the platelet surface is an opportunity for plaque rupture to result in platelet-rich thrombus at the site of injury. The unique function of the PAR-1 receptor, in being the gateway to the most potent stimuli for platelet aggregation (thrombin), represents an important pathway of prothrombotic activation during plaque rupture. PAR-1 is the mediator of thrombin's actions on the cell, such as platelet aggregation, lymphocytic mitogenesis, neuronal cellular and inflammatory responses, making it an attractive target for drug development. Understandably, PAR-1 antagonism would offer adjunctive therapy in diseases requiring antiplatelet, anti-inflammatory, and anti-proliferative effects. The presence of dual thrombin receptor system (PAR-1/PAR-4) on human platelets may be evolutionary and a mechanistic redundancy to assure adequate platelet aggregation even with high thrombin concentrations during vascular trauma.

The promising and favorable profile of the results of PAR-1 antagonists may be the next major step in the modern antiplatelet regimen. Although the clinical relevance remains under investigation, one may speculate that with a modest bleeding risk, PAR-1 antagonists as an antithrombotic and antiplatelet could mitigate some very important concerns like late drug-eluting stent thrombosis. This latter benefit alone, if proved, would provide strong rationale for the use of these drugs. The reported favorable effects will be confirmed or refuted by the results of clinical phase III trials, and will also provide a framework for further large-scale confirmatory studies to establish the role of PAR-1 receptor antagonists.

REFERENCES

1. Coughlin SR. Thrombin signalling and protease-activated receptors. Nature 2000; 407(6801): 258–264.
2. Fenton JW 2nd. Regulation of thrombin generation and functions. Semin Thromb Hemost 1988; 14(3):234–240.
3. Nelken NA, Soifer SJ, O'Keefe J, et al. Thrombin receptor expression in normal and atherosclerotic human arteries. J Clin Invest 1992; 90(4):1614–1621.
4. Barry WL, Gimple LW, Humphries JE, et al. Arterial thrombin activity after angioplasty in an atherosclerotic rabbit model: time course and effect of hirudin. Circulation 1996; 94(1):88–93.
5. Gallo R, Padurean A, Toschi V, et al. Prolonged thrombin inhibition reduces restenosis after balloon angioplasty in porcine coronary arteries. Circulation 1998; 97(6):581–588.
6. Libby P, Simon DI. Inflammation and thrombosis: the clot thickens. Circulation 2001; 103(13): 1718–1720.
7. Ruggeri ZM. Platelets in atherothrombosis. Nat Med 2002; 8(11):1227–1234.
8. Lincoff AM, Kleiman NS, Kereiakes DJ, et al. Long-term efficacy of bivalirudin and provisional glycoprotein IIb/IIIa blockade vs heparin and planned glycoprotein IIb/IIIa blockade during percutaneous coronary revascularization: REPLACE-2 randomized trial. JAMA 2004; 292(6):696–703.
9. Abrams CS. Platelet Biology. UpToDate, Inc. Accessed May 13th 2008 at http://patients. uptodate.com/topic.asp?file=platelet/7540.
10. Vu TK, Hung DT, Wheaton Coughlin SR VI. Molecular cloning of a functional thrombin receptor reveals a novel proteolytic mechanism of receptor activation. Cell 1991; 64(6): 1057–1068.
11. Rasmussen UB, Vouret-Craviari V, Jallat S, et al. cDNA cloning and expression of a hamster alpha-thrombin receptor coupled to Ca2+ mobilization. FEBS Lett 1991; 288(1–2):123–128.
12. Ishihara H, Connolly AJ, Zeng D, et al. Protease-activated receptor 3 is a second thrombin receptor in humans. Nature 1997; 386(6624):502–506.
13. Kahn ML, Zheng YW, Huang W, et al. A dual thrombin receptor system for platelet activation. Nature 1998; 394(6694):690–694.
14. Xu WF, Andersen H, Whitmore TE, et al. Cloning and characterization of human protease-activated receptor 4. Proc Natl Acad Sci U S A 1998; 95(12):6642–6646.

15. Nystedt S, Emilsson K, Wahlestedt C, et al. Molecular cloning of a potential proteinase activated receptor. Proc Natl Acad Sci U S A 1994; 91(20):9208–9212.

16. Molino M, Barnathan ES, Numerof R, et al. Interactions of mast cell tryptase with thrombin receptors and PAR-2. J Biol Chem 1997; 272(7):4043–4039.

17. Camerer E, Huang W, Coughlin SR. Tissue factor- and factor X-dependent activation of protease-activated receptor 2 by factor VIIa. Proc Natl Acad Sci U S A 2000; 97(10): 5255–5260.

18. Andersen H, Greenberg DL, Fujikawa K, et al. Protease-activated receptor 1 is the primary mediator of thrombin-stimulated platelet procoagulant activity. Proc Natl Acad Sci U S A 1999; 96(20):11189–11193.

19. Ossovskaya VS, Bunnett NW. Protease-activated receptors: contribution to physiology and disease. Physiol Rev 2004; 84(2):579–621.

20. Ramstrom S, Oberg KV, Akerstrom F, et al. Platelet PAR1 receptor density–correlation to platelet activation response and changes in exposure after platelet activation. Thromb Res 2008; 121(5):681–688.

21. Jacques SL, LeMasurier M, Sheridan PJ, et al. Substrate-assisted catalysis of the PAR1 thrombin receptor. Enhancement of macromolecular association and cleavage. J Biol Chem 2000; 275(52):40671–40678.

22. Macfarlane SR, Seatter MJ, Kanke T, et al. Proteinase-activated receptors. Pharmacol Rev 2001; 53(2):245–282.

23. Jacques SL, Kuliopulos A. Protease-activated receptor-4 uses dual prolines and an anionic retention motif for thrombin recognition and cleavage. Biochem J 2003; 376(pt 3):733–740.

24. Folts JD, Schafer AI, Loscalzo J, et al. A perspective on the potential problems with aspirin as an antithrombotic agent: a comparison of studies in an animal model with clinical trials. J Am Coll Cardiol 1999; 33(2):295–303.

25. Molino M, Blanchard N, Belmonte E, et al. Proteolysis of the human platelet and endothelial cell thrombin receptor by neutrophil-derived cathepsin G. J Biol Chem 1995; 270(19): 11168–11175.

26. Chen J, Ishii M, Wang L, et al. Thrombin receptor activation. Confirmation of the intramolecular tethered liganding hypothesis and discovery of an alternative intermolecular liganding mode. J Biol Chem 1994; 269(23):16041–16045.

27. Steinberg SF. The cardiovascular actions of protease-activated receptors. Mol Pharmacol 2005; 67(1):2–11.

28. Major CD, Santulli RJ, Derian CK, et al. Extracellular mediators in atherosclerosis and thrombosis: lessons from thrombin receptor knockout mice. Arterioscler Thromb Vasc Biol 2003; 23(6):931–939.

29. Andrade-Gordon P, Derian CK, Maryanoff BE, et al. Administration of a potent antagonist of protease-activated receptor-1 (PAR-1) attenuates vascular restenosis following balloon angioplasty in rats. J Pharmacol Exp Ther 2001; 298(1):34–42.

30. Vogel SM, Gao X, Mehta D, et al. Abrogation of thrombin-induced increase in pulmonary microvascular permeability in PAR-1 knockout mice. Physiol Genomics 2000; 4(2):137–145.

31. Derian CK, Damiano BP, Addo MF, et al. Blockade of the thrombin receptor protease-activated receptor-1 with a small-molecule antagonist prevents thrombus formation and vascular occlusion in nonhuman primates. J Pharmacol Exp Ther 2003; 304(2):855–861.

32. Damiano BP, Derian CK, Maryanoff BE, et al. RWJ-58259: a selective antagonist of protease activated receptor-1. Cardiovasc Drug Rev 2003; 21(4):313–326.

33. Cook JJ, Sitko GR, Bednar B, et al. An antibody against the exosite of the cloned thrombin receptor inhibits experimental arterial thrombosis in the African green monkey. Circulation 1995; 91(12):2961–2971.

34. Strande JL, Hsu A, Su J, et al. SCH 79797, a selective PAR1 antagonist, limits myocardial ischemia/reperfusion injury in rat hearts. Basic Res Cardiol 2007; 102(4):350–358.

35. Kosoglou T, Reyderman L, Fales RR, et al. Pharmacodynamics and pharmacokinetics of a novel protease-activated receptor (PAR-1) antagonist SCH 530348. Presented at: American Heart Association, Scientific Sessions; November 13–15, 2005; Dallas, Texas.

36. FDA Grants Fast Track Designation to Schering-Plough for its Thrombin Receptor Antagonist SCH 530348. 2006. Accessed at http://www.schering-plough.com/schering_plough/news/release.jsp?releaseID=844816.

37. Moliterno D. A Multicenter, randomized, double-blind, placebo-controlled study to evaluate the safety of SCH 530348 in subjects undergoing non-urgent percutaneous coronary intervention (TRA-PCI). In: ACC. New Orleans, LA; 2007.

38. Trial to Assess the Effects of SCH 530348 in Preventing Heart Attack and Stroke in Patients With Acute Coronary Syndrome (TRA●CER) 2007. Accessed Feb 8th 2008, at http://clinicaltrials.gov/ct2/show/NCT00527943?term=sch+530348&rank=1.

39. Trial to Assess the Effects of SCH 530348 in Preventing Heart Attack and Stroke in Patients With Acute Coronary Syndrome (TRA●CER) (Study P04736). 2008. Accessed March 3, 2008, at http://clinicaltrials.gov/ct2/show/NCT00527943?term=sch+530348&rank=1.

40. Trial to Assess the Effects of SCH 530348 in Preventing Heart Attack and Stroke in Patients With Atherosclerosis (TRA 2°P - TIMI 50). Schering-Plough, 2007. Accessed Feb 8th 2008, at http://clinicaltrials.gov/ct2/show/NCT00526474?term=sch+530348&rank=2.

41. Kai Y, Hirano K, Maeda Y, et al. Prevention of the hypercontractile response to thrombin by proteinase-activated receptor-1 antagonist in subarachnoid hemorrhage. Stroke 2007; 38(12): 3259–3565.

42. Takeuchi M. Pharmacodynamics and safety of a novel Protease Activated Receptor-1 antagonist E5555 for healthy volunteers. In: ESC Congress. Vienna, Austia, 2007.

43. Safety and Tolerability of E5555 and Its Effects on Markers of Intravascular Inflammation in Subjects with Coronary Artery Disease 2007. Accessed Feb 8th, 2008, at http://clinicaltrials.gov/ct2/show/NCT00312052?term=e5555&rank=3.

44. Safety and Tolerability of E5555 and Its Effects on Markers of Intravascular Inflammation in Subjects With Acute Coronary Syndrome. 2007. Accessed Feb 8th, 2008, at http://clinicaltrials.gov/ct2/show/NCT00548587?term=e5555&rank=2.

45. Ferraris VA, Ferraris SP, Singh A, et al. The platelet thrombin receptor and postoperative bleeding. Ann Thorac Surg 1998; 65(2):352–358.

46. Poullis M, Manning R, Laffan M, et al. The antithrombotic effect of aprotinin: actions mediated via the proteaseactivated receptor 1. J Thorac Cardiovasc Surg 2000; 120(2):370–378.

47. Shinfeld A, Zippel D, Lavee J, et al. Aprotinin improves hemostasis after cardiopulmonary bypass better than single-donor platelet concentrate. Ann Thorac Surg 1995; 59(4):872–876.

48. van der Linden J, Lindvall G, Sartipy U. Aprotinin decreases postoperative bleeding and number of transfusions in patients on clopidogrel undergoing coronary artery bypass graft surgery: a double-blind, placebo-controlled, randomized clinical trial. Circulation 2005; 112(9 suppl): I276–I280.

49. Sedrakyan A, Treasure T, Elefteriades JA. Effect of aprotinin on clinical outcomes in coronary artery bypass graft surgery: a systematic review and meta-analysis of randomized clinical trials. J Thorac Cardiovasc Surg 2004; 128(3):442–448.

50. Harmon DC, Ghori KG, Eustace NP, et al. Aprotinin decreases the incidence of cognitive deficit following CABG and cardiopulmonary bypass: a pilot randomized controlled study. Can J Anaesth 2004; 51(10):1002–1009.

51. Spiess BD, Royston D, Levy JH, et al. Platelet transfusions during coronary artery bypass graft surgery are associated with serious adverse outcomes. Transfusion 2004; 44(8):1143–1148.

52. Blood conservation using Antifibrinolytics: a Randomized Trial in a cardiac surgery population [BART (Center for Drug Evaluation and Research. Early communication about an ongoing safety review: aprotinin injection (marketed as Trasylol)]. Beltsville, MD: Food and Drug Administration, 2007.

53. Sundt TM 3rd, Bamer HB, Camillo CJ. Renal dysfunction and intravascular coagulation with aprotinin and hypothermic circulatory arrest. Ann Thorac Surg 1993; 55(6):1418–1424.

54. Schneeweiss S, Seeger JD, Landon J. Aprotinin during coronary-artery bypass grafting and risk of death. N Engl J Med 2008; 358(8):771–783.

55. Mannucci PM, Levi M. Prevention and treatment of major blood loss. N Engl J Med 2007; 356(22): 2301–2311.

56. Henry DA, Carless PA, Moxey AJ, et al., Anti-fibrinolytic use for minimising perioperative allogeneic blood transfusion. Cochrane Database Syst Rev, 2007(4):CD001886.

57. Libby P. Perplexity of plaque proteinases. Arterioscler Thromb Vasc Biol 2006; 26(10): 2181–2182.

58. van der Wal AC, Piek JJ, de Boer OJ, et al. Recent activation of the plaque immune response in coronary lesions underlying acute coronary syndromes. Heart 1998; 80(1):14–18.

59. Nikkari ST, O'Brien KD, Ferguson M, et al. Interstitial collagenase (MMP-1) expression in human carotid atherosclerosis. Circulation 1995; 92(6):1393–1398.

60. Lee RT, Schoen FJ, Loree HM, et al. Circumferential stress and matrix metalloproteinase 1 in human coronary atherosclerosis. Implications for plaque rupture. Arterioscler Thromb Vasc Biol 1996; 16(8):1070–1073.

61. Boire A, Covic L, Agarwal A, et al. PAR1 is a matrix metalloprotease-1 receptor that promotes invasion and tumorigenesis of breast cancer cells. Cell 2005; 120(3):303–313.

62. Ma L, Perini R, McKnight W, et al. Proteinase-activated receptors 1 and 4 counter-regulate endostatin and VEGF release from human platelets. Proc Natl Acad Sci U S A 2005; 102(1): 216–220.

63. Ku DD, Dai J. Expression of thrombin receptors in human atherosclerotic coronary arteries leads to an exaggerated vasoconstrictory response in vitro. J Cardiovasc Pharmacol 1997; 30(5): 649–657.

64. Damiano BP, Mitchell JA, Cheung WM, et al. Activation of vascular thrombin receptors mediates cardiac response to alpha-thrombin in isolated, perfused guinea pig heart. Am J Physiol 1996; 270(5 pt 2):H1585–H1596.

65. Antonaccio MJ, Normandin D. Role of Ca2+ in the vascular contraction caused by a thrombin receptor activating peptide. Eur J Pharmacol 1994; 256(1):37–44.

66. Tsopanoglou NE, Maragoudakis ME. On the mechanism of thrombin-induced angiogenesis. Potentiation of vascular endothelial growth factor activity on endothelial cells by up-regulation of its receptors. J Biol Chem 1999; 274(34):23969–23976.

67. Cheung WM, D'Andrea MR, Andrade-Gordon P, et al. Altered vascular injury responses in mice deficient in protease-activated receptor-1. Arterioscler Thromb Vasc Biol 1999; 19(12): 3014–3024.

68. Jacobsen AN, Du XJ, Lambert KA, et al. Arrhythmogenic action of thrombin during myocardial reperfusion via release of inositol 1,4,5-triphosphate. Circulation 1996; 93(1):23–26.

69. Yasutake M, Haworth RS, King A, et al. Thrombin activates the sarcolemmal Na(+)−H+ exchanger. Evidence for a receptor-mediated mechanism involving protein kinase C. Circ Res 1996; 79(4):705–715.

70. Sabri A, Muske G, Zhang H, et al. Signaling properties and functions of two distinct cardiomyocyte protease-activated receptors. Circ Res 2000; 86(10):1054–1061.

71. Sabri A, Short J, Guo J, et al. Protease-activated receptor-1-mediated DNA synthesis in cardiac fibroblast is via epidermal growth factor receptor transactivation: distinct PAR-1 signaling pathways in cardiac fibroblasts and cardiomyocytes. Circ Res 2002; 91(6):532–539.

31

Other Antiplatelet Agents

Catherine McGorrian
Department of Medicine, McMaster University, Hamilton, Ontario, Canada

Sonia S. Anand
CIHR and Department of Medicine, McMaster University, Hamilton,
Ontario, Canada

INTRODUCTION

This chapter aims to address the pharmacological features and the clinical and therapeutic uses of those antiplatelet agents not mentioned in detail elsewhere in this text. Specifically, we will examine the (*i*) cyclooxygenase (COX)-inhibitor group, (*ii*) the phosphodiesterase-inhibitor group, and (*iii*) other agents such as disintegrins and piracetam.

PART 1. COX INHIBITORS

Overview of Pharmacological Actions

COX is an enzyme, which regulates the conversion of arachidonic acid to various prostaglandins via its two catalytic sites and the subsequent action of various synthases. Prostaglandins are one of the primary mediators of inflammation, causing fever and pain. The COX enzyme has two isoforms, COX-1 and COX-2 (1). In conjunction with thromboxane synthase, COX-1 produces thromboxane A_2 (TXA_2) in platelets, which then in turn triggers platelet aggregation and clotting. Elsewhere, in the vascular endothelium, COX-1 produces the antithrombogenic agent prostacyclin; and in the gastric mucosa, COX-1 is responsible for producing cytoprotective prostaglandins. COX-2 closely resembles COX-1, but has a larger active catalytic site, allowing the more bulky COX-2 selective agents to selectively target this isomer. COX-1 is expressed in resting cells, whereas COX-2 appears to be induced by inflammatory states, or in response to various mitogenic factors and cytokines, making it a clear target for anti-inflammatory agents.

Aspirin and similar drugs exert their antithrombotic effect by inhibition of COX enzymes (2), and they vary in their specificity for the two isomers. Aspirin, or acetyl salicylic acid, causes irreversible inhibition of both COX-1 (via acetylation of serine-530)

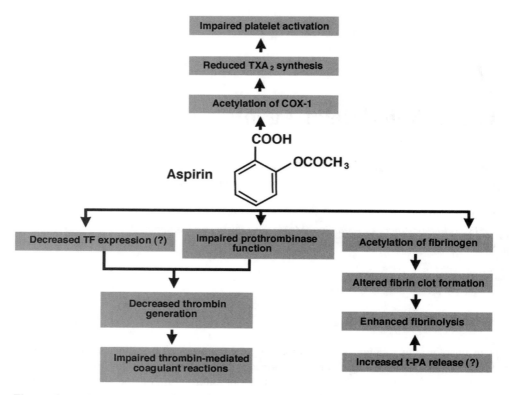

Figure 1 Antithrombotic effects of aspirin. *Source*: From Ref. 5.

and to a lesser extent COX-2 (where prostaglandin production is not fully suppressed because of the larger binding site, unless higher doses of aspirin are used). It was thought that platelets only express COX-1 proteins; however, newly formed platelets have been found also to have small amounts of COX-2 (3). A small dose of aspirin will irreversibly block platelet TXA_2 synthesis and therefore reduce platelet aggregation and clotting, although platelets may still aggregate in the presence of strong agonists such as collagen or thrombin released in response to vascular endothelial injury (4). Aspirin also has other non-COX inhibition-related effects on thrombosis, reducing thrombin generation either through decreased tissue factor production or impaired platelet function; and increasing clot permeability through changes in fibrin structure (5) (Fig. 1).

Indobufen (Ibustrin[TM], Farmitalia-Carlo Erba, Milan, Italy) is an isoindolinyl phenyl-butyric acid derivative, which is a potent COX-1 inhibitor and which causes reversible inhibition of platelet TXA_2 It reduces platelet aggregation maximally at 2 hours' post-administration of a 200 mg oral dose, with aggregation returning to normal at 24 hours, except in persons who had taken a higher (400 mg) dose (6). Indobufen has also been found to improve red cell deformability in a very small study ($n = 14$) of persons with obstructive vascular disease (7).

Triflusal is structurally similar to aspirin, but is not derived from the salicylate group. Its active metabolite, 2-hydroxy-4-trifluoromethyl benzoic acid, is an inhibitor of platelet COX-1, and triflusal also inhibits calcium-dependent platelet aggregation through inhibition of cyclic adenosine and guanosine monophosphate (cAMP and cGMP) (8). Triflusal, however, has little inhibitory effect on endothelial prostacyclin production (9). Triflusal has also been shown to increase nitric oxide production in healthy volunteers, and there is interest in its use in potentiating cognitive function in persons with Alzheimer's disease who have suffered a stroke (10).

Table 1 Overview of the COX-Inhibitor Group of Antiplatelet Agents

Agent	Method of Administration	Primary Method of Antithrombotic Action	Half-life	Clinical Uses
Aspirin	Oral	Irreversible inhibition of platelet TXA_2, through its effects on platelet COX-1 and COX-2.	2–3 hr	Primary prevention of cardiovascular events. Secondary prevention in CAD, CBVD, and PAD.
Indobufen	Oral	Reversible inhibition of platelet TXA_2, through its effects on COX-1.	7–8 hr	May be an alternative to aspirin in post-CABG patients. More data required.
Triflusal	Oral	Inhibition of platelet COX-1, cAMP, and cGMP.	1 hr (half-life of the active metabolite is 35 hr)	Similar efficacy to aspirin demonstrated in secondary prevention of noncardioembolic stroke. In combination with oral anticoagulants, it may reduce stroke risk in patients with cardioembolic stroke. Non-inferior to aspirin in secondary prevention of MI and in high-risk CVD patients. More data needed on efficacy compared with combination antithrombotic therapies.
Dipyrone	Oral/parenteral/rectal	Reversible inhibition of COX-1 and COX-2.	2.5–4.5 hr	No role in secondary prevention at present.

Abbreviations: COX, cyclooxygenase; TXA_2, thromboxane A_2; PAD, peripheral arterial disease; CABG, coronary artery bypass graft; MI, myocardial infarction; CAD, coronary artery disease; CBVD, cerebrovascular disease; PAD, peripheral arterial disease

Dipyrone is a potent analgesic agent, which also reversibly inhibits COX-1 and COX-2, either by oxidizing radical donors or sequestering activating peroxidases, and thus blocking the initiation of COX-mediated prostaglandin production (11). Indobufen, triflusal, and dipyrone are not currently available in the United States (Table 1).

Clinical and Therapeutic Uses

Aspirin
Since aspirin has been discussed in other chapters in this textbook, we will not further outline the clinical uses of aspirin in this chapter.

Indobufen

Indobufen is a platelet aggregation inhibitor that has been used to treat or prevent various thromboembolic disorders. The cardiovascular conditions in which indobufen has been most widely studied include secondary prevention in patients with cerebrovascular disease and atrial fibrillation, coronary artery bypass graft (CABG) patency, and peripheral arterial disease (PAD). However, for the most part these trials have been small and indobufen has not become commonly used in clinical practice.

In patients with atrial fibrillation, indobufen has been compared with both placebo and warfarin in the primary prevention of stroke. In a study by Fornaro et al. (12), 196 patients with cardiac risk factors for stroke (90 of whom had nonrheumatic atrial fibrillation) were randomized to either placebo or indobufen 100 mg twice daily, in a double-blind manner. Mean follow-up was 28 months. Indobufen was found to significantly reduce the primary endpoint of stroke, transient ischemic attack (TIA), embolic events, and fatal myocardial infarction (MI) [incidence 6/98 (6.1%) in the indobufen group vs. 17/98 (17.3%) in the placebo group; RR = 0.35, 95% confidence interval (CI) 0.14–0.89, $p < 0.05$] (12). The SIFA (Studio Italiano Fibrillazione Atriale) study (13) compared indobufen 100 to 200 mg twice daily with warfarin (target INR 2.0–3.5) in a prospective, randomized, open-label trial of over 12 months of treatment in 916 patients with nonrheumatic atrial fibrillation and a recent stroke or TIA (within 15 days). There was no difference between the two groups in the primary endpoint of vascular death, nonfatal stroke, or MI or embolism (incidence 10.6% in the indobufen group, 95% CI 7.7–13.5%; and 9.0% in the warfarin group, 95% CI 6.3–11.8%), with no difference noted between the Kaplan–Meier survival curves for both groups (Fig. 2).

In patients who have undergone CABG surgery, Rajah et al. (14) compared indobufen 200 mg twice daily with aspirin 300 mg plus dipyridamole 75 mg three times

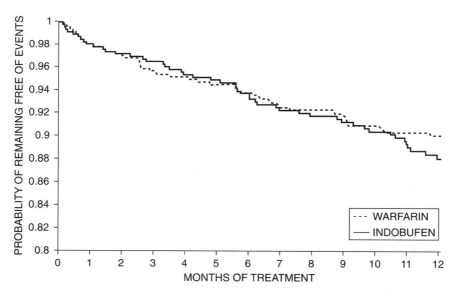

Figure 2 From the SIFA study. Survival curves for the primary outcome of vascular death, nonfatal stroke, nonfatal myocardial infarction, and nonfatal systemic or pulmonary embolism for an intention-to-treat analysis of warfarin versus indobufen. Log-rank test for the difference between the curves was $x^2 = 0.52$; $p = 0.47$. *Abbreviation*: SIFA, Studio Italiano Fibrillazione Atriale. *Source*: From Ref. 13.

daily, in 803 patients receiving saphenous vein CABGs in a prospective, randomized, double-blind study. Scheduled coronary angiography was performed on 552 patients at 12 months postsurgery. There was no significant difference in graft patency, total mortality, or recurrence of angina between the two groups. A similar study from the SINBA (Studio Indobufone nel Bypass Aortocoronarico) group also found no difference in early and one-year-graft patency between aspirin 325 mg plus dipyridamole 75 mg three times daily and indobufen 200 mg twice daily. Unfortunately, the dose of aspirin used is now nonstandard, but this was a recommended dose in use at the time the study was designed. Nevertheless, these results suggest that indobufen may remain an acceptable alternative to aspirin, although greater efficacy than aspirin has not been demonstrated (15).

The efficacy of indobufen in PAD is not well established. One randomised controlled trial (RCT) examined the efficacy of indobufen 400 mg versus aspirin 900 mg plus dipyridamole 225 mg in maintaining graft patency in 111 patients post-femoropopliteal bypass (16). A nonsignificant improvement in graft patency was noted in the indobufen group at 3 months, but the improvement was attenuated as follow-up extended to 12 months. Other RCTs have compared indobufen with placebo in patients with intermittent claudication and found significant improvements in walking distances achieved. In a blinded study of 302 patients with intermittent claudication (17), participants were randomized to either indobufen 200 mg twice daily or placebo for a period of six months. In that time, both initial claudication distance (ICD) and absolute claudication distance (ACD) improved, with ICD in the active therapy group improving from 137.9 (standard deviation or SD 68.2) to 227.9 m (SD 174.4), compared a change of 136.6 m (SD 63.2) to 153.1 m (SD 86.8) in the placebo group ($p < 0.01$). Signorini et al. (18) performed a similar unblinded RCT with a smaller sample size ($n = 52$). Again, significant improvements were noted in the ACD. However, the unblinded nature of the study makes the interpretability of these results questionable, and there is no evidence that indobufen is preferable to other antiplatelet agents in the current use in these conditions.

Finally, indobufen was examined in 1632 high-risk vascular disease patients (19) in the unblinded TISS (Ticlodipine Indobufen Stroke Study). Investigators compared indobufen 200 to 400 mg daily with ticlodipine 250 to 500 mg daily. The primary endpoint of nonfatal stroke, nonfatal MI, or vascular death was twice as common in the indobufen group as in the ticlodipine group [47 (5.8%) vs. 24 (2.9%)].

In summary, indobufen is a potent COX-1 inhibitor, with a reasonable side-effect profile. Although it may represent an alternative to aspirin in CABG patients, insufficient evidence has accrued to date to confirm this. Furthermore, evidence of greater efficacy over current standard therapy across a variety of vascular conditions has not been established.

Triflusal

Triflusal has been investigated in a number of cardiovascular conditions, including cerebrovascular diseases, atrial fibrillation, and acute coronary syndromes, in CABG and PAD patients.

Triflusal has been compared with aspirin in patients with stroke in two studies. TAPIRSS (Triflusal versus Aspirin for Prevention of Infarction: a Randomized Stroke Study) (20) randomized 431 patients who had had a recent stroke or TIA to either triflusal 600 mg or aspirin 325 mg daily. Over 586 days of follow-up, there was no significant difference between the groups in the primary endpoint of vascular death, nonfatal ischemic stroke, nonfatal acute MI, or major bleeding [30 events in the aspirin group (13.9%) vs. 27 events in the triflusal group (12.7%); odds ratio (OR) = 1.11, 95% CI 0.64–1.94]. However, there were significantly more major hemorrhage events in the aspirin group [7 (3.2%) vs.

1 (0.5%), OR = 7.10, 95% CI 1.15–43.5]. The TACIP (Triflusal versus Aspirin in Cerebral Infarction Prevention) study (21) followed a similar methodology in 2113 patients over 30.1 months of follow-up, although their primary endpoint did not include bleeding events. Again, there was no significant difference between aspirin and triflusal for the primary endpoint [incidence 138/1055 (13.1%) in the triflusal group vs. 130/1052 (12.4) in the aspirin group; hazard ratio (HR) 1.09, 95% CI 0.85–1.38], although the incidence of major bleeding was significantly higher in the aspirin group [HR for the triflusal group 0.48, 95% CI 0.28–0.82]. The efficacy of triflusal compared with a lower dose of aspirin, such as 75 to 150 mg (22), or to ASA/diyridamole combination, has not yet been assessed.

Triflusal, with and without oral anticoagulation, was compared with oral anticoagulation alone in patients with atrial fibrillation to prevent stroke in the NASPEAF (National Study for Prevention of Embolism in Atrial Fibrillation) (23) trial. This study randomized 1209 patients with atrial fibrillation and other risk factors for stroke to either triflusal 600 mg OD, acenecoumarol (target INR 2–3), or combination of triflusal and acenecoumarol (target INR 1.25–2). Patients were stratified by risk, and the higher-risk patients were randomized to either acenecoumarol or combined therapy, but not to triflusal alone. Even in the intermediate-risk group, triflusal was associated with higher rates of nonfatal stroke and TIA than the acenecoumarol groups over three years of follow-up, although bleeding was less with triflusal. For both risk groups, incidence of the primary outcome of stroke, systemic embolism, TIA, or vascular death was less in the combination group than in the acenecoumarol-only group (HR in the intermediate risk group 0.33, $p = 0.02$; and in the high risk group 0.51, $p = 0.03$) with no significant difference in bleeding between the two groups. Thus, triflusal alone does not have sufficient efficacy in stroke prevention in patients with atrial fibrillation; however it may have a role in combination with an oral anticoagulant.

Triflusal's role in acute coronary syndromes and MI has been examined in only relatively small RCTs. A 1993 study from the GEAIT (Grupo de Estudio del Triflusal en la Angina Inestable) (24) compared triflusal (300 mg three times daily) with placebo in 281 patients with unstable angina and reported a significant decrease in nonfatal MI with triflusal at six months (incidence of 4.2% in the triflusal group vs. 12.3% in the placebo group, $p = 0.013$). Further, in the TIM (Triflusal in Myocardial Infarction) trial, an RCT of 2275 patients with acute MI (25), triflusal 600 mg was non-inferior to aspirin 300 mg with respect to the primary outcome of death, nonfatal MI, and nonfatal cerebrovascular events at 35 days, and demonstrated a nonsignificant trend toward fewer bleeding events. However, further adequately powered trials would be needed to confirm this.

There is also evidence that triflusal may be an acceptable alternative to oral anticoagulation in patients with prosthetic valves. TRAC (Triflusal versus Anticoagulant in bioprosthetic valve replacement), a pilot trial by Aramendi et al. (26) randomized 193 persons with post-bioprosthetic aortic or mitral valve replacement to either triflusal 600 mg daily or acenecoumarol, target INR 2 to 3, for three months postsurgery. No difference was noted between the two groups for the primary endpoint of first episode of thromboembolism, treatment-related hemorrhage or valve-related death (HR 1.07, $p = 0.88$). Ten persons on acenecoumarol (10%) had bleeding-related complications, compared with three (3.1%) in the triflusal group. Another study randomized 209 patients undergoing CABG to either triflusal 300 mg plus dipyridamole 75 mg three times daily, aspirin 50 mg plus dipyridamole 75 mg three times daily, or placebo for six months post-saphenous vein CABG. The study was double blinded, and coronary angiograms were performed at nine days and six months postoperatively. Although there were no differences between the groups at nine days; at six months, there were trends toward fewer graft occlusions in the triflusal group than in the placebo or aspirin groups (27).

Triflusal has also been evaluated in a small RCT of 117 patients with symptomatic PAD, who were randomized to triflusal 300 mg twice daily or placebo, in which it was noted that at 24 weeks, an improvement in walking distance from baseline of at least 40% was seen in 63.6% of patients in the triflusal group, compared with 22.5% in the control group (28).

Costa et al. (29) published a Cochrane meta-analysis of triflusal in the prevention of secondary vascular events in high-risk patients, with a primary outcome of vascular death, nonfatal MI, or nonfatal stroke. Data from seven studies were included; five compared aspirin with triflusal and two compared placebo with triflusal. There was no difference in the primary outcome for the aspirin versus triflusal comparison (OR 1.04, 95% CI 0.87–1.23). The placebo versus triflusal comparison was estimated from the data of the GEAIT (24) only, and showed an increase in the primary endpoint with the placebo group (OR 2.29, 95% CI 1.01–1.23). Triflusal had significantly lower rates of hemorrhage than aspirin (incidence of any hemorrhage 336/2518 in the aspirin group vs. 212/2506 in the triflusal group, Peto OR 1.73, 95% CI 1.44–2.08, $p < 0.0001$), but more nonhemorrhagic gastrointestinal side effects (incidence of hemorrhage 1048/2611 in the aspirin group vs. 1142/2596 in the triflusal group, Peto OR 0.84, 95% CI 0.75–0.95, $p = 0.04$).

In summary, triflusal may well have a potential role as an alternative to aspirin in secondary prevention of vascular events, as it appears to be effective and reasonably safe. However, the wealth of data supporting the efficacy of aspirin means that it must remain first preference at present. In addition, triflusal has not been studied widely in the context of multiple contemporary antithrombotic and adjunctive therapies, thus the above safety and efficacy cannot be inferred to apply to the current practice. Furthermore, triflusal is not available in many countries, including North America.

Dipyrone

Dipyrone is better known as an analgesic agent than as an antiplatelet agent and is used in postoperative states and in treatment of migraine. One nonrandomized trial examined platelet aggregation in 48 patients within three days of the onset of acute MI, 36 of whom were given dipyrone. The patients who did not receive dipyrone demonstrated increased platelet aggregation (30). However, no randomized controlled trials of the efficacy of dipyrone in cardiovascular prevention could be found on searches of Medline, Embase, and the Controlled trials register of the Cochrane database.

PART 2. PHOSPHODIESTERASE INHIBITORS

Overview of Pharmacological Actions

The group of antiplatelet agents, which primarily exert their actions through phosphodiesterase inhibition, includes dipyridamole, which was developed in the late 1950s, and cilostazol. Dipyridamole is a pyrimidopyrimidine derivative, which acts to increase intraplatelet cyclic nucleotides, namely cAMP and cGMP, via inhibition of the respective phosphodiesterases and inhibition of the cell membrane adenosine transporter, which is present on erythrocytes and endothelial cells. Inhibition of this transporter leads to increased levels of plasma adenosine, which in turn causes smooth muscle cell relaxation and vasodilatation (31). Meanwhile, increasing cGMP potentiates the actions of nitric oxide, and increases cAMP increases prostacyclin production, reducing platelet aggregation.

One side effect of the adenosine-mediated vasodilatation has, however, been the phenomenon of "coronary steal," where intravenous doses of dipyridamole have been seen to precipitate hypotension and angina chest pain. This phenomenon is used to advantage in cardiac imaging studies such as thallium scans, but may have decreased the clinical usage of dipyridamole because of the fear of causing worsening angina. However, this steal phenomenon is much less common in oral dosages and has not been noted as a side effect in recent trials (32). A newer preparation of extended release (ER) dypyridamole–aspirin combination has not been observed to result in coronary steal has been shown in the ESPS (European Stroke Prevention Study)-2 trial (33) to be superior to aspirin alone in the secondary prevention of ischemic stroke.

Cilostazol (Pletal^{TM}, Otsuka America Pharmaceutical, Inc., Japan) is a selective cAMP phosphodietserase-III inhibitor. It is currently licensed for the treatment of intermittent claudication, although there has also been limited evaluation of cilostozal among patients with post-percutaneous coronary intervention (PCI) restenosis (Table 2).

Table 2 Overview of the Phosphodiesterase-Inhibitor Group of Antiplatelet Agents

Agent	Method of Administration	Primary Method of Antithrombotic Action	T1/2	Clinical Uses
Dipyridamole	Oral/parenteral	Elevates plasma adenosine, potentiates nitric oxide actions, and increases prostacyclin production.	13 hr	Used in nuclear imaging studies. In a modified release preparation, it is recommended in combination with aspirin for secondary prevention in stroke patients.
Cilostazol	Oral	Potent cyclic nucleotide phosphodiesterase III inhibitor, with weak vasodilatation and antiplatelet effects.	11–13 hr	Increases walking distances in patients with intermittent claudication. May reduce in-stent restenosis in postcoronary stenting patients, in combination with aspirin and clopidogrel.
Trapidil	Oral/parenteral	Inhibition of phosphodiesterases, causing vasodilatation. Inhibition of thromboxane A_2 and platelet-derived growth factor.	1–2 hr	May reduce angina pectoris in post-MI patients. Non-inferior to nitrates in the prevention of angina. No clear role in the prevention of in-stent restenosis in postcoronary stenting patients.

Dipyridamole

The clinical uses of dipyridamole have been a source of debate, and reviews have previously questioned its usefulness in cardiovascular therapy (34). Dipyridamole is a useful agent in stress nuclear cardiology, where it is used to provoke an ischemic response, which can then be visualized by radioisotope uptake. Intravenous dipyridamole has also been noted to improved tolerance of balloon-related ischemia (both by symptoms and by ST-segment excursion), when delivered at the time of balloon inflation in percutaneous angioplasty studies (35). However, a new role for dipyridamole in the secondary prevention of ischemic stroke has been identified by the publications of the ESPS-2 (33) and ESPRIT (European/Australian Stroke Prevention in Reversible Ischemia Trial) (36) studies, and of various meta-analyses since then.

Dipyridamole was initially used as an anti-anginal agent. Sacks et al. (37) published a meta-analysis of 11 double-blind, placebo-controlled trials of dipyridamole (doses varying from 37.5 to 224 mg/day) in angina pectoris from 1966 to 1987, and reported an OR for reduced frequency of angina with dipyridamole of 0.29 (95% CI 0.19–0.43, $p < 0.01$). However, most of the trials were of relatively short duration (2 weeks–6 months). It has been suggested that some of the anti-anginal ability of dipyridamole may be due to an increase in endothelial cell proliferation, and therefore promotion of the growth of collateral vessels (38); but more recent studies by Barbour et al. (39) and Tsuya et al. (40) have not demonstrated a consistent benefit with dipyridamole as an anti-anginal agent, although again, these were trials with small samples ($n = 15$ and 18, respectively) and short durations of treatment (1–2 week, respectively). The 2001 PISA (Persantin in Stable Angina) study (41,42) randomized 400 patients with chronic stable angina to dipyridamole 200 mg twice daily versus placebo for 24 weeks, in combination with usual anti-anginal therapy, including aspirin. There was no significant decrease in adverse events in the active therapy group, and a small increase in exercise tolerance was attributed to baseline differences between the groups. Furthermore, there is no evidence to recommend the use of dipyridamole in the emergency treatment of acute coronary syndromes (43).

The use of dipyridamole in patients post-CABG has been examined in a number of studies. Cheesebro (44) randomized patients undergoing CABG to either placebo or aspirin plus dipyridamole and found that the combination therapy group had lower rates of graft occlusions to 12 months of follow-up. However, Van der Meer et al. in the CABADAS (Prevention of Coronary Artery Bypass graft occlusion by Aspirin, Dipyridamole and Acenocoumarol/Phenprocoumon Study) study (45) compared aspirin (50 mg daily), aspirin plus dipyridamole (200 mg twice daily), and oral anticoagulants (target INR 2.8–4.8) in 912 patients undergoing CABG and found only a trend to decreased graft occlusion in the aspirin plus dipyridamole group and a trend to a higher clinical event rate in this combination group. Similarly, Goldman et al. (46) in the Veterans Affairs study in 1988 found a benefit in post-CABG saphenous graft patency with aspirin-based regimens, but the role of dipyridamole, which was included in one of the aspirin groups, was not clear. On the basis of these studies, there is insufficient information to make any recommendations on the role of dipyridamole in CABG patients.

Dipyridamole has also been used in the management of patients with prosthetic valves, and a recent Cochrane review summarized the results of 11 trials, which randomized prosthetic valve patients to oral anticoagulants versus oral anticoagulants plus antiplatelet therapy, including 6, which used dipyridamole (47). Oral anticoagulants in conjunction with antiplatelet agents were found to decrease thromboembolic events (OR 0.39, 95% CI 0.28–0.56, $p < 0.001$) and total mortality (OR 0.55, 0.5% CI 0.40–0.77, $p < 0.001$), with a twofold increase in major bleeding. However, the antiplatelet agent of choice was not clearly established, with aspirin 100 mg being no less effective than higher dose of aspirin or dipyridamole, a finding similar to that of the Antiplatelet Trialists' collaboration (48).

It is the role of dipyridamole in cerebrovascular diseases that has attracted the most attention in recent years. While older trials, such as the AICLA (Accidents Ischimiques Cerebraux Lies a l'Atherosclerose) (49) and the Persantine-Aspirin Trial (50) did not show improvements in recurrent stroke or other vascular events with the addition of dipyridamole, the ESPS-1 trial reported that antiplatelet therapy with aspirin 330 mg and dipyridamole 75 mg t.i.d. compared with placebo in 2500 stroke patients decreased recurrent stroke by 38.1% ($p < 0.01$) and all cause mortality by 30.6% ($p < 0.01$) (51). However, there was no aspirin-only arm in this trial.

Subsequent to the ESPS-1, two large-scale trials were undertaken to examine dipyridamole in secondary stroke prevention with a combination of aspirin 25 mg/dipyridamole 200 mg controlled release (Aggrenox™) twice daily: ESPS-2 and ESPRIT. The ESPS-2 (33) trial compared aspirin (50 mg), dipyridamole (400 mg modified release), aspirin and dipyridamole in combination, and placebo, in a randomized, double-blind 2×2 factorial design, in 6602 patients who had suffered a stroke or TIA within the preceding three months. The combination of aspirin and dipyridamole significantly reduced the endpoints of both stroke and stroke and death, when compared with the other regimens. Similarly, ESPRIT (36) randomized 2739 patients with a stroke within the last six months to aspirin (30–325 mg), or aspirin plus dipyridamole (200 mg twice daily). The primary endpoint of death, nonfatal stroke, or MI and major bleeding was significantly lower in the combination therapy group (HR 0.80, 95% CI 0.66–0.98), with an absolute risk reduction of 1% per year of treatment. It is notable that this improvement in clinical outcomes does not seem to come at an increased bleeding risk (52), and it may be that other effects are at play, which may also be attributable to dipyridamole, such as a potential reduction in thrombosis and atherosclerosis due to dipyridamole-induced inhibition of inflammatory gene expression in human platelet-monocyte interactions (53).

A number of surgical trials have compared the effects of dipyridamole and aspirin with control in peripheral bypass graft patency rates, with some trials showing no improvement (54,55) (though with an improvement noted in vascular event rates) (55), and another showing better patency with short-term treatment with aspirin and dipyridamole (56). Hess et al. (57) compared aspirin (330 mg), aspirin (330 mg) and dipyridamole (75 mg), and placebo in 240 patients with PAD, and found that the combination was most efficacious at reducing disease progression as assessed by angiography. However, at baseline the aspirin group had significantly more stenotic lesions than the other two groups. Do and Mahler (58) randomized patients undergoing femoral angioplasty to either oral anticoagulation (target INR 2–3) or aspirin 25 mg and dipyridamole 200 mg twice daily, and reported similar one-year vessel patency rates, and more bleeding side effects in the aspirin/dipyridamole group. At present, given the conflicting data from a small number of modest-sized studies, there seems to be no clear role for dipyridamole alone in PAD.

Given dipyridamole's vasodilatory effects, it could be postulated that it may have an effect as an antihypertensive agent. The ESPS-1 trial noted that antiplatelet therapy with aspirin and dipyridamole had increased efficacy in stroke prevention in those persons with the highest blood pressure (59); however, whether this was attributable to an effect of dipyridamole on hypertension or a postulated hypercoagulable state in the most hypertensive persons could not be ascertained. However, the ESPRIT study did not note any significant difference in blood pressure change between the aspirin and aspirin and dipyridamole groups (60), and there is no role for dipyridamole at present as an antihypertensive agent.

In summary, dipyridamole has "come in from the cold" with its reformulation to a modified release preparation with improved bioavailability, and the subsequent results of the ESPS-2 and ESPRIT trials. The use of combined aspirin and ER dipyridamole in patients with noncardioembolic stroke or TIA is now a class IIa recommendation in the most recent stroke guidelines of the American Heart Association and the American Stroke Association (61). The upcoming PRoFESS (Prevention Regimen for Effectively avoiding Second Strokes) trial (62) will compare aspirin plus dipyridamole with aspirin plus clopidogrel in this subgroup of stroke patients.

In the wider context of secondary prevention of vascular events in patients with any cardiovascular disease, the 2002 Antiplatelet Trialists' collaboration suggested that the combination of aspirin plus dipyridamole was not superior to aspirin alone (48). This was further examined in a Cochrane meta-analysis by De Schryver et al. (63), who included data from 27 studies and 23,019 participants and examined randomized trials of dipyridamole in persons with vascular disease, specifically looking at the endpoints of vascular death and vascular events (including vascular death, death from any unknown cause, nonfatal stroke, or nonfatal MI). They reported that dipyridamole alone was not superior to aspirin in preventing cardiovascular disease (CVD) death or CVD events (relative risk or RR 1.08, 95% CI 0.85–1.37, and RR 1.02, 95% CI 0.88–1.18, respectively). There was a decrease in vascular events with dipyridamole plus aspirin versus aspirin alone (RR 0.87, 95% CI 0.79–0.96), although this was only significant in the trials of patients with cerebrovascular disease. To summarize, dipyridamole has now become an established therapy in the secondary prevention of vascular events in patients with cerebrovascular disease, but has no clear role in the management of other vascular disease patients, and is not recommended as an anti-anginal agent.

Cilostazol

Cilostazol (Pletal^{TM}) is a phosphodiesterase-III inhibitor, which inhibits platelet activation and relaxes vascular smooth muscle. Apart from its role in intermittent claudication, cilostazol has also been evaluated as an adjunctive therapy to prevent stent thrombosis and in-stent restenosis in PCI.

Cilostazol is licensed for use in intermittent claudication in North America. Regensteiner et al. in a 2002 meta-analysis (64) included data from six randomized trials of cilostazol versus control ($n = 1751$) and reported that compared with pentoxifylline and placebo, cilostazol increased maximal treadmill walking, with improvements in the walking impairment questionnaire and also in health-related quality of life. More recently, a Cochrane meta-analysis synthesized data from eight trials and concluded that cilostazol was associated with an improvement in ICD and ACD, with a weighted mean difference in ICD of 31.1 m (95% CI 21.4–40.9 m) with cilostazol (65).

Cilostazol has also been proposed as an alternative to either ticlodipine (66) or clopidogrel (67) in prevention of stent thrombosis and other complications postcoronary stenting, although only short-term efficacy and safety has been evaluated. Furthermore, there is interest in the use of cilostazol as an adjunctive third agent with aspirin and a thienopyridine to reduce in-stent restenosis in coronary stenting. A number of studies have shown that such triple therapy has greater inhibition of adenosine diphospate (ADP)-induced platelet aggregation than usual therapy with aspirin and clopidogrel (68,69). The DECLARE-Long (70) RCT examined this regimen in 500 patients receiving long (≥ 32 mm) drug-eluting coronary stents and reported significant reductions in major adverse cardiovascular events (2.8% vs. 7.6%, $p = 0.016$) and target lesion revascularization (2.8% vs. 6.8%, $p = 0.036$) at six months' follow-up in the triple-therapy group compared with usual therapy. The DECLARE-DIABETES trial (71) randomized 400 diabetic patients receiving drug-eluting stents to either standard double or triple (aspirin, clopidogrel, and cilostazol) therapy and showed that late loss and restenosis were significantly less at six months in the triple-therapy group, with a trend toward lower adverse clinical events also.

In the CREST (cilostazol for restenosis) study (72), 705 patients received usual aspirin, clopidogrel for 30 days, and either cilostazol 100 mg b.i.d. or placebo. The cilostazol group had lower rates of in-stent restenosis at six months' follow-up, with a relative risk reduction of 36% ($p = 0.02$), although there were no significant reductions in clinical endpoints.

A recent meta-analysis of 23 RCTs of cilostazol in coronary stenting showed benefits associated with the cilostazol arms, with reductions in both restenosis (RR = 0.60, 95% CI 0.49–0.73, $p < 0.001$) and in the need for repeat revascularization (RR = 0.69, 95% CI 0.55–0.86, $p = 0.001$). However, the absolute number of events in the trials was small, and additional data are needed from larger-scale RCTs with contemporary therapies (e.g., high-dose, long-term clopidogrel) (73).

Cilostazol is contraindicated in patients with congestive cardiac failure and/or ventricular arrhythmias. Phosphodieserase E3 inhibition is associated with proarrhythmic activity, in such agents as milrinone, although there have been no increase seen in cardiovascular deaths with cilostazol itself (74). Furthermore, a Cochrane review did not show any increase in cardiovascular (CV) events among patients with intermittent claudication randomized to cilostazol (65); however, patients with symptomatic ischemic heart disease or who were already on antiplatelet or anticoagulant therapies were excluded.

In summary, cilostazol is indicated for use in symptomatic intermittent claudication and is also a promising third agent for use in the prevention of in-stent restenosis in coronary PCI.

Trapidil

Trapidil is a triazolopyrimidine, which acts not only as both an inhibitor of TXA_2, stimulating the synthesis and release of prostacylin, but also as an inhibitor of platelet-derived growth factor (PDGF), an enzyme found both in platelets and in vascular endothelial cells, which stimulates the proliferation of the latter cells.

Trapidil was developed as a potential therapeutic agent to prevent in-stent restenosis. Although, earlier studies both in animal models and in the STARC (Studio Trapidil versus Aspirin nella Restenosi Coronarica) trial (75) showed reductions in in-stent restenosis, the 2001 TRAPIST (Trapidil versus Placebo to prevent in-stent intimal hyperplasia) study by Serruys et al. did not replicate this finding in 312 patients undergoing Wallstent implantation who were randomized to trapidil 600 mg daily versus placebo (76). In this trial, concomitant therapy with aspirin, ticlodipine, and heparin were all permitted under study methodology. Trapidil did not reduce in-stent restenosis in TRAPIST, and there was a trend to worse outcomes in the active treatment group. Similar results to this were also seen in a trial, which used Palmaz–Schatz stents (77).

The antiplatelet action of trapidil has also encouraged interest in a potential role in patients with CAD. In JAMIS (Japanese Antiplatelet Myocardial Infarction Study), 723 Japanese patients post-MI were randomized to either aspirin 81 mg daily, trapidil 300 mg daily, or placebo (78). Both antiplatelet agents reduced the recurrence of recurrent MIs when compared with placebo, but this effect was only significant in the aspirin group. However, trapidil was noted to significantly reduce a composite endpoint of CV death, reinfarction, ischemic stroke, and uncontrolled angina pectoris—mostly mediated through its effect on the latter. A more recent non-inferiority study showed similar total exercise time using a bicycle ergonometer and similar weekly incidence of angina, in 648 patients randomized to trapidil 200 mg three times daily versus isosorbide dinitrate 20 mg twice daily for 12 weeks (79). At present, there remains no clear role for the general use of trapidil in management of cardiovascular disease.

PART 3. OTHER AP AGENTS

Disintegrins

Disintegrins are cysteine-rich, small-molecular-weight proteins, which are found in viper venom and have the ability to inhibit platelet aggregation through their binding to adhesion molecules, such as integrin receptors. These molecules have been of interest as antiplatelet agents through their ability to inhibit the $GpII_bIII_a$ receptor on the platelet surface. The $GpII_bIII_a$ receptor promotes platelet aggregation by binding fibrinogen to cause cross-linking between platelets. However, the effects of disintegrins can be unpredictable as most disintegrin agents are not only specific for the $GpII_bIII_a$ receptor but also block all argentine-glycine-aspartic acid (RGD)–dependent integrin receptors, such as those found on von Willebrand factor, fibrinogen, vitronectin, and thrombospondin. They also act as antineoplastic drugs, through the inhibition of integrins on cancer cells.

Synthetic $GpII_b$ III_a inhibitors which have been inspired by venoms include tirofiban (Aggrastat™) and eptifibatide (Integrelin™), which are discussed in another chapter. Other disintegrins include bitistatin, triflavin, piscivostatin, and barbourin. Bitistatin is an 83-amino acid monomeric disintegrin, which was first isolated from the venom of the puff adder. It is a powerful platelet inhibitor, which has been seen to accelerate tissue plasminogen activator (tPA)-induced thrombolysis and reduce rethrombosis in a canine model (80), and which is being investigated as a radiotracer agent to locate areas of thrombosis or embolism (81). Triflavin has been shown to reduce ischemic injury in a rat model of middle cerebral artery thrombosis (82). However, neither model has been assessed in large phase III trials.

Piscivostatin is a novel disintegrin, in that it is a dimeric structure, as opposed to the other agents mentioned, which are monomers. It is derived from the venom of *Agkistrodon piscivorus piscivorus*, and it has been shown to have contradictory effects of both platelet aggregation inhibition and platelet aggregate dissociation (the latter mechanism has not been clearly elucidated at this stage) (83). No clinical role has been established for piscivostatin as of yet. Barbourin is specific for the $GpII_bIII_a$ receptor on platelet membranes, unlike other disintegrins, and therefore has been the focus for the derivation of two new synthetic antiplatelet agents (84): DMP78, which has only been tested in animal models, and eptifibatide (Integrelin™), which is discussed elsewhere in this book.

In summary, the disintegrins are a complex group of compounds, some of which have made their way to clinical use (eptifibatide). However, many other agents remain to be fully evaluated.

Piracetam

Piracetam is a recognized platelet aggregation inhibitor, although its precise mode of action is not fully defined. It is thought to be a nootropic agent—an agent, which can improve cognition through alterations in neurochemicals—and acts in vitro to prevent fibrinogen binding to activated platelets. Other putative methods of action are a beneficial effect on erythrocyte deformability, potentially reducing ADP release from damaged erythrocytes, or even a rheological effect on the circulating blood or on the vessel wall (85). Despite this uncertainty in its actions, piracetam is a drug, which has been in clinical use for many years for such conditions as vertigo and cortical myoclonus, and it has a well-established safety profile (86). Piracetam was assessed in acute stroke in PASS (Piracetam in Acute Stroke Study) (87), a randomized placebo-controlled study in 927 patients within 12 hours of an acute ischemic stroke, in which the treatment group received an intravenous bolus of piracetam, followed by an oral therapy for 12 weeks. Usual care was administered concomitantly, including aspirin at the physician's discretion. The benefit of piracetam in acute stroke is thought to be its ability to increase blood flow to compromised areas of cerebral ischemia and to decrease glucose metabolism in the peri-infarct tissue. However, the groups did not differ on an assessment of functional ability at 12 weeks, with a trend toward higher 12-week mortality in the piracetam group (111/464 vs. 89/463, RR 1.24, 95% CI 0.97–1.59, $p = 0.15$). Subsequent to this, a randomized, double-blind trial was performed of piracetam 1600 mg three times daily versus aspirin 200 mg three times daily in 563 stroke patients, over two years (88). While piracetam was better tolerated than aspirin, the overall efficacy of aspirin in secondary prevention showed a trend toward superiority over piracetam. Only when the patients who were in vitro antiplatelet nonresponders were excluded, could piracetam be seen as non-inferior to aspirin.

In summary, piracetam remains of interest in the treatment of Alzheimer's disease, vertigo, and myoclonus; but it is not currently recommended in the secondary prevention of cardiovascular diseases.

TP Receptor Antagonists

The TXA_2/prostaglandin H2 or TP receptor activates phospholipase C on agonist binding and increases inositol triphosphate, diacylglycerol, and intracellular calcium levels (89). TXA_2 itself is thought to be the most potent agonists of platelet activation, and the effects of aspirin in acute coronary syndromes and others belie its role (90). Agents have been developed to target this receptor, which include GR 32191, BMS-180291 (ifetroban), S-18886 (terutroban), BM 13.177 (sulotroban), and BM-531 (a torasemide derivative). Phase II studies of these trials have been mostly disappointing (89,91), although terutroban has shown promise as an antiplatelet agent in percutaneous stenting in an animal model (92), and BM-531 has shown effective antiplatelet action, but remains to be tested in animal models (93). Ifetroban has been evaluated in animal models of myocardial ischemia, stroke, and hypertension (94), and a single double-blind, placebo-controlled study on healthy men established that it was an effective antagonist of TXA_2-dependent platelet aggregation (95). Terutroban is now undergoing phase III clinical trials in stroke patients, and further trials are awaited on these theoretically appealing agents.

CONCLUSIONS

As the knowledge of targets for antiplatelet action has increased, so too have our options for preventing platelet aggregation at different parts of the aggregation cascade. Clearly, there are a host of antiplatelet agents, which show promise in early studies; however, few have shown superior efficacy or equivalent efficacy and improved safety over the better-established therapies of aspirin and the thienopyridines. It is likely that the newer agents will have a role as adjunctive therapy, such as with ER dypyridamole–aspirin in secondary stroke prevention. In the future, pharmacogenomics may also guide us to identify those persons who will not have an adequate response to aspirin or the thienopyridines and in whom adjunctive therapy with a newer or alternative antiplatelet agent may achieve therapeutic antiplatelet activity. One difficulty is the increase in risk of bleeding as the number and/or potency of the antiplatelet agents used increases. Again, increasing knowledge of which patients are more likely to develop bleeding complications, and advances in pharmacogenomics, may in the future help us tailor our combination of drugs to achieve optimal antiplatelet action with lowest risk for individual patients.

REFERENCES

1. Xie W, Chipman J, Robertson D, et al. Expression of a mitogen-responsive gene encoding prostaglandin synthase is regulated by mRNA splicing. Proc Natl Acad Sci U S A 1991; 88: 2692–2696.
2. Vane JR. Inhibition of prostaglandin synthesis as a mechanism of action for aspirin-like drugs. Nat New Biol 1971; 231:232–235.
3. Weber AA, Zimmermann KC, Meyer-Kirchrath J, et al. Cyclooxygenase-2 in human platelets as a possible factor in aspirin resistance. Lancet 1999; 353:900.
4. McAdam BF, Catella-Lawson F, Mardini IA, et al. Systemic biosynthesis of prostacyclin by cyclooxygenase (COX)-2: the human pharmacology of a selective inhibitor of COX-2. Proc Natl Acad Sci U S A 1999; 96:272–277.
5. Undas A, Brummel-Ziedins KE, Mann KG. Antithrombotic properties of aspirin and resistance to aspirin: beyond strictly antiplatelet actions. Blood 2007; 109:2285–2292.
6. Mannucci L, Colli S, Lavessari M, et al. Indobufen is a potent inhibitor of whole blood aggregation in patients with a high atherosclerotic risk. Thromb Res 1987; 48:417–426.
7. Grasselli S, Guercioloni R, Iadevaia V, et al. In vitro and ex vivo effects of indobufen on red blood cell deformability. Eur J Pharmacol 1987; 32:207–210.
8. Murdoch D, Plosker GL. Triflusal: a review of its use in cerebral infarction and myocardial infarction, and as thromboprophylaxis in atrial fibrillation. Drugs 2006; 66:671–692.
9. De La Cruz JP, Mata JM, De La Cuesta FS. Triflusal vs aspirin on the inhibition of human platelet and vascular cyclooxygenase. Gen Pharmacol: The Vasc Syst 1992; 23:297–300.
10. Whitehead SN, Hachinski VC, Cechetto DF. Interaction between a rat model of cerebral ischemia and beta-amyloid toxicity: inflammatory responses. Stroke 2005; 36:107–112.
11. Pierre SC, Schmidt R, Brenneis C, et al. Inhibition of cyclooxygenases by dipyrone. Br J Pharmacol 2007; 151:494–503.
12. Fornaro G, Rossi P, Mantica PG, et al. Indobufen in the prevention of thromboembolic complications in patients with heart disease. A randomized, placebo-controlled, double-blind study. Circulation 1993; 87:162–164.
13. Morocutti C, Amabile G, Fattapposta F, et al. Indobufen versus warfarin in the secondary prevention of major vascular events in nonrheumatic atrial fibrillation. Stroke 1997; 28:1015–1021.
14. Rajah SM, Nair U, Rees M, et al. Effects of antiplatelet therapy with indobufen or aspirin-dipyridamole on graft patency one year after coronary artery bypass grafting. J Thorac Cardiovasc Surg 1994; 107:1146–1153.
15. Patrono C, Coller B, Dalen JE, et al. Platelet-active drugs: the relationships among dose, effectiveness, and side effects. Chest 2001; 119:39S–63S.
16. D'Addato M, Curti T, Bertini D, et al. Indobufen vs acetylsalicylic acid plus dipyridamole in long-term patency after femoropopliteal bypass. Internat Angiol 1992; 11:106–112.
17. Tönnesen KH, Albuquerque P, Baitsch G, et al. Double-blind, controlled, multicenter study of indobufen versus placebo in patients with intermittent claudication. Internat Angiol 1993; 12: 371–377.
18. Signorini GP, Salmistraro G, Maraglino G. Efficacy of indobufen in the treatment of intermittent claudication. Angiology 1988; 39:742–746.

19. Bergamasco B, Benna P, Carolei A, et al. A randomized trial comparing ticlodipine hydrochloride with indobufen for the prevention of stroke in high-risk patients (TISS study). Funct Neurol 1997; 12:33–43.

20. Culebras A, Rotta-Escalante R, Vila J, et al. For the TAPIRSS investigators. Triflusal vs. aspirin for prevention of cerebral infarction: a randomized stroke study. Neurology 2004; 62:1073–1080.

21. Matias-Guiu J, Ferro JM, Alvarez-Sabin J, et al. Comparison of triflusal and aspirin for prevention of vascular events in patients after cerebral infarction: the TACIP study: a randomized, double-blind, multicenter trial. Can aspirin ever be surpassed for stroke prevention? Stroke 2003; 34:840–848.

22. Anderson DC. Aspirin: it's hard to beat. Neurology 2004; 62:1036.

23. Perez-Gomez F, Alegria E, Berjon J, et al. Comparative effects of antiplatelet, anticoagulant, or combined therapy in patients with valvular and nonvalvular atrial fibrillation: a randomized multicenter study. J Am Coll Cardiol 2004; 44:1557–1566.

24. Plaza L, Lopez-Bescos L, Martin-Jadraque L, et al. Protective effect of triflusal against acute myocardial infarction in patients with unstable angina: results of a Spanish multicenter trial. Cardiology 1993; 82:388–398.

25. Cruz-Fernandez JM, Lopez-Bescos L, Garcia-Dorado D, et al. Randomized comparative trial of triflusal and aspirin following acute myocardial infarction. Eur Heart J 2000; 21:457–465.

26. Aramendi JI, Mestres CA, Martinez-León J, et al. Triflusal versus oral anticoagulation for primary prevention of thromboembolism after bioprosthetic valve replacement (TRAC): prospective, randomized, co-operative trial. Eur J Cardiothorac Surg 2005; 27:854–860.

27. Guiteras P, Altimiras J, Aris A, et al. Prevention of aortocoronary vein-graft attrition with low-dose aspirin and triflusal, both associated with dipyridamole: a randomized, double-blind, placebo-controlled trial. Eur Heart J 1989; 10:159–167.

28. Auteri A. Triflusal in the treatment of patients with chronic peripheral arteriopathy: multicentre double-blind clinical study vs. placebo. Internat J Clin Pharmacol Res 1995; 15: 57–63.

29. Costa J, Ferro JM, Matias-Guiu J, et al. Triflusal for preventing serious vascular events in people at high risk. Cochrane Database Syst Rev 2005; (3):CD004296.

30. Weinberger I, Joshua H, Friedmann J, et al. Inhibition of ADP-induced platelet aggregation by dipyrone in patients with acute myocardial infarction. Thromb Haemost 1979; 42:752–756.

31. Schaper W. Dipyridamole, an underestimated vascular protective drug. Cardiovasc Drugs Ther 2005; 19:357–363.

32. Diener HC. Antiplatelet drugs in secondary prevention of stroke: lessons from recent trials. Neurology 1997; 49:S75–S81.

33. Diener HC, Cunha L, Forbes C, et al. European stroke prevention study 2: dipyridamole and acetylsalicylic acid in the secondary prevention of stroke. J Neurolog Sci 1996; 143:1–13.

34. Gibbs CR, Lip GYH. Do we still need dipyridamole? Br J Clin Pharmacol 1998; 45:323–328.

35. Heidland UE, Heintzen MP, Michel CJ, et al. Intracoronary administration of dipyridamole prior to percutaneous transluminal coronary angioplasty provides a protective effect exceeding that of ischemic preconditioning. Coron Art Dis 2000; 11:607–613.

36. ESPRIT study group. Aspirin plus dipyridamole versus aspirin alone after cerebral ischaemia of arterial origin (ESPRIT): randomised controlled trial. Lancet 2006; 367: 1665–1673.

37. Sacks HS, Ancona-Berk VA, Berrier J, et al. Dipyridamole in the treatment of angina pectoris: a meta-analysis. Clin Pharmacol Therapeut 1988; 43:610–615.

38. Picano E, Michelassi C. Chronic oral dipyridamole as a 'novel' antianginal drug: the collateral hypothesis. Cardiovasc Res 1997; 33: 666–670.

39. Barbour MM, Garber WE, Agarwal KC, et al. Effect of dipyridamole therapy on myocardial ischemia in patients with stable angina pectoris receiving concurrent anti-ischemic therapy. Am J Cardiol 1992; 69:449–452.

40. Tsuya T, Okada M, Hories H, et al. Effect of dipyridamole at the usual oral dose on exercise-induced myocardial ischemia in stable angina pectoris. Am J Cardiol 1990; 66: 275–278.

41. Picano E, PISA (Persantin In Stable Angina) study group. Dipyridamole in chronic stable angina pectoris a randomized, double blind, placebo-controlled, parallel group study. Eur Heart J 2001; 22:1785–1793.

42. Jagathesan R, Rosen SD, Foale RA, et al. Effects of long-term oral dipyridamole treatment on coronary microcirculatory function in patients with chronic stable angina: a substudy of the persantine in stable angina (PISA) study. J Cardiovasc Pharmacol 2006; 48:110–116.

43. Harrington RA, Becker RC, Ezekowitz M, et al. Antithrombotic therapy for coronary artery disease: the seventh ACCP conference on antithrombotic and thrombolytic therapy. Chest 2004; 126: 513S–548S.

44. Chesebro J, Fuster V, Elveback L, et al. Effect of dipyridamole and aspirin on late vein-graft patency after coronary bypass operations. N Engl J Med 1984; 310:209–214.

45. van der Meer J, Hillege H L, Kootstra G J, et al. Prevention of one-year vein-graft occlusion after aortocoronary-bypass surgery: a comparison of low-dose aspirin, low-dose aspirin plus dipyridamole, and oral anticoagulants. The CABADAS research group of the Interuniversity Cardiology Institute of the Netherlands. Lancet 1993; 342:257–264.

46. Goldman S, Copeland J, Moritz T, et al. Improvement in early saphenous vein graft patency after coronary artery bypass surgery with antiplatelet therapy: results of a Veterans Administration cooperative study. Circulation 1988; 77:1324–1332.

47. Little SH, Massel DR. Antiplatelet and anticoagulation for patients with prosthetic heart valves. Cochrane Database Syst Rev 2003; (4):CD003464.

48. Antithrombotic Trialists' Collaboration. Collaborative meta-analysis of randomised trials of antiplatelet therapy for prevention of death, myocardial infarction, and stroke in high risk patients. Br Med J 2002; 324:71–86.

49. Bousser M, Eschwege E, Haguenau M, et al. "AICLA" controlled trial of aspirin and dipyridamole in the secondary prevention of athero-thrombotic cerebral ischemia. Stroke 1983; 14:514.

50. No authors listed. Persantine aspirin trial in cerebral ischemia. Part II: endpoint results. The American-Canadian co-operative study group. Stroke 1985; 16:406–415.

51. The ESPS Group. The European Stroke Prevention Study. Stroke 1990; 21:1122–1130.

52. Born G, Patrono C. Antiplatelet drugs. Br J Pharmacol 2006; 147(suppl 1):S241–S251.

53. Weyrich AS, Denis MM, Kuhlmann-Eyre JR, et al. Dipyridamole selectively inhibits inflammatory gene expression in platelet-monocyte aggregates. Circulation 2005; 111:633–642.

54. Kohler TR, Kaufman JL, Kacovanis G, et al. Effect of aspirin and dipyridamole on the patency of lower extremity bypass grafts. Surgery 1984; 96:462–466.

55. McCollum C, Alexander C, Kenchington G, et al. Antiplatelet drugs in femoropopliteal vein bypasses: a multicenter trial. J Vasc Surg 1991; 13:150–162.

56. Clyne CA, Archer TJ, Atuhaire LK, et al. Random control trial of a short course of aspirin and dipyridamole (persantin) for femorodistal grafts. Br J Surg 1987; 74:246–248.

57. Hess H, Mietaschk A, Diechsel G. Drug-induced inhibition of platelet function delays progression of peripheral occlusive arterial disease. A prospective double-blind arterio-graphically controlled trial. Lancet 1985; 1:415–419.

58. Do D, Mahler F. Low-dose aspirin combined with dipyridamole versus anticoagulants after femoropopliteal percutaneous transluminal angioplasty. Radiology 1994; 193:567–571.

59. Puranen J. Laakso M, Riekkinen PJ Sr, et al. Efficacy of antiplatelet treatment in hypertensive patients with TIA or stroke. J Cardiovasc Pharmacol 1998; 32:291–294.

60. De Schryver EL for the ESPRIT study group. Dipyridamole in stroke prevention: effect of dipyridamole on blood pressure. Stroke 2003; 34:2339–2342.

61. Sacco RL, Adams R, Albers G, et al. Guidelines for prevention of stroke in patients with ischemic stroke or transient ischemic attack: a statement for healthcare professionals from the American Heart Association/American Stroke Association Council on Stroke. Circulation 2006; 3:e409–e449.

62. Diener H, Sacco R, Yusuf S, et al. Rationale, design and baseline data of a randomized, double-blind, controlled trial comparing two antithrombotic regimens (a fixed-dose combination of extended-release dipyridamole plus aspirin with clopidogrel) and telmisartan versus placebo in patients with strokes: the prevention regimen for effectively avoiding second strokes trial (PRoFESS). Cerebrovasc Dis 2007; 23:368–380.

63. De Schryver EL, Algra A, van Gijn J. Dipyridamole for preventing stroke and other vascular events in patients with vascular disease. Cochrane Database Syst Rev 2003; (1):CD001820.

64. Regensteiner JG, Ware JE, McCarthy WJ, et al. Effect of cilostazol on treadmill walking, community-based walking ability, and health-related quality of life in patients with intermittent claudication due to peripheral arterial disease: meta-analysis of six randomized controlled trials. J Am Geriatr Soc 2002; 50:1939–1946.

65. Robless P, Mikhailidis DP, Stansby GP. Cilostazol for peripheral arterial disease. Cochrane Database Syst Rev 2007; (1):CD003748.

66. Hashiguchi M, Ohno K, Nakazawa R, et al. Comparison of cilostazol and ticlopidine for one-month effectiveness and safety after elective coronary stenting. Cardiovasc Drugs Ther 2004; 18:211–217.

67. Lee S, Park S, Hong M, et al. Comparison of cilostazol and clopidogrel after successful coronary stenting. Am J Cardiol 2005; 95:859–862.

68. Kim JY, Lee K, Shin M, et al. Cilostazol could ameliorate platelet responsiveness to clopidogrel in patients undergoing primary percutaneous coronary intervention. Circ J 2007; 71:1867–1872.

69. Lee B, Lee S, Park S, et al. Effects of triple antiplatelet therapy (aspirin, clopidogrel, and cilostazol) on platelet aggregation and P-selectin expression in patients undergoing coronary artery stent implantation. Am J Cardiol 2007; 100:610–614.

70. Lee S, Park SW, Kim YH, et al. Comparison of triple versus dual antiplatelet therapy after drug-eluting stent implantation (from the DECLARE-long trial). Am J Cardiol 2007; 100: 1103–1108.

71. Lee SW, Park SW, Kim YH, et al. Drug-eluting stenting followed by cilostazol treatment reduces late restenosis in patients with diabetes mellitus. The DECLARE-DIABETES Trial (a randomized comparison of triple antiplatelet therapy with dual antiplatelet therapy after drug-eluting stent implantation in diabetic patients). J Am Coll Cardiol 2008; 51:1181–1187

72. Douglas JS, Holmes DR, Kereiakes DJ, et al. Coronary stent restenosis in patients treated with cilostazol. Circulation 2005; 112:2826–2832.

73. Biondi-Zoccai GL, Lotrionte M, Anselmino M, et al. Systematic review and meta-analysis of randomized clinical trials appraising the impact of cilostazol after percutaneous coronary intervention. Am J Cardiol 2008; 155:1081–1089.

74. Pratt CM. Analysis of the cilostazol safety database. Am J Cardiol 2001; 1A:28D–33D.

75. Maresta A, Balducelli M, Cantini L, et al. Trapidil (triazolopyrimidine), a platelet-derived growth factor antagonist, reduces restenosis after percutaneous transluminal coronary angioplasty. Results of the randomized, double-blind STARC study. Studio Trapidil versus Aspirin nella Restenosi Coronarica. Circulation. 1994; 90:2710–2715.

76. Serruys PW, Foley DP, Pieper M, et al. The TRAPIST Study. A multicentre randomized placebo controlled clinical trial of trapidil for prevention of restenosis after coronary stenting, measured by 3-D intravascular ultrasound. Eur Heart J 2001; 22:1938–1947.

77. Galassi AR, Tamburino C, Nicosia A, et al. A randomized comparison of trapidil (triazolopyrimidine), a platelet-derived growth factor antagonist, versus aspirin in prevention of angiographic restenosis after coronary artery Palmaz-Schatz stent implantation. Catheter Cardiovasc Inter 1999; 46:162–168.

78. Yasue H, Ogawa H, Tanaka H, et al. Effects of aspirin and trapidil on cardiovascular events after acute myocardial infarction. Japanese antiplatelets myocardial infarction study (JAMIS) investigators. Am J Cardiol 1999; 83:1308–1313.

79. Meinertz T, Lehmacher W, Trapidil/ISDN study group. Trapidil is as effective as isosorbide-dinitrate for treating stable angina pectoris: a multinational, multicenter, double-blind, randomized study. Clin Res Cardiol 2006; 95:217–223.

80. Shebuski RJ, Stabilito IJ, Sitko GR, et al. Acceleration of recombinant tissue-type plasminogen activator-induced thrombolysis and prevention of reocclusion by the combination of heparin and the Arg-Gly-Asp-containing peptide bitistatin in a canine model of coronary thrombosis. Circulation 1990; 82:169–177.

81. Knight LC, Romano JE. Functional expression of bitistatin, a disintegrin with potential use in molecular imaging of thromboembolic disease. Protein Exp Purif 2005; 39:307–319.

82. Kaku S, Umemura K, Mizuno A, et al. Evaluation of the disintegrin, triflavin, in a rat middle cerebral artery thrombosis model. Eur J Pharmacol 1997; 321:301–305.

83. Okuda D, Morita T. Purification and characterization of a new RGD/KGD-containing dimeric disintegrin, piscivostatin, from the venom of Agkistrodon piscivorus piscivorus: the unique effect of piscivostatin on platelet aggregation. J Biochem 2001; 130:407–415.

84. Frishman WH, Burns B, Atac B, et al. Novel antiplatelet therapies for treatment of patients with ischemic heart disease: inhibitors of the platelet glycoprotein Iib/IIia integrin receptor. Am Heart J 1995; 130:877–892.

85. Stockmans F, Deberdt W, Nystrom A, et al. Inhibitory effect of piracetam on platelet-rich thrombus formation in an animal model. Thromb Haemost 1998; 79:222–227.

86. De Reuck J, Van Vleyman B. The clinical safety of high-dose piracetam—its use in the treatment of acute stroke. Pharmacopsychiatry 1999; 32(suppl 1):33–37.

87. De Deyn PP, De Reuck J, Deberdt W, et al, for Members of the Piracetam in Acute Stroke Study (PASS) Group. Treatment of acute ischemic stroke with piracetam. Stroke 1997; 28:2347–2352.

88. Grotemeyer KH, Evers S, Fischer M, et al. Piracetam versus acetylsalicylic acid in secondary stroke prophylaxis. A double-blind, randomized, parallel group, 2 year follow-up study. J Neurolog Sci 2000; 181:65–72.

89. Patrono C, Bachmann F, Baigent C, et al. Expert consensus document on the use of antiplatelet agents. The task force on the use of antiplatelet agents in patients with atherosclerotic cardiovascular disease of the European society of cardiology. Eur Heart J 2004; 25:166–181.

90. Osende JI, Shimbo D, Fuster V, et al. Antithrombotic effects of S 18886, a novel orally active thromboxane A2 receptor antagonist. J Thromb Haemost 2004; 2:492–498.

91. Husted S. New developments in oral antiplatelet therapy. Eur Heart J Suppl 2007; 9:D20–D27.

92. Vilahur G, Casani L, Badimon L. A thromboxane A(2)/prostaglandin H-2 receptor antagonist (SI8886) shows high antithrombotic efficacy in an experimental model of stent-induced thrombosis. Thromb Haemost 2007; 98:662–669.

93. Dogné JM, Rolin S, de Leval X, et al. Pharmacology of the thromboxane receptor antagonist and thromboxane synthase inhibitor BM-531. Cardiovasc Drug Rev 2001; 19:87–96.

94. Rosenfeld L, Grover GJ, Stier CT. Ifetroban sodium: an effective TxA2-PGH2 receptor antagonist. Cardiovasc Drug Rev 2001; 19:97115.

95. Swanson BN, Manning JA, Ogletree ML, et al. Effect of BMS-180291, a long-acting thromboxane A2 receptor antagonist, on platelet function in healthy men. Clin Pharm Therap 1994; 55:202 (abstr).

32

The Combination of Anticoagulants and Platelet Inhibitors Postcoronary Stent Implantation

Hussam Hamdalla and Steven R. Steinhubl
Gill Heart Institute and Division of Cardiovascular Medicine,
University of Kentucky, Lexington, Kentucky, U.S.A.

INTRODUCTION

Coronary stenting, initially introduced for the management of abrupt vessel closure and dissection, has evolved over the past decades to become applicable to a range of patients, indications, and lesions. However the initial series was met with an alarmingly high rate (~20%) of acute stent thrombosis. This was promptly reduced with a combination of anticoagulation and antiplatelet therapies. The result of this combination was associated with markedly higher rates of bleeding. Subsequently, the introduction of thienopyridines and dual antiplatelet therapy became the standard of care after percutaneous coronary intervention (PCI) with bare-metal stenting for a minimum of four weeks and was associated with a significantly lower risk of bleeding complications. With the increased utilization of PCI with stenting over the past few years, more patients are presenting with an indication for anticoagulation following PCI. Furthermore, the American College of Cardiology (ACC), the American Heart Association (AHA), and the Society for Cardiovascular Angiography and Interventions (SCAI) currently recommend a prolonged course of dual antiplatelet therapy up to one year following drug-eluting stent to prevent late stent thrombosis. (1).Because of the requirement for this prolonged antiplatelet therapy, patients with atrial fibrillation, mechanical heart valve, stroke, and venous thromboembolic disease requiring oral anticoagulation therapy represent an extremely challenging group in whom optimal antithrombotic therapy remains poorly defined.

ANTICOAGULATION VS. ANTIPLATELETS FOLLOWING PCI

The initial reports of successful stent implant for coronary stenosis were tempered with high rates of stent thrombosis. The first 105 patients to receive Wallstent reported a 24% incidence of subacute stent thrombosis at 14 days (2), and similarly the first 226 patients with a Palmaz-Schatz stent reported an 18% incidence at 14 days (3). However the

Table 1 Overview of the Dual Antiplatelet Compared to Anticoagulation Trials

	ISAR	STARS	FANTASTIC	MATTIS
Patients	517	1096	473	350
Antiplatelet therapy	T 500 mg	T 500 mg	T 500 mg	T 500 mg
	A 100 mg	A 325 mg	A 100–325 mg	A 250 mg
Anticoagulation therapy	Phenprocumon	Warfarin	OAC	OAC
	A 100 mg	A 325 mg	A 100–325 mg	A 250 mg
Target INR	3.5–4.5	2.0–2.5	2.0–2.5	2.5–3.0

Abbreviations: ISAR, intracoronary stenting and antithrombotic regimen; STARS, stent anticoagulation restenosis study; FANTASTIC, full anticoagulation versus aspirin and ticlopidine; MATTIS, multicenter aspirin and ticlopidine trial after intracoronary stenting; T, ticlopidine; A, aspirin; OAC, oral anticoagulation

addition of warfarin to a regimen of aspirin and dipyridamole reduced the rates to 0.6% at 14 days. Consequently, intense anticoagulation regimens were established including intravenous heparin and dextran, oral aspirin, dipyridamole, and warfarin. Not surprisingly, this doubled the length of hospital stay and increased the risk of hemorrhagic and vascular complications. Evidence of increased platelet surface expression of the glycoprotein (GP) IIb/IIIa receptor as a strong predictor of acute stent thrombosis led to further evaluation of anticoagulation versus antiplatelet therapy following stenting (4).

In the intracoronary stenting and antithrombotic regimen (ISAR) trial, Schömig et al. studied a dual antiplatelet regimen in patients following stent compared with anticoagulation. After successful placement of a Palmaz-Schatz stent, 257 patients were randomized to ticlopidine and aspirin combination and 260 patients to phenprocoumon and aspirin for four weeks (Table 1) (5). Dual antiplatelet therapy was associated with a remarkably lower rate of cardiac death, myocardial infarction (MI), or revascularization at 30 days (1.6% vs. 6.2%, $p = 0.01$). The risk of hemorrhagic complications was also lowered with the antiplatelet therapy from 6.5% to 0% and vascular complications from 6.2% to 0.8%. In the stent anticoagulation restenosis study (STARS), 1653 low-risk patients were randomized to one of three drug regimens after successful placement of a Palmaz-Schatz stent (6). All patients received aspirin and were then randomized to aspirin alone, or ticlopidine and aspirin, or warfarin and aspirin (Table 1). Ticlopidine and warfarin were initiated at the end of the procedure and continued for 30 days. The 30-day primary end point of death, MI, target-lesion revascularization (TLR), or stent thrombosis occurred in 3.6% assigned to aspirin alone, 2.7% to aspirin and warfarin, and 0.5% to aspirin and ticlopidine ($p = 0.001$). Overall, the risk of hemorrhagic complications was 1.8% in the group assigned to aspirin alone, 6.2% to warfarin and aspirin, and 5.5% assigned to ticlopidine and aspirin. Similarly in the full anticoagulation versus aspirin and ticlopidine (FANTASTIC) study, 236 patients were randomized to ticlopidine and aspirin and 249 patients to warfarin and aspirin (7). The primary end point of this study was the rates of bleeding at six weeks. Bleeding complications occurred in 13.5% of patients receiving antiplatelet therapy and 21% of patients receiving anticoagulation therapy ($p = 0.03$). Patients receiving antiplatelet therapy had a 5.7% risk of cardiac events and those receiving anticoagulation a risk of 8.3%. The multicenter aspirin and ticlopidine trial after intracoronary stenting (MATTIS) study evaluated the role of dual antiplatelet therapy in 350 high-risk patients (8). The primary end point of death, MI, or target-vessel revascularization (TVR) occurred in 5.6% of patients randomized to the antiplatelet arm and 11% of those randomized to the anticoagulation arm with a relative risk of 1.94 (95% CI 0.93–4.06) ($p = 0.07$). The safety end point of vascular and bleeding complication was 1.7% in the antiplatelet therapy group and 6.9% in the anticoagulation group ($p = 0.02$).

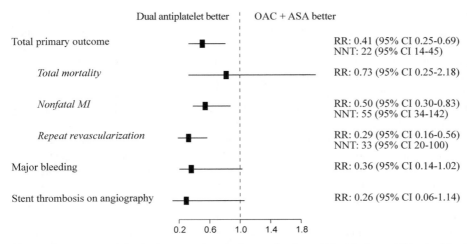

Figure 1   Relative risk of primary and secondary end points. *Abbreviations:* ASA, Aspirin; OAC, oral anticoagulation; NNT, number needed to treat. From Ref. 9.

Rubboli et al. performed a meta-analysis comparing antiplatelet therapy with anticoagulation trials (9). Taken together, these studies established the superiority and safety of dual antiplatelet therapy, with the use of aspirin in combination with a thienopyridine following coronary stent (Fig. 1). A dual antiplatelet therapy approach was associated with a 59% relative risk reduction of the combined end point of death, MI, or revascularization, as compared with an anticoagulation approach. Furthermore an antiplatelet regimen following PCI had a 64% relative risk reduction of major bleeding complication.

TRIPLE THERAPY WITH ANTIPLATELET AND ANTICOAGULATION THERAPY

The combination of antiplatelet and anticoagulation therapy has been of concern with the anticipated but poorly documented risk of bleeding. In the past, patients receiving a bare-metal stent could have dual antiplatelet therapy limited to two to four weeks to minimize the risk of stent thrombosis. For patients with an indication for long-term anticoagulation, exposure to triple antithrombotic therapy with warfarin, aspirin, and a thienopyridine could be minimized to a limited, although not insignificant, period of time. However, over the past few years, with the introduction of drug-eluting stents the risks and benefits of triple therapy have attracted more attention and concerns. The ACC/AHA/SCAI committee issued recommendations to maintain patients with a drug-eluting stent on dual antiplatelet therapy for a minimum of 12 months due to increased risk of late stent thrombosis (1). However, paucity of data and recommendations exists for the optimal antithrombotic regimen for patients with indications for dual antiplatelet therapy and anticoagulation.

In a retrospective analysis from the Mayo Clinic PCI database, Orford et al. reviewed the records of 65 consecutive patients who were discharged on dual antiplatelet therapy and anticoagulation (10). Of those 66 patients, 6 (9.2%) developed a bleeding complication by 30 days requiring medical care with 3.1% having major bleeding. Bleeding complications were seen in elderly patients >75 years or with a supratherapeutic international normalized ratio (INR) in this series. During the 30-day follow-up, there was no report of death, MI, repeat revascularization, or stent thrombosis in this small group.

Porter et al. reported on 180 patients who were on a short-term triple therapy following PCI (11). The main indication for anticoagulation in this cohort was left ventricular thrombus and atrial fibrillation. Bleeding complications were seen in 20 patients (11%) within 30 days of triple therapy with only two major bleeding events. Almost 90% of the patients maintained an INR <3.0 during triple therapy period, and this could have contributed to lower rates of major bleeding. Of interest, in 18 of the 20 patients, the bleeding event occurred during overlapping treatment with heparin. Likewise, Khurram et al. compared 107 patients on warfarin therapy who underwent PCI and were discharged on triple therapy with 107 randomly selected patients on dual therapy (12). Patients on triple therapy had more major bleeding (6.6% vs. 0.0%; $p = 0.014$) and, after adjusting for confounding variables using multivariate analysis, the hazard ratio for any bleeding was 5.44 with triple therapy ($p = 0.001$; CI 2.03–14.53) compared with dual therapy. None of the bleeding events occurred within the first 30 days, and there was no correlation between the INR levels or the aspirin dose in this series of patients. Similarly, DeEugenio et al. compared 97 patients with triple therapy to a matched control group (13). After a median follow-up of 182 days, there were 14 major bleeding events in the active group compared with 3 in the control group. As compared with the previous studies, this group had more patients with drug-eluting stents. The hazard ratio for major bleeding was 5.0 in patients receiving triple therapy (95% CI 1.4–17.8, $p = 0.012$) compared with that for the control group. Although 70% of INRs were <3.0, the median INR at the time of bleeding was 3.4 (1.19–9.89). The authors reported no difference in risk of bleeding between patients with INR goal of 3.0 and those with INR goal of 2.0 to 2.5.

A more recent report by Karjalainen et al. from Finland assessed 239 patients with an indication for anticoagulation therapy following PCI (14). They compared this group to 239 matched control patients from the PCI database. Atrial fibrillation (70%) was the most frequent indication for anticoagulation and 40% of patients received a drug-eluting stent. At the discretion of the treating physician, patients with indications for anticoagulation were prescribed different regimens—triple therapy (48%), aspirin and thienopyridine (15%), warfarin and aspirin (15%), warfarin and thienopyridine (20%). At 12 month follow-up the primary end point of death, MI, revascularization, and stent thrombosis occurred in 21.9% of patients in the anticoagulation group and 11% in the control group ($p = 0.003$). This was driven by increased mortality (8.7% vs. 1.8%), MI (10% vs. 4.8%), and stent thrombosis (4.1% vs. 1.3%) in the anticoagulation group compared with that in the control group, respectively. The secondary end point of major bleeding was also higher in the anticoagulation group 8.2% compared with that in the control group 2.6% ($p = 0.014$). Patients who were given warfarin and aspirin alone had the highest rate of stent thrombosis 15.2%, while two patients (1.9%) of those receiving triple therapy had stent thrombosis (one patient after stopping his clopidogrel). The risk of stroke was highest in patients who received dual antiplatelet therapy (8.8%) as a substitute for triple therapy; furthermore, the risk of MI was higher when patients were given anticoagulation with a single antiplatelet agent (more MIs after the discontinuation of the thienopyridine). In a multivariable analysis, predictors of major bleeding were warfarin (OR 3.4, 95% CI 1.2–9.3, $p = 0.02$), current smoking (OR 6.6, 95% CI 2.2–19.9, $p < 0.001$), female gender (OR 7.6, 95% CI 2.5–23, $p < 0.001$), and GP receptor inhibitors (OR 2.6, 95% CI 1.0–6.5, $p = 0.005$).

Atrial fibrillation is one of the most common indications for anticoagulation. Ruiz-Nodar et al. reviewed 426 patients with atrial fibrillation undergoing PCI (15). Patients had at least ≥1 risk factor according to the congestive heart failure, hypertension, age >75 years, and diabetes, and stroke (CHADS$_2$) score and ≥ 2 risk factors were present in 69%. The mean age was 71.5 ± 8.5 years, almost 75% had hypertension, and 30% had

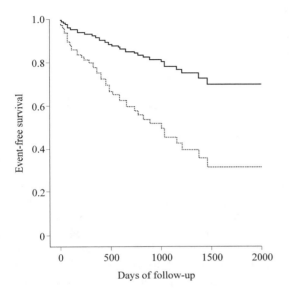

Figure 2 Kaplan-Meier Survival curves in relation to anticoagulation use at discharge. Major adverse cardiovascular events: log-rank test, $p = 0.02$. Patients were stratified according to anticoagulation use at discharge compared to nonuse. Dotted lines indicate no anticoagulation use at discharge; solid lines indicate anticoagulation use at discharge. *Source*: From Ref. 15.

ventricular function <45%. Drug-eluting stents were used in 40% of patients. Complete follow-up was available in 88% of patients with a median of 595 days. The two groups of the study were formed of 174 (40.8%) patients who were discharged on dual antiplatelet therapy and 213 (50.0%) who were discharged on triple therapy. The end point of MAE, which was defined as death, MI, TVR, major bleeding, and/or stroke occurred in 31.8% of patients with triple therapy and 41.9% in patients with dual therapy ($p = 0.03$) (Fig. 2). The risk of an embolic event was higher in patients with dual therapy than those with triple therapy (6.9% vs. 1.7%, $p = 0.02$). Mortality was also higher with patients discharged without anticoagulation (HR 3.43; 95% CI 1.61–7.54, $p = 0.002$). Among patients who were discharged on anticoagulation, there was a nonsignificant increase in risk of major bleeding with triple therapy (14.9% vs. 9.0%; $p = 0.19$) and risk of minor bleeding (12.6% vs. 9.0%; $p = 0.32$). In a Cox-regression analysis, age (HR 1.06; 95% CI 1.01–1.12, $p = 0.02$) and nonanticoagulation on discharge (HR 4.33; 95% CI 1.96–9.59, $p < 0.01$) were independent predictors of an MAE. This study does not account for possible changes in the antithrombotic and antiplatelet therapy in these patients during the follow-up period. Furthermore, there is no data available on the INR levels that were maintained in this population and possible correlation with bleeding risks.

The Global Registry of Acute Coronary Events (GRACE) is an international database that is designed to track outcomes of patients presenting with acute coronary syndromes. Nguyen et al. studied 800 patients from the GRACE registry who were discharged on warfarin following PCI (16). Of the 800 patients in this cohort, 580 (73%) received triple therapy and 220 (28%) received warfarin with a single antiplatelet agent at discharge. Among those who received a single antiplatelet agent, 49% received aspirin and 51% received a thienopyridine with warfarin. Atrial fibrillation was the main indication for warfarin therapy prior to admission; however, atrial fibrillation (24%) and ST-elevation MI (60%) were the most common indications for initiating warfarin therapy

Table 2 Stroke Risk According to CHADS$_2$ Score

Score	Annual risk (%)
0	1.9
1	2.8
2	4.8
3	5.9
4	8.5
5	12.5
6	18.2

after admission. The risk of stroke was reduced at six month follow-up with triple therapy compared with that following warfarin with single antiplatelet agent (0.7% vs. 3.4%, $p = 0.02$); however, there was no significant difference in mortality or MI. There was also no significant difference in death, MI, or stroke between patients who received aspirin or thienopyridine as the single antiplatelet agent with warfarin. The incidence of bleeding complications was not collected at follow-up. The registry also highlights the varying practices from region to region with more than 80% of patients discharged on triple therapy in the United States and just more than 60% in Europe.

CURRENT PRACTICE GUIDELINE

The ACC/AHA/SCAI committee currently recommends a minimum of four weeks of dual antiplatelet therapy in patients undergoing PCI with a bare-metal stent and preferably 12 months of dual antiplatelet therapy in patients receiving a DES. However the combination of clopidogrel and aspirin was found to be inferior to oral anticoagulation in preventing stroke and embolic events. In the atrial fibrillation clopidogrel trial with irbesartan for prevention of vascular events (ACTIVE W) trial patients with atrial fibrillation and at least one risk factor for stroke, those who received the combination of aspirin and clopidogrel had an annual risk of stroke of 2.4% compared with 1.4% in those who received oral anticoagulation ($p = 0.001$) (17). Therefore the clinical dilemma remains that while dual antiplatelets are more effective in preventing stent thrombosis than an anticoagulant-based regimen, anticoagulants are more effective than dual antiplatelets in venous thromboembolic diseases and atrial fibrillation. The utilization of the CHADS$_2$ risk score, which is based on clinical risk factors, with one point each assigned for congestive heart failure, hypertension, age >75 years, and diabetes, and two points for prior history of stroke (Table 2), might help in determining who is more likely to benefit from anticoagulation therapy (18). The ACC/AHA current guidelines for management of patients with atrial fibrillation undergoing PCI designate a class IIb for a maintenance regimen of thienopyridine with warfarin alone without an aspirin (19). The committee recommends interrupting the warfarin at the time of catheterization to avoid bleeding complications and the use of aspirin temporarily during the hiatus; however, warfarin needs to be resumed as soon as possible and the thienopyridine to be discontinued as soon as it is deemed safe.

SUMMARY

Dual antiplatelet therapy using aspirin and a thienopyridine has become the standard of care in patients after a stent implantation. The superiority of dual therapy over anticoagulation plus aspirin regimens have been established in several randomized trials making that option inadequate in stent-treated patients who require long-term anti-coagulation. In addition, only minimal, observational data exist, which provide guidance regarding the safety of triple therapy. As more patients are presenting for PCI with indications for anticoagulation, identifying the optimal antithrombotic and antiplatelet regimen to manage these patients remains a critical question. A review of all the observational studies suggests a reduced embolic event rate with the triple therapy including aspirin, thienopyridine, and anticoagulation at the expense of increased risk of bleeding. Since these studies were not randomized, it is possible that these results are not representative of the risks and benefits of triple therapy in a nonselected population.

REFERENCES

1. Grines CL, Bonow RO, Casey DE Jr., et al. Prevention of premature discontinuation of dual antiplatelet therapy in patients with coronary artery stents: a science advisory from the American Heart Association, American College of Cardiology, Society for Cardiovascular Angiography and Interventions, American College of Surgeons, and American Dental Association, with representation from the American College of Physicians. Circulation 2007; 115:813–818.
2. Sigwart U, Puel J, Mirkovitch V, et al. Intravascular stents to prevent occlusion and restenosis after transluminal angioplasty. N Engl J Med 1987; 316m 701–706.
3. Schatz RA, Baim DS, Leon M, et al. Clinical experience with the Palmaz-Schatz coronary stent. Initial results of a multicenter study. Circulation 1991; 83:148–161.
4. Neumann FJ, Gawaz M, Ott I, et al. Prospective evaluation of hemostatic predictors of subacute stent thrombosis after coronary Palmaz-Schatz stenting. J Am Coll Cardiol 1996; 27:15–21.
5. Schomig A, Neumann FJ, Kastrati A, et al. A randomized comparison of antiplatelet and anticoagulant therapy after placement of coronary-artery stents. N Engl J Med 1996; 334:1084–1089.
6. Leon MB, Baim DS, Popma JJ, et al. A clinical trial comparing three antithrombotic-drug regimens following coronary artery stenting. N Eng J Med 1998; 339:1665–1671.
7. Bertrand ME, Legrand V, Boland J, et al. Randomized multicenter comparison of conventional anticoagulation versus antiplatelet therapy in unplanned and elective coronary stenting. The Full Anticoagulation Versus Aspirin and Ticlopidine (FANTASTIC) Study. Circulation 1998; 98:1597–1603.
8. Urban P, Macaya C, Rupprecht HJ, et al. Randomized evaluation of anticoagulation versus antiplatelet therapy after coronary stent implantation in high-risk patients. The Multicenter Aspirin and Ticlopidine Trial after Intracoronary Stenting (MATTIS). Circulation 1998; 98:2126–2132.
9. Rubboli A, Milandri M, Castelvetri C, et al. Meta-analysis of trials comparing oral anticoagulation and aspirin versus dual antiplatelet therapy after coronary stenting. Clues for the management of patients with an indication of long-term anticoagulation undergoing coronary stenting. Cardiology 2005; 104:101–106.
10. Orford JL, Fasseas P, Melby S, et al. Safety and efficacy of aspirin, clopidogrel, and warfarin after coronary stent placement in patients with an indication for anticoagulation. Am Heart J 2004; 147:463–467.
11. Porter A, Konstantino Y, Iakobishvilli Z, et al. Short-term triple therapy with aspirin, warfarin, and a thienopyridine among patients undergoing percutaneous coronary intervention. Catheter Cardiovasc Interv 2006; 68:56–61.
12. Khurram Z, Chou E, Minutello R, et al. Combination therapy with aspirin, clopidogrel and warfarin following coronary stenting is associated with a significant risk of bleeding. J Invasive Cardiol 2006; 18:162–164.

13. DeEugenio D, Kolman L, De Caro M, et al. Risk of major bleeding with concomitant dual antiplatelet therapy after percutaneous coronary intervention in patients receiving long-term warfarin therapy. Pharmacotherapy 2007; 27:691–696.

14. Karjalainen PP, Porela P, Ylitalo A, et al. Safety and efficacy of combined antiplatelet-warfarin therapy after coronary stenting. Eur Heart J 2007; 28:726–732.

15. Ruiz-Nodar JM, Marin F, Hurtado JA, et al. Anticoagulant and antiplatelet therapy use in 426 patients with atrial fibrillation undergoing percutaneous coronary intervention and stent implantation implications for bleeding risk and prognosis. J Am Coll Cardiol 2008; 51:818–825.

16. Nguyen MC, Lim YL, Walton A, et al. Combining warfarin and antiplatelet therapy after coronary stenting in the Global Registry of Acute Coronary Events: is it safe and effective to use just one antiplatelet agent? Eur Heart J 2007; 28:1717–1722.

17. Connolly S, Poque J, Hart R, et al. for the ACTIVE Writing Group of the ACTIVE Investigators. Clopidogrel plus aspirin versus oral anticoagulation for atrial fibrillation in the Atrial fibrillation Clopidogrel Trial with Irbesartan for prevention of Vascular Events (ACTIVE W): a randomised controlled trial. Lancet 2006; 367:1903–1912.

18. Gage BF, Waterman AD, Shannon W, et al. Validation of clinical classification schemes for predicting stroke: Results from the National Registry of Atrial Fibrillation. JAMA 2001; 2864–2870.

19. European Heart Rhythm Assocaition, Heart Rhythm Society: Fuster V, Ryden LE, Cannom DS, et al. ACC/AHA/ESC 2006 Guidelines for the management of patients with atrial fibrillation—executive summary: A report of the American College of Cardiology/American Heart Association Task Force on Practice Guidelines and the European Society of Cardiology Committee for Practice Guidelines (Writing Committee to Revise the 2001 Guidelines for the Management of Patients With Atrial Fibrillation). J Am Coll Cardiol 2006; 48:854–906.

33
Overview of Established and New Thrombolytics

H. Roger Lijnen
*Center for Molecular and Vascular Biology, Katholieke Universiteit Leuven,
Leuven, Belgium*

INTRODUCTION

Thrombolysis consists of the pharmacological dissolution of a blood clot by administration of thrombolytic agents that activate the fibrinolytic system. This system includes a proenzyme, plasminogen, which is converted by plasminogen activators (PAs) to the active enzyme plasmin, which in turn digests fibrin to soluble degradation products. There are two physiologic plasminogen activators: the tissue-type (t-PA; EC 3.4.21.68) and the urokinase-type (u-PA; EC 3.4.21.73). Inhibition of the fibrinolytic system occurs at the level of PA by plasminogen activator inhibitors (PAI, mainly PAI-1 and in some conditions PAI-2) and at the level of plasmin by plasmin inhibitors (mainly α_2-antiplasmin) (Fig. 1). Presently available plasminogen activators include serine proteinases such as recombinant t-PA (rt-PA or alteplase) and its derivatives, two-chain u-PA (tcu-PA or urokinase) and recombinant single-chain u-PA (scu-PA or prourokinase, saruplase) as well as nonenzyme plasminogen activators such as streptokinase, anisoylated plasminogen-streptokinase activator complex (APSAC or anistreplase), and recombinant staphylokinase and derivatives. Traditionally, these were classified as fibrin-selective agents (rt-PA and derivatives, staphylokinase and derivatives, and to a lesser extent scu-PA), which digest a thrombus in the absence of systemic plasminogen activation, or as nonfibrin-selective agents (streptokinase, tcu-PA, and APSAC), which activate systemic and fibrin-bound plasminogen relatively indiscriminately (1,2). More recently, thrombolytics that act directly on fibrin have also been characterized and evaluated, including different molecular forms of plasmin as well as several fibrinolytic enzymes derived from snake venoms. In this contribution, we will review the main properties of fibrinolytic agents with therapeutic potential. Clinical experience in patients with acute myocardial infarction, deep vein thrombosis, pulmonary hypertension, and ischemic stroke will be discussed in the next chapters.

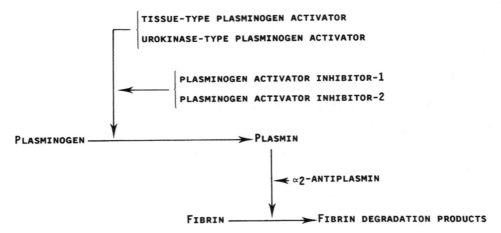

Figure 1 Schematic representation of the fibrinolytic system. The proenzyme plasminogen is activated to the active enzyme plasmin by t-PA or u-PA. Plasmin degrades fibrin into soluble fibrin degradation products. Inhibition of the fibrinolytic system may occur by PAI-1 or -2, or by the plasmin inhibitor α_2-antiplasmin. *Abbreviations*: t-PA, tissue-type plasminogen activator; u-PA, urokinase-type plasminogen activator; PAI, plasminogen activator inhibitor.

PLASMINOGEN ACTIVATORS

Enzyme Plasminogen Activators

Tissue-Type Plasminogen Activator

As early as 1947, it was reported that animal tissues contain an agent that can activate plasminogen; this factor was originally called fibrinokinase (3). Since many reports of the purification and characterization of tissue plasminogen activators from various sources, including pig heart and ovaries, and human postmortem vascular perfusates and postexercise blood have been published. The first highly purified form of human t-PA was obtained from uterine tissues (4). Using an antiserum raised against this PA, it has been shown that tissue PA, vascular PA, and blood PA are immunologically identical, but different from urokinase (5). The PA found in blood represents vascular t-PA that is released mainly from endothelial cells.

t-PA has subsequently been purified from the culture fluid of a stable human melanoma cell line (Bowes, RPMI-7272), in sufficient amounts to study its biochemical and biological properties (6). The cDNA of human t-PA has been cloned and expressed, first in *Escheria coli* and later in mammalian cell systems yielding a properly processed and glycosylated molecule (7). This rt-PA was shown to be indistinguishable from the natural activator isolated from human melanoma cell cultures, with respect to biochemical properties, turnover in vivo, and specific thrombolytic activity (8). The generation of Chinese hamster ovary cells capable of producing single-chain human t-PA has allowed the development of large-scale tissue culture fermentation and purification procedures, yielding rt-PA for commercial purposes (Activase®, Genentech Inc. South San Francisco, California, U.S.; Actilyse®, Boehringer Ingelheim Pharma GmbH, Ingelheim am Rhein, Germany). Biologically active t-PA has also been obtained by expression of cDNA in *Aspergillus nidulans* (9) and in mouse C127 cells (10).

Wild-type rt-PA (alteplase) was first obtained as a single-chain serine proteinase of 70 kDa, consisting of 527 amino acids with Ser as the NH_2-terminal amino acid; native

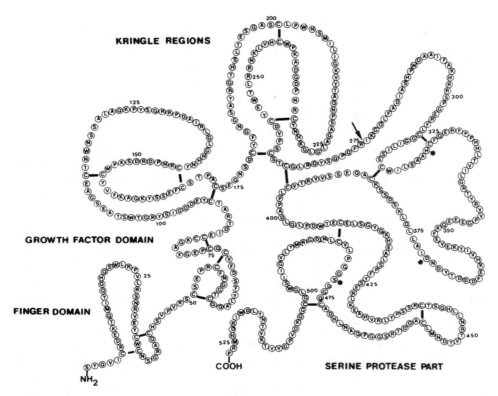

Figure 2 Schematic representation of the primary structure of t-PA. The amino acids are represented by their single letter symbols, and black bars indicate disulfide bonds. The active-site residues are indicated with an asterisk. The arrow indicates the cleavage site for conversion of single-chain to two-chain t-PA. *Abbreviation*: t-PA, tissue-type plasminogen activator.

t-PA actually contains an NH_2-terminal extension of three amino acids, but in general the initial numbering system has been maintained (Fig. 2). Limited plasmic hydrolysis of the Arg^{275}-Ile^{276} peptide bond converts t-PA to a two-chain molecule held together by one interchain disulfide bond. The t-PA molecule contains four domains: (*i*) an NH_2-terminal region of 47-residues (residues 4 to 50) that is homologous with the finger domains of fibronectin; (*ii*) residues 50 to 87 that are homologous with epidermal growth factor; (*iii*) two kringle regions comprising residues 87 to 176 and 176 to 262 that are homologous with the five kringles of plasminogen; and (*iv*) a serine proteinase domain (residues 276 to 527) with the active-site residues His^{322}, Asp^{371}, and Ser^{478} (7). In contrast to the single-chain precursor form of most serine proteinases, single-chain t-PA is enzymatically active. This was explained by the fact that true zymogens have a catalytic triad consisting of Asp^{194}, His^{40}, and Ser^{32} (chymotrypsin numbering), whereas in t-PA the His and Ser at these positions are replaced by Phe^{305} and Ala^{292}, respectively. In agreement with this hypothesis, the double mutant Phe^{305} to His and Ala^{292} to Ser was more zymogenic, as a result of the formation of a hydrogen-bonded network of Ser^{292} and His^{305} with Asp^{477}, similar to the Asp^{194}-His^{40}-Ser^{32} network that stabilizes the zymogen chymotrypsinogen (11,12). Other structural studies suggested that the formation of a salt bridge between Lys^{429} and Asp^{477} may stabilize the active conformation of single-chain t-PA (13).

t-PA has four potential glycosylation sites, of which three are occupied in type I (Asn^{117}, Asn^{184}, and Asn^{448}) and two in type II t-PA (Asn^{117} and Asn^{448}) (14). Residue 117 is predominantly N-glycosylated with oligomannose-type structures, whereas residues 184 and 448 are predominantly associated with complex-type structures in rt-PA, but with both complex- and oligomannose-type structures when isolated from melanoma cells (14). Glycosylation at residue 184 influences the biological properties of t-PA, and type II has a higher affinity for lysine (and fibrin) and a higher fibrinolytic activity (14,15). t-PA, has an O-linked fucose on Thr[61] in the epidermal growth factor domain (16) that affects cellular binding and may be relevant for clearance (17).

Structure–function analysis has revealed specific functions for the t-PA domains. Thus, high-affinity binding of t-PA to fibrin is mediated by the finger and kringle 2 domains; stimulation of its activity by fibrin also involves the finger, (kringle1?) and kringle 2 domains; in vivo clearance is regulated by the finger and growth factor domains and by the carbohydrate side chains; and the enzymatic activity resides in the serine proteinase domain (7).

t-PA is a poor enzyme in the absence of fibrin, but the presence of fibrin strikingly enhances the activation rate of plasminogen (18). During fibrinolysis, fibrinogen and fibrin are continuously modified by cleavage with thrombin or plasmin, yielding a diversity of reaction products. Optimal stimulation of t-PA is only obtained after early plasmin-cleavage in the COOH-terminal Aα-chain and the NH$_2$-terminal Bβ-chain of fibrin, yielding fragment X-polymer (19). Detailed structural studies revealed that the sequence Aα148-160 in the D-region of fibrin binds both plasminogen and t-PA, whereas the sequence γ312-324 only binds t-PA. Both these associations are of low affinity, and in the circulation, the Aα148-160 sequence will only bind plasminogen, which is present in much higher concentrations than t-PA. Other binding sites in the D-region comprise residues γ311-336 and γ337-379, which are linked by a disulfide bond (20). Studies with antibodies have identified a t-PA-binding site within the sequence γ312-324 (21). Higher-affinity binding sites for t-PA and plasminogen are located in the COOH-terminus of the α chain within the region Aα392-610 (22). The conformational changes that occur upon cleavage of fibrinogen and assembly of fibrin are associated with exposure of new sites for binding of t-PA and plasminogen, resulting in enhancement of plasminogen activation (23).

Kinetic data support this mechanism in which fibrin provides a surface to which t-PA and plasminogen adsorb in a sequential and ordered way, yielding a cyclic ternary complex (18). Formation of this complex results in an enhanced affinity of t-PA for plasminogen, yielding up to three orders of magnitude higher catalytic efficiencies for plasminogen activation. This is mediated at least in part by COOH-terminal lysine residues generated by plasmin cleavage of fibrin. Plasmin formed at the fibrin surface has both its lysine-binding sites and active site occupied and is thus only slowly inactivated by α$_2$-antiplasmin (half-life of about 10–100 seconds, as compared with about 0.1 seconds for free plasmin) (24). These molecular interactions mediate the fibrin-specificity of t-PA.

PAI-1 is the main inhibitor of both t-PA and u-PA; it is a serpin of 379–381 residues with reactive site peptide bond Arg[346]-Met[347]. Rapid inhibition of t-PA by PAI-1 involves interaction between a negatively charged region in PAI-1 (residues 350–355) and a positively charged region in t-PA (residues 296–304) (25), followed by cleavage of the reactive site peptide bond and formation of an inactive 1:1 stoichiometric complex. The positively charged loop around Arg[299] in t-PA projects out of the molecular surface as a β-hairpin and is easily accessible for interaction with PAI-1 (13). PAI-2 is a predominantly intracellular serpin that also rapidly inhibits t-PA and u-PA.

Following intravenous administration of rt-PA in humans, it is cleared from the circulation with an initial half-life of four to eight minutes. Clearance is the result of interaction with several receptor systems. Early studies showed that the uptake of t-PA by liver endothelial cells and by Kupffer cells was inhibited by ovalbumin, leading to the identification of the mannose receptor as a major t-PA receptor (26) with high affinity (Kd of 1 to 4 nM) (27). The other major pathway for t-PA clearance involves the LRP/α_2-macroglobulin receptor (28,29). The 600-kDa LRP (4525 residues) mediates the clearance of free t-PA and the t-PA/PAI-1 and u-PA/PAI-1 complexes. Complex formation of t-PA with PAI-1 increases the rate of clearance by LRP by at least one order of magnitude compared with that of free t-PA (30). The binding sites for t-PA/PAI-1 and u-PA/PAI-1 complexes are situated in the second complement-type domain cluster of LRP (31–33). The receptor-associated protein (RAP) inhibits endocytosis of most ligands to LRP (34).

Several as yet poorly characterized t-PA receptors have been identified on endothelial cells (35). In addition to actin, human umbilical vein endothelial cells (HUVEC) express 37-kDa and 45-kDa t-PA-binding proteins (36). A 20-kDa t-PA-binding protein was described, which does not interact with plasminogen, and is different from annexin II or α-enolase. In the presence of this receptor, plasminogen activation by t-PA is enhanced 90-fold. The type-II transmembrane protein p63 (CKAP4) on vascular smooth muscle cells interacts with the B-cahin of t-PA and potentiates plasminogen activation about 100-fold (37,38).

Tissue-Type Plasminogen Activator Derivates

By deletion or substitution of the functional domains, by site-specific point mutations and/or by altering the carbohydrate composition, mutants of rt-PA have been produced with higher fibrin-specificity, more zymogenicity, slower clearance from the circulation, and resistance to plasma proteinase inhibitors.

Reteplase is a single-chain nonglycosylated deletion variant consisting only of the kringle 2 and the proteinase domain of human t-PA; it contains amino acids 1–3 and 176–527 (deletion of Val^4-Glu^{175}); the Arg^{275}-Ile^{276} plasmin cleave site is maintained (39). Reteplase has a similar plasminogenolytic activity as wild-type rt-PA in the absence of a stimulator, but its activity in the presence of a stimulator is fourfold lower, and its binding to fibrin is fivefold lower. Reteplase and rt-PA are inhibited by PAI-1 to a similar degree (39). Its use in the management of occlusive thrombotic disorders has been reviewed (40).

In tenecteplase (TNK-rt-PA), replacement of Asn^{117} with Gln (N117Q) deletes the glycosylation site in kringle 1, whereas substitution of Thr^{103} by Asn (T103N) reintroduces a glycosylation site in kringle 1, but at a different locus; these modifications substantially decrease the plasma clearance rate. In addition, the amino acids Lys^{296}-His^{297}-Arg^{298}-Arg^{299} are each replaced with Ala, which confers resistance to inhibition by PAI-1 (41). Tenecteplase has a similar ability as wild-type rt-PA to bind to fibrin, and lyses fibrin clots in a plasma milieu with enhanced fibrin-specificity and delayed inhibition by PAI-1 (41).

Lanoteplase (n-PA) is a deletion mutant of rt-PA (without the finger and growth factor domains), in which glycosylation at Asn^{117} is lacking (42). Monteplase has a single amino acid substitution in the growth factor domain (Cys^{84} to Ser) (43); its therapeutic potential in treatment of acute myocardial infarction has been reviewed (44). Pamiteplase has deletion of the kringle 1 domain and substitution of Arg^{275} to Glu (rendering it resistant to conversion to a two-chain molecule by plasmin) (45). In the FAST-3 trial, monteplase and pamiteplase have been used for single bolus intravenous fibrinolysis in patients with ischemic-type chest discomfort (46).

Several of these rt-PA variants have a significantly slower clearance allowing bolus administration. Thus, reported half-lives in patients are 11 to 20 minutes for tenecteplase, 14 to 18 minutes for reteplase, 23 to 27 minutes for lanoteplase, 23 minutes for monteplase, and 30 to 47 minutes for pamiteplase (reviewed in 47,48).

Different molecular forms of the *Desmodus rotundus* salivary plasminogen activator (DSPA) have been characterized (49,50). Two high M_r forms, DSPAα$_1$ (43 kDa) and DSPAα$_2$ (39 kDa) show about 70% to 80% structural homology with human t-PA, but contain neither a kringle 2 domain nor a plasmin-sensitive cleavage site. DSPAβ lacks the finger domain, and DSPAγ lacks the finger and growth factor domains. DSPAα$_1$ and DSPAα$_2$ exhibit a specific activity in vitro that is equal to or higher than that of rt-PA, a relative PAI-1 resistance and a greatly enhanced fibrin-specificity with a strict requirement for polymeric fibrin as a cofactor (50). In several animal models of thrombolysis, DSPAα$_1$ (desmoteplase) has a 2.5 times higher potency and four- to eightfold slower clearance than rt-PA (reviewed in 47,48). In patients with acute ischemic stroke, an elimination half-life of more than two hours (up to 4.7 hr) was reported, which may have a positive impact on reocclusion rates. Desmoteplase has 70% structural homology to human t-PA, but it is a heterologous protein and may be antigenic in man.

Urokinase-Type Plasminogen Activator

u-PA is secreted as a 54-kDa single-chain molecule (scu-PA, pro-urokinase) that can be converted to a two-chain form (tcu-PA). Recombinant scu-PA (saruplase) is expressed in *E. coli* and obtained as a 45-kDa nonglycosylated molecule. u-PA is a serine proteinase of 411 amino acids, with active site triad His^{204}, Asp^{255}, and Ser^{356} located in the serine proteinase (COOH-terminal) domain (51) (Fig. 3). The molecule contains an NH$_2$-terminal

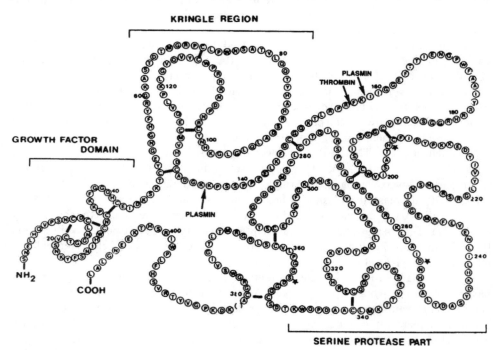

Figure 3 Schematic representation of the primary structure of scu-PA. The amino acids are represented by their single letter symbols, and black bars indicate disulfide bonds. The active-site residues are indicated with an asterisk. The arrows indicate the plasmin cleavage sites for conversion of 54 kDa scu-PA to 54 kDa tcu-PA (Lys^{158}-Ile^{159}) and of 54 kDa tcu-PA to 33 kDa tcu-PA (Lys^{135}-Lys^{136}), and for conversion of 54 kDa scu-PA to inactive 54 kDa tcu-PA by thrombin (Arg^{156}-Phe^{157}). *Abbreviations*: scu-PA, single-chain urokinase-type plasminogen activator; kDa, kilodalton; tcu-PA, two-chain urokinase-type plasminogen activator.

growth factor domain and one kringle structure homologous to the kringles of plasminogen and t-PA; it contains only one N-glycosylation site (at Asn^{302}), and is fucosylated at Thr^{18}. Phosporylation at Ser^{138} and Ser^{303} impairs the binding to cells and the interaction with PAI-1 (52). Conversion of scu-PA to tcu-PA occurs after proteolytic cleavage at position Lys^{158}-Ile^{159} by plasmin, but also by kallikrein, factor XIIa, trypsin, cathepsin B, human T cell associated serine proteainse-1, and thermolysin. A fully active tcu-PA derivative (33 kDa) is obtained after additional proteolysis by plasmin at position Lys^{135}-Lys^{136}. A low M_r form of scu-PA (32 kDa) is generated by cleavage of the Glu^{143}-Leu^{144} peptide bond. Thrombin cleaves the Arg^{156}-Phe^{157} peptide bond in scu-PA (53,54) resulting in an inactive two-chain derivative that can be reactivated by plasmin or cathepsin C (55,56).

In contrast to tcu-PA, scu-PA displays very low activity toward low molecular weight chromogenic substrates, but it appears to have some intrinsic plasminogen activating potential, which represents ≤0.5% of the catalytic efficiency of tcu-PA (57). The interaction of Lys^{300} with Asp^{335} in the flexible loop region 297–313 stabilizes the conformation of scu-PA by pulling the adjacent Ser^{356} close to the position found in the fully active enzyme (58).

In the plasma, in the absence of fibrin, scu-PA is stable and does not activate plasminogen; however, in the presence of a fibrin clot, scu-PA, but not tcu-PA, induces fibrin-specific clot lysis, although it does not bind to fibrin (59). This was explained by the finding that scu-PA is an inefficient activator of plasminogen bound to internal lysine residues on intact fibrin, but has a higher activity toward plasminogen bound to newly generated COOH-terminal lysine residues on partially degraded fibrin (60,61). The generation of small amounts of fibrin-bound plasmin, protected from α_2-antiplasmin, stimulates conversion of scu-PA to tcu-PA resulting in enhanced fibrinolysis.

The activity of scu-PA is increased by two orders of magnitude when it is bound to its receptor (uPAR) on the surface of monocytes (62,63). This is the result of colocalization with plasminogen rather than a direct effect of uPAR on the catalytic efficiency (64). This local activity may be relevant to thrombus stability, since monocytes migrate into the clot (65) and express fibrinolytic activity (66). In freshly formed clots, most of the spontaneously generated fibrinolytic activity can be inhibited by antibodies to u-PA (67).

tcu-PA, but not scu-PA, is rapidly inhibited by PAI-1 and PAI-2. Rapid inhibition by PAI-1 requires interaction with a positively-charged region in u-PA, (residues 179–184) (68). The main mechanism of removal of u-PA from the blood is, however, by hepatic clearance. scu-PA is taken up in the liver via a recognition site on parenchymal cells and is subsequently degraded in the lysosomes (69). Following intravenous infusion of recombinant scu-PA in patients with acute myocardial infarction, a biphasic disappearance was observed with initial half-life in plasma of eight minutes (70).

Amediplase, a recombinant chimeric PA consisting of the kringle 2 domain of t-PA and the COOH-terminal region of scu-PA displays a lower fibrin binding than t-PA, but has a higher clot-penetrating potency, similar to that of tcu-PA (71). In different external plasma clot lysis models, amediplase was slightly more active than tenecteplase and scu-PA (72). It is being evaluated for bolus administration to patients with acute myocardial infarction (73).

Nonenzyme Plasminogen Activators

Staphylokinase and Derivatives

Staphylokinase is a 135 amino acid protein (comprising 45 charged amino acids, no cysteine residues nor glycosylation), secreted by Staphylococcus *aureus* strains after lysogenic conversion or transformation with bacteriophages. The primary structure shows no homology with that of other plasminogen activators. Staphylokinase folds into a compact ellipsoid structure in which the core of the protein is composed exclusively of hydrophobic amino acids. It is folded into a mixed five-stranded, slightly twisted β-sheet, which wraps around a central α-helix and has two additional short two-stranded β-sheets opposing the central sheet (74). Recombinant staphylokinase is obtained by expression in *E. coli* (75,76).

Staphylokinase forms a 1:1 stoichiometric complex with plasmin. It is not an enzyme, and generation of an active site in its equimolar complex with plasminogen requires conversion of plasminogen to plasmin. During the activation process, the 10 NH_2-terminal amino acids of staphylokinase are cleaved off. In plasma, in the absence of fibrin, no significant amounts of the complex with plasmin are generated, because traces of plasmin are rapidly inhibited by α_2-antiplasmin. In the presence of fibrin, generation of the active complex is facilitated because traces of fibrin-bound plasmin are protected from α_2-antiplasmin, and inhibition of the plasmin-staphylokinase complex at the clot surface is delayed more than 100-fold. Furthermore, it does not bind to a significant extent to plasminogen in circulating plasma, but binds with high affinity to plasmin and to plasminogen, which is bound to partially degraded fibrin (77–79).

Staphylokinase, being a heterologous protein, is immunogenic in man. The wild-type protein contains three immunodominant epitopes. A comprehensive site-directed mutagenesis program resulted in the identification of variants with reduced antigenicity, but maintained fibrinolytic potency and fibrin-specificity, such as the variant with substitutions of K35A, E65Q, K74R, E80A, D82A, T90A, E99D, T101S, E108A, K109A, K130T, and K135R (code SY161) (80). Furthermore, SY161 with Ser[3] mutated into Cys was derivatized with maleimide-substituted polyethylene glycol (P) with molecular weights of 5000 (P5), 10,000 (P10), or 20,000 (P20), and characterized in vitro and in vivo (81). Staphylokinase-related antigen following bolus injection of SY161-P5, SY161-P10, or SY161-P20 in patients disappeared from plasma with an initial half-life of 13, 30, and 120 minutes and was cleared at a rate of 75, 43, and 8 mL/min, respectively, as compared with an initial half-life of 3 minutes and a clearance of 360 mL/min for wild-type staphylokinase (81).

Streptokinase and Derivatives

Streptokinase is a nonenzyme protein produced by several strains of hemolytic streptococci. It consists of a single polypeptide chain of 47 to 50 kDa with 414 amino acids (82). The region comprising amino acids 1 to 230 shows some homology with trypsin-like serine proteinases, but lacks an active site serine residue. NMR and crystallographic studies revealed a three-domain structure (83). The binding site for a kringle in plasminogen is located at the tip of a fully exposed hairpin loop in the β-domain of streptokinase (84,85).

Streptokinase activates plasminogen indirectly, following a three-step mechanism (86). In the first step, streptokinase forms an equimolar complex with plasminogen, which undergoes a conformational change resulting in the exposure of an active site in the plasminogen moiety. In the second step, this active site catalyzes the activation of plasminogen to plasmin. In the third step, plasminogen-streptokinase molecules are converted to plasmin-streptokinase complexes. The active-site residues in the plasmin-streptokinase complex are the same as those in the plasmin molecule. The main differences between the enzymatic properties of both moieties are that plasmin, in contrast to its complex with streptokinase, is unable to activate plasminogen and is rapidly neutralized by α_2-antiplasmin, which does not inhibit the complex. Since streptokinase generates free circulating plasmin when α_2-antiplasmin becomes exhausted, its use is associated with generation of a systemic lytic state.

Streptokinase is highly antigenic. Most apparently healthy persons have antibodies in their blood, due presumably to previous infections with β-hemolytic streptococci, and antibody titers may rise several 100-fold after administration to humans (87,88). After intravenous injection into humans, dogs, or mice, streptokinase is cleared from the circulation with a half-life of 15 to 30 minutes (89). Clearance mostly takes place in the liver, primarily by the α_2-macroglobulin receptor (89), which is identical to LRP (28).

APSAC (anistreplase, Eminase™, SmithKline & Beecham, Philadelphia, Pennsylvania, U.S.), is an equimolar noncovalent complex between human Lys-plasminogen and streptokinase. The catalytic center is located in the COOH-terminal region of plasminogen, whereas the lysine-binding sites (with only weak fibrin affinity) are comprised within the NH$_2$-terminal region of the molecule. Specific acylation of the catalytic center in the complex is achieved by the use of a reversible acylating agent, p-amidinophenyl-p'-anisate.HCl. This approach should prevent premature neutralization of the agent in the bloodstream and enable its activation to proceed in a controlled and sustained manner (90). Deacylation indeed uncovers the catalytic center, which converts plasminogen to plasmin (90). In experimental animal models, APSAC had a better clot specificity than streptokinase as it caused less fibrinogenolysis and consumption of plasminogen or α_2-antiplasmin and was less hypotensive (92). Clinical studies showed that APSAC is an effective thrombolytic agent, but the systemic effects are comparable with those of streptokinase.

DIRECT FIBRINOLYTICS

Plasmin(ogen) and Derivatives

Plasmin, the key enzyme responsible for degradation of fibrin, is generated by activation of the zymogen plasminogen. Human plasminogen is a 92-kDa single-chain glycoprotein, consisting of 791 amino acids; it contains 24 disulfide bonds and 5 homologous kringles (92). Its normal plasma concentration is 1.5 to 2.0 µM. It has a half-life of more than two days and is cleared via the liver. Native plasminogen has NH$_2$-terminal glutamic acid ("Glu-plasminogen"), but is easily converted by limited plasmic digestion to modified forms with NH$_2$-terminal lysine, valine, or methionine, commonly designated "Lys-plasminogen." Conversion to plasmin occurs by cleavage of the Arg^{561}-Val^{562} peptide bond, yielding a two-chain molecule stabilized by two disulfide bonds. The active site of plasmin consists of the catalytic triad His^{603}, Asp^{646}, Ser^{741}. Plasmin cleaves fibrinogen and fibrin directly, preferentially after Lys and Arg residues. Plasmin(ogen) derivatives lacking kringles 1 to 4 [mini-plasmin(ogen)] or consisting only of the proteinase domain [micro-plasmin(ogen)] have also been characterized.

The plasminogen kringles contain lysine-binding sites that mediate the specific binding of plasminogen to fibrin and the interaction of plasmin with α_2-antiplasmin; they play a crucial role in the regulation of fibrinolysis (24). The lysine-binding site in kringle 4 is formed by the hydrophobic residues Trp^{62}, Phe^{64}, and Trp^{72} surrounded by the positively charged Lys^{35} and Arg^{71} on one side and by the negatively charged side chains of Asp^{55} and Asp^{57} at a distance of about 7 Å. This structure allows ideal docking of zwitter ions, such as lysine, of which the opposite charges are also 7 Å apart (93). The lysine-binding sites in the other kringles have similar overall structure.

The main plasmin inhibitor is α_2-antiplasmin, a 70-kDa single-chain glycoprotein containing about 13% carbohydrate and 464 amino acids (94,95). α_2-Antiplasmin is a serpin with reactive site peptide bond Arg^{376}-Met^{377}. Its concentration in normal human plasma is about 1 μM. α_2-Antiplasmin forms an inactive 1:1 stoichiometric complex with plasmin. The inhibition of plasmin (P) by α_2-antiplasmin (A) can be represented by two consecutive reactions: a fast, second-order reaction producing a reversible inactive complex (PA), which is followed by a slower first-order transition resulting in an irreversible complex (PA'). This model can be represented by: P + A $\leftrightarrows$ PA → PA'. The second-order rate constant of the inhibition is very high (2 to 4 × 10^7 $M^{-1}s^{-1}$), but this high inhibition rate is dependent both upon the presence of a free lysine-binding site and an active site in the plasmin molecule, and upon availability of a plasminogen-binding site and reactive site peptide bond in the inhibitor (96). The half-life of plasmin molecules on the fibrin surface, which have both their lysine-binding sites and active site occupied, is estimated to be two to three orders of magnitude longer than that of free plasmin (97). Also plasmin moieties lacking the lysine-binding sites in kringles 1 to 4 show significantly reduced inhibition rates by α_2-antiplasmin.

Because of the rapid inhibition of plasmin by α_2-antiplasmin and the limited substrate specificity of excess circulating plasmin, systemic administration of plasmin for thrombolytic therapy was generally not considered to be a valid option. In the 1950s and 1960s intravenous plasmin for thrombolytic therapy had been investigated in pilot studies in humans. Although plasmin was generally well tolerated, these studies were discontinued, probably because of a lack of understanding of the kinetics of the inhibition of plasmin in plasma (α_2-antiplasmin was not yet discovered), the unavailability of local catheter delivery, and the lack of adequate methods for the production of stable plasmin devoid of plasminogen activators (98,99). However, recently re-examination of local administration of plasmin for arterial and venous thrombolysis was suggested. This was triggered by a study showing that plasmin induced local thrombolysis without causing hemorrhage in the rabbit (98). Hypothetical advances of plasmin over plasminogen activators would be: (*i*) no activation is needed; (*ii*) local delivery allows it to attach to and lyse thrombi; and (*iii*) after thrombolysis circulating plasmin is rapidly neutralized by α_2-antiplasmin. These considerations would suggest that local plasmin administration would not cause re-bleeding from preformed hemostatic plugs and be efficient and safe for the dissolution of long, retracted blood clots (100).

Development of adequate methods to produce highly purified natural human plasmin (98) or recombinant human microplasmin (101–103) preparations and procedures to stabilize its activity (104) has made it possible to reinvestigate the potential as a fibrinolytic agent. Studies in animal models indicate that plasmin or derivatives may be useful for treatment of ischemic stroke. Thus Nagai et al. reported a reduction in infarct size in mice with a permanent ligation of the middle cerebral artery, with a bolus of human plasmin, which was associated with neutralization of plasma α_2-antiplasmin (105,106). Microplasmin, lacking the lysine-binding sites, has no affinity for fibrin and is inhibited more slowly by α_2-antiplasmin than intact plasmin; being a truncated molecule it may be easier to obtain a pharmaceutically useful preparation. In animal models of ischemic stroke and peripheral arterial occlusion, microplasmin was comparable in potency with full-length plasmin. It did not cause a bleeding tendency or a hemostatic plug dissolution at distant sites. These data suggest that (micro)plasmin may be useful for the treatment of arterial thromboembolic disease by local catheter delivery and of ischemic stroke by systemic administration.

An engineered plasminogen variant has been constructed with an activation site, in which the P3-P1' residues were substituted by the P7-P1' residues (Thr^{363}-Ile^{370}) of factor XI. In addition, two mutations were introduced in the proteinase domain, Glu^{606} and Glu^{623} to Lys (BB-10153). The resulting plasminogen moiety is activated by thrombin. It would persist in the blood as a prodrug with long half-life and be activated to plasmin only at fresh or forming thrombi by localized thrombin (107). In the rabbit and dog, BB-10153 lysed thrombi and prevented reocclusion following bolus administration. Thrombotically active doses did not produce systemic plasmin activity and did not affect bleeding time (108). In healthy volunteers, BB-10153 was well tolerated and had a plasma half-life of three to four hours. No effects were observed on plasma levels of α_2-antiplasmin or fibrinogen, on coagulation assays or bleeding time (109).

Fibrinolytic Enzymes from Snake Venom

Two distinct classes of venom fibrin(ogen)olytic enzymes have been identified, metalloproteinases (e.g., fibrolase) and serine proteinases (e.g., β-fibrinogenolytic proteinase from *Macrovipera lebetina*). Fibrolase, isolated from the Southern Copperhead snake (*Agkistrodon contortrix contortrix*) venom has been considered as a potential agent to treat occlusive thrombi (110). A truncated form of fibrolase called alfimeprase, with NH_2-terminal sequence Ser-Phe-Pro- and molecular weight 22.6 kDa (201 amino acids), has been produced by recombinant DNA technology and expressed in *E. coli* (111) and in *Pichia pastoris* (112). Like fibrolase, alfimeprase induces direct protelytic cleavage of both α and β chains of fibrin and fibrinogen, but not of γ chains. Circulating proteinase is rapidly inhibited by α_2-macroglobulin.

Pharmacokinetic studies showed that alfimeprase is rapidly absorbed and achieves therapeutic concentrations at relatively low doses. Preclinical studies showed that adjunctive therapy with antiplatelet agents is necessary to maintain luminal patency. In phase I and II clinical trials in patients with peripheral arterial occlusion, alfimeprase effectively lysed clots with no drug-related adverse effects (113). A phase II study showed that alfimeprase restored blood flow after four hours in occluded catheters in 80% of patients, as compared with 62% with activase (114). The potential of alfimeprase remains to be confirmed in phase III clinical trials, and may require refining of its dose and administration scheme (113).

CONCLUSIONS

Thrombolytic agents are plasminogen activators that convert the zymogen plasminogen to the active enzyme plasmin, which degrades fibrin, or are direct fibrinolytic agents. All currently used thrombolytic agents have significant shortcomings, including the need for large therapeutic doses, limited fibrin-specificity, and significant associated bleeding tendency and reocclusion. Newly developed thrombolytic agents, mutants, and variants of the serine proteinases t-PA or u-PA, have reduced plasma clearance and lower reactivity with proteinase inhibitors and maintained or enhanced PA potency and/or fibrin-specificity. The nonenzyme bacterial PA staphylokinase has also shown promise for fibrin-specific thrombolysis, although neutralizing antibodies are elicited in most patients. Local delivery of plasmin or plasmin derivatives and the use of snake venom–derived direct fibrinolytics are under investigation for clinical application.

REFERENCES

1. Collen D. Thrombolytic therapy. Thromb Haemost 1997; 78:742–746.
2. Lijnen HR, Collen D. Tissue-type plasminogen activator. In: Barrett AJ, Rawlings ND, Woessner JF, eds. Handbook of Proteolytic Enzymes. London: Academic Press, 1998:184–190.

3. Astrup T, Permin PM. Fibrinolysis in animal organism. Nature 1947; 159:681–682.
4. Rijken DC, Wijngaards G, Zaal-de Jong M, et al. Purification and partial characterization of plasminogen activator from human uterine tissue. Biochim Biophys Acta 1979; 580:140–153.
5. Rijken DC, Wijngaards G, Welbergen J. Relationship between tissue plasminogen activator and the activators in blood and vascular wall. Thromb Res 1980; 18:815–830.
6. Rijken DC, Collen D. Purification and characterization of the plasminogen activator secreted by human melanoma cells in culture. J Biol Chem 1981; 256:7035–7041.
7. Pennica D, Holmes WE, Kohr WJ, et al. Cloning and expression of human tissue-type plasminogen activator cDNA in E. coli. Nature 1983; 301:214–221.
8. Collen D, Stassen JM, Marafino BJ, et al. Biological properties of human tissue-type plasminogen activator obtained by expression of recombinant DNA in mammalian cells. J Pharmacol Exp Ther 1984; 231:146–152.
9. Upshall A, Kumar AA, Bailey MC, et al. Secretion of active human tissue plasminogen activator from the filamentous fungus Aspergillus-nidulans. Biotechnology 1987; 5:1301–1304.
10. Reddy VB, Garramone AJ, Sasak H, et al. Expression of human uterine tissue-type plasminogen activator in mouse cells using BPV vectors. J Mol Biol 1987; 6:461–472.
11. Madison EL, Kobe A, Gething MJ, et al. Converting tissue plasminogen activator to a zymogen: a regulatory triad of Asp-His-Ser. Science 1993; 262:419–421.
12. Madison EL. Probing structure-function relationships of tissue-type plasminogen activator by site-specific mutagenesis. Fibrinolysis 1994; 8(suppl 1):221–236.
13. Lamba D, Bauer M, Huber R, et al. The 2.3 Å crystal structure of the catalytic domain of recombinant two-chain human tissue-type plasminogen activator. J Mol Biol 1996; 258:117–135.
14. Parekh RB, Dwek RA, Thomas JR, et al. Cell-type-specific and site-specific N-glycosylation of type I and type II human tissue plasminogen activator. Biochemistry 1989; 28:7644–7662.
15. Dwek RA. Glycobiology: "Towards understanding the function of sugars". Biochem Soc Trans 1995; 23:1–25.
16. Harris RJ, Leonard CK, Guzzetta AW, et al. Tissue plasminogen activator has on O-linked fucose attached to threonine-61 in the epidermal growth factor domain. Biochemistry 1991; 30:2311–2314.
17. Hajjar KA, Reynolds CM. α-Fucose-mediated binding and degradation of tissue-type plasminogen activator by HepG2 cells. J Clin Invest 1994; 93:703–710.
18. Hoylaerts M, Rijken DC, Lijnen HR, et al. Kinetics of the activation of plasminogen by human tissue plasminogen activator. Role of fibrin. J Biol Chem 1982; 257:2912–2919.
19. Thorsen S. The mechanism of plasminogen activation and the variability of the fibrin effector during tissue-type plasminogen activator-mediated fibrinolysis. Ann N Y Acad Sci 1992; 667:52–63.
20. Yonekawa O, Voskuilen M, Nieuwenhuizen W. Localization in the fibrinogen γ-chain of a new site that is involved in the acceleration of the tissue-type plasminogen activator-catalysed activation of plasminogen. Biochem J 1992; 283:187–191.
21. Schielen WJG, Adams HPHM, van Leuven K, et al. The sequence γ-(312-324) is a fibrin-specific epitope. Blood 1991; 77:2169–2173.
22. Tsurupa G, Medved L. Identification and characterization of novel t-PA- and plasminogen-binding sites within fibrin(ogen) αC-domains. Biochemistry 2001; 40:801–808.
23. Mosesson MW, Siebenlist KR, Voskuilen M, et al. Evaluation of the factors contributing to fibrin-dependent plasminogen activation. Thromb Haemost 1998; 79:796–801.
24. Collen D. On the regulation and control of fibrinolysis. Thromb Haemost 1980; 43:77–89.
25. Madison EL, Goldsmith EJ, Gerard RD, et al. Serpin-resistant mutants of human tissue-type plasminogen activator. Nature 1989; 339:721–727.
26. Otter M, Barrett-Bergshoeff MM, Rijken DC. Binding of tissue-type plasminogen activator by the mannose receptor. J Biol Chem 1991; 266:13931–13935.
27. Noorman F, Barrett-Bergshoeff MM, Rijken DC. Role of carbohydrate and protein in the binding of tissue-type plasminogen activator to the human mannose receptor. Eur J Biochem 1998; 251:107–113.

28. Strickland DK, Ranganathan S. Diverse role of LDL receptor-related protein in the clearance of proteases and in signaling. J Thromb Haemost 2003; 1:1663–1670.
29. Narita M, Bu G, Herz J, et al. Two receptor systems are involved in the plasma clearance of tissue-type plasminogen activator (tPA) in vivo. J Clin Invest 1995; 95:1663–1670.
30. Camani C, Bachmann F, Kruithof EKO. The role of plasminogen activator inhibitor type 1 in the clearance of tissue-type plasminogen activator by rat hepatoma cells. J Biol Chem 1994; 269:5770–5775.
31. Moestrup SK, Holtet TL, Etzerodt M, et al. α_2-Macroglobulin-proteinase complexes, plasminogen activator inhibitor type-1-plasminogen activator complexes, and receptor-associated protein bind to a region of the α_2-macroglobulin receptor containing a cluster of eight complement-type repeats. J Biol Chem 1993; 268:13691–13696.
32. Willnow TE, Orth K, Herz J. Molecular dissection of ligand binding sites on the low density lipoprotein receptor-related protein. J Biol Chem 1994; 269:15827–15832.
33. Horn IR, Van den Berg BMM, van der Meijden PZ, et al. Molecular analysis of ligand binding to the second cluster of complement-type repeats of the low density lipoprotein receptor-related protein. Evidence for an allosteric component in receptor-associated protein-mediated inhibition of ligand binding. J Biol Chem 1997; 272:13608–13613.
34. Herz J, Goldstein JL, Strickland DK, et al. 39-kDa protein modulates binding of ligands to low density lipoprotein receptor-related protein/α_2-macroglobulin receptor. J Biol Chem 1991; 266:21232–21238.
35. Redlitz A, Plow EF. Receptors for plasminogen and tPA: an update. Baillieres Clin Haematol 1995; 8:313–327.
36. Dudani AK, Ganz PR. Endothelial cell surface actin serves as a binding site for plasminogen, tissue plasminogen activator and lipoprotein(a). Br J Haematol 1996; 95:168–178.
37. Werner F, Razzaq TM, Ellis V. Tissue plasminogen activator binds to human vascular smooth muscle cells by a novel mechanism. Evidence for a reciprocal linkage between inhibition of catalytic activity and cellular binding. J Biol Chem 1999; 274:21555–21561.
38. Razzaq TM, Bass R, Vines DJ, et al. Functional regulation of tissue plasminogen activator on the surface of vascular smooth muscle cells by the type-II transmembrane protein p63 (CKAP4). J Biol Chem 2003; 278:42679–42685.
39. Kohnert U, Rudolph R, Verheijen JH, et al. Biochemical properties of the kringle 2 and protease domains are maintained in the refolded t-PA deletion variant BM 06.022. Protein Eng 1992; 5:93–100.
40. Simpson D, Siddiqui MA, Scott LJ, et al. Reteplase: a review of its use in the management of thrombotic occlusive disorders. Am J Cardiovasc Drugs 2006; 6:265–285.
41. Paoni NF, Keyt BA, Refino CJ, et al. A slow clearing, fibrin-specific, PAI-1 resistant variant of t-PA (T103N,KHRR296-299AAAA). Thromb Haemost 1993; 70:307–312.
42. Den Heijer P, Vermeer F, Ambrosioni E, et al. Evaluation of a weight-adjusted single-bolus plasminogen activator in patients with myocardial infarction: a double-blind, randomized angiographic trial of lanoteplase versus alteplase. Circulation 1998; 98:2117–2125.
43. Suzuki S, Saito M, Suzuki N, et al. Thrombolytic properties of a novel modified human tissue-type plasminogen activator (E6010): a bolus injection of E6010 has equivalent potency of lysing young and aged canine coronary thrombi. J Cardiovasc Pharmacol 1991; 17:738–746.
44. Inoue T, Nishiki R, Kageyama M, et al. Therapeutic potential of monteplase in acute myocardial infarction. Am J Cardiovasc Drugs 2005; 5:255–231.
45. Katoh M, Suzuki Y, Miyamoto T. Biochemical and pharmacokinetic properties of YM866, a novel fibrinolytic agent. Thromb Haemost 1991; 65:1193 (abstr 1794).
46. Watanabe K, Nagao K, Watanabe I, et al. Relationship between the door-to-TIMI-3 flow time and the infarct size in patients suffering from acute myocardial infarction. Analysis based on the fibrinolysis and subsequent transluminal (FAST-3) Trial. Circ J 2004; 68:280–285.
47. Lijnen HR, Collen D. Strategies for the improvement of thrombolytic agents. Thromb Haemost 1991; 66:88–110.
48. Lijnen HR, Collen D. New thrombolytic strategies and agents. Hematologica 2000; 85(suppl. 2): 106–109.

49. Gardell SJ, Duong LT, Diehl RE et al. Isolation, characterization and cDNA cloning of a vampire bat salivary plasminogen activator. J Biol Chem 1989; 264:17947–17952.

50. Krätzschmar J, Haendler B, Langer G. The plasminogen activator family from the salivary gland of the vampire bat Desmodus rotundus: cloning and expression. Gene 1991; 105:229–237.

51. Holmes WE, Pennica D, Blaber M, et al. Cloning and expression of the gene for pro-urokinase in Escherichia coli. Biotechnology 1985; 3:923–929.

52. Franco P, Iaccarino C, Chiaradonna F, et al. Phosphorylation of human pro-urokinase on Ser138/303 impairs its receptor-dependent ability to promote myelomonocytic adherence and motility. J Cell Biol 1997; 137:779–791.

53. Ichinose, Fujikawa K, Suyama T. The activation of pro-urokinase by plasma kallikrein and its inactivation by thrombin. J Biol Chem 1986; 261:3486–3489.

54. Gurewich V, Pannell R. Inactivation of single-chain urokinase (pro-urokinase) by thrombin and thrombin-like enzymes: relevance of the findings to the interpretation of fibrin-binding experiments. Blood 1987; 69:769–772.

55. Lijnen HR, Van Hoef B, Collen D. Activation with plasmin of two-chain urokinase-type plasminogen activator derived from single-chain urokinase-type plasminogen activator by treatment with thrombin. Eur J Biochem 1987; 169:359–364.

56. Nauland U, Rijken DC. Activation of thrombin-inactivated single-chain urokinase-type plasminogen activator by dipeptidyl peptidase I (cathepsin C). Eur J Biochem 1994; 223:497–501.

57. Lijnen HR, Van Hoef B, Nelles L, et al. Plasminogen activation with single-chain urokinase-type plasminogen activator (scu-PA). Studies with active site mutagenized plasminogen (Ser740→Ala) and plasmin-resistant scu-PA (Lys158→Glu). J Biol Chem 1990; 265:5232–5236.

58. Sun Z, Liu BF, Chen Y, et al. Analysis of the forces which stabilize the active conformation of urokinase-type plasminogen activator. Biochemistry 1998; 37:2935–2940.

59. Gurewich V, Pannell R, Louie S, et al. Effective and fibrin-specific clot lysis by a zymogen precursor form of urokinase (pro-urokinase). A study in vitro and in two animal species. J Clin Invest 1984; 73:1731–1739.

60. Liu JN, Gurewich V. Fragment E-2 from fibrin substantially enhances pro-urokinase-induced Glu-plasminogen activation. A kinetic study using the plasmin-resistant mutant pro-urokinase Ala-158-rpro-UK. Biochemistry 1992; 31:6311–6317.

61. Fleury V, Lijnen HR, Anglès-Cano E. Mechanism of the enhanced intrinsic activity of single-chain urokinase-type plasminogen activator during ongoing fibrinolysis. J Biol Chem 1993; 268:18554–18559.

62. Ellis V, Scully MF, Kakkar VV. Plasminogen activation initiated by single-chain urokinase-type plasminogen activator. Potentiation by U937 monocytes. J Biol Chem 1989; 264:2185–2188.

63. Manchanda N, Schwartz BS. Single chain urokinase. Augmentation of enzymatic activity upon binding to monocytes. J Biol Chem 1991; 266:14580–14584.

64. Ellis V. Functional analysis of the cellular receptor for urokinase in plasminogen activation. Receptor binding has no influence on the zymogenic nature of pro-urokinase. J Biol Chem 1996; 271:14779–14784.

65. McGuinness CL, Humphries J, Waltham M, et al. Recruitment of labelled monocytes by experimental venous thrombi. Thromb Haemost 2001; 85:1018–1024.

66. Grau E, Moroz LA. Fibrinolytic activity of normal human blood monocytes. Thromb Res 1989; 53:145–162.

67. Mutch NJ, Moir E, Robbie LA, et al. Localization and identification of thrombin and plasminogen activator activities in model human thrombi by in situ zymography. Thromb Haemost 2002; 88:996–1002.

68. Adams DS, Griffin LA, Nachajko WR, et al. A synthetic DNA encoding a modified human urokinase resistant to inhibition by serum plasminogen activator inhibitor. J Biol Chem 1991; 266:8476–8482.

69. Kuiper J, Rijken DC, de Munk GAW, et al. In vivo and in vitro interaction of high and low molecular weight single-chain urokinase-type plasminogen activator with rat liver cells. J Biol Chem 1992; 267:1589–1595.

70. Van de Werf F, Vanhaecke J, De Geest H, et al. Coronary thrombolysis with recombinant single-chain urokinase-type plasminogen activator (rscu-PA) in patients with acute myocardial infarction. Circulation 1986; 74:1066–1070.

71. Rijken DC, Barrett-Bergshoeff MM, Jie AF, et al. Clot penetration and fibrin binding of amediplase, a chimeric plasminogen activator (K2 tu-PA). Thromb Haemost 2004; 91:52–60.

72. Guimaraes AH, Barrett-Bergshoeff MM, Criscuoli M, et al. Fibrinolytic efficacy of Amediplase, Tenecteplse and scu-PA in different external plasma clot lysis models: sensitivity to the inhibitory action of thrombin activatable fibrinolysis inhibitor (TAFI). Thromb Haemost 2006; 96:325–330.

73. BioDrugs R and D Profile. . Amediplase: CGP 42935, K2tu-PA, MEN 9036. BioDrugs 2002; 16:378–379.

74. Rabijns A, De Bondt HL, De Ranter C. Three-dimensional structure of staphylokinase, a plasminogen activator with therapeutic potential. Nat Struct Biol 1997; 4:357–360.

75. Behnke D, Gerlach D. Cloning and expression in Escherichia coli, Bacillus subtilis and Streptococcus sanguis of a gene for staphylokinase: a bacterial plasminogen activator. Mol Gen Genet 1987; 210:528-534.

76. Collen D, Zhao ZA, Holvoet P, et al. Primary structure and gene structure of staphylokinase. Fibrinolysis 1992; 6:226–231.

77. Lijnen HR, Collen D. Staphylokinase, a fibrin-specific bacterial plasminogen activator. Fibrinolysis 1996; 10:119–126.

78. Collen D. Staphylokinase: a potent, uniquely fibrin-selective thrombolytic agent. Nat Med 1998; 4:279–284.

79. Collen D. The plasminogen (fibrinolytic) system. Thromb Haemost 1999; 82:259–270.

80. Laroche Y, Heymans S, Capaert S, et al. Recombinant staphylokinase variants with reduced antigenicity due to elimination of B-lymphocyte epitopes. Blood 2000; 96:1425–1432.

81. Collen D, Sinnaeve P, Demarsin E, et al. Polyethylene glycol-derivatized cysteine-substitution variants of recombinant staphylokinase for single-bolus treatment of acute myocardial infarction. Circulation 2000; 102:1766–1772.

82. Jackson KW, Tang J. Complete amino acid sequence of streptokinase and its homology with serine proteases. Biochemistry 1982; 21:6620–6625.

83. Wang X, Lin X, Loy JA, et al. Crystal structure of the catalytic domain of human plasmin complexed with streptokinase. Science 1998; 281:1662–1665.

84. Wang X, Tang J, Hunter B, et al. Crystal structure of streptokinase β-domain. FEBS Lett 199; 459:85–89.

85. Chaudhary A, Vasudha S, Rajagopal K, et al. Function of the central domain of streptokinase in substrate plasminogen docking and processing revealed by site-directed mutagenesis. Protein Sci 1999; 8:2791–2805.

86. Reddy KNN. Mechanism of activation of human plasminogen by streptokinase. In: Kline DL, Reddy KNN, eds. Fibrinolysis. Boca Raton: CRC Press, 1980:71–94.

87. Bachmann F. Development of antibodies against perorally and rectally administered streptokinase in man. J Lab Clin Med 1968; 72:228–238.

88. Ojalvo AG, Pozo L, Labarta V, et al. Prevalence of circulating antibodies against a streptokinase C-terminal peptide in normal blood donors. Biochem Biophys Res Commun 1999; 263:454–459.

89. Gonias SL, Einarsson M, Pizzo SV. Catabolic pathways for streptokinase, plasmin and streptokinase activator complex in mice: in vivo reaction of plasminogen activator with α_2-macroglobulin. J Clin Invest 1982; 7:412–423.

90. Smith RAG, Dupe RJ, English PD, et al. Fibrinolysis with acyl-enzymes: a new approach to thrombolytic therapy. Nature 1981; 290:505–508.

91. Fears R. Development of anisoylated plasminogen-streptokinase activator complex from the acyl enzyme concept. Semin Thromb Hemost 1989; 15:129–139.

92. Forsgren M, Raden B, Israelsson M, et al. Molecular cloning and characterization of a full-length cDNA clone for human plasminogen. FEBS Lett 1987; 213:254–260.

93. Wu TP, Padmanabhan K, Tulinsky A, et al. The refined structure of the ε-aminocaproic acid complex of human plasminogen kringle 4. Biochemistry 1991; 30:10589–10594.

94. Holmes WE, Nelles L, Lijnen HR, et al. Primary structure of human alpha 2-antiplasmin, a serine protease inhibitor (serpin). J Biol Chem 1987; 262:1659–1664.

95. Bangert K, Johnsen AH, Christensen U, et al. Different N-terminal forms of α_2-plasmin inhibitor in human plasma. Biochem J 1993; 291:623–625.

96. Wiman B, Collen D. On the mechanism of the reaction between human α_2-antiplasmin and plasmin. J Biol Chem 1979; 254:9291–9297.

97. Wiman B, Collen D. On the kinetics of the reaction between human antiplasmin and plasmin. Eur J Biochem 1978; 84:573–578.

98. Marder VJ, Landskroner K, Novokhatny V, et al. Plasmin induces local thrombolysis without causing hemorrhage: a comparison with tissue plasminogen activator in the rabbit. Thromb Haemost 2001; 86:739–745.

99. Collen D. Revival of plasmin as a therapeutic agent? Thromb Haemost 2001; 86:731–732.

100. Novokhatny VV, Jesmok GJ, Landskroner KA, et al. Locally delivered plasmin: why should it be superior to plasminogen activators for direct thrombolysis? Trends Pharmacol Sci 2004; 25:72–75.

101. Nagai N, Demarsin E, Van Hoef B, et al. Recombinant human microplasmin: production and potential therapeutic properties. J Thromb Haemost 2003; 1:307–313.

102. Ma Z, Lu W, Wu S, et al. Expression and characterization of recombinant human microplasminogen. Biotechnol Lett 2007; 29:517–523.

103. Medynski D, Tuan M, Liu W, et al. Refolding, purification, and activation of miniplasminogen and microplasminogen isolated from E. coli inclusion bodies. Protein Expr Purif 2007; 52:395–402.

104. Novokhatny V, Taylor K, Zimmerman TP. Thrombolytic potency of acid-stabilized plasmin: superiority over tissue-type plasminogen activator in an in vitro model of catheter-assisted thrombolysis. J Thromb Haemost 2003; 1:1034–1041.

105. Nagai N, De Mol M, Van Hoef B, et al. Depletion of circulating α_2-antiplasmin by intravenous plasmin or immunoneutralization reduces focal cerebral ischemic injury in the absence of arterial recanalization. Hemostasis, Thrombosis and Vascular Biology 2001; 97:3086–3092.

106. Nagai N, De Mol M, Lijnen HR, et al. Role of plasminogen system components in focal cerebral ischemic infarction. A gene targeting and gene transfer study in mice. Circulation 1999; 99:2440–2444.

107. Dawson KM, Cook A, Devine JM, et al. Plasminogen mutants activated by thrombin: potential thrombo-selective thrombolytic agents. J Biol Chem 1994; 269:15989–15992.

108. Comer MB, Cackett KS, Gladwell S, et al. Thrombolytic activity of BB-10153, a thrombin-activatable plasminogen. J Thromb Haemost 2005; 3:146–153.

109. Curtis LD, Brown A, Comer MB, et al. Pharmacokinetics and pharmacodynamics of BB-10153, a thrombin-activatable plasminogen, in healthy volunteers. J Thromb Haemost 2005; 3:1180–1186.

110. Swenson S, Markland FS Jr. Snake venom fibrin(ogen)olytic enzymes. Toxicon 2005; 45:1021–1039.

111. Zhang ST, Zhou YS, Lai XH, et al. Soluble expression and purification of snake venoms: fibrino(geno)lytic enzyme Alfimeprase in E. Coli. Chin Biotechnol 2006; 26:31–36.

112. Shi J, Zhang ST, Zhang XJ, et al. Expression, purification, and activity identification of Alfimeprase in Pichia pastoris. Protein Expr Purif 2007; 54:240–246.

113. Shah AR, Scher L. Drug evaluation: alfimeprase, a plasminogen-independent thrombolytic. IDrugs 2007; 10:329–335.

114. Moll S, Kenyon P, Bertoli L, et al. Phase II trial of alfimeprase, a novel-acting fibrin degradation agent, for occluded central venous access devices. J Clin Oncol 2006; 24:3056–3060.

34

Thrombolysis of Deep Vein Thrombosis

Peter Verhamme and Raymond Verhaeghe
Department of Vascular Medicine and Haemostasis, University Hospitals of Leuven, Leuven, Belgium

Geert Maleux
Department of Interventional Radiology, University Hospitals of Leuven, Leuven, Belgium

INTRODUCTION

Thrombosis of the deep veins (deep vein thrombosis; DVT) in the lower limb and pelvis is a frequent and important disorder with potentially serious clinical sequelae. Its annual incidence is estimated at 1 per 1000 in the overall population, but increases steeply after the age of 65. It thus ranks as one of the more common cardiovascular disorders. Pain and swelling of the leg secondary to venous obstruction and perivenous inflammation are the prominent early symptoms. Occasionally, extensive swelling may lead to ischemia with threatening gangrene of the extremity, a condition known as phlegmasia coerulea dolens. The detachment of fresh thrombus fragments causes pulmonary embolism (PE), the most feared short-term complication, which can be fatal. Chronic venous hypertension is the result of persisting venous obstruction and damage to the venous valves. It in turn induces chronic edema, fibrin deposition in the interstitial tissue, poor oxygen exchange, and skin changes. Episodes of painful inflammation of the perimalleolar skin develop and therapy-resistant venous ulcers follow. This is the full-blown picture of a postthrombotic syndrome (PTS), the chronic late complication of DVT of the leg.

The standard of care for acute leg vein thrombosis is conventional anticoagulation therapy, starting with heparin (either low-molecular weight or unfractionated) and relayed with oral vitamin K antagonists. The aim is to inhibit a further extension of the thromboembolic process and to prevent recurrent thrombotic events. Elastic compression stockings are advised to obviate the swelling of the leg and to reduce the risk of postthrombotic symptoms. Wells and Forster reviewed prospective cohort studies as well as randomized trials on the "natural history" of DVT, i.e., the evolution with conventional anticoagulation and with or without compression stockings. Although the incidence of PTS varied considerably across studies, severe late symptoms developed in roughly 2% to

10% if compression stockings were worn early after the initial event (1,2). Factors with an impact on the development of late postthrombotic complications are not easily recognized. Although good data are scarce, residual vein obstruction may increase the risk for PTS, whereas return to normal venous function without valvular insufficiency of the thrombosed vein may be associated with a decreased incidence of PTS (3). Return of patency is detected with ultrasound imaging in a proportion that varies from one-fourth to three-fourths of the patients treated conventionally for DVT. This evolution, however, extends over weeks to months after the initial period of thrombosis (4).

The use of thrombolytic drugs is an accepted therapy in patients with acute arterial thrombosis such as myocardial infarction and stroke. However, it always remained controversial in the initial phase of DVT. The primary goal of such therapy is to promote early vessel recanalization. In acute arterial thrombosis, early thrombus removal rescues tissue viability, and this effect is readily quantified in myocardial infarction or stroke patients as an improved survival or as salvage of myocardial or brain function. Theoretically, in DVT, early reopening of the thrombosed vein may be expected to decrease the incidence of PTS. However, randomized clinical studies to assess such a potentially beneficial effect take years of follow-up. They are tedious and thus scarce, too few patients are included, and too many are lost during follow-up. Early restoration of patency is therefore frequently considered as a surrogate endpoint.

Historically, two main periods can be distinguished in the use of thrombolytic drugs to treat DVT: from the late 1960s up to end of the 20th century, the systemic administration of lytic agents via a peripheral vein was studied, whereas the local infusion of the lytic drug via a catheter advanced into the thrombus became the main route of administration over the last 15 years.

SYSTEMIC THROMBOLYSIS

Clearance of Venous Thrombi

In DVT of the legs, thrombolytic therapy appears more effective than conventional treatment with unfractionated heparin in producing thrombus clearance assessed with serial venography. Comerota and Aldridge collected 13 controlled trials that included a total of 591 patients: in those treated with heparin, 4% had significant or complete lysis, 14% had partial lysis, and 82% failed to improve or worsened; the corresponding figures in those treated with streptokinase (SK) were 45%, 18% and 37%, respectively (5). Janssen et al. extended the overview recently. They collected 18 studies, published between 1968 and 2000, including an aggregate of 811 evaluable patients and comparing SK, urokinase (UK), and tissue-type plasminogen activator (t-PA) with standard heparin. Most of these trials resulted in higher complete or partial clot resolution rates with systemic thrombolytic than with heparin therapy, but no single study had sufficient power to prove statistical efficacy of thrombolysis in comparison with standard anticoagulation. Complete and partial lysis with lytic agents varied from 26% to 70% and from 0% to 22%, respectively (6). Goldhaber's pooled analysis, which was limited to controlled trials with strict criteria of randomization published before 1984, concluded that thrombolysis is achieved 3.7 times more often with SK than with heparin (7). Pooling of data from several trials of course assumes that treatment has a uniform effect irrespective of differences in patient selection, treatment regimens, and timing and interpretation of venograms; in other words, those differences in results between individual trials are due to chance alone. Accepted rules of meta-analysis were applied in two other reviews. Wells and Forster reviewed 12 studies in

Table 1 Significant Lysis (% of Patients) with Systemic Thrombolysis Vs. Standard Heparin Therapy in DVT in Randomized Studies

Lytic agent	Thrombolysis	Standard heparin	Odds ratio (95% CI)
SK	61.5	16.4	8.5 (4.4–16.3)
UK	10.5	11.1	1.0 (0.1–7.2)
rt-PA	29.8	3.7	11.7 (2.61–52.5)

Abbreviations: DVT, deep vein thrombosis; SK: streptokinase; UK, urokinase; rt-PA, recombinant tissue plasminogen activator.
Source: From Ref. 1.

which the short-term response could be classified as "significant" lysis (redefined from "good response," "more than 50% lysis," "moderate or substantial lysis," or "grade 3 or 4 lysis" in individual reports) and analyzed the efficacy data separately for SK, UK, and recombinant tissue-type plasminogen activator (rt-PA) (Table 1) (1). A Cochrane review analyzed complete clot lysis separately in six trials and calculated that this was more likely in the thrombolysis treatment group: although the effect varied and the data were statistically heterogeneous, a random effects model demonstrated a significant improvement (RR, 0.24; 95% CI, 0.07–0.82) (8).

Several factors may influence the early venographic result. The best documented is probably the age of the thrombus in as far as it can be estimated from the onset of clinical symptoms. Theiss published a cohort of 163 patients treated with thrombolysis: with an increasing delay of the start of thrombolytic therapy, the rate of complete lysis declined rapidly (9). Another factor reported to have some influence is a completely occluding versus an only partially occluding thrombus with a larger surface area. Lysis in response to rt-PA or to the combination rt-PA and heparin was significantly greater in venous segments involved with non-obstructive thrombi than in those with obstructive thrombi (10).

Effect on Clinical Morbidity

One of the clinical objectives for the treatment of DVT is to reduce the morbidity of the acute event. Most patients with acute DVT improve fairly rapidly when treated with rest, leg elevation, compression stockings, and standard anticoagulant therapy. Pain and leg swelling subside within hours to days, and ambulation can be resumed promptly in most of them. From the available studies, there is no evidence that symptomatic improvement occurs more rapidly with thrombolytic agents than with heparin alone in the acute phase of DVT because it was never properly evaluated. Whereas return of vein patency would be expected to lead to a prompt relief of symptoms and signs of thrombosis, the opposite is not the case: clinical experience teaches that swelling and discomfort also improve in many patients despite persistence of the venous obstruction.

A second important aim of the treatment of DVT in the legs and pelvis is the prevention of PE. The incidence of fatal or clinically significant PE is rather low once full heparin therapy followed by oral anticoagulants is started. Thrombolytic treatment can hardly be expected to achieve greater efficacy. On the contrary, embolic phenomena induced by thrombolytic treatment were initially a reason of concern, but the vast clinical experience now available indicates that PE is not an added risk with systemic thrombolytic treatment of acute DVT. In the six trials of the pooled analysis, three cases of fatal PE were reported in heparin-treated patients against one of nonfatal embolism in patients treated with thrombolysis. Four other patients had a clinical suspicion of PE in one of the six studies, but no attempts were made to confirm the diagnosis (7). In the meta-analysis of Wells and Forster, 1 patient with PE out of 263 treated with systemic thrombolysis had to be balanced against 2 with PE out of 203 receiving standard care (1). The Cochrane review mentions a relative risk of early PE with thrombolysis of 1.23 (95% CI, 0.35–4.45), dropping to 0.51 when low-quality trials were excluded (8). The most reasonable conclusion is that systemic thrombolytic therapy has no influence on the incidence of PE in either direction.

Long-Term Follow-Up: Influence on PTS

The ultimate objective of thrombolysis is to prevent late postthrombotic venous problems. As pointed out above, the reported incidence of the PTS in patients with leg DVT varies enormously with standard care: from 20% to almost 80%. Reasons for the discrepancy are the absence of an exact definition of PTS, variable duration of follow-up, and loss of patients over time. In addition, Prandoni et al. reported that whereas the cumulative incidence of severe PTS first increased (from 2.6% after 1 year to 9.3% after 5 years of follow-up), half of those recovered to a milder form with ongoing follow-up (11,12). It is intuitively expected that valvular incompetence of the popliteal, femoral, or iliac veins resulting from damage by the thrombotic process could be avoided by a timely lysis of venous thrombi. Long-term venographic evaluation of thrombolytic versus anticoagulant therapy of DVT in rather small trials was reviewed by Francis and Marder (13). Normal venograms were noted in 57% of 76 patients treated with SK versus 7% of those treated with anticoagulants alone. Also, the large majority of the latter group indeed had postthrombotic changes, including residual fibrosis, collateral flow, or incompetent venous valves between 2 and 76 months after initial therapy. In general, patients with a normal venogram tended to be asymptomatic at long-term follow-up. The problems of evaluating the long-term clinical efficacy are well illustrated in the more recent overview of Janssen et al. (6). They considered eight studies that included 423 patients. However, long-term clinical data were available for only 222 patients, and the duration of follow-up varied across studies from a few months to several years. In addition, the authors note that the assessment of PTS was not based on a validated uniform scoring system but relied on clinical examination performed at variable intervals by investigators who were not always blinded. When aggregating the data from these studies, the long-term risk of developing postthrombotic symptoms with thrombolysis varied from 0% to 80%, whereas it was 40% to 90% in the heparin group. Wells and Forster retained only five of these studies, all comparing SK and heparin, and found an incidence of PTS of 42.5% with SK versus 69.6% with heparin, the difference not being significant (OR, 0.3; 95% CI, 0.2–0.7) (1). Few trials reported PTS and leg ulceration separately; when the data were combined, no statistically significant difference was obtained for either element (8). Many years ago, Widmer et al. took an alternative look at the problem and evaluated upon therapeutic response rather than to assigned treatment group; in their patients, thrombolytic treatment was of real benefit if early clearance was obtained, with the exception of very extensive thrombosis from the lower leg to the pelvic veins (14). Similarly, two years after thrombolytic treatment with rt-PA, the PTS was less-often observed (25%) in patients in whom more than 50% lysis was achieved than in those with less than 50% lysis (56%) (15). To sum up, although a beneficial effect of systemic thrombolysis on the late complications of DVT would be a crucial element to favor this type of treatment, it was never definitely demonstrated and is unlikely to ever be demonstrated.

Safety: The Bleeding Problem

The potential advantage of rapid clot dissolution and prevention of the PTS must be balanced against the potential hazards of thrombolytic therapy. Straub collected data on bleeding in 550 patients treated with SK—the data originated from uncontrolled as well as controlled series—and calculated an incidence of major bleeding of 11% and fatal bleeding of 0.7% (16). According to these calculations, a major bleeding event may be expected for every 92 hours of SK infusion. Aggregating the data from their overview, Janssen et al. found that 9% (range 0–38%) had a major bleeding event compared with only 5% (range 0–22%) of patients receiving heparin. Hemorrhage most commonly occurred at vascular puncture sites, but spontaneous internal bleeding in different tissues did occur (6).

In the six strictly randomized studies of Goldhaber's pooled analysis, the incidence of major bleeding with thrombolytic treatment was 20.2% versus 6.6% in patients treated with heparin. In these six trials, no fatal bleeding was observed. In their meta-analysis, Wells and Forster calculated the major bleeding incidence in 13 trials and reported separately for the three major thrombolytic agents studied in DVT (Table 2). Major bleeding was defined as any bleeding requiring a transfusion or cessation of therapy, or clinically overt intracerebral, intra-articular, intraocular, retroperitoneal, or gastrointestinal hemorrhage. Two of two hundred forty-four patients suffered an intracranial hemorrhage (1%) (1). The Cochrane review analyzed major bleeding data (excluding cerebral bleeding) in 668 patients in 12 trials and calculated that those receiving thrombolysis were significantly more likely to experience major bleeding (RR, 1.73; 95% CI, 1.04–2.88). Restricted to high-quality trials, the difference was no longer significant (RR, 1.24; 95% CI, 0.65–2.36) (8).

Bleeding from vascular puncture sites frequently results from hemostatic plug resolution. This is an expected effect of thrombolysis because thrombolytic agents do not distinguish between fibrin in pathological thrombi and in hemostatic plugs. No definite correlation exists between laboratory derangements of clotting tests and bleeding manifestations, but the risk appears to increase with duration of the thrombolytic therapy.

If, despite the theoretical advantage of rapidly dissolving thrombi, systemic thrombolysis for acute DVT did not fulfill its promises and never gained wide clinical acceptance, it is mainly because of the inherent bleeding risk relative to its use (17).

Table 2 Major Bleeding (% of Patients) with Systemic Thrombolysis Vs. Standard Heparin Therapy in DVT in Randomized Studies

Lytic agent	Thrombolysis	Standard heparin	Odds ratio (95% CI)
SK	16	4.8	3.9 (1.5–10.3)
UK	0	22.2	—
rt-PA	8.4	3.3	2.52 (0.48–13.3)

Abbreviations: DVT, deep vein thrombosis; SK: streptokinase; UK, urokinase; rt-PA, recombinant tissue plasminogen activator.
Source: From Ref. 1.

Choice of Thrombolytic Agent, Dosage Scheme, and Infusion Procedure

Most published experience on systemic thrombolysis in DVT was initially with SK. A loading dose of 250,000 IU of this agent was infused over 30 minutes followed by 100,000 IU/hr for up to 72 hours or longer depending on the obtained lysis and followed by heparin and conventional anticoagulant treatment. The loading dose was able to overcome the possible neutralizing effect on therapeutically administered SK of antistreptococcal antibodies resulting from prior streptococcal infections. This SK dosage scheme resulted in a marked plasma lytic state with systemic plasminemia, depletion of plasminogen, and degradation of fibrinogen. This standard continuous infusion scheme was compared first to intermittent SK infusion and later to ultrahigh doses of SK (1.5 million units/hr for 6 hours, repeated, if necessary, every day for up to 5 days). The lytic success rate was similar, but appeared more rapidly obtained with the ultrahigh dose (18,19).

There is less published experience with UK. Various dosage schemes have been used in small clinical studies, although frequently a systemic loading dose of 2200 or 4400 IU/kg followed by a maintenance dose of 2200 or 4400 IU/kg was advocated. D'Angelo and Mannucci found similar results with four different UK schemes varying from 1500 to 4000 IU/kg given over a period of two to seven days (20). UK was compared to SK in a few non-randomized trials: the general impression is that the rate of venographic lysis with the two agents is roughly similar, but the infusion period with UK may be longer, and this agent is often said to cause less bleeding complications. In a randomized trial with blind evaluation of the venograms, van de Loo et al. compared two dosage regimens of intermittently administered UK with the standard continuous infusion of SK (21). The rate of lysis achieved after three days was equivalent in the two UK groups to that observed in the SK group. The incidence of major bleeding was the same in the three treatment groups, but minor bleeding occurred less frequently with the lower dose of UK.

Published experience with alteplase (rt-PA) is limited and also uncertainty prevails over the optimal dosage regimen. Three studies on 21, 65, and 83 patients, respectively, used short (4–24 hours, if necessary repeated once) infusion regimens with variable doses of alteplase. Venographic lysis appeared superior to that observed with heparin alone, but the success was limited (15,22,23). A continuous infusion of alteplase in fairly low dosages (0.25 mg/kg/24 hr vs. 0.5 mg/kg/24 hr) over three to seven days gave rather disappointing results (24). In these four trials, major bleeding occurred in 12 of 103 patients who received alteplase and heparin simultaneously, in 1 of 36 patients who received alteplase alone, and in 1 of 61 patients on heparin alone or with placebo. Safety and efficacy of pro-UK (single-chain UK-type plasminogen activator; saruplase) was investigated in an open, uncontrolled, pilot trial. Fifteen patients received an infusion of 800,000 IU (5 mg/hr) over 24 hours together with unfractionated heparin. Significant lysis was demonstrated on repeat venography. One retroperitoneal bleeding was observed four days after the end of pro-UK infusion (25). The available evidence does not definitely favor a particular agent or dosage scheme.

Thrombolytic agents infused for DVT are usually administered intravenously via a peripheral vein. Each additional puncture site is a potential bleeding site and should be avoided as much as possible. Major bleeding is frequently associated with invasive procedures. Deep venous or arterial catheters are best not inserted before lysis is started or, if present, preferably not removed, and carefully observed. Patients with recent surgery (in last 2 weeks) are not candidates for systemic thrombolysis if they develop DVT because of the higher risk of bleeding. An alternative infusion procedure is regional administration of the thrombolytic agent. This is achieved, e.g., with infusion of the drug in a superficial vein on the foot and application of a tourniquet above the ankle or even with infusion in the femoral artery. Infusion via the femoral artery has been advocated in patients with phlegmasia coerulea dolens, as an alternative to surgical thrombectomy. All these alternative infusion procedures have a rather historical interest. They are currently replaced by direct intraclot infusion.

CATHETER-DIRECTED THROMBOLYSIS

Technique

Catheter-directed thrombolysis (CDT) refers to pharmacological thrombolytic treatment delivered through an infusion catheter that is positioned in the thrombosed vein (26,27). Percutaneous venous access in a patient with lower limb DVT can be obtained through the ipsilateral popliteal vein (antegrade), the contralateral femoral vein (retrograde), or, more rarely, the tibial vein or the internal jugular vein. Ultrasound guidance facilitates percutaneous access and avoids complications resulting from repeated needle punctures. Guide wire and catheter manipulations are guided by fluoroscopy. Venography (through contrast injection via the inserted catheter) establishes the exact extent of the thrombosis. A prophylactic inferior vena cava filter is sometimes deployed before starting the thrombolytic therapy when a large free-floating thrombus is visible during venography. After positioning of the infusion catheter (multiside hole or end-hole) into the thrombus, the thrombolytic agent is infused through the catheter directly into the clot. The progression of clot lysis is monitored by repeated venograms with an interval of 12 to 24 hours. The position of the catheter can be altered if needed according to the progress of clot lysis in order to maintain its position embedded within the thrombosed vein. Thrombolysis is halted if no residual thrombus is visible or if lysis has not progressed between two angiographic controls. On restoration of venous patency, there is usually prompt clinical amelioration. The main advantage of CDT over systemic thrombolysis is the higher drug concentration in the clot, which enhances local lysis. Furthermore, catheter access enables the use of angioplasty and stents to treat underlying venous anomalies that hamper venous return and may predispose to rethrombosis. Although it is tempting to speculate on a potential reduction of systemic effects with CDT, currently used thrombolytic agents for CDT all have a systemic effect and, thus, are not deprived of systemic bleeding complications.

Patient Selection

The strict selection of patients for whom CDT may offer a long-term clinical benefit over standard anticoagulation without a too high risk of periprocedural complications is an essential step for the successful outcome of this invasive procedure. Patients with a high bleeding risk because of a history of bleeding complications, a recent cerebrovascular event, or a recent surgical intervention, patients with significant comorbidities or renal insufficiency, or patients with limited life expectancy are at increased risk for periprocedural complications and are less likely to benefit from the (possible) reduction in long-term postthrombotic symptoms. These patients should therefore not be considered for CDT.

Patients with phlegmasia coerulea dolens present with a limb-threatening thrombosis because of massive swelling that can lead to arterial insufficiency and venous gangrene. Treatment is an emergency and should include thrombus removal by means of CDT or contemporary surgical thrombectomy because of the high risk of limb loss in these patients. The use of CDT is supported by case reports and small series (27).

Small case series have also reported on the successful use of CDT for patients with acute inferior caval vein thrombosis. CDT can relieve the acute and often invalidating bilateral symptoms and might reduce the risk of late debilitating venous insufficiency. CDT may also reduce the risk of thrombus progression and extension into the renal and hepatic veins, thereby preserving visceral organ function. CDT often reveals an underlying anatomic predisposition for inferior vein cava thrombosis because of congenital aplasia or hypoplasia of caval vein segments.

CDT is mostly used for acute ileofemoral DVT. Acute ileofemoral DVT is defined as thrombosis of any part of the iliac vein and/or common femoral vein with or without associated femoropopliteal DVT, in which symptoms have been present for 14 days or less (28). These patients are considered at highest risk for significant long-term disabilities resulting from persistent venous obstruction and/or insufficiency. In a recent study of patients with ileofemoral DVT, 44% experienced significant symptoms of PTS during a follow-up of five years (29). Important factors to take into account when considering a patient for CDT are the duration of the symptoms and antecedents of venous thrombosis. Patients with signs or symptoms of DVT of more than two weeks or patients with acute on chronic DVT have considerably less chance of a successful procedure.

Patients with femoropopliteal thrombosis are considered to have a lower risk of PTS, and although CDT is able to remove the thrombus and provide symptom relief in the acute setting, the long-term benefits over anticoagulation are even more unclear than for patients with ileofemoral DVT, the reason why these patients are considered less suitable candidates for CDT.

Upper limb DVT (ULDVT) refers to thrombosis of the subclavian and/or axillary vein. The major risk factor for primary ULDVT, also called "Paget-Schroetter," is subclavian vein compression in the thoracic outlet. Often, a strenuous effort or repetitive overhead activities causing vessel wall damage precede occluding thrombosis. Also for ULDVT, the long-term complication of concern is the PTS (30). Sustained venous obstruction can result in chronic edema, which interferes with occupational productivity in this generally young population. A multimodal approach with CDT, surgical decompression, and endovascular repair of the vein is advocated to reduce the risk of postthrombotic symptoms in young and previously healthy patients for whom it is of the utmost importance to avoid any form of disability (31). This approach is supported by a few case series but not by any randomized trial, and controversy still exists regarding the indications and timing of thrombolytic therapy, decompression surgery, and adjunctive endovascular procedures.

Since most experience with CDT exists for ileofemoral DVT, the immediate and long-term results will only be discussed in more detail for ileofemoral DVT.

Immediate Results: Effect on Venous Patency and Symptom Relief

A number of case series have been published that report on the immediate success rate of CDT. The overall results are reviewed by Vedantham (32), Comerata (33), and Alesh (34).

Mewissen has reported on the results of the National Venous Registry, the largest multicenter study to date that included 312 infusions of UK in 287 patients treated in academic and community medical centers. The majority of these patients had acute ileofemoral DVT. Immediate success (complete or partial clot lysis) was obtained in 83% of patients (35). Grade III (complete) lysis was achieved in 31%, and grade II (50–99% lysis) in 52%. Grade III lysis was more frequent in cases of acute than in cases of chronic DVT (34% vs. 19%). The mean duration of the UK infusion was 53 hours. At 12 months, 60% of patients were free from recurrent thrombosis. Patients with incomplete clot lysis (grade I, <50%) were at increased risk of reocclusion of the vein.

Table 3 Published Case Series of CDT for Acute Ileofemoral DVT with More Than 20 Patients

Study	Year	Drug	Patients	Immediate anatomical major bleeds	success
Semba (55)	1994	Urokinase	21	85%	0%
Bjarnason (56)	1997	Urokinase	77	79%	7%
Verhaeghe (57)	1997	t-PA	25	76%	23%
Raju (58)	1998	Urokinase	24	88%	8%
Mewissen (35)	1999	Urokinase	287	83%	11%
O'Sullivan (45)	2000	Urokinase	39	87%	0%
Shortell (59)	2001	Urokinase/t-PA	31	80%	10%
AbuRahma (37)	2001	Urokinase/t-PA	51	89%	11%
Razavi (42)	2002	Tenecteplase	16	89%	6%
Sugimoto (40)	2003	Urokinase/t-PA	54	85%	0%
Grunwald (41)	2004	Urokinase/ t-PA/RPA	74	98%	5%
Kim (52)	2006	Urokinase	37	82%	7%
Protack (60)	2007	Urokinase/ t-PA/RPA	57	94%	2%

Abbreviations: t-PA tissue-plasminogen activator; RPA, reteplase.
Source: From Ref. 32.

Numerous smaller case series have reported on the favorable outcome of CDT for acute DVT. Table 3 summarizes the immediate results of other reports that included at least 20 patients. Although published case series are probably subject to publication bias, with only the most successful case series being published, it does demonstrate that in well-experienced centers, with appropriate patient selection, one can expect successful lysis and restoration of venous patency in approximately 80% of patients. This immediate success rate appeared quite similar in the different cohort studies, despite a huge variation in outcomes assessment, endovascular treatment, and DVT population that confounds an accurate comparison between these studies (also see Table 3). Differences in evaluating the rate of acute clot lysis have been addressed in a recent standardization report (28).

In a pooled analysis by Vedantham, immediate anatomical success (defined as restoration of venous patency) was observed in 88% of 860 analyzed limbs. Success rate was lower for chronic DVT. Rethrombosis occurred in 20% of patients.

In a systematic review comparing CDT with systemic thrombolysis (34), immediate restoration of venous patency was observed in more than 75% with CDT, whereas venous patency was only restored in 20% to 30% with systemic or loco-regional administration of thrombolytic agents.

In general, restoration of venous patency promptly improves symptoms, but few studies have compared early symptom relief in patients that underwent CDT versus patients on anticoagulation (33).

Long-Term Results: Effect on PTS and Recurrent Venous Thromboembolism

The use of CDT aims mainly at reducing the long-term sequelae of DVT, particularly PTS.

As already mentioned, the major problem in evaluating the long-term benefits of CDT and the effect of CDT on PTS in particular has been the absence of well-designed randomized trials and the lack of well-validated and standardized criteria for diagnosing PTS. Many cohort studies did not report on PTS, used different definitions and instruments, or used venous patency and venous function as surrogate markers of a successful outcome. Obviously, this complicates the comparison between studies, and results of pooled analysis should be interpreted with caution. Uncertainty in the true extent of the problem and the true extent of the benefit fuels the ongoing discussion on the appropriate use of CDT in the medical community. In 2006, the Society of Interventional Radiology recognized this problem and established reporting standards for endovascular treatment of lower extremity DVT and for assessing the PTS and quality of life (QOL) (28) using more appropriate scores and questionnaires.

Overall, data on the preservation of venous function in the long term are scarce, and no reasonably sized comparative trials with conventional anticoagulation are available. The only published randomized trial by Elsharawy was with SK. In this trial, venous function was assessed with duplex ultrasound and plethysmography at six months. This single-center, randomized trial demonstrated a higher rate of normal venous function in patients treated with CDT when compared with conventional anticoagulation (36). Normal venous function after six months was reported in 13 of 18 patients treated with CDT and in only 2 of 17 controls. In another prospective, non-randomized study, Aburahma and colleagues reported fewer symptoms at five-year follow-up in patients that underwent CDT compared with patients treated only with anticoagulation (37). Primary iliofemoral venous patency rates at one, three, and five years were 24%, 18%, and 18%, respectively, in patients that received anticoagulation alone and 83%, 69%, and 69%, respectively, in patients that underwent multimodal treatment that consisted of CDT with adjunctive endovascular treatment when needed. Long-term symptom resolution was achieved in 10 of 33 patients (30%) without CDT compared with 14 of 18 patients (78%) that received multimodal treatment, including CDT.

In a retrospective case-control study published by Comerota and Mewissen that used data of a prospective multicenter registry, patients treated with CDT showed a decreased incidence of PTS and enjoyed a significantly better QOL after two years of follow-up when compared with patients who received anticoagulation alone (38,39). The improved QOL results were related to the initial success of thrombolysis: patients who had a successful lytic outcome ($\geq$50% lysis) reported a significantly better physical functioning and fewer overall postthrombotic symptoms. Patients failing CDT had similar outcomes to patients treated with anticoagulation alone.

Case series have been combined, and pooled data were compared with historical data. These pooled analyses suggest that CDT may reduce long-term postthrombotic morbidity and improve the QOL. In the systematic review by Alesh, the prevalence of PTS was lower with CDT (26%) compared with systemic thrombolytic therapy (56%) (34).

The few studies with methodological limitations still evoke a controversy within the medical community regarding the use of thrombolysis for patients without signs of impending circulatory compromise. The limited available evidence suggests however a long-term benefit of CDT in a selected subgroup of patients with ileofemoral DVT. Ongoing trials should more clearly establish the risk-benefit ratio of CDT in patients with acute ileofemoral DVT.

Choice of Thrombolytic Agent, Dosage Scheme, and Infusion Procedure

Dosing schemes for venous CDT have been derived from small dose-finding studies but mainly from experience with catheter-directed local thrombolysis in peripheral arterial occlusion. There is no defined optimal agent nor dose for endovascular thrombolytic therapy. Currently, t-PA and UK are the thrombolytic agents most frequently employed for CDT and appear to have a similar efficacy and safety profile in small studies where both agents were used (40,41). SK has been used in only one study (36). Small cohort studies have recently reported on the successful use of tenecteplase (42), reteplase (41), and staphylokinase (43) in CDT. Overall, there is no evidence that the available thrombolytic drugs differ in efficacy or safety. The choice of the lytic agent and the dosage scheme is dictated by local preference rather than by scientific data. With t-PA, the dosage schemes vary from 0.025 to 0.1 mg/kg/hr (or from 0.25 to 10 mg/hr), although there is no obvious benefit from using the higher doses. For UK, 1.500 to 3.000 units/kg/hr (or 120,000–240,000 units/hr) are acceptable doses. A front-loaded regimen is sometimes applied in which a higher dose is administered for the first hours, but such initial lacing dose is less commonly used in venous than in arterial thrombosis (27).

The thrombolytic agent is administered via a continuous infusion in most treatment centers. The use of a multiside whole catheter is currently standard of care. A pulse-spray regimen with repeated forceful injection is an alternative, but clinical advantages of this delivery strategy over continuous infusion are unclear (44). The need of concomitant anticoagulant therapy to enhance thrombolytic activity and prevent new thrombus formation is often discussed. Unfractionated heparin is administered in parallel through the infusion catheter or through a peripheral catheter, but the optimal heparin-dosing scheme is unclear and may differ among the different thrombolytic agents.

Complications of CDT

The potential advantage of prevention of the PTS must be balanced against the well-known hazards of thrombolytic therapy. Major bleeding is the most significant clinical risk associated with any thrombolytic therapy. CDT does not remove this risk.

Intracranial bleeding is the most feared complication of CDT. On the basis of the descriptive series that have been published, the risk of hemorrhagic stroke is estimated at 0.2%. The risk of severe systemic bleeding varied from 0% to 23% in the different case series (Table 3). In a pooled analysis, major bleeding was around 8%, with most bleeding events confined to the vascular access site (32). In the large registry published by Mewissen, major bleeding complications occurred in 11% of patients, most often at the puncture site. One patient died of intracranial hemorrhage (35).

The use of thrombolytic agents may cause cleavage of thrombus and embolization of partially lysed fragments to the pulmonary circulation. The phenomenon of embolization is well known in arterial occlusion where approximately 10% to 15% of limbs undergoing intra-arterial thrombolysis develop distal embolism. In case series of CDT for DVT, the incidence of clinical PE is not much higher than 1% and does not appear to exceed the incidence of PE in patients treated with anticoagulation alone. Most emboli probably are of little clinical significance and will dissolve during CDT, since all currently used thrombolytic agents have a systemic effect. Although routine use is not deemed necessary, (temporary) inferior vein cave filters are sometimes placed when a major floating thrombus is visualized during venography or in patients in which PE is strictly to be avoided because of poor cardiopulmonary reserve. In a recent pooled analysis by Vedantham, looking at 19 published studies, the use of a filter was only reported in 1% of patients (32).

Other problems with CDT are related to catheter placement, angiographic monitoring, long duration of treatment, and subsequent (endovascular) interventions of underlying stenosis.

Adjunctive Endovascular Therapies

After complete or near-complete clot lysis, a repeat venogram often reveals underlying stenotic lesions that may have predisposed to the acute thrombosis. These obstructive lesions can be relieved with angioplasty with or without insertion of a stent. This endovascular treatment helps to restore normal venous return and probably reduces the risk of recurrent thrombosis. Because elastic recoil is frequent after balloon dilatation of fibrotic stenotic lesions, stents are often deployed to prevent early restenosis. Stent placement can also be used upon incomplete clot lysis to exlude residual thrombus from the vein lumen. In a recent review, it was estimated that adjunctive endovascular procedures were performed in approximately 60% of patients that underwent CDT (34).

A frequent anomaly is a stenosis of the left common iliac vein; also referred to as the May-Thurner syndrome. This originates from chronic compression of the left common iliac vein between the right common iliac artery and the sacrum. This anatomic predisposition explains why the majority of ileofemoral thrombosis are left-sided (45). Use of thrombolysis can also reveal congential hypoplasia or aplasia or duplicated vein segments as an underlying and probably underestimated predisposing factor for ileofemoral and caval vein thrombosis.

FUTURE DEVELOPMENTS

More Conclusive Trials?

Case series have documented the technical, thrombolytic, and clinical success of CDT. However, the available studies have methodological limitations. Reporting standards and quality improvement guidelines on the appropriate utilization of endovascular treatment for DVT will help to streamline clinical trials (28). Unfortunately, no randomized studies have clearly evaluated the long-term clinical effects of venous CDT. The ongoing CaVenT study aims at better defining the role of venous CDT by evaluating its clinical efficacy and safety compared with conventional treatment alone in patients with acute iliofemoral DVT. The CaVenT study is an open, randomized, controlled, clinical trial that will include over 200 patients. The primary outcome measures patency at six months and prevalence of PTS at two years (46). The TOLEDO trial (Thrombolysis Of Lower Extremity Deep vein thrombosis Oral anticoagulation) is another multicenter randomized trial that compares CDT followed by anticoagulation versus standard anticoagulation alone (47).

Better Drugs?

All currently used fibrinolytic agents are plasminogen activators. All have a systemic effect and thus a systemic bleeding risk, even when administered intra-thrombus. In the early days of thrombolytic therapy, systemic infusion of plasmin was evaluated as a direct fibrinolytic enzyme but quickly abandoned (48). There is renewed interest in the intrathrombus application of direct fibrinolytic agents such as alfimeprase and plasmin derivatives (49,50). Direct fibrinolytic agents are expected to have a local clot lysis that is at least as effective as plasminogen activators. Since plasminogen activators depend on the endogenous plasminogen system, direct fibrinolytic agents may be more effective in chronic, plasminogen-depleted clots. The systemic inactivation of plasmin derivatives by α-2-antiplasmin (and by α-macroglobulin for alfimeprase) should reduce the bleeding risk, since these agents are thought to have less or no clinically significant systemic effects.

Pharmacomechanical Clot Removal?

Different strategies that combine mechanical and pharmacological methods for clot removal are currently under investigation.

Percuteaneous mechanical thrombectomy (PMT) refers to a catheter-based strategy for thrombus removal through mechanical thrombus fragmentation and aspiration. Different mechanical thrombectomy techniques have been proposed for fast mechanical debulking of the thrombus mass, but concerns exist for vessel wall damage and for embolic particles that are generated by the mechanical maceration of the clot (51).

More recently, strategies that combine pharmacological thrombolytic therapy with mechanical thrombectomy have been developed.

The AngioJet rheolytic thrombectomy system is a high-tech mechanical thrombus removal system in which high-velocity saline jets are used to create a low-pressure zone at the distal catheter tip, resulting in the maceration and removal of thrombus through an exhaust lumen. Rheolytic PMT can be used in addition to CDT in order to reduce infusion time. Several case series have demonstrated the effectiveness of (adjunctive) rheolytic PMT and have compared adjunctive PMT with CDT for iliofemoral DVT (52). The power-pulse spray technique allows local delivery of fibrinolytics into the clot before mechanical removal. This softens the clot before removal with the thrombectomy catheter. Lin compared retrospectively rheolytic PMT with adjunctive thrombolytic therapy and CDT in a single-center study. PMT was as effective for acute thrombus removal as CDT (75% vs. 70% in 46 and 52 procedures, respectively). Venous patency at one year was also similar in both groups (64% and 68%, respectively). Reduction of the long infusion time with CDT could be a major advantage of pharmacomechanical approaches. In the study by Lin, combined pharmacomechanical thrombectomy reduced ICU and hospital stay significantly (2.4 days vs. 8.4 days, respectively) (53).

Another promising infusion system is designed for enclosed thrombolysis. The Trellis infusion catheter isolates a vein segment between two occluding balloons. Thrombolytic agents are infused through infusion holes into the space between the two balloons. Thrombolysis is enhanced through mechanical drug dispersion. Targeted delivery in between the balloons avoids a systemic effect. Aspiration before deflation of the distal balloon should avoid embolization (54). O'Sullivan published a retrospective analysis of 19 consecutive patients with acute above-knee DVT treated by PMT with the Trellis device followed by venous angioplasty and stent placement. Isolated thrombolysis with low-dose t-PA was used in all patients. Restoration of rapid inline venous flow was achieved in all cases.

Pilot studies of these pharmacomechanical approaches have been presented and need to be repeated on a larger scale. These strategies could, once efficacy and safety is appropriately investigated, open the perspective for a safe and fast, single-session clot-removal strategy in patients with DVT.

CONCLUSIONS

CDT is more effective than systemic thrombolysis in eliminating the acute clot and providing immediate symptom relief. CDT efficiently removes the thrombus and restores venous patency in up to 85% of patients with acute DVT and preserves valvular function in more patients than conventional anticoagulant therapy alone. Furthermore, CDT allows adjunctive therapies to relieve underlying venous stenosis.

Small studies suggest that CDT may reduce long-term disabilities and improve QOL because of less PTS (33). Besides its potential benefits, CDT also increases the bleeding risk, although in well-selected patients and well-selected centers, the risk of major bleeding, especially intracranial hemorrhage, is low.

CDT remains an interesting but labor-intensive approach in expert hands for patients with massive DVT, but a definite place in the management of venous thrombosis remains to be established. Combination of pharmacological thrombolysis and mechanical thrombectomy warrants further investigation.

REFERENCES

1. Wells PS, Forster AJ. Thrombolysis in deep vein thrombosis: is there still an indication?Thromb Haemost 2001; 86(1):499–508.
2. Prandoni P, Lensing AW, Prins MH, et al. Below-knee elastic compression stockings to prevent the post-thrombotic syndrome: a randomized, controlled trial. Ann Intern Med 2004; 141(4): 249–256.
3. Prandoni P, Lensing AW, Prins MR. Long-term outcomes after deep venous thrombosis of the lower extremities. Vasc Med 1998; 3(1):57–60.
4. Prandoni P, Lensing AW, Prins MH, et al. Residual venous thrombosis as a predictive factor of recurrent venous thromboembolism. Ann Intern Med 2002; 137(12):955–960.
5. Comerota AJ, Aldridge SC. Thrombolytic therapy for deep venous thrombosis: a clinical review. Can J Surg 1993; 36(4):359–364.
6. Janssen MC, Wollersheim H, Schultze-Kool LJ, et al. Local and systemic thrombolytic therapy for acute deep venous thrombosis. Neth J Med 2005; 63(3):81–90.
7. Goldhaber SZ, Buring JE, Lipnick RJ, et al. Pooled analyses of randomized trials of streptokinase and heparin in phlebographically documented acute deep venous thrombosis. Am J Med 1984; 76(3):393–397.
8. Watson LI, Armon MP. Thrombolysis for acute deep vein thrombosis. Cochrane Database Syst Rev 2004; (4):CD002783.
9. Theiss W. Thrombolysis or not in deep vein thrombosis. Thromb Res 1988; (suppl IX):57.
10. Meyerovitz MF, Polak JF, Goldhaber SZ. Short-term response to thrombolytic therapy in deep venous thrombosis: predictive value of venographic appearance. Radiology 1992; 184(2): 345–348.
11. Prandoni P, Lensing AW, Cogo A, et al. The long-term clinical course of acute deep venous thrombosis. Ann Intern Med 1996; 125(1):1–7.
12. Prandoni P, Lensing AW, Prins MH, et al. Which is the outcome of the post-thrombotic syndrome? Thromb Haemost 1999; 82(4):1358.
13. Francis CW, Marder VJ. Fibrinolytic therapy for venous thrombosis. Prog Cardiovasc Dis 1991; 34(3):193–204.
14. Widmer LK, Zemp E, Widmer MT, et al. Late results in deep vein thrombosis of the lower extremity. Vasa 1985; 14(3):264–268.
15. Turpie AG, Levine MN, Hirsh J, et al. Tissue plasminogen activator (rt-PA) vs heparin in deep vein thrombosis. Results of a randomized trial. Chest 1990; 97(4 suppl):172S–175S.
16. Straub H. [Fatal complications of fibrinolysis]. MMW Munch Med Wochenschr 1982; 124(1): 57–61.
17. O'Meara JJ III, McNutt RA, Evans AT, et al. A decision analysis of streptokinase plus heparin as compared with heparin alone for deep-vein thrombosis. N Engl J Med 1994; 330(26): 186–1869.
18. Theiss W, Baumann G, Klein G. [Fibrinolytic treatment of deep venous thromboses with streptokinase at an ultrahigh dosage]. Dtsch Med Wochenschr 1987; 112(17):668–674.
19. Martin M, Fiebach BJ. Short-term ultrahigh streptokinase treatment of chronic arterial occlusions and acute deep vein thromboses. Semin Thromb Hemost 1991; 17(1):21–38.
20. D'Angelo A, Mannucci PM. Outcome of treatment of deep-vein thrombosis with urokinase: relationship to dosage, duration of therapy, age of the thrombus and laboratory changes. Thromb Haemost 1984; 51(2):236–239.

21. van de Loo JC, Kriessmann A, Trubestein G, et al. Controlled multicenter pilot study of urokinase- heparin and streptokinase in deep vein thrombosis. Thromb Haemost 1983; 50(3): 660–663.

22. Verhaeghe R, Besse P, Bounameaux H, et al. Multicenter pilot study of the efficacy and safety of systemic rt-PA administration in the treatment of deep vein thrombosis of the lower extremities and/or pelvis. Thromb Res 1989; 55(1):5–11.

23. Goldhaber SZ, Meyerovitz MF, Green D, et al. Randomized controlled trial of tissue plasminogen activator in proximal deep venous thrombosis. Am J Med 1990; 88(3):235–240.

24. Bounameaux H, Banga JD, Bluhmki E, et al. Double-blind, randomized comparison of systemic continuous infusion of 0.25 versus 0.50 mg/kg/24 h of alteplase over 3 to 7 days for treatment of deep venous thrombosis in heparinized patients: results of the European Thrombolysis with rt-PA in Venous Thrombosis (ETTT) trial. Thromb Haemost 1992; 67(3):306–309.

25. Moia M, Mannucci PM, Pini M, et al. A pilot study of pro-urokinase in the treatment of deep vein thrombosis. Thromb Haemost 1994; 72(3):430–433.

26. Vedantham S, Millward SF, Cardella JF, et al. Society of Interventional Radiology position statement: treatment of acute iliofemoral deep vein thrombosis with use of adjunctive catheter-directed intrathrombus thrombolysis. J Vasc Interv Radiol 2006; 17(4):613–616.

27. Verhaeghe R, Maleux G. Endovascular local thrombolytic therapy of ileofemoral and inferior caval vein thrombosis. Semin Vasc Med 2001: 1(1):123–128.

28. Vedantham S, Grassi CJ, Ferral H, et al. Reporting standards for endovascular treatment of lower extremity deep vein thrombosis. J Vasc Interv Radiol 2006; 17(3):417–434.

29. Delis KT, Bountouroglou D, Mansfield AO. Venous claudication in iliofemoral thrombosis: long-term effects on venous hemodynamics, clinical status, and quality of life. Ann Surg 2004; 239(1):118–126.

30. Sevestre MA, Kalka C, Irwin WT, et al. Paget-Schroetter syndrome: what to do? Catheter Cardiovasc Interv 2003; 59(1):71–76.

31. Kreienberg PB, Chang BB, Darling RC III, et al. Long-term results in patients treated with thrombolysis, thoracic inlet decompression, and subclavian vein stenting for Paget-Schroetter syndrome. J Vasc Surg 2001; 33(2 suppl):S100–S105.

32. Vedantham S, Thorpe PE, Cardella JF, et al. Quality improvement guidelines for the treatment of lower extremity deep vein thrombosis with use of endovascular thrombus removal. J Vasc Interv Radiol 2006; 17(3):435–447.

33. Comerota AJ, Gravett MH. Iliofemoral venous thrombosis. J Vasc Surg 2007; 46(5):1065–1076.

34. Alesh I, Kayali F, Stein PD. Catheter-directed thrombolysis (intrathrombus injection) in treatment of deep venous thrombosis: a systematic review. Catheter Cardiovasc Interv 2007; 70(1):143–148.

35. Mewissen MW, Seabrook GR, Meissner MH, et al. Catheter-directed thrombolysis for lower extremity deep venous thrombosis: report of a national multicenter registry. Radiology 1999; 211(1):39–49.

36. Elsharawy M, Elzayat E. Early results of thrombolysis vs anticoagulation in iliofemoral venous thrombosis. A randomised clinical trial. Eur J Vasc Endovasc Surg 2002; 24(3):209–214.

37. AbuRahma AF, Perkins SE, Wulu JT, et al. Iliofemoral deep vein thrombosis: conventional therapy versus lysis and percutaneous transluminal angioplasty and stenting. Ann Surg 2001; 233(6):752–760.

38. Comerota AJ, Throm RC, Mathias SD, et al. Catheter-directed thrombolysis for iliofemoral deep venous thrombosis improves health-related quality of life. J Vasc Surg 2000; 32(1):130–137.

39. Comerota AJ. Quality-of-life improvement using thrombolytic therapy for iliofemoral deep venous thrombosis. Rev Cardiovasc Med 2002; 3(suppl 2):S61–S67.

40. Sugimoto K, Hofmann LV, Razavi MK, et al. The safety, efficacy, and pharmacoeconomics of low-dose alteplase compared with urokinase for catheter-directed thrombolysis of arterial and venous occlusions. J Vasc Surg 2003; 37(3):512–517.

41. Grunwald MR, Hofmann LV. Comparison of urokinase, alteplase, and reteplase for catheter-directed thrombolysis of deep venous thrombosis. J Vasc Interv Radiol 2004; 15(4):347–352.

42. Razavi MK, Wong H, Kee ST, et al. Initial clinical results of tenecteplase (TNK) in catheter-directed thrombolytic therapy. J Endovasc Ther 2002; 9(5):593–598.

43. Heymans S, Verhaeghe R, Stockx L, et al. Feasibility study of catheter-directed thrombolysis with recombinant staphylokinase in deep venous thrombosis. Thromb Haemost 1998; 79(3): 517–519.

44. Chang R, Cannon RO III, Chen CC, et al. Daily catheter-directed single dosing of t-PA in treatment of acute deep venous thrombosis of the lower extremity. J Vasc Interv Radiol 2001; 12(2):247–252.

45. O'Sullivan GJ, Semba CP, Bittner CA, et al. Endovascular management of iliac vein compression (May-Thurner) syndrome. J Vasc Interv Radiol 2000; 11(7):823–836.

46. Enden T, Sandvik L, Klow NE, et al. Catheter-directed Venous Thrombolysis in acute iliofemoral vein thrombosis—the CaVenT study: rationale and design of a multicenter, randomized, controlled, clinical trial (NCT00251771). Am Heart J 2007; 154(5):808–814.

47. Baldwin ZK, Comerota AJ, Schwartz LB. Catheter-directed thrombolysis for deep venous thrombosis. Vasc Endovascular Surg 2004; 38(1):1–9.

48. Moser KM. Thrombolysis with fibrinolysin (plasmin)-new therapeutic approach to thromboembolism. J Am Med Assoc 1958; 167(14):1695–1704.

49. Shah AR, Scher L. Drug evaluation: alfimeprase, a plasminogen-independent thrombolytic. IDrugs 2007; 10(5):329–335.

50. Novokhatny VV, Jesmok GJ, Landskroner KA, et al. Locally delivered plasmin: why should it be superior to plasminogen activators for direct thrombolysis? Trends Pharmacol Sci 2004; 25(2):72–75.

51. Comerota AJ, Paolini D. Treatment of acute iliofemoral deep venous thrombosis: a strategy of thrombus removal. Eur J Vasc Endovasc Surg 2007; 33(3):351–360.

52. Kim HS, Patra A, Paxton BE, et al. Adjunctive percutaneous mechanical thrombectomy for lower-extremity deep vein thrombosis: clinical and economic outcomes. J Vasc Interv Radiol 2006; 17(7):1099–1104.

53. Lin PH, Zhou W, Dardik A, et al. Catheter-direct thrombolysis versus pharmacomechanical thrombectomy for treatment of symptomatic lower extremity deep venous thrombosis. Am J Surg 2006; 192(6):782–788.

54. O'Sullivan GJ, Lohan DG, Gough N, et al. Pharmacomechanical thrombectomy of acute deep vein thrombosis with the Trellis-8 isolated thrombolysis catheter. J Vasc Interv Radiol 2007; 18 (6):715–724.

55. Semba CP, Dake MD. Iliofemoral deep venous thrombosis: aggressive therapy with catheter-directed thrombolysis. Radiology 1994; 191(2):487–494.

56. Bjarnason H, Kruse JR, Asinger DA, et al. Iliofemoral deep venous thrombosis: safety and efficacy outcome during 5 years of catheter-directed thrombolytic therapy. J Vasc Interv Radiol 1997; 8(3):405–418.

57. Verhaeghe R, Stockx L, Lacroix H, et al. Catheter-directed lysis of iliofemoral vein thrombosis with use of rt-PA. Eur Radiol 1997; 7(7):996–1001.

58. Raju S, Fountain T, McPherson SH. Catheter-directed thrombolysis for deep venous thrombosis. J Miss State Med Assoc 1998; 39(3):81–84.

59. Shortell CK, Queiroz R, Johansson M, et al. Safety and efficacy of limited-dose tissue plasminogen activator in acute vascular occlusion. J Vasc Surg 2001; 34(5):854–859.

60. Protack CD, Bakken AM, Patel N, et al. Long-term outcomes of catheter directed thrombolysis for lower extremity deep venous thrombosis without prophylactic inferior vena cava filter placement. J Vasc Surg 2007; 45(5):992–997.

35

Thrombolysis for Acute Pulmonary Embolism

Gregory Piazza
Cardiovascular Division, Department of Medicine, Beth Israel Deaconess Medical Center, Harvard Medical School, Boston, Massachusetts, U.S.A.

Samuel Z. Goldhaber
Cardiovascular Division, Department of Medicine, Brigham and Women's Hospital, Harvard Medical School, Boston, Massachusetts, U.S.A.

INTRODUCTION

Venous thromboembolism (VTE), including deep vein thrombosis (DVT) and pulmonary embolism (PE), is the third most common cardiovascular disorder in the United States after coronary artery disease and stroke. The incidence of VTE rises sharply after age of 60 years in both men and women, with PE accounting for the majority of the increase (1,2). The mortality rate for acute PE exceeds 15% in the first three months after diagnosis, surpassing that of myocardial infarction (3). Nearly 25% of patients with acute PE present with sudden death as the initial clinical manifestation (4). The majority of deaths from acute PE are due to acute right ventricular (RV) failure (5). Among those who survive acute PE, up to 4% may develop disabling chronic thromboembolic pulmonary hypertension (6).

Acute PE represents a constellation of clinical syndromes. Those with normal systemic arterial blood pressure and no evidence of RV dysfunction have an excellent prognosis with anticoagulation alone. Normotensive patients with PE and evidence of RV dysfunction are classified as having submassive PE and represent a subset of patients at increased risk for adverse events and early mortality (7). Massive PE describes patients presenting with syncope, systemic arterial hypotension, cardiogenic shock, or cardiac arrest. Primary therapy with thrombolysis is used for massive PE but remains controversial for submassive PE (8).

This chapter will review the rationale for thrombolysis in acute PE. The pharmacology of thrombolytic agents used to treat PE will be described, and the clinical experience with each will be discussed. Practical recommendations for the administration of thrombolytic therapy in acute PE will be provided. Finally, alternative therapies to thrombolysis for acute PE will be discussed.

Table 1 Rationale for Thrombolytic Therapy in Acute Pulmonary Embolism

- Achieves a "head start" in pulmonary reperfusion compared with standard anticoagulation.
- Reverses acute RV failure due to pressure overload and restores systemic arterial perfusion pressure.
- Prevents hemodynamic collapse due to worsening RV dysfunction.
- Reduces clot burden in pelvic and deep leg veins as well as in pulmonary arteries.
- Improves pulmonary capillary blood flow.
- Decreases the risk of developing chronic thromboembolic pulmonary hypertension.

Abbreviation: RV, right ventricular.

RATIONALE FOR THROMBOLYSIS IN ACUTE PULMONARY EMBOLISM

The rationale for thrombolytic therapy is to reverse hemodynamic compromise and gas exchange derangements associated with acute PE (Table 1). In patients with massive PE, thrombolysis restores systemic arterial perfusion pressure by relieving RV pressure overload. Short-term mortality rates for patients presenting shock or requiring cardiopulmonary resuscitation range from 25% to 65% (9). Normotensive patients with acute PE and echocardiographic evidence of RV dysfunction have submassive PE and demonstrate an increased risk of systemic arterial hypotension, cardiogenic shock, and death compared with those with normal RV function (7). Thrombolytic therapy is administered to avert hemodynamic collapse because of worsening RV dysfunction and to help prevent the development of chronic thromboembolic pulmonary hypertension.

Successful thrombolysis can be conceptualized as a "medical embolectomy" that reduces clot burden and results in more rapid reduction in RV afterload than could be achieved with anticoagulation alone. The rapid decrease in pulmonary vascular resistance results in early recovery of RV function (10,11). Furthermore, restoration of pulmonary capillary blood flow improves ventilation and oxygenation (12).

THROMBOLYTIC AGENTS USED IN PULMONARY EMBOLISM

Several thrombolytic agents have been evaluated in the treatment of patients with acute massive and submassive PE. Early experience in thrombolysis for acute PE used the first-generation agents, streptokinase and urokinase. The second generation of thrombolytic agents includes tissue plasminogen activator (t-PA) and pro-urokinase. Third-generation thrombolytic drugs, reteplase, tenecteplase, and staphylokinase, have been less thoroughly studied.

Thrombolytic agents vary in molecular structure and function, fibrin specificity, and mode of administration (Table 2). Only three agents, streptokinase, urokinase, and t-PA, are currently Food and Drug Administration (FDA)-approved. Furthermore, their availability varies widely by medical center, region, and country.

First-Generation Agents

Streptokinase

Streptokinase's half-life does not appear to be dose dependent and is approximately 80 minutes (13). Its activity declines in a monoexponential manner (13). Clearance averages 10.8 mL/min, and the apparent volume of distribution averages 1.1 L (13). The

Table 2 Comparison of the Different Agents Utilized in the Thrombolytic Therapy of Acute Pulmonary Embolism

Agent	Metabolism	Fibrin specific	Major adverse effects	Dosing	FDA-approved for PE
Streptokinase	Hepatic	No	Bleeding, allergic reactions, neutralizing antibodies may form	250,000-IU bolus over 30 min, followed by 100,000 IU/hr for 24 hr[a]	Yes
Urokinase	Hepatic	No	Bleeding, allergic reactions	4400 IU/kg bolus over 10 min followed by 4400 IU/kg/hr over 12 to 24 hr[b]	Yes
t-PA	Hepatic	Yes	Bleeding	100-mg IV infusion over 2 hr	Yes
Pro-urokinase	Hepatic	Yes	Bleeding	20-mg IV bolus followed by an infusion of 60 mg over 1 hr	No
Reteplase	Renal, hepatic	Yes (weaker relative to other fibrin-specific agents)	Bleeding	2 IV bolus injections of 10 units given 30 min apart	No
Tenecteplase	Hepatic	Yes	Bleeding	Weight-based single IV bolus of 30 to 50 mg (6000 to 10,000 units) over 5 sec	No
Staphylokinase	Renal	Yes	Bleeding	Ideal dosing for PE thrombolysis has not been determined	No

[a]The low-dose continuous infusion regimen of streptokinase is no longer used. Although not FDA-approved for PE, the acute myocardial infarction dose of 1.5 million units administered over 1 hr is usually employed.
[b]A shorter protocol using a 2-hr infusion of 3,000,000 IU of urokinase with the first 1,000,000 IU given as a bolus over 10 min has been evaluated but is not FDA-approved.
Abbreviations: FDA, Food and Drug Administration; IU, international units; IV, intravenous; kg, kilogram; PE, pulmonary embolism; t-PA, tissue plasminogen activator.

pharmacokinetics of streptokinase demonstrate that levels decline progressively during continuous prolonged infusion (13). Drug resistance due to neutralizing antibodies resulting from prior streptococcal infections reduces the effectiveness of streptokinase over time (14). Streptokinase is largely metabolized by the liver.

Relative to other fibrin-specific thrombolytic agents, streptokinase has weak fibrin specificity (14). As fibrin specificity decreases, circulating plasminogen becomes more likely to be converted to plasmin, resulting in degradation of other plasma proteins and a systemic fibrinolytic state (15).

Plasminogen activator inhibitor (PAI-1) is an inhibitor of both endogenous and exogenous fibrinolysis and mediator of thrombolytic resistance (15). Failure of thrombolysis with streptokinase for patients with myocardial infarction appears to be significantly associated with high pretreatment levels of PAI-1 (16).

The FDA has approved streptokinase 250,000 IU as a loading dose over 30 minutes followed by 100,000 units/hr for 24 hours as thrombolytic therapy for acute PE since 1977 (17). However, this low-dose continuous infusion regimen is no longer used. Instead, the acute myocardial infarction dose of 1.5 million units administered over one hour is usually employed. Streptokinase can cause allergic reactions, including fever, rash, and, rarely, anaphylaxis.

Several initial clinical trials validated the safety and efficacy of streptokinase for the thrombolytic therapy of acute PE (18–22). The largest of these early trials, the Urokinase-Streptokinase PE Trial (USPET), randomized 167 patients with angiographically documented PE to urokinase infusion for 12 hours, urokinase infusion for 24 hours, or streptokinase infusion for 24 hours (22). Although thrombus resolution was greater with urokinase regimens than streptokinase, all three regimens were more effective in accelerating PE thrombolysis as detected by ventilation-perfusion lung scanning than intravenous unfractionated heparin anticoagulation alone (22). Morbidity and mortality rates were similar among all three thrombolytic regimens (22).

A substudy of patients enrolled in the Urokinase Pulmonary Embolism Trial (UPET) and USPET evaluated 40 patients with acute PE who had been randomized to either intravenous unfractionated heparin followed by oral anticoagulation or a regimen of streptokinase or urokinase followed by anticoagulation (12). While pulmonary capillary blood volume remained abnormally low at two weeks and one year among patients treated with intravenous unfractionated heparin, pulmonary-capillary blood volume was normal at both time intervals in patients receiving thrombolytic therapy (12). In addition, pulmonary-diffusing capacity was significantly improved at two weeks and one year among patients undergoing thrombolysis compared with patients receiving anticoagulation alone (12). In a follow-up study of these patients, 23 of the 40 patients were studied after a mean of seven years to evaluate hemodynamic parameters and response to exercise (23). At rest, mean pulmonary artery pressures and pulmonary vascular resistance were significantly higher in the heparin-only group compared with patients receiving thrombolytic therapy (23). After supine bicycle ergometry, both mean pulmonary artery pressures and pulmonary vascular resistance rose significantly in the heparin-only group but not in the thrombolytic group (23). These data suggest that thrombolytic therapy may preserve the normal hemodynamic response to exercise in the long term after acute PE.

Urokinase

Urokinase has a relatively short half-life of 14 to 20 minutes and therefore must be administered as an intravenous bolus followed by a continuous infusion (24). The elimination of urokinase occurs in a biexponential manner (25). The apparent volume of distribution is approximately 11.5 L. Because it is significantly less antigenic than streptokinase, neutralizing antibodies to urokinase are rare and do not limit thrombolytic efficacy even on repeat administration. Urokinase is rapidly metabolized by the liver.

Although not fibrin specific, urokinase results in less of a systemic fibrinolytic state than other thrombolytic agents (26). Urokinase has been associated with bleeding complications and allergic reactions. However, because of its decreased antigenicity, allergic reactions to urokinase are less common than with streptokinase.

The FDA has approved a weight-based regimen of urokinase 4400 IU/kg administered as a loading dose over 10 minutes followed by 4400 IU/kg/hr over 12 to 24 hours (17). However, urokinase is often administered in a high concentration over a short period, such as a two-hour infusion of 3,000,000 IU (27).

Several early trials established the safety and efficacy of urokinase for the thrombolytic therapy of acute PE (22,28–30). In these studies, urokinase was associated with early angiographic and hemodynamic improvement as well as reduction in the extent of perfusion defects (22,28–30). In patients with massive PE, treatment with urokinase resulted in both improvements in degree of angiographic obstruction as well as in hemodynamics (31–33).

In USPET, 12- and 24-hour regimens of urokinase were compared with a 24-hour regimen of streptokinase in 167 patients with angiographically documented acute PE (22). Resolution of pulmonary emboli as measured by pulmonary angiography and perfusion lung scanning was similar between the two urokinase regimens (22). Among patients with massive PE, urokinase was associated with a significant improvement in perfusion defects compared with streptokinase (22).

The European cooperative study group investigators compared 100 mg of t-PA administered over two hours with a 12-hour weight-based regimen of urokinase (4400 IU/ kg as a bolus dose over 10 minutes followed by 4400 IU/kg/hr), with a primary endpoint of reduction in total pulmonary resistance (34). By six hours, there was no significant difference in total pulmonary resistance or angiographic severity scores between the two treatment groups (34).

Second-Generation Agents

Tissue Plasminogen Activator

The pharmacokinetics of t-PA demonstrate very little inter-patient variability and have a linear correlation between the administered dose and plasma concentration (14,35). Plasma concentrations decrease in a biphasic manner, with a prominent initial phase accounting for up to 85% of total drug elimination (15). Compared with other thrombolytic agents, t-PA has a short half-life of approximately 3.5 minutes (14). Pharmacokinetic studies demonstrate a plasma clearance of 620 mL/min and an apparent volume of distribution of 8.1 L (35). Because it is a nonantigenic molecule homologous to its endogenous form, recombinant t-PA is not associated with the development of neutralizing antibodies that may limit its thrombolytic efficacy on repeat administration. The major mechanism of clearance for t-PA is hepatic.

The FDA has approved t-PA 100 mg as an intravenous infusion administered over two hours for the thrombolytic therapy of patients with acute massive PE (17). This is the most commonly administered contemporary dosing regimen for acute PE. t-PA is nonantigenic and does not cause allergic reactions.

The safety and efficacy of t-PA have been widely evaluated in PE trials (11,27,34,36–44). In the Plasminogen Activator Italian Multicenter Study 2 (PAIMS-2), 36 patients with angiographically confirmed PE were randomized to t-PA 100 mg infused over two hours followed by unfractionated heparin infusion versus heparin alone (42). While there was no change in the heparin-only group, patients receiving t-PA plus heparin demonstrated significant angiographic thrombus resolution (42). Furthermore, mean pulmonary artery pressure decreased significantly in patients treated with t-PA and, in contrast, increased in the heparin-only group (42).

A subsequent trial tested the hypothesis that thrombolytic therapy with t-PA followed by intravenous unfractionated heparin more rapidly improves RV function and pulmonary perfusion than standard anticoagulation alone (11). One hundred one patients with hemodynamically stable acute PE randomized to either t-PA (100 mg over 2 hours) plus heparin or heparin anticoagulation alone underwent transthoracic echocardiography at baseline and at 3 and 24 hours after thrombolysis (11). In addition, pulmonary perfusion scans were performed at baseline and 24 hours (11). Among patients receiving heparin alone, RV function improved in 17% and worsened in 17% by 24 hours (11). In contrast, only 2% receiving t-PA worsened, while 39% demonstrated improvement (11). Furthermore, pulmonary perfusion was significantly improved in patients treated with t-PA compared with those receiving heparin alone (11). While no patients who had received thrombolysis with t-PA suffered recurrent PE, there were two fatal and three nonfatal PEs in those treated with heparin only (11).

In the subsequent Management Strategies and Prognosis of Pulmonary Embolism-3 (MAPPET-3) study, 256 hemodynamically stable patients with acute PE and either pulmonary hypertension or RV dysfunction were randomized to receive t-PA 100 mg over two hours followed by unfractionated heparin infusion or placebo plus heparin anticoagulation (37). The primary endpoint was in-hospital death or clinical deterioration requiring an escalation of therapy (defined as catecholamine infusion, rescue thrombolysis, mechanical ventilation, cardiopulmonary resuscitation, or emergency surgical embolectomy) (37). Compared with heparin anticoagulation alone, thrombolysis with t-PA was associated with a significant reduction in the primary endpoint (37). This difference was attributable to a high frequency of treatment escalation in patients receiving heparin alone compared with those treated with t-PA (24.6% vs. 10.2%, $p = 0.004$) (37). The frequency of major bleeding events was low in both groups (37).

Pro-Urokinase

Pro-urokinase is administered as an intravenous bolus followed by a short infusion period. It has a biexponential elimination curve, with an initial half-life of 7 minutes followed by a second-phase half-life of approximately 26 minutes (45,46). Up to 90% of pro-urokinase is eliminated by the second-phase half-life (46). The clearance of pro-urokinase averages 500 mL/min, and the apparent volume of distribution is 9 L (47). Similar to urokinase, pro-urokinase is not associated with the development of neutralizing antibodies. Therefore, patients may receive repeat administration of pro-urokinase without concern for decreased efficacy because of an antibody response. Pro-urokinase is rapidly metabolized by the liver.

Clinical experience with pro-urokinase for acute PE is limited. In a single center pilot study, 20 patients with angiographically confirmed massive PE were administered pro-urokinase as a 20-mg bolus followed by a 60-mg infusion over one hour (48). Pro-urokinase resulted in decreased total pulmonary resistance by as early as 30 minutes and continuing through 12 hours, as well as improvement in angiographic scores (48). Of note, two patients suffered recurrent PE despite thrombolytic therapy and another two suffered major bleeding complications, including a hemorrhagic stroke (48). Larger-scale trials are warranted to better assess the safety and efficacy of pro-urokinase for acute PE.

Third-Generation Agents

Reteplase

Compared with t-PA, reteplase has a relatively longer half-life that averages 14 minutes (14). Because it has a longer half-life, reteplase may be administered as a bolus injection. Plasma concentrations increase in a linear manner according to dose and decrease in a biphasic manner (14). Reteplase has an estimated plasma clearance of 280 mL/min and an apparent volume of distribution of 40 L (14). Because it is nonantigenic, reteplase is not associated with the development of neutralizing antibodies that may limit efficacy upon repeat administration (24). Reteplase undergoes combined renal and hepatic mechanisms of elimination (14).

Reteplase has decreased affinity for fibrin and endothelial cells compared with t-PA (49). The decreased fibrin specificity of reteplase results in an increased rate of systemic fibrinogenolysis compared with t-PA (49,50). Characteristics favoring reteplase's safety include low affinity for endothelial cells, low-efficacy lysis of older, platelet-rich thrombi, and short presence in the plasma after bolus administration (51,52).

Reteplase for acute PE is administered as two intravenous bolus injections of 10 units given 30 minutes apart. In clinical trials comparing reteplase to t-PA for the thrombolytic therapy of patients with acute myocardial infarction (53) and acute PE (54), reteplase and t-PA demonstrated similar rates of major bleeding.

In a randomized trial of 36 patients with massive angiographically confirmed PE, reteplase (2 bolus injections of 10 units given 30 minutes apart) was compared with t-PA (100-mg intravenous infusion over 2 hours) (54). Decreases in total pulmonary resistance were noted in both treatments groups for up to 24 hours (54). Larger-scale randomized trials will be required to further evaluate reteplase in acute PE.

Tenecteplase

Tenecteplase's longer half-life compared with t-PA (averaging 20 to 24 minutes compared with 3.5 minutes) permits single bolus injection (14). Plasma concentrations of tenecteplase decline in a biphasic manner, with the initial phase accounting for almost 70% of total elimination (15). Women, patients with lower body weights, and older patients have demonstrated slower plasma clearance of tenecteplase (55). On average, the plasma clearance of tenecteplase is 105 mL/min, which is fourfold slower than that of t-PA (56). Hepatic metabolism is the major clearance mechanism for tenecteplase. Because it is nonantigenic, drug resistance due to neutralizing antibodies does not limit the efficacy of tenecteplase upon repeat administration. Tenecteplase is administered as a weight-based single intravenous bolus of 30 to 50 mg (6000–10,000 units) for acute PE (57,58).

In the Thrombolysis in Myocardial Infarction (TIMI) 10B trial, tenecteplase was associated with a 5% to 10% decrease in fibrinogen compared with a 40% reduction in patients receiving t-PA (59). Furthermore, consumption of α_2-antiplasmin, a potent endogenous neutralizer of plasmin, was four to five times greater with t-PA than tenecteplase (59). The clinical evaluation of tenecteplase for the thrombolytic therapy of patients with acute PE has been limited (57,58).

Staphylokinase

Clearance of staphylokinase occurs in a biphasic manner (60). The elimination half-life averages 36 minutes (61). Staphylokinase has a plasma clearance of 270 mL/min and an apparent volume of distribution of 4 L (61). Staphylokinase is largely cleared by the kidney. Neutralizing antibodies may develop one to two weeks after exposure to staphylokinase and may persist for several months, resulting in reduced efficacy upon re-administration (62). Although allergic reactions to streptokinase may be encountered due to preformed antibodies from previous streptococcal infections, major allergic reactions to staphylokinase are rare (60).

Clinical experience with staphylokinase is limited. While small clinical studies have been performed evaluating staphylokinase in the treatment of venous access catheter thrombosis (63), DVT (64), and acute PE (65), larger-scale trials are required.

THROMBOLYSIS IN SPECIAL POPULATIONS

Thrombolysis in Massive Pulmonary Embolism

For massive PE, thrombolysis is generally considered to be a life-saving intervention (8,66). In a small prospective clinical trial, patients with acute PE and cardiogenic shock were randomized to thrombolysis with peripherally administered streptokinase (1,500,000 units over 1 hour) plus anticoagulation with heparin versus anticoagulation with heparin alone (67). The trial was terminated after only 8 patients of a planned 40 patients were enrolled, because the first 4 patients treated with heparin alone died within a few hours of arrival to the emergency department (67). All four patients treated with streptokinase demonstrated rapid improvement within the first hour and survived (67). Three of the four patients treated with heparin underwent postmortem examination and were found to have right ventricular infarction in addition to massive PE (67).

A meta-analysis of 11 randomized controlled trials comparing thrombolysis with anticoagulation with heparin alone for acute PE demonstrated that thrombolytic therapy was associated with a significant reduction in recurrent PE or death (9.4% vs. 19%; OR, 0.45; 95% CI, 0.22–0.92; number needed to treat = 10) in five trials that included patients with massive PE (68). Despite general consensus guidelines (69,70) supporting thrombolysis in massive PE, an analysis of the International Cooperative Pulmonary Embolism Registry (ICOPER) found that only one-third of massive PE patients received thrombolytic therapy (71). In addition, the magnitude of clinical benefit among massive PE patients undergoing thrombolysis remains unclear (71).

Thrombolysis in Submassive Pulmonary Embolism

Use of thrombolytic therapy in submassive PE continues to be controversial because of a lack of conclusive randomized controlled trials. The largest to date, MAPPET-3, compared normotensive patients with RV dysfunction who were randomized to t-PA plus standard heparin anticoagulation versus placebo plus heparin (37). The primary endpoint was in-hospital death or clinical deterioration requiring escalation of therapy, defined as vasopressor infusion, secondary thrombolysis, mechanical ventilation, cardiopulmonary resuscitation, or emergency surgical or catheter-assisted embolectomy (37). The results favored t-PA because the heparin-only group received more frequent administration of open-label thrombolysis because of "clinical deterioration" (37). The decision to administer secondary thrombolysis was at the discretion of the treating clinician not the trial investigator. A megatrial of submassive PE thrombolysis has just begun in Europe. The Pulmonary Embolism International Thrombolysis (PEITHO) trial is designed to enroll 1100 patients in 12 countries. For now, thrombolytic therapy for submassive PE should be individualized.

Thrombolysis in The Elderly

Risk of hemorrhagic complications of thrombolytic therapy appears to increase with advancing age (72). Careful screening for contraindications to thrombolysis and minimizing early invasive procedures in the peri-thrombolytic period are critical when considering thrombolytic therapy in elderly patients with acute PE.

Thrombolysis in Women

Whether women receive the same degree of benefit and are subject to a similar risk of bleeding after administration of thrombolytic therapy for acute PE remains unclear. Data from five trials of thrombolysis in acute PE were analyzed to determine whether there were any gender differences in the efficacy or safety of thrombolytic therapy (73). The degree of reperfusion after thrombolytic therapy as measured by ventilation-perfusion lung scanning, pulmonary angiography, or mean pulmonary artery pressure was similar between genders (73). In addition, the risk of major hemorrhage was similar (73). More recently, an analysis of a large prospective multicenter registry demonstrated that while men with submassive PE experienced a dramatic reduction in rate of death with early thrombolysis (2.7% vs. 11%, $p = 0.03$), women with submassive PE did not receive a significant survival benefit from thrombolytic therapy (6.3% vs. 11.1%, $p = 0.18$) (74). Furthermore, women receiving thrombolytic therapy experienced a threefold increase in the frequency of major hemorrhage (74). Because of these conflicting data, larger prospective studies will be required to definitively determine whether gender should be considered in the decision to administer thrombolytic therapy.

Thrombolysis in Cancer Patients

Thrombolytic therapy may not carry a greater risk of major bleeding in carefully selected cancer patients compared with those who do not have cancer (75). However, a comprehensive assessment should be undertaken for occult metastases that may cause catastrophic bleeding. The magnitude of benefit as measured by ventilation-perfusion lung scanning among cancer patients appears to attenuate after 24 hours compared with non-cancer patients despite similar initial angiographic responses (75). This finding suggests that cancer patients should receive immediate maximal intensity anticoagulation after undergoing thrombolytic therapy for acute PE to preserve their initial reperfusion benefit (17).

PATHOPHYSIOLOGY OF ACUTE PULMONARY EMBOLISM

The majority of pulmonary emboli originate from thrombus in the deep veins of the lower extremities and pelvis. These thrombi embolize through the inferior vena cava (IVC) and right heart, eventually lodging in the pulmonary arterial tree where they result in hemodynamic and gas exchange abnormalities.

Hemodynamic Changes

The degree of hemodynamic compromise imposed by acute PE depends upon the size of the embolus, the patient's underlying cardiopulmonary reserve, and the extent of compensatory neurohumoral adaptations. Direct physical obstruction of the pulmonary arteries, hypoxemia, and release of potent pulmonary arterial vasoconstrictors associated with PE cause an acute increase in pulmonary vascular resistance and RV afterload. The sudden elevation in RV afterload may result in RV dilatation and hypokinesis, tricuspid regurgitation, and ultimately acute RV failure. Patients with acute PE and RV failure may rapidly decompensate to systemic arterial hypotension, cardiogenic shock, and cardiac arrest. Because of pericardial constraint, acute RV dilatation and increase in diastolic pressure result in flattening of the interventricular septum with deviation toward the left ventricle (LV) in diastole and subsequent impairment of LV filling. This phenomenon of interventricular dependence can be demonstrated on Doppler echocardiography as abnormal transmitral flow. In patients with acute PE and RV dysfunction, left atrial contraction, represented by the A wave on transmitral Doppler, makes a greater contribution to LV diastole than passive filling, represented by the E wave. Furthermore, RV pressure overload may also result in increased wall stress and ischemia by increasing myocardial oxygen demand while concurrently limiting its supply (Fig. 1). Severe imbalance between RV myocardial oxygen demand and supply in the setting of RV pressure overload can lead to concomitant RV infarction.

Gas Exchange

Gas exchange abnormalities in the setting of acute PE are most often due to a combination of ventilation-to-perfusion mismatch, increases in total dead space, and right-to-left

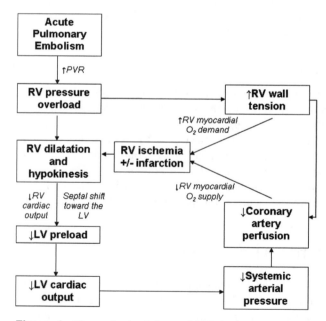

Figure 1 The pathophysiology of RV dysfunction due to acute PE. An acute elevation in RV afterload due to PE may result in RV dilatation and hypokinesis. A subsequent decrease in right-sided cardiac output and deviation of the interventricular septum toward the LV may limit LV preload and, ultimately, left-sided cardiac output. Resultant systemic arterial hypotension may impact coronary artery perfusion and thereby limit RV myocardial oxygen supply, while RV pressure overload simultaneously increases RV wall tension and myocardial oxygen demand. This imbalance between RV myocardial oxygen demand and supply can lead to concomitant RV ischemia and infarction. *Abbreviations*: PVR, pulmonary vascular resistance; PE, pulmonary embolism; RV, right ventricular; LV, left ventricule; O_2, oxygen.

shunting. Arterial hypoxemia and an increased alveolar-arterial oxygen gradient are the most commonly observed abnormalities of gas exchange in acute PE. Acute PE patients, especially those with normal underlying pulmonary function, may hyperventilate, leading to hypocapnea and respiratory alkalosis. The finding of hypercapnea may suggest massive PE, resulting in increased anatomical and physiological dead space with reduced minute ventilation.

DETECTION OF RIGHT VENTRICULAR DYSFUNCTION

Identification of patients with submassive PE remains a critical component of risk assessment, prognostication, and management. Persistent RV dysfunction at the time of hospital discharge has been associated with an increased risk of recurrent VTE (76). Clinical examination, electrocardiography, cardiac biomarker determination, chest computed tomography (CT), and echocardiography are important tools in the detection of RV dysfunction and risk stratification of patients with acute PE (Table 3).

Clinical Signs

The history and physical examination can often provide important clinical clues for the risk stratification of patients with acute PE. An analysis from the ICOPER described several clinical predictors of increased 30-day mortality, including congestive heart failure, chronic lung disease, cancer, systolic blood pressure less than or equal to 100 mmHg, age

Table 3 Tools for the Risk Stratification of Patients with Acute Pulmonary Embolism

- Clinical clues associated with increased mortality
  - Congestive heart failure
  - Chronic lung disease/pneumonia
  - Cancer
  - Systolic blood pressure less than or equal to 100 mmHg
  - Age greater than 70 yr
  - Heart rate greater than 100 beats/ min
- Electrocardiographic findings suggestive of right ventricular (RV) dysfunction
  - Sinus tachycardia
  - Incomplete or complete right bundle branch block (RBBB)
  - T-wave inversions in leads V1–V4
  - S wave in lead I, Q wave in lead III, and T-wave inversion in lead III (S1Q3T3)
- Cardiac biomarkers elevation suggestive of RV dysfunction
  - Cardiac troponins
  - Brain-type natriuretic peptide (BNP)
- Chest computed tomography (CT) evidence of RV enlargement
- Echocardiographic findings in patients with RV pressure overload
  - RV dilatation and hypokinesis
  - Interventricular septal flattening and paradoxical motion toward the left ventricle (LV)
  - Left atrial contraction (A wave) makes a greater contribution to LV diastole than passive filling (E wave) resulting in abnormal transmitral Doppler flow
  - Tricuspid regurgitation
  - Pulmonary hypertension as identified by a peak tricuspid regurgitant jet velocity of greater than 2.6 m/sec
  - Loss of inspiratory collapse of the inferior vena cava (IVC)
  - Patent foramen ovale

greater than 70 years, and heart rate greater than 100 beats/min (7). A risk stratification model incorporating prognostic variables of age, gender, comorbid conditions, including cancer, heart failure, and chronic lung disease, as well as clinical physical examination findings has been shown to accurately classify patients with acute PE into categories of increasing risk for mortality, recurrent VTE, and major bleeding (77).

Electrocardiogram

The electrocardiogram may be one of the earliest indicators of RV dysfunction in the setting of acute PE (78). Signs of RV strain include incomplete or complete right bundle branch block (RBBB), T-wave inversions in leads V1–V4, and the combination of an S wave in lead I, Q wave in lead III, and T-wave inversion in lead III (S1Q3T3) (79). In an analysis of the MAPPET-1 registry, presence of any electrocardiographic abnormality (atrial arrhythmias, complete RBBB, low voltage in the limb leads, Q waves in leads III and aVF, or ST segment changes across the precordium) was associated with an elevated risk of in-hospital mortality (9). Resting sinus tachycardia may be commonly observed and suggests increased adrenergic tone. Of note, the electrocardiogram may be entirely normal or nonspecific despite the presence of RV dysfunction in some patients with acute PE, especially those who are young and previously healthy.

Cardiac Biomarkers

Cardiac biomarkers including troponin and brain-type natriuretic peptide (BNP) have become important tools for risk stratification. Elevations in cardiac biomarkers correlate with the presence of RV dysfunction, a powerful independent predictor of adverse outcomes and early mortality in acute PE patients (7). RV pressure overload results in release of cardiac troponin because of RV microinfarction and secretion of BNP in response to increased RV shear stress (80). Elevations in levels of cardiac troponins and BNP are associated with increased short-term mortality and adverse outcomes among hemodynamically stable patients with acute PE (81,82). Because elevations in cardiac troponins and BNP may also be associated with LV ischemia and dysfunction, echocardiography should be performed to confirm the presence of RV dysfunction. The combination of cardiac biomarker determination followed by echocardiography identifies both low- and high-risk subsets of patients with acute PE (8,83).

Chest Computed Tomography

RV enlargement on chest CT is detected by comparing the RV-to-LV diameter and is usually defined as a ratio of greater than 0.9 (84). Its presence predicts an increased 30-day mortality (84,85). Detection of RV enlargement by chest CT is a particularly convenient tool for risk stratification, because it uses data acquired from the initial diagnostic scan.

Echocardiography

Echocardiography remains the imaging study of choice for detection of RV dysfunction in the setting of acute PE and is the central component of risk stratification algorithms (Fig. 2). While normotensive patients with acute PE and normal RV function generally have a benign clinical course, patients with normal blood pressures and echocardiographic evidence of RV dysfunction have an increased risk of systemic arterial hypotension, cardiogenic shock, cardiac arrest, and death (7,86). Characteristic echocardiographic

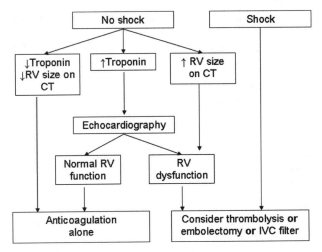

Figure 2 An algorithm for the risk stratification of patients with acute pulmonary embolism. *Abbreviations*: BNP, brain-type natriuretic peptide; CT, computed tomography; IVC, inferior vena cava; RV, right ventricular.

findings in patients with acute PE and RV pressure overload include RV dilatation and hypokinesis, interventricular septal flattening and paradoxical motion toward the left ventricle, abnormal transmitral Doppler flow, tricuspid regurgitation, pulmonary hypertension as identified by a peak tricuspid regurgitant jet velocity greater than 2.6 m/sec, and loss of inspiratory collapse of the IVC (86). Echocardiography is warranted in patients with acute PE and clinical evidence of RV failure, elevated levels of cardiac biomarkers, and unexpected clinical decompensation (5).

MANAGEMENT OF PATIENTS UNDERGOING THROMBOLYSIS FOR PULMONARY EMBOLISM

Successful thrombolytic therapy requires careful consideration of the indications and contraindications to maximize the benefits and minimize the risks. The objectives of thrombolysis should be to rapidly reduce RV afterload and thereby improve RV function, reestablish hemodynamic stability, and restore normal ventilation and oxygenation. When considering thrombolysis, the risk of major bleeding, especially intracranial hemorrhage, must be weighed against the possible benefits.

Indications

Primary therapy with thrombolysis is generally accepted as a life-saving intervention in patients presenting with acute PE and syncope, systemic arterial hypotension, cardiogenic shock, or cardiac arrest (massive PE). Although consensus is lacking, thrombolytic therapy may be considered in appropriately selected patients with acute PE, normal blood pressure, and RV dysfunction or enlargement combined with troponin elevation (submassive PE).

Contraindications

All patients should be meticulously screened for contraindications that make the bleeding risk prohibitive (Table 4) (70).

Table 4 Principal Contraindications to Thrombolytic Therapy in Patients with Acute Pulmonary Embolism

- Intracranial malignancy or tumor
- History of intracranial hemorrhage
- Cerebrovascular event or neurosurgical procedure within the prior 2 mo
- Surgery, invasive procedure, or internal organ biopsy
- Recent major trauma
- Active or recent respiratory tract, gastrointestinal, or genitourinary bleeding
- Severe uncontrolled hypertension
- Recent prolonged cardiopulmonary resuscitation
- Thrombocytopenia with under 50,000 platelets/μL
- Acute pericarditis or pericardial effusion
- Ongoing suspicion for aortic dissection

Predictors of Efficacy

Thrombolytic therapy is most successful when used early in the course of acute PE. While the efficacy of thrombolytic therapy appears to be inversely proportional to the duration of symptoms, effective thrombolysis can be achieved up to two weeks after an acute PE (87,88). In addition, patients with anatomically extensive PE have been demonstrated to achieve a greater response to thrombolytic therapy than those with smaller and often peripherally located thrombi (88).

Catheter-Directed Thrombolysis

Local, catheter-directed administration of thrombolytic agents has been evaluated with the hypothesis that drug delivery directly into the pulmonary artery may result in more rapid or complete thrombolysis because of higher local drug concentrations and fewer bleeding complications (89). Small clinical series have demonstrated successful thrombus resolution with local administration of thrombolytic therapy (90–93). However, in a study comparing catheter-directed thrombolysis to peripheral administration of thrombolytic agents, local therapy did not improve efficacy or safety (94). On the basis of the limited data available, there is insufficient evidence to support the use of catheter-directed thrombolysis over peripherally administered thrombolytic therapy (89).

Management of Immediate Anticoagulation

Because it can be discontinued and reversed quickly, intravenous unfractionated heparin is preferred in patients undergoing thrombolysis or embolectomy. In patients with massive PE, standard doses of unfractionated heparin often fail to achieve adequate therapeutic anticoagulation, with potentially fatal consequences (66). The majority of massive PE patients will require a minimum 10,000-unit bolus of unfractionated heparin followed by a continuous infusion of at least 1250 units/hr with a target activated partial thromboplastin time (aPTT) of at least 80 seconds (66).

Complications of Thrombolysis

Bleeding, in particular intracranial hemorrhage, is the most feared complication of thrombolytic therapy. Thrombolytic agents cannot differentiate between pathological and physiological clot. An analysis of data from five clinical trials of thrombolysis in acute PE reported a 1.9% risk of intracranial hemorrhage (95). A subsequent analysis from

ICOPER) reported that the risk of intracranial hemorrhage may be as high as 3% among patients receiving thrombolytic therapy for acute PE (3). Data from a center with particular expertise in thrombolysis for acute PE has suggested that the overall rate of major bleeding may approach 20% (96). These studies emphasize the importance of meticulous patient screening before administration of thrombolytic therapy.

Advancing age appears to increase the risk of hemorrhagic complications with one study demonstrating a 4% increase in risk of bleeding with each incremental year of age (72). Increasing body mass index and use of pulmonary angiography were also significant predictors of major bleeding (72). In another study, diastolic blood pressure was found to be significantly elevated among the patients that suffered intracranial bleeding compared with those who did not (95). Other predictors of hemorrhagic complications include the administration of vasopressors for systemic arterial hypotension, cancer, diabetes mellitus, and an elevated international normalized ratio (INR) before thrombolysis (96).

If a patient develops major bleeding during or after thrombolysis, thrombolytic therapy or heparin should be discontinued immediately (17). In the case of intracranial hemorrhage, both neurological and neurosurgical consultation should be obtained emergently (17). Clinicians should maintain a high index of suspicion for retroperitoneal hemorrhage, especially in patients with unexplained decreases in hematocrit, because bleeding is frequently sustained, brisk, and difficult to treat (17). Retroperitoneal hemorrhage may result from inadvertent arterial puncture during femoral vein catheterization for pulmonary angiography (17).

In the event of brisk or potentially life-threatening hemorrhage, administration of cryoprecipitate and fresh frozen plasma (FFP) may be required (17). In addition, protamine sulfate may be required if the patient has received intravenous unfractionated heparin (97). Protamine is given as a slow infusion in a dose of 1 mg for every 100 units of heparin administered over the preceding four hours up to a maximum dose of 50 mg (97). Clinicians should be mindful of a potentially severe allergic reaction that may develop to protamine in patients who have been exposed to neutral protamine hagedorn (NPH) insulin.

Other types of bleeding such as gross hematuria can generally by managed by discontinuing thrombolytic therapy or heparin (17). Trivial superficial oozing at venipuncture or arterial catheter site can often be managed with manual compression and, if needed, a pressure dressing (17).

Allergic reactions to streptokinase and, less often, urokinase may be occasionally encountered. Most often manifested as fever and rigors, this reaction may be suppressed by premedication with intravenous steroids, diphenhydramine, and oral acetaminophen (17). Rigors may be effectively treated with intravenous meperidine (17).

ALTERNATIVES TO THROMBOLYTIC THERAPY

Alternatives for primary therapy of acute PE should be considered when contraindications to thrombolytic therapy exist or when patients have failed to respond to thrombolysis. Major contraindications to thrombolytic therapy are present in nearly 30% of patients with massive PE (9). Alternative options to thrombolysis include surgical embolectomy, catheter-assisted embolectomy, and IVC filter insertion. Each of these alternative techniques has distinct strengths and limitations (Table 5).

Surgical Embolectomy

Surgical embolectomy may be considered in select patients with massive or submassive PE in whom thrombolysis has failed or is contraindicated. Rescue surgical embolectomy

Table 5 Alternative Options for Massive or Submassive Pulmonary Embolism Patients with Contraindications to Thrombolytic Therapy or in Whom Thrombolysis Has Failed

Alternative	Strengths	Limitations
Surgical embolectomy	• Effective in patients with large centrally located thrombi • Preferred after failed thrombolysis • Preferred for patients with paradoxical embolism, persistent right heart thrombi, "clot-in-transit," and hemodynamic or respiratory compromise requiring CPR • Should be performed at experienced centers	• May not be effective for smaller peripherally located thrombi • May not be widely available • Requires median sternotomy and cardiopulmonary bypass
Catheter-assisted embolectomy	• Effective in patients with large centrally located thrombi • Useful in patients with contraindications to thrombolysis and surgical embolectomy • Useful if surgical embolectomy is unavailable	• Requires the use of iodinated contrast • Volume of contrast administered may worsen right ventricular (RV) failure • Associated with risk of pulmonary hemorrhage due to arterial dissection or rupture, especially in smaller caliber vessels • Associated with vascular access site complications • Data are lacking in patients with hemodynamically stable pulmonary embolism (PE) • Hemolysis
Inferior vena cava (IVC) filter	• Effective for the prevention of recurrent PE • Useful in patients with contraindications to thrombolysis and surgical or catheter-assisted embolectomy • Retrievable filters offer temporary protection from recurrent PE	• Associated with an increased incidence of deep vein thrombosis (DVT) • Does not address the initial PE or its hemodynamic effects • May be associated with vascular access site complications

after failed thrombolytic therapy is preferred over repeat thrombolysis because of a decreased incidence of in-hospital adverse events (98). Other indications for surgical embolectomy include paradoxical embolism, persistent right heart thrombi, "clot-in-transit," and hemodynamic or respiratory compromise requiring cardiopulmonary resuscitation (97). Surgical embolectomy requires a median sternotomy and cardiopulmonary bypass and is most effective in patients with large centrally located thrombi. Perioperative mortality for patients undergoing surgical embolectomy has decreased in the last two decades (99). In specialized centers with experience in the care of such patients, surgical embolectomy has been shown to be a safe and effective technique in the treatment of massive PE (100,101). In an analysis of hemodynamically unstable patients with severe pulmonary hypertension and RV dysfunction due to acute PE, surgical embolectomy was associated with a significantly improved in-hospital mortality compared with thrombolytic therapy followed by intravenous heparin or heparin anticoagulation alone (102).

Catheter-Assisted Embolectomy

Catheter-assisted pulmonary embolectomy is an emerging technique for the primary therapy of acute PE (103–107). Catheter-assisted techniques should be considered in patients with massive PE and in whom thrombolysis and surgical embolectomy are contraindicated. Catheter-assisted embolectomy may also be considered in select cases of failed thrombolysis with ongoing hemodynamic compromise. In general, catheter-assisted techniques, such as thrombus fragmentation and aspiration, are most effective for large centrally located thrombi and when applied to fresh thrombi within the first five days of symptoms.

Inferior Vena Cava Filter Insertion

IVC filter insertion should be considered for massive or submassive PE patients in whom primary therapy, including thrombolysis and embolectomy, is contraindicated or unavailable. In addition, IVC filters are routinely placed in patients undergoing surgical embolectomy. While they significantly reduce the incidence of recurrent PE in the short term, IVC filters have not been clearly shown to lower mortality in patients with acute DVT (108). However, in an observational analysis of patients with massive PE, IVC filter insertion was associated with a reduction in 90-day mortality (hazard ratio, 0.12; 95% CI, 0.02–0.85) (71). Further prospective studies are required to validate this finding.

IVC filters do not halt ongoing thrombosis, and their insertion may be associated with vascular access site complications. In addition, IVC filters are associated with an increased rate of DVT (108). Retrievable IVC filters offer a safe and effective alternative to permanent filters and may be removed up to several months after insertion (109). Randomized trials should be performed to determine whether retrievable filters can provide a short-term reduction in recurrent PE and, possibly, improved mortality without increasing the long-term risk of DVT (110).

CONCLUSIONS

Mortality rates for patients with acute PE, especially those with hemodynamic compromise and RV dysfunction, remain high despite current options for primary therapy. The use of thrombolysis continues to be limited by a paucity of clinical trials evaluating its safety and efficacy and by significant concerns regarding bleeding complications. Large randomized controlled trials are necessary to better define the benefit of thrombolytic therapy and to identify the patients most likely to benefit. Future-generation thrombolytic agents hold promise for more site-specific thrombolysis and improved safety profiles. In the meantime, patients with massive and submassive PE may be best served by rapid triage to medical centers with expertise in the administration of thrombolytic therapy and the ability to offer alternative therapies such as embolectomy.

REFERENCES

1. Silverstein MD, Heit JA, Mohr DN, et al. Trends in the incidence of deep vein thrombosis and pulmonary embolism: a 25-year population-based study. Arch Intern Med 1998; 158:585–593.

2. Cushman M, Tsai AW, White RH, et al. Deep vein thrombosis and pulmonary embolism in two cohorts: the longitudinal investigation of thromboembolism etiology. Am J Med 2004; 117:19–25.

3. Goldhaber SZ, Visani L, De Rosa M. Acute pulmonary embolism: clinical outcomes in the International Cooperative Pulmonary Embolism Registry (ICOPER). Lancet 1999; 353: 1386–1389.

4. Heit JA. The epidemiology of venous thromboembolism in the community: implications for prevention and management. J Thromb Thrombolysis 2006; 21:23–29.

5. Piazza G, Goldhaber SZ. The acutely decompensated right ventricle: pathways for diagnosis and management. Chest 2005; 128:1836–1852.

6. Pengo V, Lensing AW, Prins MH, et al. Incidence of chronic thromboembolic pulmonary hypertension after pulmonary embolism. N Engl J Med 2004; 350:2257–2264.

7. Kucher N, Rossi E, De Rosa M, et al. Prognostic role of echocardiography among patients with acute pulmonary embolism and a systolic arterial pressure of 90 mm Hg or higher. Arch Intern Med 2005; 165:1777–1781.

8. Konstantinides S. Pulmonary embolism: impact of right ventricular dysfunction. Curr Opin Cardiol 2005; 20:496–501.

9. Kasper W, Konstantinides S, Geibel A, et al. Management strategies and determinants of outcome in acute major pulmonary embolism: results of a multicenter registry. J Am Coll Cardiol 1997; 30:1165–1171.

10. Nass N, McConnell MV, Goldhaber SZ, et al. Recovery of regional right ventricular function after thrombolysis for pulmonary embolism. Am J Cardiol 1999; 83:804–806, A810.

11. Goldhaber SZ, Haire WD, Feldstein ML, et al. Alteplase versus heparin in acute pulmonary embolism: randomised trial assessing right-ventricular function and pulmonary perfusion. Lancet 1993; 341:507–511.

12. Sharma GV, Burleson VA, Sasahara AA. Effect of thrombolytic therapy on pulmonary-capillary blood volume in patients with pulmonary embolism. N Engl J Med 1980; 303:842–845.

13. Grierson DS, Bjornsson TD. Pharmacokinetics of streptokinase in patients based on amidolytic activator complex activity. Clin Pharmacol Ther 1987; 41:304–313.

14. Caron MF, White CM. Fundamental concepts in pharmacokinetics and pharmacodynamics of fibrinolytic agents. In: Becker RC, Harrington RA, eds. Clinical, Interventional, and Investigational Thrombocardiology. Boca Raton, FL: Taylor & Francis Group, LLC: 2005: 107–120.

15. Tsikouris JP, Tsikouris AP. A review of available fibrin-specific thrombolytic agents used in acute myocardial infarction. Pharmacotherapy 2001; 21:207–217.

16. Paganelli F, Alessi MC, Morange P, et al. Relationship of plasminogen activator inhibitor-1 levels following thrombolytic therapy with rt-PA as compared to streptokinase and patency of infarct related coronary artery. Thromb Haemost 1999; 82:104–108.

17. Goldhaber SZ. A contemporary approach to thrombolytic therapy for pulmonary embolism. Vasc Med 2000; 5:115–123.

18. Tibbutt DA, Davies JA, Anderson JA, et al. Comparison by controlled clinical trial of streptokinase and heparin in treatment of life-threatening pulmonay embolism. Br Med J 1974; 1:343–347.

19. Miller GA, Sutton GC, Kerr IH, et al. Comparison of streptokinase and heparin in treatment of isolated acute massive pulmonary embolism. Br Med J 1971; 2:681–684.

20. Ly B, Arnesen H, Eie H, et al. A controlled clinical trial of streptokinase and heparin in the treatment of major pulmonary embolism. Acta Med Scand 1978; 203:465–470.

21. Hirsh J, McDonald IG, Hale GA, et al. Comparison of the effects of streptokinase and heparin on the early rate of resolution of major pulmonary embolism. Can Med Assoc J 1971; 104:488–491.

22. Urokinase-streptokinase embolism trial. Phase 2 results. A cooperative study. JAMA 1974; 229:1606–1613.

23. Sharma GV, Folland ED, McIntyre KM, et al. Long-term benefit of thrombolytic therapy in patients with pulmonary embolism. Vasc Med 2000; 5:91–95.

24. Ohman EM, Harrington RA, Cannon CP, et al. Intravenous thrombolysis in acute myocardial infarction. Chest 2001; 119:253S–277S.

25. Ueno T, Kobayashi N, Maekawa T. Studies on metabolism of urokinase and mechanism of thrombolysis by urokinase. Thromb Haemost 1979; 42:885–894.

26. Baruah DB, Dash RN, Chaudhari MR, et al. Plasminogen activators: a comparison. Vascul Pharmacol 2006; 44:1–9.

27. Goldhaber SZ, Kessler CM, Heit JA, et al. Recombinant tissue-type plasminogen activator versus a novel dosing regimen of urokinase in acute pulmonary embolism: a randomized controlled multicenter trial. J Am Coll Cardiol 1992; 20:24–30.

28. Marini C, Di Ricco G, Rossi G, et al. Fibrinolytic effects of urokinase and heparin in acute pulmonary embolism: a randomized clinical trial. Respiration 1988; 54:162–173.

29. Dickie KJ, de Groot WJ, Cooley RN, et al. Hemodynamic effects of bolus infusion of urokinase in pulmonary thromboembolism. Am Rev Respir Dis 1974; 109:48–56.

30. Urokinase pulmonary embolism trial. Phase 1 results: a cooperative study. JAMA 1970; 214:2163–2172.

31. Schwarz F, Stehr H, Zimmermann R, et al. Sustained improvement of pulmonary hemodynamics in patients at rest and during exercise after thrombolytic treatment of massive pulmonary embolism. Circulation 1985; 71:117–123.

32. Petitpretz P, Simmoneau G, Cerrina J, et al. Effects of a single bolus of urokinase in patients with life-threatening pulmonary emboli: a descriptive trial. Circulation 1984; 70:861–866.

33. The UKEP study: multicentre clinical trial on two local regimens of urokinase in massive pulmonary embolism. The UKEP Study Research Group. Eur Heart J 1987; 8:2–10.

34. Meyer G, Sors H, Charbonnier B, et al. Effects of intravenous urokinase versus alteplase on total pulmonary resistance in acute massive pulmonary embolism: a European multicenter double-blind trial. The European Cooperative Study Group for Pulmonary Embolism. J Am Coll Cardiol 1992; 19:239–245.

35. Tanswell P, Seifried E, Su PC, et al. Pharmacokinetics and systemic effects of tissue-type plasminogen activator in normal subjects. Clin Pharmacol Ther 1989; 46:155–162.

36. Levine M, Hirsh J, Weitz J, et al. A randomized trial of a single bolus dosage regimen of recombinant tissue plasminogen activator in patients with acute pulmonary embolism. Chest 1990; 98:1473–1479.

37. Konstantinides S, Geibel A, Heusel G, et al. Heparin plus alteplase compared with heparin alone in patients with submassive pulmonary embolism. N Engl J Med 2002; 347:1143–1150.

38. Goldhaber SZ, Vaughan DE, Markis JE, et al. Acute pulmonary embolism treated with tissue plasminogen activator. Lancet 1986; 2:886–889.

39. Goldhaber SZ, Kessler CM, Heit J, et al. Randomised controlled trial of recombinant tissue plasminogen activator versus urokinase in the treatment of acute pulmonary embolism. Lancet 1988; 2:293–298.

40. Goldhaber SZ, Agnelli G, Levine MN. Reduced dose bolus alteplase vs conventional alteplase infusion for pulmonary embolism thrombolysis. An international multicenter randomized trial. The Bolus Alteplase Pulmonary Embolism Group. Chest 1994; 106:718–724.

41. Diehl JL, Meyer G, Igual J, et al. Effectiveness and safety of bolus administration of alteplase in massive pulmonary embolism. Am J Cardiol 1992; 70:1477–1480.

42. Dalla-Volta S, Palla A, Santolicandro A, et al. PAIMS 2: alteplase combined with heparin versus heparin in the treatment of acute pulmonary embolism. Plasminogen activator Italian multicenter study 2. J Am Coll Cardiol 1992; 20:520–526.

43. Cuccia C, Campana M, Franzoni P, et al. Effectiveness of intravenous rTPA in the treatment of massive pulmonary embolism and right heart thromboembolism. Am Heart J 1993; 126:468–472.

44. Tissue plasminogen activator for the treatment of acute pulmonary embolism. A collaborative study by the PIOPED Investigators. Chest 1990; 97:528–533.

45. Rutherford JD, Braunwald E. Thrombolytic therapy in acute myocardial infarction. Chest 1990; 97:136S–145S.

46. Kohler M, Sen S, Miyashita C, et al. Half-life of single-chain urokinase-type plasminogen activator (scu-PA) and two-chain urokinase-type plasminogen activator (tcu-PA) in patients with acute myocardial infarction. Thromb Res 1991; 62:75–81.

47. Cohen AF, Koster RW. The clinical pharmacokinetics of saruplase. Rev Comtemp Pharmacother 1998; 9:363–370.

48. Pacouret G, Barnes SJ, Hopkins G, et al. Rapid haemodynamic improvement following saruplase in recent massive pulmonary embolism. Thromb Haemost 1998; 79:264–267.

49. Waller M, Mack S, Martin U, et al. Clinical and preclinical profile of the novel recombinant activator reteplase. In: Sasahara AA, Loscalzo J, eds. New Therapeutic Agents in Thrombosis and Thrombolysis. 2nd ed. New York: Marcel Dekker, Inc., 2003:479–500.

50. Hoffmeister HM, Kastner C, Szabo S, et al. Fibrin specificity and procoagulant effect related to the kallikrein-contact phase system and to plasmin generation with double-bolus reteplase and front-loaded alteplase thrombolysis in acute myocardial infarction. Am J Cardiol 2000; 86:263–268.

51. Stockinger H, Kubbies M, Rudolph R, et al. Binding of recombinant variants of human tissue-type plasminogen activator (t-PA) to human umbilical vein endothelial cells. Thromb Res 1992; 67:589–599.

52. Simpson D, Siddiqui MA, Scott LJ, et al. Reteplase: a review of its use in the management of thrombotic occlusive disorders. Am J Cardiovasc Drugs 2006; 6:265–285.

53. A comparison of reteplase with alteplase for acute myocardial infarction. The Global Use of Strategies to Open Occluded Coronary Arteries (GUSTO III) Investigators. N Engl J Med 1997; 337:1118–1123.

54. Tebbe U, Graf A, Kamke W, et al. Hemodynamic effects of double bolus reteplase versus alteplase infusion in massive pulmonary embolism. Am Heart J 1999; 138:39–44.

55. Modi NB, Eppler S, Breed J, et al. Pharmacokinetics of a slower clearing tissue plasminogen activator variant, TNK-tPA, in patients with acute myocardial infarction. Thromb Haemost 1998; 79:134–139.

56. Modi NB, Fox NL, Clow FW, et al. Pharmacokinetics and pharmacodynamics of tenecteplase: results from a phase II study in patients with acute myocardial infarction. J Clin Pharmacol 2000; 40:508–515.

57. Melzer C, Richter C, Rogalla P, et al. Tenecteplase for the treatment of massive and submassive pulmonary embolism. J Thromb Thrombolysis 2004; 18:47–50.

58. Kline JA, Hernandez-Nino J, Jones AE. Tenecteplase to treat pulmonary embolism in the emergency department. J Thromb Thrombolysis 2007; 23:101–105.

59. Cannon CP, Gibson CM, McCabe CH, et al. TNK-tissue plasminogen activator compared with front-loaded alteplase in acute myocardial infarction: results of the TIMI 10B trial. Thrombolysis in Myocardial Infarction (TIMI) 10B Investigators. Circulation 1998; 98:2805–2814.

60. Collen D. Staphylokinase: a potent, uniquely fibrin-selective thrombolytic agent. Nat Med 1998; 4:279–284.

61. Collen D, Van de Werf F. Coronary thrombolysis with recombinant staphylokinase in patients with evolving myocardial infarction. Circulation 1993; 87:1850–1853.

62. Vanderschueren S, Collen D, van de Werf F. A pilot study on bolus administration of recombinant staphylokinase for coronary artery thrombolysis. Thromb Haemost 1996; 76:541–544.

63. Verhamme P, Goossens G, Maleux G, et al. A dose-finding clinical trial of staphylokinase SY162 in patients with long-term venous access catheter thrombotic occlusion. J Thromb Thrombolysis 2007; 24:1–5.

64. Heymans S, Verhaeghe R, Stockx L, et al. Feasibility study of catheter-directed thrombolysis with recombinant staphylokinase in deep venous thrombosis. Thromb Haemost 1998; 79: 517–519.

65. Delcroix M, Verhaeghe R, Mortelmans L, et al. Recombinant staphylokinase thrombolysis in patients with acute pulmonary embolism. Am J Respir Crit Care Med 1998; 157:A768.

66. Kucher N, Goldhaber SZ. Management of massive pulmonary embolism. Circulation 2005; 112:e28–e32.

67. Jerjes-Sanchez C, Ramirez-Rivera A, de Lourdes Garcia M, et al. Streptokinase and heparin versus heparin alone in massive pulmonary embolism: a randomized controlled trial. J Thromb Thrombolysis 1995; 2:227–229.

68. Wan S, Quinlan DJ, Agnelli G, et al. Thrombolysis compared with heparin for the initial treatment of pulmonary embolism: a meta-analysis of the randomized controlled trials. Circulation 2004; 110:744–749.

69. Buller HR, Agnelli G, Hull RD, et al. Antithrombotic therapy for venous thromboembolic disease: the Seventh ACCP Conference on Antithrombotic and Thrombolytic Therapy. Chest 2004; 126:401S–428S.

70. Guidelines on diagnosis and management of acute pulmonary embolism. Task Force on Pulmonary Embolism, European Society of Cardiology. Eur Heart J 2000; 21:1301–1336.

71. Kucher N, Rossi E, De Rosa M, et al. Massive pulmonary embolism. Circulation 2006; 113:577–582.

72. Mikkola KM, Patel SR, Parker JA, et al. Increasing age is a major risk factor for hemorrhagic complications after pulmonary embolism thrombolysis. Am Heart J 1997; 134:69–72.

73. Patel SR, Parker JA, Grodstein F, et al. Similarity in presentation and response to thrombolysis among women and men with pulmonary embolism. J Thromb Thrombolysis 1998; 5:95–100.

74. Geibel A, Olschewski M, Zehender M, et al. Possible gender-related differences in the risk-to-benefit ratio of thrombolysis for acute submassive pulmonary embolism. Am J Cardiol 2007; 99:103–107.

75. Mikkola KM, Patel SR, Parker JA, et al. Attenuation over 24 hours of the efficacy of thrombolysis of pulmonary embolism among patients with cancer. Am Heart J 1997; 134:603–607.

76. Grifoni S, Vanni S, Magazzini S, et al. Association of persistent right ventricular dysfunction at hospital discharge after acute pulmonary embolism with recurrent thromboembolic events. Arch Intern Med 2006; 166:2151–2156.

77. Aujesky D, Roy PM, Le Manach CP, et al. Validation of a model to predict adverse outcomes in patients with pulmonary embolism. Eur Heart J 2006; 27:476–481.

78. Geibel A, Zehender M, Kasper W, et al. Prognostic value of the ECG on admission in patients with acute major pulmonary embolism. Eur Respir J 2005; 25:843–848.

79. Piazza G, Goldhaber SZ. Acute pulmonary embolism, part I: epidemiology and diagnosis. Circulation 2006; 114:e28–e32.

80. Kucher N, Goldhaber SZ. Cardiac biomarkers for risk stratification of patients with acute pulmonary embolism. Circulation 2003; 108:2191–2194.

81. Pieralli F, Olivotto I, Vanni S, et al. Usefulness of bedside testing for brain natriuretic peptide to identify right ventricular dysfunction and outcome in normotensive patients with acute pulmonary embolism. Am J Cardiol 2006; 97:1386–1390.

82. Becattini C, Vedovati MC, Agnelli G. Prognostic value of troponins in acute pulmonary embolism: a meta-analysis. Circulation 2007; 116:427–433.

83. Binder L, Pieske B, Olschewski M, et al. N-terminal pro-brain natriuretic peptide or troponin testing followed by echocardiography for risk stratification of acute pulmonary embolism. Circulation 2005; 112:1573–1579.

84. Schoepf UJ, Kucher N, Kipfmueller F, et al. Right ventricular enlargement on chest computed tomography: a predictor of early death in acute pulmonary embolism. Circulation 2004; 110:3276–3280.

85. van der Meer RW, Pattynama PM, van Strijen MJ, et al. Right ventricular dysfunction and pulmonary obstruction index at helical CT: prediction of clinical outcome during 3-month follow-up in patients with acute pulmonary embolism. Radiology 2005; 235:798–803.

86. Goldhaber SZ. Echocardiography in the management of pulmonary embolism. Ann Intern Med 2002; 136:691–700.

87. Parker JA, Drum DE, Feldstein ML, et al. Lung scan evaluation of thrombolytic therapy for pulmonary embolism. J Nucl Med 1995; 36:364–368.

88. Daniels LB, Parker JA, Patel SR, et al. Relation of duration of symptoms with response to thrombolytic therapy in pulmonary embolism. Am J Cardiol 1997; 80:184–188.

89. Arcasoy SM, Kreit JW. Thrombolytic therapy of pulmonary embolism: a comprehensive review of current evidence. Chest 1999; 115:1695–1707.
90. Vujic I, Young JW, Gobien RP, et al. Massive pulmonary embolism: treatment with full heparinization and topical low-dose streptokinase. Radiology 1983; 148:671–675.
91. Molina JE, Hunter DW, Yedlicka JW, et al. Thrombolytic therapy for postoperative pulmonary embolism. Am J Surg 1992; 163:375–380.
92. Leeper KV Jr., Popovich J Jr., Lesser BA, et al. Treatment of massive acute pulmonary embolism. The use of low doses of intrapulmonary arterial streptokinase combined with full doses of systemic heparin. Chest 1988; 93:234–240.
93. Gonzalez-Juanatey JR, Valdes L, Amaro A, et al. Treatment of massive pulmonary thromboembolism with low intrapulmonary dosages of urokinase. Short-term angiographic and hemodynamic evolution. Chest 1992; 102:341–346.
94. Verstraete M, Miller GA, Bounameaux H, et al. Intravenous and intrapulmonary recombinant tissue-type plasminogen activator in the treatment of acute massive pulmonary embolism. Circulation 1988; 77:353–360.
95. Kanter DS, Mikkola KM, Patel SR, et al. Thrombolytic therapy for pulmonary embolism. Frequency of intracranial hemorrhage and associated risk factors. Chest 1997; 111:1241–1245.
96. Fiumara K, Kucher N, Fanikos J, et al. Predictors of major hemorrhage following fibrinolysis for acute pulmonary embolism. Am J Cardiol 2006; 97:127–129.
97. Piazza G, Goldhaber SZ. Venous Thromboembolism Guidebook, Fifth Edition. Crit Pathw Cardiol 2006; 5:211–227.
98. Meneveau N, Bassand JP, Schiele F, et al. Safety of thrombolytic therapy in elderly patients with massive pulmonary embolism: a comparison with nonelderly patients. J Am Coll Cardiol 1993; 22:1075–1079.
99. Stein PD, Alnas M, Beemath A, et al. Outcome of pulmonary embolectomy. Am J Cardiol 2007; 99:421–423.
100. Leacche M, Unic D, Goldhaber SZ, et al. Modern surgical treatment of massive pulmonary embolism: results in 47 consecutive patients after rapid diagnosis and aggressive surgical approach. J Thorac Cardiovasc Surg 2005; 129:1018–1023.
101. Aklog L, Williams CS, Byrne JG, et al. Acute pulmonary embolectomy: a contemporary approach. Circulation 2002; 105:1416–1419.
102. Sukhija R, Aronow WS, Lee J, et al. Association of right ventricular dysfunction with in-hospital mortality in patients with acute pulmonary embolism and reduction in mortality in patients with right ventricular dysfunction by pulmonary embolectomy. Am J Cardiol 2005; 95:695–696.
103. Kucher N, Windecker S, Banz Y, et al. Percutaneous catheter thrombectomy device for acute pulmonary embolism: in vitro and in vivo testing. Radiology 2005; 236:852–858.
104. Kucher N. Catheter embolectomy for acute pulmonary embolism. Chest 2007; 132:657–663.
105. Goldhaber SZ. Percutaneous mechanical thrombectomy for acute pulmonary embolism: a double-edged sword. Chest 2007; 132:363–365.
106. Goldhaber SZ. Percutaneous mechanical thrombectomy for massive pulmonary embolism: improve safety and efficacy by sharing information. Catheter Cardiovasc Interv 2007; 70:807–808.
107. Chauhan MS, Kawamura A. Percutaneous rheolytic thrombectomy for large pulmonary embolism: a promising treatment option. Catheter Cardiovasc Interv 2007; 70:121–128.
108. Decousus H, Leizorovicz A, Parent F, et al. A clinical trial of vena caval filters in the prevention of pulmonary embolism in patients with proximal deep-vein thrombosis. Prevention du Risque d'Embolie Pulmonaire par Interruption Cave Study Group. N Engl J Med 1998; 338:409–415.
109. Mismetti P, Rivron-Guillot K, Quenet S, et al. A prospective long-term study of 220 patients with a retrievable vena cava filter for secondary prevention of venous thromboembolism. Chest 2007; 131:223–229.
110. Emmerich J, Meyer G, Decousus H, et al. Role of fibrinolysis and interventional therapy for acute venous thromboembolism. Thromb Haemost 2006; 96:251–257.

36

Acute Thrombolysis in Ischemic Cerebrovascular Disease

Gregory J. del Zoppo
Department of Medicine (in Hematology), Department of Neurology, University of Washington, Seattle, Washington, U.S.A.

INTRODUCTION

Antithrombotic agents play a central role in the treatment of ischemic cerebrovascular disease. Of these, select plasminogen activators (PAs) have been shown to mediate reperfusion of thrombus-occluded brain-supplying arteries when applied acutely (within the first 3 to 6 hours after ischemic stroke onset). However, work over the last decade has not substantially improved the outcomes from the original reports. This chapter addresses the use of fibrinolytic agents in the treatment of ischemic stroke and several related conditions and considers factors underlying their limited development and potential future use.

CHARACTERISTICS OF ISCHEMIC STROKE

Stroke is a syndrome of cerebral vascular disorders that present with neurological sequelae. Stroke consists of fixed or transient neurologic deficits resulting from atherothrombotic events, thromboemboli, lacunar events, subarachnoid hemorrhage, intracerebral hemorrhage, and other causes. The vascular anatomy, thrombotic or embolic sources, target arteries, timing of the stroke, and collateral protection contribute to the extent of injury during cerebrovascular ischemia. Thrombotic and thromboembolic events account for 60% to 80% of ischemic strokes in the carotid artery territory (Table 1) (1–3). For the anterior circulation, these often arise when platelet-fibrin thrombi on atheroma within the extracranial portion of the internal carotid artery (ICA, at the carotid artery bifurcation), the aortic arch, or the origin of the middle cerebral artery (MCA) embolize downstream. Thromboemboli also originate from segments of dyskinesia in the left ventricular wall formed during myocardial ischemia, atrial thrombi formed in association with (nonvalvular) atrial fibrillation, and valvular injury caused by rheumatic disease or from prosthetic valves. Lacunae, which appear in white matter and can accompany hypertension, are associated with occlusion by lipohyalinosis of small, penetrating cerebral arteries. In the posterior circulation, thrombi form at the subclavian-vertebral

Table 1 Etiologies of Focal Cerebral Ischemia

Source	Frequency
Ischemic stroke	
atherothrombotic events	40–57%
thromboembolism	16–23%
lacunae	14%
Hemorrhagic stroke	
intracerebral hemorrhage	4–18%
subarachnoid hemorrhage	10–19%

Source: The event frequencies are taken from databases provided by the Harvard Stroke Registry and the Framingham study (1–3).

artery junction and embolize into the basilar artery. In situ thrombosis of the basilar artery can occur independently in association with atheroma and can obstruct penetrating arterioles, thereby producing brain stem ischemia.

In both the carotid and vertebral-basilar territories, the ischemic lesion stabilizes into an infarction by 24 hours after arterial occlusion (4–9). Evolution of the ischemic lesion entails complex processes including local flow cessation, microvascular occlusion, inflammatory processes that involve cellular activation (e.g., of endothelial cells, platelets, and PMN leukocytes), neuron dysfunction and demise, cytokine generation, chemokines, complement activation, the transmigration of PMN leukocytes and mononuclear cells, microglial activation, and other processes initiated within the early moments following occlusion of the principal artery(ies). Interspersed within and around the evolving infarction are metastable, potentially reversible zones of glial and neuron injury in the ischemic vascular territory supplied by the occluded cerebral artery (10,11). The extent of the ischemic lesion depends upon vascular factors including the "territory-at-risk" affected (e.g., with proximal occlusions of the MCA resulting in larger lesions than those of penetrating arteries from the basilar artery), the location and length of occlusion of the arterial supply, the presence and integrity of the collateral protection, and intrinsic vulnerability of the target tissues, among other factors. During the evolving ischemic injury, the permeability barrier of the microvasculature is breached and its integrity is lost (i.e., via loss of the basal lamina matrix components). These events are also important contributors to the success and limitations of contemporary acute intervention strategies. It should be pointed out that the volume of injury relative to hemispheric volume in models of MCA occlusion may not reflect the extent or consequences of injury found in humans, owing to differences in neuroanatomy (e.g., the position of the hippocampus), vascular supply, and white matter content, for instance. Also, small lesions in the brain stem can have devastating effects compared with those of similar size lesions in the cerebral hemispheres.

In the anterior circulation, the circle of Willis allows retrograde flow for perfusion of anterior cerebral arteries when an MCA is occluded proximally. Protection of the MCA and its distal branches is achieved by patent collaterals from pial anastomoses. This element has been postulated to reduce the injury field and to extend the time to infarction (7).

The microvessel beds within the cortical gray matter and striatum have interconnections that allow reversal of flow should a portion of the bed be obstructed (12,13). The reversal occurs because the central nervous system beds are low-pressure high-flow systems. Activation or injury to the microvasculature by sustained

Table 2 Recanalization Outcome: Carotid Territory Ischemia, Intravenous Delivery

Study	Agent	Patients n	Δ(T-0) hr	Recanalization n	Recanalization %	Citation
del Zoppo	rt-PA	93 (104)	<8	32	34	(20)
Mori	rt-PA	19	<6	9	47	(21)
	C	12		2	17	
von Kummer	rt-PA	22	<6	13	59	(22)
Yamaguchi	rt-PA	47	<6	10	21	(23)
	C	46		2	4	

Abbreviations: Δ(T-0), interval from onset to treatment; rt-PA, recombinant tissue plasminogen activator; C, control.

hyperglycemia, hypertension, or inflammatory injury has been associated with increased stroke severity (14). This has been postulated to occur by compromising flow beyond the ability of the capillary beds to allow flow reversal.

Angiographic studies have demonstrated that in the carotid artery territory the incidence of large artery occlusion depends on the time from the onset of ischemic symptoms. By 72 hours after symptom onset, this frequency has dropped from ~80% at 6 hours to only 57% (15–18). The acute use of PAs accelerates the reduction in arterial occlusions (18,19). In prospective controlled trials, spontaneous perfusion of documented occlusions of the middle cerebral artery (MCA) was 17% by six hours (Table 2).

CLASSIFICATION OF CEREBROVASCULAR DISEASE

The initial symptoms experienced by the patient depend on the brain tissue regions affected by the occluded artery. The vascular supply and individual cell functions of the cortex, subcortex (striatum), and brain stem contribute to the ischemic vulnerability of the functions controlled by these regions. As an example, proximal M1 segment MCA occlusion produces significant striatal injury and cortical dysfunction; both vascular beds lie in the downstream territory. It is also known that cells of the CNS display differential sensitivity to ischemia. The endothelium of cerebral vessels is most resistant compared to astrocytes and then neurons, which are most sensitive to ischemia. Subtle differences in neuron resistance to focal and to global ischemia have been reported. Thalamic and striatal cholinergic neurons appear more resistant to ischemia than GABA (γ-aminobutyric acid) ergic neurons (24,25). In the striatum, GABAergic neurons are significantly more likely to display injury (26), but GABAergic neurons are not equally sensitive to ischemia throughout the brain (27).

The severity, injury volume, and location of the evolving lesion also depend upon the integrity of the collateral arterial supply formed by the circle of Willis and the pial arterial anastomoses, which protect the cerebral hemispheres. The striatum does not have an obvious vascular protection that has been defined so far; although one must exist, as demonstrated by residual flow above nil when the MCA is occluded (10).

Patient selection for acute intervention trials of ischemic stroke is primarily made on clinical grounds. Assessment of baseline neurological deficits and their severity [as with the National Institutes of Health Stroke Scale (NIHSS) score] give a semi-quantitative indication of stroke status, but the constellation of deficits provides an indication of the location of the lesions(s) (17). There can be substantial variability in the stroke severity in a population of patients presenting with the first stroke. Radiographic and magnetic resonance (MR) imaging methods can indicate the location and extent of the evolving lesion. CT cerebral scanning is employed to rule-out the presence of hemorrhage at the time of initial assessment, the appearance of detectable hemorrhage being an absolute contraindication to the use of a plasminogen activator for any treatment purpose. Angiography (whether four-vessel contrast or MR-based) can be used to define patient populations by location of the arterial occlusion (18). Very recently studies have asserted that MR imaging can define the extent of evolving injury in relation to the perfusion defect (PWI) underlying the deficits, and can therefore be used as a measure of determining the extent of the regions of potentially reversible injury ["ischemic penumbra" (10)] (28). Although theoretically attractive, the assertion, an untested hypothesis, failed a recent series of intervention trials (29). The DEFUSE (diffusion and perfusion imaging evaluation for understanding stroke evolution) study demonstrated that the defect volumes required to provide sufficient reversibility would be quite large compared with those asserted (see below) (30). Hence, for the moment MR detection of putative regions of lesion reversibility is not being used routinely for patient selection, as the appropriate criteria have not been developed. Progressive refinement of the methodologies for patient selection is inherent in the history of clinical testing of acute plasminogen activator use in ischemic stroke.

HEMOSTASIS AND CEREBROVASCULAR ISCHEMIA

Migrating retinal arterial thromboemboli and refractile bodies, and thrombi in cortical arteries during cerebral ischemia support the pathogenic role of platelet-fibrin thrombi in thrombosis and thromboembolic ischemic stroke (31–35). The frequency of occlusions of a cerebral artery in the carotid territory that causes symptoms decreases from 81% within 8 hours of symptom onset to 59% at 24 hours, and in 41% at 1 week (15–18,36).

Indirect evidence for the involvement of thrombi in cerebrovascular ischemia comes from studies of platelet, coagulation, and fibrinolytic system activation in patients with thrombotic stroke or with transient ischemic attacks (TIAs) (37–48). TIAs can be a manifestation of ongoing platelet activation, thrombin generation, and vascular injury in brain-supplying arteries (15–18,31,33,36,41,46,49,50).

Experimental studies also indicate that focal ischemia is associated with changes in hemostasis. Fibrin and activated platelets are deposited in microvessels within the ischemic regions shortly after MCA occlusion (51–56). The combination of heparin and an antiplatelet agent significantly reduced the density of microvascular occlusions following MCA occlusion in the nonhuman primate (52). A separate set of experiments demonstrated that acute intervention with enoxaparin could limit the volume of cerebral injury in the ischemic territory and reduce persistent neurological deficits (57). Those observations implicate local activation of hemostasis by ischemia.

THE NEUROVASCULAR UNIT

The ability of neurons to dictate the microvascular flow by altering microvessel diameter (neurovascular coupling) has been known for nearly a century (58). More recent studies have defined some of the communication pathways involved (58,59). Neurons can activate signals within astrocytes that initiate responses in microvessels and glial cells participate in this transfer of information. There is increasing evidence that interactions between endothelial cells and astrocyte end-feet (via the intervening matrix) are required to maintain the integrity of the microvessel and the permeability barriers.

The "neurovascular unit" is a conceptual framework that links microvessel and neuron injury, and their responses to injury. It is also a structural arrangement that links neurons to the components of their proximate microvessels through the common intervening astrocytes. The neurovascular unit consists of microvessels (endothelial cell-basal lamina matrix-astrocyte end-feet and pericytes), astrocytes, neurons, and their axons, in addition to other supporting cells (e.g., microglia and oligodendroglia) (26,60). The intersecting and branching microvascular network, the dendritic interconnections of neurons, and the astrocyte syncytium provide for inter-communication at several levels, and protected perfusion.

Focal ischemia exposes a discrete and highly ordered arrangement of neurons to their proximate microvessels in the striatum (26). Neurons most distant from their nearest microvessel are differentially injured compared to those nearer.

NATURAL HISTORY OF CEREBRAL ARTERY THROMBOSIS

Patients presenting with an ischemic stroke are at risk for recurrence, often within the same arterial territory. The five-year cumulative incidence of secondary stroke was 42% among males in one prospective study. A separate study noted a 32% seven-year cumulative incidence for recurrent stroke (61). The highest recurrence of ischemic stroke is within the first year following the initial event. In patients suffering a first ischemic stroke, the rate of these ischemic events, MI, or death is 10% to 12% per year (62–64).

TIAs have prognostic significance. In the carotid artery territory, completed stroke occurs in 40% to 75% of individuals with one or more TIAs, with a prevalence of approximately 30% per year (65,66). About 50% of individuals with a premonitory TIA will have a stroke within the first year (67). Stroke-related death and cardiac death have been reported to occur in 28% and 37% of TIA patients, respectively, indicating that cardiovascular mortality is significant in the stroke population (67). More recent evaluations, which have included data from placebo groups in large trials of antithrombotic efficacy, suggest a lower mortality. For example, 14% of placebo-treated individuals displayed the combined outcome events of stroke, MI, and death over two years in the United Kingdom TIA Study Group trial (68).

Mortality alone, however, is not a suitable outcome in stroke intervention trials because of its low incidence and many causes. Cerebral edema from large, hemispheric ischemic lesions can lead to transtentorial herniation and death in nearly 80% of individuals who succumb within seven days of a stroke (69).

With the development of ischemic stroke as a niche for acute intervention, outcome measures have been developed to (semi-)quantitate neurological and functional (e.g., activities of daily living) responses to the intervention. The NIHSS score and related instruments including the Scandinavian Stroke Scale, the European Stroke Scale, and others, provide primarily motor-weighted measures of neurological deficits, during anterior circulation stroke (70,71). Wityk et al. have shown the value of the NIHSS instrument in characterizing the course of both large artery and lacunar lesions over time (72), while the NINDS-funded prospective blinded safety outcome trial of recombinant tissue plasminogen activator (rt-PA) in ischemic stroke demonstrated the utility of this scale in the acute setting (17). In contemporary studies, ordinal scales used to assess activities of daily living, such as the modified Rankin Scale (mRS) and the Barthel Index, have been applied as quantitative measures of outcome.

HEMORRHAGIC TRANSFORMATION IN CEREBRAL ISCHEMIA

Hemorrhage within the brain accounts for approximately 10% of all strokes, which consist of primary intracerebral hemorrhage, subarachnoid hemorrhage, subdural hemorrhage, and hemorrhagic transformation of a primary ischemic lesion. Hemorrhagic transformation of the evolving injury is classified as hemorrhagic infarction (HI), parenchymal hematoma (PH), or both (20,73–76). PHs occur naturally during thromboembolic stroke and have been attributed, on the basis of neuropathology studies, to fragmentation and distal migration of thromboemboli that expose ischemic vessels to arterial pressure (74). Angiographic studies of thrombolytic agents in patients with thrombotic stroke have broadened this notion (17,19,21,77), suggesting that hemorrhage in the absence of reperfusion can occur from other vascular sources (e.g., collateral channels) (73,74,78). Localized (petechial) hemorrhage is associated with loss of the basal lamina from microvessels within the ischemic territory as demonstrated in animal models (50). The basal lamina constitutes one of the two barriers of the blood-brain barrier. Postmortem studies have described HI as a spectrum from scattered petechiae to more confluent hemorrhage within a region of infarction in 50% to 70% of ischemic stroke patients (73–75). HI occurs more commonly in association with cardioembolic stroke, but not with in situ atherothrombotic vascular occlusion (79). Radiographically, PH is a homogeneous, discrete circumscribed mass of blood, often associated with shift of midline structures and ventricular extension.

The frequency of detectable hemorrhage in the neuraxis is affected by the use of antithrombotic agents (1,17,18,80–86). The risk of symptomatic hemorrhage within the ischemic lesion in stroke patients increases with exposure to antiplatelet agents, anticoagulants, and PAs, in that order. Normal platelet function is essential for maintaining the integrity of the cerebrovascular bed and for preventing hemorrhage. Many reports of PH in patients suffering cerebral embolism are associated with anticoagulant treatment (87,88). With anticoagulant use increased risk of intracerebral hemorrhage is related to advanced age (>75 years), the intensity of anticoagulation, and the concomitant use of other antithrombotic agents (89).

Antiplatelet agents and anticoagulants have been used to limit the consequences of recent transient ischemia or fixed neurologic deficits associated with stroke, or as prophylaxis against second ischemic events (i.e., secondary prevention). PAs are used for acute intervention. Fibrinolytic agents are thus far the only antithrombotics successfully used to treat symptomatic focal cerebral ischemia acutely.

Antiplatelet Agents and CNS Hemorrhage

Antiplatelet agents have become a central therapeutic approach in patients with TIAs or prior stroke. These include aspirin (ASA), the combination ASA/extended-release dipyridamole (e.g., Aggrenox) (90–94), the thienopyridines (e.g., clopidogrel) (95), and other agents that can alter platelet reactivity (e.g., sulfinpyrazone, cilostazol). ASA is the agent most prevalently used for secondary prevention and to reduce cardiac risk. It can increase the incidence of symptomatic intracerebral hemorrhage following an ischemic stroke. For instance, the International Stroke Trial (IST) demonstrated a significant 0.1% increase in the incidence of symptomatic intracerebral hemorrhage in the ASA arms (82,83,96). The UK-TIA study and the European Stroke Prevention Study-2 (ESPS-2) trial demonstrated that ASA increases the incidence of symptomatic intracerebral hemorrhage (94). The combination of clopidogrel and ASA increases the incidence of major hemorrhage (intracerebral and/or transfusion-requiring) [c.f., the management of atherothrombosis with clopidogrel in high-risk patients (MATCH) trial] (97,98).

Several experimental studies have shed light on the clinical conditions that can augment the incidence of hemorrhagic transformation. Well-performed studies of two different integrin $\alpha_{IIb}\beta_3$ inhibitors demonstrate a significant dose-dependent increase in major ischemia–associated hemorrhage in two relevant focal ischemia models (mouse, primate) when given acutely (53,56). That data was largely ignored in the run-up to the development of the pan-β_3 inhibitor abciximab as a treatment for ischemic stroke. While a prospective, open phase II study of abciximab within 24 hours of stroke onset produced no apparent difference in the risk of brain hemorrhage from control (99), a subsequent phase III trial was halted because of excessive safety concerns and lack of efficacy.

Anticoagulant Agents and CNS Hemorrhage

Anticoagulant use in transient ischemia also carries an increased risk of intracerebral hemorrhage (100,101). Oral anticoagulants (e.g., the coumarins, warfarin) are used for prophylaxis against thromboembolic risk in nonvalvular atrial fibrillation [e.g., the stroke prevention in atrial fibrillation (SPAF), the atrial fibrillation aspirin and anticoagulation (AFASAK)-1, and European Atrial Fibrillation Trial (EAFT) studies] (94,102–106), prosthetic valve replacement (107–112), and unusually in the treatment of ischemic stroke. The risk of symptomatic intracranial hemorrhage among patients with TIAs receiving anticoagulants is in accord with the increased incidence of fatal hemorrhagic complications observed among elderly individuals receiving anticoagulation (113). The IST suggested an increase in symptomatic hemorrhage in patients given subcutaneous heparin (at doses not usually associated with hemorrhage) (82). However, among the few controlled, level I studies, the Warfarin-Aspirin Recurrent Stroke Study (WARSS) found no difference in outcome between TIA and ischemic stroke patients treated with tightly controlled oral anticoagulation or aspirin (114). There was no increase in intracerebral hemorrhage in the anticoagulated group. The result suggests that the risk of cerebral hemorrhage in the ischemic stroke population could be acceptably limited by rigid management of anticoagulation (114). However, the risk of intracerebral hemorrhage is increased for patients receiving oral anticoagulants at INRs in excess of 3.0 to 4.5.

Plasminogen Activators and CNS Hemorrhage

The use of PAs in ischemic stroke significantly increases the incidence of detectable intracerebral hemorrhage in a dose- and time-dependent fashion. The observation of symptomatic intracerebral hemorrhage in the small series of patients treated late following stroke onset with streptokinase (SK) or urokinase (u-PA) raised fears that application of these agents with the goal of establishing flow would lead to excessive demise. That experience led to abolition of the use of PAs in ischemic stroke. Subsequent experience with SK, u-PA, rt-PA, and recombinant pro-urokinase have refined our understanding of hemorrhagic transformation and the risks of extending intracerebral hemorrhage in the setting of ischemic stroke (see below). In short, the risk (frequency) of hemorrhagic transformation can be increased by exposure to antiplatelet agents, anticoagulants, and PAs in that order.

THE CONTEMPORARY CONCEPTUAL BASIS
FOR THE USE OF PLASMINOGEN ACTIVATOR

It is ironic that, despite the successful use of several PAs in the acute settings of myocardial ischemia, pulmonary embolism with cardiopulmonary collapse, peripheral arterial thrombosis, retinal artery occlusion, venous sinus thrombosis, and others, it is the acute use in ischemic stroke that sustains a focus on thrombolytic agents. In the setting of ischemic stroke, early attempts to achieve neurological improvement were characterized by (*i*) systemic infusion of urokinase or streptokinase, (*ii*) relatively late treatment, (*iii*) limited application of clinical trial design principles, (*iv*) a limited understanding of the natural history of ischemia-associated hemorrhage, (*v*) lack of quantitative outcome measures, (*vi*) lack of acute imaging modalities in all centers, (*vii*) lack of dose-finding strategies, and (*viii*) the absence of controls.

Plasminogen Activators Applied to Ischemic Stroke

PAs are obtained from human plasma or tissue in which the PA plays a biological role (*endogenous* PAs), or by purification from nonhuman animals or via recombinant forms of compounds derived from simpler organisms (e.g., bacteria, eukaryotic cells) (*exogenous* PAs).

Early experience with PAs in the setting of stroke employed the endogenous u-PA and the exogenous agent, SK. u-PA directly converts plasminogen to plasmin, while SK generates both free plasmin and complexes of [SK/plasmin(ogen)] in the circulation. In both cases excess plasmin degrades fibrin, circulating fibrinogen, and inactivates factors II, V, and VIII, yielding an anticoagulant state (115). Because of the complex kinetics of SK and its variable inhibition in many individuals by circulating anti-streptococcal antibodies, a dose relationship to arterial thrombus lysis cannot be derived (116). To generate a more thrombus-selective and dose-predictable agent, the stably inactive acylated plasminogen-SK activator complex (APSAC) was developed. But, only a few patients were treated with that agent.

These agents have been superseded by the recombinant single (alteplase) and two-chain (duteplase) forms of the endogenous tissue plasminogen activator (rt-PA), exogenous derivatives of rt-PA [including r-PA, teneteplase (TNK)], and other exogenous PAs. Several other exogenous agents [including staphylokinase (117,118), microplasmin (119), and others] have been examined experimentally in model systems. Because of their use in recent clinical trials of ischemic stroke and the need to explain the outcomes of those trials, three agents already employed in clinical trials will be considered in some detail.

Tissue-Type Plasminogen Activator

t-PA is synthesized as a 527 amino acid single chain, that is converted to the two-chain form by plasmin cleavage of the Arg275-Isoleu276 linkage (120,121). In the presence of fibrin in vitro the catalytic efficiencies of the single-chain and the two-chain forms are quite similar (122–124). The kinetically preferential cleavage of fibrin (in the presence of fibrin-bound plasminogen) over fibrinogen underlies the impression that both forms of rt-PA are "fibrin-selective" (120,121). The advantages of this feature have been questioned by a number of trials. The half-life ($t_{1/2}$) of both forms of rt-PA is approximately three to eight minutes in humans following a single infusion, although the biologic $t_{1/2}$ is believed to be somewhat longer, accounting for delayed hemorrhage from hemostatic thrombi (124).

Notably, equipotent thrombus-lytic activities of rt-PA in plasmas from a number of nonhuman species from rodents to primates require 10-fold higher doses/concentrations than in humans (125). In experiments in a number of small animal models of stroke, the higher concentrations have been equated with human-relevant doses for safety effects, particularly on neurons (see below).

Teneteplase

A tetra-alanine mutation at amino acids 296–299 in the t-PA sequence produces a PA relatively resistant to the principal t-PA inhibitor PAI-1. Addition of an Asn to Aln mutation at position 117 and substitution of Thr by Asn at position 103 results in a molecule with prolonged $t_{1/2}$ (126,127). The thrombus selectivity and catalytic efficiency are very similar to rt-PA (128). These characteristics allow for a single bolus injection. Additionally, no changes in fibrinogen and a modest decrease in plasminogen accompany bolus TNK. Overall, in the setting of myocardial ischemia the ASSENT-2 (assessment of the safety and efficacy of a new thrombolytic-2) trial demonstrated nearly equivalent safety judged by intracerebral hemorrhage frequency between weight-adjusted TNK and rt-PA (129). Limited studies in the CNS have been pursued so far.

Desmoteplase

Derived from the saliva of the vampire bat (*Desmodus* species), DS-PA has properties distinct from t-PA. Four DS-PA forms (α_1, α_2, β, and γ) have been isolated from *Desmodus rotundus* salivary glands that have distinct fibrinolytic activities. αDS-PA has a single kringle-like domain, a finger (F) domain, and an epidermal growth factor (EGF) domain that are similar to those of t-PA. βDS-PA lacks the F-domain and γDS-PA lacks both F- and EGF-domains. The fibrin binding of the αDS-PAs depends entirely upon the presence of the F-domain, hence the catalytic efficiency of plasminogen activation by α_1DS-PA is nearly 200-fold greater than t-PA when fibrin was added (130). In rat pulmonary embolism studies α_1DS-PA was found to be more potent and more thrombus selective than t-PA (131). Additional model studies suggested reduced hemorrhage from regions of vascular injury with α_1DS-PA compared with rt-PA (132). Few model studies for focal cerebral ischemia have been reported.

Clinical Experience with Plasminogen Activators

The association of atherothrombosis with focal cerebral ischemia provided the basis for the early trials of PAs in patients suffering ischemic stroke. As the biochemistry of PAs was under study at the time, the possibility of using those agents for recanalization of cerebral arteries leading to ischemic symptoms was of some interest. Hence, a number of small studies of the effects of the PAs available were undertaken. While ambitious, significant drawbacks to those experiments included the absence of imaging techniques with which to judge either hemorrhage or injury extent and the absence of a realization that time is an important element in injury evolution.

Among the very early reports of strategies to effect benefit with elements of the PA system, two small series of (7 and 13 respectively) ischemic stroke patients who received plasmin indicated equivocal outcome (133,134). In a series of angiographically controlled studies comparing SK or Thrombolysin® (Merck, Sharpe & Dohme, West Point, Pennsylvania, U.S.) with placebo, Meyer et al. found no significant difference in the incidence of recanalization or in clinical outcome when individuals with stable symptoms were treated within 72 hours (135). In an angiography-based study, Araki et al. demonstrated only an 8% incidence of recanalization when systemic infusion u-PA was given with 35 days of the onset of symptoms (136). In a small defining study, Fletcher et al. also observed no benefit in 31 patients treated with u-PA within 10–12 hours of symptoms (137). Four patients suffered symptomatic intracranial hemorrhage, while five patients died. That study led to a general proscription on the use of PAs in any format in individuals suffering ischemic stroke (138). Review of that experience in preparation for more acute formats suggested that the long interval to treatment after stroke onset and the possibility that some neurologic deficits were caused by undiagnosed intracerebral hemorrhage could have been major contributors to the failure of those trials (139). In addition, the application of currently accepted clinical design techniques in evaluating antithrombotics in a number of disease settings had not been developed.

Some of these issues arose in the setting of two further prospective randomized placebo-controlled trials of intravenous (IV) u-PA in patients with stable focal neurologic deficits of up to five days' duration (140,141) and two separate prospective randomized comparisons of rt-PA and u-PA in patients treated within three or five days of symptom onset, respectively (142,143). No differences in clinical outcome or in symptomatic intracranial hemorrhage were observed. Those studies, based in part on the low dose-rates employed, at least suggested that conditions could be found under which administration of a PA might be safe in the setting of focal cerebral ischemia.

Summary

Early studies, most often uncontrolled, failed to demonstrate efficacy when symptomatic improvement and death were considered as the primary outcomes. Most studies were associated with an unacceptable increase in symptomatic intracerebral hemorrhage (137). A central question was whether, given the long interval to treatment after stroke symptom onset, neurologic deficits were caused by undiagnosed hemorrhage. In the absence of proper imaging studies, these events could not be excluded. Low doses of PAs were not felt to be efficacious. PAs, hence, are contraindicated for use in patients with completed stroke.

PLASMINOGEN ACTIVATORS IN THE ACUTE TREATMENT OF ISCHEMIC STROKE

Two concepts that address injury reduction are now applied to stroke patients: (*i*) to salvage tissue, recanalization of the occluded artery must occur immediately after symptom onset, and (*ii*) the incidence/severity of hemorrhage can be limited with acute intervention (<6 to 8 hours from symptom onset) (139). Consequently, successful intervention with PAs in patients selected by strict CT and clinical criteria has shown benefit (17–20,23,84,211).

Delivery Systems for PAs to the Cerebral Vasculature

Presentation of the PA at the thrombus surface is a prerequisite for managing return of flow in the occluded segment. For complete occlusion of a brain-supplying artery (e.g., the carotid "T") lack of flow in the proximal segment must be overcome (20).

Both systemic and direct infusion approaches have been undertaken. Early studies of acute PA intervention by IV delivery employed angiographic proof of occlusion and occlusion resolution (18,19,77). For direct intra-arterial delivery angiography is obligatory for localization of the occlusion(s), measurement of outcome, and patient selection criteria.

Table 3 Hemorrhagic Transformation: Carotid Territory Ischemia, Intravenous Delivery

Study	Agent	Patients *n*	Hemorrhage		With Deterioration[a]	Citation
			HI	PH	%	
del Zoppo	rt-PA	93 (104)	21	11	31	(20)
Mori	rt-PA	19	8	2	53	(21)
	C	12	4	1	42	
von Kummer	rt-PA	22	9	3	10	(22)
Yamaguchi	rt-PA	47 (51)	20	4	47	(23)
	C	46 (47)	17	5	47	

[a]Percentage of total number of patients who demonstrated hemorrhagic transformation.
Abbreviations: HI, hemorrhagic infarction (see text); PH, parenchymatous hemorrhage (see text).

Intravenous Systemic Infusion

Recanalization of carotid artery territory occlusions by PAs using IV infusion techniques has been achieved in 34% to 59% of patients treated within eight hours of symptom onset (Tables 2 and 3) (17,21,144,145). However, recanalization of ICA occlusions is unusual (0–25%), possibly because of the low flow in the occluded arterial segment, the thrombus length, and compromised distal run-off (17,20,21,145). One prospective, open, multi-center dose-rate study of IV rt-PA (duteplase) demonstrated that early reperfusion of MCA division and branch occlusions occurred more frequently than ICA occlusions (20). Mori and colleagues first demonstrated that patients treated with rt-PA (duteplase) had improved recanalization and a significantly better clinical improvement at 30 days than those treated with placebo in a prospective blinded study (21). This was followed by a similar study conducted by Yamaguchi and colleagues (23). Hemorrhagic transformation occurred in 29% to 53% of treated patients among those studies (17,21,144,145). Both feasibility and safety of systemic PA infusion were apparent, which set the stage for larger phase III intervention trials of safety and efficacy.

rt-PA

The National Institute of Neurological Disorders and Stroke (NINDS) undertook a two-part, four-armed, placebo-controlled double-blind outcome study of rt-PA (alteplase) in patients entered within three hours after the onset of symptoms attributable to ischemic stroke (Table 4) (17). Patients were stratified and randomized into two time cohorts: <90 minutes and 90 to 180 minutes from symptom onset. In the second part of that study, rt-PA recipients displayed a significant 11% to 13% absolute increase over placebo in the number of patients with no or minimal disability/deficit in Barthel index, mRS score, Glasgow outcome scale score, and NIHSS, at 3 months and at 12 months (17). The frequency of symptomatic hemorrhage within three months was significantly greater for those patients receiving rt-PA (6.4%) than those who received placebo (0.6%). While stroke-related mortality was unchanged, intracerebral hemorrhage did contribute to demise in the rt-PA group (17,153). That study supports the current acute use of rt-PA in ischemic stroke.

Three further contemporaneous phase III prospective, blinded, randomized safety and efficacy studies of IV rt-PA (alteplase) broaden these impressions (Table 5). The European Cooperative Acute Stroke Study (ECASS) compared rt-PA (alteplase) with

Table 4 Efficacy and Hemorrhagic Transformation: Carotid Territory Ischemia, Intravenous Delivery

Study	Agent	Patients n	Δ(T-0) hr	Outcome	% Improved	Hemorrhage HI	Hemorrhage PH	Hemorrhage %[a]	Citation
Abe	u-PA	57	<720	N[b]	70	0	0		(146,147)
	C	56			47	0	0		
Atarashi	u-PA	191	<120	N[b]	45	2	0	1.0	(140)
	C	94C			44	1	0	1.1	
Otomo	u-PA	176	<120	N[b]	52	2	0	1.1	(141)
	C	188			41	1	0	0.5	
Otomo	rt-PA	171	<120	N[b]	59	2	0	1.1	(143)
	u-PA	184			55	3	0	1.6	
Abe	rt-PA	145	<72	N[b]	66	3	0	2.0	(142)
	u-PA	77			45	6	0	7.8	
Haley	rt-PA	10	<1.5	N[c]	60[g]	0	0		(148)
	C	10			10	0	0		
	rt-PA	4	1.5–3.0	N[c]	50	0	0		
	C	3			67	0	1		
MAST-E	SK	156	<6.0	M[d]	34[g]	63	33	21.0[g]	(149)
	C	154			18	57	4	3.0	
ASK	SK	165	<4.0	M[c]	36[g]	33	23	13.2[g]	(150)
	C	163			21	23	5	3.1	
MAST-I	SK	313	<6.0	M[d]	25[g]	60	21	6.7[g]	(151)
	C	309			12	27	2	0.7	
ECASS	rt-PA	313	<6.0	D[f]	36	72	62	19.8[g]	(84)
	C	307			29	93	30	6.5	
NINDS I	rt-PA	144	0–3.0	N[c]	47	–	13	5.6[g]	(17)
	C	147			39	–	3	0.0	
NINDS II	rt-PA	168	0–3.0	D[f]/N[c]	48	–	21	7.1[g]	(17)
	C	165			39	–	81	2.1	
ECASS-II	rt-PA	409	<6.0	N[c]	40	142	48	11.7[g]	(152)
	C	391			37	141	12	3.1	
ECASS-III	rt-PA	418	3.0–4.5	D[f]	53	91	22	5.3[g]	(211)
	C	403			45	82	9	2.2	

[a]Percentage with hemorrhagic transformation (most often PH) and deterioration.
Outcomes of note to each study:
N[b], neurological outcome
N[c], neurological outcome according to scoring instrument.
M[d], early mortality.
M[e], mortality (3 or 6 mo).
D[f], best disability outcome (3 mo).
[g]Statistically significant.
Abbreviations: >Δ(T-0), interval from onset to treatment; C, control; HI, hemorrhagic infarction, or asymptomatic intracranial hemorrhage (see text); PH, parenchymatous hemorrhage, or symptomatic intracranial hemorrhage (see text); SK, streptokinase; rt-PA, recombinant tissue plasminogen activator; u-PA, urokinase plasminogen activator.

placebo within six hours from symptom onset among 75 centers. There was, at three months, no significant difference between the two groups in disability outcome in median mRS (84). Post hoc analysis of the "target population" suggested an 11% to 12% absolute improvement in no or minimal disability (mRS = 0 or 1) in the rt-PA-treated group over the placebo group. In that study, there was also a significantly higher proportion of

Table 5 Recanalization Outcome: Carotid Territory Ischemia, Intra-Arterial Delivery

Study	Agent	Patients n	Δ(T-0) hr	Recanalization[a] n	%	Citation
del Zoppo	SK/u-PA	20	1–24	18	90	(77)
Mori	u-PA	22	0.8–7	10	45	(19)
Theron	SK/u-PA	12	2–504	12	100	(154)
Matsumoto	u-PA	40	1–24	24	60	(155)
Zeumer	rt-PA/u-PA	31	<4	29	94	(156)
Overgaard	rt-PA	17	<6	12	71	(157)
Barnwell	u-PA	10	<10	7	70	(158)
Lee	u-PA	20	<24?	9	45	(159)
Sasaki	rt-PA/u-PA	35	<8	16	46	(160)
Freitag	rt-PA/u-PA	22	<6	14	64	(161)
	PA + Lys-Plg	14	<6	12	86	
Gönner	u-PA	33	<4	19	58	(162)
Endo	rt-PA/u-PA	21	<6	8	38	(163)
PROACT	rscu-PA	26	<6	15	58	(18)
	Placebo	14	<6	2	14	
PROACT-2	rscu-PA + H	121	<6	80	66	(164)
	H only	59	<6	11	18	
IMS	IV + IA rt-PA	17	<3	9	53	(165)
	Placebo + IA rt-PA	18	<3	5	28	

[a]Percentage of total number of patients with recanalization.
Abbreviations: Δ(T-0), interval from onset to treatment; H, heparin; Lys-Plg, lys-plasminogen; PA, u-PA or rt-PA; plac, placebo; rscu-PA, recombinant pro-urokinase; SK, streptokinase; rt-PA, recombinant tissue plasminogen activator; u-PA, urokinase plasminogen activator; IV, intravenous; IA, intra-arterial.

patients with serious intracerebral hemorrhage (PH2, parenchymal hemorrhage with clinical deterioration) among those who received rt-PA (6.1%) compared to placebo (2.6%). The subgroup of patients with early evidence of ischemia on CT scans who should have been excluded had increased early (7-day) and late (30-day) mortality that was further increased by treatment with rt-PA. Hence, a subpopulation of patients at increased risk for severe injury and hemorrhage was identified that should have been excluded from exposure to rt-PA. The characteristics of those populations(s) will be considered below.

To reduce the number of patients at risk of intracerebral hemorrhage, careful review of the baseline CT scans for "early signs of ischemia" was performed for the follow-up study ECASS-II (152,166). Patients with early defects exceeding 33% of the hemisphere were to be excluded. A favorable outcome (mRS = 0 or 1) was observed in 40.3% of rt-PA patients compared with 36.6% of placebo patients (167). This study was effectively underpowered to detect the projected outcome because of the inclusion of mild patients. Cerebral hemorrhage causing death or deterioration (PH2) was significantly more frequent in the rt-PA group than the placebo group (11.7% versus 3.1%), but less than in ECASS. While the outcome differences were not statistically significant, the trends (in ECASS and ECASS-II) and benefits (NINDS) were consistent. The STARS (standard treatment with alteplase to reverse stroke) group completed a further prospective phase IV evaluation of rt-PA use in ischemic stroke and confirmed the NINDS results. Beneficial outcome was associated with age <75 years and the absence of "early signs" of ischemic injury (168).

The unpublished thrombolytic therapy in acute thrombotic/thromboembolic stroke (TTATTS) study of rt-PA (single chain) versus placebo by IV infusion within six hours of stroke onset was stopped by the sponsor early for the stated fear of increased hemorrhagic risk, although the prespecified safety threshold had not been broached. Questions arose about the proper arrangement of hypertension control in the patients suffering intracerebral hemorrhage early following rt-PA infusion.

Those and other studies suggested significant contributors to the risk of symptomatic intracerebral hemorrhage from IV PAs. Contributors include excessive time from the onset of symptoms to treatment, low body mass index, diastolic hypertension, older age, and the use of rt-PA (20,169,170). The appearance of "early signs of ischemia" on the initial CT scan is also associated with an increased risk of hemorrhage and demise (84,170–173). Taken together, the results of the ECASS and NINDS studies indicate the enormous importance of patient selection to reduce the hemorrhagic risk accompanying the use of PAs in acute stroke (17,84,85).

In view of the success in defining a population of patients who could be treated within three hours of symptom onset, but the failure to license rt-PA in Europe based on the ECASS and ECASS-2 datasets, a study to determine the benefit to patients treated with 4.5 hours, was undertaken in Europe. The feasibility of this study format and the timing were initially examined in a prospective registry confined to European centers (SITS-MOST) (174). ECASS-3 was conducted to determine whether the potential window for treatment efficacy with safety could be extended to 4.5 hours. The time extension is based upon earlier studies and suggested by a meta-analysis of data derived from the NINDS-sponsored trial, ECASS, and ECASS-2 (175). ECASS-3 was initiated to license rt-PA in Europe in the 3.0-hour window. ECASS-3 demonstrated a 7.2% increase in patients displaying an mRS = 0–1 at 90 days when treated with rt-PA within 3.0–4.5 hours compared to placebo (211).

Streptokinase

In contrast, experience with SK in patients with ischemic stroke was more problematic. Three symptom-based, randomized, placebo-controlled trials of acute IV delivery were terminated because of unacceptable outcome results (176,150,151). The Multicenter Acute Stroke Trial Europe (MAST-E) and the Australia Streptokinase (ASK) trials were terminated because of excessive early mortality and symptomatic intracranial hemorrhage (176,150), while the Multicentre Acute Stroke Trial-Italy (MAST-I) was terminated because of excessive early case-fatality (151). No dose-finding study preceded those trials, so a safe SK dose was not determined (177,178). Of interest was the observation that ASA increased the case-fatality of patients treated with SK when it was co-administered. Their observation has not been explained, and it has not been shown to occur when patients were exposed to ASA in conjunction with other PAs acutely. The development of SK for ischemic stroke has not been pursued since those studies.

Recent efforts have turned to PAs with other properties than rt-PA and to adjunctive treatments intending to decrease the dose of rt-PA or extend the window of successful treatment. Among the alternate PAs used in trials of ischemic stroke are TNK and DS-PA.

Teneteplase

On the basis of the apparent safety and recanalization efficacy of TNK in patients acutely suffering myocardial ischemia, TNK was examined in an open dose-escalation safety study of patients entered with qualifying strokes compatible with the criteria for the NINDS-sponsored rt-PA study (179). Patients were entered into one of four dose tiers consisting of 0.1 mg/kg ($n = 25$), 0.2 mg/kg ($n = 25$), 0.4 mg/kg ($n = 25$), or 0.5 mg/kg ($n = 13$) TNK as a single bolus within three hours of symptom onset. The dose-escalation was terminated when 2 of 13 patients suffered symptomatic intracerebral hemorrhage in the 0.5 mg/kg tier (compared with no hemorrhages in the others). To determine whether 0.4 mg/kg will produce neurological efficacy, a prospective head-to-head trial comparing TNK with rt-PA is required.

Desmoteplase

Desmoteplase (rDS-PA) has fibrin-selective properties. The program to develop recombinant DS-PA (rDS-PA) for acute intervention rested on the assumption that relative thrombus-selectivity could produce enhanced perfusion by systemic application. No dose-equivalency studies comparing rDS-PA with rt-PA have been performed. An opportunity to extend the window of treatment was pursued by linking MR technology with the timing of the intervention. Here, on the basis of the assumption that a circumferential territory of potentially reversible injury around the core exists (termed a "penumbra" by the investigators), defined by a prespecified difference between the region of perfusion (PWI) and the region of diffusion (DWI) abnormality on the initial MR imaging studies, the assertion was made that a perfusion/diffusion ratio of >1.2 ("mismatch") was sufficient to define patients capable of improvement if recanalization of the territory occurred. Instead of selecting patients on the basis of injury progression within a time limit (e.g., 3 or 6 hours as determined by experimental and clinical trials) patients not receiving rt-PA within nine hours of symptom onset but displaying a mismatch >1.2 (assumed to have salvageable tissue) were entered. While a potentially novel approach, there was little supporting data for the concept or the thresholds chosen.

Nonetheless, a series of studies of rDS-PA was mounted. The first (DIAS) was a phase II blinded placebo dose-finding efficacy trial that initially compared fixed doses of 37.5 mg and 50 mg ($n = 13$), then 25 mg ($n = 17$) of rDS-PA with placebo ($n = 16$) in a "dose-down" arrangement among patients entered from three to nine hours after symptom onset if they demonstrated a PWI/DWI ratio >1.2. The primary outcome event was symptomatic hemorrhage, with co-primary outcomes of demonstrated recanalization and an NIHSS of 0 or 1, or a change of 8 (28). The study was halted for safety reasons when it became apparent that both the lower and upper doses produced unacceptable symptomatic hemorrhage [frequencies of 23.5% (4 of 17) and 30.8% (4 of 13), respectively]. Restored perfusion was marginally greater at the lower dose (56.3%). After evaluation of the data, a second trial phase (part 2) was initiated dosing on a "per-weight" basis. In a proper dose-escalation study 62.5 µg/kg, 90 µg/kg, and 125 µg/kg ($n = 15$ each) of rDS-PA were compared with placebo ($n = 11$). A single symptomatic hemorrhage was observed at the middle dose, and recanalization occurred in 10 of 15 patients at the 125 µg/kg dose. A second phase II blinded placebo-controlled three-arm dose-finding efficacy study was performed [dose escalation of desmoteplase for acute ischemic stroke (DEDAS)] comparing 90 µg/kg ($n = 14$) rDS-PA, 125 µg/kg ($n = 15$) rDS-PA, and placebo ($n = 8$) under the same conditions as DIAS (desmoteplase in acute ischemic stroke). The primary outcome was symptomatic intracerebral hemorrhage, and co-primary outcomes of reperfusion at four to eight hours post infusion, and clinical outcomes of NIHSS of 0 or 1, mRS of 0 to 2, or Barthel index of 75 to 100 at 90 days. Prior to unblinding the data, an MR "target population" was defined (29). In the intention-to-treat analysis, no hemorrhages were observed and 8 of 15 patients demonstrated recanalization at the 125 µg/kg dose, supporting the observations of DIAS, part 2. It was claimed that in the "target population," "significant improvement in 90 day good outcome" was observed at the higher dose ($p = 0.022$). On the basis of both sets of observations, a phase III blinded three-arm placebo-controlled dose-finding efficacy trial (DIAS-2) was performed comparing 90 µg/kg ($n = 57$) rDS-PA, 125 µg/kg ($n = 66$) rDS-PA, and placebo ($n = 57$) under the same entry conditions as DIAS and DEDAS. Here the primary outcome was judged to be the difference in percentage composite outcomes between the rDS-PA patients and the placebo patients. On May 31, 2007, the sponsor reported no efficacy from this trial.

In summary, so far rt-PA (alteplase) remains the only agent approved for acute therapeutic treatment of ischemic stroke in appropriately selected individuals within three hours of symptom onset in the United States, Canada, and other countries. SK by IV delivery is not used in ischemic stroke. Extension of the treatment window to 4.5 hours awaits regulatory approval. rDS-PA has not proven efficacious in studies conducted so far, however a further phase III program by a new sponsor taking into account the weaknesses of the previous work is underway. TNK is undeveloped for ischemic stroke.

Intra-Arterial Local/Direct Delivery

The impetus to examine whether local infusion of a PA could re-establish flow through an occluded brain-supplying artery began with the realization that acute angiographic studies (within hours of symptom onset) were not accompanied with the morbidity once feared. In consequence, intra-arterial infusion studies have provided considerable information about both cerebrovascular anatomy and the treatment outcomes with thrombolytic agents. Early studies reported recanalization of symptomatic carotid artery territory occlusions in 46% to 90% of patients treated with intra-arterial local infusion of SK or u-PA within eight hours of symptom onset (Table 6) (19,77,155). In those studies, 18% to 33% of treated patients suffered hemorrhagic transformation within the ischemic territory (19,77,155). But, that frequency was consistent with historical observations from untreated patient populations. Clinical improvement was observed in a substantial number

Table 6 Hemorrhagic Transformation: Carotid Territory Ischemia, Intra-Arterial Delivery

Study	Agent	Patients n	Hemorrhage HI	Hemorrhage PH	With deterioration[a] %	Citation
del Zoppo	SK/u-PA	20	4	0	20	(77)
Mori	u-PA	22	1	3	18	(19)
Theron	SK/u-PA	12	1	2	25	(154)
Matsumoto	u-PA	40	9	4	32	(155)
Zeumer	rt-PA/u-PA	31	6	0	19	(156)
Overgaard	rt-PA	17	2	0	12	(157)
Barnwell	u-PA	10	3	0	30	(158)
Lee	u-PA	20	5	4	20	(159)
Sasaki	rt-PA/u-PA	35	7	1	23	(160)
Gönner	u-PA	33	5	2	21	(162)
PROACT	rscu-PA	26	11[b]		42	(18)
	Placebo	14	1[b]		7	
PROACT-2	rscu-PA + h	108	27	11	25	(164)
	h only	54	6	1	11	
IMS	IV + IA rt-PA	17	4	2	24	(165)
	Placebo + IA rt-PA	18	1	1	6	

[a]Percentage of total number of patients who demonstrated hemorrhagic transformation.
[b]HI + PH.
Abbreviations: HI, hemorrhagic infarction or asymptomatic hemorrhage (see text); PH, parenchymatous symptomatic hemorrhage (see text); h, heparin; IV, intravenous; IA, intra-arterial.

of those patients, although the outcomes were not quantitatively assessed and placebo comparisons were not yet undertaken.

In the vertebral-basilar artery territory thrombotic occlusions can produce significant ischemia-related disability. A retrospective comparison of clinical outcomes indicated that stroke patients who received u-PA or SK by direct intra-arterial infusion had apparent survival benefit over those who received conventional therapy (i.e., heparin) when recanalization was documented (180). Hemorrhagic transformation occurred in four patients treated with u-PA or SK; of these two deteriorated and died from the hemorrhage. That experience suggested that re-establishing flow through an occluded vertebral or basilar artery causing symptoms could arrest deterioration or perhaps improve survival and functional outcome. Given the relative scarcity of these lesions, prospective studies were not pursued and no placebo or comparative treatment study has been performed to date.

Until recently, no randomized, controlled studies of intra-arterial direct infusion had been undertaken. Two prospective studies of intra-arterial PA delivery in patients with acute thrombotic stroke have now been reported (Tables 5 and 6) (18,164). The first prospective double-blind placebo-controlled dose-finding study to be performed (prourokinase in acute cerebral thromboembolism, PROACT) compared recombinant single chain u-PA (scu-PA or pro-UK) at two doses against placebo (using 2:1 randomization) in patients treated within six hours of symptom onset for recanalization of M1 and M2 segment MCA occlusions and safety outcomes (18). Owing to restrictions by the sponsor, only one dose (6 mg) was compared with placebo. A significant increase in MCA recanalization was observed in the scu-PA group (15 of 26) (57.7%) patients versus 2 of 14 (14.3%) patients in the placebo group). During that study an increase in the frequency of hemorrhagic transformation was also observed, that prompted a review of the anticoagulation regime. The increases in both recanalization and hemorrhage proved to be heparin dependent. That study was the first to demonstrate the feasibility and efficacy of PA delivery by direct infusion.

A follow-on study, PROACT-2, prospectively tested the effect of intra-arterial recombinant scu-PA (9 mg) against no intervention for recanalization and disability outcome in an unblinded fashion. Patients with proximal MCA occlusion were openly randomized, but both groups received IV heparin, and no instrumentation was performed on "placebo" patients (164). Recanalization was marginally significantly increased with recombinant scu-PA (65.7%) compared with no intervention (18.0%), and the frequency of symptomatic intracerebral hemorrhage also increased. Disability outcome measured as $mRS = 0 - 2$ improved in the scu-PA cohort ($p = 0.046$), but was not significantly different from the control group when measured as $mRS = 0 - 1$. Hence, both recanalization and hemorrhage were dependent upon the use of the PA and the anticoagulant in those studies. A third study has not yet been performed.

In summary, two prospective trials of direct intra-arterial infusion PAs, one blinded and controlled and the other open, indicate the feasibility and relative safety of this approach. The agent under study is not available, and no PA has yet been approved for the intra-arterial approach in thrombotic stroke patients.

Local infusion thrombolysis with rt-PA (single chain) or u-PA (when it was available) has been performed at centers with the technical expertise. Dosing differs with center and among patients and is not standardized. This interventional approach now competes with the use of IV rt-PA, revascularization, and stent placement for accessible arteries. All of these approaches require demonstration of safety, with well-formed interventional/clinical teams, and appropriate, approved protocols. In the absence of a standard approved approach, there is much individual variability in agent dosing and duration, variability in the quality of PA application among centers, and little quantitative data with which to judge outcomes or safety, and to improve approaches. The approach remains experimental. Limited registries have been undertaken to evaluate the frequency and outcomes of procedures developed in communities where the procedures are being newly applied (181,182). So far these have not led to establishment of any procedure as safe or efficacious. Future efforts in this arena will require prospective properly controlled and randomized studies of the methods.

Combined Intra-Arterial and Intravenous Delivery

On the basis of the observation that the set-up for angiography (required for intra-arterial infusion) can require nearly one hour from the arrival of the patient to medical attention, the notion that initial systemic infusion of rt-PA with subsequent local infusion of an occlusion persistent was examined. There is little precedent for this approach and no pre-clinical data. The interventional management of stroke (IMS) studies examined the feasibility of combined intravenous-intra-arterial (IV-IA) infusion of rt-PA (IMS) (165), and the comparability of this approach to rt-PA alone (IMS-II) (183,184). The latter was undertaken in 81 patients, segregated into the IV rt-PA only arm ($n = 26$) and the combined treatment arm ($n = 55$). There was no difference in mortality or in the incidence of symptomatic intracerebral hemorrhage compared with the NINDS-supported trial of rt-PA (184). On the basis of that study a randomized open-label multi-center trial of the combination IV-IA regimen against "recanalization" regimens is planned (IMS-III). The proposed outcome measure is mRS 0 to 2 at three months after treatment (termed "favorable outcome"), and the study is intended to detect an absolute difference of 10% in the proportion of favorable outcomes between the two groups.

HEMORRHAGIC TRANSFORMATION WITH THROMBOLYSIS

Exposure of patients with ischemic stroke to PAs in the acute setting carries the risk of increased symptomatic hemorrhagic transformation (PH) (17,20). The NINDS-sponsored study indicated that the decrease in mortality associated with rt-PA was offset by an increase in mortality due to the PHs (17). In contrast, other studies have been contaminated by excess mortality associated with intracerebral hemorrhage (84,151). The conditions that contribute to PH in this setting have been elucidated by experimental and clinical data.

Mechanisms of Hemorrhagic Risk

Studies with stroke models indicate that hemorrhagic transformation is associated with degradation of the microvessel basal lamina matrix in the ischemic core (50). Hemorrhage occurs beginning within hours of MCA occlusion in the nonhuman primate, indicating that the risk is present from the early moments (185). Exposure of this model to rt-PA (two-chain or single-chain) within the three-hour period of MCA occlusion did not increase the frequency or severity of ischemia-related hemorrhage (186). However, in a rabbit model of focal ischemia the incidence of hemorrhage increased significantly when the PA (SK) was given later (~24 hours) after ischemia onset (187). The observation that the timing of PA delivery in relation to the onset of ischemia determines the incidence of PH has been variously confirmed in subsequent models (188–190). One explanation for that observation is the roles that matrix degradation and loss of microvessel integrity must play in erythrocyte extravasation. PAs generate plasmin from circulating plasminogen, that can degrade laminins, collagen IV, and fibronectin in matrix, as well as myelin basic protein (MBP) in the white matter, in addition to fibrin(ogen) (191,192). PAs can similarly increase microvessel permeability and hemorrhage in model preparations (193,194). A common theme is plasmin generation and its effects. So far there is no strategy available for limiting the extent of hemorrhage in the presence of PAs.

Clinical Setting of Hemorrhagic Risk

A second contributor to the extent of hemorrhage appears to be the inability to abort fibrin degradation in the presence of unopposed PA (plasmin) action. Marder had suggested that "hemostatic plugs" are necessary to limit hemorrhage from an ischemic bed in the CNS (195), but there has been little evidence to support this notion until recently. Inhibitors of the platelet fibrinogen receptor (integrin $\alpha_{IIb}\beta_3$) increase the incidence and severity of hemorrhage in the ischemic territory in a dose-dependent manner (53,56). This indicates the necessity for normal platelet function to limit hemorrhage caused by ischemic injury to the microvascular bed (53). Anecdotal clinical evidence suggests that extension of hemorrhage can occur when a PA is on board, consistent with the inability of the hemostatic apparatus to generate hemostatic plugs or a functional fibrin network. Approximately 90% of PHs observed in the setting of acute rt-PA exposure in one study were within the ischemic bed (20). This is consistent with the notion that it is microvascular injury that mediates hemorrhage.

Depth of Injury

Ueda et al. demonstrated by SPECT (*single photon emission computed tomography*) that the depth and duration of the fall in regional cerebral blood flow (rCBF) was relevant to the presence of symptomatic hemorrhage in ischemic stroke patients treated acutely with u-PA or rt-PA (196). That is, a threshold of rCBF can be determined below which the risk of a clinically significant hemorrhage (e.g., PH) in the presence of a PA is predictable. That work has not yet been applied in a prospective manner, but is consistent with the increased incidence of hemorrhage seen in ECASS (84).

Time to Treatment

One dose-escalation study of rt-PA (duteplase) demonstrated that with increasing time from symptom onset to rt-PA treatment, there was a monotonically increase in hemorrhage risk, for both HI and PH (Fig. 1) (20). This argues for earliest possible intervention, and is consistent with the data from nonhuman primate studies demonstrating the time-dependence of matrix degradation and matrix protease generation (185).

Other Contributors to Hemorrhagic Transformation

In addition to the risk with late time to treatment, symptomatic hemorrhage has been directly associated with increased diastolic blood pressure, advanced age, low body mass (hence increased dose/weight of rt-PA), and rt-PA itself (17,20,170,171). Management of blood pressure is necessary to reduce the risk of PA-associated PH.

Relation to the Patient Population

Comparison of the incidence of PH among the placebo groups from prospective controlled studies of thrombolysis in ischemic stroke indicates a highly significant linear relationship between the incidence of hemorrhage in treated patents and that of placebo patients (17,18,152,164,185). In other words, the exact incidence of symptomatic

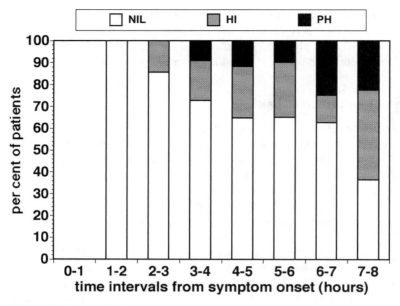

Figure 1 Increase in frequency of HI and PH with time of rt-PA (duteplase) treatment from symptom onset. *Source*: Ref. 20. *Abbreviations*: HI, hemorrhagic infarction; PH, parenchymal hemorrhage.

intracerebral hemorrhage among patents exposed to a PA within six hours of symptom onset is a function of the inherent risk among stroke patients in that population and varies from population to population. This indicates that there are yet undefined characteristics of the patients within a population that must exist that are fundamental to the risk of hemorrhage when exposed by the PA. Patient-related factors have contributed to liabilities (risk) within a number of studies (e.g., ECASS, PROACT-2, MAST-I, ASK, and others) that have eroded their potential success.

In summary, there is concordance between observations in experimental models and clinical outcomes of ischemic stroke patients with regard to PH risk in the setting of acute and delayed PA exposure. This concordance suggests that the two principal mechanisms of hemorrhage, exposure of the arterial limb in the ischemic territory to full pressure on restitution of flow and ongoing degradation of the structure of the microvasculature at risk also operate in patients. Several clinical factors that could augment that risk have been recognized, but there are other unseen characteristics also contribute to the varied risk among patient populations not described by baseline stroke severity. Defining those factors is necessary for further progress in this arena.

ADJUNCTIVE APPROACHES TO ACUTE INTERVENTION

The acute use of non-PA antithrombotic agents in the setting of ischemic stroke has been confined to two general approaches: (*i*) patients already receiving antiplatelet agents when stricken by the signal stroke and (*ii*) the addition of an antithrombotic agent to enhance some activity of the PA. The former situation is common, as in some series nearly 50% of the candidates for acute intervention rt-PA are exposed to ASA (17,20). The use of antithrombotic agents as adjuncts to PAs seems predicated on the notion that blocking thrombin generation or platelet activation could in some way extend the window for safe and effective treatment with rt-PA, or that a lower dose of the PA might be chosen. Some experience exists with experimental models that could assist here, but most of the data rests on separate trials with the antithrombotic agent alone, and the assertion that a PA + antithrombotic is additive. Experimental studies of focal ischemia have suggested that interventions with antiplatelet agents and anticoagulants, as well as agents active on nonvascular cells, could be associated with microvascular recanalization and tissue salvage (53,56).

Antiplatelet Agent A Priori

In the prospective dose-ranging study of rt-PA (duteplase), there was no relationship between the incidence of hemorrhagic transformation (or PH specifically) and contemporaneous exposure to ASA at any dose chosen (20). Similarly, the NINDS-sponsored study of rt-PA (alteplase) demonstrated no relationship of ASA to hemorrhage (17). No subsequent study has indicated an increased risk of ASA use in this setting. Similarly, although the fixed combination of ASA with extended release dipyridamole is in common use, there is no published data on hemorrhagic risk with PA exposure so far. Clopidogrel (with or without ASA) is frequently used off-indication. The MATCH study demonstrated an increased incidence of major hemorrhage (including CNS) and gastrointestinal hemorrhage alone, without an improvement in efficacy, in patients presenting with a TIA or ischemic stroke (97,98). Again there is little formal data to indicate the degree of hemorrhagic risk in the setting of acute intervention rt-PA; however it would be expected to be greater than ASA alone. In summary, there does not appear to be any added risk to patients already taking ASA who suffer a stroke when they are treated acutely with rt-PA.

Antiplatelet Exposure with the Plasminogen Activator

An interesting and disturbing outcome derived from the study of SK. All three prospective trials were halted because of excessive risk of intracerebral hemorrhage. Of these, the MAST-I study examined the impact of IV SK with or without added ASA on safety and efficacy (151). The combination resulted in a significant increase in early (7-day) mortality and in hemorrhage. The reasons for this unexpected outcome have not been explained, and no interaction between ASA and SK was known hitherto.

Addition of Anti-platelet Agent to rt-PA

Recently, interest has arisen in the possibility that concomitant use of an antiplatelet agent with rt-PA could extend the window for rt-PA treatment, improve outcome, or reduce the amount of rt-PA required and hence the risk of hemorrhage. The rationale for this approach appears to stem from experience in cardiology with the use of the pan-β_3 inhibitor abciximab with rt-PA in patients with acute MI. So far there is little preclinical evidence supporting any of these rationales, mostly because they have not been specifically tested. The known effect of complete blocking of platelet-fibrinogen receptors in focal ischemia in animal MCA:O (see above) (53,56), the unknown dose-effect in the setting of ischemic stroke, unknown interactions with rt-PA, and the lack of proper dose-equivalency studies with abciximab in the preclinical testing should have suggested extreme caution with this approach.

One phase II study (AbESTT-1) of abciximab given within 24 hours of stroke onset did not produce significant improvement or intracerebral hemorrhage in 74 patients at the doses tested (99). The relatively low incidence of hemorrhage in that study was taken as an indication of safety, and supported the undertaking of a prospective phase III study of this agent (AbESTT-2). However, that study has been terminated for reasons of safety.

In contrast, a phase II dose-escalation study [the CLEAR (combined approach to lysis utilizing eptifibatide and rt-PA in acute ischemic stroke) trial] of the integrin $\alpha_{IIb}\beta_3$ antagonist eptifibatide (integrilin) in the setting of acute rt-PA infusion demonstrated, so far, no excessive risk of hemorrhage among the ischemic stroke patients tested (197). This study has now been extended with a prospective study of modified rt-PA dosing.

In short, there is as yet no evidence that a specific $\alpha_{IIb}\beta_3$ antagonist can decrease the amount of rt-PA required or extend the window of treatment. At this writing, a single carefully performed study program of eptifibatide + rt-PA is still underway to find a safe dose of the combination.

Addition of Anticoagulant to rt-PA

There have been no studies of the acute use of anticoagulants or antithrombins in ischemic stroke patents at present. Although, experimental evidence supports the use of the low-molecular-weight heparin, enoxaparin, prior to or early following induction of MCA occlusion in rodent models of focal cerebral ischemia (57). Significant reduction in injury volume and improvement in behavioral outcome ensued.

However, there have been no attempts to combine an anticoagulant with rt-PA or another PA in the acute setting of focal cerebral ischemia. While the rationale might be the same as that offered for the adjunctive use of antiplatelet agents, it remains weak and without experimental support. Furthermore, given the increase in intracerebral hemorrhage attending the use of anticoagulants in treatment settings with thromboembolic risk (e.g., nonvalvular atrial fibrillation), the combination with a PA could unduly increase risk, with questionable benefit. That risk and benefit might be inter-related was observed in PROACT (18).

COMPLETED STROKE

At this writing, there is no rationale for the use of fibrinolytic agents in patients with stable neurological deficits produced by focal cerebral ischemia of >3 hours' duration. As noted above, patients with completed stroke are at significantly increased risk of intracerebral hemorrhage in this setting. The use of rt-PA is contraindicated in these patients.

RETINAL VASCULAR THROMBOSIS

Ischemia of the retina can be caused by thrombotic or embolic occlusion of the retinal artery or, second most commonly, by central retinal vein or branch retinal vein occlusions. Acute therapeutic options for both situations are quite limited. Kwann suggested the use of PAs to reduce ischemic injury in both settings (198). A number of anecdotal reports have documented that partial recovery of form vision was possible in some patients with retinal artery occlusion following acute intervention (199,200). Central retinal vein occlusion with visual acuity loss has been treated hours to days following onset of the deficit. In addition to conservative measures (e.g., corticosteroids), PAs have been used by systemic infusion, intravitreal infusion, direct infusion into the retinal vein, and via the ophthalmic artery (201). The use of the supraorbital arteries as ports for thrombolytic agents has been suggested (202). A number of reports have indicated the feasibility of vitrectomy with direct injection of a branch occlusion with rt-PA, including a prospective series of 28 patients (203,204). Partial visual recovery has been witnessed in select patients, even among those delayed from symptom onset. Among the complications of these approaches are vitreous hemorrhage that could lead to permanent vision loss. Overall, however, despite increased interest in the acute use of PAs, prospective studies are few, and prospective competing studies performed in acceptably controlled fashion are lacking.

FIBRINOGEN-MODULATNG STRATEGIES

Among their effects, certain PAs (e.g., u-PA, SK) can reduce circulating fibrinogen levels via degradation of the molecule. The impact of the lowered fibrinogen level on flow in the cerebral circuit is not known. However, there has been long-standing interest in the possibility that lowered blood viscosity, by reducing fibrinogen content, could increase flow within the circuit. Certain snake venoms can induce defibrinogenation when infused intravenously into humans (205). Ancrod, a purified preparation of the venom of the Malayan pit viper, *Ankistrodan rhodostoma*, infused acutely has been shown to be relatively safe in patients with ischemic stroke, when a reduction in fibrinogen of 100 mg/dL was maintained (206). According to prespecified covariate-adjusted analysis (taking into account baseline stroke severity), favorable outcomes were observed significantly more frequently in the ancrod group (42.2%) than in the placebo group (34.4%) (206,207). Severe disability was less frequent and mortality was unchanged. Intracranial hemorrhage was moderately more frequent in the ancrod group. The novel design of the Stroke Treatment with Ancrod Trial (STAT) demonstrated that careful intervention with this agent could produce a favorable benefit-risk profile (207). In contrast, no advantage to ancrod was observed in the European Stroke Treatment with Ancrod Trial (ESTAT), whose study design and patient recruitment were unlike STAT (208). A retrospective analysis of the delivery of ancrod and the subsequent fibrinogen levels in both studies suggested that the rapidity of the hypofibrinogenemia and the plateau fibrinogen levels achieved could be related to beneficial patent outcome and lowered risk of hemorrhage. Two prospective double-blind trials of ancrod with the adjusted dosing have been undertaken, the Ancrod Stroke Program (ASP)-I and ASP-II.

SAGITTAL VEIN THROMBOSIS

Thrombosis can occur in the venous drainage systems of the cerebral vasculature, including the sagittal sinus, the transverse sinuses, the great vein of Galen, or a combination of these. The presentation of thrombosis of the cerebral venous sinus(es) can be insidious or subacute, or can mimic a thrombotic stroke of the arterial tree, with motor or sensory deficits. The etiologies can include the presence of a prothrombotic state, oral hormonal replacement, local infection, and others. The appearance of peri-sagittal hemorrhage (on CT scan) suggests progression and demands rapid attention. The use of rt-PA or other PAs in the acute treatment of superior sagittal sinus thrombosis has been the subject of very few reports (209).

SUMMARY

The development of PAs as an acute treatment for thrombotic and thromboembolic stroke has depended upon the development of acceptable clinical trial strategies for acute intervention in ischemic stroke. On the basis of acute angiography, both systemic and direct infusion of PAs can increase the perfusion of an occluded brain-supplying artery of the symptomatic territory. IV infusion of rt-PA within three hours of symptom onset in ischemic stroke patients increases the probability of minimal or no disability by 11% to 13%. Current practice guidelines recommend this approach in appropriately selected patients (210). A series of clinical trials and phase IV series have confirmed this approach. To date, no other PA has, in well-conducted clinical trials, displayed benefit. While two prospective clinical trials suggest that direct infusion for scu-PA can recanalized acutely occluded arteries, no consistent demonstration of benefit has resulted. This agent is not available for clinical use. In addition, intra-arterial approaches in general are still considered experimental. Importantly, these and other recent studies have underscored the need for careful patient selection and use of the highest level of clinical trial conduct. When employed appropriately, rt-PA results in improvement in the outcome of select patients that exceeds the risk of symptomatic intracerebral hemorrhage.

REFERENCES

1. Mohr JP, Caplan LR, Melski JW, et al. The Harvard Cooperative Stroke Registry: A prospective registry of patients hospitalized with stroke. Neurology 1978; 28(8):754–762.
2. Sacco RL, Wolf PA, Kannel WB, et al. Survival and recurrence following stroke: The Framingham Study. Stroke 1982; 13:290–295.
3. Mohr JP, Barnett HJM. Classification of ischemic strokes. In: Barnett HJM, Stein BM, Mohr JP, et al., eds. Stroke: Pathophysiology, Diagnosis and Management. Vol. 1. New York: Churchill Livingstone, 1986:281–291.
4. Garcia JH, Liu K-F, Ho K-L. Neuronal necrosis after middle cerebral artery occlusion in Wistar rats progresses at different time intervals in the caudoputamen and the cortex. Stroke 1995; 26: 636–643.
5. Tagaya M, Liu K-F, Copeland B, et al. DNA scission after focal brain ischemia. Temporal differences in two species. Stroke 1997; 28(6):1245–1254.
6. Zülch K-J. The Cerebral Infarct: Pathology, Pathogenesis, and Computed Tomography. 1st ed. Berlin: Springer-Verlag, 1985.
7. Baron JC, von Kummer R, del Zoppo GJ. Treatment of acute ischemic stroke. Challenging the concept of a rigid and universal time window (editorial). Stroke 1995; 26:2219–2221.
8. von Kummer R, Meyding-Lamade U, Forsting M, et al. Sensitivity and prognostic value of early CT in occlusion of the middle cerebral artery trunk. AJNR 1994; 15:9–15.
9. Warach S, Gaa J, Siewert B, et al. Acute human stroke studied by whole brain echo planar diffusion-weighted magnetic resonance imaging. Ann Neurol 1995; 37:231–241.
10. Astrup J, Siesjö BK, Symon L. Thresholds in cerebral ischemia: the ischemic penumbra. Stroke 1981; 12(6):723–725.
11. Baron JC. Perfusion thresholds in human cerebral ischemia: historical perspective and therapeutic implications. Cerebrovasc Dis 2001; 11(suppl 1):2–8.
12. Bär T. Morphometric evaluation of capillaries in different laminae of rat cerebral cortex by automatic image analysis: Changes during development and aging. In: Cervos-Navarro J, ed. Advances in Neurology. 20th ed. New York: Raven Press, 1978:1–9.
13. Bär T, Wolff JR. The formation of capillary basement membranes during internal vascularization of the rat's cerebral cortex. Z Zellforsch Mikrosk Anat 1972; 133:231–248.
14. Johansson BB. Hypertension. In: Welch KM, Caplan LR, Reis DJ, et al., eds. Primer on Cerebrovascular Diseases. San Diego, CA: Academic Press, 1997:142–144.
15. Solis OJ, Roberson GR, Taveras JM, et al. Cerebral angiography in acute cerebral infarction. Rev Interam Radiol 1977; 2:19–25.
16. Fieschi C, Argentino C, Lenzi GL, et al. Clinical and instrumental evaluation of patients with ischemic stroke within the first six hours. J Neurol Sci 1989; 91(3):311–321.

17. The National Institutes of Neurological Disorders and Stroke rt-PA Stroke Study Group. Tissue plasminogen activator for acute ischemic stroke. N Engl J Med 1995; 333:1581–1587.
18. del Zoppo GJ, Higashida RT, Furlan AJ, et al. PROACT: a phase II randomized trial of recombinant pro-urokinase by direct arterial delivery in acute middle cerebral artery stroke. PROACT Investigators. Prolyse in Acute Cerebral Thromboembolism. Stroke 1998; 29(1): 4–11.
19. Mori E, Tabuchi M, Yoshida T, et al. Intracarotid urokinase with thromboembolic occlusion of the middle cerebral artery. Stroke 1988; 19:802–812.
20. del Zoppo GJ, Poeck K, Pessin MS, et al. Recombinant tissue plasminogen activator in acute thrombotic and embolic stroke. Ann Neurol 1992; 32(1):78–86.
21. Mori E, Yoneda Y, Tabuchi M, et al. Intravenous recombinant tissue plasminogen activator in acute carotid artery territory stroke. Neurology 1992; 42:976–982.
22. von Kummer R, Hacke W. Safety and efficacy of intravenous tissue plasminogen activator and heparin in acute middle cerebral artery. Stroke 1992; 23:646–652.
23. Yamaguchi T. Intravenous tissue plasminogen activator in acute thromboembolic stroke: A placebo-controlled, double-blind trial. In: del Zoppo GJ, Mori E, Hacke W, eds. Thrombolytic Therapy in Acute Ischemic Stroke II. Heidelberg: Springer-Verlag, 1993: 59–65.
24. Nyberg P, Waller S. Age-dependent vulnerability of brain choline acetyltransferase activity to transient cerebral ischemia in rats. Stroke 1989; 20(4):495–500.
25. Gonzales C, Lin RCS, Chesselet MF. Relative sparing of GABAergic interneurons in the striatum of gerbils with ischemia-induced lesions. Neurosci Lett 1992; 135:53–58.
26. Mabuchi T, Lucero J, Feng A, et al. Focal cerebral ischemia preferentially affects neurons distant from their neighboring microvessels. J Cereb Blood Flow Metab 2005; 25(2):257–266.
27. Francis A, Pulsinelli W. The response of GABAergic and cholinergic neurons to transient cerebral ischemia. Brain Res 1982; 243:271–278.
28. Hacke W, Albers G, Al-Rawi Y, et al. The Desmoteplase in Acute Ischemic Stroke Trial (DIAS): a phase II MRI-based 9-hour window acute stroke thrombolysis trial with intravenous desmoteplase. Stroke 2005; 36(1):66–73.
29. Furlan AJ, Eyding D, Albers GW, et al. Dose Escalation of Desmoteplase for Acute Ischemic Stroke (DEDAS): evidence of safety and efficacy 3 to 9 hours after stroke onset. Stroke 2006; 37(5):1227–1231.
30. Albers GW, Thijs VN, Wechsler L, et al. Magnetic resonance imaging profiles predict clinical response to early reperfusion: the diffusion and perfusion imaging evaluation for understanding stroke evolution (DEFUSE) study. Ann Neurol 2006; 60(5):508–517.
31. Denny-Brown D. Recurrent cerebrovascular episodes. Arch Neurol 1960; 2:194–210.
32. Russell RWR. Atheromatous retinal embolism. Lancet 1963; 2:1354–1356.
33. Hollenhorst RW. Vascular status of patients who have cholesterol emboli in the retina. Am J Ophthalmol 1966; 77:1159–1165.
34. Barnett HJM. The pathophysiology of transient cerebral ischemic attacks: Therapy with platelet antiaggregants. Med Clin North Am 1979; 63:649–679.
35. Marshall J. The Management of Cerebrovascular Diseases. Oxford: Blackwell Scientific Publications, 1976.
36. Irino T, Taneda M, Minami T. Angiographic manifestations in post-recanalized cerebral infarction. Neurology 1977; 27:471–475.
37. Dougherty JH, Levy DE, Weksler BB. Platelet activation in acute cerebral ischemia. Lancet 1977; 3:821–824.
38. Mettinger KL, Nyman D, Kjellin K-G, et al. Factor VIII related antigen, anti-thrombin III, spontaneous platelet aggregation and plasminogen activator in ischemic cerebrovascular disease. J Neurol Sci 1979; 41:31–38.
39. de Boer AC, Turpie AG, Butt RW, et al. Plasma beta thromboglobulin and serum fragment E in acute partial stroke. Br J Haematol 1982; 50:327–334.
40. Cella G, Zahavi J, de Haas HA, et al. β-thromboglobulin, platelet production time, and platelet function in vascular disease. Br J Haematol 1979; 43:127–136.

41. Feinberg WM, Bruck DC, Ring ME, et al. Hemostatic markers in acute stroke. Stroke 1989; 20:592–597.
42. van Kooten F, Ciabattoni G, Patrono C, et al. Evidence for episodic platelet activation in acute ischemic stroke. Stroke 1994; 25:278–281.
43. Feinberg WM, Pearce LA, Hart RG, et al. Markers of thrombin and platelet activity in patients with atrial fibrillation: Correlation with stroke among 1531 participants in the stroke prevention in atrial fibrillation III study. Stroke 1999; 30:2547–2553.
44. Fisher M, Zipser R. Increased excretion of immunoreactive thromboxane B2 in cerebral ischemia. Stroke 1985; 16:10–14.
45. van Kooten F, Ciabattoni G, Koudstaal PJ, et al. Increased platelet activation in the chronic phase after cerebral ischemia and intracerebral hemorrhage. Stroke 1999; 30:546–549.
46. Iwamoto T, Kubo H, Takasaki M. Platelet activation in the cerebral circulation in different subtypes of ischemic stroke and Binswanger's disease. Stroke 1995; 26:52–56.
47. Shah AB, Beamer N, Coull BM. Enhanced in vivo platelet activation in subtypes of ischemic stroke. Stroke 1985; 16:643–647.
48. Booth WY, Berndt MC, Castaldi PA. An altered platelet granule glycoprotein in patients with essential thrombocythemia. J Clin Invest 1984; 73:291–297.
49. Russell RWR. Observations on the retinal blood vessels in monocular blindness. Lancet 1961; 2:1422–1428.
50. Hamann GF, Okada Y, del Zoppo GJ. Hemorrhagic transformation and microvascular integrity during focal cerebral ischemia/reperfusion. J Cereb Blood Flow Metab 1996; 16(6):1373–1378.
51. Okada Y, Copeland BR, Fitridge R, et al. Fibrin contributes to microvascular obstructions and parenchymal changes during early focal cerebral ischemia and reperfusion. Stroke 1994; 25(9):1847–1853.
52. del Zoppo GJ, Copeland BR, Harker LA, et al. Experimental acute thrombotic stroke in baboons. Stroke 1986; 17(6):1254–1265.
53. Abumiya T, Fitridge R, Mazur C, et al. Integrin alpha(IIb)beta(3) inhibitor preserves microvascular patency in experimental acute focal cerebral ischemia. Stroke 2000; 31(6): 1402–1410.
54. del Zoppo GJ, Schmid-Schönbein GW, Mori E, et al. Polymorphonuclear leukocytes occlude capillaries following middle cerebral artery occlusion and reperfusion in baboons. Stroke 1991; 22:1276–1284.
55. Garcia JH, Liu KF, Yoshida Y, et al. Influx of leukocytes and platelets in an evolving brain infarct (Wistar rat). Am J Pathol 1994; 144:188–199.
56. Choudhri TF, Hoh BL, Zerwes HG, et al. Reduced microvascular thrombosis and improved outcome in acute murine stroke by inhibiting GP IIb/IIIa receptor-mediated platelet aggregation. J Clin Invest 1998; 102:1301–1310.
57. Stutzmann JM, Mary V, Wahl F, et al. Neuroprotective profile of enoxaparin, a low molecular weight heparin, in in vivo models of cerebral ischemia or traumatic brain injury in rats: a review. CNS Drug Rev 2002; 8:1–30.
58. Iadecola C. Neurovascular regulation in the normal brain and in Alzheimer's disease. Nat Rev Neurosci 2004; 5(5):347–360.
59. Parri R, Crunelli V. An astrocyte bridge from synapse to blood flow. Nat Neurosci 2003; 6(1): 5–6.
60. del Zoppo GJ. Stroke and Neurovascular Protection. N Engl J Med 2006; 354(6):553–555.
61. Schmidt EV, Smirnov VE, Ryabova VS. Results of the seven-year prospective study of stroke patients. Stroke 1988; 19:942–949.
62. Gent M, Blakely JA, Easton JD, et al. The Canadian-American Ticlopidine Study (CATS) in thromboembolic stroke. Lancet 1989; 1:1215–1220.
63. Britton M, Helmers C, Samuelsson K. High-dose acetylsalicylic acid after cerebral infarction. A Swedish Cooperative Study. Stroke 1987; 18:325–334.
64. Gent M, Blakeley JA, Hachinski V, et al. A secondary prevention, randomized trial of suloctidil in patients with a recent history of thromboembolic stroke. Stroke 1985; 16:416–424.

65. Marshall J. The natural history of transient ischemic cerebrovascular attacks. Q J Med 1964; 33:309–324.
66. Wolf PA, Kannel WB, McGee DL, et al. Duration of atrial fibrillation and imminence of stroke: The Framingham Study. Stroke 1983; 14:664–667.
67. Whisnant JP, Matsumoto N, Elveback LR. Transient cerebral ischemic attacks in a community, Rochester, Minnesota, 1955 through 1969. Mayo Clin Proc 1973; 48:194–198.
68. UK-TIA Study Group. United Kingdom transient ischemic attack (UK-TIA) aspirin trial: Interim results. Br Med J 1988; 296:316–320.
69. Shaw C-M, Alvord EC Jr., Berry RG. Swelling of the brain following ischemic infarction with arterial occlusion. Arch Neurol 1959; 1:161–177.
70. Muir KW, Grosset DG, Lees KR. Interconversion of stroke scales: implications for therapeutic trials. Stroke 1994; 25:1366–1370.
71. De Haan R, Horn J, Limburg M, et al. A comparison of five stroke scales with measures of disability, handicap, and quality of life. Stroke 1993; 24:1178–1181.
72. Wityk RJ, Pessin MS, Kaplan RF, et al. Serial assessment of acute stroke using the NIH stroke scale. Stroke 1994; 25:362–365.
73. Fisher CM, Adams RD. Observations on brain embolism with special reference to hemorrhage infarction. In: Furlan AJ, ed. The Heart and Stroke. Exploring Mutual Cerebrovascular and Cardiovascular Issues. 1st ed. New York: Springer-Verlag, 1987:17–36.
74. Fisher CM, Adams RD. Observations on brain embolism with special reference to the mechanism of hemorrhagic infarction. J Neuropathol Exp Neurol 1951; 10:92–94.
75. Jörgensen L, Torvik A. Ischaemic cerebrovascular diseases in an autopsy series. Part 2. Prevalence, location, pathogenesis, and clinical course of cerebral infarcts. J Neurol Sci 1969; 9: 285–320.
76. Kwa VI, Franke CL, Verbeeten B Jr, et al. Silent intracerebral microhemorrhages in patients with ischemic stroke. Amsterdam Vascular medicine Group. Ann Neurol 1998; 44:372–377.
77. del Zoppo GJ, Ferbert A, Otis S, et al. Local intra-arterial fibrinolytic therapy in acute carotid territory stroke: A pilot study. Stroke 1988; 19(3):307–313.
78. Ogata J, Yutani C, Imakita M, et al. Hemorrhagic infarct of the brain without a reopening of the occluded arteries in cardioembolic stroke. Stroke 1989; 20:876–883.
79. Yamaguchi T, Minematsu K, Choki J, et al. Clinical and neuroradiological analysis of thrombotic and embolic cerebral infarction. Jpn Circ J 1984; 48:50–58.
80. Bogousslavsky J, Van Melle G, Regli F. The Lausanne Stroke Registry: Analysis of 1,000 consecutive patients with first stroke. Stroke 1988; 19:1083–1092.
81. Foulkes MA, Wolf PA, Price TR, et al. The stroke data bank: Design, methods, and baseline characteristics. Stroke 1988; 19:547–554.
82. International Stroke Trial Collaborative Group. The International Stroke Trial (IST): a randomised trial of aspirin, subcutaneous heparin, both, or neither among 19,435 patients with acute ischaemic stroke. Lancet 1997; 349:1569–1681.
83. Chen ZM, Sandercock P, Pan HC, et al. Indications for early aspirin use in acute ischemic stroke: a combined analysis of 40,000 randomized patients from the Chinese acute stroke trial and the international stroke trial. On behalf of the CAST and IST collaborative groups. Stroke 2000; 31:1240–1249.
84. Hacke W, Kaste M, Fieschi C, et al. Intravenous thrombolysis with recombinant tissue plasminogen activator for acute hemispheric stroke. The European Cooperative Acute Stroke Study (ECASS). JAMA 1995; 274(13):1017–1025.
85. del Zoppo GJ. Acute stroke: on the threshold of a therapy? N Engl J Med 1995; 333:1632–1633.
86. Albers GW, Amarenco P, Easton JD, et al. Antithrombotic and thrombolytic therapy for ischemic stroke. Chest 2008; 133:630S–669S.
87. Cerebral Embolism Study Group. Immediate anticoagulation of embolic stroke: brain hemorrhage and management options. Stroke 1984; 15:779–789.
88. Babikian VL, Kase CS, Pessin MS, et al. Intracerebral hemorrhage in stroke patients anticoagulated with heparin. Stroke 1989; 29:1500–1503.

89. Levine MN, Raskob G, Landefeld S, et al. Hemorrhagic complications of anticoagulant treatment. Chest 2001; 119:108S–121S.

90. Harker LA. Antiplatelet drugs in the management of patients with thrombotic disorders. Semin Thromb Hemost 1986; 12:134–155.

91. Fitzgerald GA. Dipyridamole. N Engl J Med 1987; 316:1247–1257.

92. Fitzgerald GA. Dipyridamole. N Engl J Med 1987; 317:1734–1736.

93. Harker LA, Slichter SJ. Arterial and venous thromboembolism: kinetic characterization and evaluation of therapy. Thromb Diath Haemorrh 1974; 31:188–203.

94. Diener H, Cunha L, Forbes C, et al. European Stroke Prevention Study 2. Dipyridamole and acetylsalicylic acid in the secondary prevention of stroke. J Neurol Sci 1996; 143:1–13.

95. CAPRIE Steering Committee. A randomised, blinded, trial of clopidogrel versus aspirin in patients at risk of ischaemic events (CAPRIE). Lancet 1996; 348:1329–1339.

96. CAST (Chinese Acute Stroke Trial) Collaborative Group. CAST: a randomised placebo-controlled trial of early aspirin use in 20,000 patients with acute ischaemic stroke. Lancet 1997; 349:1641–1649.

97. Diener H-C, Bogousslavsky J, Brass LM, et al. Aspirin and clopidogrel compared with clopidogrel alone after recent ischaemic stroke or transient ischaemic attack in high-risk patients (MATCH): randomised, doubled-blind, placebo-controlled trial. Lancet 2004; 364:331–337.

98. Diener H-C, Bogousslavsky J, Brass LM, et al. Management of atherothrombosis with clopidogrel in high-risk patients with recent transient ischaemic attack or ischaemic stroke (MATCH): study design and baseline data. Cerebrovasc Dis 2004; 17:253–261.

99. The Abciximab in Ischemic Stroke Investigators. Abciximab in acute ischemic stroke: a randomized, double-blind, placebo-controlled, dose-escalation study. Stroke 2000; 31:601–609.

100. Baker RN, Broward JA, Fang HC, et al. Anticoagulant therapy in cerebral infarction. Neurology 1962; 12:823–835.

101. Siekert RG, Whisnant JP, Millikan CH. Surgical and anticoagulant therapy of occlusive cerebrovascular disease. Ann Intern Med 1963; 58:637–641.

102. Stroke Prevention in Atrial Fibrillation Study Group Investigators. Preliminary report of the Stroke Prevention in Atrial Fibrillation Study. N Engl J Med 1990; 322:863–868.

103. Stroke Prevention in Atrial Fibrillation Investigators. Warfarin versus aspirin for prevention of thromboembolism in atrial fibrillation: Stroke Prevention in Atrial Fibrillation II Study. Lancet 1994; 343:687–691.

104. Stroke Prevention in Atrial Fibrillation Investigators. Adjusted-dose warfarin versus low-intensity, fixed-dose warfarin plus aspirin for high-risk patients with atrial fibrillation: stroke prevention in atrial fibrillation III randomised clinical trial. Lancet 1996; 348:633–638.

105. Petersen P, Boysen G, Godtfredsen J, et al. Placebo-controlled randomized trial of warfarin and aspirin to prevention of thromboembolic complications in chronic atrial fibrillation. The Copenhagen AFASAK Study. Lancet 1989; 1:175–179.

106. EAFT European Atrial Fibrillation Trial Study Group. Secondary prevention in non-rheumatic atrial fibrillation after transient ischaemic attack or minor stroke. Lancet 1993; 342:1255–1262.

107. Barnhorst DA, Oxman HA, Connolly DC, et al. Long-term follow-up of isolated replacement of the aortic or mitral valve with the Starr-Edwards prosthesis. Am J Cardiol 1975; 35:228–233.

108. Moggio RA, Hammond GL, Stansel HL Jr, et al. Incidence of emboli with cloth-covered Starr-Edwards value without anticoagulation and with varying forms of anticoagulation. J Thorac Cardiovasc Surg 1978; 75:296–299.

109. Akbarian M, Austen WG, Yurchak PM, et al. Thromboembolic complications of prosthetic cardiac valves. Circulation 1986; 37:826–831.

110. Saour JN, Sleek JO, Mamo LAR, et al. Trial of different intensities of patients with prosthetic heart valves. N Engl J Med 1990; 322:428–432.

111. Loeliger EA. Therapeutic target values in oral anticoagulation: justification of Dutch policy and a warning against the so-called moderate-intensity regimens. Ann Hematol 1992; 64: 60–65.

112. Turpie AGG, Gunstensen J, Hirsh J, et al. Randomized comparison of two intensities of oral anticoagulant therapy after tissue heart valve placement. Lancet 1988; 1:1242–1245.

113. Walker AM, Jick H. Predictors of bleeding during heparin therapy. JAMA 1980; 244: 1209–1212.

114. Mohr JP, Thompson JL, Lazar RM, et al. A comparison of warfarin and aspirin for the prevention of recurrent ischemic stroke. N Engl J Med 2001; 345:1444–1451.

115. Collen D. The plasminogen (fibrinolytic) system. Thromb Haemost 1999; 82:259–270.

116. Brogden RN, Speight TM, Avery GS. Streptokinase: A review of its clinical pharmacology, mechanism of action, and therapeutic uses. Drugs 1973; 5:357–445.

117. Lijnen HR, de Cock F, Matsuo O, et al. Comparative fibrinolytic and fibrinogenolytic properties of staphylokinase and streptokinase in plasma of different species in vitro. Fibrinolysis 1992; 6:33–37.

118. Jespers L, Vanwetswinkel S, Lijnen HR, et al. Structural and functional basis of plasminogen activation by staphylokinase. Thromb Haemost 1999; 81(4):479–484.

119. Nagai N, De Mol M, Lijnen HR, et al. Role of plasminogen system components in focal cerebral ischemic infarction: a gene targeting and gene transfer study in mice. Circulation 1999; 99:2440–2444.

120. Robbins KC, Summaria L, Hsieh B, et al. The peptide chains of human plasmin. J Biochem 1967; 242:2333–2342.

121. Rijken DC. Structure/function relationships of t-PA. In: Kluft C, ed. Tissue Type Plasminogen Activator (t-PA): Physiological and Clinical Aspects. Vol. 1. Boca Raton, FL: CRC Press, 1988: 101–122.

122. Ranby M, Bergsdorf N, Nilsson T. Enzymatic properties of the one- and two-chain form of tissue plasminogen activator. Thromb Res 1982; 27:175–183.

123. Rijken DC, Hoylaerts M, Collen D. Fibrinolytic properties of one-chain and two-chain human extrinsic (tissue-type) plasminogen activator. J Biol Chem 1982; 257:2920–2925.

124. Ranby M, Bergsdorf N, Norrman B, et al. Tissue plasminogen activator kinetics. In: Davison JF, Bachmann F, Bouvier CA, et al., eds. Progress in Fibrinolysis. Vol. 6. New York: Churchill-Livingstone, 1982:182.

125. Korninger C, Collen D. Studies on the specific fibrinolytic effect of human extrinsic (tissue-type) plasminogen activator in human blood and in various animal species in vitro. Thromb Haemost 1981; 46:561–565.

126. Paoni NF, Chow AM, Pena LC, et al. Making tissue-type plasminogen activator more fibrin specific. Protein Eng 1993; 6(5):529–534.

127. Guzzetta AW, Basa LJ, Hancock WS, et al. Identification of carbohydrate structures in glycoprotein peptide maps by the use of LC/MS with selected ion extraction with special reference to tissue plasminogen activator and a glycosylation variant produced by site directed mutagenesis. Anal Chem 1993; 65(21):2953–2962.

128. Stewart RJ, Fredenburgh JC, Leslie BA, et al. Identification of the mechanism responsible for the increased fibrin specificity of TNK-tissue plasminogen activator relative to tissue plasminogen activator. J Biol Chem 2000; 275(14):10112–10120.

129. Assessment of the Safety and Efficacy of a New Thrombolytic (ASSENT-2) Investigators. Single-bolus tenecteplase compared with front-loaded alteplase in acute myocardial infarction: the ASSENT-2 double-blind randomised trial. Lancet 1999; 354(9180):716–722.

130. Schleuning W-D, Donner P. Desmodus rotundus (Common Vampire Bat) salivary plasminogen activator. In: Bachmann F, ed. Fibrinolytics and Antifibrinolytics. Berlin: Springer-Verlag, 2001:451–472.

131. Witt W, Baldus B, Bringmann P, et al. Thrombolytic properties of Desmodus rotundus (vampire bat) salivary plasminogen activator in experimental pulmonary embolism in rats. Blood 1992; 79:1213–1217.

132. Gulba DC, Praus M, Witt W. DSPA alpha: properties of the plasminogen activators of the vampire bat *Desmodus rotundus*. Fibrinolysis 1995; 9(suppl 1):91–96.
133. Clarke RL, Cliffton EE. The treatment of cerebrovascular thrombosis and embolism with fibrinolytic agents. Am J Cardiol 1960; 30:546–551.
134. Herndon RM, Meyer JS, Johnson JF, et al. Treatment of cerebrovascular thrombosis with fibrinolysin. Preliminary report. Am J Cardiol 1960; 30:540–545.
135. Meyer JS, Gilroy J, Barnhart MI, et al. Therapeutic thrombolysis in cerebral thromboembolism. Neurology 1963; 13:927–937.
136. Araki G, Minakami K, Mihara H. Therapeutic effect of urokinase on cerebral infarction. Rinsho to Kenkyu 1973; 50:3317–3326.
137. Fletcher AP, Alkjaersig N, Lewis M, et al. A pilot study of urokinase therapy in cerebral infarction. Stroke 1976; 7:135–142.
138. NIH Consensus Conference. Thrombolytic therapy in treatment. Br Med J 1980; 280:1585–1587.
139. del Zoppo GJ, Zeumer H, Harker LA. Thrombolytic therapy in stroke: possibilities and hazards. Stroke 1986; 17(4):595–607.
140. Atarashi J, Otomo E, Araki G, et al. Clinical utility of urokinase in the treatment of acute stage of cerebral thrombosis: Multi-center double-blind study in comparison with placebo. Clin Eval 1985; 13:659–709.
141. Otomo E, Araki G, Itoh E, et al. Clinical efficacy of urokinase in the treatment of cerebral thrombosis. Clin Eval 1985; 13:711–751.
142. Abe T, Terashi A, Tohgi H, et al. Clinical efficacy of intravenous administration of SM-9527 (t-PA) in cerebral thrombosis. Clin Eval 1990; 18:39–69.
143. Otomo E, Tohgi H, Hirai S, et al. Clinical efficacy of AK-124 (tissue plasminogen activator) in the treatment of cerebral thrombosis: Study by means of multi- center double blind comparison with urokinase. Yakuri To Chiryo 1988; 16:3775–3821.
144. von Kummer R, Forsting M, Sartor K, et al. Intravenous recombinant tissue plasminogen activator in acute stroke. In: Hacke W, del Zoppo GJ, Hirschberg M, eds. Thrombolytic Therapy in Acute Ischemic Stroke. Heidelberg: Springer-Verlag, 1991:161–167.
145. Yamaguchi T. Intravenous rt-PA in acute embolic stroke. In: Hacke W, del Zoppo GJ, Hirschberg M, eds. Thrombolytic Therapy in Acute Ischemic Stroke. Heidelberg: Springer-Verlag, 1991:168–174.
146. Abe T, Kazama M, Naito I, et al. Clinical evaluation for efficacy of tissue culture urokinase (TCUK) on cerebral thrombosis by means of multicenter double- blind study. Blood Vessels 1981; 12:321–341.
147. Abe T, Kazawa M, Naito I, et al. Clinical effect of urokinase (60,000 units/day) on cerebral infarction–Comparative study by means of multiple center double blind test. Blood Vessels 1981; 12:342–358.
148. Haley EC Jr, Brott TG, Sheppard GL, et al. Pilot randomized trial of tissue plasminogen activator in acute ischemic stroke. Stroke 1993; 24:1000–1004.
149. The Multicenter Acute Stroke Trial–Europe Study Group. Thrombolytic therapy with streptokinase in acute ischemic stroke. N Engl J Med 1996; 335:145–150.
150. Donnan GA, Davis SM, Chambers BR, et al. Trials of streptokinase in severe acute ischaemic stroke. Lancet 1995; 345:578–579.
151. Multicenter Acute Stroke Trial-Italy (MAST-I) Group. Randomised controlled trial of streptokinase, aspirin, and combination of both in treatment of acute ischaemic stroke. Lancet 1995; 346:1509–1514.
152. Hacke W, Kaste M, Fieschi C, et al. Randomised double-blind placebo-controlled trial of thrombolytic therapy with intravenous alteplase in acute ischaemic stroke (ECASS II). Lancet 1998; 352(9136):1245–1251.
153. Kwiatkowski TG, Libman RB, Frankel M, et al. Effects of tissue plasminogen activator for acute ischemic stroke at one year. National Institute of Neurological Disorders and Stroke Recombinant Tissue Plasminogen Activator Stroke Study Group. N Engl J Med 1999; 340:1781–1787.

154. Theron J, Courtheoux P, Casaseo A, et al. Local intra-arterial fibrinolysis in the carotid territory. AJNR 1989; 10:753–765.
155. Matsumoto K, Satoh K. Topical intraarterial urokinase infusion for acute stroke. In: Hacke W, del Zoppo GJ, Hirschberg M, eds. Thrombolytic Therapy in Acute Ischemic Stroke. Heidelberg: Springer-Verlag, 1991:207–212.
156. Zeumer H, Freitag HJ, Zanella F, et al. Local intraarterial fibrinolytic therapy in stroke patients: Urokinase versus recombinant tissue plasminogen activator rt-PA. Neuroradiology 1993; 35:159–162.
157. Overgaard K, Sperling B, Boysen G, et al. Thrombolytic therapy in acute ischemic stroke. A Danish pilot study. Stroke 1993; 24:1439–1446.
158. Barnwell SL, Clark WM, Nguyen TT, et al. Safety and efficacy of delayed intraarterial urokinase therapy with mechanical clot disruption for thromboembolic stroke. AJNR 1994; 15: 1817–1822.
159. Lee BI, Lee BC, Park SC, et al. Intra-carotid thrombolytic therapy in acute ischemic stroke of carotid arterial territory. Yonsei Med J 1994; 35:49–61.
160. Sasaki O, Takeuchi S, Koike T, et al. Fibrinolytic therapy for acute embolic stroke: intravenous, intracarotid, and intra-arterial local approaches. Neurosurgery 1995; 36:246–252.
161. Freitag HJ, Becker VU, Thie A, et al. Lys-plasminogen as an adjunct to local intra-arterial fibrinolysis for carotid territory stroke: laboratory and clinical findings. Neuroradiology 1996; 38(2):181–185.
162. Gönner F, Remonda L, Mattle H, et al. Local intra-arterial thrombolysis in acute ischemic stroke. Stroke 1998; 29(9):1894–1900.
163. Endo S, Kuwayama N, Hirashima Y, et al. Results of urgent thrombolysis in patients with major stroke and atherothrombotic occlusion of the cervical internal carotid artery. AJNR Am J Neuroradiol 1998; 19(6):1169–1175.
164. Furlan A, Higashida R, Wechsler L, et al. Intra-arterial prourokinase for acute ischemic stroke. The PROACT II Study: a randomized controlled trial. JAMA 1999; 282:2003–2011.
165. Lewandowski CA, Frankel M, Tomsick TA, et al. Combined intravenous and intra-arterial r-TPA versus intra-arterial therapy of acute ischemic stroke: Emergency Management of Stroke (EMS) Bridging Trial. Stroke 1999; 30(12):2598–2605.
166. von Kummer R, Allen KL, Holle R, et al. Acute stroke: Usefulness of early CT findings before thrombolytic therapy. Radiology 1997; 205:327–333.
167. Hacke W, Bluhmki E, Steiner T, et al. Dichotomized efficacy end points and global end-point analysis applied to the ECASS intention-to-treat data set: post hoc analysis of ECASS I. Stroke 1998; 29:2073–2075.
168. Albers GW, Bates VE, Clark WM, et al. Intravenous tissue-type plasminogen activator for treatment of acute stroke: The Standard treatment with alteplase to reverse stroke (STARS) study. JAMA 2000; 283:1145–1150.
169. Levy DE, Brott TG, Haley EC Jr., et al. Factors related to intracranial hematoma formation in patients receiving tissue-type plasminogen activator for acute ischemic stroke. Stroke 1994; 25: 291–297.
170. Larrue V, von Kummer R, del Zoppo GJ, et al. Hemorrhagic transformation in acute ischemic stroke: potential contributing factors in the European Cooperative Acute Stroke Study. Stroke 1997; 28(5):957–960.
171. Larrue V, von Kummer RR, Muller A, et al. Risk factors for severe hemorrhagic transformation in ischemic stroke patients treated with recombinant tissue plasminogen activator: a secondary analysis of the European-Australiasian Acute Stroke Study (ECASS II). Stroke 2001; 32(2):438–441.
172. Dubey N, Bakshi R, Wasay M, et al. Early computed tomography hypodensity predicts hemorrhage after intravenous tissue plasminogen activator in acute ischemic stroke. J Neuroimaging 2001; 11:184–188.
173. Kalafut MA, Schriger DL, Saver JL, et al. Detection of early CT signs of >1/3 middle cerebral artery infarctions: Interrater reliability and sensitivity of CT interpretation by physicians involved in acute stroke care. Stroke 2000; 31:1667–1671.

174. Wahlgren N, Ahmed N, Davalos A, et al. Thrombolysis with alteplase for acute ischaemic stroke in the Safe Implementation of Thrombolysis in Stroke-Monitoring Study (SITS-MOST): an observational study. Lancet 2007; 369(9558):275–282.

175. Hacke W, Donnan G, Fieschi C, et al. Association of outcome with early stroke treatment: pooled analysis of ATLANTIS, ECASS, and NINDS rt-PA stroke trials. Lancet 2004; 363 (9411):768–774.

176. Hommel M, Boissel JP, Cornu C, et al. Termination of trial of streptokinase in severe acute ischemic stroke. Lancet 1995; 345:578–579.

177. Gruppo Italiano Per Lo Studio Della Streptochinasi Nell'Infarto Miocardico (GISSI). Effectiveness of intravenous thrombolytic treatment in acute myocardial infarction. Lancet 1986; 1:397–401.

178. Gruppo Italiano Per Lo Studio Della Streptochinasi Nell'Infarto Miocardico (GISSI). GISSI-2: a factorial randomized trial of alteplase versus streptokinase and heparin versus no heparin among 12,490 patients with acute myocardial infarction. Lancet 1990; 336:65–71.

179. Haley EC Jr., Lyden PD, Johnston KC, et al. A pilot dose-escalation safety study of tenecteplase in acute ischemic stroke. Stroke 2005; 36(3):607–612.

180. Hacke W, Zeumer H, Ferbert A, et al. Intra-arterial thrombolytic therapy improves outcome in patients with acute vertebrobasilar occlusive disease. Stroke 1988; 19(10):1216–1222.

181. Kim D, Ford GA, Kidwell CS, et al. Intra-arterial thrombolysis for acute stroke in patients 80 and older: a comparison of results in patients younger than 80 years. AJNR Am J Neuroradiol 2007; 28(1):159–163.

182. Nedeltchev K, Fischer U, Arnold M, et al. Long-term effect of intra-arterial thrombolysis in stroke. Stroke 2006; 37(12):3002–3007.

183. The IMS Study Investigators. Combined intravenous and intra-arterial recanalization for acute ischemic stroke: the Interventional Management of Stroke Study. Stroke 2004; 35(4):904–911.

184. The IMS II Trial Investigators. The Interventional Management of Stroke (IMS) II Study. Stroke 2007; 38(7):2127–2135.

185. Heo JH, Lucero J, Abumiya T, et al. Matrix metalloproteinases increase very early during experimental focal cerebral ischemia. J Cereb Blood Flow Metab 1999; 19(6):624–633.

186. del Zoppo GJ, Copeland BR, Anderchek K, et al. Hemorrhagic transformation following tissue plasminogen activator in experimental cerebral infarction. Stroke 1990; 21(4):596–601.

187. Silvka A, Pulsinelli WA. Hemorrhagic complications of thrombolytic therapy in experimental stroke. Stroke 1987; 18:1148–1156.

188. del Zoppo GJ. Fibrinolytic agents in animal models of cerebrovascular ischemia. Fibrinolysis 1990; 4(suppl 2):3–7.

189. del Zoppo GJ. Relevance of focal cerebral ischemia models. Experience with fibrinolytic agents. Stroke 1990; 21(12 suppl):IV155–IV160.

190. del Zoppo GJ. Why do all drugs work in animals but none in stroke patients? A. Drugs promoting cerebral blood flow. J Intern Med 1995; 237(1):79–88.

191. Rifkin DB. Plasminogen activator expression and matrix degradation. Matrix 1992; (suppl. 1): 20–22.

192. Lijnen HR. Plasmin and matrix metalloproteinases in vascular remodeling. Thromb Haemost 2001; 86:324–333.

193. Marder VJ, Shortell CK, Fitzpatrick PG, et al. An animal model of fibrinolytic bleeding based on the rebleed phenomenon: Application to a study of vulnerability of hemostatic plugs of different age. Thromb Res 1992; 67(1):31–40.

194. Kimura Y, Tani T, Kanbe T, et al. Effect of cilostazol on platelet aggregation and experimental thrombosis. Arzneimittelforschung 1985; 35(7A):1144–1149.

195. Marder VJ. Fibrinolytic agents: Are they feasible for stroke therapy? In: Plum F, Pulsinelli WA, eds. Cerebrovascular Diseases, Fourteenth Research Conference. New York: Raven Press, 1986:241–247.

196. Ueda T, Sakaki S, Yuh WT, et al. Outcome in acute stroke with successful intra-arterial thrombolysis and predictive value of initial single-photon emission-computed tomography. J Cereb Blood Flow Metab 1999; 19:99–108.

197. CLEAR trial Investigators. The Combined Approach to Lysis Utilizing Eptifibatide and rt-PA in Acute Ischemic Stroke (The CLEAR Stroke Trial). Stroke 2008; 39:3268–3276.

198. Kwaan HC. Thromboembolic disorders of the eye. In: Comerota AC, ed. Thrombolytic Therapy. Orlando: Grune and Stratton, 1988:153–163.

199. Freitag H-J, Zeumer H, Knospe V. Acute central retinal artery occlusion and the role of thrombolysis. In: del Zoppo GJ, Mori E, Hacke W, eds. Thrombolytic Therapy in Acute Ischemic Stroke II. Heidelberg: Springer-Verlag, 1993:103–105.

200. Schmidt D, Schumacher M, Wakhloo AK. Microcatheter urokinase infusion in central retinal artery occlusion. Am J Ophthalmol 1992; 113:429–434.

201. Shahid H, Hossain P, Amoaku WM. The management of retinal vein occlusion: is interventional ophthalmology the way forward? Br J Ophthalmol 2006; 90(5):627–639.

202. Schwenn OK, Wustenberg EG, Konerding MA, et al. Experimental percutaneous cannulation of the supraorbital arteries: implication for future therapy. Invest Ophthalmol Vis Sci 2005; 46(5): 1557–1560.

203. Christodoulakis EV, Tsilimbaris MK. The role of vitrectomy assisted rt-PA injection for the management of branch retinal vein occlusion: case report. Semin Ophthalmol 2007; 22(2):89–93.

204. Weiss JN, Bynoe LA. Injection of tissue plasminogen activator into a branch retinal vein in eyes with central retinal vein occlusion. Ophthalmology 2001; 108(12):2249–2257.

205. Bell WR Jr. Defibrinogenating enzymes. Drugs 2001; 54(suppl 3):18–30.

206. The Ancrod Stroke Study Investigators. Ancrod for the treatment of acute ischemic brain infarction. Stroke 1994; 25:1755–1759.

207. Sherman DG, Atkinson RP, Chippendale T, et al. Intravenous ancrod for treatment of acute ischemic stroke: the STAT study: a randomized ocntrolled trial. Stroke Treatment with Ancrod Trial. JAMA 2000; 283:2395–2403.

208. Orgogozo JM, Verstraete M, Kay R, et al. Outcomes of ancrod in acute ischemic stroke. Independent Data and Safety Monitoring Board for ESTAT. Steering Committee for ESTAT. European Stroke Treatment with Ancrod Trial. JAMA 2000; 284:1926–1927.

209. Niwa J, Ohyama H, Matumura S, et al. Treatment of acute superior sagittal sinus thrombosis by t-PA infusion via venography: direct thrombolytic therapy in the acute phase. Surg Neurol 1998; 49(4):425–429.

210. Adams H, del Zoppo GJ, Alberts MJ, et al. Guidelines for the early management of adults with ischemic stroke: a guideline from the American Heart Association/American Stroke Association Stroke Council, Clinical Cardiology Council, Cardiovascular Radiology and Intervention Council, and the Atherosclerotic Peripheral Vascular Disease and Quality of Care Outcomes in Research Interdisciplinary Working Groups: the American Academy of Neurology affirms the value of this guideline as an educational tool for neurologists. Stroke 2007; 38(5):1655–1711.

211. Hacke W, Kaste M, Bluhmki E, et al. ECASS Investigators. Thrombolysis with alteplase 3 to 4.5 hours after acute ischemic stroke. N Engl J Med 2008; 359(13):1317–1329.

37

Fibrinolysis for Acute Myocardial Infarction

Cheuk-Kit Wong
Department of Medical and Surgical Sciences, Dunedin School of Medicine, University of Otago, Dunedin, New Zealand

Harvey D. White
Green Lane Cardiovascular Service, Cardiology Department, Auckland City Hospital, Auckland, New Zealand

INTRODUCTION

The most important therapeutic goal in the management of acute myocardial infarction is the early restoration of complete epicardial infarct artery patency and normal myocardial perfusion. The mechanisms of reduction in mortality with fibrinolysis include clot lysis resulting in myocardial salvage, preservation of left ventricular function, and improved left ventricular remodelling. When epicardial flow is restored within 30 minutes of occlusion, myocardial infarction can be aborted. If flow is achieved within two hours, considerable myocardial salvage can occur with beneficial effects on ventricular function and survival. When reperfusion is achieved after two to three hours, myocardial salvage is progressively reduced, and recovery of ventricular function is dependent on established collateral flow. Beyond six hours, myocardial salvage is minimal (1).

Myocardial infarction can be prevented by early fibrinolysis (2). The incidence of aborted infarction has been reported as 25% in patients treated within one hour of symptom onset (3). In the MITI trial (myocardial infarction triage and intervention) tissue plasminogen activator (t-PA) (4) administered within 70 minutes was associated with a mortality of 1.2% with a greater than 30% reduction in infarct size compared with administration after three hours.

Reperfusion can be achieved with either fibrinolysis or primary percutaneous coronary intervention (PCI). In a meta-analysis (5) of 22 trials that compared fibrinolytic therapy with placebo or control treatment ($n = 50{,}246$), the proportional mortality reduction was 48% in patients treated within one hour (95% CI, 31–61%), and patients treated within two hours had a significantly greater mortality reduction (44%; CI, 32–53%) than those treated later (20%; CI, 15–25%) (Fig. 1).

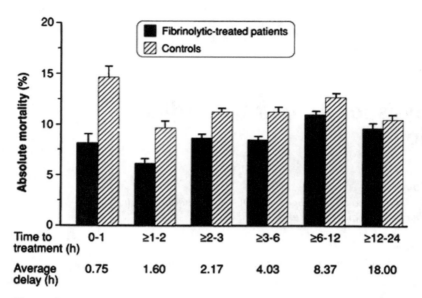

Figure 1 Mortality among fibrinolytic-treated and control patients according to treatment delay. *Source*: Adapted from Ref. 5.

The results of a meta-analysis comparing fibrinolysis with primary PCI (6) show that within centers capable of offering either catheter-based reperfusion or pharmacologic reperfusion, primary PCI appears to offer superior clinical outcomes. It is to be noted however that the meta-analysis combined treatments that have been shown to have different effects on mortality, e.g., accelerated t-PA administered over 90 minutes and streptokinase. In the GUSTO I trial, (global use of strategies to open occluded coronary arteries) t-PA given in an accelerated regimen resulted in a 14% relative and an absolute 1% mortality reduction at 30 days as compared with streptokinase given IV over one hour (7). In the meta-analysis of the 11 trials of accelerated t-PA versus PCI, the reduction in mortality with PCI was not significant, $p = 0.08$ (8).

Any incremental benefit of PCI over fibrinolysis is dependent on timely implementation, with some analyses suggesting that the incremental benefit is lost with a relative delay (door to balloon time vs. door to needle time) of between 60 minutes and 114 minutes, with lesser tolerance among high-risk patients (9,10). Importantly, there is a complex interplay between factors such as, patient age, infarct site, and initial delay in presentation and the acceptable relative delay between primary PCI and fibrinolysis (Fig. 2). In general, the superiority of primary PCI over fibrinolysis is lost early among patients <65 years and those presenting within 120 minutes of symptom onset, and the time difference could be as little as 40 minutes, in which PCI loses superiority to fibrinolysis.

For patients presenting within one hour of symptom onset, fibrinolysis appears superior to PCI. Justification of the superiority of catheter-based reperfusion over fibrinolysis is predicated on efficient and effective clinical systems of care that are able to deliver timely reperfusion in a consistent manner. In the United States, more than two-thirds of patients with ST-elevation myocardial infarction (STEMI) present to hospitals without PCI capability (11). Worldwide, PCI capability is less than in the United States (12) and fibrinolysis remains the most common reperfusion strategy.

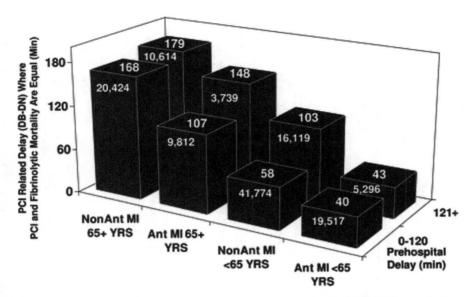

Figure 2 Adjusted analysis illustrating the heterogeneity in the DB-DN (door to balloon minus door to needle) time for which the hospital mortality rates of primary PCI versus fibrinolysis were comparable. Note that in young patients with anterior infarct a PCI related delay of 40 minutes or more could negate the treatment benefit of primary PCI compared with fibrinolysis. *Source:* Adapted from Ref. 9.

In the 2007 AHA/ACC update (13), the recommendations are as follows:

Class 1: STEMI patients presenting to a hospital without PCI capability and who cannot be transferred to a PCI center and undergo PCI within 90 minutes of first medical contact should be treated with fibrinolytic therapy within 30 minutes of hospital presentation as a systems goal unless fibrinolytic therapy is contraindicated. (*Level of Evidence: B.*)

No fibrinolytic trial since GUSTO I has demonstrated a further reduction in mortality with newer regimens (14–19), although some treatments have been found to restore thrombolysis in myocardial infarction (TIMI) grade 3 (i.e., normal) flow (20) to the infarct-related coronary artery in a higher proportion of patients (21–23).

FIBRINOLYTIC AGENTS

Comparisons of the properties and therapeutic regimens of the different fibrinolytic agents are shown in Table 1.

Streptokinase

Streptokinase is the classical agent and remains a commonly used fibrinolytic agent worldwide because of its lower cost and lower risk of intracranial hemorrhage than fibrin-specific agents. Streptokinase is associated with less intracerebral hemorrhage than t-PA. In GUSTO I, the rates were 0.5% streptokinase versus 0.7% t-PA, $p = 0.03$. Even when t-PA was provided free (and therefore cost was not an issue) in the GUSTO IIB trial (24), streptokinase was chosen as the fibrinolytic agent in 30% of patients by international investigators. It is not known why t-PA has higher rates of intracranial bleeding, but it may

Table 1 Comparison of Different Fibrinolytic Agents in Patients with Acute Myocardial Infarction

	Streptokinase	Alteplase (t-PA)	Tenecteplase (TNK-t-PA)	Reteplase (r-PA)
Administration		Bolus dose of 15 mg, then infusion of 0.75 mg/kg over 30 min (to max of 50 mg), then 0.5 mg/kg over the next 60 min (to max of 35 mg) Overall maximum dose of 100 mg Total duration of infusion of 90 min	Single-bolus dose of 0.5 mg/kg	2 bolus doses of 10 u 30 min apart
Molecular weight (kDa)	47	70	70	39
Plasma half-life (min)	23–29	4–8	20	15
Fibrin specificity	–	+++	+++	+
Plasminogen activation	Indirect	Direct	Direct	Direct
Dose	1.5 Mu over 60 min	100 mg over 90 min	0.5 mg/kg bolus	2 boluse doses of 10 u 30 min apart
Antigenicity	+	–	–	–
Hypotension	+	–	–	–
Patency at 90 min	+	+++	+++	+++
Hemorrhagic stroke	+	++	++	++
Mortality reduction	+	++	++	++
Cost	+	+++	+++	+++

Abbreviation: Mu, million units.

Note: +, Reflects the relative strength of the evidence; u, Units.

relate to t-PA crossing the blood-brain barrier (25). The standard dose of streptokinase is 1.5 million units given over 30 to 60 minutes. It should not be re-administered because of the risk of allergy and decreased efficacy (26).

TISSUE PLASMINOGEN ACTIVATOR

t-PA is manufactured by the recombinant DNA technology to produce the naturally occurring enzyme. It has a short half-life of 5 to 10 minutes. The standard intravenous dose is a bolus of 15 mg, 50 mg over 30 minutes, and then 35 mg over one hour. Gentamycin is used in its preparation and therefore sensitivity to gentamycin is a contraindication.

Reteplase

Reteplase (also known as r-PA is a deletion mutant of t-PA, with a longer half-life but lesser fibrin specificity. It is administered as two 10 u boluses given 30 minutes apart. In the RAPID-2 trial (reteplase versus alteplase patency investigation during acute myocardial infarction), r-PA achieved TIMI-3 flow in a higher proportion of patients than accelerated t-PA (59.9% vs. 45.2%, $p < 0.01$) (22). However, in the GUSTO III trial, r-PA had similar efficacy to t-PA, with 30-day mortality rates of 7.47% versus 7.24%, respectively ($p = 0.54$). Death or disabling stroke occurred in 7.89% of r-PA-treated patients versus 7.91% of t-PA-treated patients ($p = 0.97$) (15).

Tenecteplase

Tenecteplase (also known as TNK-t-PA) is a genetically engineered triple-combination mutant of t-PA, with amino acid substitute at three sites. It has a longer half-life and greater fibrin specificity than t-PA. It also has increased resistance to plasminogen activator inhibitor (PAI)-1 and causes less depletion of fibrinogen and plasminogen. A single-bolus, weight-adjusted tenecteplase regimen produced TIMI-3 flow in 63% of patients by 90 minutes (similar to t-PA) (27).

The ASSENT-2 trial (assessment of the safety and efficacy of a new thrombolytic agent) (19) found that tenecteplase did not reduce mortality (6.18% vs. 6.15% with t-PA), but was associated with less non-cerebral major bleeding (4.66% vs. 5.94%, respectively, $p = 0.0002$), particularly in the high-risk subgroups of elderly patients (>75 years) and low-bodyweight (<67 kg) females (28). Intracranial hemorrhage and stroke rates were similar.

Despite these innovations, incremental reductions in 30-day or late mortality have not been demonstrated. However, simpler treatment regimens should translate to broader application, timelier administration, and fewer treatment errors.

CHOICE OF FIBRINOLYTIC

In choosing a fibrinolytic, a fibrin-specific agent is most effective in the following situations:

- Patients < 84 years with anterior infarctions who present within 12 hours of symptom onset (29).
- Patients who have previously received streptokinase (26).

For all other patients with STEMI, streptokinase can be used.

CONTRAINDICATIONS TO FIBRINOLYSIS

There are a number of contraindications to fibrinolysis. It is important that the risk and benefit is carefully considered for each individual patient. A potential risk may be judged as less important if the patient is suffering a large anterior MI, but would be considered important if the patient was suffering a small inferior infarction. Some contraindications are considered absolute, as the potential harm caused by administration of fibrinolysis would always outweigh the benefit of fibrinolysis. These include any previous history of hemorrhagic stroke, history of stroke, dementia, or central nervous system (CNS) damage within one year; head trauma or brain surgery within six months; known intracranial neoplasm, suspected aortic dissection, internal bleeding within six weeks; active bleeding or known bleeding disorder, major surgery, trauma, or bleeding within six weeks; and traumatic cardiopulmonary resuscitation within three weeks. Whereas for relative contraindications the risk has to be carefully balanced against the potential benefit of fibrinolytic therapy. These situations include oral anticoagulant therapy, acute pancreatitis, pregnancy, or within one week postpartum; active peptic ulceration, transient ischemic attack within six months; and dementia, infective endocarditis, active cavitating pulmonary tuberculosis, advanced liver disease, intracardiac thrombi, uncontrolled hypertension (systolic blood pressure >180 mm Hg, diastolic blood pressure >110 mm Hg), puncture of non-compressible blood vessel within two weeks, and previous streptokinase therapy (only contraindicated for streptokinase re-administration).

THE ELDERLY

The number of elderly is increasing (30,31) accounting for much of the mortality and morbidity with fibrinolysis and antithrombotic treatment. A meta-analysis of 11 trials in older patients ranging from >65 to >75 years as compared with younger patients showed that older patients had 4.4-fold higher mortality and almost three-fold higher intracranial hemorrhage rates with fibrinolytic therapy (32). Fibrinolysis is markedly underutilized in older patients, and in fibrinolytic-eligible patients >75 years and <85 years only 40% of patients may receive it, and in patients aged ≥85 years only 20% may be administered fibrinolytic therapy (30).

The fibrinolytic therapy trialists (FTT) overview (33) showed that for patients >75 years there was a nonsignificant reduction in 30-day mortality from 25.3% to 24.3% CI (16–36). However, this included outcomes in patients presenting up to 24 hours after symptom onset and patients with normal ECGs, ST-depression, or T-wave inversion. A reanalysis evaluating only fibrinolytic-eligible elderly patients with ST-elevation or bundle branch block and presenting within 12 hours ($n = 3222$) of symptom onset showed a significant 35-day mortality reduction; 29.4% versus 26%. There was a larger absolute mortality reduction of 34 lives saved per 1000 elderly patients randomized in patients >75 years versus 16 lives saved per 1000 patients randomized in those <55 years. Although the elderly are at higher risk of intracranial hemorrhage, the number who survived with a nonfatal disabling stroke is low, <3% in those >85 years, and is not much increased over the rate in younger patients (34). In GUSTO I, reduction in death or disabling stroke was greater with accelerated t-PA in patients aged ≤85 years but patients >85 years randomized to streptokinase did better, and streptokinase may be the agent of choice in the very elderly (29).

There have been several small trials comparing fibrinolysis with PCI in the elderly (35,36). In the GUSTO IIB angioplasty sub study, there was no interaction between age and treatment. In the SENIOR PAMI trial (senior primary angioplasty in myocardial infarction), there was no difference in the primary endpoint of death or disabling stroke; 11.3% with PCI and 13% with fibrinolysis. The elderly may have precipitation of renal failure by contrast agents with PCI, and the optimal therapy has not been defined. Clearly early initiation of reperfusion therapy is mandatory. Older age by itself should not be regarded as a contraindication to fibrinolysis. There is a clear need for clinical trials in the elderly.

ADJUNCTIVE ANTIPLATELET THERAPIES

While modification in fibrinolytic therapies have improved early TIMI-3 flow rates, they have failed to translate into better clinical outcomes, whereas modification of adjunctive therapy to reduce reocclusion has led to improved sustained patency and reduction in reinfarction rates.

Since the early fibrinolytic studies (37), aspirin 150 to 325 mg has been a mainstay therapy for all patients undergoing either pharmacologic or catheter-based reperfusion. Aspirin should be given as early as possible and continued indefinitely (38,39).

The administration of clopidogrel 300 mg loading dose and 75 mg daily to patients <75 years undergoing fibrinolysis in the clarity-TIMI-28 trial resulted in greater rates of preserved vessel patency at angiography three to five days later TIMI 0 or 1 flow (11.7% vs. 18.4%, $p<0.001$), and a trend for reduced rates of recurrent MI (2.5% vs. 3.6%, $p = 0.08$), but not death (2.6% vs. 2.2%, $p = 0.49$) (40). These observations are supported by the CCS-2 (Chinese cardiac study)of 45,852 patients, where clopidogrel 75 mg/day without a loading dose was added to aspirin regardless of reperfusion status and compared with placebo (41). The composite primary endpoint of death, reinfarction, or stroke was reduced from 10.1% in the placebo group to 9.2% in the clopidogrel group [OR 0.91 (95% CI 0.86–0.97); $p = 0.002$], with trends of benefit observed both in patients receiving or not receiving fibrinolytic therapy. All-cause mortality was reduced from 8.1% in the placebo group to 7.5% in the clopidogrel group [OR 0.93 (95% CI 0.87–0.99) $p = 0.03$; NNT=167]. The rate of cerebral and major non-cerebral bleeding was 0.55% in the placebo group and 0.58% in the clopidogrel group ($p = 0.59$).

Trials of half-dose fibrinolytics and glycoprotein IIb/IIIa inhibition have demonstrated improved vessel patency and more rapid ST-segment resolution, but the adequately powered GUSTO V study of r-PA and abciximab demonstrated no reduction in mortality but reductions in recurrent infarction (42).

ANTITHROMBOTIC THERAPIES

Among patients receiving fibrin-specific fibrinolytic agents (t-PA, r-PA, and TNK-t-PA), unfractionated heparin (UFH) commenced early after fibrinolysis has been recommended, though the independent effect of UFH in this context has not been fully defined. The use of adjunctive UFH with streptokinase has been controversial (43,44). In an analysis of 68,000 patients treated with streptokinase and aspirin randomized to receive UFH or placebo, UFH reduced deaths by five and reinfarctions by three per 1000 patients treated with no increase in stroke (45).

Compared with high-dose UFH (5000 U bolus and 1000 U/hr), lower-dose regimens (4000 U bolus and 800 U/hr) are associated with lower rates of bleeding complications. Administration of UFH has been recommended for 24 to 48 hours, with no clear benefit for treatment beyond 48 hours. There are many well-known issues with the use of UFH, including variable therapeutic responses depending on age, weight and variable protein binding, and weight-adjusted dosing and frequent aPTT monitoring is required (46). New antithrombotic agents may overcome some of these limitations.

Low molecular weight heparins (LMWHs) have anti-Xa as well as anti-IIa activity, high bioavailability, and provide more consistent anticoagulation than UFH (46). No anticoagulant monitoring is necessary, and the risk of developing heparin-induced thrombocytopenia (HIT) is less than with UFH.

The enoxaparin and thrombolysis reperfusion for acute myocardial infarction treatment (ExTRACT)-TIMI 25 trial in 20,479 patients demonstrated the superiority of enoxaparin for four to seven days over UFH for 48 hours in reducing death and nonfatal MI at 30 days (9.9% vs. 12%, RR-0.83, $p < 0.001$), with an increase in major bleeding, (2.1% vs. 1.4%, RR-1.53, $p < 0.001$) (47). There was no effect on mortality (6.9% enoxaparin vs. 7.5% UFH). Results were similar regardless of the fibrinolytic administered. Enoxaparin also significantly reduced the rate of death, recurrent MI, recurrent myocardial ischemia, or stroke, regardless of whether patients were treated with clopidogrel without an increase in major bleeding or intracerebral hemorrhage (48). Enoxaparin was also superior to UFH in patients undergoing rescue or routine PCI after fibrinolysis for STEMI (49).

In ExTRACT, elderly patients ($\geq$75 years) received a novel enoxaparin-dosing regimen, with omission of the 30 mg IV bolus and, reduction of the subcutaneous bid dose from 1 mg/kg to 0.75 mg/kg (50). Once daily dosing of enoxaparin was given in patients with creatinine clearance <60 mL/min. The rate of the primary endpoint of death or nonfatal MI was significantly lower in patients <75 years (7.9% vs. 9.9%, $p < 0.0001$) and tended to be lower in patients $\geq$75 years (24.8% vs. 26.3%, $p = 0.10$) treated with enoxaparin compared with UFH. The rates of intracranial hemorrhage were similar in patients $\geq$75 years on enoxaparin (1.6%) or UFH (1.7%). Enoxaparin is thus an appropriate choice in the management of patients of all ages with STEMI.

The HERO-2 trial (hirulog and early reperfusion or occlusion) compared the direct thrombin inhibitor, bivalirudin to heparin among patients receiving streptokinase (17). As with other trials of adjunctive antithrombotic therapies with reperfusion, bivalirudin was not associated with reduced mortality, but lower rates of recurrent MI were demonstrated.

In the Organization to Assess Strategies for Ischaemic Symptoms (OASIS) 6, the synthetic factor X inhibitor fondaparinux reduced 30-day death or MI compared with UFH or placebo in patients receiving a fibrinolytic (10.9% vs. 13.6%, $p < 0.05$) and in patients not receiving fibrinolysis (12.2% vs. 15.1%, $p < 0.01$) (51). In patients undergoing primary PCI, there was no benefit (4.9% UFH vs. 6.0% PCI) due to an excess of catheter thrombosis. However, this appears to be largely avoided by adding UFH.

Overall mortality was reduced at 30 days from 8.9% to 7.8%, $p = 0.03$, and there were similar rates of severe bleeding in both randomized groups in patients receiving fibrinolysis as well as in patients not receiving a fibrinolytic. Thus, fondaparinux decreases mortality and reinfarction without increasing the risk of bleeding. Fondaparinux should not be used in primary PCI in preference to UFH.

INVASIVE MANAGEMENT FOLLOWING FIBRINOLYSIS

Among patients who receive fibrinolysis, accumulating evidence now supports the role of emergent angiography and PCI or "rescue PCI" for failed reperfusion, defined as ongoing chest-pain, hemodynamic instability, and/or failure of ST-segment resolution by > 50% at 90 minutes following fibrinolysis. In a meta-analysis of eight trials involving 1117 patients, rescue PCI was associated with lower rates of death, heart failure, and re-infarction by six months (29.2% vs. 41.0%, 11% absolute reduction, 95% CI 5–18%, $p < 0.001$), though a statistically significant reduction in mortality alone was not reached (odds ratio 0.69, 95% CI 0.23–1.05, $p = 0.09$). However, rescue PCI was associated with a 3% (95% CI 0–5%, $p = 0.02$) absolute increase in the risk of stroke (52). PCI for reinfarction following fibrinolysis is superior to readmission of fibrinolysis (53).

Facilitated PCI

Extending this rationale to routine emergent PCI following fibrinolysis, or "facilitated PCI" has not been associated with similar benefits. While early reports from small studies suggested that routine very early invasive management of these patients may be able to "consolidate" the benefits of pharmacologic reperfusion, in the ASSENT-4 PCI study among 1667 patients there was an increase in the risk of death, heart failure, and shock compared with primary PCI alone (18.6% vs. 13.4%, $p = 0.005$) (54), with a meta-analysis of the data dominated by the ASSENT-4 PCI study reaching the same conclusions (Fig. 3) (55). Also the recent FINESSE trial (facilitated intervention for enhanced reperfusion speed to stop events) showed no benefit of facilitated PCI following half-dose r-PA and abciximab (a potentially more robust antithrombotic approach) compared with primary PCI among 2653 patients (56). Whether a facilitated PCI strategy has a role in clinical settings where primary PCI is associated with substantial delays requires more study (57).

In the 2007 AHA/ACC update (13), the recommendations were as follows:

Class 2B: Facilitated PCI using regimens other than full-dose fibrinolytic therapy might be considered as a reperfusion strategy when all of the following are present: (*i*) Patients are at high risk, (*ii*) PCI is not immediately available within 90 minutes, and (*iii*) Bleeding

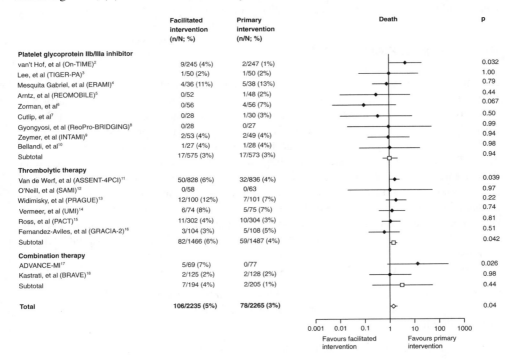

Figure 3 Short-term death in patients treated with facilitated or primary percutaneous coronary intervention. *Source:* Adapted from Ref. 55.

risk is low (younger age, absence of poorly controlled hypertension, normal body weight). (*Level of Evidence: C.*)

Class 3: A planned reperfusion strategy using full-dose fibrinolytic therapy followed by immediate PCI may be harmful. (*Level of Evidence: B.*)

Routine PCI Following Fibrinolysis

The effect of a routine early invasive strategy following successful reperfusion, but within 24 hours of onset, was examined in the GARCIA-1 study (Grupo de Análisis de la Cardiopatia Isquémica Aguda) (58). Five hundred patients were randomized to angiography and possible PCI compared with an ischemia-driven approach. At 12 months, the early invasive approach was associated with a nonsignificant reduction in death or re-infarction (7% vs. 12%, $p = 0.07$) but a lower rate of repeat revascularization (58).

Meta-analysis of three trials that compared routine PCI with stenting post fibrinolysis versus ischemia-guided stenting after administration of fibrinolysis showed a trend for a reduction in death 3.8% versus 6.7%, $p = 0.07$, and a significant reduction in death and MI at six months, 7.4% versus 13.2%, $p < 0.01$ (59). Routine PCI following fibrinolysis may achieve similar results to primary PCI as observed in GRACIA-2, where 212 patients were randomized to full-dose tenecteplase and enoxaparin and routine PCI within 3 to 12 hours (median 4–6 hours) or to primary PCI with stenting and abciximab (60). Patients randomized to tenecteplase and routine PCI had higher TIMI grade 3 flow following PCI and significantly better tissue perfusion; TIMI perfusion grade 3, 55.3% versus 25.3%, $p < 0.01$. This parameter has been shown to correlate closely with mortality (61). However, there was no difference in the rate at six-months of death, recurrent MI, stroke, or revascularization (10% vs. 12%, $p = 0.57$). Major bleeding rates were similar: 1.9% fibrinolysis versus 2.8% primary PCI, $p = 0.99$.

PRE-HOSPITAL FIBRINOLYSIS

Recent controlled trials such as the CAPTIM (comparison of the angioplasty and pre-hospital thrombolysis in acute myocardial infarction) (62) and WEST (which early ST-elevation myocardial infarction therapy) (63) trials have compared pre-hospital fibrinolysis with primary PCI. In CAPTIM patients treated by pre-hospital fibrinolysis within two hours of symptom onset had better outcome with lower mortality (2.2% vs. 5.7%, $P = 0.058$) and incidence of cardiogenic shock (1.3% vs. 5.3%, $P = 0.032$) than those treated by primary PCI (64). In WEST (63), there was a three-armed comparison of pre-hospital TNK with usual care, pre-hospital TNK with mandatory angiography, and primary PCI. The primary composite outcome of 30-day death, re-infarction, refractory ischemia, congestive heart failure, cardiogenic shock, and major ventricular arrhythmia, was not different between the randomized treatment strategies (25% pre-hospital TNK vs. 24% usual care vs. 23% pre-hospital TNK with mandatory angiography).

In the 2007 AHA/ACC update (13), the recommendations were as follows:

Class 1: A strategy of coronary angiography with intent to perform PCI (or emergency CABG) is recommended for patients who have received fibrinolytic therapy and have any of the following:

    i. Cardiogenic shock in patients <75 years who are suitable candidates for revascularization (*Level of Evidence: B.*)

ii. Severe congestive heart failure and/or pulmonary edema (Killip class III) (*Level of Evidence: B.*)

iii. Hemodynamically compromising ventricular arrhythmias (*Level of Evidence: C.*)

Similar recommendations were made for patients ≥75 years developing cardiogenic shock, provided that they were suitable candidates for revascularization.

There continues to be large treatment gaps for the use of fibrinolytic therapy in eligible patients (12,65). The GRACE study reported that 30% of eligible patients receive no reperfusion therapies. Older age, race, and diabetes have been associated with underuse of fibrinolysis (66–68).

Appropriate underuse of fibrinolysis occurs when there is delay of > 12 hours after symptom onset, there is a high risk of intracranial hemorrhage or there is marked associated comorbidity. However, there continues to be an inappropriate treatment-risk care gap where the survival benefits of fibrinolysis are denied patients on the basis of other criteria, including high risk baseline characteristics such as increasing TIMI mortality risk index (69). In an analysis of 3994 patients in a Canadian registry for each 1% increase in the TIMI risk index (which does not take into account the risk of intracranial hemorrhage) (70) there was a 3% fall in use of reperfusion therapy, which highlights the paradox that higher risk patients, who are those likely to gain more from reperfusion, were more often denied fibrinolysis.

FUTURE PERSPECTIVES

The future management of patients with STEMI depends on the development of the health care systems to deliver timely reperfusion therapy to as many patients as possible. Development of clinical networks may provide further mortality benefits to a broader population of patients presenting with STEMI (71). This may include pre-hospital fibrinolysis, in-hospital fibrinolysis followed by high rates of rescue and systematic PCI, or primary PCI. The most important approach is to reduce times from symptom onset to reperfusion. The major challenge is the translation of the enormous evidence base for the effectiveness of fibrinolytic therapy to individual patient care and to decrease the care gap in patients at higher risk so that more patients can gain the benefits of fibrinolysis worldwide. This is particularly so in places where primary PCI is not a realistic alternative for providing timely perfusion.

REFERENCES

1. Giugliano RP, Braunwald E. Selecting the best reperfusion strategy in ST-elevation myocardial infarction: it's all a matter of time. Circulation 2003; 108(23):2828–2830.
2. Davies GJ, Chierchia S, Maseri A. Prevention of myocardial infarction by very early treatment with intracoronary streptokinase. Some clinical observations. N Engl J Med 1984; 311(23): 488–1492.
3. Taher T, Fu Y, Wagner GS, et al. Aborted myocardial infarction in patients with ST-segment elevation: insights from the assessment of the safety and efficacy of a new thrombolytic regimen-3 trial electrocardiographic substudy. J Am Coll Cardiol 2004; 44(1): 38–43.
4. Weaver WD, Cerqueira M, Hallstrom AP, et al. Prehospital-initiated vs hospital-initiated thrombolytic therapy. JAMA 1993; 270:1211–1216.
5. Boersma E, Maas ACP, Deckers JW, et al. Early thrombolytic treatment in acute myocardial infarction: reappraisal of the golden hour. Lancet 1996; 348(9030):771–775.

6. Keeley EC, Boura JA, Grines CL. Primary angioplasty versus intravenous thrombolytic therapy for acute myocardial infarction: a quantitative review of 23 randomised trials. Lancet 2003; 361 (9351):13–20.

7. The GUSTO Investigators. An international randomized trial comparing four thrombolytic strategies for acute myocardial infarction. N Engl J Med 1993; 329:673–682.

8. Massel D. Primary angioplasty or thrombolysis for acute myocardial infarction? Lancet 2003; 361(9361):967–968.

9. Pinto DS, Kirtane AJ, Nallamothu BK, et al. Hospital delays in reperfusion for ST-elevation myocardial infarction: implications when selecting a reperfusion strategy. Circulation 2006; 114 (19):2019–2025.

10. Nallamothu BK, Bates ER. Percutaneous coronary intervention versus fibrinolytic therapy in acute myocardial infarction: is timing (almost) everything? Am J Cardiol 2003; 92(7): 824–826.

11. Jollis JG, Mehta RH, Roettig ML, et al. Reperfusion of acute myocardial infarction in North Carolina emergency departments (RACE): study design. Am Heart J 2006; 152(5):851–11.

12. Eagle KA, Goodman SG, Avezum A, et al. Practice variation and missed opportunities for reperfusion in ST-segment-elevation myocardial infarction: findings from the global registry of acute coronary events (GRACE). Lancet 2002; 359(9304):373–377.

13. Canadian Cardiovascular Society, American Academy of Family Physicians, American College of Cardiology et al. 2007 focused update of the ACC/AHA 2004 guidelines for the management of patients with ST-elevation myocardial infarction: a report of the American College of Cardiology/American Heart Association Task Force on Practice Guidelines. Developed in collaboration with the Canadian Cardiovascular Society endorsed by the American Academy of Family Physicians: 2007 Writing Group to Review New Evidence and Update the ACC/AHA 2004 Guidelines for the Management of Patients with ST-Elevation Myocardial Infarction, Writing on Behalf of the 2004 Writing Committee. J Am Coll Cardiol 2008; 51(2):210–247.

14. The Assessment of the Safety and Efficacy of a New Thrombolytic Regimen (ASSENT)-3 Investigators. Efficacy and safety of tenecteplase in combination with enoxaparin, abciximab, or unfractionated heparin: the ASSENT-3 randomised trial in acute myocardial infarction. Lancet 2001; 358(9282):605–613.

15. The Global Use of Strategies to Open Occluded Coronary Arteries (GUSTO-III) Investigators. A comparison of reteplase with alteplase for acute myocardial infarction. N Engl J Med 1997; 337(16):1118–1123.

16. The GUSTO V Investigators. Reperfusion therapy for acute myocardial infarction with fibrinolytic therapy or combination reduced fibrinolytic therapy and platelet glycoprotein IIb/ IIIa inhibition: the GUSTO V randomized trial. Lancet 2001; 357(9272):1905–1914.

17. The Hirulog and Early Reperfusion or Occlusion (HERO)-2 Trial Investigators. Thrombin-specific anticoagulation with bivalirudin versus heparin in patients receiving fibrinolytic therapy for acute myocardial infarction: the HERO-2 randomised trial. Lancet 2001; 358(9296): 1855–1863.

18. The InTIME-II Investigators. Intravenous NPA for the treatment of infarcting myocardium early: InTIME-II, a double-blind comparison of single-bolus lanoteplase vs accelerated alteplase for the treatment of patients with acute myocardial infarction. Eur Heart J 2000; 21(24):2005–2013.

19. The Assessment of the Safety and Efficacy of a New Thrombolytic Regimen (ASSENT)-2 Investigators. Single-bolus tenecteplase compared with front-loaded alteplase in acute myocardial infarction: the ASSENT-2 double-blind randomised trial. Lancet 1999; 354(9180): 716–722.

20. Chesebro JH, Knatterud G, Roberts R, et al. Thrombolysis in myocardial infarction (TIMI) trial, phase I: a comparison between intravenous tissue plasminogen activator and intravenous streptokinase: clinical findings through hospital discharge. Circulation 1987; 76(1): 142–154.

21. White HD, Aylward PE, Frey MJ, et al. Randomized, double-blind comparison of hirulog versus heparin in patients receiving streptokinase and aspirin for acute myocardial infarction (HERO). Circulation 1997; 96(7):2155–2161.

22. Bode C, Smalling RW, Berg G, et al. Randomized comparison of coronary thrombolysis achieved with double-bolus reteplase (recombinant plasminogen activator) and front-loaded, accelerated alteplase (recombinant tissue plasminogen activator) in patients with acute myocardial infarction. Circulation 1996; 94:891–898.

23. Antman EM, Giugliano RP, Gibson CM, et al. Abciximab facilitates the rate and extent of thrombolysis: results of the Thrombolysis in Myocardial Infarction (TIMI) 14 trial. Circulation 1999; 99:2720–2732.

24. The Global Use of Strategies to Open Occluded Coronary Arteries (GUSTO) IIa Investigators. Randomized trial of intravenous heparin versus recombinant hirudin for acute coronary syndromes. Circulation 1994; 90:1631–1637.

25. Benchenane K, Berezowski V, Ali C, et al. Tissue-type plasminogen activator crosses the intact blood-brain barrier by low-density lipoprotein receptor-related protein-mediated transcytosis. Circulation 2005; 111(17):2241–2249.

26. Elliott JM, Cross DB, Cederholm-Williams SA, et al. Neutralizing antibodies to streptokinase four years after intravenous thrombolytic therapy. Am J Cardiol 1993; 71:640–645.

27. Cannon CP, Gibson CM, McCabe CH, et al. TNK-tissue plasminogen activator compared with front-loaded alteplase in acute myocardial infarction: results of the TIMI 10B trial. Circulation 1998; 98(25):2805–2814.

28. Van de Werf F, Barron HV, Armstrong PW, et al. Incidence and predictors of bleeding events after fibrinolytic therapy with fibrin-specific agents: a comparison of TNK-tPA and rtPA. Eur Heart J 2001; 22(24):2253–2261.

29. White HD, Barbash GI, Califf RM, et al. Age and outcome with contemporary thrombolytic therapy: results from the GUSTO-I trial. Circulation 1996; 94:1826–1833.

30. Alexander KP, Newby LK, Armstrong PW, et al. Acute coronary care in the elderly, part II: ST-segment-elevation myocardial infarction: a scientific statement for healthcare professionals from the American Heart Association Council on Clinical Cardiology: in collaboration with the Society of Geriatric Cardiology. Circulation 2007; 115(19):2570–2589.

31. White HD, Aylward PEG, Huang Z, et al. Mortality and morbidity remain high despite captopril and/or valsartan therapy in elderly patients with left ventricular systolic dysfunction, heart failure, or both following acute myocardial infarction: results from the Valsartan. In: Acute Myocardial Infarction (VALIANT) trial. Circulation 2005; 112:3391–3399.

32. Ahmed S, Antman EM, Murphy SA, et al. Poor outcomes after fibrinolytic therapy for ST-segment elevation myocardial infarction: impact of age (a meta-analysis of a decade of trials). J Thromb Thrombolysis 2006; 21(2):119–129.

33. Fibrinolytic Therapy Trialists' (FTT) Collaborative Group. Indications for fibrinolytic therapy in suspected acute myocardial infarction: collaborative overview of early mortality and major morbidity results from all randomised trials of more than 1000 patients. Lancet 1994; 343(8893):311–322.

34. White HD. Thrombolytic therapy in the elderly [commentary]. Lancet 2000; 356(9247):2028–2030.

35. Grines, CL. A prospective randomized trial of primary angioplasty and thrombolytic therapy in elderly patients with acute myocardial infarction—SENIOR PAMI. 2005 Washington D.C., USA. TCT Conference, Washington D.C. 16-10-2005. (GENERIC) Ref Type: Conference Proceeding

36. Holmes DR Jr., White HD, Pieper KS, et al. Effect of age on outcome with primary angioplasty versus thrombolysis. J Am Coll Cardiol 1999; 33(2):412–419.

37. ISIS-2 (Second International Study of Infarct Survival) Collaborative Group. Randomised trial of intravenous streptokinase, oral aspirin, both, or neither among 17 187 cases of suspected acute myocardial infarction: ISIS-2. Lancet 1988; ii:349–360.

38. Antiplatelet Trialists' Collaboration. Collaborative overview of randomised trials of antiplatelet therapy—I: prevention of death, myocardial infarction, and stroke by prolonged antiplatelet therapy in various categories of patients. Br Med J 1994; 308:81–106.

39. Antithrombotic Trialists' Collaboration. Collaborative meta-analysis of randomised trials of antiplatelet therapy for prevention of death, myocardial infarction, and stroke in high risk

patients. Erratum Available at: http://bmj.com/cgi/content/full/324/7329/71/DC2. Br Med J 2002; 324(7329):71–86.

40. Sabatine MS, Cannon CP, Gibson CM, et al. Addition of clopidogrel to aspirin and fibrinolytic therapy for myocardial infarction with ST-segment elevation. N Engl J Med 2005; 352(12): 1179–1189.

41. Chen ZM, Jiang LX, Chen YP, et al. Addition of clopidogrel to aspirin in 45,852 patients with acute myocardial infarction: randomised placebo-controlled trial. Lancet 2005; 366(9497): 1607–1621.

42. Topol EJ, Ohman EM, Armstrong PW, et al. Survival outcomes 1 year after reperfusion therapy with either alteplase or reteplase for acute myocardial infarction: results from the Global Utilization of Streptokinase and t-PA for Occluded Coronary Arteries (GUSTO) III trial. Circulation 2000; 102(15):1761–1765.

43. White HD, Yusuf S. Issues regarding the use of heparin following streptokinase therapy. J Thromb Thrombolysis 1995; 2:5–10.

44. White HD. Further evidence that antithrombotic therapy is beneficial with streptokinase: improved early ST resolution and late patency with enoxaparin. Eur Heart J 2002; 23(16): 1233–1237(editorial).

45. Collins R, MacMahon S, Flather M, et al. Clinical effects of anticoagulant therapy in suspected acute myocardial infarction: systematic overview of randomised trials. Br Med J 1996; 313:652–659.

46. Hirsh J, O'Donnell M, Eikelboom JW. Beyond unfractionated heparin and warfarin: current and future advances. Circulation 2007; 116(5):552–560.

47. Antman EM, Morrow DA, McCabe CH, et al. Enoxaparin versus unfractionated heparin with fibrinolysis for ST-elevation myocardial infarction. N Engl J Med 2006; 354(14):1477–1488.

48. Sabatine MS, Morrow DA, Dalby A, et al. Efficacy and safety of enoxaparin versus unfractionated heparin in patients with ST-segment elevation myocardial infarction also treated with clopidogrel. J Am Coll Cardiol 2007; 49(23):2256–2263.

49. Gibson CM, Murphy SA, Montalescot G, et al. Percutaneous coronary intervention in patients receiving enoxaparin or unfractionated heparin after fibrinolytic therapy for ST-segment elevation myocardial infarction in the ExTRACT-TIMI 25 trial. J Am Coll Cardiol 2007; 49(23):2238–2246.

50. White HD, Braunwald E, Murphy SA, et al. Enoxaparin vs. unfractionated heparin with fibrinolysis for ST-elevation myocardial infarction in elderly and younger patients: results from ExTRACT-TIMI 25. Eur Heart J 2007; 28(9):1066–1071.

51. Yusuf S, Mehta SR, Chrolavicius S, et al. Effects of fondaparinux on mortality and reinfarction in patients with acute ST-segment elevation myocardial infarction: the OASIS-6 randomized trial. JAMA 2006; 295(13):1519–1530.

52. Wijeysundera HC, Vijayaraghavan R, Nallamothu BK, et al. Rescue angioplasty or repeat fibrinolysis after failed fibrinolytic therapy for ST-segment myocardial infarction: a meta-analysis of randomized trials. J Am Coll Cardiol 2007; 49(4):422–430.

53. Gershlick AH, Stephens-Lloyd A, Hughes S, et al. Rescue angioplasty after failed thrombolytic therapy for acute myocardial infarction. N Engl J Med 2005; 353(26): 2758–2768.

54. Assessment of the Safety and Efficacy of a New Treatment Strategy with Percutaneous Coronary Intervention (ASSENT-4 PCI) investigators. Primary versus tenecteplase-facilitated percutaneous coronary intervention in patients with ST-segment elevation acute myocardial infarction (ASSENT-4 PCI): randomised trial. Lancet 2006; 367(9510):569–578.

55. Keeley EC, Boura JA, Grines CL. Comparison of primary and facilitated percutaneous coronary interventions for ST-elevation myocardial infarction: quantitative review of randomised trials. Lancet 2006; 367(9510):579–588.

56. Kindermann M, Adam O, Werner N, et al. Clinical Trial Updates and Hotline Sessions presented at the European Society of Cardiology Congress 2007: (FINESSE, CARESS, OASIS 5, PRAGUE-8, OPTIMIST, GRACE, STEEPLE, SCAAR, STRATEGY, DANAMI-2, ExTRACT-TIMI-25, ISAR-REACT 2, ACUITY, ALOFT, 3CPO, PROSPECT, EVEREST,

COACH, BENEFiT, MERLIN-TIMI 36, SEARCH-MI, ADVANCE, WENBIT, EUROASPIRE I-III, ARISE, getABI, RIO). Clin.Res.Cardiol 2007; 96(11):767–786.

57. Gersh BJ, Stone GW, White HD, et al. Pharmacological facilitation of primary percutaneous coronary intervention for acute myocardial infarction: is the slope of the curve the shape of the future? JAMA 2005; 293(8), 979–986.

58. Fernandez-Aviles F, Alonso JJ, Castro-Beiras A, et al. Routine invasive strategy within 24 hours of thrombolysis versus ischaemia-guided conservative approach for acute myocardial infarction with ST-segment elevation (GRACIA-1): a randomised controlled trial. Lancet 2004; 364(9439):1045–1053.

59. Collet JP, Montalescot G, Le May M, et al. Percutaneous coronary intervention after fibrinolysis: a multiple meta-analyses approach according to the type of strategy. J Am Coll Cardiol 2006; 48(7):1326–1335.

60. Fernandez-Aviles F, Alonso JJ, Pena G, et al. Primary angioplasty vs. early routine post-fibrinolysis angioplasty for acute myocardial infarction with ST-segment elevation: the GRACIA-2 non-inferiority, randomized, controlled trial. Eur Heart J 2007; 28(8):949–960.

61. Gibson CM, Cannon CP, Murphy SA, et al. Relationship of TIMI myocardial perfusion grade to mortality after administration of thrombolytic drugs. Circulation 2000; 101(2):125–130.

62. Steg PG, Bonnefoy E, Chabaud S, et al. Impact of time to treatment on mortality after prehospital fibrinolysis or primary angioplasty: data from the CAPTIM randomized clinical trial. Circulation 2003; 108(23):2851–2856.

63. Armstrong PW. A comparison of pharmacologic therapy with/without timely coronary intervention vs. primary percutaneous intervention early after ST-elevation myocardial infarction: the WEST (which early ST-elevation myocardial infarction therapy) study. Eur Heart J 2006; 27(13):1530–1538.

64. Bonnefoy E, Lapostolle F, Leizorovicz A, et al. Primary angioplasty versus prehospital fibrinolysis in acute myocardial infarction: a randomised study. Lancet 2002; 360(9336):825–829.

65. Canto JG, Zalenski RJ, Ornato JP, et al. Use of emergency medical services in acute myocardial infarction and subsequent quality of care: observations from the National Registry of Myocardial Infarction 2. Circulation 2002; 106(24):3018–3023.

66. Krumholz HM, Murillo JE, Chen J, et al. Thrombolytic therapy for eligible elderly patients with acute myocardial infarction. JAMA 1997; 277(21):1683–1688.

67. Manhapra A, Canto JG, Barron HV, et al. Underutilization of reperfusion therapy in eligible African Americans with acute myocardial infarction: role of presentation and evaluation characteristics. Am Heart J 2001; 142(4):604–610.

68. Franklin K, Goldberg RJ, Spencer F, et al. Implications of diabetes in patients with acute coronary syndromes. The Global Registry of Acute Coronary Events. Arch Intern Med 2004; 164(13):1457–1463.

69. Alter DA, Ko DT, Newman A, et al. Factors explaining the under-use of reperfusion therapy among ideal patients with ST-segment elevation myocardial infarction. Eur Heart J 2006; 27(13):1539–1549.

70. Morrow DA, Antman EM, Giugliano RP, et al. A simple risk index for rapid initial triage of patients with ST-elevation myocardial infarction: an InTIME II substudy. Lancet 2001; 358(9293):1571–1575.

71. White HD, et al. Systems of care: hub and spoke for both primary PCI and angioplasty following fibrinolysis. Circulation 2008; 118(3):219–222.

38

Epilogue: The Evolution of Therapeutic Management of Thrombotic and Cardiovascular Disease

Jane E. Freedman
Department of Medicine and Pharmacology, Boston University School of Medicine, Boston, Massachusetts, U.S.A.

Joseph Loscalzo
Department of Medicine, Brigham and Women's Hospital, Harvard Medical School, Boston, Massachusetts, U.S.A.

Development in the areas of anticoagulants, platelet inhibitors, and fibrinolytics has continued with the growth in the number of patients with diseases complicated by thrombosis. New groups of therapeutics are being developed, while existing therapies are being further studied for expanding indications, beneficial combinations, and optimized dosing. In addition, therapies are being explored utilizing evolving techniques in the fields of proteomics and transciptomics. Much of the recent excitement has been centered on the potential for individual and targeted dosing in the use of anticoagulants and other antithrombotics. All of these goals hold the promise of diminished side effects and complications, particularly with bleeding.

A major goal in the use of these therapies is the development of useful tools that will guide treatment while maintaining vascular patency and minimizing bleeding complications. Laboratory monitoring and the use of surrogates, such as inflammatory biomarkers, in the setting of clinical thrombosis is a rapidly developing area of investigation. For example, while there are known advantages and disadvantages of the many available platelet function tests, they are being used to determine mechanisms of action, optimize dosing, monitor treatment failure (resistance), and compare different therapies. As anticoagulants and other antithrombotics are developed and utilized in new clinical situations, many of the new therapies have variable effects on the usual tests of coagulation and may not be useful for monitoring. How and if we monitor our patients in the setting of various thrombotic diseases and with the use of newer antithrombotics is an ongoing issue.

An example is the use of warfarin, as optimal dosing requires international normalized ratio (INR) measurement and dose titration. Pharmacogenomic analysis may personalize warfarin dosing using routine genetic testing. Currently under development are dosing nomograms devised to integrate genetic testing results with clinical variables, such as age, gender, weight, nutrition, other medications, and medical comorbidities. While there has been some utility in the setting of venous thromboembolic disease, the use of genetic testing in arterial thrombosis continues to evolve. Clearly, not all pharmacological agents have equivalent efficacy and toxicity for individuals, and genetic variability is one component that contributes to this variability. The hope is that pharmacogenetic testing may contribute to the development of personalized medicine by identifying groups of individuals who will both benefit from a particular dose of a drug and/or are at risk for suffering a drug-dependent adverse event.

The many antithrombotics used in the treatment and prevention of both arterial and venous thromboembolism have multiple limitations, including variable dose response, concerns about weight adjustment, parenteral administration, and coagulation monitoring. Currently, the primary available oral anticoagulants are limited to vitamin K antagonists known to have a slow onset of action and difficulty in dosing consistency. New developments in anticoagulants include thrombin inhibitors, antithrombotics, and novel heparins that are being developed to address these concerns. In addition, expanded indications for existing agents continue as novel effects of these agents are defined, including modulation of the tissue factor pathway inhibitor, inhibition of inflammation, and alterations of cellular adhesion. A complication of many antithrombotics is heparin-induced thrombocytopenia, and treatment for this problem continues to be refined.

There has been great excitement and progress in the area of oral anticoagulant development, including the development of both factor Xa and thrombin inhibitors (with several therapeutic agents) now into phase III testing. Direct thrombin inhibitors are a powerful alternative to traditional anticoagulants. They can specifically bind circulating and fibrin-bound thrombin and lack an obligate cofactor. Direct thrombin inhibitors do not have natural inhibitors, and they appear to have a broad therapeutic window; they have already been introduced in the areas of coronary intervention, thromboprophylaxis, and in the management of heparin-induced thrombocytopenia. Challenges that remain are concerns about monitoring and a lack of antidote.

Factor IX plays a fundamental role in coagulation reactions triggered by either TF–factor/VIIa or contact-initiated activation, and oral inhibitors in this class are undergoing clinical trials for multiple clinical thrombotic disorders. Factor XII and factor XI deficiency or inhibition affects the stability of platelet-rich thrombi, suggesting that targeting these proteases may be beneficial in patients with a history of coronary artery disease, stroke, or atrial fibrillation with the potential for a lower risk of bleeding complications.

The protein C anticoagulant pathway consists of several proteins whose mechanisms of action are distinct from other antithrombotic agents and, therefore, offers potentially novel approaches to the treatment of thrombotic diseases. The protein C pathway is particularly important in the control of microvascular thrombosis, and might provide an optimal target for the treatment of these diseases. The protein C system also elicits anti-inflammatory activity as inferred from basic and physiological studies, and regulation of this pathway may constitute an interesting approach to diminish morbidity associated with stroke and inflammatory diseases.

There have been significant advances in the development of platelet inhibitors, much due to the continuing success of aspirin and clopidogrel for the treatment of cardiovascular diseases. The primary focus has been on the development of new targets and additional therapies in successful classes that will lead to enhanced efficacy and parallel safety profiles; however, owing to the success of these drugs, a primary limitation in their development is the prohibitive cost of clinical trials demonstrating significant differences to current antiplatelet therapies.

To maximize efficacy while minimizing adverse effects, the combination of dual antiplatelet therapies has been tested in various clinical populations. Aspirin has been combined with clopidogrel in different doses and durations to assess its effectiveness compared with aspirin alone. Unfortunately, dual antiplatelet therapy often carries a significant hemorrhagic risk. Another important area of investigation has been the study of duration of therapy. Lastly, a prolific area of investigation has been the study of platelet function testing with the goal of its use in the guiding of drug development and dosing. However, platelet function measurement is confounded by factors such as redundant activation pathways; the interaction with coagulation proteins, platelets, and other vascular cells; and technical issues distinct to platelets. Additionally, while platelet function can be estimated, it may not be a reliable surrogate for thrombus formation.

In the area of adenosine diphosphate (ADP) receptor antagonists, agents have been developed that have rapid onset and shorter half-lives or are reversible and would allow for urgent surgical procedures, thus overcoming the limitations of clopidogrel. New direct and reversible $P2Y_{12}$ antagonists (cangrelor, which can only be given intravenously, and AZD6140, which can be given orally) might be attractive alternatives to thienopyridines, especially when rapid inhibition of platelet aggregation or its quick reversal is required. A recent study of prasugrel has shown that using an agent that achieved a faster, higher, and more consistent level of platelet inhibition than standard therapy could improve clinical ischemic outcomes. As with many new agents, success in preventing ischemia may come with the problem of additional bleeding.

Newer platelet inhibitory targets include agents that work via collagen receptors, serotonin receptors, or thrombin receptors, as these would complement current antiplatelet therapy. The protease activated receptor 1 (PAR-1), the target for thrombin-induced platelet aggregation, represents an important pathway of prothrombotic activation during plaque rupture. PAR-1 is the mediator of thrombin's actions on other cells as well, including lymphocytic mitogenesis and inflammatory responses, making it an attractive target for drug development. During the last decade, there has been growing development of therapies that target platelet adhesion and activation mediated through interactions of von Willebrand factor with platelet GPIb and collagen with platelet GPVI. Most of the specific antagonists directed toward these pathways have been soluble ligands, soluble receptors, and antibodies. The hope is that these specific targets will allow for separation of platelet inhibition from bleeding. One unique approach to blocking the GPIb/VWF A1 domain interaction has been through the use of a nucleic acid aptamer that binds to the A1 domain of VWF with high affinity. The field of NO-donor drugs, which can favor site-specific delivery as platelet inhibitors, continues to develop, although many targets are still in development and at preclinical stages.

While the development of thrombolytic agents is no longer the primary emphasis in this field, great strides have been made in expanding the clinical use of these therapies. This greater use occurred because the mortality rates for patients with acute pulmonary embolism, especially those with hemodynamic compromise and RV dysfunction, remain high despite current therapeutic options. In addition, there has been great interest in the use of thrombolytics for ischemic stroke. These trials have highlighted the importance of careful platelet inhibitor selection and meticulous trial design. However, the use of thrombolysis continues to be limited by a paucity of clinical trials evaluating its safety and efficacy. In addition, there have been significant issues in regard to bleeding complications. Proper dosing and timing with fibrinolytics is crucial and more information examining the use of pre-hospital or in-hospital fibrinolysis has led to increased success. As has been pointed out in section IV, large, randomized, controlled trials are necessary to define better precise risk:benefit for the use of thrombolytic therapy in these expanded clinical areas. Lastly, future development of additional thrombolytic agents may hold promise for more site-specific thrombolysis and improved safety profiles.

In summary, for fibrinolytics, anticoagulants, and platelet inhibitors, clinical utility is tightly linked to the balance between thrombosis and bleeding. New therapies and therapeutic combinations must demonstrate efficacy, but also need to have a favorable safety profile compared with currently available therapies. Some drugs are being developed with antidotes, but most are not. In addition, as new therapies are developed and new targets are utilized, off-target side effects need to be considered, such as the hepatic toxicity seen with ximelagatran. In closing, the diseases that lead to thrombotic occlusion are a major source of morbidity and mortality, and enormous strides have been made during the past decade in the development of a vast number of therapies, including antithrombotics, platelet inhibitors, and fibrinolytics.

Index

NOTE: Page numbers followed by f and t indicate figures and tables, respectively.